Contact Lenses

Contact Lenses

A Textbook for Practitioner and Student

Combined Second Edition

Edited by

JANET STONE
FBOA HD, FSMC, FAAO, DCLP

Contact Lens Practitioner, Shrewsbury. Formerly Senior Lecturer, The London Refraction Hospital

and

ANTHONY J. PHILLIPS
MPhil, FBOA HD, FSMC, FAAO, DCLP

Contact Lens Department, Flinders Medical Centre, Adelaide, South Australia. Formerly Contact Lens Practitioner, Loughborough, Leicestershire

Butterworths
London   Boston   Durban   Singapore   Sydney   Toronto   Wellington

First published 1972
Reprinted 1976
Second edition (2 vols) 1980, 1981
Combined second edition 1984
Reprinted 1985
Reprinted 1986

© **Butterworth & Co (Publishers) Ltd, 1984**

British Library Cataloguing in Publication Data

Contact lenses.–2nd ed.
   1. Contact lenses
   I. Stone, Janet   II. Phillips, Anthony J.
   (Anthony John)
   617.7'523   RE977.C6

ISBN 0-407-93274-7

Library of Congress Cataloging in Publication Data

Main entry under title:

Contact lenses.

   Reprint. Originally published: London:
   Butterworths, 1980-1981.
   Includes bibliographies and index.
   1. Contact lenses.
   I. Stone, Janet.   II Phillips, Anthony John.
   RE977.C6C59 1983   617.7'523   83-23238

ISBN 0-407-93274-7

Typeset by Butterworths Litho Preparation Department
Printed in England by Butler & Tanner Ltd., Frome, Somerset

Preface to the Second Edition

The writing of a scientific textbook has one particular frustration. This is, of course, the fact that by the time it has passed through the various stages of production, the proofs read and the final corrections made, over a year will have passed since the manuscript was submitted to the publisher. During this time, scientific progress will have continued to advance at a phenomenal pace. Thus, whilst the manuscript may be completely up to date at the time of submission to the publisher, it is, of unfortunate necessity, that much out of date by the time it reaches the reader. For example, in the twelve months between submission of manuscript and publication of the *First Edition*, hydrophilic lenses came to the forefront of contact lens development.

The *Second Edition* has been largely re-written to incorporate not only current knowledge on hydrophilic lenses but several new topics not dealt with in the *First Edition*. This has been done to provide both a greater compass of this rapidly increasing science and also to cover more completely the examination syllabuses in contact lenses as laid down by the British Optical Association, now the British College of Ophthalmic Opticians (optometrists).

The Editors would like to welcome the several new Contributors to the book and to take the opportunity of thanking all the Contributors for the work they have put in, not only into their own chapters but often for advice and comments on other chapters where they may also have had a special interest. In addition, we would like to thank the many prescription laboratories and solution manufacturers who have provided information and photographs as well as Mr W. S. Hodges of the British Standards Institution. Tony Phillips would also like to record his appreciation to four members of his staff — Linda Cholerton, Anne Collison, Julie Perrin and Pamela Bates — who dealt with much of the enormous volume of correspondence and the typing of illegible manuscripts at the Loughborough end of the editorial link. In particular, he would like to thank his wife, Susan, for her forebearance.

We would also like to acknowledge the great help of Miss J. M. Taylor, BA, ALA, Librarian and Museum Curator of the British Optical Association, in providing many of the references to other works used by various Contributors. Without the availability of this service to the profession the production of a text of this nature, much of it written by people in practice without the facilities of a university library available to them, would be extremely difficult, if not impossible.

Finally, we would like to acknowledge the assistance of the British Optical Association without whose backing the book would not have come into being.

London and Loughborough

Janet Stone and Tony Phillips

Introduction

Since the publication of the First Edition of *Contact Lenses, A Textbook for Practitioner and Student* the fitting techniques, materials and applications of contact lenses have developed very considerably, so too have methods of fabrication and, most important, the art and science of patient after-care has been accorded its rightful prominence.

Hence, the necessity for a new edition which will be welcomed by the established practitioner as well as by the student new to the subject.

This edition has the great merit that it covers basic fields of importance to those who fit contact lenses as well as the fitting techniques themselves, and progress in our understanding of the former — for example, physiology of the cornea — has played a large part in the advancement of this department of ophthalmic optics. No one would deny, for instance, that a primary aim in fitting most contact lenses is to interfere as little as possible with *normal* corneal metabolism, and our notion of what this represents is clearer today than it was only a few years ago.

Twenty-three authors have contributed, each an expert in his or her own field and yet a coherence of expression and approach has been attained by close co-operation between these workers, and the careful editorial work undertaken by Miss Stone and Mr Phillips. The chapters are in excellent order, and progress from fundamental aspects to clinical techniques. In every phase of the work a real attempt has been made, wherever possible, to avoid the unreasoned rule-of-thumb approaches which, unfortunately, have been a feature of some earlier contributions to the subject.

Undoubtedly, this work will occupy a prominent place amongst the works of reference and revision used by contact lens practitioners throughout the world. No student of ophthalmic optics can afford to be without it. Not least of all, it should appeal to the many manufacturing companies and laboratories who play no small part in caring for the ocular and visual welfare of the public.

London

G. M. Dunn
Professor of Clinical Optometry,
The City University, London

Contents

CONTENTS

CONTENTS

B. J. Tighe, BSc., PhD., CChem., FRIC
Senior Lecturer in Polymer Science, Department of Chemistry,
The University of Aston in Birmingham

A. P. Gasson, FBOA., FSMC., FAAO., DCLP
Contact Lens Practitioner, London

D. F. C. Loran, MSc., FBOA., DCLP., AMCT
Clinical Director and Senior Lecturer, Department of Opthalmics Optics,
The University of Manchester Institute of Science and Technology

F. A. Burnett Hodd, FBOA; HD., FSMC., DOrth., DCLP
Contact Lens Practitioner, London

With an Addendum on Soft Lens Flexure, by M. W. Ford, FBOA., FSMC., FAAO., DCLP.
Contact Lens Practitioner, North Shields, Tyne and Wear

CONTENTS

xii

Chapter 1

The History of Contact Lenses

A. G. Sabell

INTRODUCTION

A study of the history of contact lenses is necessary if only to appreciate how fruitful of ideas were our predecessors. The greatest achievement for which most of us can hope, is to revive a previously described idea which may have been abandoned because of some missing component of technical knowledge or prowess, and to pursue this to success within the framework of present-day technology. It is hoped, therefore, that readers will not pass over this chapter as having little relevance to modern contact lens practice, for it is upon the foundations of the past that we operate today. Likewise, the contributions which we may make, help to cement the structure upon which our successors will continue to build.

Look, therefore, very carefully at what has gone before and think deeply on these past efforts; their successes and their failures, for few ideas are completely new and the dividing line between success and failure may be very fine and may well depend, not on one's own efforts, but on the availability of supporting technology.

GENERAL DEVELOPMENTS IN THE CONTACT LENS FIELD

OPTICAL PRINCIPLES

Several well defined periods of development are recognizable from a survey of the broader aspects of contact lens history. The first of these hinges on theorizing about the optics of neutralization of the corneal surface in water. Experimental work of this period does little more than illustrate something of the optical theory which underlies the use

of the contact lens as a vision aid. This period begins with our earliest known reference, by Leonardo da Vinci, and the reader is referred to the detailed papers by Ferrero (1952) and by Hofstetter and Graham (1953) for a fuller description of this work. A useful general paper on Leonardo is that by Gasson (1976). The actual work by Leonardo da Vinci, claimed by some authors to pertain to the history of contact lenses, appears to consist of the construction of a large transparent globe intended to form a model of the human eye. This globe being filled with water, into which the observer immersed his face, resulted in the optical neutralization of the observer's corneas. Other than the fact that the corneal surface is neutralized it is difficult to see precisely what relevance this has to the history of the contact lens.

The work of René Descartes (1637) (*Figure 1.1*) has been well described by Enoch (1956) and does perhaps begin, if somewhat remotely, to have some bearing on the contact lens. The elongated water-filled tube used by Descartes to enlarge the size of the retinal image would certainly have been impossible to wear as an appliance for the correction of vision. Duke Elder (1970) also cites the experiments of Philip de la Hire around 1685 as having relevance to the history of contact lenses.

The contribution of Thomas Young (1801) provided the immediate stimulus leading to the first optical correction of astigmatism by Airy (1827) and in turn triggered the now famous speculation by Sir John F. W. Herschel (1845) (*Figure 1.2*). Herschel's far-seeing comments link the early period associated with optical theories with the beginnings of the clinical struggle. To this man, therefore, should go the honour of envisaging the more important of the present-day areas of

1

DISCOURS SEPTIESME. 79

Il ne reste plus plus qu'vn autre moyen pour augmenter la grandeur des images, qui est de faire que les rayons qui vienent de diuers points de l'obiet, se croisent le plus loin qu'il se pourra du fonds de l'œil, mais il est bien fans cõparaison, le plus important & le plus confiderable de tous. Car c'est l'vnique qui puisse seruir pour les obiets inaccessibles, aussi bien que pour les accessibles, & dont l'effet n'a point de bornes: en forte qu'on peut en s'en feruant augmenter les images de plus en plus iufques a vne grandeur indefinie. Comme par exemple, d'autāt que la premiere des trois liqueurs dont l'œil est rempli, cause a peu prés mesme refraction que l'eau commune, fi on applique tout contre vn tuyau plein d'eau, comme EF, au bout du quel il y ait vn verre G H I, dont la figure foit toute femblable a celle de la peau B C D qui couure cette liqueur, & ait mefme rapport a la distance du fonds de l'œil; il ne fe fera plus aucune refraction a l'entrée de cet œil, mais celle qui s'y faifoit auparauant, & qui estoit cause que tous les rayons qui venoient d'vn mefme point de l'obiet commencoient a fe courber dés cet endroit-

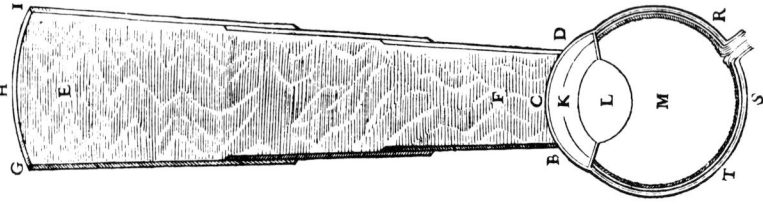

LA DIOPTRIQUE

78

plus prés de luy; ou mesme quelque peu d'auantage, a cause que ce ne sera plus sur la superficie de l'œil qu'ils commenceront a fe croiser, mais plustost sur celle du verre, dont l'obiet fera vn peu plus proche; ils formeront vne image, dont le diametre fera douze ou quinze fois plus grand qu'il ne pourroit estre si on ne fe feruoit point de ce verre: & par confequent fa fuperficie fera enuiron deus cens fois plus grande, ce qui fera que l'obiet paroi-ftra enuiron deux cent fois plus diftinctement. au moyen de quoy, il paroistra auffy beaucoup plus grand, non pas deus cent fois iustement, mais plus ou moins a propor-tion de ce qu'on le iugera estre esloigné. Car par exem-ple, si en regardant l'obiet X au trauers du verre P, on difpofe fon œil C, en mefme forte qu'il deuroit estre pour voir vn autre obiet, qui feroit a 20 ou 30 pas loin de luy, & que n'ayant d'ailleurs aucune cognoiffance du lieu ou est cet obiet X, on le iuge estre veritablement a trente pas, il femblera plus d'vn milion de fois plus grand qu'il n'est. en sorte qu'il pourra deuenir d'vne puce vn elephant; car il est certain que l'image que for-me vne puce au fonds de l'œil, lors qu'elle en est si pro-che, n'est pas moins grande, que celle qu'y forme vn ele-phant, lors qu'il en est a trente pas. Et c'est fur cecy feul qu'est fondée toute l'inuention de ces petites lunetes a puce compofées d'vn feul verre, dont l'vfage est par tout assés commun: bien qu'on n'ait pas encores connu la vraye figure qu'elles doiuent auoir: & pource qu'on sçait ordinairement que l'obiet est fort proche, lors qu'on les employe a le regarder, il ne peut paroistre si grand, qu'il feroit, fi on l'imaginoit plus efloigné.

Voiés en la page 74.

II

Figure 1.1—Pages from the seventh Discours of René Descartes (1637) showing his contact appliance

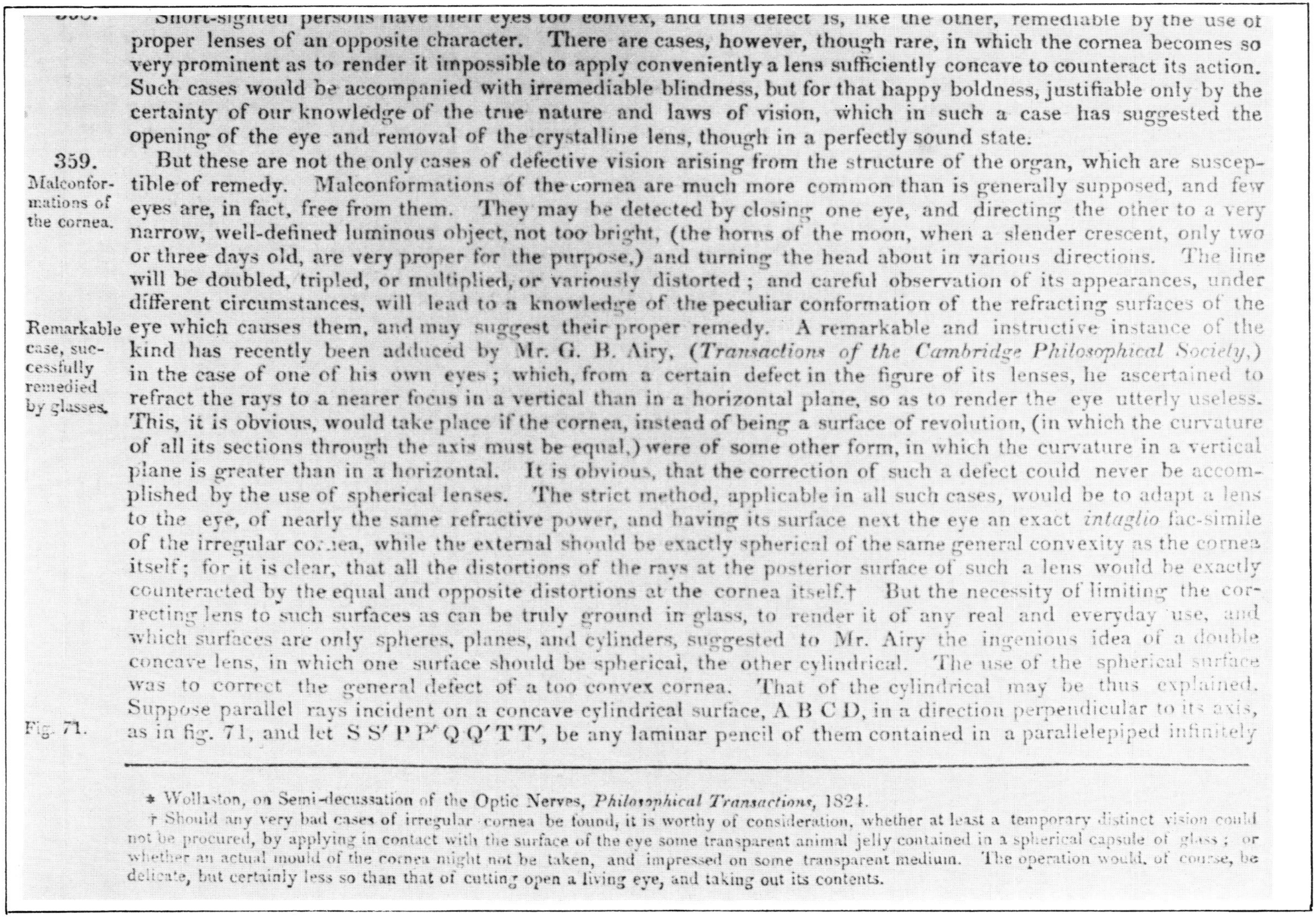

Short-sighted persons have their eyes too convex, and this defect is, like the other, remediable by the use of proper lenses of an opposite character. There are cases, however, though rare, in which the cornea becomes so very prominent as to render it impossible to apply conveniently a lens sufficiently concave to counteract its action. Such cases would be accompanied with irremediable blindness, but for that happy boldness, justifiable only by the certainty of our knowledge of the true nature and laws of vision, which in such a case has suggested the opening of the eye and removal of the crystalline lens, though in a perfectly sound state.

359.

Malconformations of the cornea.

But these are not the only cases of defective vision arising from the structure of the organ, which are susceptible of remedy. Malconformations of the cornea are much more common than is generally supposed, and few eyes are, in fact, free from them. They may be detected by closing one eye, and directing the other to a very narrow, well-defined luminous object, not too bright, (the horns of the moon, when a slender crescent, only two or three days old, are very proper for the purpose,) and turning the head about in various directions. The line will be doubled, tripled, or multiplied, or variously distorted; and careful observation of its appearances, under different circumstances, will lead to a knowledge of the peculiar conformation of the refracting surfaces of the eye which causes them, and may suggest their proper remedy. A remarkable and instructive instance of the kind has recently been adduced by Mr. G. B. Airy. (*Transactions of the Cambridge Philosophical Society.*) in the case of one of his own eyes; which, from a certain defect in the figure of its lenses, he ascertained to refract the rays to a nearer focus in a vertical than in a horizontal plane, so as to render the eye utterly useless. This, it is obvious, would take place if the cornea, instead of being a surface of revolution, (in which the curvature of all its sections through the axis must be equal.) were of some other form, in which the curvature in a vertical plane is greater than in a horizontal. It is obvious, that the correction of such a defect could never be accomplished by the use of spherical lenses. The strict method, applicable in all such cases, would be to adapt a lens to the eye, of nearly the same refractive power, and having its surface next the eye an exact *intaglio* fac-simile of the irregular cornea, while the external should be exactly spherical of the same general convexity as the cornea itself; for it is clear, that all the distortions of the rays at the posterior surface of such a lens would be exactly counteracted by the equal and opposite distortions at the cornea itself.† But the necessity of limiting the correcting lens to such surfaces as can be truly ground in glass, to render it of any real and everyday use, and

Remarkable case, successfully remedied by glasses.

which surfaces are only spheres, planes, and cylinders, suggested to Mr. Airy the ingenious idea of a double concave lens, in which one surface should be spherical, the other cylindrical. The use of the spherical surface was to correct the general defect of a too convex cornea. That of the cylindrical may be thus explained.

Fig. 71.

Suppose parallel rays incident on a concave cylindrical surface, A B C D, in a direction perpendicular to its axis, as in fig. 71, and let S S′ P P′ Q Q′ T T′, be any laminar pencil of them contained in a parallelepiped infinitely

---

* Wollaston, on Semi-decussation of the Optic Nerves, *Philosophical Transactions*, 1824.

† Should any very bad cases of irregular cornea be found, it is worthy of consideration, whether at least a temporary distinct vision could not be procured, by applying in contact with the surface of the eye some transparent animal jelly contained in a spherical capsule of glass ; or whether an actual mould of the cornea might not be taken, and impressed on some transparent medium. The operation would, of course, be delicate, but certainly less so than that of cutting open a living eye, and taking out its contents.

Figure 1.2 – The footnote in Sir John Herschel's dissertation on Light (1845) which constituted the beginning of modern thinking on contact lenses

clinical application of the contact lens. The reason for some confusion over the dates of Herschel's publications, whether 1827 or 1845, have been discussed by Bennett (1961). Although undoubtedly of great optical significance, the work of this period contributes nothing to the subsequent struggle to achieve toleration of a corrective appliance which must be worn on the eye of a visually handicapped individual. It might well be claimed that the earlier work had greater relevance to the development of the hydrodiascope by Lohnstein (1896) and Siegrist (1916).

EARLY PRACTICAL TRIALS

The second phase, that of practical clinical development, began with the work of Fick (1888), an English translation of which was made by May in the same year. This publication was preceded by two loosely related occurrences. The first was an idea put forward in 1886 by Galezowsky that a gelatin disc might be applied to the cornea immediately following cataract extraction. This disc was to be impregnated with cocaine and sublimate of mercury which would provide corneal anaesthesia to relieve post-operative pain and an antiseptic cover to prevent infection. This suggestion has been quoted by Mann (1938) although she gives no specific reference to the publication. Despite the horrifying implications of such a procedure, we may see in the proposal not only the first use of a soft and hydrophilic contact appliance but also the forerunner of the hydrophilic lens as a dispenser of ophthalmic medication. The second event preceding Fick's publication was, of course, the frequently described work by the firm of F.Ad. Müller Sohne at Wiesbaden for Dr Theodore Saemisch's patient. This consisted of the supplying of a protective contact device and does not appear to have been intended primarily as a visual aid. This contribution has been described by many authors amongst whom Nissel (1965) published a description of the origins of the firm of Müller and Sons of Wiesbaden. He quotes extensively from the work by Müller (1920) and also that of Müller and Müller (1910), both documents of great interest to the contact lens historian.

There also appeared in 1889 the inaugural thesis of August Müller of Gladbach, presented at the University of Kiel for his degree of Doctorate in Medicine and entitled 'Spectacle Lenses and Corneal Lenses'. This work incorporates the first known use of the expression 'corneal lens'. August Müller's interests (*Figure 1.3*) lay in the correction of high myopia, while Fick had been eager to produce usable vision for keratoconus patients.

Almost simultaneously Eugene Kalt in Paris was investigating contact lenses which were undoubtedly of corneal lens form, as 'orthopaedic appliances' in the treatment of keratoconus. This we may regard as laying down the groundwork which has led to the consideration of the contact lens as a means of myopia control and to its use in orthokeratology.

To return to the paper by Fick (1888); this is undoubtedly worthy of being read and re-read by all contact lens practitioners since it contains some astonishingly accurate observations and one wonders, in the light of some of Fick's observations, why the subsequent development of contact lenses took place so slowly. For example, in addition to recommending the use of contact lenses for keratoconus, Fick suggested their potential usefulness in aphakia, as prosthetic/cosmetic lenses and also postulated the use of pinhole contact lenses. He clearly foresaw the future high cosmetic demand for the wearing of contact lenses. Fick is, of course, best remembered for his description of what became called much later, Sattler's veil or, less commonly, Fick's phenomenon. He recognized that an adaptational process occurred enabling the wearer to become more tolerant, due to the regular usage of the contact lens, and even recognized that air trapped behind the contact lens on insertion retarded the onset of visual clouding. Fick was aware that the cause of this clouding lay in the epithelium.

Thus, by 1890 the foundations had been laid for: correction of visual errors, protection of the exposed cornea, remoulding of corneal shape, neutralization of corneal irregularity and the use of the contact lens as an applicator of ophthalmic drugs. Within this period also, the successes and failures of ocular toleration had been recognized and the pattern of events set which were to last until about 1930. This second period of development was therefore characterized by a lack of ability to ensure both good toleration and good vision by the majority of contact lens patients. The underlying reasons for such lack of success are to be found in the limited understanding of detailed topography, of the physiology of the anterior segment of the eye and of its responses to the contact lens. Although Fick had, in 1888, made a succession of very relevant observations, it appears that before many years were to pass he would have lost much of his interest in the contact lens. In his textbook *Diseases of the Eye and Ophthalmoscopy* (1896) he devoted only eight lines to the use of contact lenses. August Müller (1889) had described his own disappointing tolerance of contact lenses. He believed that the discomfort arose from pressure of the haptic portion of the lens on the conjunctiva. He also described the difficulty found in applying his contact lenses without air bubbles and his avoidance of this problem by inserting the lenses under water. From our understanding of the osmotic principles involved, this factor alone would account

lenses, that he was doomed to failure by such physiological factors.

It should be noted that Fick (1888) had pronounced on the subject of suitable fluids for inserting contact lenses and had settled on 2 per cent grape sugar solution, which he claimed was

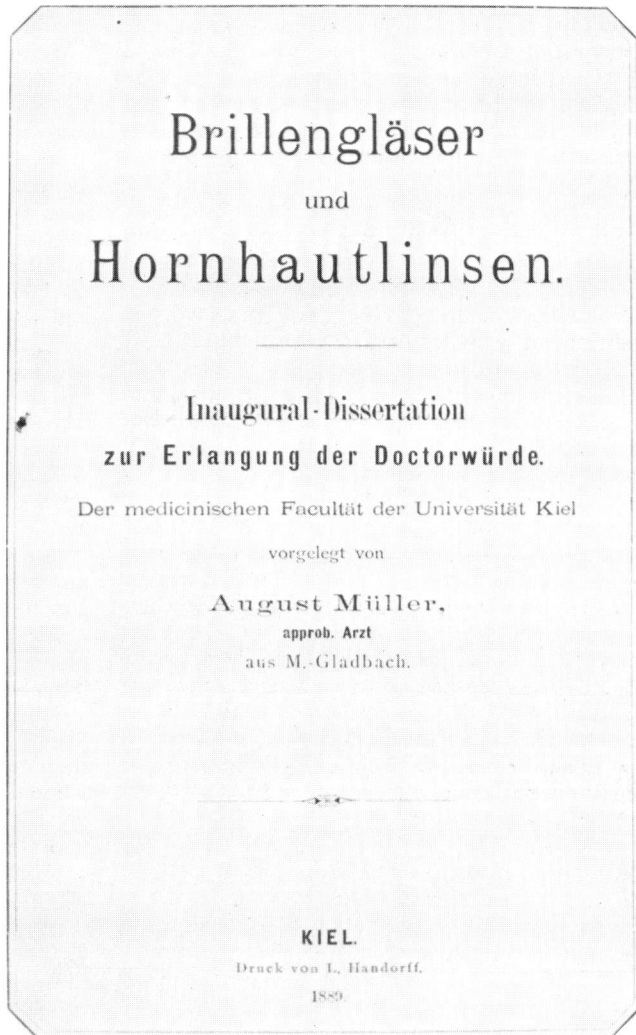

Brillengläser

und

Hornhautlinsen.

Inaugural-Dissertation

zur Erlangung der Doctorwürde.

Der medicinischen Facultät der Universität Kiel

vorgelegt von

August Müller,

approb. Arzt

aus M.-Gladbach.

KIEL.

Druck von L. Handorff.

1889.

Figure 1.3 – Title page of August Müller's doctoral thesis (1889) using, for the first time, the term 'Corneal Lenses'

for a very limited toleration since corneal oedema would develop within about fifteen minutes. Indeed, the physical discomfort which must have resulted from the marked hypotonicity of the liquid behind the contact lens probably accounts for Müller's use of cocaine eyedrops prior to inserting his lenses. It would seem, therefore, quite apart from any defects in physical fit of Müller's

capable of giving 8–10 hours wear by his rabbits before corneal clouding developed. It seems likely, had a slit lamp been available at this time, even of the level of sophistication of that used by Sattler (1938), that he would have observed the corneal clouding at an earlier stage. Fick stressed the need for sterilization of his dextrose solution by boiling prior to use and also pronounced on the need carefully to disinfect the lenses them-selves. Dor (1892) of Paris recommended the use of physiological saline solution as an insertion medium for contact lenses and this seems to have remained a popular choice up to the early 1940's. Perusal of Fick's 1888 paper shows that he had experimented with 'salt solutions, with various organic additions' and had discarded these in favour of his 2 per cent dextrose. Personal ex-periences of various contact lens solutions around 1946 convinced the author that sodium chloride solutions of various concentrations between 0.5 and 1.5 per cent were usually rejected by patients who complained of smarting sensation and redness of the eyes.

It seems, therefore, that from about 1895 until around 1930 an impasse was reached in terms of patient usage of contact lenses. Over this period the choice lay between the blown glass lenses produced by the firm of Müller's of Wiesbaden and the ground glass contact lenses such as those made by Carl Zeiss of Jena. The former were inferior in consistency of optical quality, but superior to the latter in comfort and duration of wearing. This lack of progress in achievement of longer wearing times with good vision did not prevent the development of ideas for utilization of contact appliances requiring only short-term application. Thus, the use of the contact splint to retain a corneal graft in position during healing has been attributed by Mann (1938) to de Weckers in 1900. Ideas progressed on the use of contact lenses in keratoconus and the classic form of the ground Zeiss lens began to emerge. Possibly the development by Koeppe (1918) of contact lenses for gonioscopy and for slit lamp microscopy of the fundus best illustrate the exploitation of short application potential of contact lenses.

PREFORMED FITTING SETS

During the 1920—30 period the trial fitting set as we know it today began to emerge, although Fick had in fact established the principles of preformed fitting on his rabbits around 1887 saying 'after many trials I abandoned the use of the casts and satisfied myself with obtaining glass vesicles, 21, 20, and 19 mm in diameter . . . From a large number of such small glass shells I selected the best-fitting one for each individual rabbit.' The Zeiss preformed development of the 1920—30 period began with Dr W. Stock's four lens set and developed to the massive afocal lens sets devised by Professor Leopold Heine (1929). It would seem then, although many attempts had been made from way back in the 1880's to produce good impressions of the eye surface, a lack of achievement in this quarter had allowed the preformed lens method to be developed to a reasonable level of sophistication by 1930.

OPHTHALMIC IMPRESSIONS

It was, therefore, the development of successful methods of making eye impressions to produce accurate casts of the eye surface which opened up the next phase in contact lens development. From this point, around 1930, considerably more information on ocular topography began to accumulate, although one should note that Fick in 1888, from his plaster of Paris impressions of the eyes of human cadavers had described the aspheric character of the scleral contours with considerable accuracy. In his paper of 1937, Obrig, while conscious of the potential of impression lenses, still appeared to favour the Zeiss preformed lens. He commented on the improved knowledge of ocular topography which by this time had indicated the need for larger back optic diameters. This he felt had made the use of the Zeiss lens preferable to the less consistent Müller lenses. Such views were in contrast to the opinions expressed five years earlier by Sitchevska. Obrig did, however, have certain reservations, commenting for instance 'raised corneal portions on Zeiss lenses are to be avoided wherever possible'. In the light of modern contact lens procedures, as recommended by the makers of one of the proprietary brands of hydro-philic contact lenses, it is interesting to read Obrig's (1937) recorded thoughts regarding the afocal lens system of Heine: 'Heine's method of fitting contact lenses has one decided disadvantage. It requires the investment of from $1,000 to $3,500 in trial lenses. This fact alone would prevent many ophthalmologists from working with these interesting and practical devices.'

Obrig (1938a) reported rapid strides in the use of moulded contact lenses. By this time he con-sidered the moulded lens to be 'the ideal conception of the perfect contact lens'. He clearly recognized that much intolerance was due to limbal pressure, especially at the nasal and temporal positions. This had been confirmed by the measurement of eye casts and hed realized the inaccuracy of trying to assess corneal diameter by direct measurement of the eye itself. In some cases the cast dimensions of the cornea were 3 mm larger than those given by the measurement of visible horizontal iris diameter. From the measurement of a large number of impression casts, Obrig produced his famous table showing average corneal dimensions, which set the pattern of full corneal clearance fitting during the following decade.

Curiously, although Obrig referred to clouding of the contact lens fluid by accumulation of mucous and sebaceous secretions inside the optic portion, he makes little reference to Sattler's veil, other than the mention in passing of 'transient corneal opacities' which may or may not be a part of that phenomenon. He was certainly aware of corneal clouding, since this was mentioned in his case summaries. The occurrence of limbal pressure from contact lenses was made more easily recognizable by Obrig's discovery (1938b) of the value of blue light with fluorescein solution in the fitting of contact lenses. Prior to this, the method of checking corneal clearance had been by use of the slit lamp; a technique requiring considerable expertise with this instrument.

This improvement in understanding of ocular topography and the gradual refinement of methods of fitting and observation constitute the main elements in contact lens progress prior to World War II. The pendulum was swinging from progress in the preformed field as depicted by the development of Zeiss fitting sets, to exploitation of the possibilities offered by the impression lens. Treissman and Plaice (1946) compared the advantages and disadvantages of impression and preformed lenses, and it should be remembered that their concept of the latter at that time was based on the Zeiss contact lens of the pre-war period and the Dixey plastics lens of very similar design which was developed in Britain during the early war years.

OCULAR TOPOGRAPHY AND PHYSIOLOGY

The 1930's then, was a period in which the comfort of contact lenses was improved by the realization that sustained corneal pressure from the lens was undesirable. From this stemmed the large optic portion giving initially, enhanced comfort to the wearer. This full clearance method of fitting scleral lenses was initiated by Obrig in the United States and became widely accepted in that country and also in Great Britain in the first half of the 1940's. The technique has been thoroughly discussed by Dickinson and Hall (1946), especially in relation to the Dixey preformed lenses of that period. Unfortunately, the advantages gained in comfort by a wide corneal clearance are rapidly eroded by concomitant disadvantages. First, the cosmetic appearance of this type of contact lens leaves something to be desired. Secondly, the full clearance optic must remain fluid-filled if visual performance is to be unimpaired. This calls for a glove-like seal by the haptic portion of the lens since loose channels offer the possibility of air

seepage and the resultant growth of an air bubble behind the optic portion. This zone, in this type of lens, was often fitted steeper than the cornea with a positive liquid lens which encouraged the location of any such air bubble in front of the pupil. The third and major adverse effect of the full clearance optic was the revealing of all the implications of Sattler's veil. It may seem curious that epithelial oedema induced by the wearing of contact lenses which had been observed as early as 1888 should have attracted little detailed attention until the investigation by Sattler around 1936. A possible explanation may lie in the physical discomfort induced by the ground spherical contact lenses which would often force removal of the lens long before the visual phenomena associated with Sattler's veil became pronounced. If a lens is wearable only for one hour, there is insufficient time for Sattler's veil to become objectionable (provided of course that an isotonic or slightly hypertonic solution is used to start with). The Müller lenses, on the other hand, appear to have been relatively untroubled by Sattler's veil for two possible reasons. First, the very hit and miss methods of selection of these lenses and the characteristic aspheric shapes of their haptic portions no doubt allowed loose channels for the relatively free passage of fresh tears. Secondly, such channels would be highly likely to allow seepage of air which would accumulate in the optic portion and help retard the onset of veiling. Consider the method in use at this time for detecting loose channels beneath the haptic portion. This was the application of a small quantity of 2 per cent fluorescein solution to the upper edge of the lens and the observation in white light (blue or ultra-violet light not being introduced until later) of the amber liquid tracking behind the haptic portion. But remember, the Müller blown lenses (*Figure 1.4*) were commonly made with white haptic portions akin to artificial eyes and such observations on these lenses would have been difficult.

As seen previously, such an accumulation of air behind the optic portion is likely to affect vision adversely unless of course that portion of the lens has been fitted with such a relationship to the cornea as to ensure that the air remains in the limbal region at all times. Such fine control of the fit of the optic portion was certainly not possible with the blown Müller lenses. But what if the inherent optical quality of the lens itself was poor, as were many of these blown lenses? Might not the presence of air go relatively unnoticed along with the general mediocre visual performance? Moreover, if the patient had a markedly irregular or hazy cornea and, thus, very low spectacle visual acuity, even a poor optical quality contact lens might effect considerable improvement, and a little disturbance such as that resulting from the presence of an air bubble might be regarded as of very secondary importance.

With the enhanced comfort offered by the full clearance optic it was hoped that longer wearing times might be possible. However, the new limiting factor of Sattler's veil was now revealed and indeed remained as the major cause of reduced contact lens toleration until the late 1940's. In a totally

Sattler's veil, led to considerable time being wasted during the late 1930's and early 1940's in the search for the ideal contact lens solution. Obrig and Salvatori (1957) describe vividly the wide range of possibilities which were explored. Changes noted in pH of the contact lens liquid during wear led to the trial of buffered solutions such as those formulated by Gifford and Smith (1933), Gifford (1935), and by Feldman (1937). This in turn led to the adoption by contact lens practitioners of the term 'buffer solution', used

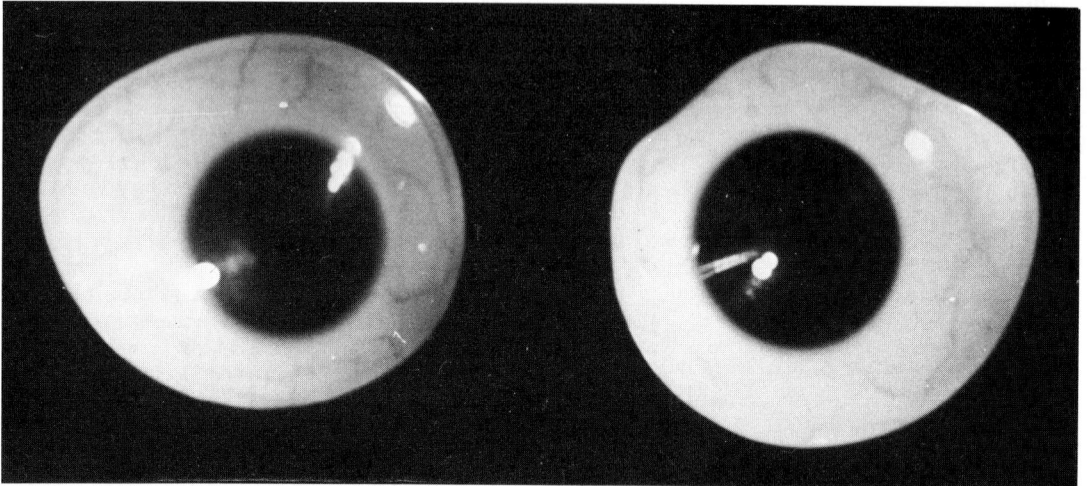

Figure 1.4–Blown glass contact lenses made by Müller's of Wiesbaden (c. 1900) showing the white haptic portions. From the museum, Department of Ophthalmic Optics, University of Aston in Birmingham

sealed lens, Sattler's veil would commence after some two hours of wear, visible to the wearer more readily indoors, as a faint blue haze resembling tobacco smoke. This haze became gradually more noticeable but without any gross reduction in visual acuity in the early stages. Shortly after onset, the classic rainbow rings resembling glaucoma haloes would become apparent. Few patients were able to pursue contact lens wear for more than about thirty minutes after the onset of these symptoms because the developing corneal oedema brought gradual onset of photophobia, blepharospasm, and an unpleasant sensation of heat to the eyes.

CONTACT LENS SOLUTIONS

The observation that tonicity and pH of solution may have some bearing on the onset time of

incorrectly to mean any suitable fluid used to form the liquid lens behind an unfenestrated contact lens, a term now rarely heard. It seems likely that this adoption of the term arose out of the supposed mechanical cushioning effect of the reservoir of liquid held behind the contact lens.

However, not all workers were led astray by the apparent comfort of wide corneal clearance, and the search for the 'elixir' of an ideal contact lens solution. Two notable exceptions in the 1930's were A. Mueller-Welt and Joseph Dallos, the latter laying down principles for the fitting of scleral contact lenses which have not been improved on since. Working on the assumption that the natural body fluid offers the best chance of success, Dallos in the 1930's set out to conserve the tears reservoir and to allow for its interchange by fresh tears. This process is discussed more fully later.

ACRYLIC CONTACT LENSES

Several other developments at this time were to stimulate interest in contact lenses and to herald in the current era of widespread contact lens usage. First, the gradual introduction of plastics materials to largely, but not yet completely, replace glass. Early attempts with plastics in the United States failed principally through unsuitability of available materials. The compromise introduced by Feinbloom (1937) of a plastics haptic portion holding a glass optic zone presents us with the 'half-way house'. The final introduction of the all-acrylic moulded lenses in the United States by Obrig Laboratories and of acrylic lathe-turned preformed lenses by the firm of C. W. Dixey in Great Britain, led not only to easier lens modification, but also opened the way to the development of successful corneal lenses. A second development at this time, also attributed to Obrig (1943), was the modification of existing cold dental alginates to produce the first specifically ophthalmic impression material.

A third step forward, perhaps at the time appearing to be of relatively minor significance, was the discovery by Obrig, referred to earlier, of the value of cobalt blue light for viewing fluorescein solution behind the contact lens. Solutions of fluorescein had been used in ophthalmology since first introduced by Straub in 1885, for the investigation of corneal lesions. In the fitting of scleral lenses, whilst white tungsten light was adequate for detecting the presence of the amber concentrated fluorescein solution tracking through loose channels beneath the haptic portion, the interpretation of varying depths of dilute fluorescein within the optic portion was not possible with this illumination. Corneal clearance had been determined by viewing the lens *in situ* by slit lamp microscopy. It was during such an inspection that Obrig (1938b) fortuitously discovered the value of the cobalt blue filter and thus provided a more ready means of detecting limbal pressure in his scleral lenses. This method of observation must have contributed greatly to the comfort of many patients. The enormous value of this discovery, leading as it did in later years to considerable improvements in the activating light source, is undeniable. It is hard to envisage the handicap to the development of corneal lenses had this simple step not been taken.

CORNEAL LENSES

By 1948, therefore, the way lay open to the attainment of all-day tolerance for the contact lens wearer. The principles of tears interchange in scleral lenses derived from Dallos's minimum clearance principles, over the next five years allowed the widespread achievement of long tolerance for many scleral lens wearers.

It should be emphasized that for most contact lens practitioners, there occurred, in the late 1940's, a great boost to morale as the work of Dallos (1946) and of Bier (1948) in developing the fenestrated method of fitting scleral lenses began to be widely applied. The difference in duration of wear between the unfenestrated scleral lens as fitted by most practitioners of the time and that of the minimum clearance fenestrated contact lens had to be seen to be believed. Lenses of full corneal clearance rarely allowed longer wearing time than three hours without removal to allow the subsidence of Sattler's veil. Scleral lenses, unfenestrated, but with a suitable minimum clearance optic and a suitably loose scleral fitting, might, by accident or design, allow eight to ten hours to be achieved without removal. However, more frequently the figure for this type of lens would be around four to six hours. Overnight as it seemed, patients could be transferred into all-day-long wearers of contact lenses for the very first time. The development, as with all others, revealed several minor problems not previously of great consequence; annoying clicking sounds produced in some lenses by the fenestration and frothing, often accompanied by 'dimple veil' causing visual inconvenience to the patient (*see* Chapter 10; and Chapter 16, Volume 2).

The introduction of acrylic materials around 1938 allowed, from 1948 onwards, the development of corneal lenses, eventually capable of giving all-day wear. The gradual refinement of lens design of these two forms of contact lenses has allowed them to cater for nearly all potential users. The progressive development in design of contact lenses is discussed later. One more radical innovation remains to be mentioned. The announcement in the *New Scientist* on 18th January, 1962, that O. Wichterle and D. Lim in Prague had developed contact lenses made of a new 'hydrocolloid' material, did not give rise to any great elation here in Great Britain. The short report announced that the Czechs had, with the new soft lenses, been able to achieve wearing times of up to eight hours in 10 per cent of patients fitted. By this time, the bi-curve hard corneal lenses of the late 1950's had been even further improved by multi-curve designs similar to those in wide use today. Some 75 per cent of patients were able to achieve 12–16 hours of continuous daily wear with such lenses. The prospect, therefore, of eight hours tolerance from the hydrophilic lens did not raise much enthusiasm (Wichterle, Lim and Dreifus,

1961). The hidden potential in the Czechoslovakian lens lay in the ability, by employing mass production methods, to provide 'off the peg' contact lenses which might be fitted in a matter of minutes. If the life span of these new contact lenses was only a few weeks, why worry, the mass production methods would soon bring down the manufacturing costs so low that we would all have disposable 'throw away and get replacement' type contact lenses.

Where has the happy vision gone to? It gradually emerged that apart from some restriction in toleration, reasonable vision with a gel lens was confined to those with strictly limited levels of corneal astigmatism. Microbiological problems also began to emerge and these three factors demanded long years of continued development. Restricted toleration problems were largely eliminated by further purification of the lens material and by development work on lens design. Optical prescription limitations, however, are still very much present despite some improvements. The problems of disinfecting these lenses still give rise to much heart searching and it is true to say that many practitioners and research workers are by no means satisfied with the currently available methods of disinfecting soft lenses. Likewise, the relatively complicated maintenance procedures necessary for patient use of soft lenses do not compete well with the more simple handling methods of the acrylic corneal or scleral lens. As a result of huge sums of money poured into soft lens research in 'reaching for the carrot' of large profits from a vastly expanded contact lens wearing populace, the manufacturing costs became so prohibitive as to totally destroy any image of 'throw away' contact lenses. Despite some recent reductions in supply costs in some quarters, hydrophilic lenses remain poor competitors financially and optically with conventional acrylic corneal lenses. Their greatest potential at the present time lies in their use for medical indications, and in particular in their ability to enable a relatively safe 24 hour-a-day wearing. This opens up the field of therapeutic use in various corneal disorders and also offers a contact lens correction to many aged or disabled patients who might have extreme problems in handling the other forms of contact lens.

THE DEVELOPMENT OF EYE IMPRESSION PROCEDURES

The concept of reproducing a cast or model of the eye surface as a means of manufacturing contact lenses is a natural one. Indeed, Herschel (1845), had said '. . . or whether an actual mould of the cornea might not be taken, and impressed on some transparent medium'. It is natural that Fick should have explored this possibility and he refers in the 1888 paper to his plaster of Paris eye impressions of rabbits and also of human cadavers. With respect to the rabbits, Fick described his technique in the following terms: 'In one of these animals, I drew the lids and nictitating membrane from the eyeball and filled the resulting sac with plaster of Paris of fluid consistence.' No mention is made of the use of a shell and since the plaster would set to a completely rigid state, such an appliance would seem unnecessary.

August Müller (1889) also makes mention of living eye impressions taken in plaster of Paris, and regarded it as a potentially suitable technique. From the present viewpoint the setting characteristics of plaster of Paris make it obvious to most that it is an unsuitable material for reproducing accurately the shape of a living and potentially mobile organ which can be distorted by pressure or indeed from its own movement. This factor apart, the absorbent qualities of the drying plaster must create marked disturbance of the epithelial surface and its mucin coating. Additionally, these very early workers would have had only cocaine eyedrops available as a local anaesthetic, a drug which, because of local cellular toxicity is now regarded as unsuitable for eye impressions even in conjunction with the greatly improved modern impression materials. From around 1890, although various attempts at refining the technique were made, little progress was achieved until after 1930.

Among the methods which had been tried were those of von Csapody (1929). He tried plaster of Paris on animal eyes but was unable to prevent it adhering and damaging the eye on removal. After trying other materials such as cocoa butter, whale fat and the paraffins, he settled for paraffin wax adjusted to a setting temperature around 40°C. This he poured in molten state into a glass cylinder which rested on the eye surface and which served to hold the eyelids apart. As the wax began to set, Csapody poured on top, a layer of iced liquid paraffin to render the paraffin wax sufficiently rigid to avoid distortion while being removed. After removal, a plaster of Paris positive cast was made as a stage towards making a metal positive die over which a glass shell could be blown. Von Csapody is also credited by Mann (1938) with attempting to make eye impressions in a material called Dentakoll.

In 1927, Joseph Dallos, approaching final qualification as a physician, joined the staff of the No.1 Eye Clinic at the Royal Hungarian Peter Pázmány University at Budapest (*Figure 1.5*). Dallos quickly developed an interest in the use of

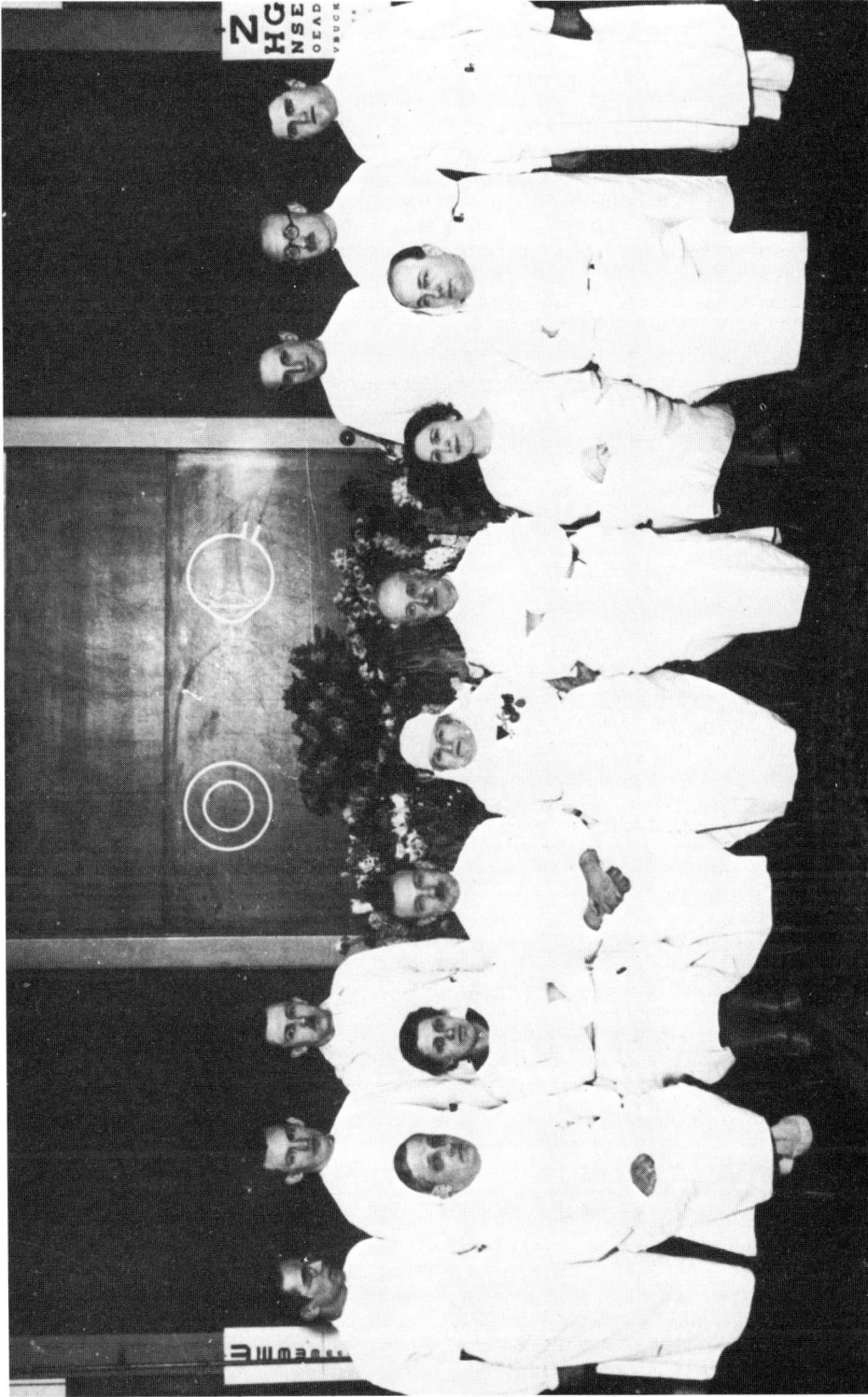

Figure 1.5—The staff of the No.1 Eye Clinic at the Royal Hungarian Peter Pázmány University, Budapest (c. 1930). Dr Joseph Dallos is standing, second from the right

contact lenses for correction of visual defects, but was frustrated by the limited choice afforded between the ground Zeiss lenses and blown Müller lenses of the time. Around 1931, Dr Alphons Poller of Zurich, had described a material derived from seaweed which was intended for preparation of surface impressions to make anatomical models. Shortly afterwards, in turning his thoughts towards eye impressions, Dallos's attention was drawn to Poller's Negocoll. His first trial with this material was made on a cadaver, the skin of the face, nose and eyelids being reproduced. Between the partially closed eyelids, a section of the corneal surface was reproduced with a smooth polished texture.

years he accumulated a large enough collection of glass shells made from his earlier impressions to enable him to avoid, with most patients, the necessity of taking further impressions. Gradually this set of 'type shells' grew until it contained several thousand shells from which a very near fit could be selected for almost any eye. As Dallos has demonstrated, it is not the initial selection nor the initial impression which provides the finished lens, but the careful tailoring of this preliminary form to the precise requirements of the individual eye. To this modification procedure Dallos gave the title 'haptics', which he described in 1936, as 'a new branch of prosthetics'.

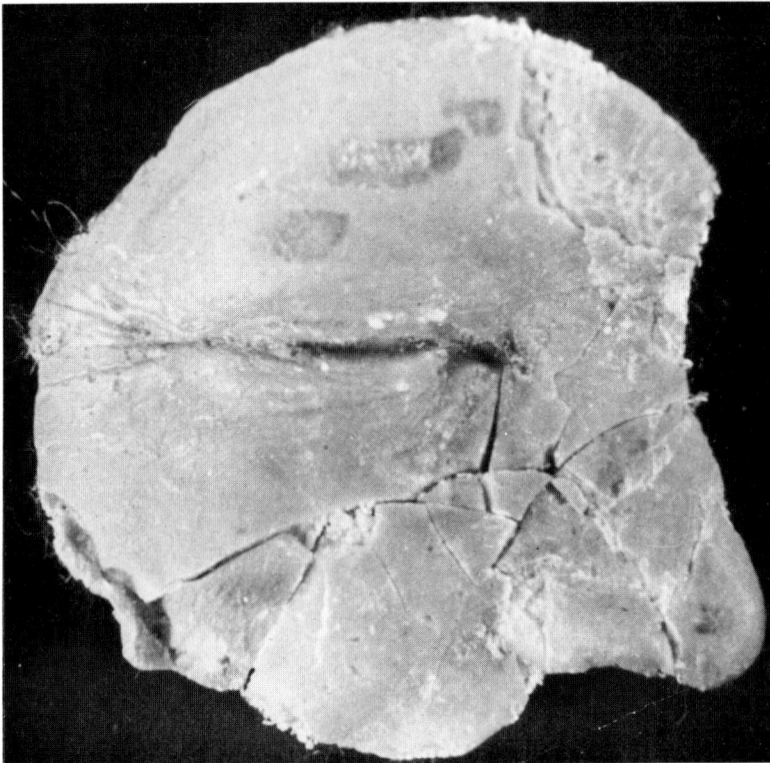

Figure 1.6 – The original Hominit cast made from the first impression made by Dallos using the new material 'Poller's Negocoll' (c. 1932). The right eyelids and nasal profile of the cadaver are clearly visible. From the museum, Department of Ophthalmic Optics, University of Aston in Birmingham

Dallos prepared a positive cast of this impression in the wax-like substance Hominit (*Figure 1.6*) and the smooth appearance of the visible corneal segment convinced him that Negocoll would be a suitable medium for ophthalmic impressions. Dallos went on to evolve a satisfactory impression routine by using Müller contact lenses as impression trays. Although he was the originator of the modern impression technique, he was never completely satisfied with the results achieved. After a few

Despite the apparent sound footing on which Dallos had placed Negocoll eye impressions, a few workers still attempted to use wax by various methods. Such a technique was described by Prister (1933) who devised an instrument in which a thin sheet of dental modelling wax could be suspended for application to the eye surface. The application of hot wet packs of cotton wool were used to soften the wax sheet and mould it to the shape of the eye. After this had been achieved, cold swabs were applied before the wax impression and its carrier were removed. Prister recommended making two plaster models from each wax impression, the cornea of one being varnished so that keratometry on the varnished cast could be compared with direct keratometry of the patient's cornea. This he suggested would act as an index of distortion resulting from the impression procedure.

A modification of this method using dental wax was, in fact, still being recommended by Feinbloom (1937) and also by Town as late as 1940. In Town's method, thin sheets of dental modelling wax approximately 0.7 mm thick were employed to make a shell by moulding over a hemisphere of the same radius of curvature as a preformed contact lens of approximately correct fit. Town, while agreeing that the Negocoll method resulted in the best impression of the cornea and limbus, nevertheless believed that as good an approximation of the somewhat variable shape of the scleral portion was to be obtained by the wax shell method. Having moulded his wax shell, he removed the central portion and substituted a small glass optic segment of 12 mm diameter. He then cut the external dimensions of the wax shell to an approximate size between 20 × 22 mm and 24 × 26 mm. This he placed on the anaesthetized eye for a period of 15 minutes. The eye was then sprayed with iced water to ensure rigidity of the wax model during removal.

Stevens (1936) described a method of eye impressions using Negocoll. In contrast to Dallos's use of a Müller lens as an impression tray, she reverted to the use of aluminium tubes used in the same manner as von Csapody's glass cylinders. These metal tubes, about 1 inch in length, were squeezed to form an oval section corresponding more nearly to the palpebral aperture. The technique resulted in a good impression of the cornea and limbus but the area of sclera reproduced was minimal and to this end it was an unsatisfactory method for the contact lens practitioner. In all fairness it should be added that the procedure was employed for making corneal models as part of an investigation into keratoconus and was not primarily intended as a basis for contact lens fitting.

Obrig (1937) described a technique for eye impressions essentially similar to that of Dallos, using Müller contact lenses as trays to hold Negocoll. He regarded the use of a speculum, recommended by Stevens, as unnecessary and undesirable and believed that the lens would achieve its natural centration if the lids were allowed to resume their normal position. Obrig did, however, recommend irrigation of the Negocoll impression with cold water to aid setting before

attempting to remove it from the eyes. He attributed the idea of specially designed shells or trays for eye impressions to Dr Harry Eggers who suggested the attachment of a fixed handle to a Müller type contact lens. Obrig at this time was himself employing a funnel-shaped blown glass shell, some 22 mm in diameter and 7 mm deep, having a handle about 25 mm long. He recommended plugging the hollow blown handle with cotton wool to aid retention of the Negocoll. These shells were marked with coloured spots or lines, red for right and light blue for left, which also served to indicate the position of the nasal canthus on the otherwise round shell. A problem was encountered when too much Negocoll was inserted with the shell. This tended to flow out beneath the lids extending away from the shell and encouraged the Negocoll to adhere to the eye surface so that it pulled away from the impression tray during removal. These early glass trays had no perforations to encourage the material to key on.

It is interesting to note that the early Zeiss moulded lenses introduced about 1936, which Obrig (1937) envisaged ordering from his casts, were stated to be oval in shape with dimensions of 20 × 19 mm. Another curiosity of the time is a recommendation that right and left markers on the finished lenses be placed at the nasal side of the haptic portion to aid correct positioning of the lenses. These markers were recommended to consist of coloured lines and one cannot help thinking that such marks would not be very acceptable cosmetically. Obrig mentioned incidentally, that delivery time of the moulded glass lenses from Jena was some two months, rather longer than the time taken for them to supply their ground preformed lenses.

Obrig's 1938a paper described a new design of impression tray and recognized the need to have a range of different sizes to cater for variations in eye size, palpebral aperture, lid tension, etc. Obrig's choice of material was still Negocoll, but his impression trays, although still of blown glass, were now oval in a range of sizes from 22 × 24 mm to 24 × 26 mm, the bowl being much nearer in shape to that of the Müller contact lens. He reported having performed well over four hundred impressions and had obviously resolved many of the points of difficulty encountered by earlier workers. He did, however, remark on the necessity in several instances to take up to three impressions of each eye in order to achieve a successful result. The time scale for these impressions is interesting when the various techniques are compared. Obrig (1938a) for instance, allowed his shell of Negocoll to remain on the eye for about five minutes before removal was attempted. The actual removal time averaged two to three minutes, but he reported one case in which he required nine minutes to achieve successful removal. Against such problems should be judged therefore, the slightly earlier decision by Dallos to abandon the impression method in favour of using 'type shells'. Although the 'type shell' approach may appear potentially lengthy and tedious, it should not be judged against the very easy and successful impressions made possible by modern materials and by the accumulated experience of the subsequent years, but against the less reliable methods of that time.

It is clear that, with the use of such non-perforated shells, excess Negocoll would be forced outwards into the fornices and it does appear that large particles had to be sought for and extracted following the removal of the impression itself. This problem has been largely eliminated with modern impression materials and perforated trays (see Chapter 9). Although attention was paid to the improvement of impression techniques by various workers, for example, Chisholm (1940) in developing methods and ideas for fixation and positioning of the eye, it is probably in the field of improved impression materials that most progress has been made. Maisler (1939) described the adaptation to ophthalmic use of 'a reversible hydrocolloid gel' introduced some months earlier by a San Francisco dental surgeon. This material – Kerr's hydrocolloid – was manufactured by the Detroit Dental Manufacturing Company, and was packaged in collapsible toothpaste-type tubes. The tube was immersed in hot water and kneaded to soften the consistency of the material. The hydrocolloid was employed on the eye between $104°F$ and $100°F$. After removal, dental plaster or stone was used to make the positive eye cast. Maisler found that the blown glass impression trays as recommended by Obrig (1938a) were too fragile and described his own trays made in silver which could be made sufficiently thin as to be malleable and therefore adjusted in contour to suit the individual eye. Maisler's shells were described as having perforations 'to obtain a better fixation between the gel and the moulding shell'. This may well be the origin of this design feature which is almost universally applied today. Maisler claimed a very fast setting time for Kerr's hydrocolloid – 'it is possible to obtain a hard gel within a minute's time by flushing the highly conductable silver shell with iced water from an undine'. He postulated the idea of a double-walled silver shell with inlet and outlet so that iced water could pass through the tray itself instead of being run over the patient's face and lids.

The introduction of cold-water mixed impression materials provided a considerable improvement in

this method of fitting contact lenses. Obrig (1943) introduced the first cold alginate impression material intended specifically for ophthalmic work. This was Ophthalmic Moldite, a material available until comparatively recently and therefore used by practitioners over nearly thirty years. Obrig had received the first supplies of this new material in the summer of 1942 and had made a considerable number of impressions before the publication of his paper. By this time, he was employing acrylic impression trays in place of his earlier blown glass ones. These new shells also had hollow tubular handles but had perforations around the bowl and he would appear, therefore, to have adopted this feature of the Maisler shells. From experience with Ophthalmic Moldite it would not appear to be a very suitable material for use with an unperforated shell after the manner in which Negocoll had been employed. On the other hand, Moldite did not seem so likely to leave large particles behind in the fornices. Essentially the routine described by Obrig (1943) is the classic 'insertion method' as used earlier with Negocoll and as still preferred by some practitioners to this day.

Obrig's 1943 paper, however, was not the first to describe the use of a cold alginate impression material. Boshoff earlier that year, had described his experience using the dental alginate Zelex (Figure 1.7), manufactured in London by the Amalgamated Dental Manufacturing Company. Curiously, Boshoff recommended that after anaesthetization, 'the soft paste is now ladled into the conjunctival sac while the lids are retracted and lifted slightly off the eyeball'. After this, he filled 'a large contact glass with the paste' and applied this also to the eye. He made the point that if the eye moves the paste and contact lens move with it. This principle of the natural centration of a handleless shell had been advocated by Obrig (1937) and was obviously to form the basis for the so-called 'concentric moulding' technique described later by Jessen and Wesley (1949). The contact lens used seems to have employed no perforations to aid adhesion of the Zelex, and Boshoff applied a rubber suction holder to the 'contact glass' to facilitate removal of the impression. He claimed that one advantage of Zelex lay in the shorter setting time – some three to six minutes as compared to that of Negocoll. Obrig, in describing Ophthalmic Moldite, also claimed a five-minute time from the mixing to the gelling points.

Sugar (1943), referred to recent improvements in dental impression materials and related these to developments in eye impressions. He surveyed the advantages and disadvantages already discussed and introduced another dental alginate, 'Coe-Loid powder', manufactured by Coe Laboratories of Chicago. This material was mixed at room temperature using water in which was dissolved a chemical retarder. Sugar was apparently using perforated impression trays as described by Obrig (1943). Setting time with Coe-Loid varied from five minutes at 65°F to two and a half minutes at 80°F in very much the same way as currently used alginate materials. Like Moldite, immersion in a fixing solution after removal from the eye was deemed necessary.

By the end of World War II (that is, 1945), therefore, cold setting impression materials were

whilst the impression material was being applied and avoid unseen contact between the cornea and the impression shell. The author was a subject for a demonstration of this non-anaesthetic method by one of Obrig's staff shortly after the opening of the London branch. It was certainly not a painful process but would have been unsuitable for use on the more apprehensive type of patient since good relaxation is an essential feature of first class impressions.

Shortly after this time, Jessen and Wesley (1949) published their account of what was claimed to be a new method of taking eye impressions, which they called 'concentric molding'.

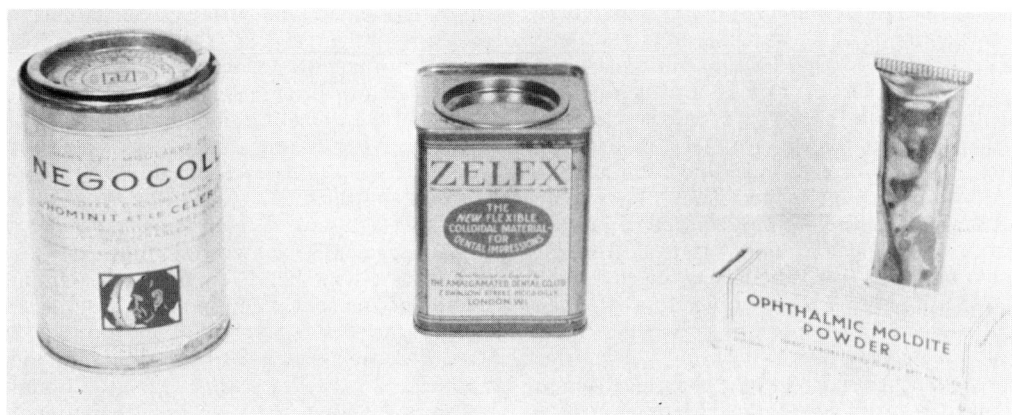

Figure 1.7 – The principal eye impression materials in use between 1933 and 1950. From the museum, Department of Ophthalmic Optics, University of Aston in Birmingham

firmly established. Dental Zelex was commonly employed in Great Britain until about 1947 when Obrig Laboratories opened a London branch and Moldite became readily available. Along with the arrival of Obrig Laboratories, came an impression technique new to Britain. This was the so-called 'injection method' still widely used.

Steele (1948) drew attention to the development by American optometrists of the technique of taking eye impressions without using any form of anaesthetization. The need for this variation in procedure was brought about by the drugs laws in the United States which necessitated the presence of a physician to instil the local anaesthetic drops. (The same legal restriction also led to the development by United States' optometrists of the technique of scleral tonometry.) It would seem logical that the injection method was developed so that the patient's eye could remain stationary

The technique hinged on the use of a contact lens-like impression tray with no handle. A description was given of the design for such an impression tray, no perforations being mentioned and the description of the procedure suggests that none were employed. The inside of the tray was 'scored or grooved' for good adhesion of the Moldite. The photograph of trays for concentric moulding published in Wesley and Jessen's later book (1953) shows a pair of impression trays each having four large perforations through the haptic portion. This would support the contention that Ophthalmic Moldite did not adhere well to an unperforated tray. The theory behind the concentric method was that provided the impression tray has the same dimensions and proportions as that required in the finished lens, it will centre itself accurately with its optic portion corresponding to the patient's cornea. Therefore, the positioning of

the eye by means of visual fixation of the contra-
lateral eye will be unnecessary. The patient may
either look straight ahead or may, in fact, close
both eyes while the impression material gels.

Over more recent years the method of using
trays without handles has been developed to a
very high level of efficiency by F. A. B. Hodd and
provides, in certain circumstances, a technique
superior to the use of trays with fixed handles.
It is interesting to speculate that this technique
has evolved from what was undoubtedly the very
first method to give a successful impression. It is
possible with the correct application of this type
of impression tray, to reach the point where little
or no modification to the haptic portion of the
resultant shell is required.

Returning to the subject of impression materials,
the introduction in Great Britain around 1950 of a
specifically prepared Ophthalmic Zelex packaged
into single-dose plastic tubes is worthy of note.
Ophthalmic Moldite had always been available in
multiple dose metal foil packages; so that the introduction of the correctly measured amount of
Ophthalmic Zelex supplied in a tube which could
be used as a measure for the correct volume of
water, did offer a great attraction at first. However,
it should be noted that materials packaged in such
small quantities appear to suffer loss of their
setting characteristics more rapidly than when
packaged in greater bulk.

In more recent years there has been a reversion to
dental alginates as shown by the current popularity
of materials such as Tissutex and Kromopan.
Storey (1972) has also published some observations
on the possible use of polysulphide rubber impression materials.

In retrospect, therefore, rapid progress in understanding ocular topography and the principles of
'haptics' followed close on the successful eye
impressions first achieved by Dallos around 1932.
Although much time and effort has been expended
on preformed lens designs by many workers over
three-quarters of a century of contact lens history,
the good eye impression still remains an unrivalled
basis for the fitting of scleral contact lenses. As a
final observation on eye impressions, the reader's
attention is drawn to the work of Dallos (1964)
in attempting to apply the technique of precise
corneal impressions to the fitting of acrylic corneal
lenses. It is appropriate to conclude this section
on the development of eye impressions by quoting
Obrig and Salvatori (1957). 'The original work of
Dallos in discovering and proving the use of
Negocoll as a practical, satisfactory medium for
making accurate molds of the living human eye
has done more than anything else to make modern
contact lenses a reality.'

DEVELOPMENT IN CONTACT LENS DESIGN

The gradual progress in contact lens design is, to a
great extent, the product of developing knowledge
of ocular topography and of ocular physiology.
A starting point may be taken as the words of
Herschel (1845) '. . . spherical capsules of glass'.
No simpler concept could be expressed than this
and it would seem to represent the commencement
of contact lens design.

Fick (1888) had begun by describing the
contact lens as 'a thin glass shell bounded by
concentric and parallel spherical segments'. Graham
(1959) contends that this description can only be
interpreted as 'the simple form characteristic of
corneal lenses'. Fick, in fact, goes on to describe
his initial experiment using large rabbits and,
from his plaster casts of these animals' eyes he
concluded that 'the radius of curvature of the
cornea did not differ materially from that of the
sclera, and the eyeball of the rabbit is pretty nearly
a sphere'. After having a number of shells blown
over the rabbit casts, Fick 'abandoned the use of
the casts and satisfied myself with obtaining glass
vesicles 21, 20 and 19 mm in diameter and with
having a segment separated from these, the base of
which was distant but a few millimetres from the
equator of the sphere'. From these stock sizes he
selected the best fit for each individual rabbit.
Thus, Fick was the first to use a preformed lens
approach.

The author has some doubts, therefore, over
Graham's contention that Fick's description of
a contact lens was necessarily that of a corneal
lens. It seems equally feasible that such a description fits his scleral lenses for rabbits. It is some
four pages later, after discussing the effects of
contact lens wear on the eyes of rabbits, that
Fick turns his attention to the human eye. He
concluded, from his plaster casts of the eyes of a
cadaver that 'the cast of a human eye shows very
plainly that the cornea is the segment of a sphere
of smaller radius of curvature than the rest of the
globe'. He then described having a glass sphere
made and then 'a portion of this small glass globe
was heated and a protrusion blown out'. Fick
himself wore this first human lens for two hours
and described his observations. Later, other
subjects repeated these wearing trials. It would
seem, therefore, that his first human lenses were
of scleral form and that single segment types
were, in fact, scleral lenses for rabbits and not
corneal lenses for human eyes. Indeed, Fick's
first paper on the subject was published before
any of his patients were actually wearing a
contact lens and was concerned with the results of
his preliminary experiments and with speculation

as to useful fields of application for the appliance. The lenses which he subsequently requested Professor Abbe to make for him are described as having an optic radius of curvature of 8 mm with a diameter of 14 mm and a scleral band of 3 mm width having a radius of curvature of 15 mm. This made an overall size of just under 20 mm – decidedly a scleral contact lens.

What is certainly interesting and has a bearing on contact lens design, is that Fick recognized the following features, many of which were not utilized until many decades later.

(1) From the cast of the human eye 'the radius of curvature of the conjunctiva increases steadily from before, backwards as we would naturally expect when we consider that only in the immediate neighbourhood of the cornea does the conjunctiva lie directly on the globe, while further back it is separated from this by a constantly thickening layer of tendons, connective tissue, fat and muscles.'

(2) 'Concerning the clouding of the cornea, it was easily demonstrated that it was produced solely by the liquid. For if a glass be applied without filling it with liquid, the cornea will remain clear.'

Thus, Fick recognized the factor which has provided the limitation to usefulness of scleral lenses with spherical haptic portions. He had observed the crucial feature on which the fenestrated scleral lens was to be based many decades later as a means of solving the very phenomenon of corneal clouding with which his name was to be associated. Fick is usually, and rightly, credited with an interest in correcting the sight of keratoconus patients. Such patients may have central corneal opacification for which he described the treatment of iridectomy, often followed at that time by corneal tattooing. He described the potential usefulness of a pinhole contact lens, saying 'a contact lens which has been rendered opaque except opposite the artificial pupil'. This device he suggested as an alternative to corneal tattooing which too often resulted in severe infection of the eye.

Several authors have attributed the suggestion of contact lenses for aphakia to later writers, but Fick in 1888 wrote 'at the same time the high degree of hypermetropia in aphakia could be diminished by increased curvature of the glass cornea'. Fick described also the potential use of the cosmetic (prosthetic) contact shell 'by the use of a contact lens upon which the iris and a black pupil is painted'. In retrospect, therefore, Eugen Fick showed an astonishing insight into the future of the contact lens field.

SCLERAL LENSES

If we follow, first, the development of the scleral contact lens, practitioners were, for the next few decades, confined either to the blown lens such as that made at Wiesbaden, or to the solid ground lens being made primarily by Carl Zeiss of Jena. We may gain some concept of the former type by reference to the writings of Sitchevska (1932). In this paper, which compared the design of the two forms of contact lens, she drew attention to the empirical fitting procedure necessary for the Müller lenses. The necessity to try very large numbers of lenses was tedious both to the patient and the practitioner and if subsequently the lens should break or become roughened, the whole process had to be repeated. Sitchevska reported several cases fitted with Müller contact lenses around 1929 to 1931. The numbers of lenses tried in during the fitting sessions were as follows: '100 trials to select lenses for a pair of eyes, 20 tried for one eye, 45 for one eye and 20–30 for the other, 35 lenses tried for one eye.'

The problems in selecting a suitably fitting Müller lens become very apparent. Nevertheless, toleration was often surprisingly good, Sitchevska quoting 8–10 hours, 12–14 hours, 6–9 hours, 10–12 hours, 4–5 hours, 8–9 hours, and 6–8 hours in successive patients. In contrast, a number of these patients had already tried wearing the ground Zeiss lenses with typical wearing times recorded as 'could not wear, 1–2 hours or half to one hour'. The chances of good visual correction, however, were much higher when using the Zeiss lens.

To what can we attribute the greater toleration of the Müller lenses? Sitchevska quoted a weight of 0.5 g for the Zeiss and a little more for the Müller lens, so weight seems not to provide the answer. She described the classic design of the Zeiss lens 'the glass until recently was standardized to four precise corneal curvatures, the radii of which are 6.5, 7.1, 8.1 and 9 mm. The diameter of the corneal segment is 12 mm and the height of the corneal segment or its depth varies with the various radii – 3.0, 4.0, 4.5 and 5.0 mm respectively'. Therein lies the reason for the choice of such a curious range of back optic radii. If we remember that up to this time no method had been devised for obtaining detailed impressions of the cornea, and what dimensions had been obtained were the result of optically measuring the visible iris diameter, the reasons for regarding a back optic diameter of 12 mm as satisfactory, become apparent.

Duke-Elder (1961) quotes the average corneal diameter from the findings of many different workers as 11.7 mm horizontally by 10.6 mm vertically and slightly less in females. From these figures, an optic diameter of 12 mm seems more than adequate. It was not until 1938 when Obrig first published his table of corneal dimensions as determined from the measurements of several hundred eye casts resulting from Negocoll impressions, that the inadequacy of back optic diameter of the Zeiss lens became completely apparent. The reader should remember that the means of determining lack of corneal touch at this time lay in slit lamp examination of the contact lens on the eye. The slit lamps of this period had nowhere near reached the present level of sophistication and ease of use. Moreover, the assessment of clearance at the limbal region would have been more uncertain with the slit lamp than would apical clearance. Fluorescein solution, long used for the detection of corneal lesions, had been recommended as an aid to detection of loose channels under the haptic portion of contact lenses. Von der Heydt and Gradle (1930) had recommended the slit lamp in conjunction with fluorescein for these observations. The examination, however, was made with white tungsten light so the fluorescence of the dye was only poorly activated. It was not until 1938 that Obrig drew attention to the value of using cobalt blue light for this work. Thus, it is not surprising that the significance of the small back optic diameter of the Zeiss contact lens was not recognized earlier.

In contrast to the Zeiss lens, with its haptic portion of about 4.5 mm wide, Sitchevska described the Müller lens as having a haptic band nasally of 4–5 mm, superiorly and inferiorly of 7–8 mm and temporally of 10–12 mm and comments on its 'gradual transition from the corneal into the scleral part'. Here then were reasons for the greater acceptability of the blown Müller lens. Obrig and Salvatori (1957) cite both Sommer (1927) and Gill (1928) as attributing the greater comfort of the Müller lens in part to its natural fire polish as a consequence of the techniques of its manufacture. Having examined the quality of finish on Zeiss lenses of the period, the author does not accept this factor as being sufficient to account for the marked discrepancy. We must look to the design of the back surfaces to account for the better toleration and to the greater likelihood of loose channels in the Müller lens allowing tears interchange. One should remember that in those days of restricted tolerance, high ametropes often managed to use the Müller contact lenses throughout the day, by wearing monocularly and alternating between right and left lenses.

The development of design in the Zeiss ground lens is in itself an interesting study. Mann (1938) claims that the Zeiss ground lens was first produced in 1911. The first vestiges of a preformed fitting set approach were seen around 1920 with the introduction of the four lens set already referred to. Dr W. Stock, its originator, was himself a sufferer from keratoconus and intended this four lens set primarily for the investigation of that condition. Dallos (1936) credits Professor Hans Hartinger with the idea of blending the sharp junction between optic and haptic portions of the Zeiss lens and Zeiss trade literature of around 1933 offers the option of a totally blended transition. Over the course of the 1920's, an increasing range of back haptic radii were added to the original 12 mm standard radius. First, a choice of three radii 11.0 mm, 12.0 mm and later 13.0 mm. Later, the half millimetre steps and ultimately, according to Dallos (1936), a full range in 0.25 mm steps from 10.0 mm to 14.0 mm were available.

Around this time was also being evolved the 'afocal lens approach' of Professor Leopold Heine. This offered a choice of a large range of afocal Zeiss lenses of varying back optic radii with which a wide range of ametropia could be corrected purely by means of the liquid lens. The ultimate range of back optic radii extended from 5.0 mm to 11.0 mm and eventually these could be procured in steps of 0.1 mm. Towards 1930 it had become the practice to grind some optical power on to the Zeiss prescription lens so that a total correction could be achieved partly from the liquid lens and partly from the optical power of the contact lens. However, such optical power was limited to the order of ±7.00 D. It was not until Dallos in 1933 made the suggestion that if the front optic diameter be restricted to some 8 mm, much higher optical values would become possible and a great saving effected in thickness and weight. Despite this technical progress, Dallos (1936), remarking that the University of Kiel Eye Clinic had a set of over 300 different Zeiss lenses, voiced the opinion that these were able to satisfy only a very small percentage of those who needed to be fitted with contact lenses. Dallos went on to survey the developing topographic knowledge of the eye which was accruing from successful eye impressions, noting the changes in scleral curvature from one meridian to another and naturally concluding that a lens construction based on segments of a sphere, could not possibly result in the uniform contact necessary to achieve a high level of comfort.

Another of the major contributions by Dallos to contact lens technology in the early 1930's was the development of glass moulding as a means of producing the initial contact shell. It became necessary to perfect a series of stages by which the Negocoll impression and its resultant Hominit positive could be transposed via plaster of Paris into a brass die suitable for the glass moulding procedure. Moreover, it was important that such shells should be capable of being optically ground and polished in the central portion in order to form the clinically important link between the wearable but optically imperfect Müller lens and the optically good but less well tolerated Zeiss lens. The attempts at optically grinding the Müller lenses by Erggelet and von Hippel, reported by

with bunsen burner to heat the glass plate (*Figure 1.8*). The metal die, which is an essential feature in the process of moulding a glass contact lens was held by means of forceps, or some other suitable attachment, in the hand of the technician. When the glass had reached a suitable temperature as judged by its colour the metal die was quickly thrust through the softened glass plate and the source of heat removed. On removal

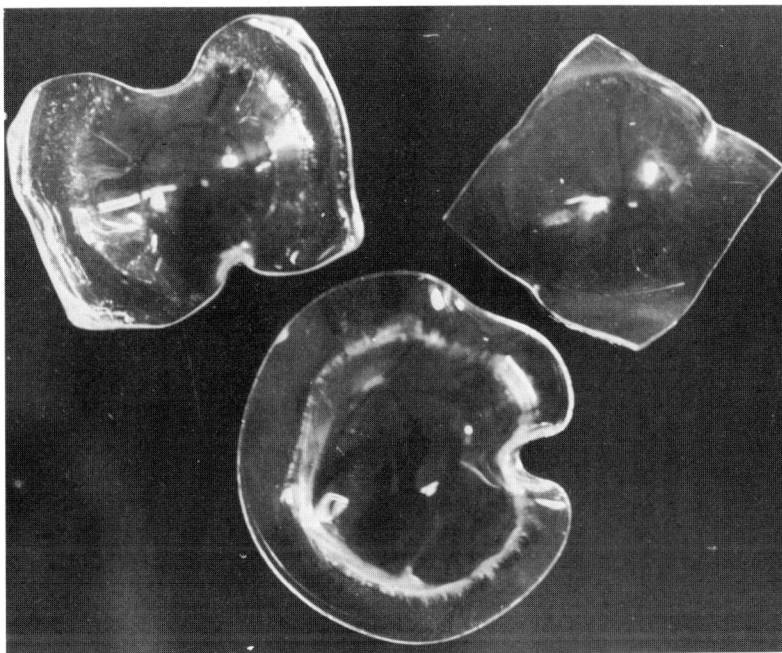

Figure 1.8 – The results of initial experiments at moulding sheet glass made by Dallos in Budapest (c. 1932). From the museum, Department of Ophthalmic Optics, University of Aston in Birmingham

Sitchevska (1932), had all ended in complete failure. That this process is not intrinsically impossible was later demonstrated by Dallos, although for normal scleral lens production it would not appear to be a sound production method. From this point on, therefore, a third method of manufacturing contact lenses had begun, a method which was to dominate the field until well into the 1950's. It was a method equally applicable to the new acrylic materials which were to be introduced some ten years later.

Dallos's earlier attempts at glass moulding were made in the bacteriology laboratory of the No.1 Eye Clinic, Budapest, and were begun using sections of cleaned photographic plates. The earliest attempts were made with equipment no more elaborate than a standard laboratory tripod

of the heat, the glass solidifies so rapidly that unlike moulding acrylic materials it is not strictly necessary that the die should be held in a mechanically rigid clamp. Later, presses as developed by Dallos and his team became rather more sophisticated and an example of one produced in the early 1940's is shown in *Figure 1.9*.

It was from this time on that Dallos established what he referred to as 'haptics, a new branch of prosthetics'. It was this establishment of rules for the modification of casts and shells leading systematically to the achievement of a well balanced contact lens, that placed Dallos at the forefront of contact lens practitioners of the inter-war years. Dallos himself said in 1936 'one does not now select at random among the ready made shells or bowls and trust a patient's judgement as to the best one to use; but with the same precision with which the dioptric requirements are prescribed one forms the shells for the individual patient'.

It is interesting, however, that by 1938, Dallos, although still thoroughly disenchanted with the Zeiss lens, was also showing signs of moving away from eye impressions. With respect to the Zeiss fit could be achieved by using even the very narrow haptic portion of the 20 mm Zeiss lens, he had become sceptical of the necessity of taking eye impressions for each individual patient. Dallos (1938) went on to say 'you start every case with an approximately fitting shell. If you have got a set consisting of 30 pairs of differently shaped

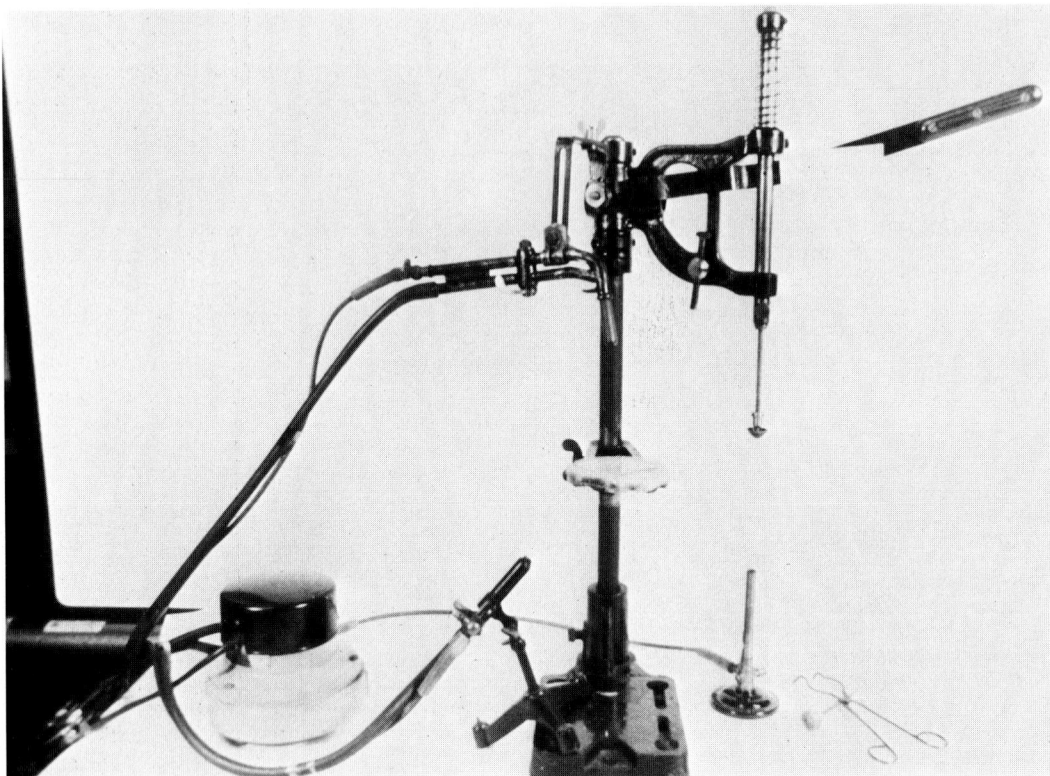

Figure 1.9–A Dallos gas operated press for the moulding of glass contact shells (c. 1942). Two gas jets heat the glass blank from above and below simultaneously, whilst the bunsen burner heats the brass die in readiness for the moulding process. From the museum, Department of Ophthalmic Optics, University of Aston in Birmingham

lens he said '. . . the scleral periphery of these spherical glass bowls will reach the conjunctiva and touch it, but only over certain circumscribed areas. These areas are always at the edge of this ring-shaped scleral part, either on the peripheral margin, or on the limbus inside, so that even if the glass does rest on the scleral conjunctiva it never fits with its surface, but rather with sharp edges'. We were later to see, using this same reasoning, the introduction by Forknall (1948) of the 'offset scleral lens'. Although Dallos did not for one instant accept that a uniform scleral forms, you will very probably find a type that will not differ or differs only slightly from the eye to be fitted. If you have not got this set, then you had better take a mould from the eye'. We see therefore that by 1938 Dallos had firmly established his technique of fitting from 'type shells' in preference to making new impressions for each patient.

There followed the development of this unique approach to the fitting of scleral contact lenses, a method which comparatively few practitioners have learned and fewer still have mastered. It was an achievement which for years to come, set Dallos far ahead of his contemporaries in the achievement of long toleration combined with good visual results. The natural outcome of these complexities in scleral lens fitting was to encourage rather than to discourage an interest in the potentialities of the spherical preformed lens.

Impetus was given to the preformed lens following the introduction of acrylic materials. In the United States this development occurred predominantly in the field of the moulded impression lenses pioneered by Obrig, although Feinbloom (1937) had, some years earlier, introduced a contact lens with a plastics haptic portion and a glass optic. In England, by contrast, the early moves were made in the preformed field. C. W. Dixey and Co., made their first experiments which led to their 'flexible contact lenses' in 1938. Although these were at first plastics replicas of the Zeiss lens, their manufacturing process was unique and marks the introduction of the fourth major lens-making process. According to Ridley (1946), Dixey's were the first to use a precision lathe for cutting contact lenses from solid blocks of I.C.I. Transpex material. This lathe-cutting process allowed much greater variability in dimensions than was readily obtainable from the glass-grinding methods of Zeiss. The Dixey lenses were of the same order of thickness as the Zeiss lens but could readily be made thinner (down to 0.3 mm) without becoming excessively fragile. Thus, a saving of about 60 per cent on the weight of the glass Zeiss lens could be achieved.

The image of this almost infinite variety of sizes and shapes offered by the 'Dixey flexible contact lens' encouraged an increase in the number of contact lens practitioners, especially in the non-medical sphere. Names like Frank Dickinson and Keith Clifford Hall began to be closely associated with the fitting of this form of lens. Their textbook in 1946 contained considerable information on the development from the Zeiss to the Dixey forms of contact lens. In the medical sphere, Ridley (1946) came out with enthusiasm on the side of the Dixey lens. He presented an analysis of results of two hundred consecutive patients and said 'it is believed that this series justifies a revival of interest in the spherical or regular types of lens'. Ridley believed that 80 per cent of contact lens patients were suitable for fitting by this method and that the lens could be prescribed by an opthalmologist in the same way that prescriptions for spectacles were handed out.

Dallos's message of the direct involvement of the contact lens practitioner in the achievement of a personally tailored contact lens seemed unattractive to seekers after an easier road. It should be remembered that in Great Britain, for the period between the introduction of the Dixey lens, until about 1947, the only plastics contact lenses available were of preformed design. Patients for whom impressions were necessary still had to be supplied with glass lenses. This factor swung preference somewhat artificially towards the preformed lens approach.

This interest in preformed lenses was further accentuated by the introduction, between 1945 and the end of 1948, of a number of apparently new ideas. From America came a new concept by Feinbloom who had pioneered the early transition from glass to plastics. Feinbloom (1945) discarded the concept that the weight of a scleral lens was best supported over as broad an area as possible. He felt that a minimal tangential touch would not only evoke less sensation but would enable a better balance on the toroidally shaped sclera, and he introduced the 'Feincone lens'. At this time, no toroidal preformed scleral lenses were in regular production and the only alternative lay in the impression. It has been suggested in the section on development of impression techniques that this limitation of choice in the United States may have placed the optometrist in an embarrassing situation *vis-a-vis* the drugs' laws. Thus, any preformed lens able to make further inroads into the 20 per cent or so of patients for whom impressions seemed the only answer must have been welcomed. The 'Feincone lens' offered a preview of the apparent simplicity of fitting which was to reappear in the corneal lens sphere in later years as a result of similar tangential designs. Certainly lack of the sharp corneo-scleral junction caused by making the conic scleral portion tangential to the optic, resulted in an initially favourable sensory response. It was, however, in the American tradition set by Obrig, a full clearance lens and therefore did nothing to reduce the effects of Sattler's veil. Watson (1947) commented on its prominent appearance and, introducing his 'Kelvin lens' he described his attempts at improving cosmetically on this American design. Curiously, a second conical design was announced in the same issue of the *Optician*, by Cohen (1947), whose design was also manifestly based on Feinbloom's lens. These designs were reviewed by McKellen (1949).

By far the best known design in Great Britain said to be based on the Feincone lens is the 'wide angle lens' of Nissel, introduced in 1947. This and the other two conical designs mentioned had one aim in common, to reduce the vast numbers of permutations introduced by the Dixey system. In theory, it was possible to order well over 3,000 different Dixey lenses without repeating oneself, and this did not include variations in optical power. By standardizing the diameter of the optic portion and relating the apical cone angle of its transition region to a fixed relationship with the back central optic radius, a considerable reduction in permutations was achieved by the wide angle design. For specific detail of the construction of wide angle lenses and of typical fitting sets the reader is referred to Chapter 10 on preformed fitting techniques.

This post-war period saw the introduction of two other concepts worthy of note. The first, by Bier and Cole (1948), was introduced as a small set of preformed fitting shells intended to supplement the fitting sets of Dixey lenses then in use. Once again, the rationale was one of simplification of the processes of scleral lens fitting to reduce the number of fitting lenses needed by the less experienced practitioner. This was the 'transcurve lens' and its originators claimed cosmetic superiority by virtue of a larger overall size than that of the Dixey type preformed lens. The most significant contribution associated with the transcurve lens was the introduction of the separate corneal measuring caps now referred to as FLOMS (Fenestrated Lenses for Optic Measurement). In the author's opinion, these provide one of the most useful aids for teaching students the fundamental principles of the optic fit. Again, the design features of these measuring lenses are dealt with in Chapter 10.

The second of these post-war concepts was the 'offset lens' of Forknall (1948), designed with an aspheric haptic portion to obtain a more even pressure on the sclera. This also aided simplification of fitting by the elimination of the necessity to adjust haptic radius when overall size was changed. As McKellen (1963) later pointed out, this design was neglected by most contact lens practitioners and the concept achieved wider prominence only after its re-introduction by Ruben within the sphere of corneal lenses around 1966. The use of 'offset scleral lenses' is also dealt with under Preformed Fitting in Chapter 10.

One should not end this account of aspheric scleral lens development without reference to the lenses of A. Mueller-Welt. Starting with experience of making and fitting artificial eyes, Mueller-Welt established the ability to grind optical surfaces on blown lenses and later, using acrylic materials, expressed a preference for polymerization in making the initial shell rather than cutting or grinding. Mueller-Welt (1950) described the design of his lenses as having a capillary tears layer over the cornea and retaining an air cushion beneath the haptic portion. This part of the lens may incorporate several areas of differing curvature, seeking to take account of the anatomy of the insertions of the four recti muscles. Thus, with these two designs we can see the preformed advocates attempting to reproduce in mathematical terms, the natural asphericity achieved by the practitioners using the impression or 'type-shell' approach to fitting.

The design of scleral lenses and the principles on which their fitting is based has therefore changed little over the past 30 years. One or two more recent developments are worthy of note, such as the methods of Marriott (1967, 1970) for the manufacture of impression shells and also the scleral lens design developed by Lewis (1970) both of which are particularly useful in hospital eye service contact lens work.

CORNEAL LENSES

For some time after 1948, corneal lenses were believed by many to have originated with those devised by Tuohy and by Woehlk. These lenses have been described by Bier (1957) and it is interesting to note that while the name of Tuohy is much more widely known as a corneal lens pioneer, the lenses being used at that time by Woehlk more nearly conform in size to those corneal lenses in use today.

However, Obrig and Salvatori (1957) and Graham (1959) have put forward evidence of the attempted use of corneal lenses from as early as 1888. According to Graham, one of the first to draw attention to earlier usage of corneal lenses was Emerich Rakoss, who published a paper entitled 'How New is the Corneal Lens?' in May 1950. Both authors refer to the lenses by Kalt of Paris as being of corneal lens design. Obrig and several other authors have described M. Kalt as an optician. This seems unlikely in view of his participation in meetings of the Société Francaise d'Ophtalmologie, as reported (in the discussion following a paper) by Chevallereau (1893). It would seem likely that this was Eugene Kalt of Paris whose photograph is published by Duke-Elder (1969). In addition, Graham presents reasons for supposing that Fick's early lenses were also of corneal design and this point has already been discussed.

There can be little doubt, however, that August Müller of Kiel University was the first to use the name corneal lenses — 'Hornhautlinsen', although it is doubtful whether this is an accurate description of the type of lens which he employed since it is described as having a scleral radius of 12.0 mm.

Experimental corneal lenses were made by Carl Zeiss and were described by von Rohr and Stock (1912). Erggelet also used such lenses experimentally and Obrig and Salvatori (1957) published a letter from Dr Hans Hartinger confirming this. The purpose of these lenses was to induce artificial ametropia for subjective testing of various designs of spectacle lens.

Some years later, H. J. M. Weve used glass corneal lenses to aid observation of the retina during detachment surgery. This lens was referred to by Mann (1938), and Obrig and Salvatori (1957) again published a letter from Weve on their use. These authors also quoted Zeiss records as showing a number of companies and institutions to whom glass corneal type contact lenses were supplied in the 1935/36 period.

It is safe to assume that, while these early glass corneal lenses may have been of value for experimental work or as aids to eye surgery, they were unsuccessful as routine corrective appliances for ametropia. Obrig and Salvatori (1957) quote from a letter by Dr L. L. Forchheiner saying that these lenses could not be worn satisfactorily owing to their weight. Graham (1959) published a comparison of dimensions between a Zeiss-made 1932 glass corneal lens of thickness 0.6 mm and a 1948 variety acrylic lens of thickness 0.3 mm. Since apart from thickness, these lenses were of similar dimensions and allowing for the specific gravity of the two materials, it would appear that the glass lens would be at least four times the weight of the plastics one. One must also bear in mind the surface characteristics of the two materials. Glass wets more readily and has a more slippery surface when on the eye. This factor has been quoted to account for a preference for glass artificial eyes by patients who have changed over to wearing an acrylic prosthesis. Since successful performance and comfort of a corneal lens depends on the ability of the upper lid to raise the lens on the cornea after each blink, it seems unlikely that glass would offer a suitable material for a corneal lens. Thus, the key factor necessary for successful development of corneal lenses was the development of polymethyl methacrylate around 1936 and its introduction as a contact lens material around 1938 by Obrig in the United States and by C. W. Dixey and Company in England. Indeed, it may well be claimed that Dixey's development of the first precision lathes for cutting contact lenses also played indirectly a major part in the success of this type of lens.

By 1952, the Tuohy lens had become well known and yet was still a poor competitor with the scleral lenses of that period. This may be judged by reference to the American Army Report which is quoted extensively by Obrig and Salvatori (1957). It was not until the introduction of the single curve 'microlens' in 1954 that corneal lenses appeared to offer an effective alternative to scleral lenses. This lens (Dickinson, 1954), devised jointly by W. P. Soehnges in Germany, Frank Dickinson in England and John C. Neill in the United States, proved a considerable improvement on the larger Tuohy lenses. Reference to *Table 1.1* will make clear the design differences.

Table 1.1–Comparison of Parameters of the Tuohy and Microlens Corneal Lenses

Parameters	Tuohy lens	'Microlens'
Overall size	11–12 mm	9.5 mm
Centre thickness	0.25–0.35 mm	0.20 mm (afocal)
BCOD	8.0–9.0 mm	9.5 mm
Back surface peripheral curve	One	None
Width of peripheral curve	1.5 mm	Nil
Relationship of peripheral curve to BCOR	0.3–0.6 mm flatter	Identical

For comparison of fit, the reader should consider only the zone of constant curvature. Thus, we are effectively comparing a 'microlens' of overall size 9.5 mm fitted 0.3–0.6 mm flatter than the corneal keratometer reading, with a Tuohy lens effectively of 8.5 mm diameter fitted about 0.35 mm flatter than the keratometer reading. The central bearing zone was therefore similar in size in both cases. The Tuohy lens being considerably larger, the resultant fluorescein band of edge clearance was broader. This, in turn, limited the application of this larger lens for the fitting of astigmatic eyes and Bier (1957) considered 2.00 D of corneal astigmatism to represent the limit of usefulness for the Tuohy lens. By contrast, the 'microlens' allowed fitting of up to 4.00 D of corneal toricity. Both designs, having a hard apical pressure zone tended to result in apical corneal erosions. With this factor in mind, the smaller and thinner microlens had obvious advantages and its designers specified that centre thickness should be calculated on the basis of an afocal lens of centre thickness of 0.2 mm. This is a realistic standard which could still be usefully followed by many of todays corneal lens manufacturers.

About this time, an interesting, if unproductive, design of corneal lens was introduced by de Carle (1953) which was designated the 'corneal flange lens'. This was a peripheral bearing lens having minimal central clearance and a fairly large fenestration. It was an interesting attempt to apply scleral lens principles to the fitting of corneal lenses. As such it was unsuccessful through inability to control air bubble movement.

Concern over corneal apical erosion and corneal curvature changes resulting from long periods of microlens wear led to the establishment by Bier (1956a, 1956b) of a new principle of fitting. His 'contour lens' of similar size and thickness to the 'microlens' could, by virtue of its smaller BCOD, be fitted nearly in alignment with the central zone of the cornea, thereby minimizing to a considerable degree the central erosion problem. Edge clearance was still maintained by a peripheral curve some 1.25 mm wide. Bier postulated that flatter corneas were likely to require a greater peripheral curve flattening relative to BCOR than steeper corneas. He therefore recommended fitting sets in which the degree of peripheral flattening ranged from 0.3 mm at the 7.3 mm BCOR region to 0.7 mm at the 8.5 mm end of the range. This system does make for some complications in using such a set and from about 1960 it became more common to employ fitting sets with a standard peripheral flattening throughout the full lens range. It is interesting to note that with recent trends to establish fitting sets having a constant edge lift, we may be moving back towards the principle established loosely by Bier in 1956. With his introduction of the contour lens, Bier also laid down the principles of apical clearance fitting, producing a slightly modified design of lens for this purpose. The mode of fit, however, was not popular and did not gain acceptance until later design changes allowed its full exploitation.

Two main changes in design paved the way to apical clearance fitted corneal lenses. The first of these was the addition of a flat edge bevel or narrow peripheral curve of some 12 mm radius. This feature was introduced into the United Kingdom by de Carle, with the Sphercon corneal lenses which were modifications of a slightly earlier American design of the same name. The popularity of these lenses developed in Great Britain over the early 1960's and established firmly the multicurve principle.

The second feature, also seen in the Sphercon range of lenses, which helped to establish successful apical clearance fitting, was the reduction of overall size. This resulted from the manufacturing of fitting sets of standard lenses around 9.20 mm and smaller lenses of 8.70 mm.

The trend towards narrower intermediate and peripheral zones in tricurve, tetracurve and pentacurve corneal lenses at this time led, via various degrees of blending of transitions, to the manufacturing of various continuous back surface designs. Thus, the late 1960's were characterized by the establishment of a series of aspheric corneal lenses ranging from the tangential conic periphery designs of Thomas (1968) and Stek (1969) through the continuous offset bicurve principle (Ruben, 1966; Nissel, 1967), to the lathe-cut continuous aspheric lens of Nissel (1968). We have thus reached the present-day period with a wide range of corneal lens designs including toric and multifocal lenses available for selection by practitioners in order to fit successfully the vast majority of prospective patients.

A discussion of hard corneal lenses should not end without reference to the 'Apex lens' of Fraser and Gordon (1967). This, like the scleral design of Lewis (1970) was a lens designed specifically for the hospital service. The name 'Apex' — said to be derived from 'aphakic experiment' — not perhaps the most tactful of designations, nevertheless clearly defines its area of application. It is a large corneal/perilimbal design which in an aphakic prescription is necessarily fairly thick and heavy. It is a design likely to be tolerated well only by corneas which have suffered a fair depletion of sensibility as is commonly the case following cataract surgery. The great advantage of this design which has been discussed by Ruben (1967) lies, for aphakics, in the great stability of vision resulting from the limbal locating characteristics.

SOFT CONTACT LENSES

The final section of this contact lens history must relate to the designs in various soft contact lenses. As stated in the first section of this chapter, the early Czechoslovakian hydrophilic lenses were introduced in the belief that manufacturing costs would be so low as to provide disposable contact lenses. The second hope was that, being a very flexible material, a single back surface curve, steeper than the human cornea would suffice and such a lens could be pressed into place and would conform to the corneal contours.

The original lenses therefore had an aspheric rear surface derived from the centrifugal force employed in their spin-casting mode of fabrication. Visual instability rapidly forced the multiplication of back surface curves and led to lens design studies such as that of Larke and Sabell (1971). From around 1967, the availability of buttons of the dehydrated Hema material allowed development of lathe-cutting techniques and the application of conventional back surface designs as had been employed in various hard corneal and perilimbal lenses. The characteristics of soft lens materials and the various lens designs which are in current use will be dealt with in later chapters (see Volume 2, Chapters 13 and 14).

The history of any subject is, to a considerable extent, a story of human endeavour. In the field of contact lenses, two names stand out above all others. A. Eugen Fick made so many significant observations and predictions in his paper of 1888 that one is left with the feeling that all subsequent work has been tying up the loose ends which he indicated. Fick seems to have provided so many of the clues necessary to assist later workers.

The second of these great names is that of Joseph Dallos, for what other worker in the field of ophthalmology has devoted an entire working life to the furtherance of contact lenses? The work of Dallos from 1927, reopened a somewhat static field and from then on he made a series of practical contributions which carried the contact lens from the status of an interesting novelty to that of a routinely applied correction. Indeed, when one looks at the maintenance routine which todays patient has to apply daily to hydrophilic contact lenses one wonders whether Dallos had not reached the optimum point by 1936, when he said: 'its care is simple. In the evening after it is removed it is washed in water, dried with a clean cloth and put away in a padded box'. When one considers the present-day dependence of the contact lens wearer and, indeed, of the contact lens practitioner on technologists in many spheres, which in turn usually ends in inconvenience to both patient and practitioner, one may look back with nostalgia to the period during which contact lenses were truly regarded as 'solutionless lenses'.

We find, therefore, from study of the past events, that a recurrent pattern emerges. Initial concepts often represent over-simplification and the uncovering of problems leads to increasing complexity in design, materials and procedures in order to solve these problems. This increasing complexity may eventually reach proportions which become self-restrictive and which therefore call for attempts at re-simplification, at the same time retaining those features proven to be useful during the phase of increasing complexity. The overall trend is towards greater intricacy but conscious effort should be made to limit unnecessary technical complication. This is also true of contact lens economics; the most widespread application and usage of contact lenses will be aided by striving for simplicity of maintenance and handling procedures since in the end, each appliance must be used by a lay person with very limited supervision. Development work aimed at reducing both supply and manufacturing costs of contact lenses is also important if maximum use is to be achieved. To these ends, the processes of re-simplification become important.

No attempt has been made in this chapter to deal with the history of contact lens instrumentation. Neither has any detailed consideration been possible of development of knowledge relating corneal physiology and pathology to the use of contact lenses. One day, perhaps a detailed history of contact lens manufacturing will be written, but such items must wait for the future and it is time for the reader to turn to a consideration of present-day knowledge and techniques.

ACKNOWLEDGEMENTS

I am indebted to the following persons for guidance and assistance in the preparation of this chapter.

Dr Joseph Dallos for many hours spent in discussion and for the most generous donation of many items of great historic interest to the Museum of the Department of Ophthalmic Optics at Aston University. Mr George Nissel for most useful advice and suggestions. The University of Kiel Library for the loan of August Müller's dissertation 'Brillengläser und Hornhautlinsen'. The University of Durham Library for the loan of Volume 4 of Encyclopaedia Metropolitana (1845). Mr Richard Hildred of the Birmingham and Midland Eye Hospital for photographic assistance. Last but by no means least to: Mrs Brenda Phillips of the Department of Ophthalmic Optics, University of Aston, for great patience over typing.

REFERENCES

Airy, G. B. (1827). 'On a peculiar defect in the eye, and a mode of correcting it.' *Trans. Camb. Phil. Soc.* **2**, 267–271

Bennett, A. G. (1961). 'Contact lenses: origin.' *Optician* **141**(3663), 644

Bier, N. (1948). 'The practice of ventilated contact lenses.' *Optician* **116**, 497–501

Bier, N. (1956a). 'A study of the cornea.' *Am. J. Optom.* **33**, 291–304

Bier, N. (1956b). 'The contour lens – a new form of corneal lens.' *Optician* **132**(3422), 397–399

Bier, N. (1957). *Contact Lens Routine and Practice*, 2nd ed. London: Butterworths

Bier, N. and Cole, P. J. (1948). 'The "transcurve" contact lens fitting shell.' *Optician* **115**(2987), 605–606

Boshoff, P. H. (1943). 'Use of Zelex in making impressions of the eye for molded contact glasses.' *Archs Ophthal. N.Y.* **29**, 282–284

de Carle, J. (1953). 'Corneal flange contact lenses.' *Optician* **125**(3248), 616–620

Chevallereau, M. A. (1893). 'Traitement du kératocone.' *Bull. Mëm. Soc. fr. Ophtal.* **11**, 385–392

Chisholm, J. F. (1940). 'Corneal molding for contact lenses.' *Archs Ophthal. N.Y.* **24**, 552–553

Cohen, L. B. (1947). 'The new "Lewcone" contact lens.' *Optician* **114**, 226–227

von Csapody, I. (1929). 'Abgusse der lebenden augapfelo-berfläche für verordnung von kontaktgläsern.' *Klin. Mbl. Augenheilk* **82**, 818–822

Dallos, J. (1933). 'Ueber haftgläser und kontaktschalen.' *Klin. Mbl. Augenheilk* **91**, 640–659

Dallos, J. (1936). 'Contact glasses, the "invisible" spectacles.' *Archs Ophthal. N.Y.* **15**, 617–623

Dallos, J. (1938). 'The individual fitting of contact glasses.' *Trans. Ophthal. Soc. U.K.* **57**, 509–520

Dallos, J. (1946). 'Sattler's veil.' *Br. J. Ophthal.* **30**, 607–613

Dallos, J. (1964). 'Individually fitted corneal lenses made to corneal moulds.' *Br. J. Ophthal.* **48**, 510–512

Descartes, R. (1637). *Discours de la Methode,* Discours No. 7, *La Dioptrique* p.79

Dickinson, F. (1954). 'Report on a new corneal lens.' *Optician* **128**(3303), 3–6

Dickinson, F. and Hall, K. G. C. (1946). *An Introduction to the Prescribing and Fitting of Contact Lenses.* London: Hammond and Hammond

Dor, H. (1892). 'Sur les verres de contact.' *Revue Gén. Ophtal.* **11**, 493–497

Duke-Elder, S. (1961). *The Anatomy of the Visual System, System of Ophthalmology.* **2**, 93. London: Kimpton

Duke-Elder, S. (1969). *Diseases of the Lens and Vitreous: Glaucoma and Hypotony, System of Ophthalmology.* **11**, 260. London: Kimpton

Duke-Elder, S. (1970). *Ophthalmic Optics and Refraction, System of Ophthalmology.* **5**, 713. London: Kimpton

Enoch, J. M. (1956). 'Descartes' contact lens.' *Am. J. Optom.* **33**, 77–85

Feinbloom, W. (1937). 'A plastic contact lens.' *Am. J. Optom.* **14**, 41–49

Feinbloom, W. (1945). 'The tangent cone contact lens series.' *Optom. Wkly* **36**, 1159–1161

Feldman, J. B. (1937). 'pH and buffers in relation to ophthalmology.' *Archs Ophthal. N.Y.* **17**, 797–810

Ferrero, N. (1952). 'Leonardo da Vinci: of the eye.' *Am. J. Ophthal.* **35**, 507–521

Fick, A. E. (1888). 'A contact lens.' Translation by C. H. May. *Archs Ophthal.* **19**, 215–226

Fick, A. E. (1896). *Diseases of the Eye and Ophthalmoscopy.* Translation by A. B. Hale. (1902). p.261. Manchester: King

Forknall, A. J. (1948). 'Offset contact lenses.' *Optician* **116**(3006), 419–421

Fraser, J. P. and Gordon, S. P. (1967). 'The "apex lens" for uniocular aphakia.' *Ophthal. Optician* **7**, 1190–1194 and 1247–1253

Gasson, W. (1976). 'Leonardo da Vinci – ophthalmic scientist.' *Ophthal. Optician* **16**, 393–541

Gifford, S. R. (1935). 'Reaction of buffer solution and ophthalmic drugs.' *Archs Ophthal. N.Y.* **13**, 78–82

Gifford, S. R. and Smith, R. D. (1933). 'Effect of reaction on ophthalmic solutions.' *Archs Ophthal. N.Y.* **9**, 227–233

Gill, R. R. (1928). 'Korrektion des keratokonus durch kontaktgläser.' *Klin. Mbl. Augenheilk.* **80**, 100

Graham, R. (1959). 'The evolution of corneal contact lenses.' *Am. J. Optom.* **36**, 55–72

Heine, L. (1929). 'Die korrektur saemtlicher ametropien durch geschliffene kontaktschalen.' *Ber. 13' Congr. Ophthal. Amst.* **1**, 232–234

Herschel, J. F. W. (1845). ' "Light" Section XII "Of the structure of the eye, and of vision".' *Encyclopaedia Metropolitana* **4**, 396–404

von der Heydt, R. and Gradle, H. (1930). 'Concerning contact glasses.' *Am. J. Ophthal.* **13**, 867–868

Hofstetter, H. W. and Graham, R. (1953). 'Leonardo and contact lenses.' *Am. J. Optom.* **30**, 41–44

Jessen, G. N. and Wesley, N. K. (1949). 'Concentric molding.' *Optom. Wkly* **40**, 753

Koeppe, L. (1918). 'Die mikroskopie des lebenden augenhintergrundes mit starken vergrösserungen im fokalen lichte der Gullstrandschen Nernstspaltlampe.' *Albrecht v. Graefes Arch. Ophthal.* **95**, 282–306

Larke, J. R. and Sabell, A. G. (1971). 'Some basic design concepts of hydrophilic gel contact lenses.' *Br. J. physiol. Optics* **26**, 49–60

Lewis, E. M. T. (1970). 'A haptic lens design.' *Ophthal. Optician* **10**, 56–59 and 86

Lohnstein, T. (1896). 'Zur gläserbehandlung des unregelmässigen hornhaut-astigmatismus.' *Klin. Mbl. Augenheilk.* **34**, 405–423

McKellen, G. D. (1949). 'Conicai contact lenses.' *Br. J. Ophthal.* **33**, 120–127

McKellen, G. D. (1963). 'The "offset" haptic lens.' *Optician* **14**(3479), 105–107

Maisler, S. (1939). 'Casts of the human eye for contact lenses.' *Archs Ophthal. N.Y.* **21**, 359–361

Mann, I. (1938). 'The history of contact lenses.' *Trans. Ophthal. Soc. U.K.* **58**, 109–136

Marriott, P. J. (1967). 'The construction of impression haptic lenses.' *The Contact Lens,* **1**(3), 8–14

Marriott, P. J. (1970). 'The use of acrylic laminates in fitting impression haptic lenses.' *Br. J. physiol. Optics* **25**, 29–43

Mueller-Welt, A. (1950). 'The Mueller-Welt fluidless contact lens.' *Optom. Wkly* **41**, 831–834

Müller, A. (1889). 'Brillengläser und hornhautlinsen.' *Inaugural Diss. Univ. Kiel* **20**

Müller, F. A. and Müller, A. C. (1910). *Das Kunstliche auge,* 68–75. Wiesbaden: J. F. Bergmann

Müller, F. E. (1920). 'Ueber die korrektion des keratokonus und anderer brechungsanomalien des auges mit müllerschen kontaktschalen.' *Inaugural Diss. Univ. Marburg*

Nissel, G. (1965). 'The Müllers of Wiesbaden.' *Optician* **150**(3897), 591–594

Nissel, G. (1967). 'Off-set corneal contact lenses.' *Ophthal. Optician* **6**, 857–860

Nissel, G. (1968). 'Aspheric contact lenses.' *Ophthal. Optician* **7**, 1007–1010

Obrig, T. E. (1937). 'Fitting of contact lenses for persons with ametropia.' *Archs Ophthal. N.Y.* **17**, 1089–1120

Obrig, T. E. (1938a). 'Molded contact lenses.' *Archs Ophthal. N.Y.* **19**, 735–758

Obrig, T. E. (1938b). 'A cobalt blue filter for observation of the fit of contact lenses.' *Archs Ophthal. N.Y.* **20**, 657–658

Obrig, T. E. (1943). 'A new ophthalmic impression material.' *Archs Ophthal. N.Y.* **30**, 626–630

Obrig, T. E. and Salvatori, P. L. (1957). *Contact Lenses.* 3rd ed. pp.340–345. New York: Obrig Laboratories Inc.

Prister, B. (1933). 'I vetri adesivi ed il calco del segmento anteriore del bulbo.' *Boll. Oculist.* **12**, 149–160

Rakoss, E. (1950). 'How new is the corneal lens?' *Ophthal. Dispenser* May 1950, cited by Graham, R. (1959)

Ridley, F. (1946). 'Recent developments in the manufacture, fitting and prescription of contact lenses of regular shape.' *Proc. R. Soc. Med.* **39**, 842–848

von Rohr, M. and Stock, W. (1912). 'Ueber eine methode zur subjektiven prüfung von brillenwirkungen.' *Albrecht v. Graefes Arch. Ophthal.* **83**, 189–205

Ruben, M. (1966). 'The use of conoidal curves in corneal contact lenses.' *Br. J. Ophthal.* **50**, 642–645

Ruben, M. (1967). 'The apex lens.' *The Contact Lens* **1**(4), 14–28

Sattler, C. H. (1938). 'Erfahrungen mit haftgläsern.' *Klin. Mbl. Augenheilk.* **100**, 172–177

Siegrist, A. (1916). 'Die behandlung des keratokonus.' *Klin. Mbl. Augenheilk.* **56**, 400–421

Sitchevska, O. (1932). 'Contact glasses in keratoconus and in ametropia.' *Am. J. Ophthal.* **15**, 1028–1038

Sommer, F. (1927). 'Ueber kontaktgläser zur korrektion des keratokonus.' *Inaugural Diss. Univ. Freiburg*

Steele, E. (1948). 'American modifications of the contact lens moulding technique.' *Optician* **115**(2968), 87

Stek, A. W. (1969). 'The Percon contact lens – design and fitting techniques.' *The Contact Lens* **2**(2), 12–14

Stevens, C. L. (1936). 'A method for making casts of the human cornea.' *Am. J. Ophthal.* **19**, 593–595

Stock, W. (1920). 'Ueber korrektion des keratokonus durch verbesserte geschliffene kontaktgläser. *Ber. 42 Versamml. dt. ophthal. Ges.*

Storey, J. K. (1972). 'The possible use of polysulphide rubber impression material in contact lens work.' *Ophthal. Optician* **12**, 1017–1018

Straub (1885). Paper published in *Centralblatt f. Augenheilk* (Title, vol. and page unknown) cited in Benson, A. H. (1902). 'A note on the value of the fluorescein test.' *Ophthal. Review* **21**, 121–130

Sugar, H. S. (1943). 'A new material for anterior-segment impressions.' *Am. J. Ophthal.* **26**, 1210–1212

Thomas, P. (1968). 'The prescribing and fitting of conoid contact lenses.' *Contacto* **12**(1), 66–69

Town, A. E. (1940). 'Impression technic for contact glasses.' *Archs Ophthal. N.Y.* **23**, 822–824

Treissman, H. and Plaice, E. A. (1946). *Principles of the Contact Lens.* pp.64–65. London: Kimpton

Watson, R. K. (1947). 'The "Kelvin" contact lens.' *Optician* **114**(2948), 228–230

Wesley, N. K. and Jessen, G. N. (1953). *Contact Lens Practice.* p.86. Chicago: Professional Press

Wichterle, O., Lim, D. and Dreifus, M. (1961). 'A contribution to the problem of contact lenses.' *Cesk. Oftal.* **17**, 70–75

Young, T. (1801). 'On the mechanism of the eye.' *Phil. Trans. R. Soc.* **16**, 23–88

Chapter 2

Anatomy and Physiology of the Cornea and Related Structures

G. L. Ruskell

So much new information on the structure and function of the cornea has been produced recently that it becomes a considerable task to keep up to date. For a variety of reasons, the contact lens practitioner probably has more need to be aware of new information on these subjects than anyone else engaged in eye care, and in this chapter an attempt is made to refer to all recent significant advances in knowledge and to emphasize those items which are of most interest to the clinician. Indeed, a large part of recent work has been triggered by the desire to know of the structural and functional changes that may be produced by placing a lens in contact with the eye.

THE EPITHELIUM (*Epithelium anterius corneae*)

The outermost of the five layers of the cornea consists of stratified epithelium mounted on a fine basement membrane. Next to the membrane are the basal cells, which are columnar and possess an approximately spherical nucleus which is displaced towards the anterior pole or the head of the cell. Two or three rows of smaller interlocked wing or umbrella cells are mounted on the basal cells. Their nuclei differ from those of the basal cells in being smaller, more oval in section and in having their long axes orientated in the plane of the cornea. The wing cells become thinner with increased displacement from the basal cells and they are in turn capped by two or three layers of surface squamous cells (*Figure 2.1*).

The epithelium is of regular thickness (about 70 μm in the fixed adult eye) and it is continuous with that of the conjunctiva where it thickens and becomes folded. Generation of new cells by mitosis occurs mainly in the basal cell layer but also to a limited extent in the second layer (Machemer, 1966). Epithelial mitosis appears to display a circadian distribution in rats, being most common at 7 a.m. and least common at 7 p.m. (Cardoso *et al.,* 1968). Basal cells make room for new ones by migrating to the next layer and they subsequently move up to the surface of the cornea, becoming squamosed and sloughed away by the action of the eyelids.

Autoradiographic studies of epithelial cell nuclei labelled with tritiated thymidine indicate that the life cycle of cells lasts between three and a half and seven days in a variety of young animals (Hanna and O'Brien, 1960; Süchting, Machemer and Welz, 1966). By arresting the division of cells at metaphase with colchicine, Bertanlanffy and Lau (1962) determined that 14.5 per cent of epithelial cells are renewed daily in rats. Assuming that surface cells desquamate at the same rate, then the epithelium would be totally regenerated in a period of seven days. The life cycle of corneal epithelial cells in man was estimated, from the results of isotope studies of enucleated eyes, to take about seven days (Hanna, Bicknell and O'Brien, 1961).

Adrenaline (epinephrine) and sympathectomy were each found to decrease the mitotic rate in rats (Friedenwald and Buschke, 1944*b*). This interesting phenomenon has not been explained satisfactorily. If, as seems probable, this decrease is related to innervation and not simply to circulating adrenaline, then it may not occur in man because adrenergic terminals are not present in the corneas of primates as they are in those of rats (Ehinger, 1964, 1971).

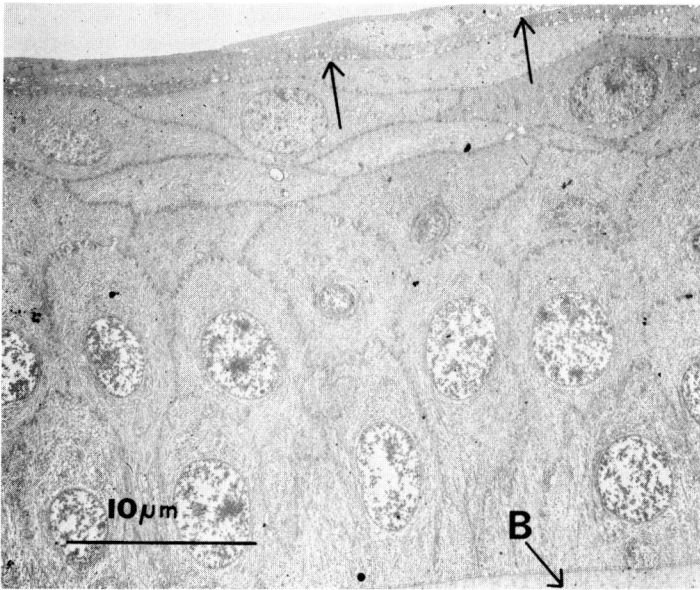

Figure 2.1–Electron micrograph of epithelium taken from close to the centre of the cornea. The cell borders are pronounced because of the presence of numerous desmosomes which have a high electron density. Relatively wide intercellular spacings (arrows) occur between the desmosomes of the flat, surface epithelial cells; this feature is a preliminary stage in desquamation. This and all subsequent electron micrographs illustrating this chapter were taken from monkey material. (B) Bowman's layer or anterior limiting layer. Lead citrate

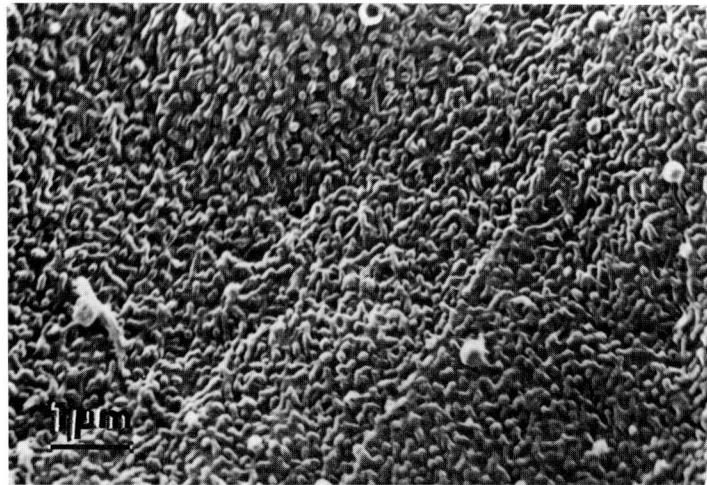

Figure 2.2–Scanning electron micrograph of the surface of the cornea showing the microvilli with a line marking the borders of adjacent epithelial cells

In contrast to the surface cells of skin, those of the cornea are unkeratinized and they retain their organelles — which suggests that metabolic processes are still functioning. Superficially, the cells present a smooth regular surface as seen through an optical microscope but, as Jakus (1964) has shown with the electron microscope, the shallowest of furrows exist between adjacent surface cells which, she suggests, offer a favourable surface for the adherence of tears. However, the most prominent irregularity is caused by the so-called microvilli (*Figure 2.2*), which range up to 0.75 μm in length in man (Ehlers, 1965a; Payrau *et al.*, 1967). Pedler (1962) described surface processes or microvilli in kitten corneas and he considered them to be remaining components of desmosomes previously attached to desquamated cells, a view supported by observations on the epithelium of perilimbal conjunctiva in monkeys (Macintosh, 1968). *Figure 2.3* illustrates the commencement of surface cell sloughing; protrusions of cytoplasm and the consequent development of microvilli occur as a result of desmosome resistance to sloughing. It therefore seems inappropriate to ascribe any function to the microvilli, even that of facilitating the adherence of tears.

If the eye has been bandaged, or if pressure is exerted through the lids, the epithelium wrinkles (Bron, 1968). This gives rise to a quickly fading mosaic, which is made visible with fluorescein staining.

The space between epithelial cells is uniformly very narrow. The apposed cell membranes are remarkable for their steep, short and fairly regular undulations (*Figure 2.1*). These occur at all cell interfaces except between apposed basal cells.

membrane to detach with the epithelium; but experimental lesions of rabbit corneal epithelium revealed that basement membranes were commonly left in place (Khodadoust *et al.,* 1968).

Another type of epithelial cell, the dendritic or polygonal cell, has been described (Sugiura, 1965). In man, these cells were identified mostly at basal cell level in both the central and peripheral cornea (Segawa, 1964). Their existence has been questioned by Perera (1969), who attributed the dendritic form to fixation artefacts in a careful study of human and monkey epithelium. He concluded that '. . . the normal human epithelium consists of cells of one lineage only'.

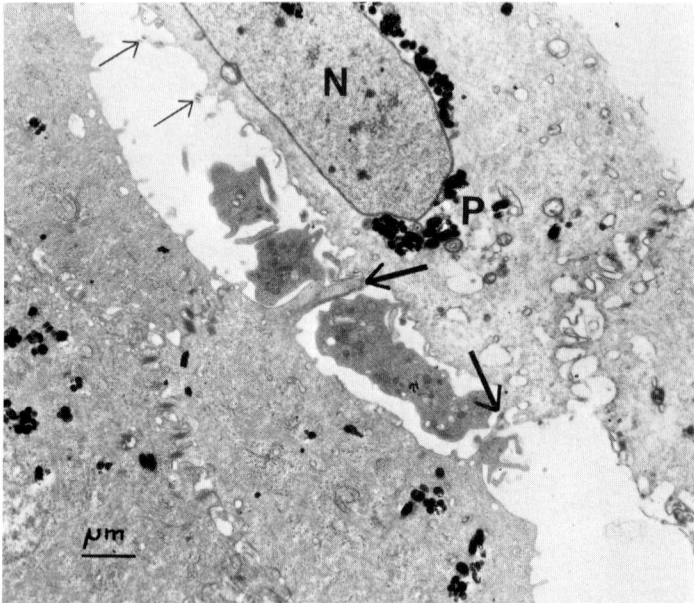

Figure 2.3–Electron micrograph showing partial detachment of surface cells from the perilimbal epithelium prior to sloughing. Cytoplasmic extrusions opposite desmosomes (thick arrows) mark the persisting attachment zones. Desmosomes have broken away from the attached cells and are suspended from microvilli of the detaching cell (thin arrows). (N) nucleus; (P) pigment granules. Lead citrate

The cell membrane is modified by the frequent occurrence of attachment zones or desmosomes, which appear as electron-dense plaques, and each one is paired by a similar modification of the apposed cell membrane (*Figures 2.1, 2.2* and *2.3*). A fine fibrillar substance occupies part of the intercellular space between the plaques. The interlocking of cells, together with the abundant desmosomes, might offer an explanation for the commonly occurring clean detachment of the full-thickness of epithelium as opposed to an irregular excavation of the cells following trauma. However, basal cells also possess numerous desmosomes linking them to the basement membrane, and consequently one might expect the basement

The nerve fibre terminals of the epithelium are described on pages 38 and 39, together with other nerve fibres of the cornea.

EPITHELIAL DAMAGE

In the context of this book, it is appropriate to consider at some length the reactions of corneal epithelium to damage. The smallest corneal wounds – such as a pin-prick – are covered in about three hours by the neighbouring basal cells, which send out pseudopodia to cover the excavated area (Friedenwald and Buschke, 1944a). Normal mitosis is inhibited and plays no part in healing. Although these observations were made on rats, a similar time course probably obtains in man: a small lesion observed by fluorescein staining one day and absent on the next is a common clinical observation. If a somewhat larger area of the cornea is denuded, cells from all layers of the surrounding epithelium migrate and flatten to cover the wound. In this event, mitosis is again at first inhibited; but after a few hours, it recommences and takes an active part in repair. In experiments on rabbits, Mann (1944) found that an area 2–3 mm in diameter will become covered within twenty-four hours, and in three days the area will have a normal appearance as determined by fluorescein staining. The time course of repair is independent of the cause of the lesion except in the case of thermal burns, when it is delayed, and the time course applies whether or not the underlying tissues are affected. Other experiments on rabbits have shown that the establishment of a tight adhesion of newly regenerated epithelium takes only a few days if the basement membrane is largely intact, but initially the new epithelium is very susceptible to damage (Khodadoust et al., 1968). The results of this study serve to emphasize the need to discontinue wearing contact lenses for a few days after incurring significant epithelial damage. On theoretical grounds at least, the concept that continued wearing of lenses will afford protection to the regenerating epithelium is questionable. If the lesion lies close to the limbus, conjunctival cells will take part in the migration, as may be ascertained by the movement into the cornea of pigment cells from the limbus in rabbits; and the same process was confirmed in man by observations on Negro patients (Mann, 1944). After massive or total denudation of the corneas of rabbits, it was found that 50 per cent coverage occurs after twenty-four hours, 75 per cent after forty-eight hours (Langham, 1960), and total coverage takes from four to twelve days (Mann, 1944; Heydenreich, 1958; Khodadoust et al., 1968). On completion of coverage of the cornea, the epithelium is one or two cells thick (Khodadoust et al., 1968), and after two weeks it is two to three cells thick (Heydenreich, 1958); but several weeks pass before the epithelium is of normal thickness. Langham found that normal thickness may be attained in one region of a previously completely denuded cornea whilst another remains uncovered.

Three hours following epithelial abrasions in rabbits, polymorphonuclear leucocytes appeared in the basal lamina and at the edge of the abrasion. Epithelial cells bordering the abrasion were flattened and they developed surface ruffles and filopodia at their free edges (Pfister, 1975). The ruffles and the long, fine filodopia extended to

form attachments to the basal lamina giving the impression of a capacity to draw the cells forward into the area of the defect.

One might expect that epithelial repair slows with age, and Marré (1967) found that this was so in rabbits; but the difference in rate of repair in 4–6 month old and 4–6 year old animals was very slight.

There is evidence to suggest that chemotactic substances liberated from the epithelium are responsible for initiating the early stages of healing both in the epithelium and in the stroma (Weimar, 1960). Immediately after deep corneal wounding in rats, a period of proteolytic activity gives rise to the invasion of the cornea by polymorphonuclear leucocytes and to phagocytic activity by the stromal cells. The epithelium appears to be the source of the proteolytic enzymes which trigger these early responses to injury.

Anaesthetics — being protoplasmic poisons — necessarily alter cellular metabolism, and Freidenwald and Buschke (1944a) showed that if these or other agents such as adrenergic drugs are applied locally in experimental animals mitosis is inhibited. Gunderson and Liebman (1944) found that the epithelial healing process in guinea-pigs was delayed by anaesthetics. Healing was retarded by inhibition of both mitosis and migration. This effect varied with concentration and tonicity but not with pH. If local anaesthetics are applied excessively, epithelial and possibly stromal opacification is caused, accompanied by the eruption of cells and bleb formation. The whole cornea will stain in this condition. Certain synthetic anaesthetics have a less toxic effect on the epithelium than cocaine (Gunderson and Liebman, 1944; Boozan and Cohen, 1953; Rycroft, 1964), but with prolonged use they are all capable of producing serious corneal damage (Epstein and Paton, 1968).

Imprinting of the corneal epithelium by corneal contact lenses has been reported by Dixon (1964) and others in a small proportion of patients. Imprinting usually takes the form of a raised crescent inferiorly. It has been argued by Cochet that the softness or fragility of the epithelium is variable, and he observed a marked fragility in 5 per cent of patients seeking to wear contact lenses (Guilbert, 1963). Fragility was determined by fitting an engraved spherical cone to the Goldman applanation tonometer and assessing the extent of imprinting of the epithelium when applied to the cornea. Apparently, in France fragility testing is widely used in determining the suitability of patients for wearing contact lenses.

Imprinting in rabbit corneal epithelium was accompanied by the loss of a wing cell layer and increased mitosis (Greenberg and Hill, 1973).

BOWMAN'S LAYER (*Laminar limitans anterior*)

Beneath the fine basement membrane of the epithelium is a layer of uniform thickness of about 12 μm which, histologically, appears homogeneous. Recently with the aid of electron microscopy, a very fine unorientated fibrillar meshwork has been resolved, the elements of which resemble the collagen fibrils of the stroma, suggesting a common origin for the two layers (*Figure 2.4*). Microscopic

THE STROMA (*Substantia propria cornea*)

The stroma constitutes 90 per cent of the corneal thickness and gives the cornea its strength. It is remarkable for its regular structure and the absence of blood vessels, which are the two basic features on which corneal transparency rests. The stroma consists of about two hundred layers or lamellae of collagen fibrils. The fibrils, which are buried in a mucoid matrix, have a periodicity which is

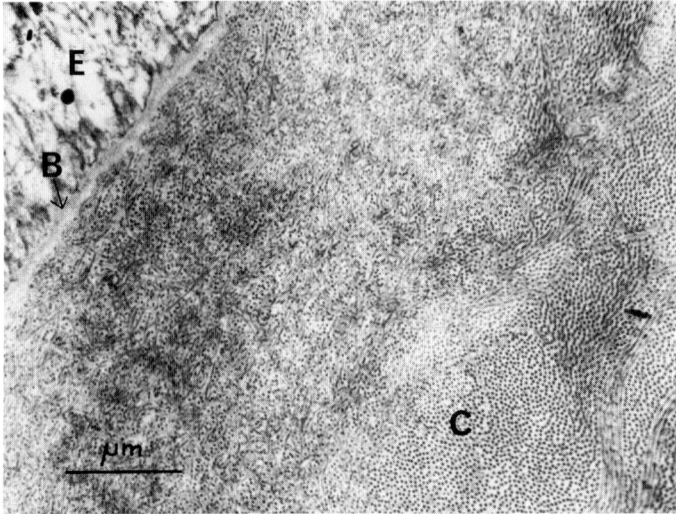

Figure 2.4–Electron micrograph of Bowman's layer. Note the lack of orientation of the collagen fibrils. Bowman's layer merges with the stroma (below and right), in which the collagen fibrils are orientated. (B) basement membrane; (C) collagen fibrils of the stroma; (E) epithelium. Lead citrate

inspection reveals that the anterior limiting layer terminates abruptly at the limbus, but short, fine extensions to the conjunctiva have been described by a number of authors. Over the whole of its area, the layer is penetrated by fine unmyelinated nerve fibres which pass from the stroma to the epithelial cells; the nerve fibres lose their Schwann cell sheaths as they leave the stroma.

The frequency of epithelial damage without involvement of this layer is evidence of its relative toughness; but if it does become damaged, fibrous scar tissue is laid down, resulting in a permanent opacity – although some reduction of the initial scar area usually occurs. To ascribe a stronger tendency for this layer to retain scar tissue compared with the underlying stroma is questionable in view of their similar structural elements. Significant mechanical damage to Bowman's layer by a contact lens, however grossly mishandled, is an unlikely occurrence.

characteristic of collagen. Despite several earlier light microscopic descriptions of elastic fibres in the stroma, they have not been observed with the electron microscope except in areas immediately adjacent to the trabecular meshwork. The fibril diameters are of a regular size at any given depth in the stroma but they vary between an average of 19 nm in the anterior layers and 34 nm in the posterior layers in man (Jakus, 1961).

A majority of the lamellae have a similar thickness (1.5–2.5 μm) and they lie parallel to each other, but the fibrillar orientation of adjacent lamellae is angled (Jakus, 1964). A randomness of lamellar orientation is widely accepted but there is evidence that corneal collagen is predominantly orientated diagonally upward and outward (Schute, 1974). The lamellae probably extend uninterrupted across the cornea without lateral changes in direction, and they are continuous with lamellae of the sclera. Their widths are difficult to assess, but some appear to be in excess of 1 mm. A few lamellae are extremely thin, as may be seen with the electron microscope. Although an impression of separateness of adjacent lamellae prevails when viewing the ultrastructure of the stroma, here and

At the corneo-scleral margin, the stromal lamellae undulate, branch and probably interweave. The fibrils of single lamellae remain parallel to each other but their diameters vary tenfold or more (*Figure 2.6*), and some variation in diameter

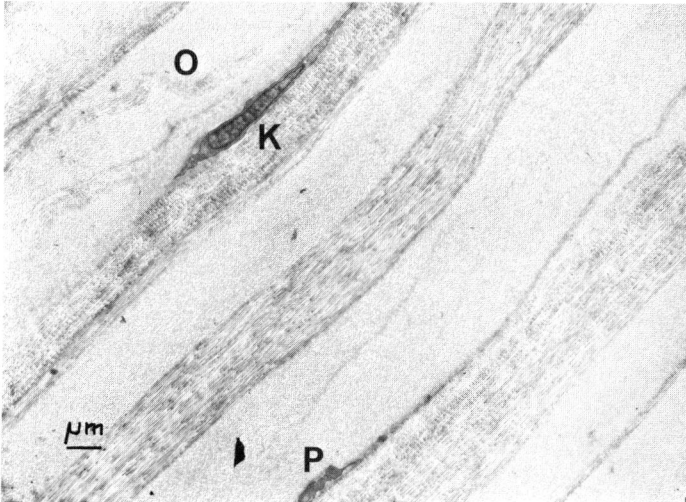

Figure 2.5–Electron micrograph of the lamellae of the stroma. Alternate lamellae are of similar fibril orientation but have different thicknesses. Thin, oblique fibril bundles (O) connect alternate lamellae in places. A dense keratocyte (K) is sectioned transversely through its nucleus and lies in a lamellar interface. The narrow intercellular space between adjacent keratocyte cell processes (P) is also shown. Phosphotungstic acid

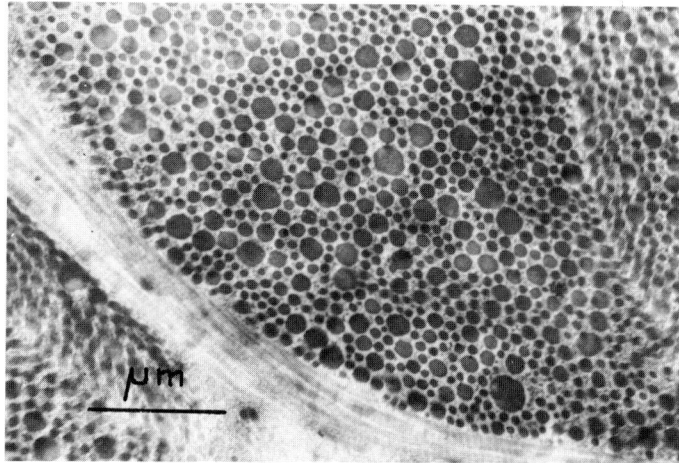

Figure 2.6–Electron micrograph of a transverse section through collagen fibrils of the scleral spur. The difference between adjacent collagen fibril diameters is marked. Lead citrate

there, thin, slightly oblique branches connect one lamella with another (*Figure 2.5*). This general arrangement explains the ease with which the stroma may be slit along its thickness, as in preparation for lamellar corneal grafting. Towards the periphery of the cornea, some lamellae lie approximately concentric with the limbus (Kokott, 1938; Polack, 1961); these are responsible, in part, for the peripheral thickening of the cornea.

is present throughout the sclera. At the deep surface of this region, the canal of Schlemm and the corneo-scleral meshwork are located; a description of their structure and relations is beyond the scope of this chapter.

The main cellular element of the stroma is the keratocyte (corneal fibrocyte, corpuscle or fixed cell), which is a flattened, dendritic cell disposed in the interface between adjacent lamellae (*Figure*

2.5). In a single interface, the cell bodies are well spaced across the cornea; but their thin, lengthy processes are so extensive that many come into contact with processes from neighbouring cells, giving the appearance of a delicate wide-mesh network. This is repeated at each lamellar interface. The nuclei of these cells are flat, approximately oval discs embedded in a sparse perikaryon. More than one nucleus may be present.

There is good evidence that the fibrocytes of the cornea are exceptional in displaying a phagocytic function. Klintworth (1969) has reviewed and extended the literature in which phagocytosis of a wide variety of foreign particulate substances by these cells has been described. Polymorphonuclear leucocytes and mast cells are present in the periphery of the stroma. Autoradiographic studies of thymidine labelled nuclei reveals little or no evidence of DNA synthesis among the keratocytes, which indicates that they seldom divide (Hanna and O'Brien, 1961; Machemer, 1966).

DESCEMET'S LAYER (*Lamina limitans posterior*)

The posterior limiting layer is about half the thickness of the anterior limiting layer and similarly appears devoid of internal structure in section under the light microscope. It thickens slightly in the periphery, and becomes thicker with age. Electron microscopical examination reveals that in man the anterior part of this layer has a fine regular organization. In tangential sections, it has a two-dimensional lace network appearance with a repeating hexagonal unit with seven dense nodes marking the angles; these are connected by fine filaments of equal length. The networks are stacked in depth in register as revealed by transverse sections; dark bands are discernible perpendicular to the plane of the cornea consisting of columns of dark granules, which are the nodes of the tangential section network (Jakus, 1964). The posterior part of this layer has the same fine granular appearance in whichever plane it is sectioned and it shows no signs of a patterned organization.

THE ENDOTHELIUM (*Endothelium camerae anterioris*)

This deepest layer of the cornea lacks the thin basement membrane usually associated with endothelia. The endothelium consists of a single thin layer of predominantly hexagonal cells which present a smooth surface to the anterior chamber. Seen in tangential sections, the cell borders are ill-defined because of the oblique cell interfaces and the interdigitation of broad processes of adjacent cells. The nucleus may have an oval or a kidney shape and the cytoplasm often appears granular and vacuolated. The cells are well stocked with organelles, especially mitochondria, and the endoplasmic reticulum is prominent. The electron microscope reveals that the vacuolization seen in light microscopic sections is due to swelling of mitochondria, with destruction of their internal membranes; it is therefore a swift post-mortem change or a fixation artefact. Near the posterior border of this layer, the intercellular space is reduced to form a tight junction of 10 nm width which presumably restricts the movement of substances in and out of the cornea between the endothelial cells (Iwamoto and Smelser, 1965). A few mitotic patterns occur in very young but not adult animals (Sallmann, Caravaggio and Grimes, 1961) nor adult man (Machemer, 1966). Cells increase in size during growth of the eye and probably spread to cover damaged areas when injured.

THE CONJUNCTIVAL SAC AND THE EPITHELIAL SURFACE

The conjunctiva is a mucous membrane which lines the posterior surface of each eyelid, reflecting sharply at the fornix to line the anterior eyeball where it becomes continuous with the corneal epithelium. The opposite faces of the conjunctiva are presumably in contact, apart from a very thin liquid film. Estimates of the depth of the sac vary, and the measurements of the sac superiorly and inferiorly presented in *Figure 2.7* are those of Ehlers (1965*b*). The circumference of the sac has a mean value of about 9.5 cm, and Ehlers showed that the circumference varies with the width of the palpebral fissure. The conjunctiva covering the eyeball (bulbar), and especially that of the fornix, is thrown into numerous horizontal folds and consequently the sac is potentially larger than is shown in *Figure 2.7*. Ehlers found that the sac may be distended inferiorly to 14–16 mm and superiorly to 25–30 mm, which is more than enough to lodge a displaced contact lens.

The following description of the histology of the conjunctiva is largely restricted to the epithelium. The form of the conjunctival epithelium varies considerably with position. At the limbus, and again at the lid margin, the epithelium is stratified, unkeratinized and several cells thick. In these positions, the cellular arrangement is quite similar to that of the cornea except that the flat-surfaced epithelium varies in thickness because of the undulations of the basement membrane and because — at least in the limbal conjunctiva — the intercellular spaces are larger. Goblet cells are occasionally present in the limbal epithelium, but

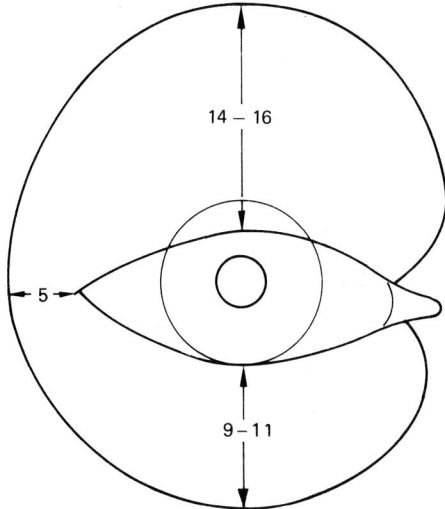

Figure 2.7–Approximate contours of the fornix and the dimensions of the unextended conjunctival sac in millimetres when the eye is open. Based on the data of Whitnall (after Baker) and Ehlers

these become gradually more numerous through the bulbar conjunctiva increasing to a maximum at the fornix and plica semilunaris. The epithelium of the bulbar conjunctiva becomes thinner with increasing distance from the limbus until at the fornix it is only two cells thick. Surface squamous

cells are present at the limbus but not at the fornix. The intercellular spaces are greatest at the fornix except towards the surface, where the bulky goblet cells lie in close apposition to the adjacent, tall, narrow supporting cells (*Figure 2.8*). The concentration of goblet cells continues into the palpebral conjunctiva as far as the tarsal plate (the so-called orbital conjunctiva).

The palpebral conjunctival epithelium opposite the tarsal plate of the upper eyelid consists of two layers of flat cells, and goblet cells are absent. According to Wolff (1948), the palpebral conjunctiva is three or four cells thick in an equivalent position in the lower eyelid.

No information is available regarding the turnover rate of cells in the conjunctival epithelium except at the limbus, where tritiated thymidine labelled basal cells are sloughed away after 132–154 hours in rats — which according to Süchting, Machemer and Welz (1966), is rather slower than in the corneal epithelium. It is likely that the turnover rate of cells is much reduced in the glandular parts of the conjunctiva. The goblet cells, which are apocrine glands, probably survive total evacuation of their secretion granules and become recharged, as appears to be the case in goblet cells of the gut (Freeman, 1962).

Slight elevations of the bulbar conjunctiva may occur opposite the palpebral aperture. These are known as pingueculae and are probably due to sub-epithelial degenerative processes. They are yellow with a fatty appearance and are roughly triangular with the apex away from the cornea. Pingueculae are uncommon in young eyes but they occur frequently in elderly people, especially

Figure 2.8–Electron micrograph of the apex of a conjunctival goblet cell. Nearly all the cytoplasm consists of secretion granules (G). The goblet cell borders are indicated by arrows where apposed cell processes are discernible. The conjunctival surface is indicated by the microvilli of adjacent supporting cells (S). The material extruding from the apex of the cell includes secretion granules and other organelles of which granular endoplasmic reticulum can be recognized. Lead citrate

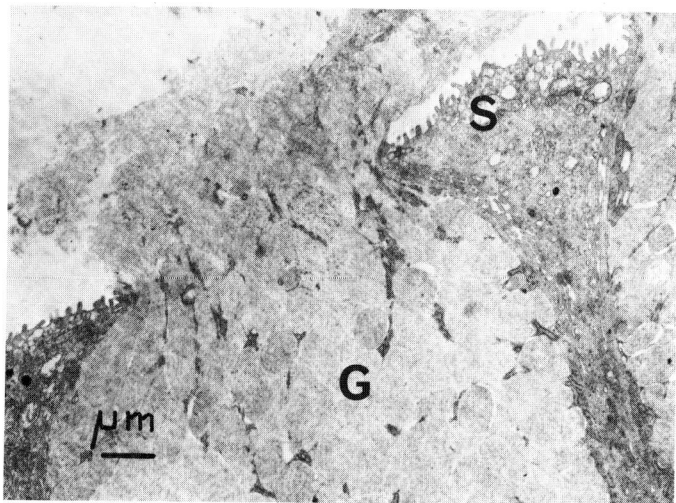

among those exposed to dust and wind. Exposure to ultra-violet radiation is also a contributary factor. Among other age changes is a reduction in the number of epithelial cells including goblet cells (Gornig and Pommer, 1971).

The blood vessels of the bulbar conjunctiva tend towards a radial arrangement. Arterioles pass from the anterior ciliary arteries before they penetrate the sclera and others pass round the fornix from arterioles of the palpebral conjunctiva. At the limbus, capillaries are again radially disposed mainly between the palisades (radial thickenings of epithelium) and form fine vascular loops at the margin of the cornea. Venules pass back, converge and anastomose frequently and many of the larger venules lie adjacent to the arterioles. The sclera overlaps the cornea anteriorly about the vertical meridian so that transparency loss is gradual across the transition. Consequently, the limbal vessels may give the impression of penetrating the cornea. Many of the conjunctival capillaries are closed in the normal eye but irritation of the cornea or conjunctiva will increase the number and size of blood-bearing vessels.

Small lymphatic vessels are present in the conjunctiva including fine lymphatic capillaries that extend to the corneo-scleral border. They drain into larger sub-conjunctival vessels.

The conjunctiva is served by sensory nerves that branch from certain divisions of the ophthalmic nerve and the infra-orbital nerve. Most of them probably terminate in the sub-epithelial tissues but some pass into the epithelium and lie on the basement membrane or between basal cells. A few terminals penetrate closer to the surface. Although special forms of terminal including encapsulated endings have been reported in the conjunctiva in the past, it now appears that practically all sensory fibres form free nerve endings. Sympathetic nerves are also present in the conjunctiva and parasympathetic terminals of pterygopalatine ganglion origin were described recently in monkeys (Macintosh, 1974); both are probably exclusively vasomotor.

EYELIDS

The skin of the eyelids is very thin. The epidermis consists of only six or seven layers of epithelial cells beneath the keratinized surface layer. At the lid margin, the epithelium thickens and becomes moist and the keratinized layer terminates in front of the orifices of the tarsal glands. Here the epithelium is continuous with that of the marginal conjunctiva where the epithelium is the thickest in the eyelid. The elastic dermis contains small sweat glands. The hairs of the skin are extremely fine and short and most of them fail to extend beyond their follicles. Sebaceous glands associated with the hairs are commensurately small.

Nearly a third of the thickness of the eyelid is made up of the striated orbicularis oculi muscle, which is bordered anteriorly and posteriorly by loose non-adipose connective tissue. The orbicularis is a thin muscle surrounding the palpebral aperture and extending well beyond the orbital margin on to the face. Structurally and functionally, the muscle is divisible into orbital and palpebral portions. Most of the orbital portion lies beyond the orbital margin and its border describes a horizontal ellipse approximately. It is continuous with the palpebral portion, which itself is clearly divisible into preseptal (lying in front of the orbital septum) and pretarsal parts, the latter terminating near the palpebral margins. Jones (1961) described the orbicularis muscle with considerable precision. He showed that the fascicles of the pretarsal muscle are broadest in the central region of the eyelid, tapering laterally to terminate just beyond the outer canthus. In contrast, the fascicles of the preseptal muscle maintain a regular width, terminating laterally in the raphé, where fibres of the upper and lower eyelids meet. A weak lateral palpebral ligament joins the posterior face of the raphé to the lateral orbital margin at the orbital tubercle. The upper fascicles of the orbital division are continuous with the lower ones laterally. The palpebral furrows or sulci mark the transition from pretarsal to preseptal portions. The divisions of the orbicularis oculi taper and fuse medially and they are anchored to the orbital margin by the strong medial palpebral ligament. Jones distinguished separate ligaments of the three portions of the muscle, and each of them possessed a deep and a superficial ligament or head. According to Jones, the deep heads of the inferior and superior preseptal muscles terminate in the fascial sheet bridging the lacrimal fossa laterally (the lacrimal diaphragm). This structural arrangement — which has been questioned by Brienen and Snell (1967) — figures prominently in a postulated mechanism of lacrimal liquid drainage. The whole of the orbicularis is innervated by the facial nerve.

Behind the orbicularis oculi lies the tarsal plate, which may be regarded as the skeleton of the eyelid. It consists of a very dense plate of fibrous tissue that has a base close to the lid margin. In the upper lid, it extends to the level of the superior palpebral furrow and its upper boundary describes an arc from the medial to the lateral canthus. In the lower lid the plate is only a third as deep.

If pressure is applied inwards and downwards along the superior palpebral furrow, using the fingers or a glass rod, and the lid margin is pulled upwards, the upper lid may be everted. This position is maintained without assistance by the strength of the tarsal plate, provided that the eyes are directed downwards. This manoeuvre is used to permit inspection of the palpebral conjunctiva. When the eyes look upwards, the lid reverts to its normal position. Foreign bodies are frequently lodged in the conjunctiva between the base of the upper tarsal plate and the lid margin where the sub-tarsal sulcus is formed.

Eversion of the lid reveals the tarsal (Meibomian) glands, which are buried within the tarsal plate. The glands run nearly the full length of the tarsus and, in fact, beyond the tarsus at the lid margin, and they are arranged approximately parallel. There are about twenty-five in the upper eyelid and about twenty in the lower eyelid. The openings of the gland ducts are disposed in a single row along the lid margin, behind the lashes. The glands are sebaceous and holocrine, the ruptured pyknotic cells forming the oily secretion. Overflow of tears is prevented by a coating of tarsal gland secretion along the lid margins, and this is extended in a thin film across the precorneal tears layer (*see* Tears, page 51).

Tarsal glands quite commonly become infected, forming a chalazion or internal stye. Although not painful itself, the chalazion frequently produces a small, hard, discrete elevation of the inner surface of the eyelid, and irritation of the cornea may ensue. Irregularity of the tarsal conjunctiva of whatever cause potentially presents a problem for the contact lens wearer. Hodd, in a personal communication, considers that in numerous cases of lens intolerance a chalazion is the culprit.

The palpebral conjunctiva lines the posterior face of the eyelids. It is firmly attached to the tarsal plate by a thin fibrous sub-epithelial layer that is rich in capillaries and venules. There is good evidence that the vessels nourish the cornea when the lids are closed. Some small lymphatic vessels are also present in this layer, and they communicate with other lymphatics of the eyelids at the upper and lower margins of the tarsal plate. The epithelium is described on pages 34–35.

The levator palpebrae superioris is a striated muscle with the function of elevating the upper eyelid. It therefore opposes the action of the orbicularis oculi. The levator passes above the superior rectus muscle within the orbit and it has a broad tendonous insertion in the lid. Part of the insertion terminates at the upper border of the tarsus, and the remainder passes in front of the tarsus between the fascicles of the orbicularis to the skin. The levator is innervated by the oculomotor nerve.

A thin layer of smooth muscle — the superior tarsal muscle of Müller — contributes to the elevation of the eyelid. It is a short muscle connecting the inferior fascial sheath of the levator with the upper margin of the tarsus. The superior tarsal muscle is innervated by sympathetic nerve fibres, and it has a weak action compared to that of the levator. This is suggested by the difference in the sizes of the two muscles and by the observation that sympathectomy produces a modest depression of the upper lid compared with the marked ptosis after oculomotor neurectomy. The specific role of the superior tarsal muscle in effecting elevation of the lid is uncertain. An inferior tarsal muscle is found in the lower lid with attachments to the fascial sheaths of the inferior rectus and inferior oblique muscles and to the inferior tarsus. No counterpart to the levator palpebrae superioris is present in the lower lid. The limited capacity to depress the lid is therefore produced by contraction of the inferior rectus muscle and the inferior tarsal muscle.

STRUCTURE OF THE EYELID MARGINS

The line of tarsal gland orifices at the margins of the lids marks the sharp transition from unkeratinized epithelium of the conjunctiva posteriorly to the keratinized epithelium of the skin. Two or three irregular rows of cilia, or eyelashes, emerge from the skin in front of the tarsal gland orifices. The lashes are thick and strong, and those of the upper eyelid are longer and more numerous. The lash follicles are disposed between the terminations of the pretarsal portion of the orbicularis muscle and the lid margin and they lack arrectores pilorum. Lashes are replaced two or three times a year and regrow quickly after epilation. They are normally curved outwards, but in rare instances they may grow inwards to touch the cornea and give rise to pain.

Paired sebaceous glands (of Zeis) open into the lash follicles, and their oily secretion moistens the lashes. Sweat glands (of Moll) are also present in small numbers in the lid margins. Unlike sweat glands elsewhere, they are uncoiled and possess a wide lumen. Although they sometimes open into lash follicles, they usually exhibit the common feature of sweat glands of opening directly on to the skin.

Small bundles of striped muscle fibres (of Riolan) are present immediately beneath the skin of the lid margins. Most of these lie anterior to the tarsal gland ducts but a few are present posterior to the ducts. In general, they run approximately parallel to the lid margins but some fibres pass obliquely between the ducts. It has been postulated that these fibres control the lumina of the ducts. However, this appears unlikely other than as an occurrence incidental to their function of maintaining the lid margins in apposition to the eye during lid closure.

The eyelid sometimes catches the edge of a corneal contact lens. This problem is caused by the lens periphery standing off from the cornea, but an unusual configuration of the posterior margin of the eyelid might be a predisposing factor. However, Shanks (1965) employed a moulding technique to examine this feature in a small group and found little variation between individuals.

LID MOVEMENTS

In waking hours, the upper eyelid is very active as a result of reflex blinking. A basic rhythm of blinking occurs at a frequency of twelve blinks a minute according to King and Michels (1957), or rather more than this according to others. Alterations of the rate of blinking are produced by many factors such as anxiety, noise or a stuffy atmosphere — but, interestingly, not by a dry atmosphere. A blink is completed in less than one-third of a second. During this period, the eye makes a rapid upwards and inwards movement and returns. Ginsborg (1952) found this movement to be between 20 and 100 minutes of arc nasally and between 40 and 70 superiorly when the eyes were initially in the primary position; but the direction and extent varies with the initial position of the eyes. In secondary positions of gaze, there is a tendency for the eye to move towards the primary position during blinking (Ginsborg and Maurice, 1959). This small displacement is insufficient to account for the movement of a contact lens relative to the eye during a blink; clearly it is the traction of the eyelid that causes the lens movement.

If closure of one eye is prevented by holding the lid when a person attempts to shut both eyes, a movement upwards and outwards is usually seen. This displacement is known as Bell's phenomenon, and it is most strikingly displayed in some cases of facial paralysis (Bell's palsy). The movement is far greater than that induced by blinking as measured by Ginsborg.

Closure in blinking is produced by relaxation of the levator followed by contraction of the palpebral portion of the orbicularis oculi. The whole orbicularis and frequently the accessory muscles contract when the eyes are squeezed shut. This may occur reflexly (optical blinking or menace reflex) together with a backward movement of the head when, for example, the eyes are exposed to a dazzling light, or when a tonometer or contact lens approaches the eye. All contact lens practitioners, however considerate their manner, must have faced the problem of a patient's prolonged blepharospasm prior to the initial insertion of a contact lens.

Gordon (1951) held that in downward gaze, as in reading, the orbicularis muscle plays no active part and that relaxation of the levator is alone responsible for the partial closure of the palpebral aperture. In upward gaze, contraction of both the levator and the frontalis muscle occurs.

CORNEAL INNERVATION

The cornea is served by seventy to eighty small sensory nerves which are derived from the ciliary nerves which branch from the ophthalmic division of the trigeminal nerve. Nerves enter the sclera from the uvea at the level of the ciliary body and pass anteriorly to enter the cornea radially and predominantly in the middle layers. A few nerves enter the corneal stroma superficially from the episcleral and conjunctival layers, and some of these travel concentrically with the limbus and remain close to it. The myelin sheaths of axons terminate at the limbus or within 0.5 mm of entering the cornea. Occasionally, myelin persists a little further and, exceptionally, even to the centre of the cornea; such fibres are, of course, opaque and they present a striking picture when viewed through a biomicroscope. The perineurium and the fibres and cells of the endoneurium also terminate at the limbus. Only the unmyelinated nerve fibre bundles advance into the cornea. Each bundle consists of several axons enclosed by a Schwann cell (Matsuda, 1968). Hence, complete nerve trunks are not present in the cornea.

Initially, the nerve fibre bundles of the cornea are grouped together; but these separate to give rise to the plexiform arrangement which is the characteristic form seen in the full thickness of the cornea under low magnification with intravital methylene blue staining (Zander and Weddell, 1951a; Oppenheimer, Palmer and Weddell, 1958). The plexus is particularly dense beneath the anterior limiting layer.

Axons separate and possibly divide at intervals and form fine terminal branches, some of which may lose their Schwann cell investment; the terminal axons follow a lengthy, tortuous course between the stromal fibrils. They bear a large number of small bead-like varicosities, with a larger one at each terminal.

Fibres from single nerve bundles at the limbus may be distributed to as much as two-thirds of the area of the cornea. Consequently, there is a considerable overlapping by nerve fibres from different nerve bundles. Measurements of receptive fields of the cornea of the cat recorded from ciliary nerves are consistent with the anatomical arrangement of nerve fibre bundles and, indeed, overlapping of receptive fields of single nerve fibres has been demonstrated (Tower, 1940; Lele and Weddell, 1959). This arrangement explains why sensitivity persists in all areas of the cornea subsequent to large, full-penetration, perilimbal incisions as undertaken in the surgical treatment of cataract and glaucoma (Schirmer and Mellor, 1961). It also explains inability to localize stimuli on the cornea.

The epithelium receives a prolific supply of terminal nerve fibres which pass perpendicularly from the dense plexus underlying the anterior limiting layer. This layer is penetrated by the nerve fibre bundles, which lose their Schwann cell investment at this stage. On entering the epithelium, the fine naked axons separate and possibly divide as they pass between the basal and wing cells. Varicosities similar to those present in the stroma occur in the epithelium. These have been demonstrated in silver impregnated (Wolter, 1957) and methylene blue stained (Zander and Weddell, 1951a) material and by electron microscopy (Whitear, 1960; Jakus, 1962; Matsuda, 1968). Matsuda showed that varicosities of fibre terminals in the epithelium are of two types in rabbits and man. One contains mitochondria and the other contains both mitochondria and vesicles. Varicosities without vesicles probably serve a sensory function, and those with vesicles are probably motor, he suggested. But it appears unlikely that sympathetic motor terminals are regularly present in primate eyes as Ehinger (1971) using the catecholamine fluorescence technique observed just one terminal in a study of 142 primate eyes. There is no reliable evidence of the presence of parasympathetic motor terminals in the cornea. Perhaps the primate cornea contains sensory fibres alone but this matter awaits clarification.

If the sensory nerves of the cornea are destroyed by ophthalmic or trigeminal neurectomy, changes in corneal structure occur and a neuro-paralytic keratitis usually develops. This has led to the concept of a trophic function of corneal nerves which parallels that of cutaneous nerves. The mechanism of the trophic function is not understood, but a popular hypothesis is that it is dependent on antidromic stimulation of sensory nerves.

SENSITIVITY OF THE CORNEA AND CONJUNCTIVA

Common experience and the earliest measurements of surface sensitivity indicate that the sensitivity of the cornea is probably unsurpassed by that of any other part of the body. The measurement of threshold sensitivity has been practised throughout this century, but it is probably true to state that progress has only recently been made in calibrating the stimulus with accuracy. Notwithstanding, the technique of aesthesiometry remains blunted by uncertainties, and the data it provides — whether absolute or relative — can only be accepted with caution in so far as it applies to the cornea and conjunctiva. The stimulus employed was classically a fine hair or a series of hairs of different lengths and weights applied to the surface of the cornea; but more recently, a nylon monofilament has been used. The force exerted is measured in weight per unit area of contact; the area of contact is assumed to remain constant and the weight or pressure is varied. The method of varying the unsupported length of monofilament between the holder and the point of contact is usually employed in corneal aesthesiometers. Pressure on the instrument is increased until the monofilament bends and this end-point for each length of monofilament is pre-calibrated. The length of monofilament is decreased until a threshold response is elicited. The shorter the length of monofilament the greater is the pressure required to bend it. In experimental animals, threshold and differential responses may be measured electrophysiologically.

The sensitivity of the cornea varies from a maximum apically to a minimum peripherally. The threshold value increases slowly, then more quickly, to a maximum of 2.0 g/mm^2 at the periphery. Von Frey and Strughold, pioneers in this field, used hairs in determining the apical threshold to be 0.2 g/mm^2 (Strughold, 1953). A considerable drop in sensitivity was measured in crossing to the limbal conjunctiva (30–35 g/mm^2) and sensitivity increased towards the fornix and again at the lid margins. Corneal sensitivity was found to be rather greater in the horizontal meridian than in the vertical meridian. Recently, studies in which various nylon monofilament aesthesiometers have been used have furnished results in sharp contrast to those of Strughold (Boberg-Ans, 1955; Cochet and Bonnet, 1960; Schirmer and Mellor, 1961). With such instruments, a central threshold of about 15 mg/mm^2 is found, which is considerably lower than earlier assessments. The peripheral threshold reduces to only half the central threshold. According to Cochet, in a personal communication, Sédan observed an annular zone of raised sensitivity about 4 mm from the centre of the cornea in 30 per cent of cases.

Boberg-Ans (1955) found the threshold of limbal, bulbar and fornix conjunctiva to vary between 72 and 200 mg/mm^2. Similar results have been recorded from the palpebral conjunctiva, but at the lid margin the level of sensitivity approaches that of the central cornea (Dixon, 1964; Lowther and Hill, 1968).

according to Cochet. Nylon and hair are both affected by humidity.

Sensitivity varies with age. In a study of 150 patients whose ages ranged between 10 and 90 years, Boberg-Ans (1956) found a peak sensitivity in young patients three times that of his oldest patients. Most of the sensitivity reduction occurs between the ages of 50 and 65 years (Jalavisto,

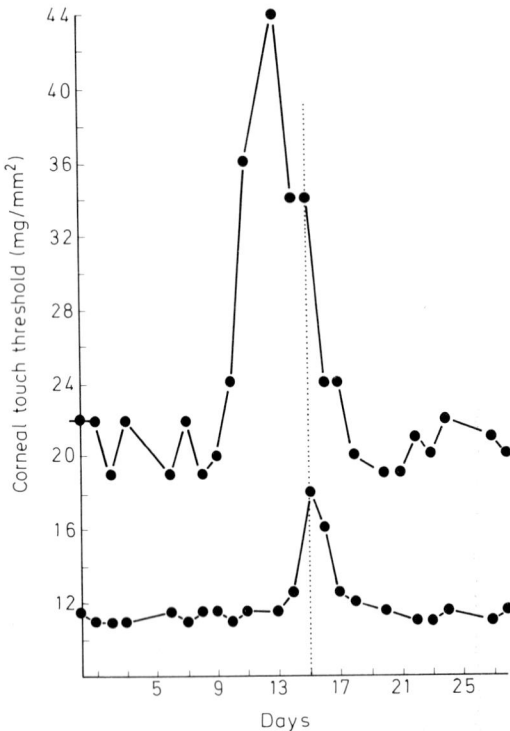

Figure 2.9–Relationship between corneal touch threshold and number of days of the menstrual cycle in women. Days are numbered from the assumed occurrence of ovulation and the dotted line represents onset of menstruation (from Millodot, M., 1974, Br. J. Ophthal. 58, 752–756 by kind permission of the author and publishers)

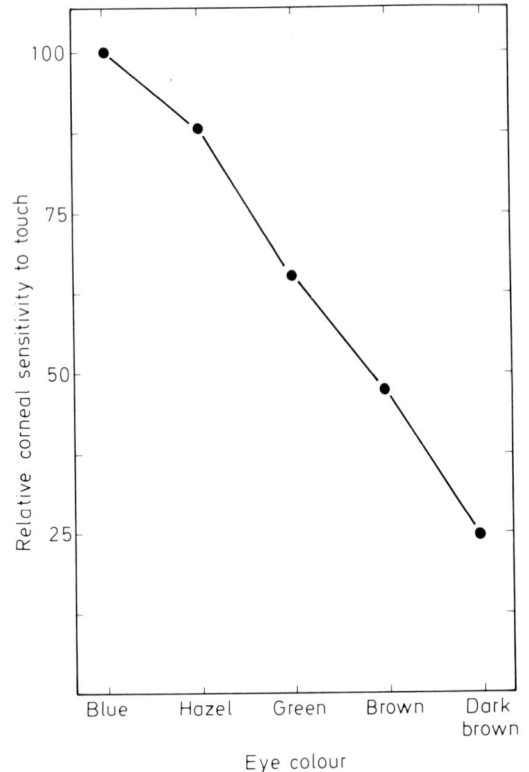

Figure 2.10–Relative corneal sensitivity to touch as a function of the colour of the iris (112 subjects). The dark brown group consists of non-white subjects. The sensitivity is the reciprocal of the touch threshold measured in mg/mm^2 and the group with greatest sensitivity has been assigned 100 (from Millodot, M., 1975b, by kind permission of the author and publishers)

The agreement among the results of these more recent studies is impressive. Presumably, the nylon monofilament instruments are more reliable than hairs. Certainly, control of the form of the monofilament tip becomes possible, and this must be important for accuracy. Lately, the diameter of the nylon monofilament has been reduced from rather less than 12 to 8/100 mm^2 in the popular Cochet-Bonnet instrument. This change has brought about a significant improvement in its performance,

Orma and Tawast, 1951) or even later (Sédan, Farnarier and Ferrand, 1958). Sensitivity is usually approximately the same in both eyes, and there is no reliable evidence to indicate a difference in sensitivity between the sexes but it is worth noting Millodot and Lamont's (1974) observation that the average sensitivity in nine women was approximately halved during the premenstruum and at the onset of menstruation (Figure 2.9). Corneas display a diurnal variation in sensitivity with about a third greater sensitivity as the day progresses from morning to evening (Millodot, 1972). Perhaps the most striking variation is that displayed between people of different iris colour. Millodot (1975*b*) found that blue-eyed people have a greater sensitivity than those with dark-brown irises (*Figure 2.10*). Non-white people with dark-brown irises have less sensitive corneas than Caucasians with similar iris colour. On average, non-white people have four times less sensitive corneas than blue-eyed people and half as sensitive corneas as brown-eyed Caucasians.

Depression of corneal sensitivity as a consequence of limbal transection for cataract extraction is surprisingly slight. The threshold value adjacent to the incision is raised to little more than twice the normal (Schirmer and Mellor, 1961); but recovery of sensitivity was found to be negligible over a period of two years. The survival of nerve fibres entering the cornea across half its circumference is adequate to maintain a high degree of sensitivity over the whole of the cornea. One might expect some recovery of sensitivity subsequent to a limbal incision if one is free to extend Zander and Weddell's (1951*b*) observations on rabbits to man. They found that normal innervation was recovered in favourable cases nine months after keratotomy of up to one-third of the corneal circumference; but the speed of regeneration of corneal nerve fibres is related to age, being more rapid in the young (Rexed and Rexed, 1951).

Corneal sensitivity is usually reduced subsequent to the wearing of hard corneal contact lenses. A measurable loss of sensitivity occurs after one or two hours wear and may depress to one-third of the original, according to Boberg-Ans (1955). Byron and Weseley (1961), using von Frey hairs, found that the sensitivity loss varied remarkably between different persons. A few patients showed no changes whilst others showed sensitivity losses up to 25 times the normal; 79 of 97 eyes were less sensitive after four hours wear. Similarly, Dixon (1964) measured an average 13 times increment in the threshold stimulus strength using a nylon aesthesiometer after full adaptation to corneal contact lenses. Fewer than half of Edmund's (1967) patients displayed sensitivity loss. More recently, Millodot (1975*a*), using a Cochet-Bonnet nylon aesthesiometer under carefully controlled conditions, found that the touch threshold value was doubled on average in eleven young people after wearing their corneal contact lenses for eight hours (*Figure 2.11*). The sensitivity reduction was approximately the same for the central and peripheral cornea. The fact that Millodot's patients had been wearing contact

lenses for 14 months (median) suggests that sensitivity changes persist, although the contrary view has been expressed on several occasions. Indeed, when examined a year later under similar circumstances elevation of touch threshold persisted at nearly the same level (Millodot, 1976).

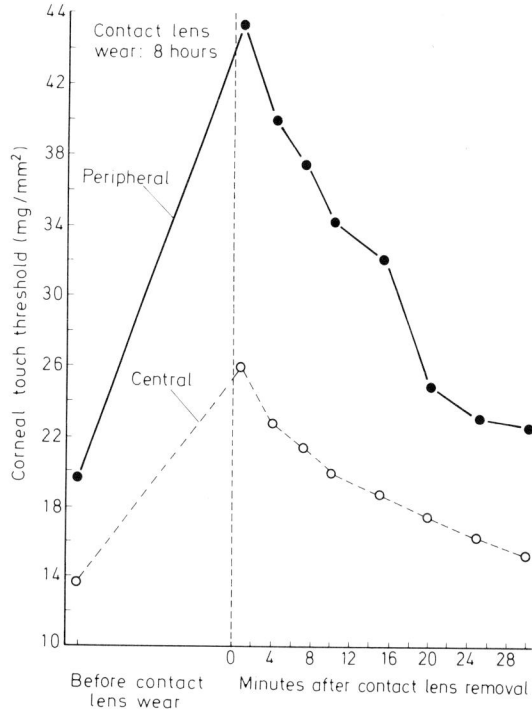

Figure 2.11–The effect of hard contact lenses on corneal touch threshold averaged from the eyes of eleven subjects. Thresholds before lens insertion and at frequent intervals after eight hours wear are plotted. Threshold at the centre of the cornea is about half that at the periphery. Recovery of sensitivity after contact lens removal is comparable in both positions (after Millodot, 1975a)

It is unlikely that a correlation exists between adequacy of fit and the maintenance of sensitivity. A negative correlation may exist between sensitivity and corneal oedema. Eyelid margin sensitivity is also reduced by wearing corneal contact lenses (Lowther and Hill, 1968).

It is generally agreed that on removal of contact lenses corneal sensitivity gradually recovers to the level measured before insertion. Most of the recovery is effected in half an hour (*Figure 2.11*) and is complete in two hours.

Soft contact lenses induce little sensitivity reduction; Larke and Sabell (1971) found none while Knoll and Williams (1970) observed a loss that was not statistically significant. However, when sensitivity was measured subsequent to the removal of soft contact lenses a small but significant increase was found (Millodot, 1974). Evidently sensitivity had been reduced. This loss was probably obscured in earlier studies by the diurnal increment of sensitivity as the day progresses.

Schirmer (1963) has suggested that in determining the suitability of patients before prescribing contact lenses corneal sensitivity should be taken into account; but in particular, he values the degree of tolerance of a sustained stimulus as a better criterion. High tolerance and low sensitivity, as Schirmer suggests, would appear to be suitable features for successful contact lens wear on the evidence of his data using his instrument. But others take a different view (for example, Cochet and Bonnet, 1960), and the general value of these criteria has yet to be demonstrated. At the present time, there appears to be little reason to promote the routine use of aesthesiometry in contact lens practice: and it must be remembered that the technique is not without hazard.

SENSIBILITY OF THE CORNEA AND CONJUNCTIVA

One associates the sensations of pain and irritation with the cornea, possibly to the exclusion of any others. Von Frey and his co-workers proposed and maintained this view over several decades against the evidence of other groups who claimed that the cornea exhibits several sensibilities. The problem is of broad interest in that von Frey postulated the well-known correlation between specific forms of cutaneous sensory end-organs with particular functions. Free nerve endings mediate pain sensitivity, according to this hypothesis; and, as we have seen, the cornea is populated exclusively by them. The qualitative evaluation of sensitivity is of limited practical importance to the contact lens practitioner, but he is dealing with a structure which is at the centre of an engaging physiological dispute and he may be interested in a brief account of the views of the opponents of von Frey's conception of cutaneous sensitivity.

Lele and Weddell (1956) claimed that the sensibilities of touch, cold, warmth and pain may be experienced if the cornea is suitably stimulated. Strughold (1953) himself, although a principal proponent of the von Frey concept, appeared to concede the possibility of touch sensibility as distinct from irritation. Nafe and Wagoner (1937) claimed that either touch or pain sensations may be elicited from the cornea according to the intensity of the stimulus. Based on the under-standing that pain impulses conducted by the trigeminal nerve — and therefore including those initiated in the cornea — are chiefly presented at the caudal end of the nucleus of the spinal trigeminal tract in the lower brainstem, Sjoqvist (1938) incised the tract at this level in cases of trigeminal neuralgia. This procedure effectively reduces the sensibility of pain whilst sufficient tactile sensibility is retained to avoid the possibly blinding consequences associated with total anaesthesia which results from the alternative operation of trigeminal neurectomy (Rowbotham, 1939; Grant, Groff and Lewy, 1940). Patients treated by this procedure experience no discomfort if the cornea is moderately stimulated, and they recognize the predominating sensation as touch.

One is, perhaps, at liberty to conclude from this evidence that the sensation of touch is fully differentiated from pain, but it is noteworthy that in cats the representation of pain sensation is spread throughout the nucleus of the spinal trigeminal tract (Eisenman, Landgren and Novin, 1963; Kerr, 1963). The separate representation of pain in the trigeminal nerve nucleus is inconsistent with the 'gate control' theory of Melzack and Wall (1965). They argue that pain is experienced as a consequence of increased strength of any form of stimulation sufficient to release the central inhibition set up by activity of cells of the substantia gelatinosa. On this basis Sjoqvist's incision may be considered to so reduce total sensory input that the threshold for pain is not reached or the gate is not opened.

Perhaps the most controversial aspect of corneal sensibility is that of temperature. Von Frey concluded, from experiments in which he stimulated the cornea with cooled and heated rods, that temperature sensations were absent. He also noted the absence of Ruffini endings and Krause endbulbs. In the adjacent conjunctiva, Strughold and Karbe (1925) found many warm and cold spots. Employing intravital staining of nerves and the low magnification level of the biomicroscope, they concluded that warm spots related to Ruffini endings and cold spots to Krause end-bulbs. These observations supported their view that warmth and cold sensibilities are not experienced from the cornea. Subsequent studies by Weddell and Zander (1950) and Oppenheimer, Palmer and Weddell (1958) unequivocally reject this correlation in the conjunctiva. Complex nerve endings are rare and irregularly occurring, and in some species they are altogether absent. They therefore cannot be considered to relate to the function of temperature reception. This leads to the conclusion that morphologically unspecialized nerve endings are related to a variety of sensibilities, and that absence of all but free nerve endings in the cornea does not preclude the reception of stimuli giving rise to sensations other than pain.

Nafe and Wagoner (1937) concluded from their experiments that both warmth and cold sensations are absent in the cornea. Lele and Weddell (1956), in challenging the validity of these experiments, pointed out that these investigators were searching to establish that vascular receptors are responsible for the sensations of warmth and cold and that it was in their interest to find a negative response to these stimuli in the avascular cornea. Kenshalo (1960) showed that thermal changes may be recognized by the cornea, but he claimed that the quality of the sensation is irritation rather than warmth. The temperature difference required for threshold sensitivity was found to be much in excess of that necessary in the conjunctiva, lips and skin. However, the detectable temperature changes in Lele and Weddell's subjects, employing short-duration warm and cold air jets, indicated an accurate discrimination: a cold jet was never confused with a warm jet. Although the elicited sensations were equated approximately with those of warmth and cold, these workers recognized them to be somewhat singular in quality.

CORNEAL TRANSPARENCY

The most obvious and simple explanation for the transparency of the cornea is that its components all have the same refractive index; but a number of easily observed factors discount this. For instance, an anatomist might doubt the validity of this explanation because he is able to discern the structure of the cornea in unstained sections using phase contrast microscopy which is dependent on refractive index differences. Similarly, cellular detail is discernible in the living eye with a bio-microscope. The birefringence of the cornea is evident from the interference figures it displays when examined with polarized light, and this property has been examined in detail (Naylor, 1953; Stanworth and Naylor, 1953).

Cogan and Kinsey (1942b), accepting a difference in refractive index of the stromal components, proposed that refraction at their surfaces is minimized as a consequence of a limited liquid component, and one may point to the phenomenon of scleral transparency *in situ* in the dehydrated state in support of this. But this concept is at variance with the facts that the liquid component is of the order of 80 per cent by weight and collagen fibrils constitute only 18 per cent of the volume of the stroma.

Caspersson and Engström (1946) postulated that the fibrils of the stroma are positioned parallel to the surface of the cornea in rows which are perpendicular to it. Light rays would be refracted to and fro along a row of fibrils and finally emerge undeviated. The gaps between fibrils were considered to be 'plugged' by the mucoid ground substance of graduated refractive index with a peak equal and adjacent to that of the fibril, thereby avoiding reflection at interfaces. This scheme is untenable for a number of reasons — one of which is that it accounts only for light rays of normal incidence.

No satisfactory hypothesis explaining the transparency of the cornea as a whole has appeared, but Maurice (1957, 1962a) has offered an explanation of the transparency of the stroma. His hypothesis is precisely stated and does not invoke extravagant assumptions. It embraces light of all incidences and satisfactorily explains how transparency is lost in various circumstances. Maurice proposed that the stromal fibrils, which were found to have a refractive index of about 1.55 in the dry state, are so arranged to behave as a series of diffraction gratings permitting transmission through the liquid ground substance (refractive index 1.34). We have already seen that the fibrils in adjacent regions of the stroma are of remarkably regular diameter and that they are probably regularly spaced so that, neglecting the curvature of the cornea, in any plane a reasonable facsimile of a diffraction grating exists. It is of interest to note that the fibrils of the opaque sclera do not show these properties. A diffraction grating eliminates scattered light by destructive interference and permits the transmission of light energy maxima at angles θ to a normally incident beam, the angles depending on the physical characteristics of the grating and the light. Accordingly, $\sin \theta = m\lambda/d$, where m is any integer and d is the space between grating elements. The fibrils are the grating elements which, it is suggested, are disposed in an hexagonal lattice as shown in *Figure 2.12*. Only the first of the energy maxima applies because the grating or fibril interval is shorter than the wavelength of light or $\lambda/d > 1$, and the equation is only satisfied when m is zero and consequently θ is $0°$. In this manner the transmission of normally incident light through the stroma, without deviation or significant scattering, is explained. As shown in *Figure 2.12*, a light beam of other than normal incidence is covered by the hypothesis simply by considering an oblique lattice plane. Other planes can be drawn, and together they explain the transmission of light through the cornea at different incidences. The lattice theory has been questioned — for example, Smith (1969) argued that Maurice's calculations of refractive index differences were incorrect — but the theory has gained wide acceptance as a reasonable explanation of transparency of the stroma.

The slight irregularities of collagen fibril separation as seen with the electron microscope were regarded by Maurice as preparation artefacts. Others have taken them into account such as Hart and Farrell (1969) who computed the probability distribution function for the relative position of

reduced. Local pressure on the cornea reduces transparency in the compressed region, again as a result of fibril disarray, but normal transparency returns immediately the pressure is withdrawn, allowing the forces maintaining the regular fibrillar spacing to operate once more. The haze and haloes around bright lights which often become very noticeable when contact lenses are worn are the result of corneal swelling, and again this may be explained in terms of the lattice theory. Alter-

Figure 2.12–Lattice arrangement of the fibrils of the corneal stroma. If lines were drawn joining the adjacent fibrils they would describe a lattice. The parallel lines pass through rows of fibrils and represent light wave fronts. The rows of fibrils may act as diffraction gratings (Maurice, 1957) and hence, wave fronts of widely differing orientations may traverse the stroma

fibrils from electron micrographs. They found that the mathematical summation of the phases of light waves scattered by the partially ordered array gave magnitude and wavelength dependence of the scattered light in good agreement with that found experimentally. Benedek (1971) presented proof that the scattering of light is produced only by fluctuations in the index of refraction of wavelengths larger than one-half the wavelength of light in the medium. Since the index fluctuations are far shorter than this value, transparency of the stroma is explained without the need for a perfect lattice of collagen fibrils. It has the added advantage of explaining the transparency of Bowman's layer.

When the cornea is oedematous its transparency is reduced and this may be explained in terms of the lattice theory in that the regularity of the fibrillar spacing is disturbed by the excess liquid and the efficiency of fibrils as grating elements is

natively, transparency loss with oedema may be explained by the formation of spaces within the stroma free of collagen fibrils and larger than the critical size of half the wavelength of light.

If our understanding of the transparency of the stroma is satisfactory, we are still left without an explanation of transparency of other layers of the cornea. They have a different structure from that of the stroma and yet a biomicroscope reveals that the epithelium scatters less light than does the stroma. This problem awaits solution.

A most interesting study by Bernhard, Miller and Møller (1965) showed that many insects have a surface corneal nipple array which has the property of increasing light transmission. The minute nipples are shorter than the wavelength of light, as is their separation, so that they become visible only by means of electron microscopy. They are approximately cone-shaped with adjacent bases in contact, and they cover the whole surface of each ommatidium. This transmission phenomenon applies only to visible wavelengths. As noted earlier, microvillus-like structures are present on the surface of the human cornea but their irregularity and infrequency does not allow comparison with the insect nipple array — but Bernhard's studies serve to emphasize that there is still much to be learned about light transmission through cellular structures.

The maintenance of corneal transparency is clearly dependent on the forces which limit its hydration. These forces are very susceptible to disturbances such as that produced by an inserted contact lens. Corneal hydration undoubtedly follows the insertion of a contact lens; some lenses are worse offenders than others and some persons are more affected than others. The dehydrating forces are discussed in the following section.

MAINTENANCE OF CORNEAL TRANSPARENCY

The cornea functions in a liquid environment and yet it has the capacity to maintain a steady solid/liquid ratio of about 1:4. If this ratio is increased by liquid uptake, the cornea loses its transparency. As the excised or damaged cornea is remarkably hygroscopic (the excised cornea in water increases to about four times its normal thickness), we may conclude that the transparent, living cornea, as a significant part of its workload, has to pump out water.

The integrity of its surface layers is essential for maintenance of corneal transparency, indicating that the pump operates through them. It is widely accepted that the endothelium carries the major burden in this active process, and much recent evidence supports this view. The pumping function could explain the high oxygen consumption by the endothelium per unit volume compared with that of the epithelium (Freeman, 1972). In experiments on rabbits, Maurice (1972) showed that the endothelium has the capacity to pump out water up to twelve times its own thickness in an hour. But both epithelium and endothelium have been shown to act as inert partial barriers to ion and liquid influx under experimental conditions such as hypothermia or anoxia, when the pump cannot be working, and therefore one may consider the pump to complement the action of the structural barriers in effecting the detergescence of the cornea. The barrier characteristics of the limiting layers are different in that the epithelium is far more impermeable to organic ions than is the endothelium, whilst the endothelium is more resistant than the epithelium to diffusion of water (Maurice, 1951; Donn, Miller and Mallett, 1963).

The nature of the pump is uncertain but it is unlikely to be a passive process, as Cogan and Kinsey (1942a) postulated in their 'osmotic pump' theory. It has been shown that work has to be done to prevent excessive hydration of the cornea, for if metabolic processes are inhibited the cornea swells and becomes opaque due to the uptake of water. A 'metabolic pump' is therefore actively transporting substances across the surface layers. Active transport is the movement of a substance across a biological membrane against an electrochemical potential gradient, requiring the use of energy. The potential gradient is due to the inequality of distribution of electrolytes on the two sides of the membrane. A well-known example of active transport elsewhere is the maintenance of sodium and potassium gradients across the surface membrane of nerve axons, establishing an electrical charge across the membrane. A similar mechanism is thought to be partially responsible for the production of aqueous humour in the eye.

The most popular concept of the metabolic pump is that of ion expulsion from the cornea; the ion is usually considered to be sodium. The resulting excess external sodium causes anions to follow passively, creating a hypotonic stroma relative to the bathing liquids, with the result that water is drawn out of the cornea. In this way, an osmotic gradient is produced to counteract the swelling pressure of the cornea. Among studies supporting this concept is that of Mishima and Hayakawa (1972) who found an increased content of sodium together with chlorine in the stroma when metabolism was inhibited. This sodium pump theory lost ground when an active transport of sodium ions *into* the cornea through the epithelium was demonstrated in the rabbit (Donn, Maurice and Mills, 1959). It appears unlikely that the endothelium would work to counteract this movement. Alternative theories, such as a primary water pump out of the cornea or water expulsion by means of pinocytosis, have their supporters but they appear to be less substantially based than the ion pump. Donn (1966) has published a useful discussion of the possible nature of the pump.

Although the foregoing illustrates the inadequacy of present knowledge to explain the nature of corneal deturgescence, the importance of metabolic forces in this process is established by experiments such as the loss of transparency and increased thickness at temperatures low enough to inhibit metabolism, and the recovery of transparency and normal thickness when the temperature is raised (Davson, 1955; Harris and Nordquist, 1955;

Mishima, 1968). Deprivation of oxygen or the application of metabolic poisons such as iodo-acetate also produces opacification of the cornea (Philpot, 1955).

A punctate lesion of the corneal endothelium causes a well-circumscribed region of stromal opacification opposite the lesion, suggesting that liquid intake is confined to the traumatized zone by the vigorous activity of the adjacent endothelium (Langham, 1960). Removal of the epithelium *in vivo* leads to hydration of the cornea but to a lesser extent than when the endothelium is removed (Maurice and Giardini, 1951). The deep aspect of the cornea is exposed to a greater hydrostatic pressure as a consequence of the intraocular pressure, which may explain the difference (Anseth and Dohlman, 1957). If the epithelium is scraped off the rabbit cornea, the stroma swells. Regeneration of the layer progresses from the periphery, and the newly covered stroma regains its normal thickness while the remaining denuded area stays grossly swollen. This situation is maintained even after 72 hours, when 90 per cent of the cornea is covered (Langham, 1960).

At the corneo-scleral junction there is a potential liquid leak into the cornea, but Maurice (1962*b*) calculated that the endothelium has more than sufficient pumping power to deal with the influx of water from this region.

In summary, it has been shown that the surface layers of the cornea act as inert, partial barriers to water influx and that, superimposed on this, a metabolic pump opposes the swelling pressure of the cornea. The nature of the pump is uncertain, but it is vigorous – particularly across the endothelium – and it probably consumes a large proportion of the cellular energy of the cornea.

METABOLIC PROCESSES

The following description of the metabolic processes in the cornea is confined to a consideration of glucose metabolism. De Roetth (1950) has shown that carbohydrate metabolism predominates in the cornea as indicated by a respiratory quotient of unity, and glucose is the principal monosaccharide of this process. Much of the energy released in the metabolism of glucose is used in the phosphorylation of ADP (adenosine disphosphate) to ATP(adenosine triphosphate), and energy is stored in this form. The efficiency of a metabolic pathway may therefore be measured in terms of the number of ATP molecules produced. The processes of greatest importance in the metabolism of glucose are, first, the glycolytic Embden-Meyerhof pathway followed by the Krebs tricarboxylic or citric acid cycle, and, second, the oxidation of glucose directly by the pentose phosphate pathway or hexose monophosphate shunt. These will be considered in turn and then related specifically to corneal metabolism.

Embden-Meyerhof Pathway

In this complex glycolytic process, enzymes called dehydrogenases act as catalysts for each stage in the process and finally split the glucose molecule into two molecules of pyruvic acid. In the third of the four stages of the glycolytic process, liberated energy is used to form two molecules of ATP from ADP and inorganic phosphate. If glycolysis occurs under aerobic conditions, six additional molecules of ATP are formed. Thus, the total ATP molecule yield of aerobic glycolysis is eight, while anaerobic glycolysis yields only two.

Under anaerobic conditions, pyruvic acid is converted to lactic acid without significant liberation or uptake of energy. Under aerobic conditions, glucose metabolism does not stop at this point but continues until the final products are carbon dioxide and water. This further breakdown is brought about by the citric acid cycle. During the cycle, carbon dioxide and hydrogen atoms are released. The hydrogen atoms, at length, become oxidized to form water; and the total oxidative process synthesizes a further thirty ATP molecules (*Figure 2.13*).

Hexose Monophosphate Shunt

Although the glycolytic pathway just described is the principal pathway for the oxidation of glucose, others are available. Of these, the hexose monophosphate shunt is the most important. In this process, glucose 6-phosphate takes part in a cyclic mechanism in which one glucose molecule is directly oxidized to carbon dioxide and water, liberating energy to produce a net gain of thirty-five ATP molecules.

The most efficient mechanism for useful energy production is therefore the oxidation of glucose to carbon dioxide and water through the Embden-Mayerhof pathway and the citric acid cycle. Anaerobic breakdown of glucose with lactic acid as the end-product releases useful energy, but the amount is very small. The hexose monophosphate shunt rivals aerobic glycolysis in yielding thirty-five ATP molecules. There is evidence that a significant part of the energy released in this cycle is employed in biosynthesis (Bell, Davidson and Scarborough, 1965).

Carbohydrate Metabolism in the Cornea

Glycolysis is predominantly exhibited in the epithelium. The high level of enzyme and pyruvic nucleotide concentration and the rate of oxygen consumption indicate that the endothelium also has a high glycolytic activity, but the relative inaccessibility of this layer has limited studies

Meyerhof pathway followed by the citric acid cycle and 35 per cent by means of the hexose monophosphate shunt. Kuhlman and Resnick (1959) estimated that, in the total cornea of rabbits, up to 70 per cent of glucose is oxidized to carbon dioxide via the shunt mechanism. There is evidence that the metabolism of the corneal layers is interrelated. For example, it is found that lactic acid,

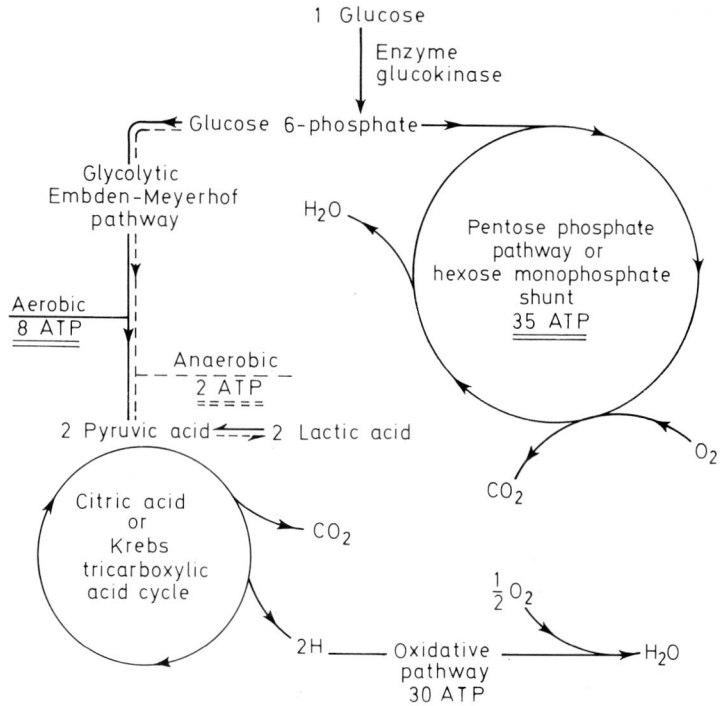

Figure 2.13–Outline of glucose metabolism showing the Embden–Meyerhof and pentose phosphate pathways

upon it. In contrast, the stroma shows very little metabolic activity. Tissues exhibiting aerobic glycolysis accumulate lactate because the Embden-Meyerhof pathway is more efficient than the aerobic mechanisms which cause the combustion of pyruvate to carbon dioxide and water (Langham, 1954).

Anaerobic glycolysis alone, with its low energy yield, is evidently inadequate to maintain the cornea in its normal state as, in the absence of oxygen, the cornea swells and loses its transparency (Heald and Langham, 1956, and many others).

Kinoshita and his colleagues have demonstrated that the hexose monophosphate shunt is unusually active in the cornea (Kinoshita and Masurat, 1959; Kinoshita, 1962). They estimated that, in the bovine corneal epithelium, about 65 per cent of the glucose is metabolized by way of the Embden-

which is produced in all layers of the cornea, cannot be utilized in the absence of the epithelium (Herrmann and Hickman, 1948).

SOURCES OF METABOLITES

The avascularity of the cornea promotes enquiry into the possible routes of metabolite supply. There are clearly three possibilities: (1) from the perilimbal blood vessels; (2) from the aqueous humour; and (3) from the tears liquid. A common method of investigation is to alter the availability of metabolites from one of these possible sources and note if the cornea shows any alteration.

There is little reason to doubt that the perilimbal blood vessels provide metabolites for the cornea — at least, for the peripheral cornea; but that this route is of limited importance is indicated by experiments and observations where blood flow has been interrupted. Gundersen (1939) noted that corneal transparency was unaltered in his patients following complete peritomy of the cornea. Scarification of the conjunctiva in cases of perilimbal melanomas, and experimental thermocoagulation of the perilimbal tissues in rabbits, fails to interfere with corneal transparency. Diffusion of radioactive substances from the limbus into the cornea following sub-conjunctival or systemic injection has been observed. These substances are found to be in greater concentration peripherally than centrally (Maurice, 1951; Pratt-Johnson, 1959). Maurice (1962b) found that large molecules are the most likely to diffuse to the central cornea, and the conditions for this occurrence are least favourable for oxygen and glucose.

The question of the relative importance of tears liquid and aqueous humour as sources of glucose for the cornea appears to be settled in favour of the aqueous, but it is still uncertain whether or not the tears liquid route is of any practical importance. Bock and Maumenee (1953) inserted thin polythene sheets between stromal lamellae in rabbits and observed a thickening of the overlying stroma with complete degeneration of the epithelium in the central zone after two days. The deep underlying stroma and the endothelium were normal during this period and the epithelium maintained its integrity when the polythene sheet was trephined with several 2 mm holes. The conclusion was reached that the epithelium and stroma are dependent on the aqueous humour for metabolites. But these results are not altogether consistent with more recent studies. For example, water impermeable polypropylene sheets inserted between stromal lamellae in cats were tolerated for more than a year without pathological changes, deep or superficial to the sheet (Pollack, 1962). In similar experiments, Knowles (1961) reported an absence of pathological changes for periods of up to ten weeks in rabbits. Clearly, the deeper layers may flourish when isolated from the anterior layers and hence the aqueous must be a source of metabolites for the cornea. It is unlikely that much glucose moves in the other direction, from the tears to the cornea, as the concentration of 2.6 mg/100 ml in tears in man (Giardini and Roberts, 1950) is far too little to be of much significance in the nourishment of the cornea (Maurice, 1962b). Glucose concentration is more than ten times as great in the aqueous (Reim et al., 1967). A reduction in epithelial glycogen and ATP as well as glucose was demonstrated following the insertion of intralamellar membrane barriers (Turss, Friend and Dohlman, 1970) and these changes could not be prevented by tarsor-

rhaphy or the topical application of glucose. Thoft and Friend (1972) observed a passive diffusion of a labelled amino acid through the endothelium. The rapid turnover of epithelial cells demands a considerable utilization of amino acids in the synthesis of protein and, as expected, the concentration was high, but it was actively accumulated by the epithelium only after it had appeared in the stroma, suggesting that none was taken up from the tears despite their rich amino acid content (Balik, 1958). It appears that epithelium has a very low permeability to amino acids and glucose.

The utilization of atmospheric oxygen by the cornea through the tears film has been demonstrated in a number of ways. In man, symptoms of corneal irritation together with the haze and haloes known as Sattler's veil (Finkelstein, 1952) were experienced when the cornea was deprived of atmospheric oxygen (Smelser, 1952; Smelser and Ozanics, 1952). These symptoms were induced two and a half hours after pumping nitrogen saturated with water vapour into tight-fitting goggles. The introduction of oxygen relieved the symptoms. Langham (1952) exposed the eyes of rabbits to a pure oxygen atmosphere for three to three and a half hours and found that the lactic acid concentration in the cornea was reduced by a third. Using a nitrogen atmosphere for the same period of time, lactic acid concentration was increased by a third. These observations indicated an increase in aerobic glycolysis in the first case and a decrease in the second, again establishing that atmospheric oxygen is utilized by the cornea. Hill and Fatt (1964) measured the rate of oxygen uptake by the corneal epithelium in man by using oxygen electrodes embedded in a tight-fitting scleral lens with an oxygen-filled reservoir between the lens and cornea. They observed a rapid reduction in the oxygen tension in the reservoir as a result of oxygen uptake by the cornea. A rate of oxygen uptake of 4.8 μl/cm^2/hr was calculated from their results. However, Farris, Takahashi and Donn (1967), using the same technique, interpreted their data differently to arrive at a figure of 1.4 μl/cm^2/hr.

Langham (1952) concluded that the rabbit cornea also utilizes aqueous oxygen. The lactic acid concentration decreased from a value of unity to 0.7, three to three and a half hours after introducing an oxygen bubble into the anterior chamber; the concentration was increased to 1.26 if nitrogen was used in place of oxygen. Fatt and Bieber (1968) and Fatt, Freeman and Lin (1974) calculated oxygen distribution profiles through the thickness of the cornea in rabbits as shown in *Figure 2.14*. The profiles were determined from measurements of the partial oxygen pressures at the surfaces and existing knowledge of stromal oxygen consumption, diffusion coefficients and solubility. The regular reduction of the partial oxygen pressures from 155 mm Hg at the anterior surface and from 55 mm Hg at the posterior surface to a minimum at the junction of the endothelium with Descemet's layer suggests that oxygen serving the endothelium is derived from the aqueous and that atmospheric oxygen serves the remainder of the cornea. Although equivalent data in man are limited, Fatt and Bieber believe that the oxygen distribution

THE EFFECTS OF CONTACT LENSES ON CORNEAL METABOLISM

A contact lens presents a barrier between the cornea and the atmosphere, and from the foregoing it follows that the most likely interference with corneal metabolism a contact lens might cause is deprivation of oxygen with a consequent reduction in aerobic glycolysis. Oxygen uptake by the tears in front of the lens would continue, but transference of oxygen to the film behind the lens may be prevented. Normally, this situation is avoided

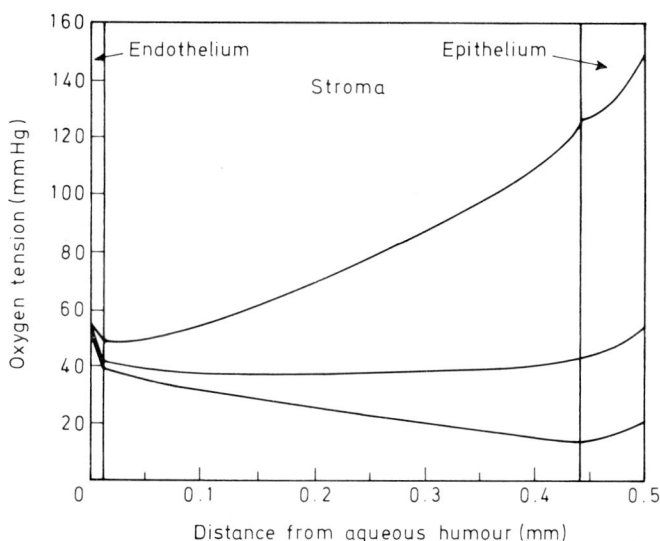

Figure 2.14–Summary of oxygen tension profiles for various conditions based on measurements made under each condition at the epithelial surface and under the normal condition at the endothelial surface in rabbits. The curves joining the surface points were calculated. The upper and middle curves represent the eye open and closed conditions respectively. The lowest curve represents the profile with a soft contact lens of low permeability on the eye (modified from Fatt, Freeman and Lin, 1974)

profiles in rabbits '. . . represent, at least qualitatively, the situation in the human cornea'. When the lids were closed long enough for equilibrium levels to be reached, the partial oxygen pressure at the epithelium reduced to the same level (55 mm Hg) measured at the endothelial surface (Figure 2.14), with a trough within the stroma. Under these circumstances, it appears, first, that the vessels of the palpebral conjunctiva must provide the epithelium with oxygen because if contact between these surfaces is prevented the partial oxygen pressure falls to zero. Earlier, Langham (1952) reached the same conclusion. Secondly, the altered profile suggests that aqueous oxygen is being used now by deeper structures of the cornea. Similar studies of the CO_2 partial pressures showed that corneal and aqueous CO_2 passed out to the tears when the lids were open, but when they were closed some passed to the aqueous from the cornea.

with hard corneal lenses because they move and produce tears circulation, permitting some degree of oxygen and carbon dioxide exchange between the cornea and atmosphere.

Soft lenses also move on the eye but the circulation of tears behind the lens is less although they have the advantage of transmitting oxygen in amounts varying with the nature and thickness of the material (Fatt and St. Helen, 1971; Morrison and Edelhauser, 1972; Peterson and Fatt, 1973). Tears exchange is least with scleral lenses; in the case of fenestrated lenses Ruben (1967) calculated the rate of tears exchange to be half that obtained with hard corneal lenses.

Presumably, the cornea can comfortably tolerate a reduction of the partial oxygen pressure at the epithelial surface from 155 to 55 mm Hg, for this occurs when the lids are closed for some length of time and there is evidence that the cornea can tolerate levels as low as 11–19 mm Hg (Polse and Mandell,

1970). Farris, Takahashi and Donn (1967), using the oxygen electrode method, observed a transient increase in oxygen uptake by the corneal epithelium measured a few seconds after comfortably fitted corneal lenses had been worn for a period of eight hours. But even after only two minutes wear, a large increase in oxygen uptake occurred (Hill and Leighton, 1968). The increased uptake of oxygen was about the same whether soft hydrophilic or hard methacrylate lenses were worn (Hill, 1967). The increase was due to the replenishment of the supply of dissolved oxygen normally present when an unlimited supply is available from the

1970; Millodot, 1975a). Increases of 20 per cent have been recorded. The increase usually takes more than one hour after insertion of a lens to reach a maximum thickness (El Hage et al., 1974) and within two hours of removing the lens normal thickness is recovered. Epithelial swelling contributes to the thickening (Farris, Kubota and Mishima, 1971) and increased curvature has been recorded (Miller, 1969). Some debate attends the question of corneal thickening with soft lenses. Although earlier measurements led to the conclusion that the cornea does not swell (Krejčí and Bíleck, 1970; Larke and Sabell, 1971) it now

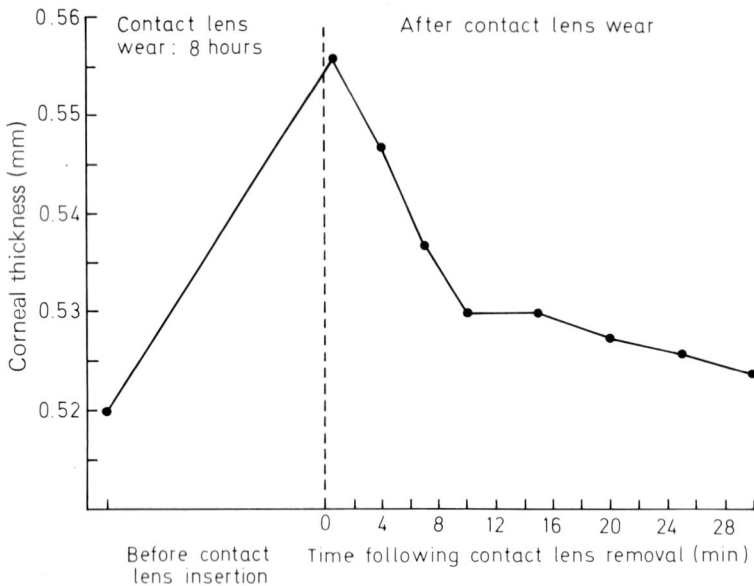

Figure 2.15–Relationship between central corneal thickness and the wearing of hard contact lenses for 8 hours. Each point represents the mean of 11 subjects (after Millodot, 1975a)

atmosphere. The level of oxygen deprivation induced by wearing corneal lenses was found to be slightly greater than that caused by lid closure for five minutes (Farris, Takahashi and Donn, 1967). Following the argument of Fatt and his colleagues. aqueous oxygen utility extends deeper than the endothelium when the level of tears liquid oxygen is depressed by the presence of a contact lens.

Interference with normal corneal metabolism will produce a thickening and a reduction of transparency of the cornea. The thickening which is observed with corneal lens wear varies between individuals. Most people show a measurable thickening and it seems likely that when none is reported the thickening is simply too little to permit detection. Increases in thickness average between 4 per cent (Honda, Sakaue and Kyoko, 1968; Farris, Kubota and Mishima, 1971) and about 7 or 8 per cent (*Figure 2.15*) (Manchester,

seems likely that some swelling does occur (El Hage et al., 1974) and it may compare with that induced by hard corneal lenses (Bailey and Carney, 1973; Polse, Sarver and Harris, 1975). Vertical striae are quite commonly present while soft lenses are worn but corneal curvature does not appear to be altered. Much has been written favouring the concept that oedema reduces as the eyes adapt to contact lenses but specific data is often lacking. Some recovery from oedema seems likely but it is probably slow (Farris, Kubota and Mishima, 1971) and possibly incomplete. Evidence of sustained oedema may be found with greater facility. In this context, it is worth noting that corneal thickening, approximately equal in amount to that induced by contact lenses, occurs normally during sleep. On awakening, the cornea gradually thins over a period of one or two hours (Mandell and Fatt, 1965; Gerstman, 1972).

Alterations in glycolysis have been measured after fitting contact lenses to experimental animals. The corneas of guinea-pigs fitted with scleral lenses became thicker and less transparent and the lactic acid content increased rapidly (Smelser and Chen, 1955). An increased lactic acid content would be expected as a result of reduced aerobic glycolysis, and Hirano's (1959) observation of depleted glycogen content in rabbit corneas fitted with corneal lenses indicates an increased consumption of glycogen by means of the less productive anaerobic glycolytic cycle in an endeavour to compensate. Morley and McCulloch (1961) also observed an increased lactic acid content in both the stroma and epithelium of rabbits fitted with contact lenses; and in addition, they observed a slight decrease of oxidized pyridine nucleotides and a decrease in the percentage of protein in the epithelium. These results suggest that both aerobic glycolysis and protein synthesis were reduced.

The loss of transparency associated with induced thickening is so slight that it cannot be measured objectively.

TEARS

The basic secretion of tears is largely derived from the lacrimal gland, with small additional contributions from the accessory lacrimal glands, the mucous conjunctival glands and the sebaceous tarsal (Meibomian) glands. A conjunctival gland or goblet cell is shown in *Figure 2.8* in the process of releasing mucin granules into the tears film. The lacrimal gland has usually been classified as a serous gland, but recent evidence shows that it is in fact a sero-mucous gland in rats (Scott and Pease, 1959) man and monkeys (Ruskell, 1969 and 1975; Allen, Wright and Reid, 1972). The watery secretion is explained by the greater activity of the serous cells. It has been proposed that the lacrimal gland does not take part in the basic secretion of tears because the eye remains moist if the lacrimal gland is congenitally absent, or when the gland is removed or its motor nerve supply is interrupted. It may be true that the eye usually remains sufficiently moist for comfort in these circumstances with retention of an optically adequate corneal surface, but denervation or removal of the gland nonetheless produces a radical reduction in the basic secretion of tears (Golding-Wood, 1964; Ruskell, 1969).

Superimposed on the basic secretion are the phasic increments in secretion induced reflexly by mechanical or chemical irritation and by psychogenic factors. To distinguish between the two, the words 'lacrimation', to describe reflex tears, and 'weeping', for psychogenic tears, have been suggested.

THE PRE-CORNEAL FILM

Wolff (1948) considered the pre-corneal film to consist of a triple-layered structure with a central watery phase made up of the serous secretion of the lacrimal gland and constituting the bulk of the film; a thin superficial oily layer was thought to issue from the tarsal glands and a deep layer of mucoproteins from the conjunctival glands.

The presence of a thin superficial oily layer is suggested by the coloured interference fringes which may be observed with a biomicroscope. Further evidence of the surface film and of its origin is provided by Mishima and Maurice (1961), who demonstrated in rabbits that tears film evaporation increases at least tenfold in the absence of tarsal gland secretion. This amount of increased evaporation is approximately that expected of water in the absence of a surface lipid film. Despite this apparently straightforward evidence for tarsal gland function, when secretion, expressed from human tarsal glands, was spread over a saline solution no significant reduction in evaporation was observed (Brown and Dervichian, 1969). Although the experimental conditions of this study are not beyond criticism, the results are at least sufficient to re-open discussion of the matter.

Wolff's assumption of a mucoid layer deepest in the film, although widely accepted, is unsupported by the evidence of Ehlers' (1965a) investigations. Ehlers showed that the outermost parts of the epithelium of the cornea are infiltrated by lipids which are probably produced by the tarsal glands, and that the mucoprotein secretion of the conjunctival glands is not disposed as a deep film but dispersed within the thick central water phase of the film.

The pre-corneal film is of nearly uniform thickness of between 6 and 9 μm (Ehlers, 1965a; Mishima, 1965). Ehlers observed that it reduces by about 20 per cent five seconds after blinking and by nearly 50 per cent after thirty seconds. There is little flow across the cornea between blinks. The limited flow and the uniform thickness are the consequences of the 'framing' function of the eyelids which is eliminated if the eyelids are withdrawn from the eyeball, causing a spotty drying of the pre-corneal film.

The spreading of the film is a function of the nature of tears. This spreading ability — that is to say, its efficiency as a wetting agent — is dependent on a low surface tension which is usually considered to be brought about by the protein content. But tears liquid is not rich in protein compared with other body liquids. Ehlers (1965a) argued that the surface-acting lipids from the tarsal glands are of most importance in lowering both the interfacial tension between the tears film and the epithelium and the surface tension. A lipid film has the property of building up more readily and has greater stability than a protein film, which renders the former more suitable for providing sharp vision immediately after blinking. It should be added that the spreading of the tears film is facilitated by the movement of the eyelids across the cornea. In the presence of a contact lens, the interfacial tension at three surfaces has to be considered. The desirable establishment of low interfacial tension at the two surfaces of the contact lens is partly related to the nature and to the condition of the lens.

FUNCTION OF TEARS

Tears liquid is essential for the maintenance of the normal optical properties of the cornea; without it, corneal metabolic processes are impaired, as noted earlier, with consequent loss of transparency. Further, the excellent refracting surface which the smooth tears film provides would be lost and an irregularly refracting, dessicated epithelial surface would be substituted. Tears liquid is the lubricant for eyelid movement over the cornea and the medium for flushing away foreign matter which potentially endangers the optical integrity of the cornea.

Lysozyme, the enzyme originally described by Fleming (1922) in tears liquid, is selectively bacteriolytic by destruction of the cell wall. Lysozyme therefore affords a degree of protection against pathogenic organisms lodged in the conjunctival sac. Thompson and Gallardo (1941) produced evidence of another native antibacterial agent of tears liquid which was characterized by its specific action against certain staphylococci.

TEARS DRAINAGE

Much of the tears liquid lies in strips (the rivus lacrimalis) along the lid margins and against the cornea, presenting a concave cylindrical free surface. Medially, the strips terminate in the so-called lacrimal lake which is often described as a reservoir of tears liquid bathing the caruncle and bounded by the inner canthus and the free edge of the plica semilunaris. This delimitation is obviously changed as the eye moves from the primary position. But, as Wolff (1948) pointed out, under normal circumstances the inner canthus is moist but does not contain a pool of fluid. The punctum lacrimale of each papilla is turned in towards the cornea and interrupts the marginal tears strips.

Drainage of tears is initiated by the movement of tears liquid from the marginal tears strips through the punctum and into the canaliculus by capillary attraction. This is facilitated by the continuous movement of liquid nasally which is effected by lid closure; closure occurs first at the outer canthus and then, progressively, to the inner canthus. If a very small spot of dye is applied to a marginal tears strip, blinking will cause the dye to spread towards the punctum. It will neither move to the fornix nor to the outer canthus (Ehlers, 1965a).

The canaliculi are embedded in the orbicularis muscle so that on contraction of the muscle the canaliculi are closed and shortened and the tears liquid is driven into the lacrimal sac. Regurgitation is prevented by the simultaneous closure of the ampulla of each canaliculus. The muscular activity amounts to a milking action rather than a peristalsis. The pre-septal portion of the orbicularis muscle is claimed to have a deep insertion from each lid to the lacrimal diaphragm which is the lateral fascial wall of the lacrimal sac, with the consequence that contraction causes a lateral movement of the lacrimal diaphragm. It follows that the sac becomes dilated, and it is thought to produce a reduction of the pressure in the sac which produces a siphoning of tears liquid. This postulated mechanism (Jones, 1961), which constitutes a lacrimal pump, would appear to demand closure of the 'valve' of Hasner which occludes the nasal exit of the naso-lacrimal duct (ostium lacrimalis), in order to create an effective vacuum for siphoning. This probably does not occur, and pressure measurements within the sac reveal no change during eyelid movement (Wright and Maurice, personal communication). Further, the existence of the necessary structures for operating the lacrimal pump, postulated by Jones, has been questioned (Brienen and Snell, 1967). Hence, it appears that an elaborate pumping mechanism may not be present and that gravitation alone may account for the movement of the tears out of the lacrimal sac.

TEARS OUTPUT

The daily output of tears is usually considered to be rather less than 1 g. This figure is based on the data of Schirmer (1903), but it has been questioned because of the probable inaccuracy of his measuring technique. Tests developed recently, that measure the rate of dilution of a stain applied to the marginal tears strip, probably introduce less error, but results are not consistent. Originally, Nover and Jaeger (1952) calculated the surprisingly high average rate of 14 g of tears secretion daily, but Kirchner's (1964) results were similar to those of Schirmer. However, Norn (1965) subsequently reported a daily tears output of 15–30 g measured from 186 eyes. The instillation of a stain (rose bengal and/or fluorescein) will obviously tend to elevate the recorded figure for basic tears secretion both by its own bulk and by its irritant effect. But the method neither involves the aspiration of tears nor neglects to account for tears escaping through the puncta, and these are important shortcomings of other tests, some of which also share the error invoked by corneal irritation. Hence, it may be tentatively concluded that the lacrimal secretion normally produced is well in excess of 1 g as suggested by Schirmer but rather less than the 15–30 g measured by Norn.

In a study of a large number of full-term infants, Penbharkkul and Karelitz (1962) encountered shedding of tears as early as five and a half hours of age and as late as 84 days. The onset of lacrimation occurred during the first four weeks in a majority of infants, and in most it occurred first with crying associated with hunger and pain. Sjögren (1955) used nasal irritants to determine the onset of reflex lacrimation in infants and found that it occurred in all but 13 per cent during the first few weeks of life.

With advancing years, basic tears secretion decreases gradually: the difference between the sexes is negligible (Norn, 1965) except in early adult life, when females have a higher rate of secretion (Henderson and Prough, 1950; de Roetth, 1953). Sex differences concerning psychogenic tears or weeping are clearly a separate matter.

Schirmer's popular tears secretion test is unsatisfactory as a precise quantitative test for tears secretion but it is of considerable value in comparing the production of tears between eyes of a pair and between eyes of different persons. The test should find a place in routine contact lens practice, according to some authorities (for example, Halberg, 1967), as an aid in determining the suitability of a patient for contact lens wear. It is argued that patients with a low rate of tears secretion are more likely than others to be intolerant of lenses. If this is too indulgent a view, it is at least reasonable that practitioners should be aware of the problems of limited or reduced lacrimal gland secretion. Lacrimal hypersecretion, induced by contact lenses, has been held responsible for corneal oedema on rather insubstantial grounds and the idea has been refuted (Uniacke and Hill, 1970; Farris, Kubota and Mishima, 1971).

In Schirmer's test, filter paper strips (Whatman's No.1 are satisfactory), 5 mm in width are folded 5 mm from one end. This short end is trimmed at the corners and inserted into the inferior conjunctival sac, displaced laterally to avoid contact with the cornea (see Figure 14.8a and b, Chapter 14, Volume 2). Anaesthesia is not used. After five minutes, the exposed length of moistened filter paper is measured to the fold. A 15 mm length is moistened, on average, in a five-minute period. Standardized sterile strips are available if preferred.* The test should not be undertaken immediately after any procedure that may induce hypersecretion of tears.

NEURAL CONTROL OF TEARS

Irritation of the cornea, conjunctiva, nasal mucosa and of any area served by the trigeminal nerve causes reflex lacrimation. The trigeminal nerve is responsible for the sensory input of the reflex pathway and if it is blocked, or surface anaesthesia applied, reflex lacrimation is abolished. The paths of the central nervous system associated with psychogenic weeping are unknown, and a knowledge of the link between the trigeminal nerve and the facial nerve in the reflex lacrimation pathway is lacking.

Both parasympathetic nerve fibres (from the pterygopalatine or sphenopalatine ganglion) and sympathetic nerve fibres (from the superior cervical ganglion) have been thought to be responsible for motor control of lacrimal gland secretion; but in recent experiments on cats and monkeys, only parasympathetic fibres could be shown to exercise this control (Botelho, Hisada and Fuenmayor, 1966; Ruskell, 1969). There is no clear evidence of motor control of the tarsal and conjunctival glands.

*Schirmer tear test (Knox Laboratories, Aylesbury, Bucks.).

REFERENCES

Allen, M., Wright, P. and Reid, L. (1972). 'The human lacrimal gland. A histochemical and organ culture study of the secretory cells.' Archs Ophthal. 88, 493–497

Anseth, A. and Dohlman, C. H. (1957). 'Influence of the intraocular pressure on hydration of the corneal stroma.' Acta Ophthal. 35, 85–90

Bailey, I. L. and Carney, L. G. (1973). 'Corneal changes from hydrophilic contact lenses.' Am. J. Optom. 50, 299–304

Balik, J. (1958). 'The amino acid content of tears.' Sborn. lék. 60, 332–336, as cited in Ophthal. Lit. 12, No.4847 (1958)

Bell, G. H., Davidson, J. N. and Scarborough, H. (1965). Textbook of Physiology and Biochemistry, p.150. Edinburgh and London: Livingstone

Benedek, G. B. (1971). 'Theory of transparency of the eye.' *Applied Optics* **10**, 459–472

Bernhard, C. G., Miller, W. H. and Møller, A. R. (1965). 'The insect corneal nipple array.' *Acta physiol. scand.* **63**, Suppl. 243

Bertanlanffy, F. D. and Lau, C. (1962). 'Mitotic rate and renewal time of the corneal epithelium in the rat.' *Archs Ophthal.* **68**, 546–551

Bock, R. H. and Maumenee, A. E. (1953). 'Corneal fluid metabolism: experiments and observations.' *Archs Ophthal.* **50**, 282–285

Boberg-Ans, J. (1955). 'Experience in clinical examination of corneal sensitivity.' *Br. J. Ophthal.* **39**, 705–726

Boberg-Ans, J. (1956). 'On the corneal sensitivity.' *Acta Ophthal.* **35**, 149–162

Boozan, C. W. and Cohen, I. J. (1953). 'Ophthaine; new topical anesthetic for eye.' *Am. J. Ophthal.* **36**, 1619–1621

Botelho, S. Y., Hisada, M. and Fuenmayor, N. (1966). 'Functional innervation of the lacrimal gland in the cat.' *Archs Ophthal.* **76**, 581–588

Brienen, J. A. and Snell, C. A. R. D. (1967). 'A new examination of the orbicularis oculi.' *Ophthalmologica* **154**, 104–113

Bron, A. J. (1968). 'Anterior corneal mosaic.' *Br. J. Ophthal.* **52**, 659–669

Brown, S. I. and Dervichian, D. G. (1969). 'The oils of the meibomian glands.' *Archs Ophthal.* **82**, 537–540

Byron, H. M. and Weseley, A. C. (1961). 'Clinical investigation of corneal contact lenses.' *Am. J. Ophthal.* **51**, 675–694

Cardoso, S. S., Ferreira, A. L., Camargo, A. C. M. and Böhn, G. (1968). 'The effect of partial hepatectomy upon circadian distribution of mitosis in the cornea of rats.' *Experentia* **24**, 569–570

Caspersson, T. and Engström, A. (1946). 'Hornhinnevävnadens transparens.' *Nord. Med.* **30**, 1279–1282, cited by D. M. Maurice (1957)

Cochet, P. and Bonnet, R. (1960). 'L'esthésia cornéenne. Sa measure clinique ses variations physiologiques et pathologiques.' *Clin. Ophtal.* **4**, 1–27

Cogan, D. G. and Kinsey, V. E. (1942a). 'The cornea. I: Transfer of water and sodium chloride by osmosis and diffusion through the excised cornea.' *Archs Ophthal.* **27**, 466–476

Cogan, D. G. and Kinsey, V. E. (1942b). 'The cornea. V: Physiological aspects.' *Archs Ophthal.* **28**, 661–669

Davson, H. (1955). 'The hydration of the cornea.' *Biochem. J.* **59**, 24–28

Dixon, J. M. (1964). 'Ocular changes due to contact lenses.' *Am. J. Ophthal.* **58**, 424–443

Donn, A. (1966). 'Cornea and sclera. Annual review.' *Archs Ophthal.* **75**, 261–288

Donn, A., Maurice, D. and Mills, N. (1959). 'Studies on living cornea *in vitro*. II: The active transport of sodium across the endothelium.' *Archs Ophthal.* **62**, 748–757

Donn, A., Miller, S. and Mallett, N. (1963). 'Water permeability of the living cornea.' *Archs Ophthal.* **70**, 515–521

Edmund, J. (1967). 'The cosmetic indication for using contact lenses.' *Acta Ophthal.* **45**, 760–768

Ehinger, B. (1964). 'Adrenergic nerves to the eye and its adnexa in rabbit and guinea-pig.' *Acta Univ. Lund.* (2), No.20

Ehinger, B. (1971). 'A comparative study of the adrenergic nerves to the anterior eye segment of some primates.' *Z. Zellforsch. mikroskop. Anat.* **116**, 157–177

Ehlers, N. (1965a). 'The precorneal film. Biomicroscopical, histological and chemical investigations.' *Acta Ophthal.* Suppl. 81

Ehlers, N. (1965b). 'On the size of the conjunctival sac.' *Acta Ophthal.* **43**, 205–210

Eisenman, J., Landgren, S. and Novin, P. (1963). 'Functional organization in the main sensory trigeminal nucleus and in the rostral subdivision of the nucleus of the spinal trigeminal tract in the cat.' *Acta physiol. scand.* **59**, Suppl. 214

El Hage, S. G., Hughes, C. C., Schlauer, K. R. and Jarell, R. L. (1974). 'Evaluation of corneal thickness induced by hard and flexible contact lens wear.' *Am. J. Optom.* **51**, 24–33

Epstein, D. L. and Paton, D. (1968). 'Keratitis from misuse of corneal anaesthetics.' *New England J. Med.* **279**, 396–399. Annotated in *Lancet,* 16 Nov. (1968)

Farris, R. L., Takahashi, G. H. and Donn, A. (1967). 'Corneal oxygen flux in contact lens wearers.' In *Corneal and Scleral Contact Lenses*, ed. by L. J. Girard, pp.413–425. St. Louis: Mosby

Farris, R. L., Kubota, Z. and Mishima, S. (1971). 'Epithelial decompensation with corneal contact lens wear.' *Archs Ophthal.* **85**, 651–660

Fatt, I. and Bieber, M. T. (1968). 'The steady-state distribution of oxygen and carbon dioxide in the *in vivo* cornea. 1: The open eye in air and the closed eye.' *Exp. Eye Res.* **7**, 103–112

Fatt, I. and St. Helen, R. (1971). 'Oxygen tension under an oxygen-permeable contact lens.' *Am. J. Optom.* **48**, 545–555

Fatt, I., Freeman, R. D. and Lin, D. (1974). 'Oxygen tension distributions in the cornea: a re-examination.' *Exp. Eye Res.* **18**, 357–365

Finkelstein, I. S. (1952). 'The biophysics of corneal scatter and diffraction of light induced by contact lenses.' *Am. J. Optom.* **29**, 231–259

Fleming, A. (1922). 'On a remarkable bacteriolytic element found in tissues and secretions.' *Proc. roy. Soc.* B **93**, 306–317

Freeman, J. A. (1962). 'Fine structure of the goblet cell mucous secretory process.' *Anat. Rec.* **144**, 341–357

Freeman, R. D. (1972). 'Oxygen consumption by the component layers of the cornea.' *J. Physiol.* **225**, 15–32

Friedenwald, J. S. and Buschke, W. (1944a). 'Mitotic and wound-healing activities of the corneal epithelium.' *Archs Ophthal.* **32**, 410–413

Friedenwald, J. S. and Buschke, W. (1944b). 'The effect of excitement of epinephrine and of sympathectomy on the mitotic activity of corneal epithelium in rats.' *Am. J. Physiol.* **141**, 689–694

Gerstman, D. R. (1972). 'The biomicroscope and Vickers image-splitting eyepiece applied to the diurnal variation in human central corneal thickness.' *J. Microsc.* **96**, 385–388

Giardini, A. and Roberts, J. R. E. (1950). 'Concentration of glucose and total chloride in tears.' *Br. J. Ophthal.*

34, 737–743

Ginsborg, B. L. (1952). 'Rotation of the eyes during involuntary blinking.' *Nature,* **169,** 412–413

Ginsborg, B. L. and Maurice, D. M. (1959). 'Involuntary movements of the eye during fixation and blinking.' *Br. J. Ophthal.* **43,** 435–437

Golding-Wood, P. H. (1964). 'The ocular effects of autonomic surgery.' *Proc. R. Soc. Med.* **57,** 494–497

Gordon, G. (1951). 'Observations upon the movement of the eyelids.' *Br. J. Ophthal.* **35,** 339–351

Gornig, H. and Pommer, G. (1971). 'Alternsveranderungen des Konjunktivalepithels.' *Z. Altensforsch.* **23,** 391–395

Grant, F. C., Groff, R. A. and Lewy, F. H. (1940). 'Section of descending spinal root of fifth cranial nerve.' *Arch. Neurol. Psychiat.* **43,** 498–509

Greenberg, M. H. and Hill, R. M. (1973). 'The physiology of contact lens imprints.' *Am. J. Optom.* **50,** 699–702

Guilbert, J. (1963). 'Contact lens fitting in France.' *J. Am. optom. Ass.* **34,** 1403–1405

Gunderson, T. (1939). 'Vascular obliteration for various types of keratitis. Its significance' regarding nutrition of corneal epithelium.' *Archs Ophthal.* **21,** 76–107

Gunderson, T. and Liebman, S. D. (1944). 'Effect of local anaesthetics on regeneration of corneal epithelium.' *Archs Ophthal.* **31,** 29–33

Halberg, G. P. (1967). 'Lacrimal function and contact lenses.' In *XXth International Congress of Ophthalmology, Munich, 1966. Contact Lens Symposium,* pp.149–154. Basel: Karger

Hamano, H. (1960). 'Topical and systemic influences of wearing contact lenses.' *Contacto* **4,** 41–48

Hanna, C. and O'Brien, J. E. (1960). 'Cell production and migration in the epithelial layer of the cornea.' *Archs Ophthal.* **64,** 536–539

Hanna, C., Bicknell, D. S. and O'Brien, J. E. (1961). 'Cell turnover in the adult human eye.' *Archs Ophthal.* **65,** 695–698

Hanna, C. and O'Brien, J. E. (1961). 'Thymidine-tritium labelling of the cellular elements of the corneal stroma.' *Archs Ophthal.* **66,** 362–365

Harris, J. E. and Nordquist, L. T. (1955). 'The hydration of the cornea. 1: The transport of water from the cornea.' *Am. J. Ophthal.* **40,** 100–110

Hart, R. W. and Farrell, R. A. (1969). 'Light scattering in the cornea.' *J. opt. Soc. Am.* **59,** 766–774

Heald, K. and Langham, M. E. (1956). 'Permeability of the cornea and blood-aqueous barrier to oxygen.' *Br. J. Ophthal.* **40,** 705–720

Henderson, J. W. and Prough, W. L. (1950). 'Influence of age and sex on flow of tears.' *Archs Ophthal.* **43,** 224–231

Herrmann, H. and Hickman, F. H. (1948). 'The adhesion of epithelium to stroma in the cornea.' *Bull. Johns Hopk. Hosp.* **82,** 182–207

Heydenreich, A. (1958). '*Die Hornhautregeneration.* Marhold: Halle

Hill, R. M. (1967). 'Effects of hydrophilic plastic lenses on corneal respiration.' *J. Am. optom. Ass.* **38,** 181–184

Hill, R. M. and Fatt, I. (1964). 'Oxygen measurements under a contact lens.' *Am. J. Optom.* **41,** 382–387

Hill, R. M. and Leighton, A. J. (1968). 'Effects of contact lens apertures on corneal respiration under dynamic conditions.' *Am. J. Optom.* **45,** 65–79

Hirano, J. (1959). 'Histochemical studies on the corneal changes induced by corneal contact lenses.' *Jap. J. Ophthal.* **3,** 1–8

Honda, Y., Sakaue, E. and Kyoko, O. (1968). 'Studies on the thickness of the cornea wearing contact lenses.' (In Japanese). *J. Jap. Contact Lens Soc.* **10,** 133–141. In *Fol. ophthal. Jap.* **19,** No.11

Iwamoto, T. and Smelser, G. K. (1965). 'Electron microscopy of the human corneal endothelium with reference to transport mechanisms.' *Invest. Ophthal.* **4,** 270–284

Jakus, M. A. (1961). 'The fine structure of the human cornea.' In *The Structure of the Eye,* ed. by G. K. Smelser. New York and London: Academic Press

Jakus, M. A. (1962). 'Further observations on the fine structure of the cornea.' *Invest. Ophthal.* **1,** 202–225

Jakus, M. A. (1964). *Ocular Fine Structure. Selected Electron Micrographs.* Retina Foundation, Inst. Biol. Med. Sci. Monographs & Conferences, Vol. 1. London: Churchill

Jalavisto, E., Orma, E. and Tawast, M. (1951). 'Ageing and relation between stimulus intensity and duration in corneal sensibility.' *Acta physiol. scand.* **23,** 224–233

Jones, L. T. (1961). 'An anatomical approach to problems of the eyelids and lacrimal apparatus.' *Archs Ophthal.* **66,** 111–124

Kenshalo, D. R. (1960). 'Comparison of thermal sensitivity of the forehead, lip, conjunctiva and cornea.' *J. appl. Physiol.* **15,** 987–991

Kerr, F. W. L. (1963). 'The divisional organization of afferent fibres of the trigeminal nerve.' *Brain* **86,** 721–732

Khodadoust, A. A., Silverstein, A. M., Kenyon, K. R. and Dowling, J. E. (1968). 'Adhesions of regenerating corneal epithelium: The role of basement membrane.' *Am. J. Ophthal.* **65,** 339–348

King, D. C. and Michels, K. M. (1957). 'Muscular tension and the human blink rate.' *J. exp. Psychol.* **53,** 113–116

Kinoshita, J. H. (1962). 'Some aspects of the carbohydrate metabolism of the cornea.' *Invest. Ophthal.* **1,** 178–186

Kinoshita, J. H. and Masurat, T. (1959). 'Aerobic pathways of glucose metabolism in bovine corneal epithelium.' *Am. J. Ophthal.* **48,** 47–52

Kirchner, C. (1964). 'Untersuchungen über das Ausmass der Tränensekretion beim Menschen.' *Klin. Monatsbl. Augenheilk.* **144,** 412–417

Klintworth, G. K. (1969). 'Experimental studies on the phagocytic capability of the corneal fibroblast.' *Am. J. Path.* **55,** 283–294

Knoll, H. A. and Williams, J. (1970). 'Effects of hydrophilic contact lenses on corneal sensitivity.' *Am. J. Optom.* **47,** 561–563

Knowles, W. F. (1961). 'Effect of intra-lamellar plastic membranes on corneal physiology.' *Am. J. Ophthal.* **51,** 274–284

Kokott, W. (1938). 'Über mechanisch funktionelle Strukturen des Auges.' *Graefes Arch. klin. exp. Ophthal.* **138,** 424–485

Krejčí, L. and Bílek, K. (1970). 'Effect of the long-term all-day use of soft gel contact lenses on the cornea.' (in Czech). *Čs. Oftal.* **26,** 23–28

Kuhlman, R. E. and Resnick, R. A. (1959). 'The oxidation

of C-14-labelled glucose and lactate by the rabbit cornea.' *Arch. Biochem. Biophys.* **8**, 29–36

Langham, M. E. (1952). 'Utilization of oxygen by the component layers of the living cornea.' *J. Physiol.* **117**, 461–470

Langham, M. E. (1954). 'Glycolysis in the cornea of the rabbit.' *J. Physiol.* **126**, 396–403

Langham, M. E. (1960). 'Corneal metabolism and its influence on corneal hydration in the excised eye and in the living animal.' In *The Transparency of the Cornea,* ed. by Sir Stewart Duke-Elder and E. S. Perkins. Oxford: Blackwell

Larke, J. R. and Sabell, A. G. (1971). 'A comparative study of the ocular responses to two forms of contact lenses.' *Optician* **162**(4187), 8–12 and (4188) 10–17

Lele, P. P. and Weddell, G. (1956). 'The relationship between neurohistology and corneal sensibility.' *Brain* **79**, 119–154

Lele, P. P. and Weddell, G. (1959). 'Sensory nerves of the cornea and cutaneous sensibility.' *Exp. Neurol.* **1**, 334–359

Lowther, G. E. and Hill, R. M. (1968). 'Sensitivity threshold of the lower lid margin in the course of adaptation to contact lenses.' *Am. J. Optom.* **45**, 587–594

Machemer, R. (1966). 'Autoradiographische Untersuchungen des Regenerationzonen der Hornhaut.' *Graefes Arch. klin. exp. Ophthal.* **170**, 286–297

Macintosh, S. R. (1968). 'The ultrastructure of conjunctival epithelium in monkeys.' Student special study, The City University, London

Macintosh, S. R. (1974). 'The innervation of the conjunctiva in monkeys. An electron microscopic and nerve degeneration study.' *Graefe's Arch. klin. exp. Ophthal.* **192**, 105–116

Manchester, P. T. (1970). 'Hydration of the cornea.' *Trans. Am. ophthal. Soc.* **68**, 425–461

Mandell, R. B. and Fatt, I. (1965). 'Thinning of the human cornea on awakening.' *Nature* **208**, 292–293

Mann, I. (1944). 'A study of epithelial regeneration in the living eye.' *Br. J. Ophthal.* **28**, 26–40

Marré, M. (1967). 'Zur Altersabhängigkeit der Heilung von Hornhautepitheldefekten.' *Graefes Arch. klin. exp. Ophthal.* **173**, 250–255

Matsuda, H. (1968). 'Electron microscopic study of the corneal nerve with special reference to its endings.' *Jap. J. Ophthal.* **12**, 163–173

Maurice, D. M. (1951). 'The permeability to sodium ions of the living rabbit's cornea.' *J. Physiol.* **122**, 367–391

Maurice, D. M. (1957). 'The structure and transparency of the cornea.' *J. Physiol.* **136**, 263–286

Maurice, D. M. (1962a). 'Clinical physiology of the cornea.' *Int. ophthal. Clin.* **2**, 561–572

Maurice, D. M. (1962b). 'The cornea and sclera.' In *The Eye,* ed. by H. Davson, Vol. 1, pp.289–368. New York and London: Academic Press

Maurice, D. M. (1972). 'The location of the fluid pump in the cornea.' *J. Physiol.* **221**, 43–54

Maurice, D. M. and Giardini, A. (1951). 'Swelling of the cornea *in vivo* after the destruction of its limiting layers.' *Br. J. Ophthal.* **35**, 791–797

Melzack, R. and Wall, P. D. (1965). 'Pain mechanisms: a new theory.' *Science* **150**, 971–979

Miller, D. (1969). 'Contact lens-induced corneal curvature and thickness change.' *Archs Ophthal.* **80**, 430–432

Millodot, M. (1972). 'Diurnal variation of corneal sensitivity.' *Br. J. Ophthal.* **56**, 844–847

Millodot, M. (1974). 'Effect of soft lenses on corneal sensitivity.' *Acta Ophthal.* **52**, 603–608

Millodot, M. (1975a). 'Effect of hard contact lenses on corneal sensitivity and thickness.' *Acta Ophthal.* **53**, 576–584

Millodot, M. (1975b). 'Do blue-eyed people have more sensitive corneas than brown-eyed people?' *Nature* **255**, 151–152

Millodot, M. (1976). 'Effect of the length of wear of contact lenses on corneal sensitivity.' *Acta Ophthal.* **54**, 721–730

Millodot, M. and Lamont, A. (1974). 'Influence of menstruation on corneal sensitivity.' *Br. J. Ophthal.* **58**, 752–756

Mishima, S. (1965). 'Some physiological aspects of the precorneal tear film.' *Archs Ophthal.* **73**, 233–241

Mishima, S. (1968). 'Corneal thickness.' *Survey Ophthal.* **13**, 57–96

Mishima, S. and Hayakawa, M. (1972). 'The function of the corneal endothelium in relation to corneal dehydration and nutrition.' *Israel J. med. Sci.* **8**, 1507–1518

Mishima, S. and Maurice, D. M. (1961). 'The oily layer of the tear film and evaporation from the corneal surface.' *Exp. Eye Res.* **1**, 39–45

Morley, N. and McCulloch, C. (1961). 'Corneal lactate and pyridine nucleotides (PNS) with contact lenses.' *Archs Ophthal.* **66**, 379–382

Morrison, D. R. and Edelhauser, H. F. (1972). 'Permeability of hydrophilic contact lenses.' *Invest. Ophthal.* **11**, 58–63

Nafe, J. and Wagoner, K. (1937). 'Insensitivity of cornea to heat and pain derived from high temperatures.' *Am. J. Psychol.* **49**, 631–635

Naylor, E. J. (1953). 'Polarised light studies of corneal structure.' *Br. J. Ophthal.* **38**, 77–84

Norn, M.S. (1965). 'Tear secretion in normal eyes estimated by a new method. The lacrimal streak dilution test.' *Acta Ophthal.* **43**, 567–573

Nover, A. and Jaeger, W. (1952). 'Kolorimetrische Methode zur Messung der Tränensekretion (Fluoreszein-Verdünnungstest).' *Klin. Monatsbl. Augenheilk.* **121**, 419–425

Oppenheimer, D. R., Palmer, E. and Weddell, G. (1958). 'Nerve endings in the conjunctiva.' *J. Anat.* **92**, 321–352

Payrau, P., Pouliquen, Y., Faure, J.-P. and Offret, G. (1967). *La Transparence de la Cornée. Les Mécanismes de ses Altérations,* p.49. Paris: Masson

Pedler, C. (1962). 'The fine structure of the corneal epithelium.' *Exp. Eye Res.* **1**, 286–289

Penbharkkul, S. and Karelitz, S. (1962). 'Lacrimation in the neonatal and early infancy period of premature and full-term infants.' *J. Pediat.* **61**, 859–863

Perera, R. N. (1969). 'Basal cells of the corneal epithelium in man and monkey.' *Br. J. Ophthal.* **53**, 592–605

Peterson, J. F. and Fatt, I. (1973). 'Oxygen flow through a soft contact lens on a living eye.' *Am. J. Optom.* **50**, 91–93

Pfister, R. R. (1975). 'The healing of corneal epithelial

abrasions in the rabbit: a scanning electron microscope study.' *Invest. Ophthal.* **14**, 648–661

Philpot, F. J. (1955). 'Factors affecting the hydration of the rabbit cornea.' *J. Physiol.* **128**, 504–510

Polack, F. M. (1961). 'Morphology of the cornea. 1: Study with silver stains.' *Am. J. Ophthal.* **51**, 179–184

Pollack, I. P. (1962). 'Corneal hydration studied in stromal segments separated by intralamellar discs.' *Invest. Ophthal.* **1**, 661–665

Polse, K. A. and Mandell, R. B. (1970). 'Critical oxygen tension at the corneal surface.' *Archs Ophthal.* **84**, 505–508

Polse, K. A., Sarver, M. D. and Harris, M. G. (1975). 'Corneal edema and vertical striae accompanying the wearing of hydrogel lenses.' *Am. J. Optom.* **52**, 185–191

Pratt-Johnson, J. A. (1959). 'Studies on the anatomy and pathology of the peripheral cornea.' *Am. J. Ophthal.* **47**, 478–488

Reim, M., Lax, F., Lichte, H. and Turss, R. (1967). 'Steady state levels of glucose in the different layers of the cornea, aqueous humor, blood and tears *in vivo*.' *Ophthalmologica* **154**, 39–50

Rexed, B. and Rexed, V. (1951). 'Degeneration and regeneration of corneal nerves.' *Br. J. Ophthal.* **35**, 38–49

de Roetth, A., Jr. (1950). 'Respiration of the cornea.' *Archs Ophthal.* **44**, 666–676

de Roetth, A., Sr. (1953). 'Lacrimation in normal eyes.' *Archs Ophthal.* **49**, 185–189

Rowbotham, G. (1939). 'Observations on effects of trigeminal denervation.' *Brain* **62**, 364–380

Ruben, M. (1967). 'Corneal changes in contact lens wear.' *Trans ophthal. Soc. U.K.* **87**, 27–43

Ruskell, G. L. (1969). 'Changes in nerve terminals and acini of the lacrimal gland and changes in secretion induced by autonomic denervation.' *Z. Zellforsch. mikroskop. Anat.* **94**, 261–281

Ruskell, G. L. (1975). 'Nerve terminals and epithelial cell variety in the human lacrimal gland.' *Cell Tiss. Res.* **158**, 121–136

Rycroft, P. V. (1964). 'Ophthaine (proparacaine hydrochloride): local anaesthetic for ophthalmic surgery.' *Br. J. Ophthal.* **48**, 102–104

Sallmann, C., Caravaggio, L. L. and Grimes, P. (1961). 'Studies on corneal epithelium of the rabbit. 1: Cell division and growth.' *Am. J. Ophthal.* **51**, 83–94

Schirmer, O. (1903). 'Studien zur Physiologie und Pathologie der Tränenabsonderung und Thränenabfur.' *Graefes Arch. klin. exp. Ophthal.* **56**, 197–291

Schirmer, K. E. (1963). 'Corneal sensitivity and contact lenses.' *Br. J. Ophthal.* **47**, 493–495

Schirmer, K. E. and Mellor, L. D. (1961). 'Corneal sensitivity after cataract extraction.' *Archs Ophthal.* **65**, 433–436

Schute, C. C. D. (1974). 'Haidinger's brushes and predominant orientation of collagen in corneal stroma.' *Nature* **250**, 163–164

Scott, B. L. and Pease, D. C. (1959). 'Electron microscopy of the salivary and lacrimal glands of the rat.' *Am. J. Anat.* **104**, 115–161

Sédan, J., Farnarier, G. and Ferrand, G. (1958). 'Contribution a l'étude de la keraesthésie.' *Ann. Oculist* **191**, 736–751

Segawa, K. (1964). 'Electron microscopic studies on the human corneal epithelium: dendritic cells.' *Archs Ophthal.* **72**, 650–659

Shanks, K. R. (1965). 'The shape of the margin of the upper eyelid, related to corneal lenses.' *Br. J. physiol. Optics* **22**, 71–83

Sjögren, H. (1955). 'The lacrimal secretion in newborn, premature and fully developed children.' *Acta Ophthal.* **33**, 557–560

Sjoqvist, O. (1938). 'Studies on pain conduction in the trigeminal nerve.' *Acta Psychiat. Neuro.* Suppl. 17, 1–139

Smelser, G. K. (1952). 'Relation of factors involved in maintenance of optical properties of cornea to contact-lens wear.' *Archs Ophthal.* **47**, 328–343

Smelser, G. K. and Chen, D. K. (1955). 'Physiological changes in cornea induced by contact lenses.' *Archs Ophthal.* **53**, 676–679

Smelser, G. K. and Ozanics, O. (1952). 'Importance of atmospheric oxygen for maintenance of the optical properties of the human cornea.' *Science* **115**, 140

Smith, J. W. (1969). 'The transparency of the corneal stroma.' *Vision Res.* **9**, 393–396

Stanworth, A. and Naylor, E. S. (1953). 'Polarised light studies of the cornea. I. The isolated cornea.' *J. exp. Biol.* **30**, 160–163

Strughold, H. (1953). 'The sensitivity of cornea and conjunctiva of the human eye and the use of contact lenses.' *Am. J. Optom.* **30**, 625–630

Strughold, H. and Karbe, M. (1925). 'Die Topographie des Kältesinnes auf Cornea und Conjunctiva, ein Beitrag zur Frage nach den spezifischen Empgängern desselben.' *Z. Biol.* **83**, 189–212

Süchting, P., Machemer, R. and Welz, S. (1966). 'Die Lebenszeit der Epithelzelle der Rattencornea und conjunctiva.' *Graefes Arch. klin. exp. Ophthal.* **170**, 297–310

Sugiura, B. (1965). 'The polygonal cell system of the corneal epithelium.' In *Die Struktur des Auges. II. Symposium,* ed. by J. Rohen, Eighth International Congress of Anatomists, Wiesbaden, pp.463–479. Stuttgart: Schattauer

Thoft, R. A. and Friend, J. (1972). 'Corneal amino acid supply and distribution.' *Invest. Ophthal.* **11**, 723–727

Thompson, R. and Gallardo, E. (1941). 'The antibacterial action of tears on staphylococci.' *Am. J. Ophthal.* **24**, 635–640

Tower, S. S. (1940). 'Unit for sensory reception in cornea. With notes on nerve impulses from sclera, iris and lens.' *J. Neurophysiol.* **3**, 486–500

Turss, R., Friend, J. and Dohlman, C. H. (1970). 'Effect of a corneal barrier on the nutrition of the epithelium.' *Exp. Eye Res.* **9**, 254–259

Uniacke, N. P. and Hill, R. M. (1970). 'Osmotic pressure of the tears during adaptation to contact lenses.' *J. Am. optom. Ass.* **41**, 932–936

Weddell, G. and Zander, E. (1950). 'A critical evaluation of methods used to demonstrate tissue neural elements, illustrated by reference to the cornea.' *J. Anat.* **84**, 168–195

Weimar, V. (1960). 'Healing processes in the cornea.' In *The Transparency of the Cornea,* ed. by Sir Stewart

Duke-Elder and E. S. Perkins, pp.111–124. Oxford: Blackwell

Whitear, M. (1960). 'An electron microscope study of the cornea in mice, with special reference to the innervation.' *J. Anat.* **94**, 387–409

Wolff, E. (1948). *The Anatomy of the Eye and Orbit,* 3rd Ed. p.166. London: Lewis

Wolter, J. R. (1957). 'Innervation of the corneal endothelium of the eye of the rabbit.' *Archs Ophthal.* **58**, 246–250

Zander, E. and Weddell, G. (1951a). 'Observations on the innervation of the cornea.' *J. Anat.* **85**, 68–99

Zander, E. and Weddell, G. (1951b). 'Reaction of corneal nerve fibres to injury.' *Br. J. Ophthal.* **35**, 61–88

Chapter 3

Drugs and Solutions in Contact Lens Practice and Related Microbiology

J. H. Stewart-Jones, G. A. Hopkins and A. J. Phillips

FORMULATION

The aim in formulating eyedrops and eye lotions is to produce a solution which is sterile, effective, stable, clear, non-toxic and comfortable. To accomplish these ideals, attention must be paid to certain physical and chemical properties of the formulated solutions, not least of which is pH. The pH of an ophthalmic solution can affect its therapeutic effect, comfort, stability, sterility and viscosity (Hind and Goyan, 1947).

Ophthalmic drugs are, in most instances, alkaloid salts, salts of weak bases and strong acids, which in a pH of above 7 (that is, an alkaline pH), become free bases, insoluble in water but soluble in lipids. The corneal epithelium (*see Figure 2.1*) is a cellular layer whose cells are joined by desmosomes. There are minimal intracellular spaces, and so to pass the epithelium, drugs must pass through the lipoprotein cell membranes; that is, they must be lipid-soluble. Thus, a high pH will facilitate passage through the epithelium. The stroma, containing few cells, favours water-soluble substances while the endothelium again is more permeable to substances soluble in lipids.

Thus, for a drug to pass through the cornea, its solubility must swing from lipid-soluble to water-soluble, to lipid-soluble, and back to water-soluble again to dissolve in the aqueous.

A high pH, therefore, although increasing passage through the epithelium, may inhibit passage through the stroma. Also, a high pH is irritating and the drug may precipitate from the eyedrops or may become unstable and be hydrolysed. Brawner and Jessop (1962) found that contact lens solutions with a neutral pH were less irritating than those with acid reactions.

Tears contain one or more buffer systems which will keep the pH between 7.2 and 7.6. When a drop is applied to the eye it will be buffered to this range irrespective of its normal pH unless it is highly buffered itself. It is therefore questionable whether buffering eyedrops is useful.

The eye can tolerate solutions with osmotic pressures between the equivalent of 0.5 and 2.0 per cent sodium chloride (0.9 per cent is isotonic) with little or no discomfort, and there is no justification for raising the tonicity of hypotonic solutions (solutions with an osmotic pressure less than the tears) to an isotonic value. Solutions of eyedrops, as normally prepared, are generally hypotonic; that is, they have an osmotic pressure less than tears. Notable exceptions are 10 per cent phenylephrine and 30 per cent sulphacetamide sodium which are hypertonic and therefore cause some stinging, initially, on instillation. Eye lotions, however, because of the larger amounts used, should be isotonic.

MICROBIOLOGY

The science of microbiology involves the study of three distinctly different types of organism – fungi, bacteria and viruses. Fungi are composed of large cells with a well-defined, multi-chromosomal nucleus surrounded by a nuclear membrane. Bacteria are smaller, simpler cells with only one chromosome and no nuclear membrane, while virus particles are not really cells at all. By far the most important group as far as the practitioner is concerned is the bacteria.

The normal diameter of a bacterial cell is of the order of 1 micrometre (μm)*, bounded by a rigid

*This used to be termed 'micron'.

cell wall. This is an important structure since it can account for up to 25 per cent of the volume of the cell and is responsible for many of the properties of the cell. It determines the shape of the cell and allows it to withstand an extreme range of hostile environments as well as determining some of the biochemical differences between species. Some of the bacteria have a structureless, gel-like, capsule surrounding the cell wall which further protects the cell, especially from phago-cytosis. Such bacteria are therefore more virulent than species without one. Below the cell wall is the protoplast which is the living part of the cell, surrounded by the cell membrane and containing many cytoplasmic structures such as ribosomes and the single bacterial chromosome.

Bacteria multiply by binary fission or the splitting of the cell into two equal daughter cells. Unlike the cell division in higher animals, there is no mitosis.

There are many characteristics which are used to classify or 'type' bacteria. One of the most common of these is the shape and form of aggre-gation. Spherical bacteria are referred to as cocci. When they are found in pairs they are called diplococci; if in fours, tetrads. Streptococci are formed of chains of cocci while staphylococci have the form of bunches of grapes.

Rod-shaped bacteria are called bacilli. Cocco-bacilli are short and stumpy in appearance while fusiform and filiform bacilli are longer and thinner. If the cell is curved or spiral in form then they are called vibrios and spirillas respectively.

Biochemical differences also assist the typing of bacteria. For example, the form of respiration of any bacterial species can fall into one of three groups: (1) aerobes, which can exist only in the presence of air; (2) anaerobes, which can exist only in the absence of air; and (3) facultative anaerobes, which can exist under either condition.

The permeability of the cell wall determines the bacterial cell's reaction to certain histological stains. Most important is Gram's stain which involves treatment with two different stains, and organisms are designated Gram-positive and Gram-negative depending on the stain that they retain.

BACTERIA AND DISEASE

Not all bacteria cause disease. In fact, many organisms are responsible for maintaining the fertility of the soil by nitrogen fixation. However, many diseases result from the invasion of bacteria into tissues. The relationship between bacteria and disease is embodied in Koch's postulates, as follows.

(1) The organism is regularly found in the lesions of the disease.

(2) It can be isolated in pure culture on artificial media.

(3) Inoculation of this culture into a healthy animal will produce lesions of the disease.

(4) The organisms can be recovered from these animals.

Bacteria cause disease by two mechanisms: (1) invasion and destruction of tissues when only the infected part shows lesions; and (2) the pro-duction of toxins which are carried by the blood and lymph systems to all parts of the body and produce widespread effects. Toxins are of two types — exotoxins and endotoxins. Exotoxins are proteins, produced principally by the Gram-positive bacteria and are released without damage to the bacterial cell. They are very potent (1 mg of botulinum toxin will kill 1 million mice) and tend to be specific for certain tissues (botulinum toxin attacks the nervous system). Endotoxins are non-protein substances, produced by many Gram-negative organisms and are only produced if the cell breaks down. These are less potent and tissue-specific than the exotoxins.

Invasiveness of bacteria depends on the organism's resistance to phagocytosis and its survival in cells. If the organism, by having a thick capsule, can resist phagocytosis, then it will behave as an extracellular parasite. If it becomes ingested by the phagocytes but stays alive inside the cell, then it will become an intracellular parasite.

The virulence of an organism depends on both the toxicity and the invasiveness of the cells. It is measured in terms of an LD_{50}; that is, the number of organisms needed to kill 50 per cent of a test group of animals.

FUNGI

Fungi are composed of more complex cells than bacteria. They grow either as single cells (yeasts) or as multi-cellular filamentous colonies (moulds or mushrooms).

Yeast cells are oval cells of about $3-5$ μm in diameter surrounded by a cell wall. Beneath the cell wall is the cell membrane containing a nucleus with a nuclear membrane and several chromosomes. The cytoplasm contains mitochondria and an endoplasmic reticulum, structures which are absent from bacteria.

Some fungi exhibit the property of dimorphism; that is, they can exist either in the form of yeast cells or as mould hyphae dependent on conditions. Some pathogens appear in tissues as cells while others grow *in vitro* as hyphae. There are four main classes of fungi, the Phycomycetes (including Mucor the bread mould), the Ascomycetes (including Penicillium, the penicillin producer), the Basidiomycetes (the mushrooms) and the Deuteromycetes (which include most of the human pathogens).

The first three classes can reproduce by a sexual method as well as asexually while the Deuteromycetes have no sexual phase and because of this are called the Fungi Imperfecti.

Fungi are less important than bacteria in causing diseases in man although their harmful effects can have far reaching results on the food supply and can produce substances which are extremely toxic; for example, muscarine and ergotamine. However, fungi can produce several diseases which range from the just irritating (athletes' foot) through to very serious and possibly lethal conditions (Madura foot). Fungal infections predominantly affect the skin and mucous membranes but systemic infections can occur which threaten all systems of the body. All fungi are aerobic or facultative anaerobes (even brewer's yeast grows better in air, although it is grown for its anaerobic effect).

VIRUSES

It is an interesting, if philosophical, question as to whether or not viruses are living organisms. They can be regarded as extremely simple organisms or very complex chemicals. They consist of a single type of nucleic acid surrounded by a protein sheath and lack the fundamental mechanisms for growth and multiplication (ribosomes, enzymes and energy-generating systems). They multiply by invading a host cell and by using its replication machinery to produce new viral nucleic acid and protein involving the death of the host cell. Their peculiar 'life-cycle' makes them obligate intracellular parasites.

Viruses are extremely small, the largest virus being approximately the same size as the smallest bacterium. Their smallness of size accounts for the term 'filtrable viruses' indicating that they can pass through filters which will retain other microorganisms.

There are three main types of virus distinguished by the type of host they invade — animal viruses, plant viruses and bacterial viruses or bacteriophages. The diseases resulting from infection by viruses include many common conditions ranging from the childhood diseases such as mumps and measles to several serious and notorious illnesses such as smallpox and rabies.

Infections directly or indirectly caused by contact lens wear are most likely to involve the cornea and conjunctiva. Fungal growth has been found on soft lenses and therefore the possibility of fungal as well as bacterial and viral infections should always be considered. The appropriate aspects of after-care and management are dealt with in Chapter 16, Volume 2. Any infection or suspected infection or allergic response requires medical treatment, preferably by an ophthalmologist who is conversant not only with contact lens fitting but also with the implications of prolonged ocular contact with the various constituents of contact lens solutions and materials.

Readers wishing to pursue further the subject of microbiology and the eye are referred to the work of Locatcher–Khorazo and Seegal (1972).

ANTIMICROBIAL AGENTS

Antimicrobial agents can be usefully divided into physical and chemical agents. Their function is to produce either sterilization which is removal or killing of all viable organisms, or disinfection which is the elimination of the possibility of infection from a material (and may not involve the removal of all viable organisms).

PHYSICAL AGENTS

The mode of action of all these agents (with the exception of filtration) is to subject the organisms to sufficient energy to produce lethal protein denaturation and cell changes. The most common physical agent is heat. While a temperature of $70°C$ will kill most vegetative organisms in a few minutes (Dallos and Hughes, 1972, reported that *Ps. aeruginosa* and *Strept. faecalis* are killed at $70°C$ in 5 minutes), spores are resistant to boiling, even for hours. To ensure complete sterilization, the autoclave is now the method of choice, exposing the material to a temperature of $121°C$ for 15–20 minutes. The medium in which the material is heated is steam, as moist heat is much more effective than dry heat in killing bacteria. To sterilize by dry heat requires a temperature of $160°C$ and a time of 2 hours and is clearly only suitable for glass or metal objects. Thermolability is always a disadvantage in heat sterilization and for some materials such as milk or wine a much lower temperature than $121°C$ is used to avoid breakdown of the material being treated. Pasteurization of milk consists of heating the milk to $62°C$ for 30 minutes.

At the other end of the temperature scale, freezing only slightly lowers the viable count of bacteria, and, indeed, freezing is a method of preserving cultures.

Irradiation by ultra-violet light is a method useful in reducing the level of airborne contamination by acting on the DNA molecules in bacteria. Apart from air sanitation, ultra-violet radiation can be used for sterilizing surfaces, but is of little use for sterilizing solutions contained in ultra-violet absorbing containers. Irradiation by gamma-rays is a popular method for sterilizing single-dose containers of eyedrops. The method of kill produced by these rays is markedly different from that produced by ultra-violet rays, involving irradiation at much higher energies. Free hydroxyl radicles are produced which are highly oxidizing and cytotoxic.

Waves of a different nature; that is, sound waves, also have a disruptive effect on bacteria — see page 77. Frequencies of between 15 kHz up to MHz are bactericidal but this effect has little practical application as yet.

One method of removal of bacteria from suspensions without killing, is filtration, using filters with a maximum pore size of 1 μm. This is the method of choice for heat-labile materials.

CHEMICAL AGENTS

Chemical agents can be divided into two different groups: the non-specific bactericidal, disinfecting agents which are mostly used *in vitro*, and the more specific bactericidal or bacteriostatic chemotherapeutic agents which are used *in vivo* to treat established infections or to act as prophylactic agents to prevent the occurrence of infections.

DISINFECTING AGENTS

There are a large number of compounds which can be lethal to microorganisms if applied in sufficiently high concentrations. However, it is a property of the common disinfecting agents that they have an antibacterial effect in low concentrations. Their effect is dependent on their concentration and the temperature. Hence, the sterilizing technique of heating with a bactericide.

Although disinfectants cover a wide group of compounds, there are two major mechanisms of action: (1) the dissolving of lipids from the cell membranes; and (2) the alteration by denaturation of proteins essential to the cell's life.

Before any antimicrobial substance is used for disinfecting or keeping solutions sterile it must, of course, be subjected to stringent *in vitro* tests to determine its potency and spectrum of activity (that is, how many different types of bacteria will be inactivated by it). Any *in vitro* test applied must bear some relationship to the actual use to which the substance is to be put; for example, a substance which is to be incorporated into contact lens solutions must be tested in a way that will to some extent mirror its practical use.

Davies and Norton (1975) suggest that the activity of an antimicrobial substance, determined by an *in vitro* test, will depend on several criteria, as follows.

(1) The organism used and the conditions under which it is grown.

(2) The method of harvesting the cells (preparing the inoculum).

(3) The volume of test solution and the size of the inoculum.

(4) The temperature of holding the experimental solution and the frequency of sampling.

(5) The recovery medium to be used and the time and temperature of incubation.

(6) The criterion of antimicrobial activity to be considered acceptable.

Brown (1968), while investigating the survival of *Ps. aeruginosa* in fluorescein sodium solutions containing phenylmercuric nitrate, found that when cells were inoculated direct from the nutrient they retained their activity longer than cells which were washed in water before inoculating into the test solution. The broth had a protective effect. Riegelman, Vaughan and Okumoto (1956) state that *in vitro* tests sometimes give a false result because of 'carry-over' from the test solution to the recovery medium.

It is apparent since the reports of Norton *et al.* (1974) and McBride and Mackie (1974) that the antimicrobial performance of some contact lens solutions is open to question. Of fourteen contact lens soaking solutions only seven inactivated the four test strains (three bacteria and one fungus) within 4 hours. They recommend some form of standard test for contact lens solutions. The mere presence of an antimicrobial substance in the formulation is no guarantee of adequate disinfecting ability.

Ganju (1974), however, felt that the tests applied by Norton *et al.* (1974) were too rigorous and a solution containing sufficient antibacterial substance to pass their tests would be too irritating to ocular tissues. He applied tests to soft contact lens soaking solutions using smaller numbers of bacteria.

Recently, Lindeman-Meester (1974) has applied the tests of Kelsey and Sykes (1969) and Maurer (1969) for soft contact lens soaking solutions.

Mercury Compounds (thiomersalate, phenyl-mercuric nitrate)

Mercury compounds kill bacteria because the mercury ions bind to sulph-hydryl groups which form important chemical groups of enzymes and proteins. Their action against Pseudomonas is slow and they are incompatible with bengal rose (Strachan, 1971) and, in certain concentrations, benzalkonium chloride (Dabezies, 1970).

Benzalkonium Chloride

This substance is a cationic detergent which even in low concentrations is active against a considerable range of bacteria. In higher concentrations it can be irritating (Sussman and Friedman, 1969) and has been reported to cause significant corneal damage (Gasset et al., 1974). It has been reported to lose its activity in the presence of cotton, polyvinyl alcohol and methylcellulose (Strachan, 1971). In concentrations above 0.01 per cent it has the disadvantage in contact lens solutions of interfering with the wetting effect of these solutions. This is because the cationic hydrophilic group binds with the lens surface leaving the hydrophobic chain 'sticking out' (Dabezies, 1970).

Cetrimide (Cetavlon, *I.C.I.*)

Like benzalkonium chloride, this is a cationic detergent, producing its bactericidal effect by dissolving the lipoprotein membrane of the bacterial cell and denaturing proteins. Some patients show a sensitivity reaction to this compound (Strachan, 1971) and the activity can be lost if the solution comes in contact with bark corks (Anderson and Keynes, 1958). In fact, Lowbury (1958) found cultures of *Ps. aeruginosa* growing in solutions of cetrimide that had been stoppered with a cork. It is often used in combination with chlorhexidine (Hibitane).

Chlorhexidine (Hibitane)

This shares the disadvantage of cetrimide in being inactivated by cork (Linton and George, 1966). It is also incompatible with many anions which prevents its use in many solutions. It is, however, one of the main antibacterial agents used in hydrophilic lens solutions due to its low 'binding' ability (*see* page 75).

Hydroxybenzoates

These compounds have fallen from use since it was found that they were inactive against *Ps. aeruginosa*.

Hugo and Foster (1964) found that strains of Pseudomonas could grow in solutions of hydroxy-benzoates without previous adaptation. Barkmar *et al.* (1969) found them very irritating. However, they are being re-introduced in the form of Nipastat in soft contact lens soaking solutions.

Chlorbutol

Chlorbutol is found in many eyedrop formulations and contact lens solutions. This volatile antimicrobial agent has antifungal and antibacterial effects.

Phenylethanol

This compound has very little activity on its own but has a synergistic action with many antibacterial substances, such as benzalkonium chloride, chlorhexidine, phenylmercuric nitrate and chlorbutol (Richards and McBride, 1972).

Sodium Edetate (EDTA)

Ethylenediaminetetra-acetic acid (EDTA) is a chelating agent which produces its effect by removing calcium ions from solution and disrupting the cell wall (MacGregor and Elliker, 1958; Brown and Richards, 1965). It is especially used with benzalkonium chloride with which it has a synergistic action. Since mercurial antimicrobials depend on their action for mercury, it would seem likely that EDTA would antagonize the action of thiomersalate. Brown (1968) found that a mixture of PMN (phenylmercuric nitrate) and EDTA was less effective than PMN alone. However, Richards and McBride (1972) found an opposite effect. Further work needs to be done to determine the reaction of EDTA with mercurial antimicrobials, since many contact lens solutions contain a mixture of these two substances.

SOLUTIONS FOR HYDROPHOBIC AND SEMI-HYDROPHILIC LENSES

The various solutions and drops available in the United Kingdom (and elsewhere) for use with hard lenses are given in Appendix E, *Table I*, at the end of this volume.

The large majority of modern corneal lenses are manufactured from polymethyl methacrylate. This material has good optical and mechanical properties which make it very suitable as a contact lens material. In addition the material is inert as far as the eye is concerned and rarely, if ever, produces an allergic response. Unfortunately polymethyl methacrylate is hydrophobic in nature as it contains a large number of hydrophobic methyl groups in proportion to its hydrophilic carboxy ester groups. This means that the lens surface is not readily wetted by the tears fluid. In order to avoid patient discomfort, therefore, the lenses need to be wetted before being placed on the eye. A second consequence of the hydrophobic nature of the plastics is that hydrophobic substances present on the eye, on the fingers, in soaps and cosmetics, readily adhere to the lens surface. These substances are therefore likely to irritate the eye by disruption of the tears film and are also likely to be present on the lenses when they are removed from the eye. Rewetting solutions for use with the lens *in situ* are often therefore necessary and, further, the lenses should always be cleaned immediately after removal from the eyes.

Despite being hydrophobic in nature, polymethyl methacrylate is, nevertheless, capable of absorbing a small quantity of liquid (around 2 per cent). This small amount of liquid has two particular effects on corneal lenses (Phillips, 1969). First, complete hydration of the lens improves its wettability. This in turn improves both patient vision and comfort and reduces adherence of mucus to the lens. Secondly, due to surface expansion, the curvature of a dehydrated corneal lens alters significantly (depending on power and thickness) over the first few hours of wear as it becomes hydrated. This again may affect patient comfort (as the fit is temporarily incorrect) and vision (as an incorrect tears lens is introduced). Further, when not in the eye there is a high risk of bacterial contamination of the lenses if they are left to dry out, and traces of mucus not cleaned from the lens provide an excellent bacterial breeding ground.

The hydrophobic nature of the lens material plus the effect of the liquid content when hydrated has necessitated the formulation of four types of contact lens solutions and gels, each with its own specific functions: (1) wetting solutions; (2) cleaning agents; (3) storage (soaking) solutions; and (4) rewetting solutions.

Each group, however, must nevertheless conform to the following prerequisites of all contact lens solutions.

(1) They must be sterile, stable and transparent.

(2) All solutions must be harmless to the eye if instilled undiluted.

(3) They must have no adverse effect on the contact lens material for which they are intended.

(4) They must be compatible with all other solutions used for the same lens material.

(5) All solutions should be sterile and, if presented in multidose form, be self-sterilizing.

WETTING SOLUTIONS

Following the discussion above, the functions of a wetting solution may be listed as follows.

(1) By acting as a lubricant between the surfaces of the lens and of the cornea and lids, its cushioning effect minimizes discomfort to the patient during initial insertion of the lens and subsequent wearing. This, in turn, encourages the prolonged wearing of lenses.

(2) By its action of encouraging even distribution of tears over the lens, it improves the optical performance.

(3) It acts as a mechanical buffer between lens and finger during the act of lens insertion and thus prevents lens contamination. This same buffer action prevents discomfort and possible corneal insult should the lens be inserted too rapidly.

(4) The wetting agents within the solution make it a suitable daily cleaning solution for many wearers for use following lens removal.

There is available to the practitioner a very wide choice of commercially produced wetting solutions. Some have fairly simple formulations, others appear more complex. However, all wetting solutions should have the following essential properties in addition to the criteria already listed above.

(1) They must have an adequate wetting effect on polymethyl methacrylate, even in high dilution.

(2) They must contain a viscous additive so that the solution adheres to the lens while it is being inserted and forms a protective cushion effect.

The constituents of a wetting solution vary with different proprietary brands, but the following include those main ingredients normally incorporated.

Preservative(s)

Those commonly used to maintain solution sterility include benzalkonium chloride (0.004–0.01 per cent), chlorbutol (0.2–0.5 per cent), phenylmercuric acetate or nitrate (0.002–0.01 per cent), thiomersalate (0.001–0.01 per cent), chlorhexidine digluconate (0.003–0.01 per cent), and cetylpyridinium chloride (0.001–0.01 per cent). Ethylenediaminetetra-acetate (EDTA) (0.01–0.1 per cent), a chelating agent, may also be incorporated to enhance the antimicrobial activity of the bactericide in the wetting solution. It was demonstrated by Gould and Inglima (1964) that solutions containing either benzalkonium chloride or chlorbutol, when compounded with a 0.1 per cent EDTA solution, displayed a marked increase in activity against *Ps. aeruginosa*. Further, by removal of metal ions from the bacterium cell wall, resistance to the bactericidal agent was prevented from building up. As previously stated (page 63) there is some doubt if the enhancing effect of EDTA is as effective with phenylmercuric nitrate (Brown, 1968). Richards and Reary (1972) showed a reduction in the efficacy of thiomersalate when EDTA was added in acid media.

Details of preservatives are given in Appendix E, *Table I*, at the end of this volume.

Viscosity-building Agent(s)

Methylcellulose, polyvinyl alcohol, hydroxypropyl-methylcellulose (hypromellose) and hydroxyethyl-cellulose may be used to increase the viscosity of the solution and act as lubricant and clinging agents.

Wetting Agent(s)

Polyvinyl alcohol, as well as having good viscosity-building properties is also often used for its good adhesive and wetting properties. Krishna and Brow (1964), using 1.4 per cent polyvinyl alcohol in isotonic saline solution, found it had a greater surface contact time than 0.5 per cent methyl-cellulose in isotonic saline solution. They also found that, unlike methylcellulose, polyvinyl alcohol does not retard regeneration of corneal epithelium. The liquid polymer polyvinyl pyrro-lidone is also often used for its good spreading and wettability on the eye and lens surfaces (Hill and Terry, 1974).

Isotonic and Buffering Agents

Sodium and potassium chloride may be added to make the solution isotonic with tears. However, the importance of isotonicity has been over-emphasized in the past — especially for the small quantities involved on a contact lens — and a range of 0.7–1.2 per cent sodium chloride solution equivalents is acceptable.

The normal range of tears liquid pH is from 7.0 to 8.5. Not only does this vary from person to person but there is also a daily temporal variation within the same individual (Carney and Hill, 1975). For this reason a solution may show a pH range of 6.0–8.5 with greater initial comfort the nearer to the physiological average of 7.2 (Brawner and

Jessop, 1962). The solution should either not be buffered or only weakly buffered in order to allow the solution to adjust to the pH of the tears liquid as quickly as possible. Borate, bicarbonate and particularly phosphate buffers are those commonly used.

Distilled Water, and Possibly a Colouring Agent

The inclusion of a bactericidal agent is obviously essential in most solutions used in contact lens practice. But of equal importance is the hygiene observed by the individual in making sure that his hands are washed thoroughly, and are free of all traces of creams and nicotine prior to the handling of the lenses.

CLEANING AGENTS

One of the most important aspects of any lens care regimen is the use of a prophylactic cleaning step in the normal daily hygiene routine to remove mucus, dirt, cosmetics and other environmental contaminants prior to overnight storage of the lens in a disinfectant solution. From a microbiological point of view, a clean lens is far easier to disinfect than a dirty lens as the removed contaminants cannot inactivate the preservative. Furthermore, these deposits can build up in time to levels sufficient to interfere with vision, lens wettability, and wearing comfort unless adequate prophylactic cleaning is carried out daily. As lens cleaning is accomplished outside the eye and the cleaning product used to effect the cleaning is not meant for direct instillation, it is possible to use slightly stronger cleaning agents than could normally otherwise be tolerated.

Although anionic, nonionic, and amphoteric (balanced positive and negative constituents) cleaning agents are currently used in contact lens cleaning products, preference seems to favour non-ionic and amphoteric cleaners (Shively, 1975a). These cleaning agents emulsify lipids, solubilize debris, and remove accumulated contaminants most favourably in an alkaline (pH 7.4 and above) environment. Following rinsing under cold running tap water the lens surface is clean and ready for overnight storage. It should be mentioned that cleaning hydrophobic and semi-hydrophobic lenses with various household cleaners such as laundry detergents, dishwashing compounds, skin cleansers and hair shampoos cannot be recommended because of their offensive and harsh actions on the lens surface or potential for damage to the cornea. This group of cleaners normally contains strong anionic detergents, caustic chemicals or detrimental solvents. Additionally, it is well known that *an*ionic detergents interact with commonly used *cat*ionic preservative agents such as benzalkonium chloride, chlorhexidine digluconate or acetate, and cetylpyridinium chloride resulting in deposition of a water-insoluble film on lenses with resultant discomfort for the wearer.

Specific itemization of constituents in various cleaning products cannot be given as most of these agents are regarded as proprietary to the lens solution manufacturer. Where the latter are not available, manufacturers should be requested to provide information to support claims made for their cleaning products.

Even though cleaning products are not meant for direct instillation, it is important that they be packaged sterile and be self-disinfecting due to repeated exposure to the environment during use. This is normally accomplished by the use of preservative agents as described in the discussion on wetting solutions.

Isotonicity is not considered necessary in cleaning products as these products are not meant for direct instillation. Viscosity agents are incorporated by some manufacturers although their function in this context is not apparent.

Finally, although these products are meant for use outside the cornea, it is important that no irreversible ocular insult occur should they be accidentally transferred to the eye.

Cleaning products are routinely used by rubbing the solution on the lens surfaces and massaging the debris and contaminants off the lens surfaces with the fingers. This is then following by a water rinse to remove the contaminants. However, various mechanical lens cleaning devices for wearer usage have emerged, mainly in the United States, which appear to facilitate this cleaning process. The use of an adjunctive cleaning solution is still, of course, required. The advantage of these devices appears to be for those wearers with poor manual dexterity and to reduce the continual surface scratching through the use of the fingers.

SOAKING SOLUTIONS

On removal from the eye and after cleaning, corneal lenses should be stored in a specially formulated soaking solution. This serves the following functions.

(1) By means of the bactericidal agent it contains, it should sterilize the lens and maintain its sterility.

(2) Maintenance of the hydrated equilibrium of the lens while it is not being worn.

(3) Prevention of the hardening of any ocular secretions remaining on the lens and to loosen the adhesion of any accumulated mucus.

Phillips (1969) has reviewed the arguments in favour of storing a corneal lens in a soaking solution. The advantages of this form of storage over dry storage include improved lens surface wetting, visual performance and patient comfort, less corneal staining and lens abrasion and greater evidence of freedom from bacterial contamination. Further, due to hydration and dehydration, the curvature of a lens stored dry fluctuates every time it is placed on or removed from the eye. A lens stored in a soaking solution retains a constant curvature.

Soaking solutions also contain the antibacterial agents listed under Wetting Solutions (page 64). Slightly higher concentrations or two synergistic agents are often employed since decontamination is one of the major functions of the storage solution. Solubilizing agents are also often incorporated to loosen the attachment of any debris attached to the lens. Soaking solutions should preferably irritate either minimally or not at all if transferred to the eye, although some manufacturers recommend that the solution be rinsed from the lens prior to the application of a wetting solution.

It is important to realize that the capability and efficacy of the solution to disinfect lenses is related to the regular changing of the storage solution every two or three days. The solution in the storage case will deplete with use as solution is removed with the lens. Further, the effectivity of the preservative will be reduced with each disinfection cycle by contaminants adhering to the lens surface such as mucus, atmospheric dust, etc., and even cellular constituents released from dead and dying cells. If too many cycles of disinfection are carried out in the same volume of solution the concentration of bactericide may be reduced to an inefficient level; or worse, to such an extent that, for example, a resistant Pseudomonad may actually grow in the solution. Responsibility for correct instruction of the lens wearer in this aspect of lens hygiene rests with the practitioner.

The importance of proper storage cases for use with soaking solutions must also be emphasized. Sufficient fluid volume must be contained to enable adequate diffusion of adsorbed contaminants into the solution and also to provide sufficient quantities of available preservative. Identification for each right and left lens must be provided, preferably also with tactile projections. Colour coding of container caps is also helpful.

Caps should be screw threaded to prevent solution loss even under such conditions as pressurized aeroplane cabins. Storage cases should not contain any materials which may be irritant to the eye such as plasticizers found in the sponge rubber inserts sometimes used. For the reasons listed above it is not sufficient to issue the patient with lens mailing containers for permanent use as storage cases.

ARTIFICIAL TEARS/REWETTING AGENTS

When no contact lens is present the precorneal film has the primary role of resurfacing the cornea with a hydrophilic coating with every blink, since there is no actual flow of tears across the cornea. Introduction of the lens disturbs this corneal resurfacing process and the lens itself becomes the surface which the precorneal film must coat with a hydrophilic layer. Further, this fluid film easily ruptures when adjacent to the boundary of a solid object such as a contact lens placed in the film. When this phenomenon is associated with incomplete blinking, corneal staining in the peripheral—horizontal (3 and 9 o'clock) regions can often be detected, presumably indicating areas of localized corneal dessication. When the precorneal film is unable to spread over the lens due to lipid contamination (presumably arising from Meibomian gland hyperactivity due to irritation of the inner lid margins) then decreased visual acuity and possible patient discomfort results.

In view of the above problems, rewetting solutions* have been designed for use with the lens *in situ*. These solutions contain wetting agents such as polyvinyl alcohol or polysorbate 80, or highly viscous solutions containing polyvinylpyrrolidone. Some are intended for use with hard lenses and some with soft lenses (as indicated in the footnotes), but those for use with soft lenses are really suitable for both types.

An artificial tears solution is indicated in conditions where natural tears liquid is reduced (*see* Chapter 7). A number of proprietary preparations* are available to the practitioner. Such solutions may contain benzalkonium chloride (0.004–0.01 per cent), chlorbutol (0.5 per cent), thiomersalate (0.02 per cent), EDTA (0.05–0.1 per cent) as preservatives; polyvinyl alcohol, hypromellose or hydroxyethylcellulose as wetting and viscosity-building agents; and sodium, potassium or magnesium chloride to provide solution isotonicity.

* Appendix E, *Tables I* and *II*, at the end of this volume, give more details of these preparations for hard and soft lenses.

Again, depending on the preservative, some of these are not suitable if soft lenses are worn. This rules out those containing chlorbutol and benzalkonium chloride.

Some cellulose acetate butyrate lenses should not be stored in solutions containing benzalkonium chloride as a slow reaction occurs with the material over a period of several months. The lens takes on a light straw colour, fluoresces a light blue under ultra-violet light, and a change in BCOR results.

MULTI-FUNCTIONAL SOLUTIONS

Multi-functional solutions are generally intended to combine the actions of cleaning and storage — or wetting, cleaning and storage — in one single product. The rationale behind the manufacture of such solutions is that some wearers will not carry out correct lens hygiene procedures due to the confusion of the multiplicity and expense of the solutions they must use. Most contact lens practitioners come across patients who omit one or more steps of the hygiene regimen simply because they run out of the appropriate solution. Often this step is then permanently omitted.

The basic components of combination cleaning and storage solutions are similar to the individual solutions with these functions. Most cleaning ingredients are nonionic or amphoteric (Shively, 1975*a*) for the reasons mentioned earlier. Most combination wetting and storage solutions are similar in formulation to wetting solutions but with a lower viscosity. The writer has found that patients with lens mucus problems have sometimes benefitted by storage of the lenses in combination solutions containing wetting agents such as polyvinyl alcohol, presumably due to surface adsorption of the wetting agent.

As might be expected, the combination of different lens hygiene functions into multi-functional solutions has elicited discussion about a possible compromise of efficacy in these products. For example, the relatively high viscosity required for a mechanical buffer action is contrary to the low viscosity required for diffusion of surface contaminants into the storage solution. Further, solution viscosity of any degree would appear to retard bactericidal activity as was shown by the poorer performance of all combination wetting and soaking solutions tested by Norton *et al.* (1974) compared to soaking solutions alone. Whilst acknowledging some compromise, the practitioner may feel that certain patients, for example, through lack of mental ability, application or responsibility, or simply because of occupational factors such as large amounts of travelling or when on holiday, should be advised to use multi-functional products.

SOLUTIONS FOR HYDROPHOBIC AND SEMI-HYDROPHILIC LENSES OTHER THAN THOSE OF POLYMETHYL METHACRYLATE

Certain lens materials such as cellulose acetate butyrate (CAB) and silicone with PMMA, as well as poly 4-methyl-pentene-1 (Larke *et al.*, 1973) have emerged to challenge the current hard lens material polymethyl methacrylate. Due to the increased gas permeability they may provide an answer to the problems associated with corneal oedema. Due to the slight hydration (2–7 per cent) of some of these materials, they may be classified as rigid semi-hydrophilic lenses although primarily hydrophobic in nature (*see* Chapter 24, Volume 2).

For some years, the use of flexible hydrophobic lens materials such as silicone rubber or other synthetic hydrophobic polymers has been undergoing evaluation in the United States and Germany in particular. Silicone rubber lenses are manufactured from approximately 40 per cent cross-linked dimethyl polysiloxane (silica) mixed with siloxane polymer as a filler, and the entire mixture heated at a high pressure in order to achieve further polymerization and cross-linking. The silica helps to determine the refractive index of the final lens which lies somewhere between 1.49 and 1.56. Although the material is highly transmissive to oxygen and other gases, water adsorption is negligible (0.4 per cent compared with 1.5–2.0 per cent for PMMA) and lens parameters are not normally affected by the storage solution characteristics (Phares, 1972*a*) the solution being used for its antibacterial function only. The extreme hydrophobic nature of silicone lenses makes them difficult to wet and maintain wettable during wearing. Wetting solutions containing polyvinyl alcohol or cellulose derivatives and formulated for conventional PMMA lenses are not adequate wetting agents for silicone lenses (Krezanoski, 1972*a*). They may be used with safety, however, with the exception of solutions containing chlorbutol as this is bound or adsorbed onto the lens surface. This concentrating effect of the preservative causes marked ocular discomfort. To overcome its hydrophobic nature, silicone lenses have been surface-coated with a more hydrophilic material (although this suffers from the expected disadvantage that it eventually wears off) or treated to produce surface molecular reorientation (Shively, 1975*a*). Special wetting agents are also being investigated in an attempt to overcome the wetting problem (Krezanoski, 1972*a*). Most cleaners

designed for PMMA lenses are only partly effective in maintaining silicone lens surfaces clean. Two manufacturers produce solutions specifically for storing silicone rubber lenses. Complementary solutions have been developed for cleaning these lenses. Details are given in Appendix E, *Table II*, at the end of this volume.

Combinations of differing classifications of material into a single lens have also been achieved, for example a polymethyl methacrylate optic portion with a polyhydroxyethylmethacrylate (polyHEMA) periphery. This appears to allow the optical quality of a rigid lens and the comfort of a flexible hydrophilic lens to be partly combined though, of course, raises potential problems from the lens sterility and wetting point of view (*see* Hydrophilic Lenses, below).

In each instance the practitioner must consult the manufacturers' literature extremely carefully to decide which solutions may or may not be used with each material. Both verbal and written instructions must be given to each patient who should also be advised not to use any unlisted solutions without first checking with his practitioner.

SOLUTIONS FOR HYDROPHILIC LENSES

Appendix E, *Table II*, at the end of this volume, gives details of the drops and solutions available in the United Kingdom (and elsewhere) for soft lenses.

During the early stages in the development of hydrophilic lenses it was thought that the hydrophilic nature of the surface would obviate the need for most solutions since wetting agents were obviously unnecessary, and for the same reason it was thought that cleaning would also be unnecessary. However, as experience has been gained over the last few years the complexities of dealing with new materials for use in contact with the eye has become increasingly apparent. Further, whilst the large majority of hydrophobic lenses are still made from a single material (PMMA), hydrophilic lenses are made from many materials, include differing additives, and with widely varying physical and physiological properties.

Perhaps the most difficult problem that has arisen with hydrophilic lenses is that of sterilization. Fortunately a considerable number of conjunctival sacs do not contain pathogenic bacteria. Smith (1954) reported 5000 cases in which swabs were taken from the conjunctival sacs of apparently normal eyes. Of these cases, 47 per cent showed no bacterial contamination in the sac. Other authors quote between 20 and 70 per cent as the incidence of sterile conjunctival sacs (Duke-Elder, 1965). In general, the majority of the conjunctival flora are harmless saprophytes involved in the destruction of dead cells. Only 25 per cent of conjunctival sacs appear to contain potential pathogens (Smith, 1954). Bacteria such as *Ps. aeruginosa* are rarely found in the sac. *Staph. aureus* is found more often but still only in a minority of cases (2–15 per cent). Even if an organism is a potential pathogen, it has been established that the conditions in the sac are likely to reduce the virulence of the organism. This is due in part to its relatively low temperature, in part to the action of the lysozyme of the tears, and in part to the mechanical action of blinking and the sluicing effect of the lacrimal secretion. In addition to the physical and chemical factors inhibiting the pathogens, non-pathogens also contribute to the protection of the eye by competing with the pathogens for nutrients. These factors combine to provide a relatively stable protective system for the eye against infection.

There are, however, many examples of how changes in the prevailing conditions can disrupt this balance; for example, keratoconjunctivitis sicca due to insufficient or inadequate tears; exposure keratitis due to the inability of the lids to sweep the cornea, and even bandaging the eye which causes an increase in the number and virulence of organisms, discharge often being noted. Contact lenses unfortunately interfere with the eyes' defence mechanisms. Hydrophilic lenses in particular prevent the lids from sweeping the cornea and interfere with the tears washing the cornea. They probably raise the corneal temperature and can also induce breaks in the corneal epithelium. In reports that appear in the literature of corneal infection occurring in otherwise 'normal' contact lens wearers, one of the main causes has been found to be the introduction of significant bacterial contamination either on the lens or via contaminated solutions. Whilst bacteria appear unable to penetrate the intermolecular 'pores' of hydrophilic lenses (Matas, Spencer and Hayes, 1972; Knoll, 1972) except possibly into defects in older lenses (Poster, 1972; Tripathi and Ruben, 1972), the tears liquid absorbed by the lenses serves as an excellent bacterial culture medium.

Further, surface irregularities in the lens occurring during manufacture (Matas, Spencer and Hayes, 1972; Filppi, Pfister and Hill, 1973) and eye secretions adhering to the lens surface may permit a nidus to form where bacteria can aggregate and possibly be protected from disinfection processes.

It was also pointed out by Ruben (1966) that fungi can grow into hydrophilic lenses and Filppi, Pfister and Hill (1973) have shown penetration by *Aspergillus fumagatus*, and Dallos and Hughes (1972) penetration by *Thrichotecium roseum* (this latter mould sometimes being found in tap water). The mechanism of penetration is probably by means of enzymes which cause degradation of the lens material and permit entry of the fungal hyphae.

Lenses which show spots on or within the lens substance should not be dispensed even though they may not necessarily be fungal growth and could, for example, be rusting ferrous particles (Loran, 1973). Even though there is no apparent damage to the lens there is always a possibility that endotoxins synthesized by the fungus are bound within the plastics. Fungi will quickly overcome the preservative in any disinfecting solution unless the solution is replaced at daily intervals. Thus, as well as antibacterial activity, any method of soft lens disinfection must also have a high fungicidal capability.

A further problem occurring with hydrophilic lenses is that of deposits adhering to the lens surfaces. The main sources of these deposits are ocular secretions, tap water contaminants which may have been absorbed by the lenses, eyedrops, finger dirt, eye make-up and contaminants introduced during manufacture and from the atmosphere. The bulk of deposits, however, are mucoproteins from the tears liquid. Also found are calcium (Ruben, Tripathi and Winder, 1975), iron and other insoluble divalent and trivalent metal salts if impure water for storage or rinsing solutions has been used. Environmental and occupational factors also affect the cleanliness of lenses. Rusting ferrous particles are commonly seen in the surface of the lenses or deeper if introduced during manufacture (or possibly from high speed projectile particles). Some eyedrops containing phenylephrine, adrenaline or berberine cause discoloration and some preservatives from sterilizing and hydrating solutions may concentrate in the matrix of soft lenses causing either discoloration or surface filming and consequently discomfort to the patient (Ganju and Cordrey, 1975). Handling the lenses may transfer a variety of contaminants such as lipstick, mascara, oily creams, detergents and nicotine to the lenses if strict personal hygiene is not observed. Further, Wilson *et al.* (1971) found fungal contamination in 12 per cent of eye make-up samples and bacterial contamination in as high as 43 per cent of samples.

Repeated disinfection by boiling and to a lesser extent with chemical disinfecting solutions denatures the surface mucoprotein, slowly building up a tenacious irregular surface layer. This may cause symptoms of discomfort, lowered acuity, lens discoloration and conjunctival injection and possibly an apparent change in fitting and power.

For these reasons the development has taken place of daily cleaning solutions to prevent surface deposits from building up and rejuvenating products to remove deposits already present.

Because of the gradual build-up of deposits on the lenses, a more effective cleaning treatment is required at periodic intervals depending on the patient, lens material, method of disinfection, etc. Ganju and Cordrey (1975) and Gasson (1975) have shown measurable drops in ultra-violet and visible light transmission through many lenses only a few months old which had not been correctly cleaned. Typically this was around 15 per cent for visible light, and Gasson noted that some 15 per cent of soft lens wearers noted a reduction in acuity after six months wear (although approximately twice as many reported an improvement). Because of the nature of the material most lenses cannot be repolished as with hard lenses, and the development of enzymatic and oxidative systems has emerged, some for use by the patient and others for use by the practitioner.

Finally, it is not uncommon for hydrophilic lens wearers to experience some discomfort or temporary drop of vision while the lenses are worn. Ignoring physical causes such as lens movement or distortion, the cause may vary from inadequate tears formation and a dirty lens, to personal idiosyncrasies. To overcome the problem, products have been developed which rehydrate and clean the lens *in situ*. These products are especially helpful in cases where the front surface of the lens has become dehydrated; for example, due to low environmental humidity, causing a change in lens curvature resulting in discomfort and impairment of vision.

The usual sequence of events during soft lens wear and care is for the lens to be cleaned on removal from the eye with a special cleaning solution. This is rinsed off with a suitable saline rinsing solution. The lens is then disinfected or sterilized by one means or another. It is then ready to wear, but sterile or preserved normal saline solution must be used to rinse the soaking solution off the lens in some cases, unless the lens has been boiled in unpreserved saline solution. Also, prior to or during wear a rewetting solution may be used. From time to time special cleaning or rejuvenating procedures become necessary, utilizing further special solutions or compounds.

The problems of sterilization, cleaning, rinsing, restoring and rehydrating hydrophilic lens materials has led to the development of four specific groups of systems and solutions: (1) disinfecting solutions or systems and rinsing solutions; (2) cleaning solutions and methods; (3) rejuvenating systems; and (4) lens conditioning and tears replacement solutions.

METHODS OF DISINFECTION

Heating Methods

The American Food and Drug Administration (F.D.A.) regulations state that methods for soft lens hygiene should fulfil the requirements for disinfection. This is defined as 'the physical or chemical process producing destruction of pathogenic microorganisms' (United States, F.D.A., 1973). This definition does not imply the destruction of bacterial spores since these are at a resistant stage but only of vegetative microorganisms. Mould spores are considered to be reproductive stages and resist heat only slightly better than vegetative forms of bacteria. Total sterility is only achieved by autoclaving for 15 minutes at 120°C and 15 lb/in^2 pressure and for this reason moist heat units which destroy vegetative microorganisms are often described as 'asepticizors' rather than 'sterilizers'.

Heating was suggested some years ago by Ruben (1966) and Morrison (1966) and was recognized by the F.D.A. in 1972 as the first approved method of disinfection for use with soft lenses. It is also the only method of lens disinfection currently permitted by the Japanese health authorities. Although the physical requirement for disinfection is 80°C for 10 minutes, the temperature achieved inside the Bausch and Lomb lens carrying case during a normal asepticizing cycle is 96°C for approximately 20 minutes (Mote, Filppi and Hill, 1972). Typical heating units are shown in *Figures 3.1, 3.2* and *3.3* and a typical heating cycle is shown in *Figure 3.4*. A small autoclave unit (the Durasoft Autoclave Sterilizer, *Wesley, Jessen Inc.*) for patient use is also available. This keeps the lenses at a temperature of 120°C, or just above, for 20 minutes (Snyder, Hill and Bailey, 1977). This is ideal for sterilization but may degrade the lens material.

Boiling, and particularly repeated boiling, may possibly cause molecular breakdown or degradation of the lens material over a period of time thereby shortening the life of the lens. Mandell (1974), however, states that the temperature at which this occurs rapidly for HEMA material is probably about 30°C higher than that normally used in the asepticizing process so that any breakdown of the molecular structure probably occurs at an extremely slow rate. Since all current lens materials are stable below 85°C, Dallos and Hughes (1972) tried to achieve sterilization by pasteurization at 70–73°C. They found that representative samples of heat resistant pathogenic bacteria were killed after heating for 2 minutes at 70°C. These writers recommended daily pasteurization with the unit heating up to 72°C (that is, slightly higher than

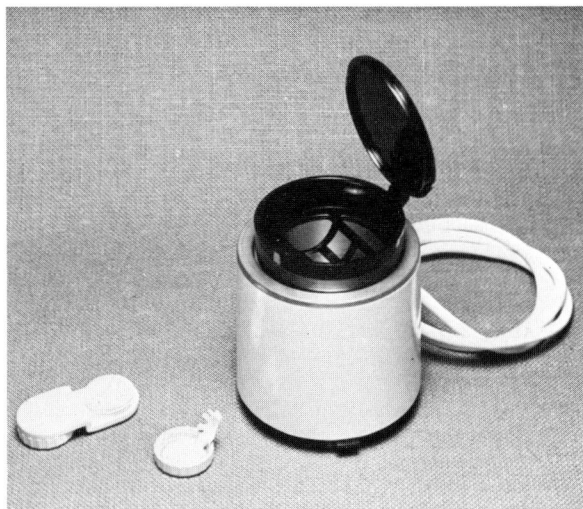

(a)

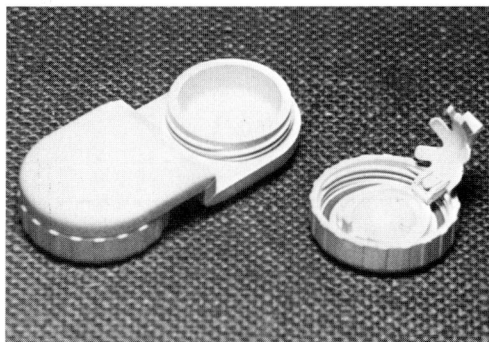

(b)

Figure 3.1–(a) Bausch and Lomb Soflens 'Aseptor Unit' showing where the flat lens container (left) fits into the black top during heating. (b) Enlargement of lens container showing the dome inside the cap on which the lens is placed and held by the hinged retainer. The container is filled with saline solution

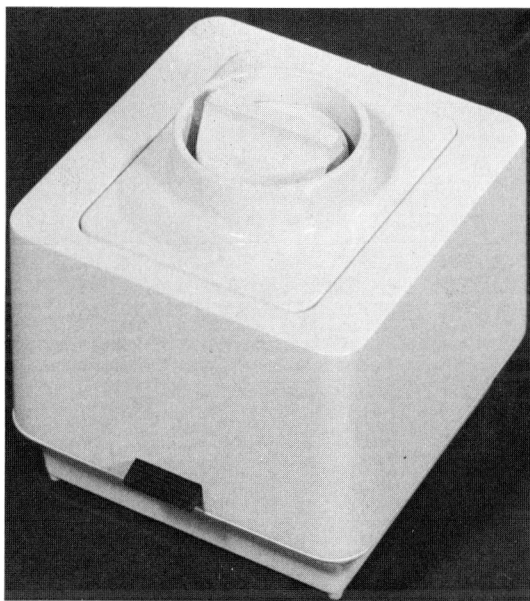

(a)

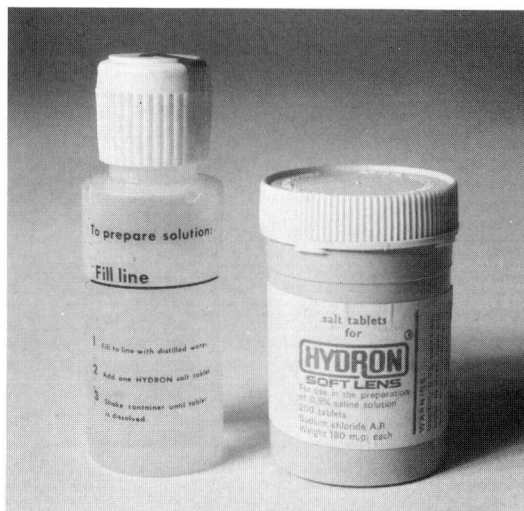

(b)

Figure 3.2–(a) Smith and Nephew Optics Aseptor Unit. (b) Salt tablets and solution bottle showing 'fill line'. (c) Lens container and lens supports

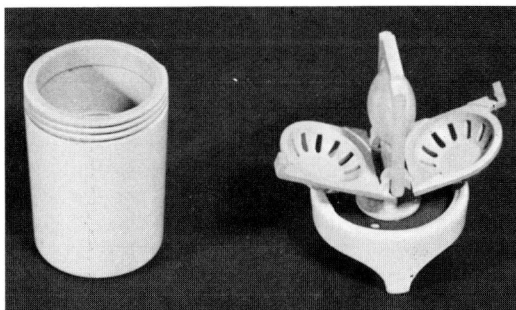

(c)

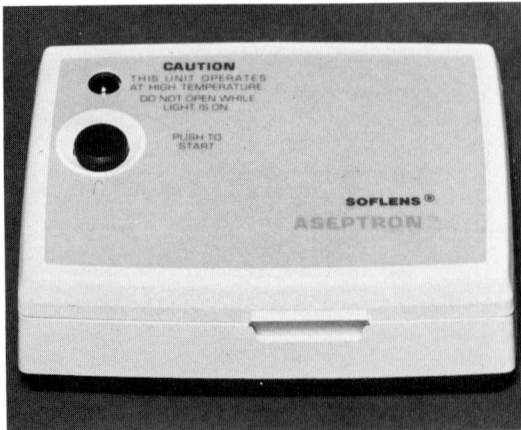

(a)

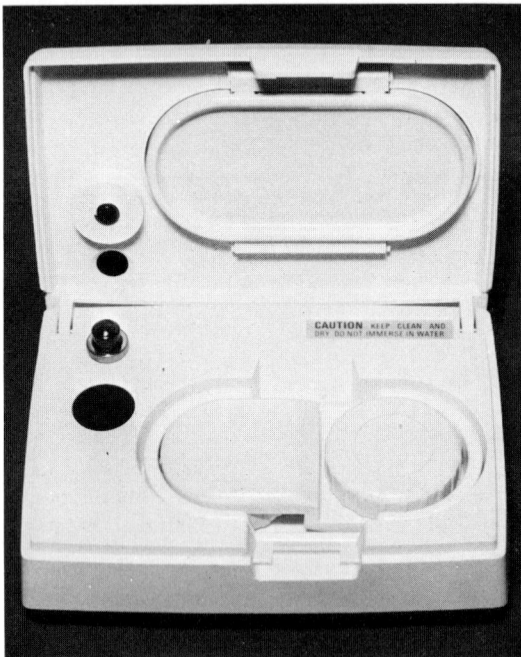

(b)

Figure 3.3—(a) Bausch and Lomb dry heat Aseptron unit. (b) Opened unit showing lens container

units has been demonstrated by Knoll (1972) using bacteria, a fungus and virus; Mote, Filppi and Hill (1972) using Gram-positive and Gram-negative bacteria, a spore former, and a fungus; Hydron Lens Ltd. (1972) using a selection of pathogenic bacteria; Filppi, Pfister and Hill (1973) using the fungus *A. fumagatus*; and Busschaert *et al.* (1974) using a selection of bacteria, fungi and bacterial spores. Busschaert and his co-workers found, however, that bacterial spores were occasionally able to survive the asepticizing cycle; Tragakis, Brown and Pearce (1973) also found the fungus *A. fumagatus* sometimes survived asepticization (possibly by sporulating); and Bernstein, Stow and Maddox (1973), in contrast with the other workers listed above, found 20 per cent of unopened Soflens cases to be contaminated after asepticization by the patient. This number increased to 86 per cent contamination of the cases a few hours after opening although presumably the lenses would normally be in the wearers' eyes by this time.

In their study, one patient showing bacterial contamination of her container and an eye infection admitted to changing the saline solution only every 2—3 days. The importance of daily asepticization and making up of fresh solution must

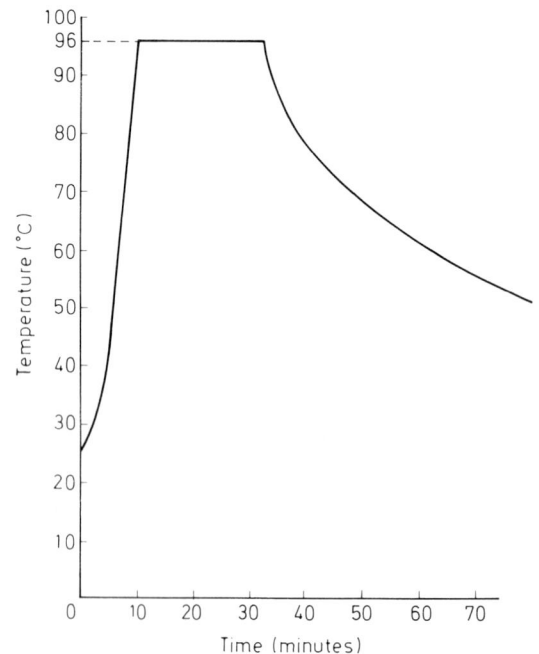

Figure 3.4—Time-temperature cycle of the saline solution contained in the contact lens case during a Bausch and Lomb Aseptor heating cycle (modified, after Mote, Filppi and Hill, 1972)

required) over a 2—3 hour period and remaining at 72°C for 30 minutes.

As stated above, units used in practice immerse the lens storage container, which keeps the lenses in a suitable saline solution (*see* page 73), in steam from boiling water. The temperature reached inside the lens case is typically around 96°C for 20 minutes. The efficacy of these asepticizing

therefore be greatly impressed on the patient. In the United States some manufacturers have now begun producing pre-prepared saline solution containing thiomersalate, as an added method of disinfection following asepticization should the container be opened and bacteria inadvertently allowed to enter. This has been approved by the F.D.A. for one particular lens system. Bacteria may also be sucked in from the outside as the container cools and patients must be advised to use the correct screw-cap container and to make sure it is firmly tightened. Similarly, a loose cap may allow loss by evaporation of the water within the container causing hypertonicity of the saline solution, alteration of the lens dimensions and subsequent discomfort on lens insertion.

Normal saline solution in which lenses are to be boiled may be made up from specially manufactured salt tablets or granules shaken up with the correct quantity of purified or distilled water. It is important that this solution is not used for rinsing the lenses prior to their insertion in the eye, for neither purified nor distilled water are sterile, and are often very far from it. Also available are sterile (unpreserved) saline solutions such as Salettes as detailed in Appendix E, *Table II*, at the end of this volume, as well as 0.9 per cent sodium chloride solution available in 1 litre and 500 ml bags intended for intravenous saline drips. Normal saline solution preserved with thiomersalate and EDTA is also suitable for the boiling of lenses, and the commercially available brands of preserved saline solution are also included in Appendix E, *Table II*.

One major problem with boiling is that mucoproteins present on the lens become coagulated or denatured on the lens surface by the asepticizing process. The film thus formed may cause lens discomfort, loss of acuity, loss of transparency, conjunctival injection and possibly a change in lens fitting and power. It may also reduce lens porosity and thereby aid the formation of corneal oedema. For this reason daily cleaning is a necessity prior to boiling (*see* below).

The instructions to be given to the patient regarding asepticizing are given in Chapter 8. Practitioners using trial lenses stored in saline solution should boil them at frequent intervals once they have been used and re-sealed in order to kill bacteria which may have survived earlier boiling by sporulating. Lenses received from the manufacturer should ideally have been autoclaved and therefore be sterile. Lenses which have been used on a patient's eye should be boiled or preferably autoclaved (Litvin, 1977), before being returned to the lens rack.

The use of autoclaving by laboratories to achieve lens sterilization would not, however, appear to be without its drawbacks. Larke (1974) has noted that the pH of lens storage saline solution is usually acidic in the region of 5.5–6.5 following autoclaving and often therefore gives rise to ocular irritation. In addition, should the lens vial remain unopened for a matter of weeks or months, the pH will continue to fall and may reach 4.0–4.5. The absorption of atmospheric carbon dioxide with the formation of weakly dissociated carbonic acid would seem a possible mechanism and this seems to be a problem in lens vials which have gas-permeable silicone rubber stoppers.

The advantages of boiling or asepticizing as a method of lens disinfection may therefore be summarized as follows.

It is generally accepted as an effective method of lens disinfection and is recognized as such by the American and Japanese Health Authorities.

After the initial purchase of the boiling unit it is the least expensive method.

Where unpreserved saline solution is used (*see* adjacent paragraph) there is no risk of allergy to any preservative.

The disadvantages may be summarized as follows.

The fees for the fitting and supply of soft lenses are higher than for corneal lenses. The additional cost of the asepticizor often makes it initially prohibitive.

There is a fairly high risk of microorganism build-up if the procedure is not carried out daily and fresh saline solution prepared daily (Brown *et al.*, 1974).

Certain bacterial spores may survive asepticizing and may cause lens damage if the boiling is not carried out daily to destroy vegetative forms of the organism.

Since some aseptors use saline solution which does not contain a preservative, there is a slight risk of microorganisms being transferred on to the lens from the fingers. Such a possible case has been cited by Storey (1973).

Of the various methods of hydrogel disinfection, heating methods cause the greatest denaturing effect of ocular secretions remaining on the lens surface with the accompanying disadvantages mentioned above.

Repeated heat disinfection may cause slow degradation of the polymer structure thereby reducing the life of the lens. It should be emphasized that this effect undoubtedly varies from material to material and that to the writer's knowledge no experimental work has yet been undertaken on this aspect.

Following from the previous paragraphs, the technique is not a universal one suitable for all lens materials and some materials degrade very quickly with repeated heat sterilization.

Although not as slow for lens disinfection as soft lens storage solutions (see below) the method is not rapid, taking approximately one hour and possibly a further hour for cooling and for the lens dimensions to return to normal (Loran, 1974). Again, although quicker than the hydrogen peroxide disinfection procedure, the method is slightly more time consuming for the patient than the use of soft lens storage solutions.

There are occasions when it is impossible to asepticize by boiling; for example, whilst travelling.

Chemical Disinfection

Hydrogen Peroxide

The first method of chemical disinfection was by means of 3 per cent hydrogen peroxide (Isen, 1972). The need for an alternative to heating methods arose because the lens material currently used by Isen did not stand up well to repeated boiling. Although tending to fall out of favour after its initial introduction (see below) it has been revived in recent years.

In the original method described by Isen, the lenses were soaked for 5 minutes in hydrogen peroxide 3 per cent which is highly acidic having a pH of 3.0. This was therefore neutralized by exposure to 0.5 per cent sodium bicarbonate in 0.9 per cent sodium chloride for 1 minute and the lenses then immersed in 0.9 per cent sodium chloride alone for 15 minutes. The lenses were then stored overnight in isotonic saline solution. Feldman (1971) stated that *hot* water should be added to dissolve the bicarbonate, otherwise residual pyrogenic material remains, followed by three rinses with sterile saline solution before storage. The technique used currently still involves placing the lens in 3 per cent hydrogen peroxide for 10–15 minutes but followed by four elution cycles in fresh, sterile, thiomersalate-preserved isotonic saline solution.

Gasset, Ramer and Katzin (1975) describe a slightly modified procedure where after soaking for 5 minutes in 3 per cent hydrogen peroxide, the lenses are rinsed once with a 2.5 per cent sodium thiosulphate solution and then soaked for a further 15 minutes in a 2.5 per cent sodium thiosulphate solution.

The procedure appears to be very effective as a method of disinfection (Phares, 1972a; Isen, 1972).

Tragakis, Brown and Pearce (1973) reported that the procedure killed a variety of organisms on lenses which had been in use, including the fungus *A. fumagatus*. However, these workers found that whilst the method was very effective when using hydrogen peroxide which had been kept in sealed glass vials, the method was largely ineffective when using solution which had been kept in plastics screw-top containers. Similar results were reported by Morrison *et al.* (1973). This breakdown of hydrogen peroxide to oxygen and water when exposed to the atmosphere or to light, or in the presence of dust or fine metallic particles undoubtedly represents a major disadvantage of the method (Charles, 1975). Stability also depends on storage at low temperatures. Other disadvantages include the relatively long time involved for the patient and the dangers of omitting the sodium bicarbonate neutralizing step. Failure to carry out this step can cause marked ocular irritation. Prior to the introduction of thiomersalate-preserved saline solution (used for overnight storage following lens disinfection), the effectiveness of the method was also suspect since there was no guarantee that the saline solution itself was sterile. The oxidizing effect of the hydrogen peroxide bleaches impurities on the lens surface usually leaving the lens optically clear. However, deposits are not actually removed from the lens, which is not therefore cleaned in the true sense of the word.

Chlorhexidine and Thiomersalate Preserved Saline Storage Solutions

Because of the inconvenience of the boiling and hydrogen peroxide disinfection routines, alternative methods were looked for with emphasis on the search for simple storage and rinsing solutions which would be non-irritant to the eye and harmless to lens materials.

The first and major problem was that of the adsorptive or binding ability of most hydrogel materials. Since hydrophilic lenses have the ability to take up water, they will of necessity absorb an aqueous solution of chemical which might be presented to them. This should not create a problem if the solution by itself is safe on the eye. A potential problem arises, however, if the soft lens adsorbs (or loosely complexes with certain molecules on the lens surface) the preservative from the solution since this will then be concentrated on the surface. Unfortunately, many of the commonly used hard lens solution preservatives are strongly bound by hydrogel materials.

These preservatives are harmful to living bacterial cells and will generally be damaging to the corneal epithelial cells if present in higher than normal concentrations.

Benzalkonium chloride (a cationic preservative) has been shown to be a strong soft lens binder whereas thiomersalate (an anionic preservative) is not (Sibley and Yung, 1973). It would appear, therefore, that electrostatic forces are involved. Chlorhexidine as a cationic preservative is also bound (Sibley, 1973, cited by Browne, Anderson and Charvez, 1974) but as it has a large molecular structure and a very weak cationic action its binding capacity is about one-sixth that of benzalkonium chloride (Hind, 1975). Various authors have shown that for most patients the amount of preservative bound to the lens is insufficient to cause ocular irritation (Krezanoski, 1972a; Phares, 1972b; Brown et al., 1974; Hind, 1975). Other workers have mentioned the binding ability of the other commonly used hard lens preservatives, phenyl-mercuric nitrate and chlorbutanol (Krezanoski, 1972b; Ganju, 1974), but EDTA does not appear to be bound to any significant degree. Surprisingly, Lerman and Sapp (1971), from laboratory and clinical experiments, determined that the concentration of benzalkonium chloride and chlorbutol normally used in ophthalmic preparations was bound to an insufficient degree to cause ocular irritation. This unexpected result may be due to the fact shown by Otten and Szabocsik (1976) that the final formulation of the solution has a significant effect on the binding ability of the preservative, although they were unable to offer any explanation for this.

Although chlorhexidine is only minimally bound to clean lens material it is very effectively bound to protein deposits on the lens surface and, unfortunately, this exacerbates the binding effect. Not only does this reduce the efficacy of the solution but the increased concentration of bound preservative causes symptoms of ocular discomfort over a period of time as the lens contaminants build up, often leading to lens rejection (Hind, 1975). Further, there is the danger of a sudden release of preservative from the lens to the cornea if there is a pH change, fluid movement across the lens or replacement by ions present in the tears liquid (Ganju, 1974). Daily cleaning of the lens is therefore of paramount importance.

Most of the soft lens storage or soaking solutions* may also be used for rinsing lenses following lens cleaning. However, any solution of normal saline

is suitable for this rinsing procedure. Ideally, unpreserved sterile saline solution should be used but non-sterile saline solution (made up from salt tablets and purified or distilled water) is permissible provided that the lens is to be boiled or disinfected by some other means, directly afterwards. Preserved saline solutions* specially formulated for lens rinsing are also available.

For the reasons discussed above it is obviously essential that patients with soft lenses must be advised not to use any hard lens solutions or medicated eyedrops utilizing preservatives. It is also important that soft lens solutions contain the least possible amount of preservative in order to minimize any binding effect to the lens material or contaminants. The use of minimal quantities of preservative has led to criticism of the antibacterial efficacy of these solutions.

Norton et al. (1974), using proprietary soft lens storage solutions, found that none was able to disinfect a standard laboratory contamination of 10^6 organisms/ml^{-1} of Ps. aeruginosa, Staph. aureus, M. luteus and C. albicans in less than 24 hours, many taking 48 hours. These workers also found discrepancies between different solutions containing similar quantities of the same preservatives and postulated two reasons for this. First, that all the solutions were packaged in plastics containers and some preservatives may be adsorbed by the plastics. This could result in reduced concentration of preservative available in the solutions and would depend on such factors as the type of plastics used and the time stored (indicating the need for manufacturers to date-stamp solution bottles). Secondly, that the solutions used are complex and usually contain viscolizers such as hydroxyethylcellulose and polyvinyl alcohol, buffering agents, electrolytes and surfactants, all of which may influence the antibacterial performance of the preservative.

Holden and Markides (1971) found that a solution of 0.001 per cent thiomersalate took over 24 hours to kill an inoculum of Staph. aureus, and 6—24 hours for an inoculum of Ps. aeruginosa. Grosvenor, Charles and Callender (1972) and Baker and Remington (1972) all found that lenses from manufacturers stored in the same solution were often received highly contaminated. Charles (in Davis et al., 1973) noted that this solution was also ineffective against clumped groups of bacteria. Similar results to those of Holden and Markides (1971) were found for Staph. aureus by Lindeman-Meester (1974) using 0.002 per cent thiomersalate plus 0.1 per cent EDTA. Tragakis, Brown and Pearce (1973) found that high concentrations (10^7/ml^{-1}) of P. vulgaris were able to survive 24 hours exposure to 0.005 per cent chlorhexidine.

* See Appendix E, Table II, for examples.

Feldman (1971) found this concentration of chlorhexidine to be effective against several bacteria but to be ineffective against the fungus *A. fumagatus*. Similar results against fungi were stated by Charles (*in* Davis *et al.,* 1973).

It would appear from the above, and the results of other workers, that of the two commonly used preservatives suitable for soft lens storage solutions – chlorhexidine and thiomersalate – chlorhexidine is the more effective but has poor fungicidal capacity. Thiomersalate is slower acting but is known to be more effective as an anti-fungal. For this reason almost all solutions utilizing these preservatives make use of both agents, chlorhexidine at 0.0005–0.005 per cent and thiomersalate at 0.001–0.0025 per cent strengths, and they may also incorporate EDTA at 0.01–0.1 per cent. The incorporation of EDTA is both for enhancement of the bactericidal effect of the main preservative, and the postulated advantage of reducing calcium ions which may eventually form deposits on the lens.

The solutions are made isotonic and may contain liquid polymers such as polyvinylpyrrolidone, and possibly surfactants to act as cleaning agents. Hampson (1973) states that lenses stored in an acidic pH solution take two to three times as long to settle and become comfortable as those stored in a slightly alkaline pH solution. For this reason most manufacturers moderately buffer solutions to a neutral or slightly alkaline pH.

As stated earlier, Holden and Markides (1971) found that a solution of 0.001 per cent thiomersalate alone took 24 hours to kill high concentrations of *Staph. aureus* and *Ps. aeruginosa*. Using a combination of 0.005 per cent chlorhexidine and 0.001 per cent thiomersalate the killing time was reduced to 2–15 minutes. Similar results were found by Toxicol Laboratories (1972) using a different proprietary solution with similar constituents. Feldman (1971) gives a decontamination time for a similar chlorhexidine-thiomersalate combination of less than 1 hour for all bacteria tested except *Staph. aureus* which was killed in under 2 hours. Phares (1972b) found a sterilizing time of 15 minutes to 3 hours for an inoculum of *Ps. aeruginosa, Staph. aureus* and *Esch. coli* using 0.005 per cent chlorhexidine alone. Tragakis, Brown and Pearce (1973), using bacteria and fungi, gave a sterilizing time of 8 hours for inocula of bacteria and fungi. Grosvenor, Charles and Callender (1972) took cultures from the cases and chlorhexidine-thiomersalate storage solutions of 125 patients wearing soft lenses. In only one case was a positive culture found and here there was serious doubt that the wearer in question was following the practitioner's instructions.

From the accumulated evidence it would appear that chlorhexidine-thiomersalate disinfecting solutions are able to cope with all levels of bacterial and fungal contamination normally encountered. There is evidence that very large levels of contamination may take several hours for disinfection although even this should be coped with during the overnight storage period. Higher levels of contamination should be greatly reduced by cleaning and rinsing prior to storage (*see* below).

Other Chemical Disinfection Solutions

Because of some of the disadvantages associated with chlorhexidine-thiomersalate storage solutions alternative methods of chemical disinfection have been examined. Specifically, greater antibacterial activity, reduced binding (especially to adsorbed protein), and greater cleaning efficiency have been looked for.

Alternative lens disinfection systems based on an iodophor in an isotonic polymeric vehicle appear to show good clinical results (Johnson and Littlewood, 1975). When the iodophor (in a phosphoric or citric acid diluent) is placed in combination with a complementary neutralizing medium preserved with sorbic acid, EDTA and sodium borate, the iodine is reduced to the iodide ion. Unique to this system is the colour indicating a disinfecting action. When the solution and the lenses have become colourless there is a remaining preservative action, but the lenses may be safely inserted direct from the solution. Disinfecting time is stated by the manufacturer to be 2 hours. The concentration of active (diatomic) iodine is 0.005 per cent, and there appears to be the definite advantage of no binding effect of the preservative (although Stone, 1976, reported pronounced stinging if first used on old, and therefore probably contaminated, lenses when disinfection should be followed by boiling to prevent this problem). Slightly more attention and co-operation is required on the part of the patient in the correct preparation of the disinfecting solution since neutralization is essential, the diluent having a pH of less than 5.0. A further disadvantage is that the cost of iodophors is high compared to other disinfectant methods.

Another overnight storage solution combines thiomersalate with a quaternary ammonium compound, alkyl triethanol ammonium chloride, to provide the disinfecting action. The disinfecting action reported by the manufacturer is slow but effective and is reported not to concentrate in the lens (Shively, 1975a). However, this combination did not achieve excellent clinical success according to Morgan (1975a). In addition to acting as an antimicrobial agent, the alkyl triethanol ammonium chloride is also used for its surfactant properties, and two other surfactants — polysorbate 80 and propylene glycol — are also included to give the solution a cleaning as well as a disinfecting action.

Ganju and Thompson (1975) have reported a disinfectant solution (see Appendix E, Table II) containing a mixture of methyl, ethyl, propyl and butyl esters of p-hydroxybenzoic acid (Nipastat) in combination with a water-soluble polymer complex and reported success in its use as a lens disinfectant. It should be noted, however, that the numbers of microorganisms challenged was low compared with other workers and that the first subculture was not taken until after 8 hours exposure to the preservative. The work of Hugo and Foster (1964) has also shown that it is not always entirely effective in eliminating contamination by Ps. aeruginosa. The p-hydroxybenzoates show a very slight tendency to concentrate on hydrophilic lens surfaces in a similar manner to chlorhexidine. The great advantage of this preservative is that it is non-mercurial and contains no quaternary ammonium compound, thereby providing a very useful alternative for patients showing a possible allergy or sensitivity to chlorhexidine-thiomersalate preserved solutions.

Charles (1975) points out the possibility of using sonic oscillation, that is, the use of sonic energy of frequencies above 200,000 Hz for cleaning and asepticizing hydrogel lenses. High frequency sound waves are used by microbiologists both for killing microorganisms and for cleaning purposes. However, in tests by Charles, sonication for periods of as long as 2—3 hours was required to kill an inoculum of Ps. aeruginosa. Spores are also somewhat resistant to this procedure.

Lastly, an American patent issued to Blank (1975) outlines the use of a solution which releases active chlorine in solution in the presence of a lens but which is non-damaging to the eye in concentrations effective for disinfection. The active chloride is generated through use of various compounds containing chlorine such as chlorinated trisodium phosphate, sodium dichlorocyanurate, potassium dichlorocyanurate and tri-chloroisocyanusic acid. This system is stated to be equally effective with all current lens materials. No lens compatability data is shown, however, and little ocular irritation data is given. Further clinical and laboratory work on these compounds must be awaited before their general usage can be recommended.

The advantages of chemical disinfecting solutions may therefore be summarized as follows.

Generally they are convenient, and for the patient who may already have hard lenses, they fit into a similar pattern.

The initial cost is low.

They are portable.

They are generally effective for all microorganisms normally encountered and this will still apply even if the wearer occasionally omits to change the solution daily or does not wear his lenses for a few days.

Sporulating bacteria are destroyed if they revert to their vegetative form.

There appears to be no effect on the life of the lenses.

There is less coagulation of mucoprotein left on the lens than with heat sterilization.

Set against these are the following disadvantages.

Chemical disinfecting solutions are more expensive in the long term.

There is a risk of some binding with certain antimicrobial agents and this applies particularly if the lens is not cleaned prior to being placed in the solution.

There is some risk of ocular irritation by solution constituents. Hind (1975) has estimated this to be 5—10 per cent for one proprietary solution, and 4 per cent for another as estimated by Trager (in Davis et al., 1973).

The solutions cannot generally cope with large influxes of microorganisms.

The solution method is slow, normally taking 6—8 hours to be certain of complete disinfection.

Many preservatives still cause slight coagulation of any mucoprotein remaining on the lens surfaces.

Most solutions have no cleaning action and still necessitate the use of separate cleaning compounds.

The possibility exists that solutions may be suitable for use with only specified lens materials.

Practitioners occasionally find that patients using heating methods of disinfection will change to chemical disinfection, for example, on holiday when mains electricity may not be available or may be the wrong voltage. Whilst many patients experience no difficulties with alternating disinfection methods it can sometimes give rise to problems. First, it has already been mentioned above that heating methods of disinfection accelerate the denaturation of proteinacious deposits on the lens surface. Chlorhexidine then binds more strongly to these deposits than to the lens surface and gives rise to a toxic or allergenic response. Secondly, there is good evidence that tear protein bound to contact lens surfaces can cause an immune response (Allansmith et al., 1977; Refojo and Holly, 1977). The present understanding of this process is that the adsorbed protein molecule undergoes changes that may be accelerated by alternating dry/wet and hot/cold conditions, as well as by mechanical rubbing from fingers and lids. The altered denatured protein may then no longer be recognized as 'self' and be capable of provoking an autoimmune response (McMonnies, 1978).

Conversely, practitioners may wish their patients to change from chemical disinfection of their lenses to heat disinfection, or from one chemical disinfection method to another; as may be done if a patient is thought to have developed an adverse reaction to a particular preservative. Before doing so all traces of the existing preservatives should be removed from the lenses by (1) soaking the lenses in at least three changes of unpreserved normal saline solution at room temperature during a period of 24 hours; or (2) boiling the lenses in distilled water followed by an overnight soak in unpreserved normal saline solution, replenishing the latter and then re-boiling; or (3) boiling in unpreserved normal saline solution, replenishing and then re-boiling.

The properties of a soft lens disinfecting solution may therefore be listed as follows (modified from Cureton and Sibley, 1974).

The solution should be capable of disinfecting the lenses in 4–6 hours or less.

The antimicrobial agents used should not easily be inactivated by small amounts of proteins, lipids or other tears components.

The solution should be isotonic and either non-buffered or lightly buffered to a pH approximating that of the average tears liquid.

The antimicrobial agents used should not bind to protein or other lens surface deposits from the eye.

The solution should not react with or adsorb to soft lens materials.

The solution should be non-irritating and non-toxic to the ocular tissues.

Two additional useful but not essential properties may also be listed.

The solution should be capable of withstanding boiling without degrading.

The combination of a cleaning action with the disinfectant/storage action would be helpful.

CLEANING SOLUTIONS AND METHODS

While the lens is on the eye, the mucin in the tears fluid is adsorbed onto the surface of the lens in the same way that it is adsorbed onto the epithelium of the cornea. Mucin and other proteins of the tears such a lysozyme remain in their natural state when attached to the soft lens surface in the eye. As long as the soft lens remains in the environment of the tears fluid the eye will usually accommodate the lens without excessive protein film build-up. However, as mentioned earlier, daily removal of the lens, over a period of time, results in the denaturing of adsorbed proteins. This process occurs very slowly when the lenses are stored in a cold sterilizing solution but more rapidly when they are boiled. The problem is compounded by lipid secretions from the Meibomian glands which can also bind to the lens surfaces, forming a lipoprotein film that is difficult to remove and which can impair visual acuity and cause discomfort. Further, chlorhexidine and other preservatives will bind to this film increasing both their concentration and contact time with the eye and causing a burning sensation (Hind, 1975). As mentioned earlier, sudden release of adsorbed preservative may also cause marked irritation.

In addition, the bound preservative loses its disinfecting ability so that the solution takes longer to sterilize the lens. The surface film may itself serve as a growth medium for bacteria and fungi and may actually protect microorganisms trapped within it. Cureton and Hall (1974), Hind (1975) and Thompson and Mansell (1976) have shown a marked improvement in the time taken for disinfection where lenses have been cleaned prior to storage. This has presumably arisen from the combined effect of physically reducing the number of microorganisms by cleaning and rinsing, and also by removing or reducing surface contaminants and thereby enhancing the disinfectant action of the boiling or chemical solution.

In addition to the lipoprotein surface film, various salts, di-valent or tri-valent ions (for example, calcium) and other contaminants such as environmental pollutants, chemical vapours, cosmetic ingredients, water impurities, nicotine, oils and dirt from the fingers and preservative and active ingredients from ophthalmic products may be present in the adsorbed or absorbed state.

The cleaning problem is further complicated by the fact that different lens materials are affected by contaminants in different ways. Some lens materials become cloudy and hazy and accumulate rough deposits which are sometimes impervious to ordinary cleaning procedures. Other lens materials become discoloured and occasionally form deposits in the form of white spots (Ganju and Cordrey, 1975). Contaminants are often visible to both patient and practitioner with the naked eye, and the patient should be instructed to cease wearing any lens showing any opaque area on its surface. Surface deposits are often best seen with the slit lamp and usually take the form of roughness of the lens surface appearing between blinks.

Cleaning solutions have therefore been developed for daily use and usually contain chemicals such as hypromellose, sodium chloride, thiomersalate and EDTA. Because of the porous nature of hydrophilic lenses and their interaction with many ionic compounds the selection of a surfactant is limited to a non-ionic block copolymer which is capable of lowering the interfacial tension at the solid-water interface (Ganju and Cordrey, 1975). The solution is often made slightly viscous to facilitate handling and is sometimes made slightly hypertonic so that any contaminants which have been absorbed by the matrix are drawn out by the osmotic pressure differential (Ganju and Cordrey, 1975). The solution may further be formulated at an alkaline pH to maximize protein removal (Hind, 1975). The cleaner* should be designed to be safe and cause minimal or no ocular discomfort if accidentally instilled into the eye; to be readily rinsed off the lens by the rinsing or storage solution; and to be compatible with all hydrophilic lens materials and accessories.

An alternative method of removing protein deposits from the lens surface has been developed for HEMA and some other materials using a proteolytic enzyme (Morgan, 1975b). The enzyme used is Papain, derived from the dried and purified latex of the pawpaw fruit (*Carica papaya*) tree and normally used as a meat tenderizer and in the manufacture of chillproof beer. Papain is an extremely effective proteolytic enzyme in the context of soft lens deposits and the results are often very dramatic. Unfortunately, the method has little or no action against lipids, waxes or cosmetic contaminants, etc. Lens structure is not affected since the enzymatic activity is specific for peptide linkages (Blanco, Curry and Boghosian, 1975). It is recommended to be used once every seven days for a two-hour period followed by the normal disinfection routine since the enzyme has no antimicrobial action. This has the minor disadvantage that the wearer must remember when to carry out the additional procedure. Further, the procedure is slightly time-consuming and in addition ocular irritation results if the (overnight) cleaning procedure is not also followed by careful lens cleaning to remove the surface debris so formed. For many patients it is not necessary to use the enzyme treatment as often as once a week, particularly if a daily cleaning solution is also used.

Other cleaners incorporating enzymes for the removal of lipids and mucin are also available, *see* Appendix E, *Table II*, at the end of the volume.

From the discussion above it can be seen that after removal of the lenses, whatever the chosen method of sterilization, the patient should be strongly advised to carry out a prophylactic daily

* *See* Appendix E, *Table II*, for examples.

cleaning step prior to lens disinfection. The relative advantage of daily cleaning solutions compared to the weekly use of proteolytic enzymes has yet to be assessed. Some practitioners may prefer to recommend the use of a cleaning solution on a daily basis and the monthly use of a proteolytic enzyme as an additional precautionary step. Such a step becomes more logical when it is appreciated that some cleaning solutions are mainly effective for lipids whereas the enzyme is effective for proteins. Patients using heat disinfection must be advised to carefully rinse cleaning solutions from the lens prior to it being placed in the asepticizor unit since certain cleaners may be baked on, forming a white film and making the lens unwearable (Davis *et al.,* 1973).

REJUVENATING SYSTEMS

Those practitioners with experience of hard lenses will be familiar with the periodic lens rejuvenation necessary, usually due to accumulated surface abrasions, and usually done by surface repolishing. Unfortunately, repolishing of hydrophilic lenses is not usually possible although the practitioner is occasionally faced with a similar problem of uncomfortable or unwearable lenses. The situation arises because the patient either does not clean his lenses (even though he may disinfect them) or does not clean them thoroughly. A gradual build-up of surface deposits then takes place until the lens becomes uncomfortable for the reasons given earlier (Sagan and Schwaderer, 1974). The usual cleaning solutions are not normally effective against marked encrusted deposits and discoloured lenses. Two rejuvenation techniques are currently available, both intended for use by the practitioner, not only because of their relatively complex method of usage but also because of the risk of ocular damage if used incorrectly. Both are based on similar oxidative cleaning principles to chemically 'scrub' the lens free of both organic and inorganic contaminants.

In the method recommended by one manufacturer the lens is boiled for 10 minutes in a solution made up with saline solution and copolymer/oxidizing agent which has been gently shaken. It is allowed to soak for a further 2 hours at a constant temperature of $70-80°C$, without which, cleaning by this treatment is incomplete. The lens is then removed, rinsed with saline solution, and boiled for half an hour with fresh saline solution to remove all traces of the copolymeric agent and to sterilize it (Ganju and Cordrey, 1975). This is followed by soaking in an associated solution to remove any remaining white spots (calcium deposits). The method used in the alternative process utilizes a two-step system (*see* Appendix E, *Table II*), the lenses being soaked for not less than 4 hours (depending on the severity and extent of the lens discoloration) in a solution of each agent. The first reagent is alkaline and breaks down organic debris such as mucoproteins, while the second, acidic reagent, removes inorganic salt deposits (Shively, 1975*b*). The lenses are cleaned between each boiling period using a proprietary cleaning solution and equilibrated in isotonic salt solution for a minimum of 2 hours at room temperature before being worn. Ideally, the pH of the solution should be checked prior to re-insertion.

A further rejuvenating system utilizing an oxidizing action uses an inorganically based active substance with electrolytic properties making it water soluble. On being raised to a temperature of 60°C the product evolves reactive oxygen which decomposes organic substances. The oxidation products are readily water soluble and easily dispersed. The lenses are heated at a constant temperature in a distilled or purified water solution of the cleaner for a period of 2–4 hours and ideally utilizing a magnetic stirrer to keep the lenses constantly agitated. After completion of the process the lenses are cleaned with a surfactant cleaner, rinsed and stored in saline or preserved storage solution for 30 minutes to allow normal tonicity and dimensions to be restored. Although suitable for most lens materials, practitioners must always confirm that the process is safe to be used with each lens type and, if requesting laboratory cleaning with the product, they must state the lens material to the laboratory. Tinted lenses may also become discoloured by this process although it does have the particular advantage that it is one of only two rejuvenating techniques claimed to remove calcium deposits. The method has the further advantage that it is both anti-bacterial and anti-fungal so that the lenses are both cleaned and disinfected at the same time.

The enzyme treatment mentioned above may also be considered a form of rejuvenating system. Its efficacy may be increased by treating the lenses during two consecutive overnight storage periods in the case of badly coated lenses. Although not as effective as the foregoing techniques it has the advantage of simplicity and the fact that it may be done by the patient.

LENS CONDITIONING, TEARS REPLACEMENT AND SIMILAR SOLUTIONS

Some soft lens wearers experience occasional discomfort or loss of acuity whilst the lens is in the eye. Assuming that no fitting problems exist, the cause may be partial dehydration of the lens or the build-up of Meibomian secretion on the lens surface. To overcome these problems solutions have been developed which clean and rehydrate lenses *in situ* (*see* Appendix E, *Table II*, at the end of this volume). One manufacturer has also developed a solution (Hydrosol, *Contactasol*) to be rubbed into the lens surface prior to insertion and which is stated to aid initial comfort and to reduce the build-up of surface deposits during subsequent wear.

Hypertonic saline (Appendix E, *Table III*) drops may be needed by patients having continuous or extended wear soft lenses. These drops are normally medically prescribed and are used to relieve oedema of the cornea, particularly on awakening. They may also be needed at regular intervals throughout the day where some pathological condition exists which necessitates continuous wear, but where oedema results. The drops are available as 2 and 5 per cent sodium chloride preserved with thiomersalate 0.002 per cent and EDTA 0.05 per cent.

Soft lenses are still developing at a rapid pace and coupled with this has been the development of related solutions. Practitioners must accept the fact that no particular solution or technique will be ideal for every patient or lens material. In the same way that careful investigation will indicate the optimum lens material and parameters for a particular patient, the practitioner must equally carefully ensure that the method of disinfection selected is both appropriate to his individual patient's temperament, occupation and available facilities as well as to the lens material to be used.

Similarly, care must be taken in choosing the lens storage case or container. Particularly with asepticizor units the practitioner may have no choice since only the one design of case will fit the unit. Where a choice is possible the practitioner should choose a container which conforms to the following ideals.

A transparent container will allow the quantity of solution to be seen.

The container should have to be everted to remove the lenses thereby ensuring that the solution is changed at least each time the lens is worn.

It should be clearly marked 'Left' and 'Right', preferably also colour-coded, possibly with identifying tactile projections.

The storage solution volume should not be so small that insufficient quantities of preservative are contained (where chemical disinfecting solutions are used). It should be large enough to allow adequate diffusion and dilution of contaminants into the solution. Conversely the container volume should not be so large that excessive quantities of solution are used which may discourage daily changing of the solution because of the cost.

The container material must be compatible with lens materials and solution constituents.

The container material must be capable of withstanding regular boiling and have leak-proof caps.

SCLERAL LENS SOLUTIONS

For a sealed scleral lens, a solution of sodium bicarbonate 2 per cent, with chlorbutol, 0.2 per cent, can be used. It is important to avoid the use of hydroxybenzoates, or phenylmercuric nitrate or acetate in a sealed scleral lens solution, as they cause intense irritation to the eye.

OPHTHALMIC PREPARATIONS*

Eyedrops are either dispensed in multiple-dose containers or in a single-dose disposable unit (*Figure 3.5*), the latter having the advantage of ensuring that a sterile solution is always available for use. Unfortunately, at the present time not all the preparations required are available in this form (*see* Appendix E, *Table III*).

Substances in solution are more likely to break down than those in a dry state. Therefore, a limit must be put on the time for which eyedrops may be used. An expiry date is shown on the labels of some preparations. This refers only to unopened bottles, stored according to the manufacturers' instructions. Usually, this means in a cool dark place. If no expiry date is shown, eyedrops can usually be stored for about one year without the need for discarding. However, once a bottle has been opened, the drops become susceptible to contamination and oxidation from the air. The storage time for opened bottles of eyedrops is therefore much less, and it is valuable to have a guide as to how long partly used bottles may be kept. The British Pharmaceutical Codex (1973) recommends that eyedrops for domiciliary use may be used for about one month after opening,

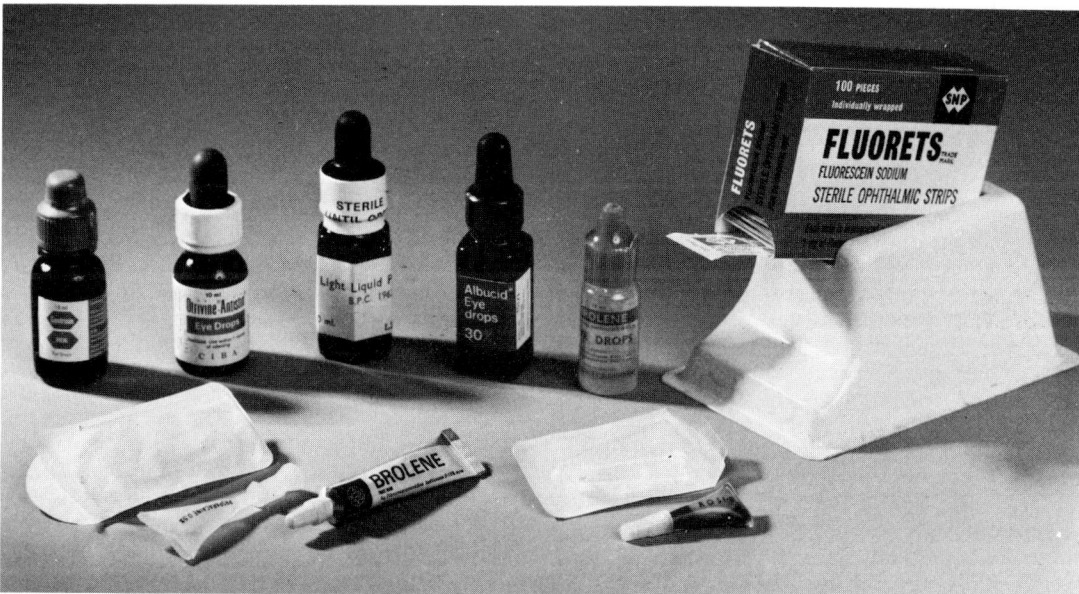

Figure 3.5–Single and multiple-dose containers for eye preparations. (Back: left to right: Gantrisin – Roche; Otrivine–Antistin – CIBA; Light Liquid Paraffin B.P.C.; Albucid – British Schering; Brolene – May and Baker; Fluorets – Smith and Nephew Pharmaceuticals. Front: left to right: Proparacaine Uni-Min – Barnes-Hind; Brolene ointment – May and Baker; Rose Bengal Minim – Smith and Nephew Pharmaceuticals)

* More details of the following ophthalmic preparations mentioned on pages 82–86 are obtainable from *Mims*, published monthly by Haymarket Publishing Limited, Medical Division, 76 Dean Street, London W1A 1BU, and the *Data Sheet Compendium* published yearly by the Association of the British Pharmaceutical Industry (Pharmind Publications). These publications give brand names and the names of the various manufacturing drug houses, as well as strengths, dosages, legal categories, contra-indications, side-effects, etc.

while those for use in hospital wards require not only a separate container for each patient but when both eyes are being treated a separate container for each eye. Further, these eyedrops should be discarded not later than one week after opening. These recommendations do not apply to multiple-dose containers of fluorescein which should be discarded after having been used only once.

The single-dose form contains about 0.5 ml of the particular eyedrop and no preservatives, bacteridical or fungicidal agents are incorporated into these preparations. Hence, these preparations must only be used for one patient and must not be stored after use. Irrespective of container form or time, any eyedrops which become discoloured or cloudy should not be used.

When using the orthodox method of instilling drops into the conjunctival sac, great care must be taken not to contaminate the end of the dropper tube by touching the lids or lashes. If this does accidentally occur, then the dropper must either be re-sterilized or discarded and replaced. This is an obvious disadvantage of the plastics-type multi-dose container, which has its dropper permanently fixed and cannot be satisfactorily sterilized if contaminated. The method using a glass rod for instillation is particularly suitable for use with fluorescein solution. The glass rod should only be used for one patient, then re-sterilized before subsequent use. Care must be taken not to damage the bulbous instilling end of the glass rod by careless handling.

Eye ointments are also frequently used, and the danger of contamination is just as great as with the use of eyedrops — particularly since no preservatives can be incorporated in these ointments. The 1973 British Pharmaceutical Codex recommends that every care should be taken to keep eye ointment in a sterile state. Whenever possible, single-dose containers should be used and the ointment can be administered either direct from the tube into the lower conjunctival sac (providing it is being used for only one patient) or by the glass rod method.

Hydrophilic lenses should be removed before any ophthalmic drugs are administered, as some therapeutic agents and preservatives can be concentrated in these lenses. This is particularly necessary with multiple-dose eyedrops containing preservatives which when released from the lens can have an irritant effect on the eye.

The following topical ophthalmic preparations are the ones most commonly used in contact lens practice: (1) topical anaesthetics; (2) conjunctival decongestants; (3) diagnostic staining agents; and (4) chemotherapeutic agents.

TOPICAL ANAESTHETICS

Topical anaesthetics are used in contact lens practice to produce surface anaesthesia of the cornea and conjunctiva by reducing the sensitivity of their sensory nerve endings. Their action, which is reversible, prevents the transmission of impulses along the nerve fibres.

The ideal requirements of a surface anaesthetic are:
Rapidity of action.
Adequate depth of anaesthesia.
Short duration.
Non-toxic.
Non-irritant.
No subsidiary actions such as cycloplegia, mydriasis or vasoconstriction.
Stability.

The depth and duration of anaesthesia depends on the strength of the drug used and the number of drops instilled at regular intervals. For this reason, onset and duration times of anaesthesia can sometimes be misleading.

All the topical anaesthetics have some effect on the corneal metabolism and increase its permeability to other drugs. Hence, adrenaline 0.1 per cent instilled into the eye normally causes no mydriatic effect, whilst if instilled after a topical anaesthetic some dilatation of the pupil may occur. This should not be confused with the pupil dilatation which occurs following the instillation of 0.1 per cent adrenaline in patients with hyper-excitability of the sympathetic system; known as Loewi's adrenaline eye test, used in the diagnosis of thyrotoxicosis. Another effect on the cornea which is frequently encountered is desquamation of the superficial epithelium, cocaine being one of the chief offenders. But all local anaesthetics have some deleterious effect on the corneal epithelium due to the insensibility produced.

The three most commonly used topical anaesthetics are amethocaine (Tetracaine; Pantocaine; Pontocaine; Decicaine), proxymetacaine (Ophthaine, *Squib*; Proparacaine, 'Uni-Mins', *Barnes-Hind*), and oxybuprocaine hydrochloride (*Smith and Nephew Pharmaceuticals;* Dorsacaine, Novesine, *Wander*). All have the advantage of causing no subsidiary actions such as cycloplegia, mydriasis or vasoconstriction. Their legal category is indicated in Appendix E, *Table III*.

Amethocaine Hydrochloride

Solutions of 0.5 or 1 per cent cause some initial discomfort on instillation, due to a stinging sensation. Onset time of anaesthesia is 10–30 seconds and duration of anaesthesia is about

10 minutes. It has no subsidiary actions, and only very rarely does it cause any toxic effects.

Amethocaine is incompatible with alkalis, bromides, silver salts and oxidizing agents, and solutions should be protected from light.

Proxymetacaine (Proparacaine) Hydrochloride

A 0.5 per cent solution is a very satisfactory all-round anaesthetic, pleasant, non-irritant, safe, effective and free from subsidiary actions (Rycroft, 1964). With a single instillation, the onset of anaesthesia occurs in an average of 13 seconds and persists for an average of 15.2 minutes (Boozan and Cohen, 1953). Its initial discomfort is considerably less than with amethocaine, and allergic manifestations have occurred only rarely. In a clinical evaluation of cocaine, Dorsacaine (Novesine), Proxymetacaine, Pontocaine and Butyn, Jervey (1955) found that Proxymetacaine seemed to produce the least discomfort. It is recommended that Proxymetacaine should be stored in a refrigerator after opening, to prevent discoloration. Once discoloured, it should be discarded.

Oxybuprocaine Hydrochloride (Benoxinate)

Oxybuprocaine hydrochloride, 0.4 per cent, is a synthetic p-aminobenzoic acid derivative incompatible with alkalis and silver salts. Onset time of anaesthesia is about 30 seconds and duration of anaesthesia about 10–15 minutes. Emmerich, Carter and Berens (1955) compared Benoxinate, 0.4 per cent, with Pontocaine, 0.5 per cent and found that sensations of irritation were significantly less with Benoxinate, and that the microscopic changes in the epithelium of the cornea were significantly less after the application of Benoxinate.

Topical anaesthetics are used primarily in contact lens practice prior to taking eye impressions. For this purpose, usually two to three drops are instilled – the first into the lower conjunctival sac, and the subsequent drops on to the superior limbal region, so allowing the anaesthetic to run gently over the whole cornea. This ensures that the whole cornea is effectively anaesthetized. One drop can also be instilled in the fixing eye to inhibit the blink reflex. Regardless of the particular anaesthetic which is used, it is of the utmost importance to ensure that either the corneal sensitivity has returned or that the eye is adequately protected by an eyepad or shade before the patient leaves the practice. The possible hazard of a foreign body becoming embedded in an insensitive cornea must not be overlooked.

Following the instillation into the conjunctival sac of a local anaesthetic, lacrimation may be reduced, and to prevent corneal epithelial drying from occurring (which is liable to cause a rapid and severe drop in vision) patients should be encouraged to blink frequently until normal sensitivity returns (about 15–20 minutes). Alternatively, an artificial tears solution may be instilled. This keeps the cornea moist. Eye-rubbing should be discouraged as the surface epithelial cells may be damaged or dislodged.

CONJUNCTIVAL DECONGESTANTS

These are drugs which may be used to prevent conjunctival injection during the impression process or during prolonged fitting procedures. The two preparations most frequently used are adrenaline (epinephrine) and naphazoline, the former being the more widely used. Both are sympathomimetics, acting as vasoconstrictors, producing only slight, if any, mydriatic effect, depending on the pigmentation of the iris, a dark iris being least affected.

More details are given in Appendix E, *Tables I* and *III* at the end of this volume.

Adrenaline Acid Tartrate *B.P.* (Epinephrine)

This is the form generally used for preparing eyedrops, though adrenaline hydrochloride is also sometimes used. Solutions are sterilized by autoclaving, with the addition of sodium metabisulphite. Adrenaline solutions must, however, be kept in well-secured amber-coloured bottles protected from the light and air. If the solution does become discoloured, it should be discarded. As a conjunctival decongestant, adrenaline, 0.1 per cent is used, one or two drops being instilled into the lower conjunctival sac, which has a time course of about 1 hour.

Adverse systemic effects from its topical administration are rare but include skin pallor, tremors, marked nervousness and increased respiratory and heart rate and blood pressure. Pupil dilatation may occur if instillation follows the use of a topical anaesthetic, or probably more likely, when there is damage to the corneal epithelium. A miotic should be used if there is considered to be any risk of precipitating an attack of acute narrow-angle glaucoma.

Naphazoline

This is available as the nitrate or hydrochloride, the nitrate being most frequently used as it is compatible with silver nitrate. It is a quick-acting, powerful and prolonged vasoconstrictor, used as a 1:1000 or 1:2000 aqueous solution, the latter strength usually being considered adequate. In action it is similar to adrenaline, but they are not chemically related. It has the advantage over adrenaline of being more stable to heat, light and air.

Adverse side-effects are not common and it has no marked effect on pupil size, amplitude of accommodation or on the ocular tension. Hurwitz and Thompson (1950), using 0.1 per cent naphazoline hydrochloride, found only a slight mydriatic effect, this occurring mainly in those subjects with lightly pigmented irides. They also found a negligible effect on accommodation.

One or two drops instilled into the lower conjunctival sac are adequate and it has a time course of about 4 hours. As with all vasoconstrictors, excessive use over long periods, particularly in chronic conditions, is not advised as the blood vessels gradually cease to react to it, and hyperaemia will persist.

A preparation which contains a vasoconstrictor (decongestant) and an antihistamine (anti-allergic) is suitable for contact lens practice, where in general the injection of the conjunctiva is due to a non-inflammatory cause. One such preparation (see Appendix E, *Table III*) contains 0.05 per cent w/v xylometazoline hydrochloride (vasoconstrictor) and 0.5 per cent w/v antazoline sulphate (antihistamine). Following instillation the effects last about 8 hours.

In addition to the preparations already mentioned there are a number of proprietary brands of decongestant solutions containing phenylephrine hydrochloride, 0.12–0.25 per cent, which have a time course of about 4 hours. These solutions (see Appendix E, *Table I* at the end of this volume) are not listed in the Poisons Rules and are therefore freely available to the general public.

The advisability of their indiscriminate use must be questioned, particularly with the inherent, if rare, danger of precipitating an attack of closed-angle glaucoma in a susceptible subject. Also, if a patient has an injected eye from wearing a contact lens, it is preferable that he seeks the advice of his practitioner so that the cause can be remedied. To instil a decongestant agent only masks the primary cause of the injection. These preparations can also cause discoloration of a hydrophilic lens if instilled into the eye with such a lens *in situ*.

DIAGNOSTIC STAINING AGENTS

Fluorescein

Fluorescein stains damaged living tissue of the cornea and conjunctiva green and yellow respectively. It is used as a means of checking the contact lens fit and for detecting corneal abrasions. It may also be used to demonstrate patency of the lacrimal drainage channels into the nose, which is essential if contact lenses are to be fitted. A few minutes after instillation of fluorescein into the conjunctival sac of one eye only, the nose should be blown into a paper tissue which should show green staining under ultra-violet light. The other side may then be checked.

The official salt is Fluorescein Sodium *B.P.* either as a 1 or 2 per cent solution, or as fluorescein-impregnated paper strips. It is essential that all solutions (other than single-dose units) are adequately protected with a bactericidal agent as *Ps. aeruginosa* can readily thrive in fluorescein (Chatoo, 1963; Doris, 1964). The impregnated strips have the advantage that they can be stored for an indefinite period without fear of deterioration or contamination, provided that they are kept dry.

For the instillation of fluorescein solution, the glass rod technique is an ideal method (*Figures 3.6* and *3.7*). It ensures sterility by the use of a fresh sterile glass rod each time, which is never directly brought into contact with the fluorescein solution in the bottle. This method also regulates more accurately the amount instilled into the eye. There is nothing more unsightly than the excess stain sometimes seen surrounding the eyes and/or the faces of patients after its use. Following the

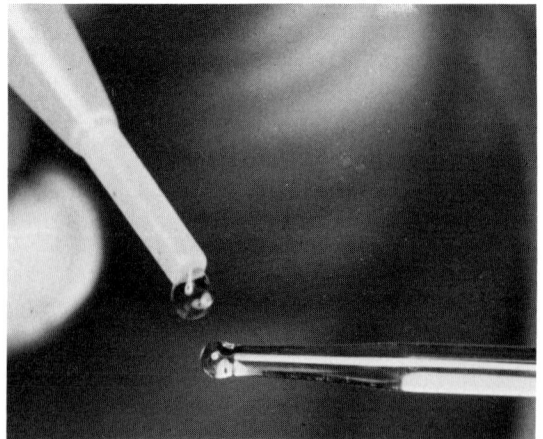

Figure 3.6—One drop of fluorescein solution is instilled onto the bulbous end of a glass rod

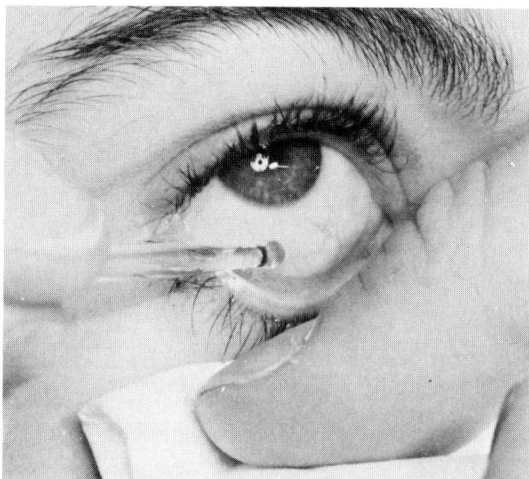

Figure 3.7–The lower eyelid is gently pulled down, and the fluorescein instilled into the conjunctival sac

instillation of fluorescein for detection of abrasions, it is usually advisable to instil a drop of normal saline solution to wash away any excess fluorescein from the normal tears film (*Figure 3.8*), which might otherwise mask any damaged areas. Such areas, if present, may then be observed with ultra-violet light, an ordinary corneal loupe, or a slit lamp biomicroscope.

Fluorescein sodium (molecular weight 376) has been used routinely for many years in contact lens practice for evaluating the fit of a hard contact lens. However, it is unsuitable for evaluating the fit of a hydrophilic lens because of its absorption and binding to the lens. If fluorescein has been instilled into the eye there should be a delay of at least 1 hour (and preferably 2) before a hydrophilic lens is inserted.

A fluorescent water-soluble dye, Fluorexon, has been described by Refojo, Miller and Fiore (1972) and Refojo, Korb and Silverman (1972). It is a derivative of fluorescein but has a molecular weight of 710 and is absorbed much more slowly than fluorescein. The stain is reversible and washes out of the lens by boiling it in a saline solution. Fluorexon can be used as a 0.5 per cent solution and stains damaged epithelium of the cornea and conjunctiva, but the fluorescence is not as effective as fluorescein. Also, solutions of Fluorexon are just as vulnerable to contamination as fluorescein (Refojo, Korb and Silverman, 1972) hence, single-dose eyedrops are advocated. Fluorexon is no longer commercially available.

Rose Bengal

This is a fat-soluble stain and is used as a 1 per cent solution to determine the presence of dried areas of corneal and conjunctival epithelium, prior to contact lens fitting, as well as the influence of facial skin conditions on contact lens tolerance. Its action differs from fluorescein in staining dead or desquamated tissue red when viewed under white light, the presence of excess desquamation being an indication of an abnormal ocular condition or skin disease, either clinical or subclinical.

The conjunctiva and skin are of the same origin; and if the palpebral or bulbar conjunctiva stain red, it is advisable to reject the patient for contact lenses until medical advice on the ocular or facial skin condition has been obtained. Otherwise, the wearing of contact lenses may only aggravate matters. Conditions in which positive staining occur are: keratoconjunctivitis sicca (Sjögrens syndrome), seborrhoeic eczema, acne vulgaris and acne rosacea.

A mixed stain of 1 per cent fluorescein and 1 per cent rose bengal has been suggested by Norn (1964) as serving a useful dual purpose in determining both epithelial lesions and degenerate epithelial cells. As mucus is also stained red by

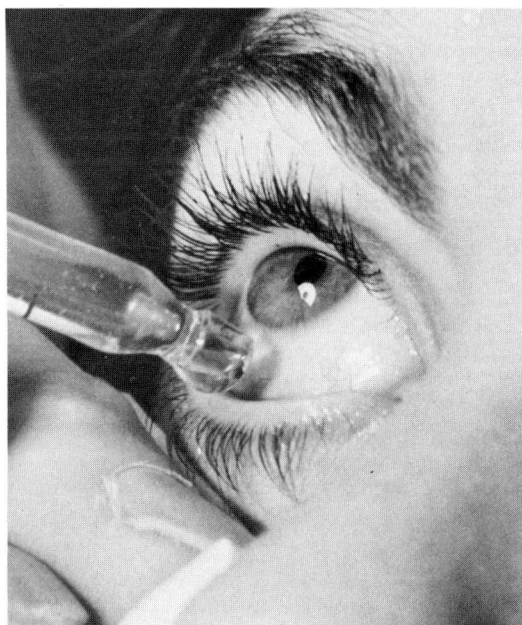

Figure 3.8–One drop of normal saline solution is instilled into the conjunctival sac prior to examination. Care is taken not to touch the globe, lids or lashes with the dropper tip

rose bengal, it can be differentiated if necessary by instilling one drop of 1 per cent alcian blue (Norn, 1964) which stains the mucus blue.

CHEMOTHERAPEUTIC AGENTS

The most effective of the chemotherapeutic agents are the broad spectrum antibiotics which with one exception (framycetin), however, are not available to the ophthalmic optician. As the use of a topical chemotherapeutic agent is purely prophylactic in contact lens practice, there are a number of preparations which meet this requirement. They are mainly preparations which belong to the sulphonamide group of drugs, and as a few patients are allergic to sulphonamides, it is advisable to exclude this possibility by questioning the patient before their use. Their legal categories are indicated in Appendix E, *Table III*.

Framycetin Sulphate

Framycetin is available as 0.5 per cent drops or ointment. It is active against many strains of Gram-positive and Gram-negative bacteria, for example *Staph. aureus*, *E. coli*, and some strains of *Ps. aeruginosa* and *Pr. vulgaris*. It is not inactivated by pus or bacteria. Resistant strains can develop with indiscriminate use. Framycetin is very similar in properties to Neomycin.

Mafenide Propionate

This is available in 5 per cent solution only, the recommendation for its use being 3 or 4 drops, 3–4 times daily. It is relatively insoluble but has the general properties of sulphonamides and has the same spectrum of action.

Sulphacetamide Sodium

This is the sulphonamide most frequently used in ophthalmic practice. It is available as 10, 15, 20 or 30 per cent eyedrops, or as a 2.5, 6 or 10 per cent eye ointment. The eyedrops must be protected from light, otherwise they deteriorate and show signs or precipitation.

Sulphacetamide Sodium and Zinc Sulphate

This contains sulphacetamide, 5 per cent, and zinc sulphate, 0.1 per cent, in an aqueous solution. Its antibacterial activity is considered equal to that of a 30 per cent solution of sulphacetamide sodium.

The range of activity of these chemotherapeutic agents is confined to the sulphonamide-sensitive organisms, which include many of the Gram-positive and some of the Gram-negative organisms.

Propamidine Isethionate

This is another useful chemotherapeutic agent; it is available as an eye ointment containing 0.15 per cent dibromopropamidine isethionate, or as eyedrops containing 0.1 per cent propamidine isethionate. The range of activity is against pyogenic cocci and some Gram-negative organisms, *Esch. coli* and *P. vulgaris*; some activity is also shown *in vitro* against *Ps. aeruginosa*. It is also liable to cause an allergic reaction in a few patients.

Care must be taken not to fall into a false sense of security in thinking that a single application of any one of these agents necessarily prevents an infection of the eye becoming established. Only repeated applications may be able to resolve an infection, then it becomes a therapeutic rather than a prophylactic measure (the former being the responsibility of a medical practitioner).

MISCELLANEOUS AGENTS

Hypertonic Saline Solution

This is useful for the relief of corneal oedema. Its continued use for therapeutic purposes to relieve corneal oedema during extended soft lens wear, necessary for some pathological ocular conditions, should be carried out under medical supervision (*see* page 80).

STATUTES AND REGULATIONS

The Medicines Act was enacted in the United Kingdom in 1968 but the orders relating to the sale and supply of drugs were not made until 1978. The appointed day was 1st February, 1978, but because of the impact of the legislation a deferment of some of its effects was made until 1st August of the same year.

The Medicines Act covers all aspects of the manufacture, testing and sale of medicinal agents and it is proposed to concentrate here on Part III which specifically deals with the sale and supply of medicinal substances.

The effect of this part of the Act is to divide products into three groups. There is a provision for setting up a General Sales List, which contains all those drugs and agents which it is thought can be safely sold to the general public without the supervision of a pharmacist. The General Sales List was published in 1978 and contains some of the pharmaceutical agents used by ophthalmic opticians, for example, hypromellose. However, in Schedule 6 of the order there is a specific exclusion from the General Sales List of all eyedrops and eye ointments.

The other list of drugs is the Prescription Only Medicines List which contains those drugs, only obtainable on the prescription of a doctor, dentist or veterinary surgeon. As with all of this type of legislation there are exemptions and special cases. However, again, eyedrops are singled out as requiring special control. For example, amethocaine hydrochloride is POM (Prescription Only Medicine) only when injected or applied to the eye.

Substances which appear on neither list are referred to as pharmacy medicines and although available for sale to anyone can only be sold under the supervision of a pharmacist. Thus, if an eyedrop is not on the POM list it is automatically a pharmacy medicine (designated as P).

The lists published in 1978 make specific provision for the use of drugs by the ophthalmic optician. In the POM list there is a provision for the registered ophthalmic optician to obtain and supply certain drugs. (The original list as published has been modified by further statutory controls and some agents have been deleted and some added.) The agents listed include mydriatic/cycloplegics, miotics and sulphonamides. There is a separate order allowing the ophthalmic optician to obtain but not supply local anaesthetics and oxyphenbutazone ointments. Appendix E, *Tables I* and *III* at the end of this volume, give details of the drugs and eyedrops used in association with contact lens fitting and wearing.

Contact lens solutions and contact lenses were brought under the Medicines Act by an order made in 1976. However, this particular order was mainly concerned with the manufacture and labelling and made no provision for subjecting them to control of sale.

In 1980, several important rules were applied to contact lens solutions which can be summarized as follows. With effect from January 1st, no new solution, not previously on the market, could be sold without a product licence. For solutions on the market by that day, data was required to be submitted to the DHSS before 1st March. Such solutions would have a transitional exemption. It is the intention of the DHSS to phase in the licensing of these products by setting different 'end dates' for such exemptions. Within 6 months of these end dates, labelling will have to conform to requirements. One interesting point is that pharmacists and holders of the DCLP will be able to relabel contact lens solutions.

No decision has been made yet as to the avenues for the sale of contact lens solutions. It is expected that this will be kept under review and orders made if it is considered necessary.

As yet the only effect of this legislation will be to slow the introduction of new products on the market. Its effects on existing solutions will occur at a later stage.

ACKNOWLEDGEMENTS

The authors wish to express their sincere thanks to the many laboratories and individuals who contributed information for use in this chapter. Especial thanks go to Dr Chuck Shiveley of Alcon Laboratories, Fort Worth, Texas and the Staff of Messrs. Smith and Nephew Research Ltd., Gilston Park, Essex.

REFERENCES

Allansmith, M. R., Korb, D. R., Greiner, J. K., Henriquez, A. S., Simon, M. A. and Finnemore, V. M. (1977). 'Giant papillary conjunctivitis in contact lens wearers.' *Am. J. Ophthal.* **83**, 697–708

Anderson, K. and Keynes, R. (1958). 'Infected cork closures and apparent survival of organisms in antiseptic solutions.' *Br. med. J.* **2**, 274–275

Baker, S. R. and Remington, J. S. (1972). 'Contamination of soft gel lenses.' *Contacto* **16**(3), 4–6

Barkmar, R., Germanis, M., Karpe, G. and Malmborg, A. S. (1969). 'Preservatives in eye drops.' *Acta Ophthal.* **47**, 461–475

Bernstein, H. N., Stow, M. N. and Maddox, Y. (1973). 'Evaluation of the asepticization procedure for Soflens hydrophilic contact lens.' *Canad. J. Ophthal.* **8**, 575

Blanco, M., Curry, B. and Boghosian, M. P. (1975). 'Studies of the effect of enzymatic cleaning on the physical structure of hydrophilic lenses.' *Contacto* **19**(5), 17–20

Blank, I. (1975). 'Sterilization of soft, hydrophilic acrylate and methacrylate copolymer materials.' U.S. Patent. 3,876,768

Boozan, W. C. and Cohen, I. J. (1953). 'A new topical anaesthetic for the eye.' Am. J. Ophthal. 36, 1619–1621

Brawner, L. and Jessop, D. G. (1962). 'A review of contact lens solutions.' Contacto 6, 49–51

Brown, M. R. W. (1968). 'Survival of Pseudomonas aeruginosa in fluorescein solution. Preservative action of PMN and EDTA.' J. Pharm. Sci. 57, 389–392

Brown, M. R. W. and Richards, R. M. E. (1965). 'Effect of ethylenediaminetetra-acetate on the resistance of Pseudomonas aeruginosa to antibacterial agents.' Nature (Lond.) 207, 1391

Brown, S. I., Bloomfield, S., Pearce, D. B. and Tragakis, M. (1974). 'Infections with the therapeutic soft lens.' Archs Ophthal. 91, 275–277

Browne, R. K., Anderson, A. N. and Charvez, B. W. (1974). 'Solving the solution problem.' Optician 167(4325), 19–24

Busschaert, S. C., Szabocik, J. M., Good, R. C. and Woodward, M. R. (1974). 'Challenging the efficacy of the Soflens Aseptor.' J. Am. optom. Ass. 45, 700–703

Carney, L. G. and Hill, R. M. (1975). 'pH profiles: part 1 – one pH, or many?' J. Am. optom. Ass. 46, 1143–1145

Charles, A. M. (1975). 'A comparison of some commercial methods for asepticizing and cleansing hydrogel lenses.' Contacto 19(3), 4–11

Chatoo, B. A. (1963). 'Fluorescein in ophthalmic practice.' Ophthal. Optician 3, 723–735

Cureton, G. L. and Hall, N. C. (1974). 'The separate functions of cleaning and sterilising soft contact lenses.' Am. J. Optom. 51, 406–411

Cureton, G. L. and Sibley, M. J. (1974). 'Soft contact lens solutions, past, present and future.' J. Am. optom. Ass. 45, 285–291

Dabezies, O. H. (1970). 'Contact lens hygiene, past, present and future.' Contact Lens med. Bull. 3(2), 3–15

Dallos, J. and Hughes, W. H. (1972). 'Sterilisation of hydrophilic contact lenses.' Br. J. Ophthal. 56, 114–119

Davies, D. J. G. and Norton, D. A. (1975). 'Challenge tests for antimicrobial agents.' J. Pharm. Pharmac. 27, 383–384

Davis, H., Charles, A. M., Trager, S. and Phares, R. E. (1973). 'The soft lens situation: solutions, sterilization and contamination.' Contacto 17(4), 8–32

Doris, J. A. (1964). 'Maintenance of sterility of eyedrops in ophthalmic practice.' Ophthal. Optician 4, 12–14, 19

Duke-Elder, S. (1965). System of Ophthalmology, Vol. VIII, pp. 141–143. Diseases of the Outer Eye, Part 1 – Diseases of the Conjunctiva and Associated Diseases of the Corneal Epithelium. London; Kimpton

Emmerich, R., Carter, G. Z. and Berens, C. (1955). 'An experimental clinical evaluation of Dorsacaine hydrochloride (Benoxinate, Novesine).' Am. J. Ophthal. 40, 841–848

Feldman, G. L. (1971). 'Sterility with soft lens solutions.' Lecture presented to the Canadian Guild of Dispensing Opticians, October 23rd, Toronto, Ontario

Filppi, J. A., Pfister, R. M. and Hill, R. M. (1973). 'Penetration of hydrophilic contact lenses by Aspergillus fumagatus.' Am. J. Optom. 50, 553–557

Ganju, S. N. (1974). 'The disinfection of hard and soft contact lenses.' Ophthal. Optician 14, 1202–1208

Ganju, S. N. and Cordrey, P. (1975). 'The physical contamination of hydrophilic contact lenses and their restoration.' Optician 170(4398), 19–25

Ganju, S. N. and Thompson, R. E. M. (1975). 'A new cold sterilising system for soft contact lenses.' Contacto 19(1), 19–23

Gasset, A. R., Ishir, Y., Kaufman, H. E. and Miller, T. (1974). 'Cytotoxicity of ophthalmic preservatives.' Am. J. Ophthal. 78, 98–105

Gasset, A. R., Ramer, R. M. and Katzin, D. (1975). 'Hydrogen peroxide sterilisation of hydrophilic contact lenses.' Archs Ophthal. 93, 412–415

Gasson, A. P. (1975). 'Visual considerations with hydrophilic lenses.' Ophthal. Optician 15, 439–448

Gould, H. L. and Inglima, R. (1964). 'Corneal contact lens solutions.' Eye Ear Nose Throat Mon. 43, 39–49

Grosvenor, T., Charles, A. and Callender, M. (1972). 'Soft contact lens bacteriological study.' Ophthal. Optician 12, 1083–1091; and Canad. J. Optom. 34, 11–18

Hampson, R. M. (1973). 'Considerations in the checking and predictability of hydrophilic lenses.' Optician 165(4328), 4–16

Hill, R. M. and Terry, J. E. (1974). 'Ophthalmic solutions: viscosity builders.' Am. J. Optom. 51, 847–851

Hind, H. W. (1975). 'Various aspects of contact lens solutions for hard and soft lenses.' Optician 169(4380), 13–29

Hind, H. W. and Goyan, F. M. (1947). 'A new concept of the role of hydrogen ion concentration and buffer systems in the preparation of ophthalmic solutions.' J. Am. pharm. Ass. 36, 33

Holden, B. A. and Markides, A. J. (1971). 'On the desirability and efficacy of chemical sterilisation of hydrophilic contact lenses.' Aust. J. Optom. 54, 325–336

Hugo, W. B. and Foster, J. H. S. (1964). 'Growth of Pseudomonas aeruginosa in solutions of esters of p-hydroxybenzoic acid.' J. Pharm. Pharmac. 16, 209

Hurwitz, P. and Thompson, J. M. (1950). 'Uses of naphazoline (Privine) in ophthalmology.' Archs Ophthal. 43, 712–717

Hydron Lens Ltd. (1972). Hydron Soft Lens Technical Report, p.19. Hydron Lens Ltd., Harold Hill, Romford, England

Isen, A. A. (1972). 'The Griffin lens.' J. Am. optom. Ass. 43, 275–286

Jervey, J. W. (1955). 'Topical anaesthetics for the eye.' Sth med. J. 48, 770–774

Johnson, D. G. and Littlewood, T. (1975). 'A clinical study to determine patient acceptance and efficiency of a new regimen of soft lens care.' Submitted to Canad. J. Ophthal. Cited by Shiveley (1975a)

Kelsey, J. C. and Sykes, G. (1969). 'A new test for the assessment of disinfectants with particular reference to their use in hospitals.' Pharm. J. 202, 607–609

Knoll, H. A. (1972). 'Microbiology and hydrophilic contact lenses.' Am. J. Optom. 48, 840

Krezanoski, J. Z. (1972a). 'Pharmaceutical aspects of cleaning and sterilizing flexible contact lenses.' Ophthal. Optician 12, 1035–1091

Krezanoski, J. Z. (1972*b*). 'The significance of cleaning hydrophilic contact lenses.' *J. Am. optom. Ass.* **43**, 305–307

Krishna, N. and Brow, F. (1964). 'Polyvinyl alcohol as an ophthalmic vehicle.' *Am. J. Ophthal.* **57**, 99–106

Larke, J. R., Smith, P. G., Pedley, D. G. and Tighe, B. J. (1973). 'A semi-rigid contact lens.' *Ophthal. Optician* **13**, 1065–1067

Larke, J. R. (1974). 'Some bacteriological considerations of soft lens wear.' *Br. J. physiol. Optics* **29**, 66–91

Lerman, S. and Sapp, G. (1971). 'The hydrophilic (Hydron) corneoscleral lens in the treatment of corneal disease.' *Canad. J. Ophthal.* **6**, 1–8

Lindeman-Meester, H. H. M. (1974). 'Fluids for soft contact lenses tested by the Kelsey-Sykes test and Maurer test.' *Contact Lens* **4**(6), 27–29

Litvin, M. W. (1977). 'The incidence of eye infections with contact lenses.' *Optician* **174**(4496), 11–14

Locatcher-Khorazo, D. and Seegal, B. (1972). *Microbiology of the Eye*. St. Louis, Missouri: Mosby

Loran, D. F. C. (1973). 'Surface corrosion of hydrogel contact lenses.' *Contact Lens* **4**(4), 3–10

Loran, D. F. C. (1974). 'Determination of hydrogel contact lens radii by projection.' *Ophthal. Optician* **14**, 980–985

Lowbury, E. J. L. (1958). 'Contamination of cetrimide and other fluids by *Ps. pyoceanea*.' *Br. J. industr. Med.* **8**, 22

MacGregor, D. R. and Elliker, P. R.(1958). 'A comparison of some properties of strains of *Pseudomonas aeruginosa* sensitive and resistant to quaternary ammonium compounds.' *Canad. J. Microbiol.* **4**, 499–503

Mandell, R. B. (1974). *Contact Lens Practice, Hard and Flexible Lenses*, p.819. Springfield, Ill: Thomas

Matas, B. R., Spencer, W. H. and Hayes, T. L. (1972). 'Scanning electron microscopy of hydrophilic contact lenses.' *Archs Ophthal.* **88**, 287–295

Maurer, I. C. (1969). 'A test for stability and long term effectiveness in disinfectants.' *Pharm. J.* **203**, 529–534

McBride, R. J. and Mackie, M. E. L. (1974). 'Evaluation of the antibacterial activity of contact lens solutions.' *J. Pharm. Pharmac.* **26**, 899–900

McMonnies, C. M. (1978). 'Allergic complications in contact lens wear.' *Int. Contact Lens Clinic* **15**, 182–189

Morgan, J. F. (1975*a*). Paper presented before the Canadian Contact Lens Association of Ophthalmologists, June, 1975. Cited by Shively, C.D. (1975*a*)

Morgan, J. F. (1975*b*). 'Evaluation of a cleaning agent for hydrophilic contact lenses.' *Canad. J. Ophthal.* **10**, 214

Morrison, R. J. (1966). 'Hydrophilic contact lenses.' *J. Am. optom. Ass.* **37**, 211–218

Morrison, R. J., Tresser, A., Vigodsky, H. S. and Pollan, S. (1973). 'The effectivity of hygiene procedures upon soft contact lens material.' *Contacto* **17**(1), 23–27

Mote, E. M., Filppi, J. A. and Hill, R. M. (1972). 'Does heating arrest organisms in hydrophilic cases?' *J. Am. optom. Ass.* **43**, 302–304

Norn, M. S. (1964). 'Vital staining in practice using a mixed stain and alcian blue.' *Br. J. physiol. Optics* **21**, 293–298

Norton, D. A., Davies, D. J. G., Richardson, N. E., Meakin, B. J. and Keall, A. (1974). 'The antimicrobial efficiencies of contact lens solutions.' *J. Pharm. Pharmac.* **26**, 841–846. Also reproduced in *Optician* **168**(4360), 14–16

Otten, M. and Szabocsik, J. M. (1976). 'Measurement of preservative binding with Soflens (polymacon) contact lens.' *Aust. J. Optom.* **59**, 277–283

Phares, R. E. (1972*a*). 'Soft lens care.' *J. Am. optom. Ass.* **43**, 308–313

Phares, R. E. (1972*b*). 'Microbiology and hygienic care of hydrophilic lenses.' *Contacto* **16**(3), 10–12

Phillips, A. J. (1969). 'Contact lens plastics, solutions and storage – some implications.' *Ophthal. Optician* **9**, 75–79

Poster, M. G. (1972). 'A preliminary study of the service life of the "Soflens".' *Am. J. Optom.* **49**, 868–870

Quinn, L. H. and Burnside, R. M. (1951). 'Gantrisin in the treatment of conjunctivitis.' *Eye Ear Nose Throat Mon.* **30**, 81–82

Refojo, M. F., Korb, D. R. and Silverman, H. I. (1972). 'Clinical evaluation of a new fluorescent dye for hydrogel lenses.' *J. Am. optom. Ass.* **43**, 321–326

Refojo, M. F., Miller, D. and Fiore, N. S. (1972). 'A new fluorescent stain for soft hydrophilic lens fitting.' *Archs Ophthal.* **87**, 275–277

Refojo, M. F. and Holly, F. J. (1977). 'Tear protein adsorption on hydrogels: a possible cause of contact lens allergy.' *Contact Lens J.* **3**(1), 23–25

Richards, R. M. E. and McBride, R. J. (1972). 'The preservation of ophthalmic solutions with antibacterial combinations.' *J. Pharm. Pharmac.* **24**, 145–148

Richards, R. M. E. and Reary, J. M. E. (1972). 'Changes in antibacterial activity of thiomersal and P.M.N. on autoclaving with certain adjuvants.' *J. Pharm. Pharmac.* **24**, (Suppl.) 84–89

Riegelman, S., Vaughan, D. G. and Okumoto, M. (1956). 'Antibacterial agents in *Pseudomonas aeruginosa* contaminated ophthalmic solutions.' *J. Am. pharm. Ass. (Sc.Ed.)* **45**, 93–98

Ruben, M. (1966). 'Preliminary observations of soft (hydrophilic) contact lenses.' *Proc. R. Soc. Med.* **59**, 531–532

Ruben, M., Tripathi, R. C. and Winder, A. F. (1975). 'Calcium deposition as a cause of spoilation of hydrophilic soft contact lenses.' *Br. J. Ophthal.* **59**, 141–148

Rycroft, P. V. (1964). 'Ophthaine (proparacaine hydrochloride) a local anaesthetic for ophthalmic surgery.' *Br. J. Ophthal.* **48**, 102–104

Sagan, W. and Schwaderer, K. N. (1974). 'A new cleaning technique for hydrophilic contact lenses.' *J. Am. optom. Ass.* **45**, 266–269

Shively, C. D. (1975*a*). *Accessory Solutions Utilized in Contact Lens Care and Practice*. Private monograph published by Alcon Universal Ltd., Fort Worth, Texas

Shively, C. D. (1975*b*). 'Hydrophilic flexible lens cleaning and chemical disinfection systems.' *Contacto* **19**(3), 33–37

Sibley, M. J. and Yung, G. (1973). 'A technique for the determination of chemical binding to soft contact lenses.' *Am. J. Optom.* **50**, 710–714

Smith, C. H. (1954). 'Bacteriology of the healthy conjunctiva.' *Br. J. Ophthal.* **38**, 719–726

Snyder, A. C., Hill, R. M. and Bailey, N. J. (1977). 'Home sterilization: fact or fiction?' *Contact Lens Forum*, February, 41–43

Stone, J. (1976). Personal communication

Storey, K. (1973). 'Question corner.' *Ophthal. Optician* **13**, 1219

Strachan, J. P. (1971). 'Physiology, pharmacology and contact lenses.' *Aust. J. Optom.* **54**(1), 3–14

Sussman, J. D. and Friedman, M. (1969). 'Irritation of rabbit eyes caused by contact lens wetting solutions.' *Am. J. Ophthal.* **68**, 703–706

Thompson, R. E. M. and Mansell, P. E. (1976). 'The cleansing and decontamination of hydrophilic contact lenses – an improved standard chemical method.' *Optician* **171**(4419), 11–15

Toxicol Laboratories Ltd. (1972). 'Hydrosoak and Hydrosol – a comprehensive study.' p.2. Independent study carried out for Messrs. Contactosol Ltd., Esher, Surrey

Tragakis, M. P., Brown, S. I. and Pearce, D. B. (1973). 'Bacteriological studies of contamination associated with soft contact lenses.' *Am. J. Ophthal.* **75**, 496–499

Tripathi, R. C. and Ruben, M. (1972). 'Degenerative changes in a soft hydrophilic contact lens.' *Ophthal. Res.* **4**, 185–192

United States Food and Drug Administration (1973). *'Microbiological Guidelines for New Contact Lenses.'* May, 1973

Wilson, L. A., Kuehne, J. W., Hall, S. W. and Ahearn, D. G. (1971). 'Microbial contamination in ocular cosmetics.' *Am. J. Ophthal.* **71**, 1298–1302

Chapter 4

Practical Optics of Contact Lenses and Aspects of Contact Lens Design

Janet Stone and J. L. Francis

This chapter has been enlarged since the first edition, to include several new features which have been requested by interested contact lens practitioners and readers. Thus, the relevant aspects of soft contact lenses have been included throughout the chapter, and worked numerical examples are given to illustrate suitable methods of calculation. To this end the booklet *Optical Tables for Contact Lens Work* by J. L. Francis, published by Hatton Press in 1968, has been incorporated in a modified and extended version. Its text is included in the substance of the chapter and its tables are amalgamated with those in the Appendices at the end of this volume. Also included are two approaches to the design of contact lenses; one being a somewhat mathematical approach involving mainly the use of sagitta to determine the necessary radii and thickness values for various portions of the lens, and the other the method of drawing out lenses to scale. Both have a place in the manufacture and specification of contact lenses, the mathematical approach being amenable to the computer treatment of lens design. Finally, some examination questions from past Visual Optics papers of the British Optical Association's Advanced Contact Lens Examination are included with their answers, so that examination candidates can satisfy themselves of the correctness of their approach to numerical questions, at least.

There are two main aspects to be considered when dealing with the optics of contact lenses — the effects on the wearer of the optical differences from spectacles; and the necessity for the practitioner to understand the components which affect the back vertex power of the contact-lens/liquid-lens system. There is some overlap of these

two aspects, but for the sake of convenience they are discussed separately in the two following sections. In the second section a set of approximate rules is included, the use of which should permit contact lens practitioners to make quick and reasonably accurate estimates of changes in power caused by altering certain lens parameters. In both sections it is assumed that the reader has an understanding of basic optics and vergence considerations. The Cartesian sign convention is used throughout. For further understanding of the basic principles involved readers are referred to the works of Bennett (1966), Obstfeld (1978) and Emsley (1955).

THE PRACTICAL EFFECTS OF OPTICAL DIFFERENCES BETWEEN CONTACT LENSES AND SPECTACLES

Again, it is convenient to subdivide this section; but it will be apparent to the reader that there is an overlap between the subdivisions. For example, a myope's eyes look bigger without negative spectacle lenses for the same reason that the myope himself sees objects larger than with spectacles — because the minifying effect of the spectacle lenses is removed.

The various differences, and similarities, between contact lenses and spectacles will now be considered.

COSMETIC APPEARANCE

Aside from the generally improved appearance that is usually achieved by doing away with spectacles, the magnification of the spectacle lenses is also eliminated. An observer therefore sees the eyes looking their normal size — smaller than with spectacles for a hypermetrope and bigger for a myope. Ugly appearances due to the prismatic effects of spectacle lenses are also removed.

FIELD OF VIEW OR FIELD OF FIXATION, AND FIELD OF VISION

The wearer of a pair of centred contact lenses has a field of view equal in size to his field of fixation, that is, limited only by the extent to which he can move his eyes. This normally gives a clear field of view of about $100°$.

the other hand, the hypermetropic spectacle wearer (*Figure 4.2*) has a real field of view smaller than $80°$. This means that, on transferring to contact lenses, the myope must move his eyes about more to see the same area of the visual field as he saw with his spectacles. The reverse applies to the hypermetrope.

The sizes of the real and apparent fields of view through the spectacle lens, are easily calculated. The angular subtense of the spectacle lens at the eye's centre of rotation, C, gives the apparent macular field of view, B. For example, size of spectacle lens, 50 mm. Thus, the semi-diameter is 25 mm. Distance from spectacle lens to C is 25 mm. Therefore $\frac{1}{2}B = \tan^{-1}\frac{25}{25} = 45°$. And thus $B = 90°$.

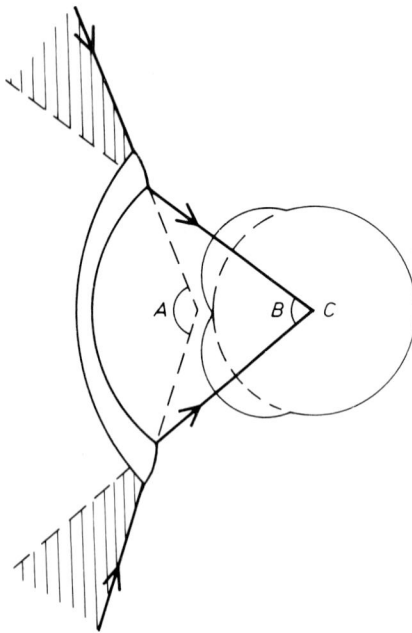

Figure 4.1–Field of view of a myope through a spectacle lens. A = Actual macular field of view. B = Apparent macular field of view. A > B. C = Centre of rotation of eye. Hatched area is seen double due to prismatic effect (doubling is minimized by the spectacle frame, if present)

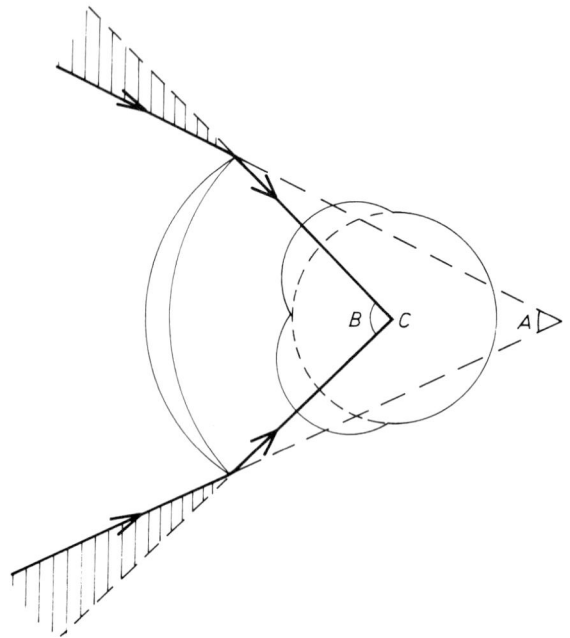

Figure 4.2–Field of view of a hypermetrope through a spectacle lens. A = Actual macular field of view. B = Apparent macular field of view. A < B. C = Centre of rotation of eye. Blind area due to prismatic effect (and spectacle frame when present) is shown hatched

By comparison, the clear field of view of the spectacle wearer is limited by the size and vertex distance of the spectacle lens and is restricted to an apparent field of about $80°$ (although blurred vision is possible beyond the limits of the spectacle lens or frame as far as the eyes can rotate). *Figure 4.1* shows that in fact the myopic spectacle wearer has a much larger real field of view than this, depending on the power of the spectacle lens. On

To obtain the size of the real macular field of view, A, requires that the position of the image of C, as formed by the spectacle lens, be found. Then A is the angular subtense of the spectacle lens at that point. Using the same example as above, if the lens has a power of -10.00 D, and making use of the usual nomenclature for object and image distances, then: $l = -25$ mm. Therefore, $L = -40.00$ D. $F = -10.00$ D. Thus, $L' = L + F =$

-50.00 D. $l' = 1000/L' = -20$ mm. C is thus imaged 20 mm from the spectacle lens, on the same side as C. Therefore, $\frac{1}{2}A = \tan^{-1}\frac{25}{20} = 51° 20'$. And thus $A = 102° 40'$.

In addition, the prismatic effects of the spectacle lenses cause blind areas in the peripheral visual field of the hypermetrope and areas of doubled vision for the myope, as illustrated in *Figures 4.2* and *4.1* respectively. The blind area experienced by a hypermetrope is enlarged due to the thickness of the spectacle frame. This prismatic effect and the blind area are particularly troublesome to aphakics owing to the high power of the spectacle lenses. Contact lenses afford great relief.

Whereas the average spectacle wearer accustoms himself to the presence of a spectacle frame in his peripheral visual field, the contact lens wearer must get used to an effect similar to some entoptic phenomena. In corneal lens wearers, this effect is a halo or partial halo in the peripheral visual field caused by refraction of light through the peripheral zone of the lens, including transitions, and through the surrounding tears film. The wearer of fenestrated scleral lenses experiences a similar effect due to the bubble, which gives rise to unusual reflections and refraction of light. In both cases, the effect subsides as the lenses settle and lacrimation decreases. However, a slight effect may always remain, particularly if the pupil is large and the anterior chamber deep (Stone, 1959). *Figure 4.3* illustrates the optical reasons for these effects.

OBLIQUE ABERRATIONS

Even best-form spectacle lenses allow objects viewed through their periphery to suffer from the effects of oblique aberrations – these being oblique astigmatism, coma, distortion, transverse chromatic aberration and curvature of field. Contact lenses remain almost centred in all directions of gaze, and any imperfections they impart to the retinal image are therefore kept to a minimum. By contrast, the visual acuity of a person wearing high-powered correcting spectacle lenses may drop slightly when the eyes are rotated to look through the most peripheral zones of the lenses.

PRISMATIC EFFECTS

Apart from the prismatic effects of spectacle lenses already mentioned, which affect both the appearance of a person and his field of view, two other factors must be considered. These are the prismatic effects of spectacle lenses during convergence and those due to the anisometropic spectacle correction, when the eyes make version movements.

Convergence

Spectacles optically centred for distance vision but which are used for all distances of gaze differ from contact lenses, which move with the eyes and thus remain centred (or nearly so) for all distances and positions of gaze.

Thus, during near vision, a spectacle-wearing myope experiences a base-in prism effect and a spectacle-wearing hypermetrope a base-out effect, as shown in *Figure 4.4*. Provided that contact lenses remain optically centred, no such prism effect is experienced by the contact lens wearer. Therefore, for a given object distance, the contact-lens-wearing myope exerts more convergence and the hypermetrope less convergence than with spectacles.

Table **4.1**–Comparison of Convergence with Spectacles and Contact Lenses

Spectacle refraction in dioptres	Convergence in prism dioptres			
	At $\frac{1}{3}$ metre from spectacle plane		At $\frac{1}{4}$ metre from spectacle plane	
	Spectacles	Contact lenses	Spectacles	Contact lenses
-20	11.11	16.66	14.56	21.66
-15	12.11	16.66	15.87	21.66
-10	13.33	16.66	17.56	21.66
-5	14.80	16.66	19.31	21.66
0	16.66	16.66	21.66	21.66
$+5$	19.03	16.66	24.67	21.66
$+10$	22.19	16.66	28.63	21.66
$+15$	26.64	16.66	34.14	21.66

Table 4.1 gives the amount of convergence in prism dioptres exerted by both eyes in various degrees of ametropia, assuming spectacles centred for a distance C.D. of 60 mm and worn 27 mm in front of the eyes' centres of rotation, and contact lenses giving an equivalent power, remaining centred for all distances of gaze and worn 15 mm in front of the centres of rotation of the eyes. *Table 4.2* is used as a basis for the graph in *Figure 4.5*.

The significance of this difference in convergence must be considered in association with changes in accommodation (*see* Accommodation,

94

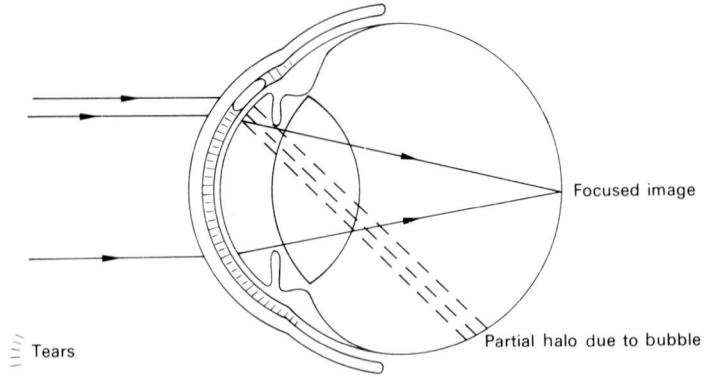

Figure 4.3–A partial halo in the visual field caused by the bubble behind a scleral lens. Similar effects occur with corneal lenses

Tears

Focused image

Partial halo due to bubble

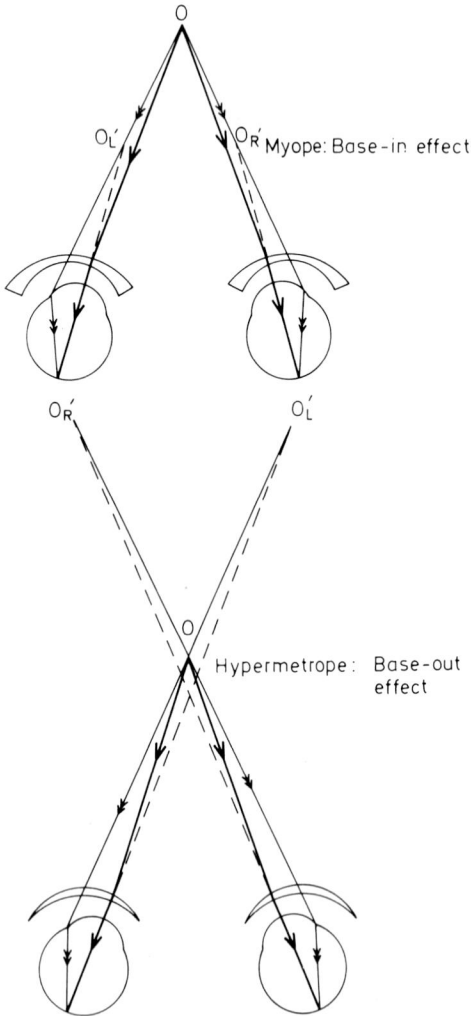

Figure 4.4–Spectacles centred for distance vision give prismatic effects when the eyes converge

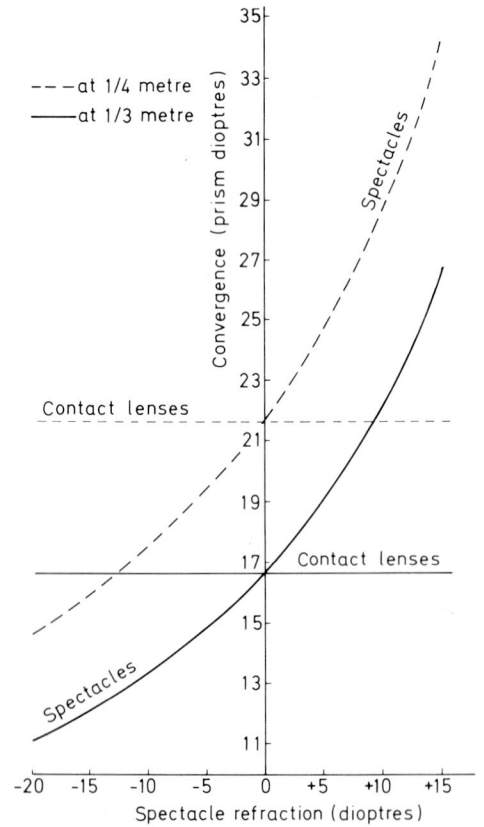

Figure 4.5–Convergence with spectacles and contact lenses

Myopic eye: Base-down effect

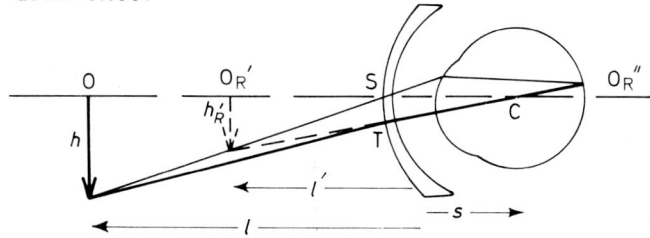

Hypermetropic eye: Base-up effect

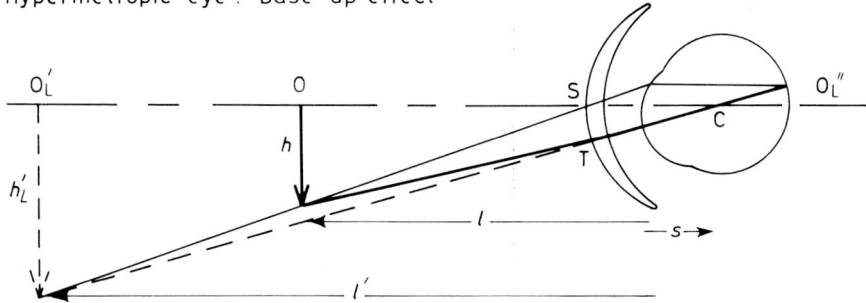

Figure 4.6—Anisometropia: during near vision when wearing spectacles the visual axis of the hypermetropic eye is depressed more than that of the myopic eye. The image seen by the hypermetropic eye is also larger than that seen by the myopic eye. O = object. O_R' and O_L' = images of O formed by the spectacle lenses. O_R'' and O_L'' = retinal images

page 106, where it is shown that the ratio between accommodation and convergence remains the same with spectacles and contact lenses). The effect of the change in convergence alone, when transferrring from spectacles to contact lenses, is only likely to be unfortunate in a myope whose near point of convergence is abnormally remote, when the removal of the base-in prism may be sufficient to disrupt binocular vision at near.

The general effect of transferring from spectacles to contact lenses for near vision, is as if the myope had brought his near task a little closer, for he must converge and accommodate more; whereas for the hypermetrope the reverse applies and it is as if he had increased his working distance.

Anisometropia

Since contact lenses move with the eyes, the visual axes always pass through their optical centres — or very close to them. Thus, differential prismatic effects which can create difficulties for anisometropic spectacle wearers are virtually removed. (The effects of contact lens movement

on the eyes are considered in the section on Incorporation of Prism, below.)

An example will serve to illustrate this:

Spectacle correction: R. −4.00 DS
L. +1.00 DS

Prismatic effect when looking down at an object 10 cm below the horizontal and 25 cm in front of the spectacle plane (assumed to be 25 mm in front of the centres of rotation of the eyes):

R. 3.33 prism dioptres, base-down.
L. 1.00 prism dioptre, base-up.

Difference between the two eyes in the vertical meridian is over 4 prism dioptres, which is too great for the patient to obtain comfortable binocular single vision. This spectacle correction would therefore necessitate vertical head movements rather than eye movements. *Figure 4.6* illustrates the difference in vertical eye rotation that would be required with this spectacle correction, in use as described, as well as the difference in magnification (*see* Relative Spectacle Magnification, page 103).

Calculation of the prismatic effect is simple. The positions and sizes of the images O_R' and O_L'

formed by the spectacle lenses are first found (*Figure 4.6*).

Thus, for the right eye, $l = -25$ cm. Therefore, $L = -4$ D.

Now $F = -4$ D, and since $L + F = L'$, $L' = -8$ D.

Therefore $l' = -12.5$ cm.

Since $\dfrac{h'}{h} = \dfrac{L}{L'}$, $h'_R = 10 \times \dfrac{-4}{-8}$ cm = 5 cm.

And for the left eye, $l = -25$ cm. Therefore, $L = -4$ D.

Now $F = +1$ D, and therefore $L' = -3$ D.

Therefore, $l' = -33.33$ cm.

And $h'_L = 10 \times \dfrac{-4}{-3}$ cm = 13.33 cm.

Then the points (T) at which the two visual axes intersect the spectacle lenses must be found.

There are for each eye, similar triangles, with apex at C and bases at O' and ST (the distance s (SC) is assumed to be 25 mm).

Thus, $\dfrac{\text{ST}}{h'_R} = \dfrac{s}{s-l'}$ and ST = $5 \times \dfrac{2.5}{15.0} = 0.833$ cm

for the right eye

And $\dfrac{\text{ST}}{h'_L} = \dfrac{2.5}{35.83}$

Thus, ST = $13.33 \times \dfrac{2.5}{35.83} = 0.930$ cm for the

left eye.

Now, from Prentice's Law (*see* page 97), the prism effect of the right lens is $-4 \times 0.833 = 3.33$ prism dioptres base-down, and that of the left lens is $+1 \times 0.930 = 0.93$ prism dioptres base-up.

As pointed out, this gives over 4 prism dioptres difference between the two eyes, the actual difference being 4.26 prism dioptres.

An alternative way of looking at this is to calculate the actual angles through which each eye rotates downwards, and then find the difference:

Thus, the right eye rotates downwards by an angle of

$$\tan^{-1} \dfrac{h'_R}{s-l'} = \tan^{-1} \dfrac{5}{2.5-(-12.5)} = \tan^{-1} \dfrac{5}{15}$$

This is an angle of $\dfrac{500}{15}$ prism dioptres = 33.33 prism dioptres.

The left eye rotates downwards by an angle of

$$\tan^{-1} \dfrac{13.33}{2.5-(-33.33)} = \tan^{-1} \dfrac{13.33}{35.83}$$

This is an angle of

$\dfrac{1333}{35.83}$ prism dioptres = 37.20 prism dioptres.

The difference between the rotation required of the two eyes is thus 3.87 prism dioptres, which as expected, differs a little from the value measured in the spectacle plane, which was 4.26 prism dioptres.

The latter method – of determining the angles through which each eye rotates – is the way in which angular values for convergence are also calculated. An object located on the midline between the two eyes (*Figure 4.4*) is then considered as an object of height (*h*) equal to half the interpupillary distance, since this is its distance from the optical axis of the spectacle lens.

Horizontal prismatic differences are more tolerable than vertical differences. In fact, during version movements of the eyes, the anisometropic spectacle wearer learns to make allowance for the increasing prismatic difference as the visual axes intersect points at increasing distances from the optical centres. This habit of allowing for the prismatic difference shows itself as a non-comitant heterophoria which may persist for some time after contact lenses are first worn, and this can at first cause difficulty on lateral rotation of the eyes. From habit, one eye moves more than the other, and objects tend to be seen double until a new extraocular muscle balance is achieved.

INCORPORATION OF PRISM

Most manufacturers of contact lenses prefer not to incorporate more than 3 prism dioptres into either a scleral or a corneal lens, as the thickness difference with such steeply curved surfaces makes more than this amount impracticable, although it can be done on lenses of high power.

Because the prism base always rotates downwards in a corneal lens, and remains down and slightly in, it is impossible to prescribe a horizontal prism satisfactorily. Vertical prism is also limited, therefore, to one lens, and so the maximum vertical prism that may be prescribed is about 3 prism dioptres but this may be be rejected due to physical discomfort. Soft lenses behave similarly to corneal lenses and have similar limitations.

In scleral lenses, it is possible to prescribe horizontal and vertical prism to a maximum of 6 prism dioptres, shared between the two eyes. This necessitates great care in fitting the haptic portion of the lens to prevent lens rotation on the eye due to the weight of the prism.

With spectacles, the difficulties of lens rotation do not arise. It is rare for more than 6 prism dioptres to be needed in a correction, and this can easily be prescribed in spectacles.

With contact lenses some unwanted prismatic effect occurs due to movement of the lenses on the eyes. One of the aims of correct fitting is to ensure that this movement is similar for both lenses so that little prismatic difference between the two eyes is experienced.

The prism effect due to such movement is given by:

$$P = F.c \text{ (Prentice's Law)},$$

where

P is prism effect in prism dioptres;

F is back vertex power, in dioptres, of contact-lens/liquid-lens system;
c is displacement in cm.

If the powers of the two lenses are the same and the movement is similar, then no prismatic difference occurs. If the two lens powers are not

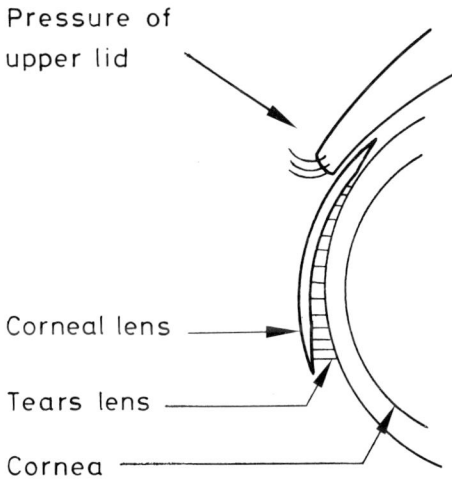

Figure 4.7–Prism base-down liquid lens: this effect is due to tilt of a corneal lens caused by pressure of the upper lid

the same, the amount of movement enables the prismatic difference to be calculated. It is worth noting that, if a person wears a negative-powered contact lens in one eye and a positive-powered lens in the other, to counteract the prismatic effects due to vertical lens movement, the negative lens should move up (prism base-down) as the positive lens moves down (also prism base-down). With corneal lenses, because of the position of the centre of gravity and the action of the lids during blinking (*see* Chapter 11), this desirable opposite movement of positive and negative lenses frequently actually occurs.

If a lens tilts due to pressure of the upper lid on a corneal lens or to downwards lag of a scleral lens, then a certain amount of extra prism base-down is introduced due to the liquid lens, as shown in *Figure 4.7*. Bennett (1966) has shown that this may be enough to counteract the prism base-up effect of a high negative scleral lens. Again, this tilt may be ignored as long as it is similar in the two eyes.

Where a contact lens has prism worked on it, then the prism power on the eye is the same as that in air. The liquid lens (unless it contains a prism element of its own due to tilt of the contact lens) has no effect on the prismatic element of the contact lens.

CYLINDER EFFECT INTRODUCED BY PRISM, SLIP AND TILT

The suggestion that a prism in a contact lens introduces a significant cylindrical element is incorrect. Although the refracted pencil is slightly oblique the amount of cylinder introduced is negligible. For example, taking a lens of BVP +10.00 D, BCOR 7.80 mm and centre thickness 0.40 mm, calculation shows that the cylindrical element introduced is only 0.023 D for a prism of $3^\triangle$. Expressed as a positive cylinder, the power is along the prism base–apex line and the axis perpendicular to it. Thus, in the example given, if the prism is base down along 90, there will be a +0.023 D cylinder axis 180.

Lenses can also tilt by slipping on the eye. If the slipping occurs as a rotation about the centre of curvature (C_2) of the back surface then C_2 will not be displaced, but C_1, the centre of curvature of the front surface, is displaced. Thus, the chief ray is deviated and is no longer normal to the front surface. This introduces a small amount of astigmatism, as shown in the following example. Taking a lens of BVP +12.00 D, BCOR 7.80 mm and centre thickness 0.44 mm, calculation shows that if the lens slips by 2.0 mm then 0.23 D of astigmatism results. The effect increases sharply with increased slip (0.52 D astigmatism with 3.0 mm slip) but only slightly with increasing curvature. The axis of the induced positive cylinder is perpendicular to the direction of slip.

In the case of negative lenses of similar numerical power, the astigmatism induced is less.

Note: In the above examples the effect of the back surface has been neglected as the refractive index change at this surface is small.

Clearly, the induced astigmatism may be increased if the lens actually tilts on the eye as well as slipping. When the whole lens tilts through a small angle the resulting astigmatism can be found approximately by the equation:

$$\text{Cylinder} = F \tan^2 \theta,$$

where θ is the angle of tilt and F is the back vertex power of the lens. The cylinder axis is perpendicular to the direction of tilt. Thus, if $F = +10.00$ D and $\theta = 5°$, the induced cylinder is $+0.0765$ D. If the direction of tilt is vertical, that is, about a horizontal axis, then the cylinder axis is horizontal. Such a lens, tilted in the vertical about a horizontal axis, due to upper lid pressure on the top of the lens is shown in *Figure 4.7*. There is also a very small change in the spherical element given approximately by the equation:

$$\text{Sphere} = F \left(1 + \frac{1}{3} \sin^2 \theta\right).$$

Thus, in the same example the sphere is increased to $+10.025$ D, which is of no significance.

Sarver (1963) has studied the effect of contact lens tilt on residual astigmatism and his experimental observations bear out the above theoretical findings.

MAGNIFICATION

Any correction, be it a spectacle lens or a contact lens, alters the size of the basic retinal image. (The basic retinal image is taken to be the size in the uncorrected eye assuming blur circles of zero diameter, that is, 'pin-point' pupils.) This change in the basic retinal image size is known as spectacle magnification, even when it is the magnification due to contact lenses. In order to make a satisfactory comparison between spectacles and contact lenses, the differences in magnification given by the two forms of correction must be considered for both spherical and toric correcting lenses. This magnification is affected by the form and thickness of the lens.

Spherical Lenses

Positive spectacle lenses magnify and negative lenses minify, and this magnification or minification increases with the vertex distance. Only if a corrective lens is worn in the plane of the eye's entrance pupil is unit magnification of the basic retinal image achieved. Thus, a contact lens worn on the cornea approaches as nearly as possible to giving unit magnification. Only an intraocular implant can be fitted closer to the entrance pupil plane. Bennett (1966) has shown that spectacle magnification may be expressed as

$$\frac{1}{1 - aF}$$

where F is the power of the correcting lens in dioptres and is assumed to be infinitely thin, and a is the distance in metres from the correcting lens to the entrance pupil plane. *Figure 4.8* shows how this expression is derived.

The size of the retinal image is proportional to the angular subtense of the object at the entrance pupil. This angular subtense is w' when the spectacle lens is present and w when it is not.

Now, $w' = \dfrac{h'}{\dfrac{1}{F} - a}$ and $w = \dfrac{h'}{\dfrac{1}{F}}$

Thus, spectacle magnification $\dfrac{w'}{w} = \dfrac{\dfrac{1}{F}}{\dfrac{1}{F} - a} = \dfrac{1}{1 - aF}$

Note: When a spectacle lens is present, a is equal to the vertex distance plus approximately 3 mm. With a contact lens a is about 3 mm, this being the approximate distance of the entrance pupil plane from the cornea.

Thus, it can be seen that myopes who change from spectacles to contact lenses see objects larger than before, and hypermetropes see objects smaller than before. This is illustrated by the graph in *Figure 4.9*, which shows the percentage increase or decrease in retinal image size given by theoretically infinitely thin contact lenses as compared with infinitely thin spectacle lenses. More realistic values are shown for typical aligning corneal lenses and typical scleral lenses, again compared with infinitely thin spectacle lenses. The slope for a soft lens would fall somewhere between the corneal and scleral lens slopes, depending on thickness.

Myopes can be expected to obtain increased visual acuity in contact lenses but may experience some disorientation when they are first worn owing to the apparent increase in the size of the external world.

Conversely, hypermetropes might expect to have poorer acuity with contact lenses than with spectacles; but since the difference in image size is only of real significance in the higher powers, it is only the high hypermetropes who are affected. Since these are aphakic, in the majority of cases, they enjoy seeing objects reduced to only slightly larger than their normal size again. The disorientation experienced by an aphakic due to the

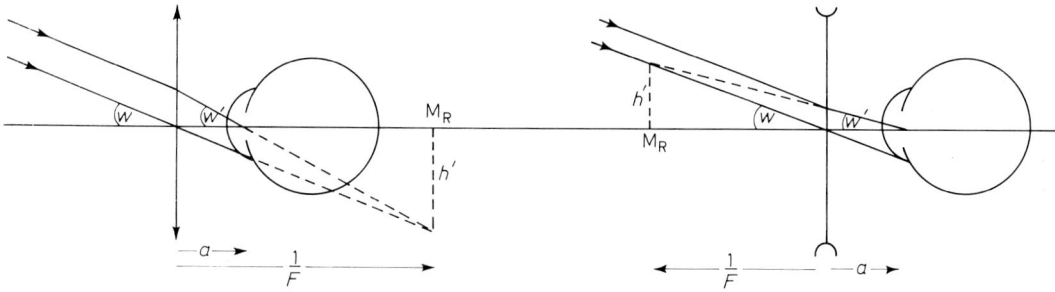

Figure 4.8–Spectacle magnification is $\frac{w'}{w}$. A distant off-axis object, subtending an angle w at the spectacle lens, is imaged by the lens of power F, in the far-point plane M_R. The image is of size h' and subtends an angle w' at the centre of the entrance pupil, which is situated at a distance of a metres from the spectacle lens. The left-hand diagram shows the situation in hypermetropia, and the right-hand diagram in myopia

magnification of his spectacles is comparable with but far worse than the disorientation felt by a high myope who transfers from spectacles to contact lenses. This is because the high positive spectacle correction causes field restriction and apparent image movement due to prismatic effects and aberrations, whereas a myope's contact lenses do not suffer from these additional defects.

The graph in *Figure 4.10* shows the different values for spectacle magnification given by four types of lenses. Theoretical values are drawn for spectacle lenses (assumed infinitely thin, and worn 12 mm from the cornea) and contact lenses (also assumed infinitely thin, and worn on the cornea, 3 mm in front of the entrance pupil) as well as more realistic values for typical corneal lenses and typical scleral lenses, taking form and thickness into account. Again, soft lenses can be expected to fall between the two, but closer to the values for corneal lenses because of the greater similarity in thickness. The latter consideration is dealt with more fully under the heading Shape Factor on page 100. The spectacle magnification of an infinitely thin contact lens should be multiplied by this factor to obtain a truer idea of the retinal image size when making comparisons with spectacles. This is borne out in *Figure 4.9*.

Toric Lenses

The graph in *Figure 4.10* shows that contact lenses cause less change in size of the basic retinal image than do spectacle lenses.

A toric spectacle lens gives different magnification in different meridians, which produces distortion of the retinal image. This is particularly noticeable in oblique astigmatism, as Bennett

(1967) pointed out. A square object seen through a toric spectacle lens may look rectangular if the principal meridians are horizontal and vertical, or diagonal like a parallelogram if the principal meridians are oblique. This distortion of shape is

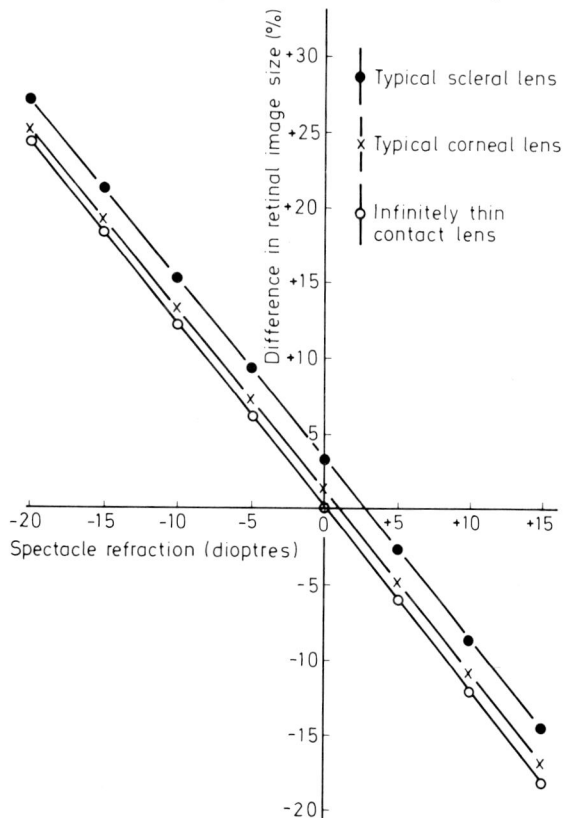

Figure 4.9–Percentage difference in retinal image size: comparison with a thin spectacle lens

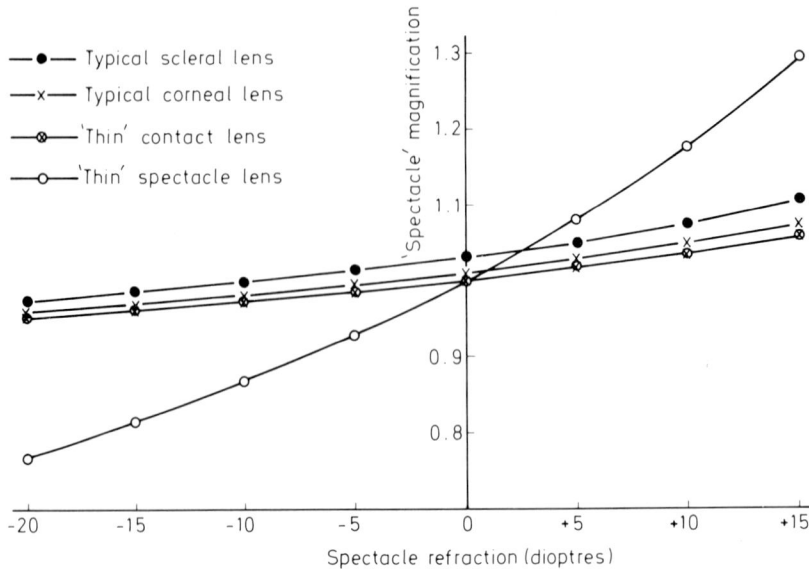

Figure 4.10–Variation of magnification with type and form of correcting lens

minimized with a contact lens because the meridional difference in magnification is reduced, as can be seen from the graph in *Figure 4.10*.

Difficulty may arise when a toric spectacle correction has been worn for many years and a perceptual allowance has been made for the distortion. On transferring to contact lenses, which give a less distorted retinal image, the perceived image may appear more distorted until the processes of perception become readjusted to the new situation. The type of effect experienced with spectacles and contact lenses is shown in *Figure 4.11* where the spectacle lens contains a high oblique cylinder.

Shape Factor

The magnification of two lenses having the same back vertex power is affected by their front surface power and thickness. Shape factor is the allowance which must be made for the increase in magnification due to the form and thickness of the lens and is given as:

$$\frac{1}{1 - tF_1/n}$$

which is the ratio between back vertex power and equivalent power, where

  n = refractive index;
  t = central optic thickness in metres;
  F_1 = front surface power in dioptres.

The values for spectacle magnification for the thin lenses in *Figure 4.10* should therefore be amended to

$$\frac{1}{1 - aF} \cdot \frac{1}{1 - tF_1/n}$$

if shape factor is to be taken into account. This expression is easily applied to spectacle lenses but a contact lens system comprises a plastics lens and a tears lens in combination. The expression for the shape factor is correspondingly more involved. Bennett (1966) has derived an approximate simplified expression for shape factor of a contact lens system, based on values which are normally known. This is:

$$1 + t(K + C) - (t_1/n_1)F_2$$

where

  t = total reduced thickness in metres, of plastics lens and liquid lens;
  K = ocular refraction in dioptres;
  C = keratometer reading in dioptres, where the index of calibration is assumed to equal that of the tears liquid (= 1.336);
  t_1 = thickness of plastics contact lens in metres;
  n_1 = refractive index of plastics material of contact lens;
  F_2 = interface power in dioptres at the back optic surface of the contact lens.

This expression was used in *Tables 4.2, 4.4* and *4.5* (pages 102 and 103) on which the graphs in

Retinal image   Perceived image

with spectacles

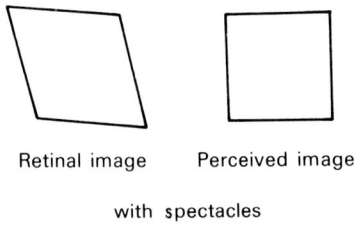

Figure 4.11–Perceptual compensation for retinal image distortion: this is acquired during spectacle wear and continues when contact lenses are first worn

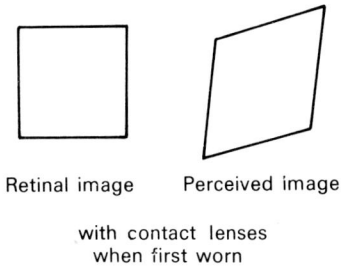

Retinal image   Perceived image

with contact lenses
when first worn

—o— Aligned scleral lens

—•— Flat scleral lens

—x— Aligned corneal lens

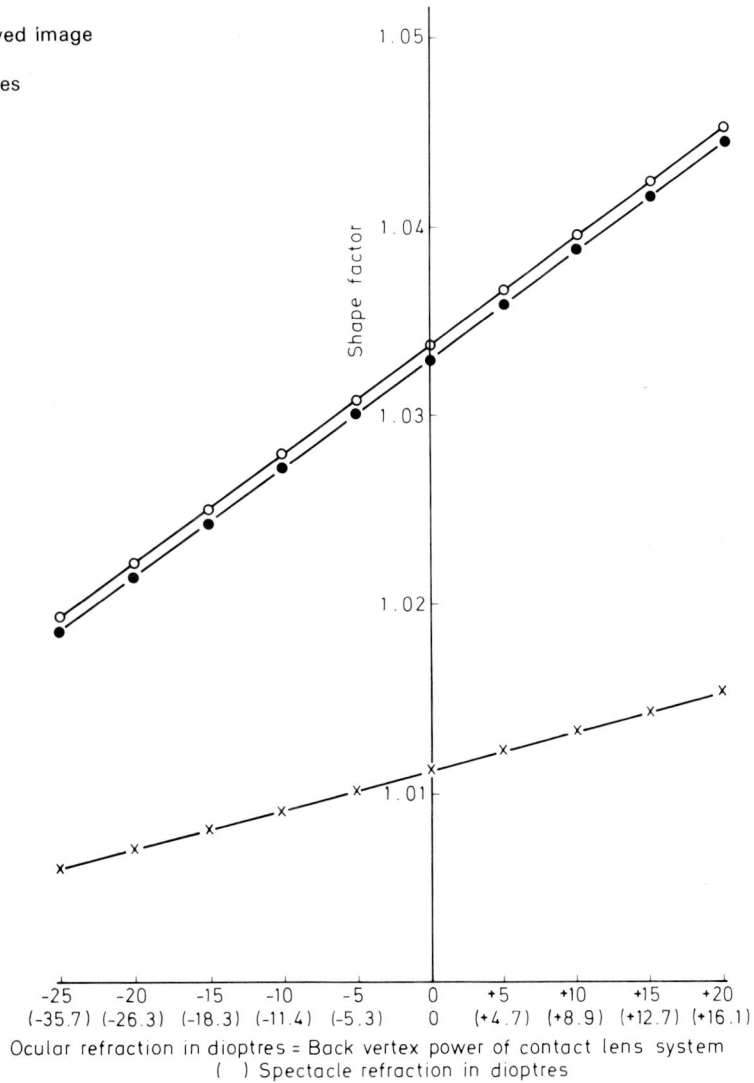

Figure 4.12–Relationship between retinal image sizes with scleral and corneal lenses

Shape factor

-25	-20	-15	-10	-5	0	+5	+10	+15	+20
(-35.7)	(-26.3)	(-18.3)	(-11.4)	(-5.3)	0	(+4.7)	(+8.9)	(+12.7)	(+16.1)

Ocular refraction in dioptres = Back vertex power of contact lens system
( ) Spectacle refraction in dioptres

Figures 4.9, 4.10 and *4.12* are based. These show that a corneal lens gives somewhat smaller retinal images than the corresponding scleral lens, because a scleral lens has a larger shape factor than a corneal lens.

Figure 4.12 shows shape factor for corneal and scleral lenses. Corneal lenses were assumed to be 0.2 mm thick and scleral lenses 0.75 mm thick, and the liquid lens was taken to be 0.1 mm thick in all cases. This is a rather broad assumption because negative lenses, especially those of high power, are normally thinner than the values stated, while positive lenses may be considerably thicker. Also the tears lens behind a corneal lens may be less than 0.1 mm thick. However, the values assumed permit sufficient illustration of the effect of thickness on shape factor. Had more accurate thickness values been used the graphs shown would have been slightly more steeply sloped. A keratometer reading (*C*) of +42 D was assumed. This gives a corneal radius of 8 mm. The corneal lenses have the same back central optic radius as the corneal radius, which is fairly typical. For comparison, values are shown for scleral lenses having the same back central optic radius. Values are also given for scleral lenses with a back central optic radius of 8.75 mm. (It is normal for the back optic of a scleral lens to be fitted about 0.50–0.75 mm flatter than the keratometer radius value.) It can be seen from the graph that this flattening has little effect on the shape factor as compared with the thickness difference between corneal and scleral lenses. Soft lenses are generally a little thicker than corneal lenses, but only slightly so. When on the eye they fit so that the back surface of the lens almost parallels the central cornea. Thus they would have a shape factor only slightly greater than corneal lenses, if at all.

Values used in the tables and graphs are:

		Aligned corneal lens	Aligned scleral lens	Flat scleral lens
n_1	=	1.49	1.49	1.49
n_2	=	1.336	1.336	1.336
t_1	=	0.2 mm	0.75 mm	0.75 mm
t_2	=	0.1 mm	0.1 mm	0.1 mm
Back central optic radius	=	8.00 mm	8.00 mm	8.75 mm
F_2 (interface)	=	−19.25 D	−19.25 D	−17.60 D
Corneal radius	=	8.00 mm	8.00 mm	8.00 mm
Keratometer reading (*C*)	=	+42.00 D	+42.00 D	+42.00 D

Shape factor is given approximately as

$$1 + t(K + C) - (t_1/n_1)F_2$$

where $t = t_1/n_1 + t_2/n_2$.

Table 4.2–Shape Factor with Corneal and Scleral Lenses

Ocular refraction (K) in dioptres = BVP of contact lens system	Shape factor		
	Aligned corneal lenses	Aligned scleral lenses	Flat scleral lenses
−25	1.006085	1.019405	1.01858
−20	1.007145	1.022295	1.02147
−15	1.008185	1.025145	1.02432
−10	1.009225	1.028025	1.02720
−5	1.010265	1.030925	1.03010
0	1.011305	1.033825	1.03300
+5	1.012345	1.036725	1.03590
+10	1.013385	1.039575	1.03875
+15	1.014445	1.042425	1.04160
+20	1.015485	1.045275	1.04445

The percentage increase in retinal image size as compared with an infinitely thin contact lens is shown bold, and then the first bold numeral should be followed by a decimal point.

Table 4.3–Shape Factor with Typical Corneal and Scleral Lenses

Spectacle refraction in dioptres	Ocular refraction (K) = BVP of equivalent contact lens system	Shape factor	
		Aligned corneal lens	Flat scleral lens
−20	−16.13	1.0079	1.0237
−15	−12.71	1.0086	1.0257
−10	−8.93	1.0095	1.0279
−5	−4.72	1.0103	1.0303
0	0.00	1.0113	1.0330
+5	+5.32	1.0124	1.0361
+10	+11.36	1.0137	1.0395
+15	+18.29	1.0151	1.0434

The percentage increases as compared with an infinitely thin contact lens system are bold as in *Table 4.3*.

Whereas *Table 4.2* gives shape factor for various values of ocular refraction, *Table 4.3* gives shape factor for various values of equivalent spectacle refraction. These values were obtained by interpolation from the graph in *Figure 4.12*.

Bennett (1968, 1972) has done a considerable amount of work in calculating realistic retinal image sizes in the aphakic eye corrected by spectacle

Table 4.4–Spectacle Magnification

Spectacle refraction in dioptres	Ocular refraction (K) = BVP of contact lens system	Spectacle magnification			
		Thin spectacle lens	Thin contact lens	Aligned corneal lens	Flat scleral lens
−20	−16.13	0.769	0.955	0.962	0.977
−15	−12.71	0.816	0.965	0.972	0.989
−10	−8.93	0.870	0.975	0.983	1.001
−5	−4.72	0.930	0.986	0.994	1.016
0	0.00	1.000	1.000	1.011	1.033
+5	+5.32	1.081	1.015	1.027	1.050
+10	+11.36	1.177	1.033	1.048	1.073
+15	+18.29	1.290	1.057	1.072	1.104

lenses and contact lenses, and in the pre-aphakic eye corrected by spectacles. He has not only taken into account the shape factor of the two types of correcting lens, but has considered the likely variations in axial length and corneal power (*Figure 4.13*). He has thereby derived some very useful values for relative spectacle magnification.

RELATIVE SPECTACLE MAGNIFICATION

This is defined as the ratio between the retinal image size in a corrected ametropic eye to that in a standard emmetropic eye. Various formulae have been given to calculate it, depending on

whether the difference between the two eyes is axial or refractive. Its main use is in determining whether or not a particular type of correction is likely to improve or disrupt binocular vision, by comparing the two retinal image sizes.

Where a person has different ocular refractions in the two eyes, the different magnification given by the two spectacles lenses (or contact lenses) may result in poor binocular vision. This is usually due to fusion difficulties resulting from unequal retinal image sizes. (Similar distribution of the

Table 4.5–Percentage Increase of Retinal Image Size by Comparison with Infinitely Thin Spectacle Lenses

Spectacle refraction in dioptres	Ocular refraction in dioptres	Percentage increase in retinal image size given by		
		Thin contact lens	Aligned corneal lens	Flat scleral lens
−20	−16.13	+24.2	+25.0	+27.0
−15	−12.71	+18.3	+19.1	+21.2
−10	−8.93	+12.1	+13.0	+15.0
−5	−4.72	+6.0	+6.9	+9.3
0	0.00	0.0	+1.1	+3.3
+5	+5.32	−6.1	−5.0	−2.9
+10	+11.36	−12.3	−11.0	−8.9
+15	+18.29	−18.1	−16.9	−14.4

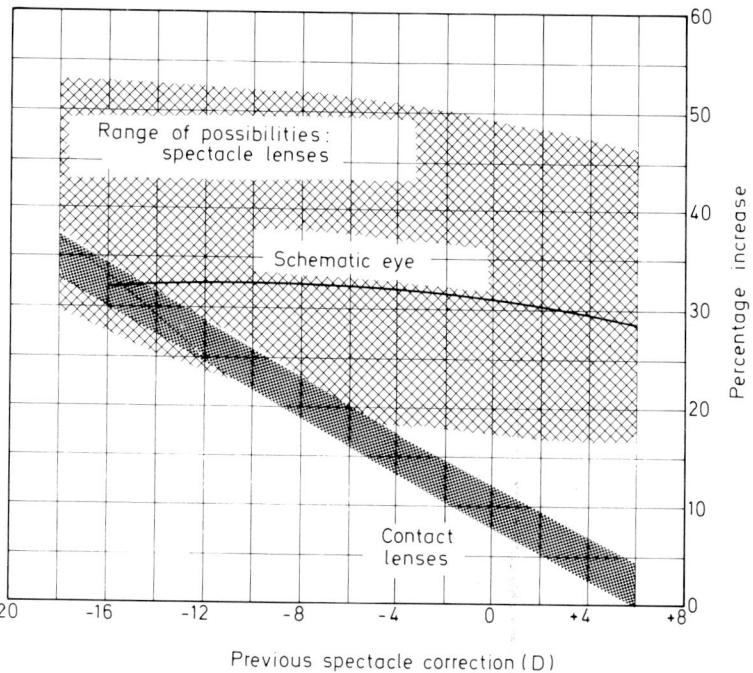

Figure 4.13–Percentage increase in the retinal image size in the aphakic eye corrected by spectacle and contact lenses. The graph indicates the possible spread of values, depending on the optical dimensions of the given eye (reproduced by kind permission of A. G. Bennett)

retinal receptors in the two eyes is assumed although this may be a false assumption.)

It is common to think of anisometropia as being either axial or refractive. Sorsby, Leary and Richards (1962) have shown that most naturally occurring anisometropia is predominantly *axial*, but this is often accompanied by a smaller refractive difference between the two eyes.

By contrast, one obvious example of *refractive* anisometropia is unilateral aphakia. It is in such cases that contact lenses give greater similarity in retinal image sizes than do spectacle lenses. As can be seen from the graphs in *Figure 4.10*, a corneal lens for the aphakic eye renders the minimum amount of magnification of the basic retinal image and therefore gives almost equal retinal image sizes in the two eyes, which are of the same length.

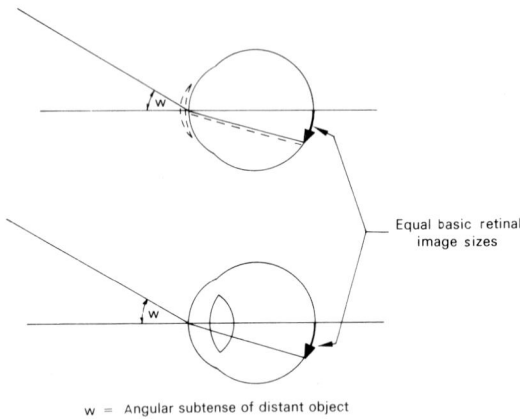

w = Angular subtense of distant object

Figure 4.14–Refractive anisometropia: corneal lenses cause minimum change in the basic retinal image size

The diagrams in *Figure 4.14* illustrate how two eyes of the same length have similar basic retinal image sizes. Contact lenses give rise to a minimum change in basic retinal image size, thereby permitting a good chance of binocular vision.

Figure 4.15 shows how eyes of unequal length have unequal basic retinal image sizes. In such cases, contact lenses – which scarcely affect this basic size – are unsatisfactory if fusion is to be achieved. A spectacle lens worn by the ametropic eye makes the retinal image in that eye closer in size to that of the other eye. Typical of such a case is unilateral myopia.

If it becomes necessary to compare or calculate retinal image sizes, it is simplest to assume a reduced eye as shown in *Figure 4.15*. The reduced eye is assumed to have a refractive index of 4/3 and a single spherical refracting surface of radius 5.55 mm giving it a power of +60 D.

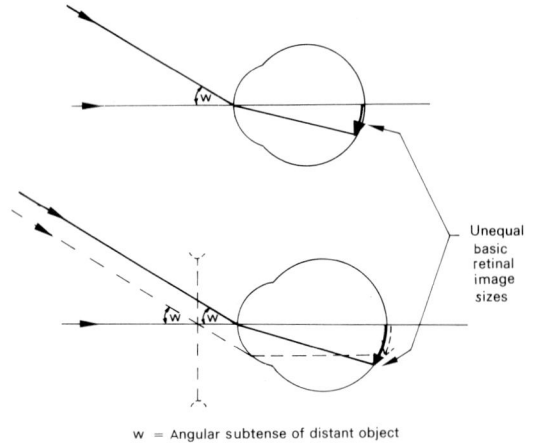

w = Angular subtense of distant object

Figure 4.15–Axial anisometropia: a spectacle lens before the ametropic eye gives equality of retinal image sizes

When the error (K) is known to be axial, then the power of the reduced eye (F'_e) is assumed as +60 D and its length is k'.

Now, $k' = \dfrac{n'}{K'}$, where $K' = K + F'_e$.

Thus, if the ocular refraction, $K = -10$ D then

$$K' = +50 \text{ D and } k' = \frac{4}{3} \times \frac{1000}{50} = 26.67 \text{ mm}.$$

A standard emmetropic eye has an axial length,

$$f'_e = \frac{n'}{F'_e} = \frac{4}{3} \times \frac{1000}{60} = 22.22 \text{ mm}.$$

When the error is known to be refractive (as in aphakia) then the power of the eye (F'_e) is determined from its length (k') and its ocular refraction (K). For example, $K = +12$ D, $k' = 22.22$ mm.

Thus, $K' = \dfrac{4}{3} \times \dfrac{1000}{22.22} = +60$ D,

and $F'_e = K' - K = 60 - 12 = +48$ D.

As can be seen from *Figure 4.15*, the principal ray determining the basic retinal image size, undergoes refraction at the principal point of the eye according to Snell's Law.

Considering this principal ray, prior to refraction the angle subtended at the eye's principal point is w, and after refraction the angle subtended by the basic retinal image is thus

$$\frac{w}{n'}.$$

(All angles are small, and the sine, tangent and angle in radians then all become equal.)

But $\dfrac{w}{n'} = \dfrac{\text{basic retinal image size}}{k'}$

Thus, basic retinal image size $= \dfrac{w}{n'}k' = \dfrac{w}{K'}$
(in metres).

Note: The principal ray may already have undergone refraction at a spectacle lens or contact lens, so that w is then equivalent to the w' of *Figure 4.8.* Thus, the spectacle magnification is taken into account in determining the angular subtense at the principal point prior to refraction by the eye. The final retinal image size then becomes

$$\dfrac{1}{1 - aF} \cdot \dfrac{w}{K'} \text{ (in metres).}$$

In the standard emmetropic eye the retinal image size is thus $w \times 60$ metres.

Two examples will serve to illustrate the differences between axial and refractive anisometropia. The vertex distance is assumed as 12 mm and the distance from cornea to entrance pupil as 3 mm. Shape factor has not been taken into account.

The first example, (1), is representative of refractive anisometropia and is a unilateral aphakic having basically equal retinal image sizes in the two eyes because the eyes are similar in length. Thus, the spectacle magnification afforded by both spectacles and contact lenses has a direct effect on the retinal image sizes. With spectacles, the difference in magnification between the two eyes is large and so, therefore, is the percentage difference between retinal image sizes. With contact lenses, it is small. Obviously, the contact lens correction allows the greater chance for binocular vision.

The second example, (2), is that of unilateral axial myopia, in which the power of both eyes is assumed to be 60 D. Thus, the basic retinal image sizes are proportional to the axial lengths (or inversely proportional to the dioptric lengths as

shown in *Table 4.6*). These basic image sizes are then affected by the spectacle magnifications; so that, with spectacles, where the difference in magnification is large there is only a small difference in the retinal image sizes. With contact lenses, the spectacle magnifications are almost the same but the retinal images are very different in size. Here, spectacles provide the better chance for binocular vision. The values found in the examples may be checked using the information given in the adjacent column, using standard reduced eye data; the values above being correct to two places of decimals.

It should be pointed out that where binocular vision is absolutely impossible the patient is free of any asthenopic symptoms. If binocular vision is made possible but difficult, symptoms may occur. This frequently arises with the unilateral aphakic. Because of the greater reduction in magnification afforded by corneal and soft lenses, these should allow slightly better binocular vision than sclerals. The aphakic also enjoys the other benefits of contact lenses over spectacles – but even so, the symptoms of difficult binocular vision have often caused the unilateral aphakic to abandon contact lenses.

The extremes of purely refractive or purely axial anisometropia, as shown in the examples in *Table 4.6*, are rare. In most anisometropes, contact lenses afford other advantages – such as absence of differential prism – which make their effects on retinal image size worth investigating before they are ruled out entirely. In the writer's experience, the perceptual process which allows fusion of different-sized images is more readily adaptable than is the extraocular musculature which has to cope with dissimilar prism effects. In spite of the fact that most anisometropia is mainly axial, contact lenses have been found to be more acceptable than spectacles to many anisometropes. This may well be due to differences in retinal receptor spacing in the two eyes.

It is as well to note that corneals or soft lenses are the better types of contact lens to use in

Table 4.6

Spectacle correction in dioptres		Ratio of basic retinal image sizes in uncorrected eyes (R/L)	With spectacle correction			With contact lenses		
			Spectacle magnification		Difference in retinal image sizes	Spectacle magnification		Difference in retinal image sizes
R.	L.		R.	L.	%	R.	L.	%
(1) +2	+12	60.00:60.00	1.03	1.22	18.29	1.01	1.04	3.75
(2) −1	−10	51.07:59.01	0.99	0.87	1.98	1.00	0.97	12.87

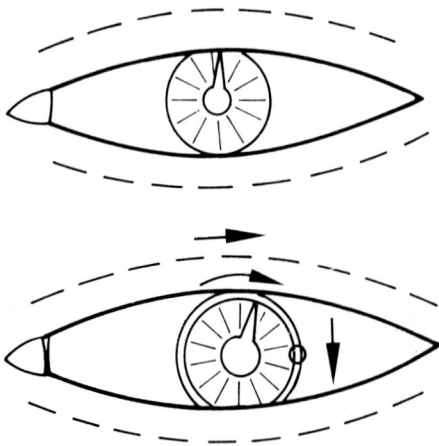

Figure 4.16 – The effect of a high positive scleral lens: there is a wider lid aperture and the eye tends to rotate in the directions shown

In order to calculate the actual amount of accommodation exerted by the eye, known as the ocular accommodation (A), it is necessary to determine the ocular refraction (K) and the distance (b) at which the near object of regard is imaged by the spectacle lens, of power F_S. For example, *Figure 4.17a* shows a myope wearing a spectacle lens of -8 D, who reads at a distance (l), 25 cm from the spectacle plane. Thus, the spectacle accommodation (A_S) is 4 D. Now if the spectacle lens is worn 12 mm from the eye, the ocular refraction (K) is -7.30 D *(see Appendix A)*.

(The method of calculating ocular refraction from spectacle refraction and vertex distance, d, should be apparent from *Figure 4.19* if K is substituted for L and k for l.)

anisometropia, as the weight difference is minimized. In scleral lenses, the weight of the high positive lens may cause hypophoria and excyclophoria of the aphakic eye *(Figure 4.16)*. This is an extreme example.

ACCOMMODATION

The accommodation exerted for a given working distance varies, depending on whether spectacles or contact lenses are worn. More accommodation is required by myopes and less by hypermetropes when they transfer from spectacles to contact lenses *(see Table 4.7 and the graph in Figure 4.18)*.

Table 4.7 – Comparison of Accommodation with Spectacles and Contact Lenses

Spectacle refraction in dioptres	Ocular accommodation in dioptres			
	At $\frac{1}{3}$ metre from spectacle plane		At $\frac{1}{4}$ metre from spectacle plane	
	Spectacles	Contact lenses	Spectacles	Contact lenses
-20	1.89	2.90	2.50	3.82
-15	2.09	2.90	2.76	3.82
-10	2.32	2.90	3.06	3.82
-5	2.58	2.90	3.40	3.82
0	2.90	2.90	3.82	3.82
$+5$	3.27	2.90	4.31	3.82
$+10$	3.72	2.90	4.89	3.82
$+15$	4.25	2.90	5.61	3.82

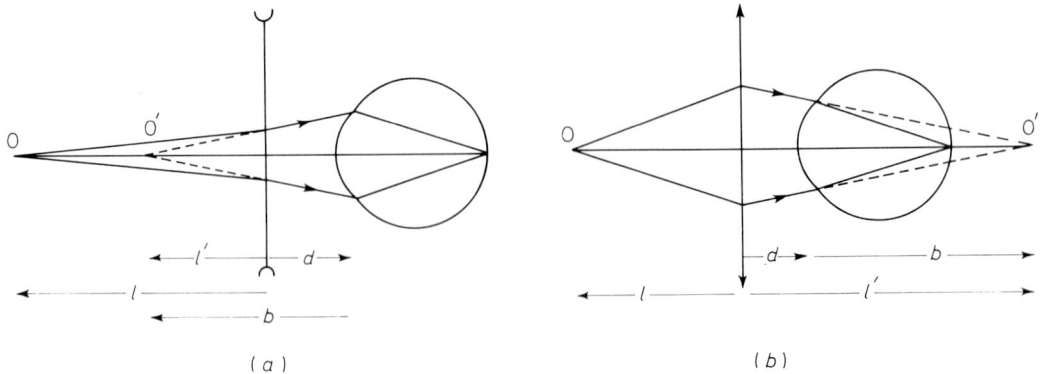

(a)

(b)

Figure 4.17 – Near vision through spectacle lenses. The near object of regard, O, is imaged at O', which is at a distance, b, from the eye. The object, image and vertex distances from the spectacle lens are l, l', and d respectively. (a) Myopia. (b) Hypermetropia

The near object, O, is imaged by the spectacle lens at O'.

Now $l = -25$ cm. Therefore, $L = -4$ D. $F_s = -8$ D. Therefore, $L' = -12$ D. Thus, $l' = -8.33$ cm. But $b = l' - d = -8.33 - 1.2 = -9.53$ cm.

$$B = \frac{1}{b \text{ (in metres)}} . \text{ Thus, } B = -10.5 \text{ D.}$$

But -7.30 D of this corrects the ocular refraction. The remaining 2.20 D must be overcome by the use of the myope's accommodation, that is, $A = K - B$.

This demonstrates the effectivity of the spectacle lens in permitting such a myope to use only 2.2 D of accommodation, whereas if a contact lens were worn the same near object would be 26.2 cm from the eye necessitating 3.82 D of accommodation.

Figure 4.17b shows a similar situation for a hypermetrope. $F_s = +8$ D, $l = -25$ cm and $d = 12$ mm. Thus, $K = +8.85$ D (*see* Appendix A).

Now $L = -4$ D, $F_s = +8$ D. Therefore, $L' = +4$ D and $l' = +25$ cm.

But $b = l' - d = +25 - 1.2 = +23.8$ cm. Therefore, $B = +4.2$ D.

Since $A = K - B$, $A = +8.85 - 4.2 = +4.65$ D.

This demonstrates how the ocular accommodation of a hypermetrope wearing spectacles is in excess of that required if contact lenses are worn. In this example 4.65 D of accommodation is required as compared to 3.82 D in contact lenses.

Table 4.8 – Ratio Between Accommodation in Dioptres, and Convergence in Prism Dioptres, with Spectacles and Contact Lenses

Spectacle refraction in dioptres	Ratio of accommodation to convergence			
	At $\frac{1}{3}$ metre from spectacle plane		At $\frac{1}{4}$ metre from spectacle plane	
	Spectacles	Contact lenses	Spectacles	Contact lenses
−20	0.170	0.174	0.172	0.176
−15	0.173	0.174	0.174	0.176
−10	0.174	0.174	0.174	0.176
−5	0.174	0.174	0.176	0.176
0	0.174	0.174	0.176	0.176
+5	0.172	0.174	0.175	0.176
+10	0.168	0.174	0.171	0.176
+15	0.160	0.174	0.164	0.176

If a comparison is made of the graphs of convergence in *Figure 4.5* and the graphs of accommodation in *Figure 4.18*, it will be noted that the slopes showing convergence and accommodation with spectacles are the same. They are also the same with contact lenses. As Westheimer (1962) has already stated, this implies that the accommodation/convergence ratio is the same with contact lenses as it is with spectacles. It has also been shown by both Stone (1967) and Bennett (1967) that if contact lenses remain centred for all working distances and a comparison is made with spectacles centred for distance vision, the accommodation/convergence ratio remains approximately the same with both forms of correction, as shown in *Table 4.8*.

The figures for the basis of this table come from *Tables 4.1* and *4.7*. Bennett (1967) has derived an expression for the accommodation/convergence ratio with spectacles to that with contact lenses by using binomial approximations.

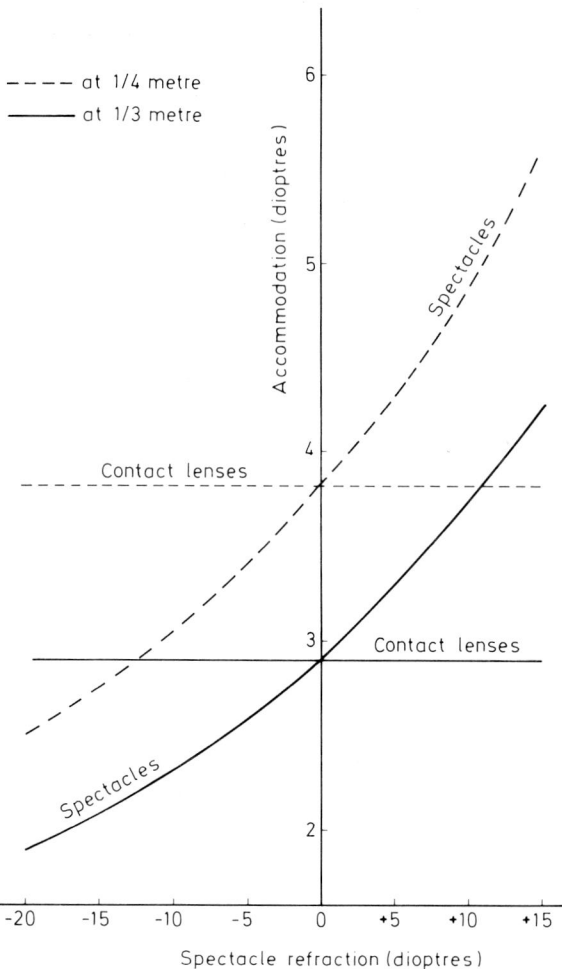

- - - - at 1/4 metre
——— at 1/3 metre

Figure 4.18 – Accommodation with spectacles and contact lenses

This is based on a theoretical analysis and shows that:

$$\frac{\text{Acc./Con. ratio with spectacles}}{\text{Acc./Con. ratio with contact lenses}} \doteqdot 1 - F(s - 2d)$$

where

F = spectacle lens power in dioptres;
s = distance from spectacle plane to centre of rotation of eye, in metres;
d = vertex distance of spectacle lens in metres.

Now, if $d = s/2$ it can be seen that the accommodation/convergence ratio is the same with both spectacles and contact lenses.

In *Table 4.8*, d was taken as 12 mm and s as 27 mm, which accounts for the slight discrepancies between the values found for the two forms of correction. But as d is always approximately $s/2$, the ratios are always approximately the same.

Changes in accommodation should therefore only cause difficulty in the presbyopic or pre-presbyopic myope, who may have trouble in exerting extra accommodation and convergence.

OPTICAL CONSIDERATIONS OF CONTACT LENSES ON THE EYE

To understand why a contact lens correction often differs considerably from a spectacle correction, the significance of the following points must be fully understood.

(1) The contribution made by the liquid (tears) lens.

(2) The effects of radius changes on back vertex power of the contact-lens/liquid-lens system.

(3) The differences between total and corneal astigmatism.

This section is intended as a practical guide in determining both scleral, soft and corneal lens powers, and it employs the method of specifying back optic radii in millimetres rather than in terms of the keratometer reading in dioptres.

To correct fully an eye's refractive error, the back vertex power of the contact-lens/liquid-lens system must equal the ocular refraction (K) — not to be confused with the keratometer reading, also often denoted as 'K'.

In the following considerations, it will be assumed that surface powers are additive provided that their separations are small. This leads to some approximations. It will also be assumed that the back vertex power of a contact lens can be directly added to the vergence of the light reaching it — although this, again, is an approximation, as the following example shows.

Example: Consider a scleral lens with the following characteristics:

Back vertex power (BVP) in air -12 D
Central optic thickness (t_c)   0.80 mm
Back central optic radius (BCOR) = (r_2) 8.75 mm
Front central optic radius (FCOR) = (r_1) 11.40 mm
Refractive index (n)   1.49
Refraction with this lens *in situ*, (F_S) +8.00 D
Vertex distance (d)   12 mm

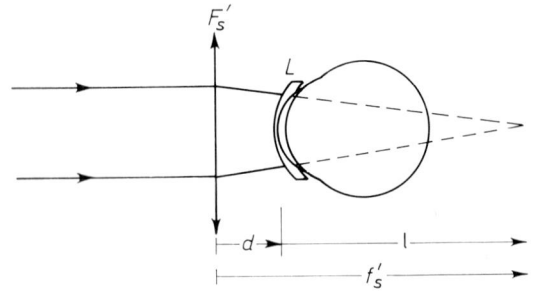

Figure 4.19–Effective power of spectacle lens at contact lens is

$$L = \frac{1}{l} = \frac{F'_s}{1 - dF'_s}$$

Reference to *Figure 4.19* shows the following:

Reduced vergences   Equivalent air distances
$F'_s = +8.00$ D $\longrightarrow f'_s = +125$ mm
               $-d = $ 12 mm
$L = +8.85$ D $\longleftarrow$ $l = +113$ mm

The effective power of the spectacle lens at the front surface of the scleral lens = $L = +8.85$ D. If it is assumed that BVP of the scleral lens may be added directly to this, then the BVP of the required scleral lens

= $+8.85$ D $- 12.00$ D
= -3.15 D

But this is only approximate, as more accurate calculations show:

Front surface power, $F_1 = \dfrac{(n - 1)1000}{r_1}$

$= \dfrac{(1.49 - 1)1000}{11.4}$

$= +43$ D

Back surface power, $F_2 = \dfrac{(1 - n)1000}{r_2}$

$= \dfrac{(1 - 1.49)1000}{8.75}$

$= -56$ D

Reduced thickness, $t/n = \dfrac{0.8}{1.49}$

$= 0.54$ mm

Reduced vergences   *Equivalent air distances*

$L_1 = +\ 8.85$ D

$+F_1 = +43.00$ D

$\overline{L'_1 = +51.85\ \text{D}} \longrightarrow +19.29$ mm

$-t/n = -\ 0.54$ mm

$L_2 = +53.30$ D $\longleftarrow +18.75$ mm

$+F_2 = -56.00$ D

$\overline{L'_2 = -\ 2.70\ \text{D}}$ This is the correct BVP of the contact lens required.

It can be seen that the error due to the use of the approximate method is an over-correction of -3.15 D $- (-2.70)$ D $= -0.45$ D.

Note: Francis (1968) has compiled some very useful tables which remove most of the hard work from accurate methods of calculation. These are now incorporated into this textbook and their use is dealt with at the end of this chapter, along with some helpful examples. The tables referred to form the appendices to this book and are incorporated at the end of this volume.

However, the approximate method is less inaccurate when the contact lens used for refraction purposes approximates closely to the power required. The example above shows why a contact lens having an entirely different back vertex power from that required should not be used for refraction.

The example above also uses a combination of positive spectacle lens and negative contact lens, which constitutes a Galilean telescope system. This should be avoided, wherever possible, since it gives a higher magnification than that obtained with the final contact lens. Hence, a false assessment of visual acuity may be made, and disappointment will follow when the final contact lens does not give the patient such a good visual acuity.

Different aspects of refraction with contact lenses will now be considered:

OCULAR REFRACTION

BVP of final contact lens in air

+ BVP of liquid lens in air (liquid lens assumed thin)

= Ocular refraction

OCULAR ASTIGMATISM

Front surface corneal astigmatism

+ Back surface corneal astigmatism

+ Crystalline lens astigmatism (referred to the corneal plane)

= Total ocular astigmatism

Note: The front surface of the cornea usually has greater positive power near the vertical meridian – that is, 'with-the-rule' astigmatism – whereas the other two contributors to total ocular astigmatism normally have 'against-the-rule' astigmatism, the total effect usually being 'with-the-rule', although this decreases with age.

ASTIGMATISM OF THE FRONT SURFACE OF THE CORNEA AND THE EFFECT OF THE LIQUID LENS

Refractive index of tears, n_t = 1.336

Refractive index of cornea, n_c = 1.376

When a hard contact lens with spherical back surface is placed on the eye, the front surface of the liquid lens is spherical because it is formed by the back surface of the contact lens. If the front surface of the cornea is toroidal, then the back surface of the liquid lens is also toroidal, with radii (r) equal to that of the cornea but having negative power.

The powers in air of the back surface of the liquid lens are given by $F = (1 - 1.336)1000/r$, and the powers of the front surface of the cornea are given by $F = (1.376 - 1)1000/r$. This means that the front surface astigmatism of the cornea is partly neutralized by the back surface astigmatism of the liquid lens. The amount neutralized is thus 336/376, which is 90 per cent. This is of importance with toroidal corneas because it is likely that the back surface of the cornea itself will neutralize the remaining 10 per cent of the front surface astigmatism.

Thus, with a hard spherical contact lens on the eye, any residual astigmatism found is almost entirely due to the crystalline lens since practically all the corneal astigmatism is corrected, that is:

Back surface astigmatism of liquid lens

+ Front surface astigmatism of cornea

+ Back surface astigmatism of cornea

= Zero (approximately)

THE EFFECTS ON ASTIGMATISM OF POWER CHANGES DUE TO SOFT LENS FLEXURE AND EQUILIBRATION

Unlike the rigid hard lens, spherical soft lenses flex to match the corneal contour. They therefore replicate the front surface corneal toricity on their own front surface. The thickness of the soft lens itself may slightly reduce the amount of toricity transferred, but as soft lenses all have a refractive index higher than that of the cornea, the amount of astigmatism transferred to the soft lens front surface is usually about the same as that of the corneal front surface. Different soft lenses have different refractive indices, and the refractive index can vary with the state of hydration at which the soft lens reaches equilibrium on the eye. When fully hydrated most soft lens materials have a refractive index in the region of 1.36–1.46. Thus, the amount

central cornea, and since the soft lens forms almost a glove fit in this region, any tears lens present is usually of zero or very low negative power.

It may be helpful at times to be able to determine the astigmatism of the front surface of a soft lens and how it may alter whilst *in situ* on the eye. *Table 4.9* shows the amount of astigmatism introduced by the toroidal surface of any lens (soft or hard) provided its radii of curvature and

Table 4.9–Rate of Change of Surface Power in Air, in Terms of Dioptres per 0.10 mm Change in Radius, for Surfaces of Various Curvatures and Various Refractive Indices (body of table shows dF/dr, in dioptres per 0.10 mm change in r)

Refractive indices	Surface radius of curvature (mm)						
	6.50	7.00	7.50	8.00	8.50	9.00	9.50
1.33	0.781	0.673	0.587	0.516	0.457	0.407	0.366
1.34	0.805	0.694	0.604	0.531	0.471	0.420	0.377
1.35	0.828	0.714	0.622	0.547	0.484	0.432	0.388
1.36	0.852	0.735	0.640	0.562	0.498	0.444	0.399
1.37	0.876	0.755	0.658	0.578	0.512	0.457	0.410
1.38	0.899	0.776	0.676	0.594	0.526	0.469	0.421
1.39	0.923	0.796	0.693	0.609	0.540	0.481	0.432
1.40	0.947	0.816	0.711	0.625	0.554	0.494	0.443
1.41	0.970	0.837	0.729	0.641	0.567	0.506	0.454
1.42	0.994	0.857	0.747	0.656	0.581	0.519	0.465
1.43	1.018	0.878	0.764	0.672	0.595	0.531	0.476
1.44	1.041	0.898	0.782	0.688	0.609	0.543	0.488
1.45	1.065	0.918	0.800	0.703	0.623	0.556	0.499
1.46	1.089	0.939	0.818	0.719	0.637	0.568	0.510
1.47	1.112	0.959	0.836	0.734	0.651	0.580	0.521
1.48	1.136	0.980	0.853	0.750	0.664	0.593	0.532
1.49	1.160	1.000	0.871	0.766	0.678	0.605	0.543

of astigmatism transferred to the front surface of the soft lens depends on a number of factors: the type of material and its flexibility, its thickness and its refractive index in the equilibrated state on the eye.

What is more important, is to realize that the astigmatism on the front surface of the soft lens is partly neutralized by the back surface astigmatism of the cornea as well as that at the cornea/soft lens interface, and possibly by crystalline astigmatism also. Bennett (1976) has shown that any soft lens fitted with its back surface flatter than the cornea very slightly corrects corneal astigmatism (*see* page 117). As it flexes to match the steeper cornea the soft lens becomes more negative in power, and this increase in negative power is greater along the steeper meridian, hence the slight correction of corneal astigmatism.

It should also be remembered that there is little, if any, liquid lens between a soft lens and the

refractive index are known. It shows the change in surface power in air for a change of radius of 0.10 mm, for refractive indices between 1.33 and 1.49 in steps of 0.01. (Interpolation would permit power changes for even smaller gradations in refractive index than 0.01 to be obtained.)

Because a change of radius of 0.10 mm induces different power changes, depending on whether the curvature of the surface is steep or flat, this is allowed for by taking surface radii in 0.50 mm steps between 6.50 mm and 9.50 mm.

Thus, for example, for a large change in radius, say from 7.00 mm to 8.00 mm, and for a refractive index of 1.45, the figure in the intermediate (r = 7.50 mm) column should be used. So, for a lens of front surface radii 7.00 mm X 8.00 mm the power difference, or astigmatism, is 10 X 0.800 = 8.00 D, which gives an error of only 0.036 D.

If there is only a moderate radius change, as for a surface of radii 7.00 mm X 7.50 mm then (using the same refractive index of 1.45) it is best to average the figures in the two relevant columns to obtain the effect of a 0.10 mm change in radius; that is, the average of 0.918 and 0.800 is 0.859 D, and for the 0.50 mm difference is 5 X 0.859 = 4.295 D of astigmatism. This gives an error of 0.009 D.

For small radius differences, as for a surface of radii 7.00 mm X 7.20 mm and of refractive index 1.44, then the value in the column applying to the nearest radius should be used; in this case it is 7.00 mm, and thus 0.898 D is the value for a 0.10 mm radius change. So the 0.20 mm difference in surface radii would give 2 X 0.898 = 1.796 D of astigmatism, an error of only 0.05 D.

If the front surface of a soft lens alters curvature while it is on the eye, as for example due to temperature changes or evaporation, then there is a surface power change which may also be obtained from Table 4.9. Suppose the front surface of a lens steepens from 9.50 mm to 9.40 mm and the lens is assumed to have a refractive index of 1.43, then its power will change by 0.476 D, and as this is a steepening of a convex surface, the power will become more positive. Changes in toricity of a surface would lead to changes in astigmatism which can be determined from Table 4.9 in the same way.

Table 4.10–Rate of Change of Surface Power in Air (F) for Changes in Refractive Index (n) of 0.01, for Various Radii of Curvature (r)

r in mm	dF/dn in D	r in mm	dF/dn in D
6.40	1.5625	8.00	1.2500
.50	1.5385	.10	1.2346
.60	1.5152	.20	1.2195
.70	1.4925	.30	1.2048
.80	1.4706	.40	1.1905
.90	1.4493	.50	1.1765
7.00	1.4286	.60	1.1628
.10	1.4084	.70	1.1494
.20	1.3699	.90	1.1236
.30	1.3889	.80	1.1369
.40	1.3514	9.00	1.1111
.50	1.3333	.10	1.0989
.60	1.3158	.20	1.0870
.70	1.2987	.30	1.0753
.80	1.2821	.40	1.0638
.90	1.2658	.50	1.0526

However, such radius changes of a soft lens occurring whilst it is on the eye are often accompanied by changes in refractive index, again due to equilibration factors such as temperature changes and evaporation from the lens. Table 4.10 shows how the surface power may alter if

this occurs. For example, evaporation might lead to a rise in refractive index from 1.39 to 1.40 for a surface of radius 8.50 mm. There is then a resultant power change of 1.1765 D, while a change from 1.39 to 1.41 would lead to twice this amount, that is, 2.353 D. For a rise in refractive index, there is always an increase in power of the surface, and a drop in refractive index leads to a decrease in surface power.

Note: In Table 4.10, as indicated in the above paragraph, the changes in power are linear at any one radius; thus for a radius of 7.50 mm, a change of refractive index of 0.06 would give a surface power change of 6 X 1.3333 = 7.9998 D; and a change of refractive index of 0.006 would give a power change of 0.79998 D.

When these factors of radius and refractive index change with equilibration are considered, it is surprising that the powers of soft lenses on the eye remain as constant as they do. Small changes in visual acuity due to alterations in power are therefore both understandable and to be expected.

THE EFFECTS OF FLEXURE ON THIN HARD LENSES

In the same way that a soft lens flexes to conform to the corneal contour there is a tendency for very thin hard lenses to flex on toroidal corneas, partially replicating the corneal astigmatism. Harris and Chu (1972) found that with lens centre thicknesses of less than 0.13 mm, the thinner the lens, the more it flexes; and the more corneal astigmatism present, the greater is the lens flexure. They found that thin lenses flexed in a predictable manner and induced astigmatism which affected the amount of residual astigmatism. Their results are summarized in Figure 4.20. As can be seen this flexure-induced astigmatism can be made use of to benefit the patient. Frequently, as explained on page 109, if the lens does not flex, all corneal astigmatism is corrected by the liquid lens and any residual astigmatism is due to the crystalline lens. The latter is normally a small to moderate amount of against-the-rule astigmatism. If such is found, and if the cornea has with-the-rule astigmatism, then obviously by fitting a thin lens the induced with-the-rule astigmatism caused by the lens flexure can be used to partially or completely neutralize the against-the-rule residual astigmatism. The standard of visual acuity and quality may thus be improved.

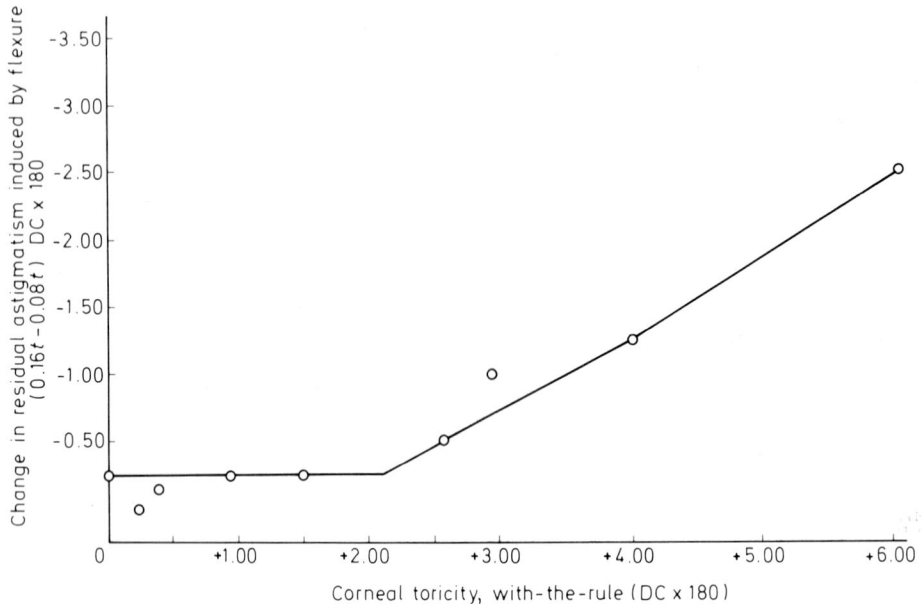

Figure 4.20—The difference in residual astigmatism between that induced by a thick lens (0.16 mm) and that induced by a thin lens (0.08 mm) for corneas of various toricities. For example, a patient has −1.25 DC X 90 residual astigmatism with a 0.16 mm thick lens, and a 4.00 D with-the-rule toric cornea. Changing the lens to one of 0.08 mm thickness induces −1.25 DC X 180 of astigmatism due to flexure, thereby eliminating the residual astigmatism (reproduced by kind permission of M. G. Harris and C. S. Chu)

KERATOMETRY AND CORNEAL ASTIGMATISM

Keratometers measure front surface corneal radii but give *total* corneal power on the assumption, given above, that the back surface of the cornea has −10 per cent of the power of the front surface.

The true refractive index of the cornea (1.376) is therefore not used to calibrate keratometers. Instead, an index of 1.3375 is usually used (n_k). This allows the instrument to read total corneal power (or approximately 90 per cent of the front surface power).

But n_k and n_t are almost the same (1.3375 and 1.336). Indeed, some keratometers are calibrated for an index of 1.336 or even 1.332. Therefore, the astigmatism measured by the keratometer is almost the same as that corrected by the back surface of the liquid lens. In fact, the use of n_k instead of n_t gives a *power* value which is slightly too high; for a radius of 8 mm the use of n_k gives F_k = 42.19 D and the use of n_t gives F_t = 42.00 D. But astigmatism is the *difference between the two principal powers*, and the error due to the slight difference in the refractive indices is then reduced to an insignificant amount. This is illustrated in the following example of a cornea with an extreme amount of astigmatism.

Example:

Keratometry	8 mm/+42.19 D along 180
$(n_k = 1.3375)$	7 mm/+48.21 D along 90
Total corneal astigmatism	+ 6.02 DC × 180
Liquid lens back surface powers	8 mm/−42.00 D along 180
$(n_t = 1.336)$	7 mm/−48.00 D along 90
Liquid lens back surface astigmatism	− 6.00 DC × 180

Even in such an extreme example it can be seen that the amount of total corneal astigmatism uncorrected by the liquid lens is an insignificant amount of +6.02 − 6.00 = +0.02 D. In this context, it is therefore valid to state that all the astigmatism measured by keratometry is corrected by the back surface of the liquid lens.

RESIDUAL ASTIGMATISM

Since the amount of astigmatism corrected by the liquid lens can be measured by keratometry (as shown above), the amount of residual astigmatism with a hard spherical contact lens may be predicted in advance, although this assumes that the lens is reasonably thick and does not flex (*see* pages 109 and 112). If this is so then:

Total ocular astigmatism
− Astigmatism measured by keratometry
= Residual astigmatism

Care must be taken when determining the total ocular astigmatism from the spectacle refraction and vertex distance as it is incorrect to calculate the effective change in power of the cylinder alone.

Example showing correct method of calculating the effective power of a cylinder at the eye:

Spectacle refraction	−6.00/−1.00 × 180
Vertex distance	12 mm
Spectacle refraction in crossed cylinder form	−6.00 × 90/−7.00 × 180
Ocular refraction in crossed cylinder form, after allowing for vertex distance (*see* Appendix A, page 306)	−5.60 × 90/−6.46 × 180
Ocular refraction	−5.60/−0.86 × 180

This shows that the 1 D cylinder is reduced to 0.86 D due to the associated sphere power, whereas if the sphere power were ignored there would be no significant change in the power of the cylinder − which is demonstrably quite incorrect. The higher the powers of sphere and cylinder are, the greater is the effect of vertex distance.

Prediction of residual astigmatism allows the effect of this amount of astigmatism to be simulated by the use of a trial cylinder in front of the patient's usual spectacle correction. The sphere power may then be adjusted to obtain the best visual acuity. If this is inadequate, it is obvious that the contact lens must incorporate a cylinder for the correction of the residual astigmatism in order to obtain a satisfactory visual acuity. A suitable lens design may then be selected at the outset of the fitting.

With spherical soft lenses, owing to their replication of corneal astigmatism, the residual astigmatism is usually almost the same as the ocular astigmatism and if this is 1 D or more a toric soft lens or a hard lens may be necessary to obtain adequate visual acuity.

Approximate Rule (1)

Generally speaking, if the corneal astigmatism and total ocular astigmatism are both 'with-the-rule' or 'against-the-rule' and the difference between them (residual astigmatism) is less than 0.75 D, this cylinder may be ignored when hard spherical lenses are to be fitted. When spherical soft lenses are to be fitted ocular astigmatism of 0.75 D or less may usually be ignored.

REFRACTION WITH A CONTACT LENS OF INCORRECT BACK CENTRAL OPTIC RADIUS

Fitting sets of corneal lenses, particularly at the extremes of the range, often have back central optic radii in steps of 0.1 mm or 0.2 mm, so that the lens required to give the best fit may fall between two fitting lenses and the refraction may have to be carried out using a lens of incorrect BCOR.

A similar situation arises with scleral lenses. Not all trial scleral shells are sighted, and the refraction may have to be done with a lens of incorrect BCOR.

In this case:

Liquid lens power in air
+ Trial contact lens BVP in air
+ Effective power at the contact lens of the additional spectacle lens
= Ocular refraction

If the BCOR is flatter than that to be ordered, the liquid lens is more negative than it will be with the final contact lens (*Figure 4.21*). The vergence

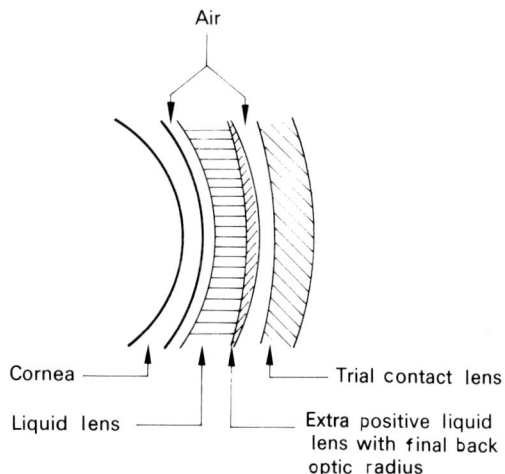

Figure 4.21–Refraction with a trial contact lens: the trial contact lens has too flat a back optic radius

of the light reaching the front surface of the liquid lens must therefore be adjusted to allow for this. Negative power must be added to counteract the extra positive power of the final liquid lens.

When fitting soft lenses, this does not apply because they conform to the central corneal contour. Only if very big radius differences between lens and cornea are used is there any effect on the liquid lens. Even then this defect is rather unpredictable as it depends on the relationship of the back surface of the lens to the peripheral corneal contour, which varies from one eye to another. If the back surface of the lens closely parallels the entire cornea, then the liquid lens will have zero power, but if the lens touches the apex region of the cornea and clears the peripheral region there is likely to be a small negative-powered liquid lens. Soft lenses fitted with BCOR 1 mm or more flatter than the keratometer readings, may therefore introduce a liquid lens of up to −0.50 D.

Approximate Rule (2)

If, when fitting hard lenses BCOR is flatter than that to be ordered, add −0.25 D to the BVP of the contact lens for each 0.05 mm that the BCOR is too flat.

When BCOR is steeper than that to be ordered, add +0.25 D to the BVP of the contact lens for each 0.05 mm that the BCOR is too steep.

This rule can be shown to be approximately correct by checking on a Heine's scale or by using radius/power tables for a refractive index of 1.336 (see Appendix B, *Table V*, page 323).

Examples: *(i)* A typical corneal lens problem

(ii) A typical scleral lens problem

		(i)	*(ii)*
BCOR used		8.10 mm	8.25 mm
BCOR ordered		8.00 mm	8.50 mm
Change in liquid lens power	from:	+41.48 D	+40.73 D
	to:	+42.00 D	+39.53 D
	by:	+0.52 D	−1.20 D
Contact lens BVP change to counteract this	Accurate method:	−0.52 D	+1.20 D
	Approximate method:	−0.50 D	+1.25 D
Error of approximate method		+0.02 D	+0.05 D

These examples show that the error of the approximate method is sufficiently small to be ignored.

BACK VERTEX POWER

This section applies particularly to scleral lenses and to high positive corneal and soft lenses.

The vergence of light reaching the eye must be the same with the final lens as when the refraction is done with a trial contact lens. Thus, BVP must be specified on orders for lenses. Sometimes only the front vertex power of the trial contact lens is known. When this is so, the laboratory must be given the central optic thickness of the trial lens so that its BVP may be calculated.

Example:

BVP of trial scleral lens	+5.62 D
t_c	0.50 mm
BOR	8.00 mm
FVP	+5.40 D

This illustrates the difference between BVP and FVP for a typical scleral lens.

If the lens were to be ordered on the basis of FVP without t_c being specified, it might be returned from the laboratory as:

FVP	+5.40 D
t_c	0.75 mm
BOR	8.00 mm
BVP (instead of +5.62 D)	+5.75 D

There is thus an error in BVP of +0.12 D, and the error increases with thickness and power (see Appendix D, page 336). Special care should therefore be taken when ordering high positive lenses, whether scleral, corneal or soft.

Corneal lenses are much thinner than sclerals, and the errors due to thickness differences are correspondingly much smaller. However, thickness should be specified with corneal lenses as it affects movement of the lens on the cornea as well as lid sensation and the rigidity of the lens itself (see Chapter 11). Soft lens thickness should also be specified for in addition to back vertex power considerations it affects the comfort, the rigidity and the gas permeability of the lens.

Spherical aberration becomes an important consideration when dealing with steeply curved surfaces, and with a contact lens on the eye the front surface of the lens suffers from positive spherical aberration which may seriously affect the BVP of the lens as it moves on the cornea. For example, a single vision corneal lens fitted as a distance prescription to an aphakic has been known to prove adequate in power for some close work. This occurs if the lens becomes displaced off-centre (usually upwards) relative to the pupil when the wearer looks down, and due to spherical aberration the effective power of the lens is increased. Unfortunately, not all spherical aberration effects are so beneficial, and a high positive lens which does not centre well on the cornea may therefore give poorer distance visual acuity than expected, possibly blurring to 6/18 from 6/6 if 1.00 D of positive spherical aberration is introduced.

Figure 4.22 shows that a decentration of 2.5 mm on the eye leads to an addition of +1.7 D for a

and its curvature (that is, its BCOR; or posterior apical radius, PAR, if the back surface is aspherical) and power should be as specified by the manufacturer.

After being placed on the eye several changes occur, all of which affect the power of the lens:

(1) The centre of the back surface takes up the same curvature as the central cornea, or almost so. This curvature change – so that the back

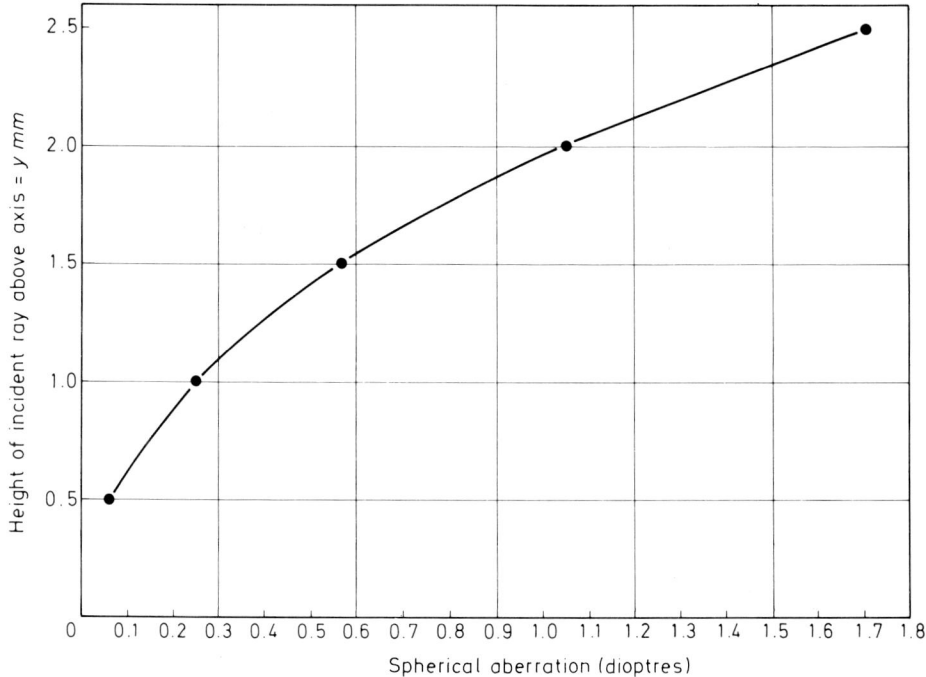

Figure 4.22– Variation of spherical aberration with aperture for a contact lens (n = 1.490) of +12.00 D BVP, BCOR of 7.80 mm and t_c of 0.35 mm. Parallel incident light is assumed

lens of BVP +12.00 D, centre thickness of 0.35 mm and BCOR of 7.80 mm.

Aspherical front surfaces can reduce these spherical aberration effects, thereby improving visual acuity. Kerns (1974) has shown that such lenses permit improved visual acuity in patients with residual astigmatism, possibly reducing the size of the circle of least confusion, due to removal of the spherical aberration effects.

POWER CHANGES OF SOFT LENSES

Before being placed on an eye a soft contact lens is normally in a fully hydrated state in normal saline solution and the refractive index is at its lowest value. The lens is also at room temperature

surface of the lens takes up a different curvature on the eye from its curvature when in an unstressed and unsupported state in saline solution – is commonly referred to as flexure. The amount of the resultant power change due to flexure, be it spherical or toroidal, is small.

Various empirical methods of predicting the power change due to this flexure have been suggested, such as assuming that the front optic radius changes by the same amount as the back optic radius (Baron, 1975), or alternatively that the two surfaces change in the same ratio. Strachan (1973) termed this ratio between the pre-wear and post-wear back optic radii, the 'wrap-factor'. The most plausible explanation and theoretical exposition has been given by Bennett (1976), who bases his argument on the criterion that the volume of the lens remains constant even though its curvature changes. This seems a valid assumption to make. He also assumes that there is no redistribution of lens thickness, that the centre thickness remains unchanged and that the front surface of the lens remains spherical if the cornea is spherical. Bearing these factors in mind he has

all materials. (The greatest error introduced would be of the order of 0.10 D for a lens of centre thickness 0.60 mm and a change in r_2 from 6.5 mm to r_2' of 6.0 mm, the value for the change in power for $n = 1.36$ being −0.68 D and that for $n = 1.46$ being −0.78 D.) It is interesting that Wichterle (1967), by a completely different method arrived

Table 4.11–Change in Power When a Soft Lens is Moulded by the Cornea to a Steeper Back Optic Radius, Refractive Index (1.43–1.44) and Volume Remaining the Same

Thickness	Back optic radius: r_2 (mm)							
t	9.5	9.0	8.5	8.0	7.5	7.0	6.5	6.0
mm	D	D	D	D	D	D	D	
0.10	−0.03	−0.05	−0.05	−0.07	−0.08	−0.10	−0.12	
0.15	−0.06	−0.07	−0.08	−0.09	−0.12	−0.15	−0.18	
0.20	−0.07	−0.09	−0.11	−0.13	−0.15	−0.20	−0.24	
0.25	−0.10	−0.11	−0.13	−0.16	−0.19	−0.24	−0.30	
0.30	−0.12	−0.13	−0.16	−0.19	−0.23	−0.28	−0.36	
0.35	−0.13	−0.15	−0.18	−0.22	−0.27	−0.33	−0.41	
0.40	−0.14	−0.18	−0.21	−0.25	−0.30	−0.37	−0.47	
0.45	−0.16	−0.19	−0.24	−0.28	−0.34	−0.41	−0.53	
0.50	−0.19	−0.21	−0.26	−0.31	−0.37	−0.46	−0.58	
0.55	−0.20	−0.24	−0.28	−0.33	−0.41	−0.51	−0.63	
0.60	−0.21	−0.26	−0.30	−0.37	−0.44	−0.55	−0.68	

Note: the change is invariably an addition of *minus* power and is virtually independent of the back vertex power of the original lens. For every 0.01 increase in refractive index over 1.44 the above figures should be increased by 1.5 per cent.

calculated that both positive and negative lenses change power with flexure, by the same amount as concentric lenses change power when they are bent. These changes are summarized in *Table 4.11* which is reproduced by kind permission of A. G. Bennett. He calculated the values from an equation he has derived, namely, that

$$F_v' = -\frac{(n-1)}{n} \cdot \frac{t}{r_2^2}$$

which for a value of n of 1.43 gives

$$F_v' = \frac{-300\, t}{r_2^2},$$

where F_v' is back vertex power, t is centre thickness, n is refractive index and r_2 is back central optic radius.

Thus,

$$\triangle F_v' = -300\, t \left(\frac{1}{r_2'^2} - \frac{1}{r_2^2} \right)$$

where r_2' is the radius to which r_2 changes after flexure. Now the refractive index of different soft lenses in their hydrated state varies between 1.36 and 1.46, but even if this variation is allowed for the values in *Table 4.11* would be altered by an insignificant amount and can safely be applied to

at a value for $\triangle F_v'$ only 10 per cent different from Bennett's, namely,

$$270\, t \left(\frac{1}{r_2'^2} - \frac{1}{r_2^2} \right).$$

Had Bennett assumed a refractive index of 1.37 for soft lens materials instead of 1.43, he and Wichterle would have arrived at exactly the same expression.

Unfortunately, these power changes are not always those found in practice and some of the differences are explicable as outlined in (2) and (3) below. It would appear from the work of Sarver, Ashley and Van Every (1974) and of Sarver, Harris and Polse (1975) that the spuncast lenses of Bausch and Lomb, which have an aspheric back surface, may have a different power change due to flexure from lathe-cut lenses. Sarver and his co-workers term the change in power induced by the flexure of the lens and any liquid lens present, the 'supplemental power effect'. They quote an example of a lens of BVP −4.00 D being required to correct the eye of a −3.00 D myope — the supplemental power effect being +1.00 D. Of 54 eyes examined wearing the Bausch and Lomb soft lens, all had a positive supplemental power effect, that is, either the lens was fitted steeper than the eye and became flatter and less negative on flexure or there was a positive liquid lens, or both.

Now the early fitting methods recommended by Bausch and Lomb did not relate the posterior apical radius (PAR) of the lens to the keratometer reading of the cornea to be fitted. Thus, many lenses were fitted which had a PAR steeper than the cornea. This accounts for the positive supplemental power effect found on many eyes, since flexure in such cases would flatten the lens. By contrast most lathe-cut lenses are fitted with BCOR considerably flatter than the central cornea (see Chapter 14, Volume 2) and so flexure induces a negative increase in power or negative supplemental power effect (see Table 4.11).

It is interesting that Sarver, Harris and Polse (1975) found a zero supplemental power effect with spuncast lenses of PAR fitted approximately 0.50 mm flatter than the keratometer reading. Indeed, from Table 4.11 it can be seen that for a centre thickness of less than 0.30 mm and for average PAR little change in power with flexure is to be expected for a change of 0.50 mm. However, Sarver and his co-workers remark that there is a large variation in the supplemental power effects found for a given corneal radius/PAR relationship. They state that lens thickness could be a factor contributing to the variation in supplemental power effects found. This is borne out by Bennett's work (Table 4.11) which shows that flexure of thicker lenses induces a greater change of lens power. They also state that peripheral corneal flattening and the shape of the back surface of the lens may be contributory factors. This seems very likely since a lens with aspherical back surface is likely to flex differently on a given cornea from a lens whose back surface is spherical.

Voerste (1976) also considered that corneal geometry influences lens flexure. He used Hydroflex/m lenses which are lathe-cut but of similar size to Bausch and Lomb lenses, and found a preponderance of zero and low negative (mainly up to −0.50 D) supplemental power effects in a study on over 200 eyes. Only a few eyes had a positive supplemental power effect. This is good clinical evidence in support of Bennett's theoretical work (Table 4.11) for the Hydroflex/m lenses are fitted up to 0.4 mm flatter than the mean keratometer reading and would thus steepen on flexure. Also, the lenses used in Voerste's study were all negative lenses and therefore very thin − between 0.1 mm and 0.2 mm centre thickness. Voerste also studied 30 eyes fitted with larger lathe-cut lenses (14.5−15.5 mm overall size) and with these there was a larger negative (mainly up to −0.75 D) supplemental power effect. This again confirms Bennett's theoretical work, for the larger Hydroflex lenses are fitted up to 1.4 mm flatter than the central cornea, thereby steepening

more with flexure and so inducing a greater increase in negative power, and possibly also retaining a small negative liquid lens.

Bennett also showed that on toroidal corneas the differential bending of a flatter spherical soft lens so that its back surface steepens to conform to the eye in both meridians, very slightly corrects the corneal astigmatism since there is a greater negative flexure effect along the steeper meridian. However, he showed that the amount of corneal astigmatism which can be corrected in this way is theoretically very small − from 2 to 13 per cent dependent on centre thickness.

(2) As the temperature of the cornea is 37°C and room temperature is about 20°C there is a change in temperature of the lens when it is put on the eye which leads to steepening with an accompanying slight increase in the negative power of the lens. (The effects on surface power of small changes in radius are shown in Table 4.9, page 110.)

(3) The increase in temperature and the fact that the front surface of the soft lens is exposed to the air which leads to evaporation, means that the water content of the lens decreases slightly when on the eye. This leads to a small increase in refractive index and further steepening of the lens, both of which tend to increase its negative power. (The changes in surface power due to alterations in refractive index are shown in Table 4.10, page 111.)

Ford (1976) terms this altered state of the lens when on the eye, 'the equilibrated state', which takes into account changes due to flexure, temperature and evaporation. He has developed tables and graphs for Sauflon material of 70 per cent water content and for lenses of different thicknesses. These permit the changes in BVP due to equilibration and flexure to be determined from the changes in thickness and BCOR. Thereby a lens of appropriate hydrated BVP can be selected. An example is given of a Sauflon 70 lens of hydrated BVP of −9.25 D and BCOR 9.00 mm being selected for an eye of ocular refraction −10.00 D and keratometer reading 7,50 mm. The hydrated lens thickness of 0.21 mm would decrease to 0.204 mm on equilibration and the BCOR would alter to 8.743 mm. The effects of flexure would contribute −0.30 D, leaving the requirement of an equilibrated BVP of −9.70 D which is obtained by a hydrated BVP of −9.25 D.

Unfortunately, as Ford (1974) has also shown, the amount of change in the lens due to evaporation depends on the tears output of the wearer. Thus, greater changes occur in those lenses worn by people with dry eyes than in those with normal or excessive tears output. According to Ford, variations in tears output alone can contribute to differences in power of over 1 D, and he has gone so far as to suggest that in order to determine the equilibrated lens power on the eye soft lens wearers should be put into one of three categories according to their tears output. An allowance could then be made for evaporation based on the tears output.

Obviously, then, the determination of the required soft lens power for a given eye is rather imprecise. It depends on whether the lens is lathe-cut or spuncast (although in general the effects of flexure are similar), on the rate of peripheral corneal flattening, on the tears output of the wearer, on the temperature and evaporation from the lens which in turn may be affected by external atmosphere and temperature as well as the lens material itself and its thickness. This section can therefore give no more than a guide as to what to expect.

ALTERATION OF THE BACK OPTIC RADIUS OF SCLERAL CONTACT LENSES

Sometimes a lens is supplied which has the correct BVP and is initially a good fit. After being worn for a few weeks, settling takes place and a heavy central corneal touch develops.

Two possibilities arise:

(1) *The back optic may be ground out using the same BCOR, thereby reducing central optic thickness.* This is usually done when the limbal clearance is also too small, as demonstrated by the fluorescein picture.

As shown by Swaine (1956), grinding substance out of the back optic surface affects the vergence reaching the eye in two ways: the reduction in plastics thickness adds negative power to the BVP of the contact lens, and the increase in liquid thickness adds positive power to the tears lens. The latter may be ignored if the liquid lens is restored to its originally satisfactory thickness.

Example:

BVP of scleral lens	+6.00 D
t_c	0.60 mm
BOR	8.50 mm
Keratometry: front corneal radius	7.75 mm

This gives central corneal touch after settling, and is ground out to:

t_c	0.40 mm
BOR	8.50 mm
This gives liquid thickness	0.10 mm

The reduction in thickness of the contact lens adds −0.54 D to its BVP, making the BVP +5.46 D.

The increase in thickness of the liquid lens from zero to 0.10 mm changes the liquid lens power from −3.83 D to −3.72 D, an addition of +0.11 D.

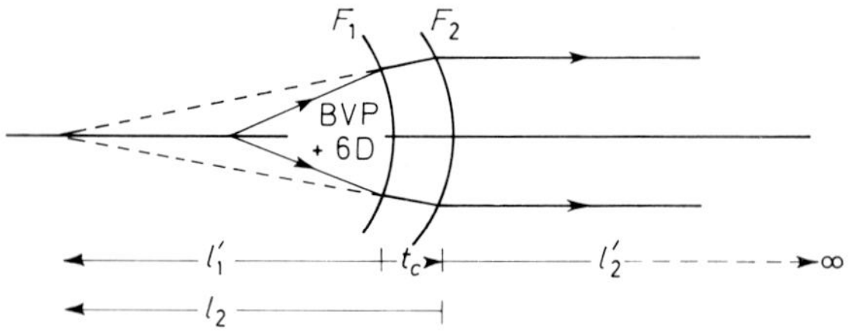

Figure 4.23—A pencil of rays traced 'backwards' through the optic portion of a scleral lens

Detailed calculations to obtain these BVP values are as follows. Tracing a pencil of rays 'backwards' through the scleral lens, as in *Figure 4.23*, the back surface power becomes F_1 and the front surface power becomes F_2. As the BOR = 8.5 mm,

$$F_1 = \frac{(1.49 - 1)\,1000}{-8.5} = -57.65 \text{ D}.$$

$$
\begin{aligned}
L_1 &= -6.00 \text{ D} \\
+F_1 &= -57.65 \text{ D} \\
\hline
L_1' &= -63.65 \text{ D}
\end{aligned}
$$

$$l_1' = \frac{1.49 \times 1000}{L_1'} = \frac{1490}{-63.65} \text{ mm} = -23.41 \text{ mm}$$

$$t_c = 0.60 \text{ mm}$$

$$l_2 = l_1' - t_c = -23.41 - 0.60 \text{ mm} = -24.01 \text{ mm}$$

$$L_2 = \frac{1.49 \times 1000}{l_2} = \frac{1490}{-24.01} \text{ D} = -62.06 \text{ D}$$

$L_2' = 0$ D (emergent rays are parallel).

$$F_2 = L_2' - L_2 = +62.06 \text{ D}$$

Now that the front surface power of the lens is known, the effect of grinding out the back surface to give a new thickness, t_c, of 0.4 mm can be determined, and the new BVP ascertained.

Tracing a pencil of rays 'forwards' through the lens as in *Figure 4.24*, $F_1 = +62.06$ D (previously F_2) and $F_2 = -57.65$ D (previously F_1).

$$
\begin{aligned}
L_1 &= 0 \text{ D (incident parallel light)} \\
+F_1 &= +62.06 \text{ D} \\
\hline
L_1' &= +62.06 \text{ D}
\end{aligned}
$$

$$l'_1 = \frac{1.49 \times 1000}{L'_1} = \frac{1490}{+62.06} \text{ mm} = +24.01 \text{ mm}$$

$$t_c = 0.40 \text{ mm}$$

$$l_2 = l'_1 - t_c = +23.61 \text{ mm}$$

$$L_2 = \frac{1.49 \times 1000}{l_2} = \frac{1490}{+23.61} \text{ D} = +63.11 \text{ D}$$

$$\frac{+F_2 = -57.65 \text{ D}}{L'_2 = \quad +5.46 \text{ D}} = \text{BVP of thinner scleral lens.}$$

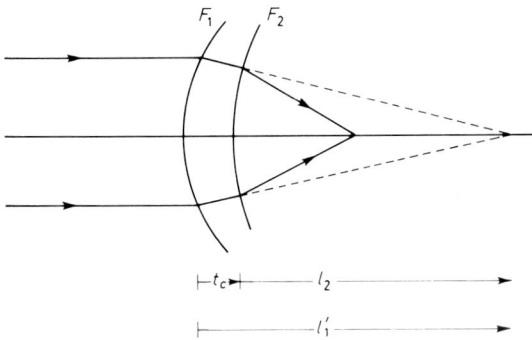

Figure 4.24–A pencil of rays traced 'forwards' through the optic portion of a scleral lens

Note: The above method of calculation, termed the 'step-along' method by W. Swaine, is an alternative to the use of reduced vergences with equivalent air distances and reduced thicknesses, as, for example, the calculations shown on pages 108 and 109.

The liquid lens power in air may be found as follows.

Its front surface radius is the BOR of the scleral lens = +8.50 mm.

Its back surface radius is the corneal radius found by keratometry = +7.75 mm.

Thus, front surface power,

$$F_1 = \frac{(1.336 - 1) \, 1000}{+8.5} = +39.53 \text{ D}$$

Back surface power,

$$F_2 = \frac{(1 - 1.336) \, 1000}{+7.75} = -43.36 \text{ D}$$

And for $t = 0$ mm, BVP = $F_1 + F_2 = -3.83$ D

After grinding out the back optic portion of the scleral lens, the liquid lens thickness, t, becomes 0.10 mm. The power of the liquid lens in air is then found thus. An incident parallel beam of light is assumed, so

$$\begin{aligned} L_1 &= 0 \\ +F_1 &= +39.53 \text{ D (as before)} \\ \hline L'_1 &= +39.53 \text{ D} \end{aligned}$$

$$l'_1 = \frac{1.336 \times 1000}{L'_1} = \frac{1336}{+39.53} \text{ mm} = +33.80 \text{ mm}$$

$$t = 0.10 \text{ mm}$$

$$l_2 = l'_1 - t = +33.70 \text{ mm}$$

$$L_2 = \frac{1.336 \times 1000}{l_2} = \frac{1336}{+33.70} \text{ D} = +39.64 \text{ D}$$

$$\frac{+F_2 = -43.36 \text{ D (as before)}}{L'_2 = \quad -3.72 \text{ D}} = \text{BVP}$$

These calculations may be simplified by the use of *Tables II, IV* and *V* of Appendix B as explained on pages 125–127.

Approximate Rule (3)

This applies to hard scleral lenses.

Reduction of 0.1 mm plastics thickness
adds   −0.25 D.
Increase of 0.1 mm liquid thickness
adds   +0.12 D.

In the example give above, the total effect on the vergence reaching the eye is −0.52 D + 0.11 D = −0.41 D, or if it is assumed that the original liquid thickness is restored by the grind-out, the vergence is changed by −0.52 D as the liquid lens is then unaltered.

For this reason, as Fletcher (1965) has stated, it is wise to order the original scleral lens a little too positive (by +0.25 D to +0.50 D, depending on the visual acuity obtainable). Even if the lens does not settle enough to require grinding out, it is bound to settle a certain amount, thereby reducing the liquid thickness and adding negative power to the liquid lens. A total settling of 0.2 mm is quite normal.

(2) *The BCOR may be steepened as well as the reduction in thickness.* This is usually done when the limbal clearance is more than adequate, as indicated by a large bubble in a fenestrated lens, surrounding the area of corneal touch.

The grinding out has the same effect described in (1) above, coupled with a further increase in negative power due to the steepened BCOR. The liquid lens is made more positive, but to a lesser extent than the negative increase of the contact lens.

Example:

BVP   +6.00 D
t_c 0.60 mm
BCOR   8.50 mm

This gives heavy central corneal touch and a large limbal bubble. 0.20 mm is to be removed centrally by grinding out, and the BCOR is to be steepened at the same time to 8.25 mm. The final apical corneal clearance required is 0.10 mm.

The effect on the plastics lens is to reduce the BVP from +6.00 D to +3.74 D, which is:

−0.52 D due to the thickness reduction
   (see (1) above)
−1.74 D due to the radius alteration (see
   Appendix B, *Table II, n* = 1.49)
−2.26 D total change in BVP

This is partially offset by the increase in positive power of the liquid lens from −3.83 D to −2.52 D, which is:

+0.11 D due to the thickness increase (see
   (1) above)
+1.20 D due to the radius change (see Appendix
   B, *Table V, n* = 1.336)
+1.31 D total change in liquid lens power

The change in vergence reaching the eye is approximately −1.00 D:

−2.26 D due to the plastics lens
+1.31 D due to the liquid lens
−0.95 D total change in vergence

The BVP of the contact lens should be changed to correct this amount, that is, from its new value of +3.74 D by +1.00 D to +4.74 D. This change must be carried out on the front surface of the lens.

Approximate Rule (4)

For each 0.05 mm that the BCOR of a sighted scleral lens is steepened, +0.12 D must be added to the altered BVP of the plastics lens (by changing the front surface power) in order to keep the BVP of the plastics/liquid system unchanged.

Applying the approximate rules to the example given results in:

Rule (4)
BCOR steepened by 0.25 mm = 5 × 0.05 mm steepening
   Compensation for negative increase at plastics/liquid interface = 5 × +0.12 D = +0.62 D to add to BVP

Rule (3)
Reduction of plastics thickness by 0.20 mm = 2 × 0.10 mm
   Compensation for negative power added = 2 × +0.25 D = +0.50 D to add to BVP

Rule (3)
Increase of liquid thickness by 0.10 mm = 1 × 0.10 mm
   Compensation for positive power added = 1 × −0.12 D = −0.12 D to add to BVP

Total change to be made to   +0.62 D
altered BVP by changing   +0.50 D
front surface power   −0.12 D
                                 +1.00 D

This yields almost the same result as that found by detailed calculation, which gave +0.95 D.

An alternative method of steepening the BCOR is to select the BCOR which will give the extra clearance required. This is done by deciding how much is to be ground out and over what diameter the BCOR is to be steepened. (This diameter is usually about 8−9 mm to allow adequate coverage of the pupil area.) Then the sagitta of the existing BCOR at this diameter may be determined (see Appendix C, page 332). The substance to be removed is added to this sagitta and gives the sagitta value at the same diameter for the steeper BCOR required. (Nomograms, as compiled by Clark, 1970, may be used as an alternative to tables for determining sagitta values.)

Example:
BCOR   9.00 mm
Diameter   9.00 mm
Sagitta   1.206 mm
Extra clearance   = 0.20 mm
Sagitta of new BCOR = 1.406 mm
Diameter as before = 9.00 mm
New BCOR required   = 7.90 mm
                    (see Appendix C)

This method of determining BCOR usually means that there is a considerable alteration over the central area alone which does not always result in a satisfactory fit. Central corneal clearance is achieved but touch may remain at the transition of the old and new back optic curves. (On the whole, it is better to steepen the BCOR by a small amount, such as 0.25 mm, after removing most of the substance required using the original BCOR.)

TORIC CONTACT LENSES
(*see* Chapter 18, Volume 2)

Both optical and fitting considerations of these lenses have been dealt with in detail by Capelli (1964), Stone (1966) and Westerhout (1969). In résumé, it may be said that if the back optic surface of a contact lens is to be made toroidal, the BVP required should be found either with a lens having the correct toroidal BCOR or with a spherical lens having a BCOR equal to the flatter meridian of the toric lens to be ordered. In the latter case, which is not as straightforward as the former, some calculation is necessary in order to determine the BVP of the final toric lens to be ordered. Since the BCOR of one meridian is to be steepened by a known amount when ordering, the calculation is the same as that for a spherical lens where a refraction has been carried out with a trial lens of incorrect BCOR, as outlined on pages 113 and 114 and summarized in *Approximate Rule (2)*. It is a simple matter of allowing for the fact that the liquid lens power in one meridian will be different with the final lens in place from the value with the spherical trial lens in place. An allowance for this difference must therefore be made on the plastics contact lens itself, as shown in the following example.

Example:

BCOR of lens to be ordered	7.50 mm along 90 8.30 mm along 180
BCOR of spherical trial lens for refraction	8.30 mm
BVP of spherical trial lens for refraction	−3.00 D
Additional spectacle lens needed	−1.00/+0.50 × 180
BVP of final contact lens along 180 is thus	−3.00 + −1.00 = −4.00
BVP of final contact lens along 90 is thus	−3.00 + −1.00 + +0.50 + allowance for radius change, of −4.00 D − *see Approximate Rule (2)* = −7.50 D in total.

(When the radius change is as large as this it is more accurate to look up the change in power of the liquid lens, remembering that this change is a change of the front surface of the liquid lens in air − *see* pages 113 and 114 and *see* Appendix B, *Table V*, for a Refractive Index Difference of 1.336 − 1. In this example, this gives a change of −4.32 D, that is, 0.32 D more than the value given by *Approximate Rule (2)*. Thus, the BVP of the final contact lens along 90 should be −7.82 D.)

It can now be established whether or not a front toroidal surface will be necessary on the final lens. This depends on whether or not the cylinder power of the back surface in air is the same as the cylinder element of the BVP in air:

BVP of final lens (in air)	−4.00/−3.82 × 180
Back surface powers (in air)	−65.33 along 90
(From Appendix B, *Table II,* for 1.490 − 1)	−59.04 along 180
Back surface cylinder in air is thus	−6.29 × 180
Front surface cylinder required	−3.82 − −6.29 × 180 = +2.47 × 180

The above example is an obvious case where a front surface cylinder is necessary to give good visual acuity. Frequently the front surface cylinder calculated in this way is quite small and the practitioner may prefer to order a lens with a spherical front surface and risk leaving the patient with a small amount of uncorrected astigmatism. In such a case the cylinder element of the BVP of the final lens must be altered by this amount, that is, the cylinder element of the BVP is then the same as the back surface cylinder in air.

It often helps in considering the optical effects of contact lenses with toroidal back surfaces, to imagine the existence of a very thick tears lens, in the centre of which is sandwiched a perfectly flat layer of air. The surfaces bounding this flat layer of air are therefore of zero power in all meridians, the tears on either side forming two liquid lenses − one whose power depends on the toroidal radii of the back surface of the contact lens, and the other quite separate one whose power depends on the corneal radii. Then the optical effect of the tears on the cornea (which is to neutralize the corneal astigmatism − *see* page 109) can be considered separately from the plastics/tears interface at the back of the contact lens. If appropriate the two can be added together. Thus, the rear portion of this tears lens corrects the corneal astigmatism, but further astigmatism is introduced by the front portion at the plastics/tears interface (*see* Chapter 18, Volume 2).

BIFOCAL CONTACT LENSES

Like bifocal spectacle lenses, contact lens bifocals are available in both solid and fused types. Chapter 19, Volume 2 deals with the various designs and methods of fitting. The two types most frequently fitted are the concentric solid bifocal with distance portion in the centre and the fused bifocal with the near segment on the back surface. The latter is shown in *Figure 4.26*. An appreciation of the optical principles of these two main types should permit a general understanding of all other designs of bifocal contact lens.

Concentric Solid Bifocals

As *Figure 4.25a* and *b* shows, these are available with the addition worked on either the front or back optic surface (and, of course, a combination of back and front surface additions could be used).

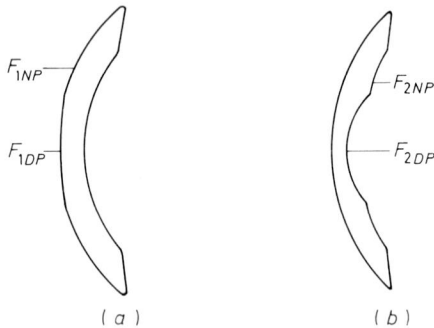

*Figure 4.25 – Concentric solid bifocal corneal lenses.
(a) Front surface addition. (b) Back surface addition*

Where the addition is on the front surface (a plastics/air interface), the front optic portion has two radii worked on it, the steeper corresponding to the near portion of the lens. Then, provided that the lens is assumed to be infinitely thin, the near addition is equal to the difference between the two front surface powers.

For example, if the near addition to be incorporated is +3.00 D and where F_{1DP} and F_{1NP} are the front surface powers of the distance and near portions respectively, then $F_{1NP} = F_{1DP} + 3.00$. Since this is a plastics/air interface the appropriate front optic radii may be obtained from Appendix B, *Table II* (a radius/power table for polymethyl methacrylate of refractive index 1.490). If, in a particular case, F_{1DP} is calculated to be +58.00 D, the nearest value to this in the table is 57.99 giving a radius, r_{1DP}, of

$$8.45 \text{ mm} \quad = \frac{(1.490 - 1)1000}{58.00}$$

For an addition of +3.00 D, F_{1NP} must therefore be +61.00 D and the nearest value to this in the table is 61.02, giving a radius of 8.03 mm.

If thickness is to be taken into account, reference to Appendix B, *Table IV* (lower figures for convergent light) should be made. In the example just given, if the centre thickness of the distance portion were 0.20 mm and that of the near portion 0.22 mm, entering the initial vergence column at 58.0 D for the distance portion, it can be seen that 0.20 mm thickness adds 0.46 D to this power. The reduced vergence reaching the back surface is thus +58.46 D. Similarly, for the near portion, entering the initial vergence column between 60.0 D and 62.0 D, 0.22 mm thickness adds between 0.54 D and 0.57 D to the reduced vergence; say, 0.56 D. The difference between 0.46 D and 0.56 D is 0.10 D and is small enough to be ignored, but it indicates that F_{1NP} should be reduced by this amount, from +61.00 D to +60.90 D, giving r_{1NP} as 8.05 mm instead of 8.03 mm. This small radius change is not really worth making as will be shown.

In fact, most practitioners agree that there is a tendency for a small negative-powered liquid lens to collect in front of the upper and lower portions of any corneal lens due to the tears rivus along the eyelid margins. The configuration of the front surface of a solid bifocal with front surface addition (*Figure 4.25a*) is such that this tears lens may slightly reduce the front surface positive power at the periphery. If anything, then, it is wise to err on the positive side, and indeed many practitioners increase the addition they have determined, by as much as +1.00 D to allow for this negative tears lens although its amount is rather variable depending as it does on the patient's tears output and the rate of evaporation in differing atmospheric conditions. Concern over the effect on the addition, of differences in thickness between the distance and near portions, is therefore seen to be unwarranted.

When the addition is on the back surface, no allowance for the effect of thickness need even be considered, but the major consideration here is that it is a plastics/tear interface, rather than a plastics/air interface.

In air the power depends on

$$\frac{1.490 - 1}{r}$$

whereas in tears it depends on

$$\frac{1.490 - 1.336}{r}.$$

This is a factor of 0.49/0.154 or approximately 3.18. Thus, the practitioner and manufacturer must make the back surface radii such as to provide approximately three times the addition on the back surface (when measured in air) that is really required, due to the neutralizing effect of the tears. This point is important to remember when checking such a lens on the focimeter.

Usually this type of bifocal is fitted with a steep BCOR (r_{2DP}) and small BCOD, with the first back peripheral optic radius (r_{2NP}) providing the near addition and fitted so as to align or be just flatter than the cornea. For example, if BP_1OR (r_{2NP}) is 8.50 mm, reference to Appendix B, *Table I* for 1.490 – 1.336 shows F_{2NP} to be −18.118 D. (It is negative in power because the medium of higher refractive index is concave.) To give a +3.00 D addition requires that F_{2DP} be −21.118 D and thus r_{2DP}, the BCOR, is seen by interpolation in the table, to be 7.27 mm. Now if this lens were measured in air on a focimeter, the radii of 8.50 mm and 7.27 mm would have surface powers, for 1.490 − 1, of −57.65 D and −67.40 D respectively (*see* Appendix B, *Table II*). Thus, the near addition measured in air is +9.75 D, which equals the near addition in tears X 3.18 (approximately), as stated above.

Fused Bifocals

These are very similar to fused bifocal spectacle lenses except that most corneal lenses have the segment on the back surface, and the refractive index of the fused segment is usually 1.56. The optical theory is easily understood if reference is made to *Figure 4.26*. Since the back surface is a negative surface and the segment has the higher

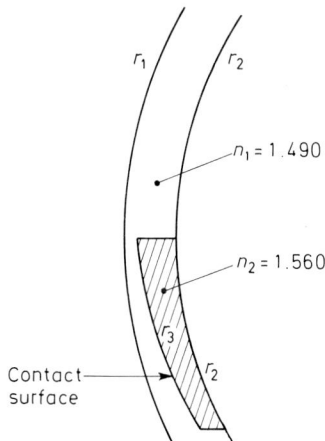

Figure 4.26−Fused bifocal corneal lens: r_1, r_2 and r_3 are the radii of the front, back and contact surfaces respectively; n_1 and n_2 are the refractive indices of the main lens and the near segment

refractive index, there is actually a gain in *negative* power at the back surface of

$$\frac{1.560 - 1.490}{r_2},$$

and where r_2 is in mm this expression becomes

$$\frac{-70}{r_2} \text{ D.}$$

For example, if the BCOR (r_2) is 8.00 mm then the back surface powers in tears are:

$$F_{2DP} = \frac{(1.336 - 1.490)1000}{8.00} \text{ D} = -19.25 \text{ D}$$

(*see* Appendix B, *Table I*).

$$F_{2NP} = \frac{(1.336 - 1.560)1000}{8.00} \text{ D} = -28.00 \text{ D}$$

(*see* Appendix B, *Table X*).

The difference,

$$F_{2NP} - F_{2NP} = -8.75 \text{ D} = \frac{-70}{8} \text{ D } (see \text{ above).}$$

This back surface power difference, due to the segment, may be obtained from Appendix B, *Table XI*, for BCOR values ranging from 5.00 mm to 9.00 mm in 0.10 mm steps (and in 0.01 mm steps, by interpolation).

It should be emphasized here that the power difference due to the segment is the same whether the power is determined in air or in tears, because the BCOR, r_2, is the same throughout (as distinct from the back surface solid bifocal where $r_{2DP} < r_{2NP}$). This is easily shown using the same value for r_2 as above. The back surface powers in air are

$$F_{2DP} = \frac{(1 - 1.490)1000}{8.00} \text{ D} = -61.25 \text{ D}$$

(*see* Appendix B, *Table II*).

$$F_{2NP} = \frac{(1 - 1.560)1000}{8.00} \text{ D} = -70.00 \text{ D}$$

(*see* Appendix B, *Table IX*).

The difference, $F_{2NP} - F_{2DP} = -8.75 \text{ D} = \frac{-70}{8} \text{ D.}$

This is exactly the same result as when the back surface powers were determined in tears (*see* above).

Because the back surface addition is the same measured in air as in tears, the addition read on a focimeter is the same as that on the eye.

Since the fused segment gives rise to a gain in negative power on the back surface, it must give rise to a gain in positive power at the contact surface sufficient to overcome the negative gain as well as to provide the near addition, that is, if the power of the contact surface is F_3, then

$$F_3 = \text{Addition} - \left(-\frac{70}{r_2}\right) = \text{Addition} + \frac{70}{r_2}$$

Now F_3 (which is convex to the medium of higher refractive index)

$$= \frac{1.560 - 1.490}{r_3} D = \frac{70}{r_3} D \text{ (where } r_3 \text{ is in mm).}$$

And since $F_3 = \text{Addition} + \dfrac{70}{r_2}$

$$r_3 = \frac{70}{\text{Add.} + \dfrac{70}{r_2}}$$

(where the addition is in D, and r_2 and r_3 are in mm).

Appendix B, *Table XII* gives r_3, the contact surface radius, for values of r_2, the BCOR, from 6.0 mm to 9.0 mm in 0.1 mm steps and additions from +1.00 D to +4.00 D in 0.50 D steps.

For example, if the addition were +3.00 D and the BCOR 8.00 mm,

then $F_3 = +3.00 - (-8.75) D = +11.75 D$

and $r_3 = \dfrac{(1.560 - 1.490)1000}{11.75} \text{mm} = 5.95 \text{ mm}$

(*see* Appendix B, *Table XI* used by looking up 11.75 D in the body of the table, and by interpolation, the corresponding radius is seen to be 5.95 mm).

However, r_3 is directly obtainable from Appendix B, *Table XII*, by reference to the BCOR (r_2) and the addition.

OPTICAL CHANGES OF THE EYE CAUSED BY CONTACT LENSES

Contact lenses may bring about curvature, thickness and refractive index changes of the cornea. These effects, both with and without the contact lenses in place, are dealt with in Chapters 16 and 17, Volume 2.

Besides the effects mentioned in these chapters it seems appropriate here to record the work of Carney (1975) who has used atmospheres of 100 per cent oxygen tension and zero oxygen tension coupled with flat-fitting and steep-fitting hard corneal lenses to study curvature and thickness changes of the cornea induced by hard corneal lenses. A summary of his results suggests that all lenses tend to mould the cornea to their own shape — flat lenses flattening and steep lenses steepening

the central cornea. In addition, those lenses which give rise to central corneal oedema cause an unequal change in corneal thickness, it being greatest in the centre which leads to steepening of the corneal front surface. Now such steepening leads to an increase in myopia, and flattening to an increase in hypermetropia.

The resulting dioptric change in air, measurable as a change in ocular refraction, is largely masked by the wearing of the contact lens because the corneal change is neutralized by the tears. The ratio:

$$\frac{\text{dioptric change in air}}{\text{dioptric change with contact lens in place}}$$

$$= \frac{9.4}{1} = \frac{1.376 - 1.0}{1.376 - 1.336} \ .$$

As can be seen it is dependent on the refractive index differences of the cornea in air relative to the cornea in tears. Thus, a person who becomes 1 D more myopic due to corneal steepening manifests less than 0.12 D of this whilst wearing his contact lenses.

The wearing of hard contact lenses tends to cause central corneal oedema and steepening, whilst the removal of the lenses results in central corneal thinning and flattening (Mandell and Polse, 1969; Polse, 1972). The mechanism of this change has been likened by Stone (1973) to the curvature change of a hard negative corneal lens during its hydration/dehydration cycle (Gordon, 1965). The resultant increases and decreases in myopia (and astigmatism) have been well documented by Rengstorff (*see* Chapter 17, Volume 2).

It is often not realized that the presence of oedema alone can lead to a small increase in myopia — the lowering of the corneal refractive index due to the imbibation of water actually increases the total power of the cornea, a decrease in index of 0.01 giving rise to a power increase of approximately +0.12 D. This surprising result occurs because the back surface of the cornea has no effect as a negative powered surface once the corneal refractive index drops to that of the aqueous (1.336). Therefore, as the corneal refractive index lowers during oedema, the corneal back surface has less and less neutralizing effect on the front surface power (Rengstorff and Arner, 1971). The small change in corneal thickness brought about by oedema has little effect on its own, on corneal power. It is the lowering of refractive index and the accompanying curvature change which affects the refractive error.

With soft lens wear the cornea often suffers an increase in thickness due to oedema, but this occurs throughout the entire cornea and is not localized to the central region only as with hard corneal lens wear. The result is dependent on the degree of oedema, but the curvature change varies from very slight steepening to very slight flattening. The associated change in refractive error is also very small (Mandell, 1975). The oedema which leads to a uniform thickness increase in the cornea and therefore to a small increase in the anterior corneal radius which would decrease myopia, also leads to a drop in refractive index which would increase myopia. Thus, although soft lenses do bring about changes of the cornea, there is very little effect on refractive error and therefore very little associated 'spectacle blur' (*see* Subjective Refraction, Chapter 16, Volume 2).

OPTICAL TABLES FOR CONTACT LENS WORK* WITH EXAMPLES TO ILLUSTRATE THEIR USE

It is hoped that the tables incorporated in the appendices to this book will help to simplify and to speed up optical calculations which occur in the contact lens field. The principles involved are well covered elsewhere (Bennett, 1966), and are therefore not dealt with in detail here.

Appendix A shows the effective power of spectacle lenses at various distances from the back surface of the spectacle lens. Thus, it can be seen from the table that a lens of back vertex power +7.00 D, has an effective power of +7.76 D, in a plane 13 mm from the back surface of the lens, while the effective power of a −7.00 D lens at the same vertex distance is −6.41 D. From this table, then, can be obtained very quickly, the effective power of a trial spectacle lens at the eye. A comprehensive table of this sort can be useful in other ways, such as comparing spectacle and ocular refraction, in assessing the correction of astigmatism in near vision and in the determination of spectacle and ocular accommodation.

THE CONTACT LENS

In Appendix B, *Table I*, the surface power, in air, corresponding to a given radius of curvature has been plotted for various refractive indices. For the refractive index differences of (1.49−1) and (1.336−1), *see* Appendix B, *Tables II* and *V* respectively, steps of 0.01 mm in radius have been used so that the corresponding steps in power are small enough for the table to be used in the reverse direction, that is, the radius required to produce a

* Adapted from *Optical Tables for Contact Lens Work*, by J. L. Francis (1968). Hatton Press.

given change in light vergence can be found with sufficient accuracy. To illustrate this, suppose a pencil of rays has been traced 'backwards' through a lens of index 1.49, and when incident on the front surface the divergence of the pencil is −71.50 D. If the light is to emerge into air as a parallel pencil then the front surface must have a power of +71.50 D. Looking down the appropriate power column of Appendix B, *Table II*, the nearest figure listed is 71.53 and the corresponding radius is 6.85 mm.

Table III is based on *Table II* but enables the change in surface power resulting from a given change of radius to be looked up directly. It applies to plastics material in air (n = 1.490) and can be helpful when it is decided to fit a contact lens with a toric surface. For example, if the BCOR chosen for one principal meridian is 8.0 mm and that of the second principal meridian is 7.1 mm, then the difference in power between the two meridians, in air, is found from *Table III* to be 7.76 D. Since it is the back surface of the contact lens which is being dealt with, it is the steeper meridian which has the greater negative power.

It should also be clear that *Table III* can be used to give an estimate of the 'thin lens' power of a contact lens in air, that is, the sum of the surface powers without allowance for thickness. So, if a lens has a front surface radius of 8.50 mm and a back surface radius of 7.80 mm, it can be seen from *Table III* that the corresponding thin lens power in air is −5.17 D, the negative sign agreeing with the fact that the back surface has the steeper radius.

Appendix B, *Table IV*, shows directly the change in reduced vergence due to thickness for a given initial vergence. This greatly reduces the labour involved in this type of calculation and eliminates reference to reciprocal tables and to tables of reduced thickness. This table covers initial vergences from 100.0 D to 40.0 D in 2.0 D steps for a range of thicknesses from 0.01 mm to 1.50 mm, the upper part of this range being included to cover the case of rather thick scleral lenses. In each cell of the table the lower figure gives the increase in vergence due to thickness for convergent light, while the upper figure indicates the decrease in vergence due to thickness for divergent light. The use of *Table IV* is best illustrated by some numerical examples:

Example:

To find the BVP in air, of a contact lens of given radii of curvature and thickness.

Take r_1 = +7.05 mm, r_2 = +8.00 mm, t = 0.6 mm

From Appendix B, *Table II*, the surface powers are found to be, F_1 = +69.50 D and F_2 = −61.25 D, so a pencil of parallel rays incident on the front surface of the lens becomes convergent after refraction to the extent of +69.50 D. Now entering the 'initial vergence' column of *Table IV* at the nearest figure to 69.50, that is, at 70.00, find at this level the cell corresponding to a thickness of 0.60 mm. Since the rays are convergent use the lower figure in the cell: +2.03. This is the increase in vergence due to the thickness. Thus, the rays incident on the second surface of the lens have a vergence of +69.50 + 2.03 = +71.53 D. Addition of the back surface power, with due regard to sign, gives the required back vertex power in air. Thus, BVP = +71.53 − 61.25 = +10.28 D. The process takes much longer to describe than to do. It can be conveniently set out as follows:

Sum of the surface powers	+69.50
	−61.25
	+ 8.25
Add thickness allowance	+ 2.03
BVP =	+10.28 D

It will be appreciated that some degree of approximation is involved owing to the steps used in the vergence column of Appendix B, *Table IV*, but errors due to this are small. In the above example, more accurate calculations give a result of +10.25 D, so the error in the approximate result is 0.03 D, nearly 0.3 per cent. If greater accuracy in using *Table IV* is desired, it is not difficult to interpolate between the rows.

Example:

To find the front surface power, in air, of a contact lens of given BVP, BCOR and thickness.

Consider a lens 0.50 mm thick, of BVP = −20.00 D and BCOR = 7.80 mm

From Appendix B, *Table II*, the back surface power = −62.82 D.

Now tracing backwards through the lens, take a pencil of rays, which initially converges towards the posterior focus of the lens, that is, a pencil with an incident vergence of +20.00 D.

Incident vergence at back surface	+20.00
Back surface power to be added	−62.82
Vergence after refraction	−42.82 D

Entering Appendix B, *Table IV*, at 42.0 D the thickness allowance where t = 0.5 mm is 0.58 D

(upper figure for divergent light), but for 44.0 D the allowance is 0.64. By interpolation therefore take 0.61 as the allowance for an initial vergence of 42.82 D. So adding 0.61 to −42.82 D gives the vergence of light reaching the front surface as −42.21 D. Clearly the front surface power required is of equal amount but opposite sign, namely, +42.21 D. From Appendix B, *Table II*, the corresponding radius of curvature is seen to be +11.61 mm.

This type of calculation can easily be applied to each principal meridian in turn when the lens considered has a toroidal back surface.

As a further example of the use of the tables discussed so far, consider the following. In a particular case, a choice of BCOR has been made and an afocal lens of this radius is placed on the eye. It is then found that a trial spectacle lens of +5.00 D placed 12 mm in front of the contact lens is necessary to correct the residual refractive error. The problem is: What BVP should be ordered for the finished contact lens? The liquid lens is not involved here as this is assumed to be the same in the trial set up as with the finished lens. If the BCOR chosen is 7.90 mm and the afocal lens used is 0.25 mm thick, first it is necessary to find the characteristics of the afocal lens. From Appendix B, *Table II*, F_2 = 62.03 D. Using Appendix B, *Table IV*, the thickness allowance for divergent light is 0.64 D so the front surface power of the afocal lens is − (−62.03 + 0.64) = +62.03 − 0.64 = +61.39 D, and *Table II* gives the corresponding radius as 7.98 mm. Tracing a pencil of parallel rays through the spectacle trial lens and the afocal contact lens:

Vergence after refraction at +5.00 D spectacle trial lens	+ 5.00
Effective power at 12 mm (from Appendix A)	+ 5.32
Front surface power of afocal contact lens to be added	+61.39
	+66.71
Allowance for thickness (from Appendix B, *Table IV*)	+ 0.76
Incident vergence at second surface	+67.47
Back surface power of contact lens to be added	−62.03
Vergence in air after refraction	+ 5.44 D

The BVP to be ordered for the finished lens is thus +5.44 D. Should the trial contact lens employed not be afocal, the calculation is entirely similar, the characteristics of the trial contact lens being determined as in the previous example.

THE LIQUID LENS

Tables V and *VI* of Appendix B are of similar type to *Tables II* and *III*, but are applicable to the liquid lens in air and are therefore based on a refractive index of 1.336. To find the power of the liquid lens in air the procedure is as follows. In a particular case let the BCOR of the contact lens be 8.00 mm, and the radius of curvature of the cornea be 7.80 mm. The surface powers of the liquid lens are obtained from *Table V*. These are F_1 = +42.00 D and F_2 = −43.08 D, so considered as a thin lens the power of the liquid lens is the sum of these two powers = 1.08 D. If the thickness of the liquid lens is 0.10 mm the effect of this can be found from *Table VII*. Entering this table at 42.0 D the allowance for a thickness of 0.10 mm is 0.13 D, and in this case is to be added. The BVP of the liquid lens in air thus = +42.00 − 43.08 + 0.13 = −0.95 D.

The quantity which matters most in the correction of an ametropic eye is, of course, the back vertex power of the contact lens and liquid lens combined. A good approximation to this is obtained simply by adding the BVP of the contact lens to that of the liquid lens. For instance, if the contact lens in the example just quoted had a BVP in air of −10.00 D, then the combination of contact lens plus liquid lens has a BVP of approximately −10.95 D. If greater accuracy is required then the procedure is as follows.

With a contact lens of BVP = −10.00 D the vergence of light incident on the first surface of the liquid lens = −10.00 D. Vergence after refraction at the first surface of the liquid lens = +42.00 − 10.00 = +32.00 D.

Entering Appendix B, *Table VII*, at 32.0 D, the thickness allowance for 0.10 mm = 0.08 D, so the BVP of the combined contact and liquid lens is +32.00 − 43.08 + 0.08 = −11.00 D in air. This result differs by only 0.05 D from the approximate one obtained earlier. A greater difference may arise in cases having a thicker liquid lens and a contact lens of considerable back vertex power. It should be remembered that nowadays when most cases are fitted with corneal lenses, the tears thickness is so small that sufficient accuracy is obtained by ignoring any thickness allowance for the liquid lens. (Soft lenses, also, retain a liquid lens of negligible thickness.) In these cases the power of the liquid lens is obtained by adding the two surface powers or perhaps more quickly, by using *Table VI* as outlined below.

Table VI gives directly the change in surface power resulting from a given change in radius for the liquid lens in air. This is probably the quickest way of estimating the liquid lens power, the effect of thickness being ignored. Thus, if the liquid lens has a front surface radius of 7.70 mm and a back surface radius of 7.60 mm, then the thin lens power is obtained directly from *Table VI* as −0.57 D. The table may also be used when a toroidal surface is involved.

The right-hand column of *Table I* in Appendix B also gives interface powers for various radii of the back surface of the contact lens when in contact with the liquid lens (that is, 1.49 − 1.336 and relative index = 0.154), and *Table VIII* needs little explanation. It gives the change in power resulting from a change of radius (also for n_R = 0.154). Thus, a decision to alter the back optic radius of the contact lens from 8.00 mm (r_1 in the table) to 7.90 mm (r_2 in the table) changes the power of the contact surface by 0.24 D, and since the surface of higher refractive index is a negative surface (the back surface of the contact lens) the effect of the modification is to add −0.24 D. This type of modification is often made to final sighted scleral lenses in order to improve the fit of the optic portion, and may then necessitate an alteration to the front surface power of the contact lens in order to compensate for the change in interface power and keep the combination BVP of the contact lens/liquid lens the same.

FUSED BIFOCAL CONTACT LENSES

Tables IX to *XII* of Appendix B relate to fused bifocal corneal lenses. The underlying theory has already been explained (*see* pages 123−124, and *Figure 4.26*).

Table IX gives surface powers in air for plastics material of refractive index 1.560, the material of which the fused segment is made. Thus, it can be used for determining the power of the back surface of the segment in air for BCOR values between 5.00 mm and 9.00 mm in 0.10 mm steps (and in 0.01 mm steps, by interpolation using the difference column). For example, if the BCOR is 8.05 mm, power F for r = 8.00 mm, is 70.0000 D. The difference for a 0.01 mm change in r is 0.0886 D, and therefore for a 0.05 mm change in r the difference is 5 X 0.0886 D. This difference is thus 0.443 D and evidently must be subtracted from 70.0000 D giving F = 69.557 D. This may be verified by calculating the power value midway between the powers for r = 8.00 mm and r = 8.10 mm, which gives 69.568 D. This gives a small discrepancy of 0.01 D in the second place of decimals, which is of no significance. Having determined the power value, it must be ascribed a sign, and since it is a concave surface, the power is −69.57 D.

Table X is similar to *Table IX*, but gives the surface powers in tears (1.560 − 1.336) and may therefore be used for determining the back surface power of the fused segment when on the eye. Again, this is a negative power since the surface is concave to the medium of higher refractive index. Used with *Tables II* and *I* for (1.490 − 1) and (1.490 − 1.336) respectively, *Tables IX* and *X* permit the power of the back surface of the segment to be compared with the back surface power of the main lens, both in air (*Tables IX* and *II*) and in tears (*Tables X* and *I*). Differences in power on the back surface between the segment and the main lens may thus be determined, but this information is directly obtainable from *Table XI* for (1.560 − 1.490). *Table XI* can also be used for determining contact surface powers for radii (r_3 in *Figure 4.26*) from 5.00 mm to 9.00 mm in 0.10 mm steps (and again by interpolation, in 0.01 mm steps).

Table XII allows the radius, r_3, of the contact surface to be determined for various near additions and values of the BCOR. Thus, for a BCOR of 8.00 mm and a near addition of +3.00 D, a contact surface radius, r_3, of 5.9574 mm, say, 5.96 mm is required (cf page 124).

ASPECTS OF CONTACT LENS DESIGN

The main purpose of this section is to give some guidelines to those contact lens practitioners who wish to design their own lenses. It is hoped that they can then avoid the pitfall of ordering a lens of such thickness that it is impossible to manufacture. Whilst intended primarily for the design of hard corneal lenses, the principles outlined in this section may be applied to any type of contact lens.

Readers are referred to Creighton's *Contact Lenses Fabrication Tables* (1964) for a more detailed exposition on this subject.

Sagitta of Front and Back Surfaces

It should be obvious from *Figure 4.27a* and *b* that for both positive and negative lenses the sagitta or sag value, s, of the front surface of a lens plus the edge thickness, t_e, must equal the primary sag (of the back surface), p, plus the centre thickness, t_c.

Thus, $s + t_e = p + t_c$

For a positive lens there is a danger of ordering the centre thickness too small to permit adequate

edge thickness, and for a negative lens the attempt to keep the edge thickness reasonably small may result in the centre of the lens becoming excessively thin.

The values for p and s may be found as follows.

Primary Sag, p

From *Figure 4.28a* it can be seen that the primary sag of the back surface of a tricurve corneal lens is $I + II + III$, where I is the sag of the BCOR at the BCOD. II and III may be determined by studying *Figure 4.28b* and *c*.

Thus, $II = x_1 − y_1$ where x_1 is the sag of BP_1OR at BP_1OD and y_1 is the sag of BP_1OR at BCOD.

III is determined in exactly the same manner as II (see *Figure 4.28c*).

Thus, $III = x_2 − y_2$ where x_2 is the sag of BP_2OR at OS (or BP_2OD if the lens has more than three back surface curves) and y_2 is the sag of BP_2OR at BP_1OD.

It can be seen, then, that the primary sag of a C3 lens is given by $p = I + (x_1 − y_1) + (x_2 − y_2)$ and for a C4 lens $p = I + (x_1 − y_1) + (x_2 − y_2) + (x_3 − y_3)$.

All the individual sag values may be obtained directly or by interpolation from Appendix C. For example, the tricurve corneal lens C3/8.00:7.0/9.05:7.8/10.80:8.6 has a primary sag, p, which can be calculated as follows.

I = sag of BCOR of 8.00 mm at BCOD of 7.0 mm = **0.806 mm.**

$II = x_1 − y_1$.

Now x_1 = sag of 9.05 mm (BP_1OR) at 7.8 mm (BP_1OD) = 0.884 mm (by interpolation in Appendix C).

y_1 = sag of 9.05 mm (BP_1OR) at 7.0 mm (BCOD) = 0.704 mm (by interpolation in Appendix C).

Thus, II = 0.884 − 0.704 = **0.180 mm,**
$III = x_2 − y_2$.

Now x_2 = sag of 10.80 mm (BP_2OR) at 8.6 mm (OS) = 0.893 mm,

and y_2 = sag of 10.80 mm (BP_2OR) at 7.8 mm (BP_1OD) = 0.729 mm.

So III = 0.893 − 0.729 = **0.164 mm.**

And primary sag, $p = I + II + III$ = 0.806 + 0.180 + 0.164 = **1.150 mm.**

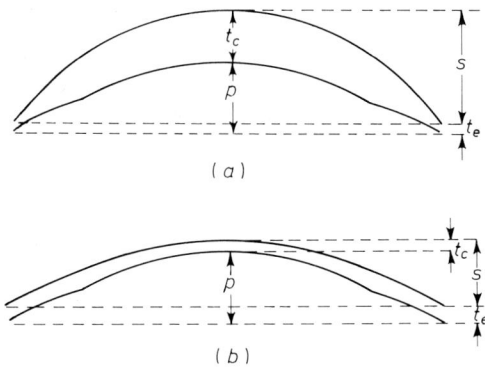

Figure 4.27—$s + t_e = p + t_c$ (a) Positive lens. (b) Negative lens

Front Surface Sag, s

Now suppose the lens with the above primary sag value of 1.150 mm is to be made up with BVP of +2.00 D. It is then necessary to determine the front optic radius in order to calculate the sag, s, of the front surface. To obtain the front optic radius, r_1, necessitates guessing a value for the centre thickness, t_c. In this case, suppose t_c = 0.21 mm. Then r_1 may be calculated as described on page 126.

Taking a pencil of rays backwards through the lens:

Incident vergence at back surface	$= -$ 2.00 D
Power of back surface to be added	$= -61.25$ D
(see Appendix B, Table II)	
Vergence after refraction	$= -63.25$ D
Allowance for 0.21 mm t_c	$= +$ 0.56 D
(see Appendix B, Table IV)	
Vergence reaching front surface	$= -62.69$ D
Front surface power	$= +62.69$ D
Front surface radius, r_1	$=$ 7.815 mm
(see Appendix B, Table II)	
And sag, s, of r_1 at OS of 8.6 mm	$=$ **1.289 mm**
(by interpolation in Appendix C).	

Edge Thickness, t_e

Continuing the above example it is known that $s + t_e = p + t_c$ (Figure 4.27).

Thus, $1.289 + t_e = 1.150 + 0.21$

and $t_e = $ **0.071 mm.**

Bearing in mind that this is an edge thickness value measured parallel to the primary axis of the lens and not perpendicular to the surface (which would give a slightly lower value), this would be too small an edge thickness to allow adequate

rounding to be carried out. It may be decided, therefore, to increase the edge thickness by 0.10 to 0.171 mm. If this is done the centre thickness will obviously be altered by a similar amount to 0.31 mm. This involves recalculating the front optic radius to allow for the new centre thickness. Hence, a new value will be obtained for s, and ultimately a slightly modified value for t_e. The calculation is as follows.

Incident vergence at back surface	$= -$ 2.00 D	
Power of back surface to be added	$= -61.25$ D	(As before)
Vergence after refraction	$= -63.25$ D	
Allowance for 0.31 mm t_c (see Appendix B, Table IV)	$= +$ 0.82 D	
Vergence reaching front surface	$= -62.43$ D	
Front surface power	$= +62.43$ D	
Front surface radius, $r_1 =$ (see Appendix B, Table II)	7.85 mm	

With this new value for r_1 of 7.85 mm, sag, s, at 8.6 mm OS = **1.2825 mm** (Appendix C).

Again, since $s + t_e = p + t_c$,
$$1.2825 + t_e = 1.150 + 0.31$$
$$\text{and } t_e = 0.1775 = \textbf{0.178 mm.}$$

This edge thickness is slightly greater than that required above (0.171 mm), but is probably near

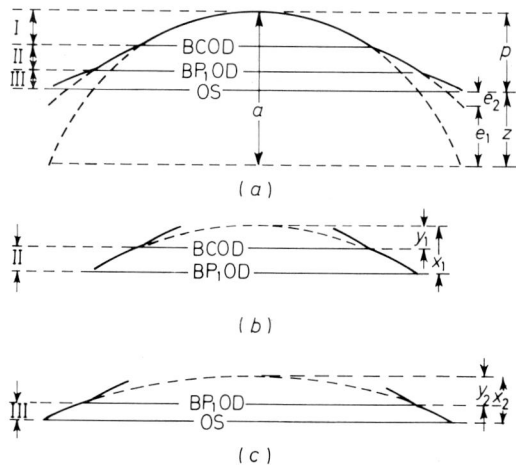

Figure 4.28—Back surface of lens.
(a) $p = I + II + III$ (b) $II = x_1 - y_1$
      $z = a - p$ (c) $III = x_2 - y_2$
      $z = e_1 + e_2$

enough from a clinical and manufacturing stand-point, particularly as this measurement is for a value determined parallel to the axis of the lens, and edge thicknesses are normally measured perpendicular to the surface which would result in a smaller value of, say, 0.15–0.16 mm. However, if this value for edge thickness is now greater than required further calculation could be done, reducing t_e and t_c by a similar amount, recalculating s and obtaining a final value for t_e.

Lenticular Lenses

If, in the above example, it is felt that the t_c value of 0.31 mm is too great, but the edge thickness (parallel to the axis) of 0.178 mm is desirable, then a lenticular front surface may be designed. Its central and peripheral radii may be determined as follows.

Remembering that $s + t_e = p + t_c$

suppose a t_c value of 0.21 mm is desired, then the sag of the front surface,

$$s = p + t_c - t_e$$
$$= 1.15 + 0.21 - 0.178$$
$$= \mathbf{1.182\ mm}$$

If a lenticular front surface is to be made, then its total sag, s, will be composed of two portions, A

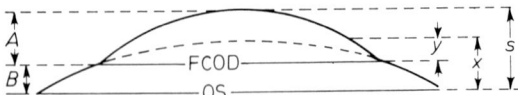

Figure 4.29–Front surface of lenticular lens.
$$s = A + B \qquad B = x - y$$

and B (*Figure 4.29*), where A is the sag of the FCOR, r_1, at FCOD; and $B = x - y$
x = sag of FPOR at OS
y = sag of FPOR at FCOD.

Now in the example being used, r_1 has already been calculated for a t_c value of 0.21 mm, and $r_1 = 7.815$ mm (*see* page 129).

It is convenient to make the lenticular diameter the same as the back central optic diameter, that is, let FCOD = BCOD = 7.0 mm.

Thus, A = sag of r_1, 7.815 mm, at FCOD, 7.0 mm = **0.827 mm** (by interpolation in Appendix C). But, $s = 1.182$ mm, and as $B = s - A$, then $B = $ **0.355 mm**.

Determination of Front Peripheral Radius

Now a front peripheral optic radius (FPOR) must be found which gives a value for B of **0.355 mm** = $x - y$.

At first this value must be guessed, but some idea of where to start 'guessing' is obtained by taking a mean of the back peripheral radii, erring if anything on the flat side. In the example being used the back peripheral radii are 9.05 and 10.80 mm, the mean being 9.925 mm. Guessing the FPOR as 10.00 mm gives:

x = sag of 10.00 mm FPOR at 8.6 mm OS
    = 0.972 mm
y = sag of 10.00 mm FPOR at 7.0 mm BCOD
    = 0.633 mm.

Thus, $B = x - y = $ **0.339 mm**.

Now this is slightly smaller than the value of 0.355 mm required for B. Therefore, 10.00 mm must be slightly too flat a radius to use for the FPOR. A second guess is therefore made, say 9.80 mm, the steeper radius giving a greater sag value. Using 9.80 mm for the FPOR x and y are again calculated:

Thus, x = sag of 9.80 mm at 8.6 mm OS
        = 0.994 mm

and y = sag of 9.80 mm at 7.00 mm BCOD
        = 0.646 mm,

so $B = x - y = $ **0.348 mm**.

This is within 0.007 mm of the required value for B.

Trying yet again and using 9.60 mm for the FPOR gives:

x = sag of 9.60 mm at 8.6 mm = 1.017 mm

y = sag of 9.60 mm at 7.0 mm = 0.661 mm

And $B = x - y = $ **0.356 mm** which is only 0.001 mm greater than the required value.

This is near enough to be used, and the front surface sag value, s, which equals $A + B$ is therefore 0.827 mm + 0.356 mm. Hence, $s = 1.183$ mm. As this is 0.001 mm greater than originally required, the edge thickness (measured parallel to the axis) will be reduced by this amount from 0.178 mm to 0.177 mm. Obviously this is of no significance.

Form of the Carrier Zone

It is of interest here to know how the edge thickness, t_e, compares to the junction thickness, t_j, at the edge of the lenticular portion (both being measured parallel to the axis of the lens).

The form of the carrier zone of a lenticular lens affects the position which the lens takes up on the eye. A lens is said to have a negative carrier zone when its edge thickness is greater than the junction thickness and a positive carrier zone when the reverse applies, the thickness relationship being similar to that of negative and positive lenses. Now lenses having negative and parallel surfaced carrier zones have been found to provide better attachment of the lens to the upper eyelid than positive carrier zones, which encourage the lens to drop. It is therefore desirable for the edge thickness to be equal to or greater than the junction thickness in order to provide a parallel surfaced or negative carrier zone, respectively.

In the example already calculated, *Figure 4.30* shows the central portion of the lens. Evidently $I + t_c = A + t_j$.

Thus, $t_j = I + t_c - A$

$$= 0.806 + 0.21 - 0.827$$

$$= \textbf{0.189 mm}$$

Now the edge thickness is 0.177 mm, and since the junction thickness is greater than the edge thickness the lens has a positive carrier zone, which, in most cases, is not desirable.

To ensure either a negative or else a parallel surfaced carrier zone, a minimum junction thickness of about 0.14 mm (measured parallel to the axis) is usually desirable on positive lenticular lenses. (If thinner than this lenses of polymethyl methacrylate material are liable to crack around the edge of the lenticular zone if subjected to any accidental squeezing between the fingers.) However, in the example used, reducing the junction thickness from 0.189 mm by 0.049 mm to 0.14 mm would necessitate reducing the centre thickness from 0.21 mm, by the same amount, 0.049 mm, to 0.161 mm.

This involves recalculating the entire front surface of the lens. Therefore, let t_c now be 0.16 mm.

Tracing a pencil of rays backwards through the lens gives:

Incident vergence at back surface	$= -2.00$ D
Power of back surface to be added	$= -61.25$ D
(As before – *see* page 129)	
Vergence after refraction	$= -63.25$ D
Allowance for 0.16 mm t_c	$= +0.43$ D
(*see* Appendix B, *Table IV*)	
Vergence reaching front surface	$= -62.82$ D
Front surface power	$= +62.82$ D
Front surface radius	$= 7.80$ mm
(*see* Appendix B, *Table II*)	
Sag A of 7.80 mm at FCOD 7.0 mm	$= 0.829$ mm

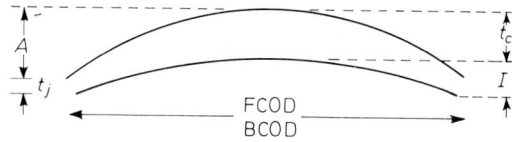

Figure 4.30–Central portion of lenticular lens.
$A + t_j = t_c + I$

Now $s + t_e = p + t_c$

Thus, $s + t_e = 1.150 + 0.16 = 1.31$ mm.

Obviously, having decided on a lenticular design any edge thickness can be chosen. If a parallel surfaced carrier zone is required, which should provide attachment to the upper lid with minimum edge thickness, then a t_e value of 0.14 mm is indicated – the same as the junction thickness.

Thus, $s + 0.14 = 1.31$ and so $s = 1.17$ mm

But $s = A + B$ (*see Figure 4.29*)

Thus, $B = 1.17 - 0.829 = 0.341$ mm.

Now a value for FPOR must be found which yields a value for B of 0.341 mm.

Referring to previous calculations (*see* page 130) shows that a value for FPOR of 10.00 mm gives $B = 0.339$ mm. Evidently then, since this value for B is only 0.002 mm less than that required, a value of 10.00 mm for the FPOR would be adequate and would give an edge thickness (measured parallel to the axis) of 0.142 mm, resulting in a lens with a very slightly negative carrier zone.

Negative Lenses

An entirely similar approach may be used for determining the front radii of negative lenses and if excessive edge thickness would be a problem a reduced optic design can be employed. The front peripheral radius of the carrier zone may then be determined in order to arrive at the desired edge thickness (*Figure 4.31*). With negative lenses of high power, a desirable edge thickness frequently results in the lens having a positive carrier zone because the edge thickness is less than the junction thickness. This positive carrier zone encourages the lens to drop whereas it may be more desirable for the lens to attach to the upper lid. Since 'lid attachment' is more likely to be achieved with a negative or parallel surfaced carrier zone some way must be found of reducing the junction thickness of these high minus lenses. By creating a front junction radius (FJR) the junction thickness may be reduced so that it is equal to or less than the

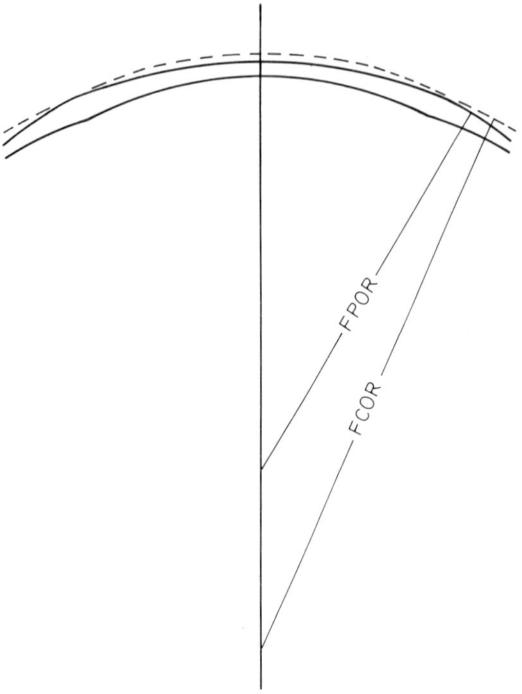

Figure 4.31–Lenticular negative lens

edge thickness, the carrier zone thereby becoming parallel surfaced or negative, respectively. Such a FJR is shown in *Figure 4.32*.

Occasionally, with very highly powered negative lenses a front junction radius is necessary anyway to join the FCOR to the FPOR. From *Figure 4.32* it can be seen that the FJR is a shorter radius than either the FCOR or FPOR.

If, for example, the FCOD and BCOD are the same (say, 7.0 mm) and the junction thickness at that diameter is 0.20 mm (t_{j1}), but really a junction thickness of 0.14 mm is desired, then a radius is determined which will give this value of 0.14 mm (t_{j2}) at a diameter of, say, 7.6 mm (FC$_2$OD) as a compromise.

Reference to *Figure 4.32* shows that sag, j, of the junction radius $= b - c$

where b = sag of FJR at FC$_2$OD

and c = sag of FJR at FC$_1$OD.

Also sag, v, of BP$_1$OR at the width of the FJR = $x_j - y_j$

where x_j = sag of BP$_1$OR at FC$_2$OD

and y_j = sag of BP$_1$OR at FC$_1$OD
(*Note:* FC$_1$OD = BCOD)

Now $t_{j1} = u + j$ or $j = t_{j1} - u$

and $t_{j2} = u + v$ or $u = t_{j2} - v$.

What is required is that $t_{j2} = 0.14$ mm

x_j = sag of 9.05 mm (BP$_1$OR) at 7.6 mm (FC$_2$OD)
     = 0.837 mm

y_j = sag of 9.05 mm (BP$_1$OR) at 7.0 mm (FC$_1$OD)
     = 0.704 mm

and $x_j - y_j = v = $ **0.133 mm**

Since $u = t_{j2} - v$

$$u = 0.14 - 0.133 = \textbf{0.007 mm}$$
and since $j = t_{j1} - u$

$$j = 0.20 - 0.007 = \textbf{0.193 mm.}$$

Thus, a radius (FJR) must be found for which $j = 0.193$ mm and, as $j = b - c$ (*Figure 4.32*), then $b - c$ also equals 0.193 mm. At first the radius must be guessed, say, FJR = 6.00 mm.

Thus, b = sag of 6.00 mm (FJR) at 7.6 mm (FC$_2$OD)
     = 1.357 mm

and c = sag of 6.00 mm (FJR) at 7.0 mm (FC$_1$OD)
     = 1.127 mm,

so $j = b - c = 0.230$ mm.

This is too large a value for j and therefore 6.00 mm must be slightly too steep a value for FJR. A flatter value for FJR is therefore selected, say, 7.00 mm.

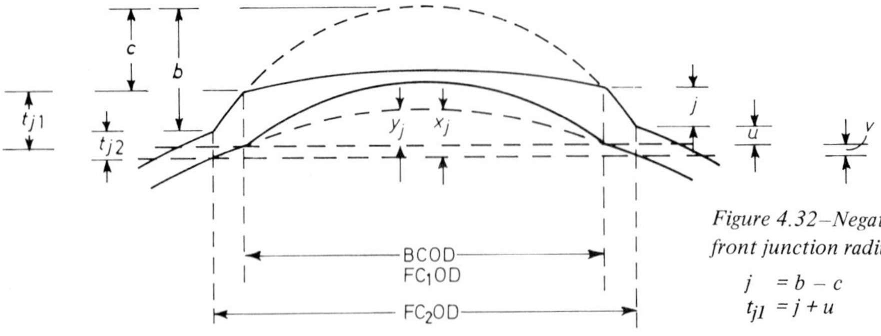

Figure 4.32–Negative lenticular lens with front junction radius.

$$j = b - c \qquad t_{j2} = u + v$$
$$t_{j1} = j + u \qquad v = x_j - y_j$$

Again b = sag of 7.00 mm (FJR) at 7.6 mm (FC$_2$OD)
= 1.121 mm

and c = sag of 7.00 mm (FJR) at 7.0 mm (FC$_1$OD)
= 0.938 mm

so $j = b - c$ = 0.183 mm.

This is now too small a value for j, which needs to be 0.193 mm, and therefore 7.00 mm is too flat a value for FJR. However, 7.00 mm is obviously much closer to the right value for FJR than was 6.00 mm (which gave a value for j of 0.230 mm). Guessing again at a value nearer 7.00 mm than 6.00 mm, 6.75 mm can be tried for FJR.

Now b = sag of 6.75 mm (FJR) at 7.6 mm (FC$_2$OD)
= 1.171 mm

and c = sag of 6.75 mm (FJR) at 7.6 mm (FC$_1$OD)
= 0.978 mm

so $j = b - c$ = 0.193 mm which is exactly the value required.

Thus, a junction radius of 6.75 mm is necessary on the front surface to join FCOR to FPOR and reduce the junction thickness from 0.20 mm to 0.14 mm. This then allows a suitable carrier zone to be designed.

Axial Edge Lift

Another aspect of lens design is to create peripheral curves which will give a desired axial edge lift. This may be done by calculation in the following manner.

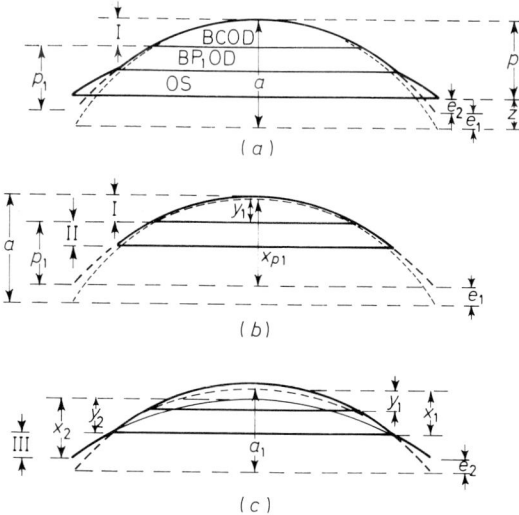

Figure 4.33–(a) Axial edge lift $z = e_1 + e_2 = a - p$.
(b) $e_1 = a - (I + p_1)$ and $p_1 = x_{p1} - y_1$.
(c) $e_2 = a_1 - x_1 - III$ and $III = x_2 - y_2$

From *Figure 4.33a* it is seen that for a tricurve lens, the axial edge lift $z = a - p$ where p is the primary sag and equals $I + II + III$ (*see Figure 4.28a*). If the two peripheral curves are to contribute equally to the edge lift then e_1 must be equal to e_2 where $e_1 + e_2 = z$.

For example, a lens has a BCOR of 8.00 mm. The BCOD is 7.0 mm, BP$_1$OD is 7.8 mm and OS is 8.6 mm. An axial edge lift of 0.12 mm is required, of which 0.06 mm is to be contributed by BP$_1$OR and 0.06 mm by BP$_2$OR. The values for BP$_1$OR and BP$_2$OR to give the necessary edge lift are determined as follows.

BP$_1$OR

From *Figure 4.33b* it can be seen that the lens is treated first as if it were a bicurve lens with BP$_1$OR extending out to the OS.

Then $e_1 = a - (I + p_1)$ where $p_1 = x_{p1} - y_1$

x_{p1} and y_1 are the sags of BP$_1$OR at OS and BCOD respectively.

From above, $a = e_1 + I + p_1$ and so $p_1 = a - I - e_1$

Now a = sag of 8.00 mm (BCOR) at 8.6 mm (OS)
= 1.254 mm

I = sag of 8.00 mm (BCOR) at 7.0 mm (BCOD)
= 0.806 mm

and $p_1 = a - I - e_1$ = 1.254 − 0.806 − 0.06
= **0.388 mm**

It is now necessary to guess a value for BP$_1$OR which will permit x_{p1} and y_1 to be determined so as to give a value for p_1 as near to this value of 0.388 mm as possible, because $p_1 = x_{p1} - y_1$. So, let BP$_1$OR = 9.00 mm.

Then x_{p1} = sag of 9.00 mm (BP$_1$OR) at 8.6 mm (OS)
= 1.094 mm

y_1 = sag of 9.00 mm (BP$_1$OR) at 7.0 mm (BCOD)
= 0.708 mm

giving $p_1 = x_{p1} - y_1$
= 1.094 − 0.708
= **0.386 mm**

This value for p_1 is close enough to the value for p_1 found above (from $a - I - e_1$) not to require further calculation. Hence, BP$_1$OR can be taken as 9.00 mm. Had the value for p_1 found from $x_{p1} - y_1$ been considerably different from 0.388 mm then it would have been necessary to recalculate using another value for BP$_1$OR. A figure much smaller than 0.388 mm would have indicated that too flat a value had been selected for BP_1OR and that recalculation using a steeper value is necessary. Conversely, a value much greater than 0.388 mm would have indicated that too steep a value had been selected for BP_1OR and that recalculation using a flatter value is necessary. As it is, the use of 9.00 mm for BP_1OR leads to a very small error of 0.002 mm in p_1 indicating that e_1 will be 0.062 mm instead of 0.060 mm (because $e_1 = a - I - p_1$). Now the remainder of the edge lift, z, is contributed by BP_2OR and is e_2. But $e_2 = z - e_1 = 0.12 - 0.062 = 0.058$ mm.

BP_2OR

Thus, a value for BP_2OR must now be guessed at, which will, after calculation yield a result of 0.058 mm for e_2.

Calculations to determine e_2 are similar to those for e_1. From *Figure 4.33c*, $e_2 = a_1 - x_1 - III$, where a_1 is the sag of BP_1OR at OS, x_1 is the sag of BP_1OR at BP_1OD and III is now $x_2 - y_2$ (*see Figure 4.33c*). x_2 is the sag of BP_2OR at OS, and y_2 is the sag of BP_2OR at BP_2OD. Thus, $III = a_1 - x_1 - e_2$.

Thus, $a_1 =$ sag of 9.00 mm (BP_1OR) at
8.6 mm (OS)
$= 1.094$ mm

$x_1 =$ sag of 9.00 mm (BP_1OR) at
7.8 mm (BP_1OD)
$= 0.889$ mm

e_2 is assumed to be 0.058 mm

Since $III = a_1 - x_1 - e_2$ then III
$= 1.094 - 0.889 - 0.058$
$= \mathbf{0.147}$ **mm.**

It is necessary to guess a value for BP_2OR which will permit x_2 and y_2 to be determined so as to give a value for III as near to this figure of 0.147 mm as possible, because $III = x_2 - y_2$. So let BP_2OR be 11.00 mm.

Then $x_2 =$ sag of 11.00 mm (BP_2OR) at
8.6 mm (OS)
$= 0.875$ mm

$y_2 =$ sag of 11.00 mm (BP_2OR) at
7.8 mm (BP_1OD)
$= 0.715$ mm

giving $III = x_2 - y_2 = 0.875 - 0.715.$
$= 0.160$ mm

Since this value for III is bigger than 0.147 mm, then 11.00 mm must be too steep a radius for BP_2OR. Therefore, another guess is made for BP_2OR, say, 11.50 mm.

Again $x_2 =$ sag of 11.50 mm (BP_2OR)
8.6 mm (OS)
$= 0.834$ mm

$y_2 =$ sag of 11.50 mm (BP_2OR)
7.8 mm (BP_1OD)
$= 0.681$ mm

giving $III = x_2 - y_2 = 0.834 - 0.681$
$= 0.153$ mm

This is nearer the value required, but still too large, and indicates that BP_2OR must be even flatter. Guessing yet again, let BP_2OR be 12.00 mm.

Now $x_2 =$ sag of 12.00 mm (BP_2OR) at
8.6 mm (OS)
$= 0.797$ mm

$y_2 =$ sag of 12.00 mm (BP_2OR) at
7.8 mm (BP_1OD)
$= 0.651$ mm

giving $III = x_2 - y_2 = 0.797 - 0.651$
$= 0.146$ mm

This is near enough to 0.147 mm for it to be unnecessary to recalculate using another value for BP_2OR, which may therefore be taken as **12.00 mm.** The small error of 0.001 mm in III means that e_2 is 0.059 instead of 0.058, (because $e_2 = a_1 - x_1 - III$).

The total axial edge lift, $z = e_1 + e_2 = 0.062 + 0.059 = 0.121$ mm, just 0.001 mm greater than originally required.

The value of z arrived at in the above manner may be checked by reference to *Figure 4.28* where it is seen that $z = a - (I + II + III)$.

Now $a =$ sag of 8.00 mm (BCOR) at
8.6 mm (OS)
$= \mathbf{1.254}$ **mm**

$I =$ sag of 8.00 mm (BCOR) at
7.0 mm (BCOD)
$= \mathbf{0.806}$ **mm**

$II = x_1 - y_1$

and $x_1 =$ sag of 9.00 mm (BP_1OR) at
7.8 mm (BP_1OD)
$= 0.889$ mm

$y_1 =$ sag of 9.00 mm (BP_1OR) at
7.0 mm (BCOD)
$= 0.708$ mm

Thus, $II = x_1 - y_1 = 0.889 - 0.708$
$= \mathbf{0.181}$ **mm**

$III = x_2 - y_2$ and has been calculated above,
thus $= \mathbf{0.146}$ **mm**

and $z = 1.254 - (0.806 + 0.181 + 0.146)$
$= \mathbf{0.121}$ **mm**

Any lens of known back surface specification may thus have its axial edge lift determined by this method. However, it should be remembered that blending transitions inevitably alters the value somewhat. If a computer is being used to make such calculations, it is simple enough to allocate a radius and width to the blends and treat these as extra back surface curves, thereby permitting more accurate determination of axial edge lift values.

Details of five corneal lens fitting sets with constant axial edge lift, designed by Rabbetts (1976) and the author (Stone, 1975) for The London Refraction Hospital, are shown below. Sets 1, 3 and 4 are useful where fitting is by the central alignment or minimal apical clearance techniques, whereas sets 2 and 5 are usually more appropriate to central apical clearance fitting (which reduces the peripheral clearance).

Set 1

Corneal lenses with 0.12 mm axial edge lift, 8.6 mm overall size

7.00:7.00/	7.85:7.80/	9.00:8.60
7.10	8.00	9.25
7.20	8.10	9.50
7.30	8.25	9.65
7.40	8.40	9.90
7.50	8.50	10.30
7.60	8.70	10.40
7.70	8.80	10.65
7.80	9.00	10.90
7.90	9.15	11.20
8.00	9.25	11.40
8.10	9.40	11.70
8.20	9.55	11.90
8.30	9.75	12.20
8.40	9.90	12.75
8.50	10.05	13.00
8.60	10.30	13.50

Set 2

Corneal lenses with 0.15 mm axial edge lift, 9.0 mm overall size

7.00:7.00/	7.40:7.80/	8.40:8.60/	10.00:9.00
7.10	7.55	8.60	10.20
7.20	7.70	8.80	10.40
7.30	8.85	9.10	10.40
7.40	8.10	9.30	10.50
7.50	8.30	9.50	10.60
7.60	8.40	9.70	10.80
7.70	8.55	9.90	11.00
7.75	8.65	10.00	11.10
7.80	8.75	10.10	11.30
7.85	8.80	10.20	11.40
7.90	8.85	10.40	11.50
8.00	9.00	10.60	11.70
8.10	9.20	10.80	11.90
8.20	9.30	11.00	12.10
8.30	9.45	11.30	12.40
8.40	9.60	11.60	12.60
8.50	9.80	11.70	12.90
8.60	10.00	11.90	13.10
8.70	10.40	12.00	13.20

Set 3

Corneal lenses with 0.15 mm axial edge lift, 9.2 mm overall size

7.00:7.00/	7.55:7.80/	8.20:8.60/	8.65:9.20
7.10	7.70	8.35	8.85
7.20	7.80	8.60	9.10
7.30	7.95	8.70	9.30
7.40	8.10	8.90	9.50
7.50	8.20	9.05	9.70
7.60	8.30	9.20	10.00
7.70	8.45	9.40	10.30
7.80	8.55	9.60	10.60
7.90	8.70	9.75	10.80
8.00	8.80	9.90	11.00
8.10	8.95	10.10	11.25
8.20	9.05	10.30	11.45
8.30	9.25	10.50	11.70
8.40	9.30	10.70	12.00
8.50	9.50	10.80	12.25
8.60	9.60	11.10	12.50

Set 4

Corneal lenses with 0.175 mm axial edge lift, 9.5 mm overall size

7.00:7.50/	7.70:8.20/	8.40:9.00/	9.00:9.50
7.10	7.85	8.60	9.20
7.20	8.00	8.80	9.50
7.30	8.15	9.00	9.90
7.40	8.25	9.20	10.00
7.50	8.40	9.40	10.30
7.60	8.50	9.60	10.60
7.70	8.70	9.80	10.80
7.80	8.90	10.00	11.15
7.90	9.00	10.20	11.50
8.00	9.10	10.40	11.70
8.10	9.30	10.60	11.95
8.20	9.40	10.85	12.40
8.30	9.55	11.05	12.70
8.40	9.65	11.35	13.00
8.50	9.85	11.55	13.40
8.60	9.95	11.75	13.65
8.70	10.10	12.00	14.05
8.80	10.25	12.20	14.50
8.90	10.40	12.55	15.00
9.00	10.55	12.85	15.25

Set 5

Corneal lenses with 0.19 mm axial edge lift,
9.5 mm overall size

7.00:7.50/	7.80:8.20/	8.60:9.00/	9.25:9.50
7.10	7.90	8.80	9.50
7.20	8.05	9.00	9.85
7.30	8.25	9.20	10.15
7.40	8.35	9.40	10.40
7.50	8.50	9.65	10.70
7.60	8.65	9.85	11.00
7.70	8.80	10.05	11.30
7.80	9.05	10.30	11.60
7.90	9.15	10.50	11.85
8.00	9.30	10.70	12.30
8.10	9.40	11.00	12.70
8.20	9.50	11.30	13.00
8.30	9.70	11.50	13.50
8.40	9.80	11.80	13.80
8.50	10.00	12.00	14.20
8.60	10.15	12.20	14.50
8.70	10.25	12.55	15.00
8.80	10.50	12.70	15.50
8.90	10.60	13.00	16.00
9.00	10.70	13.55	16.30

Drawing Lenses to Scale

Another way to design lenses is to draw them to scale at $X40$ full size as recommended by Mackie (1973), who has described the method in detail. Graph paper, 56×38 cm, a drawing board and beam compass (preferably 50 cm long) are essential, as well as a contact lens slide rule or tables such as those in the appendices to this book, or an electronic calculator. Only half the lens need be drawn, as shown in *Figure 4.34* and one side of the graph paper is taken as the primary axis of the lens. It is helpful to mark up the graph paper with mm (4 cm at the chosen scale) markings both along and perpendicular to the axis, as this eases the measurement of lengths during the drawing process.

First, the BCOR is measured off and drawn as shown in *Figure 4.34* with centre, C_1, to extend from A on the axis to B representing the overall size of the lens. Point D, indicating the limit of the BCOD can then be marked off by measurement on the graph paper. The axial or radial edge lift desired may then be measured off from B and the final edge position, E, of the lens thus located. If the lens is only to have one back surface peripheral curve, its radius is found by bisecting the line DE at right-angles and finding where the perpendicular bisector intersects the axis at C_2. The BPOR is then C_2D or C_2E and can be measured off with the compasses on the graph paper.

Should two peripheral curves be required then a point between B and E is marked off, say F, and

a radius C_2D or C_2F is then found as above, but by locating its centre where the perpendicular bisector of DF cuts the axis. Then on the arc DF (which is now BP_1OR) the limit of BP_1OD is marked where required by measurement on the graph paper. This point is denoted here as G. To obtain BP_2OR, GE is now bisected perpendicularly and the centre, C_3, for the final peripheral curve is located where this perpendicular bisector of GE cuts the axis. The radius of this curve is C_3G or C_3E and can be measured with the compasses on the graph paper. Obviously any number of peripheral curves may be drawn in this fashion, contributing to the edge lift just as the lens designer wishes.

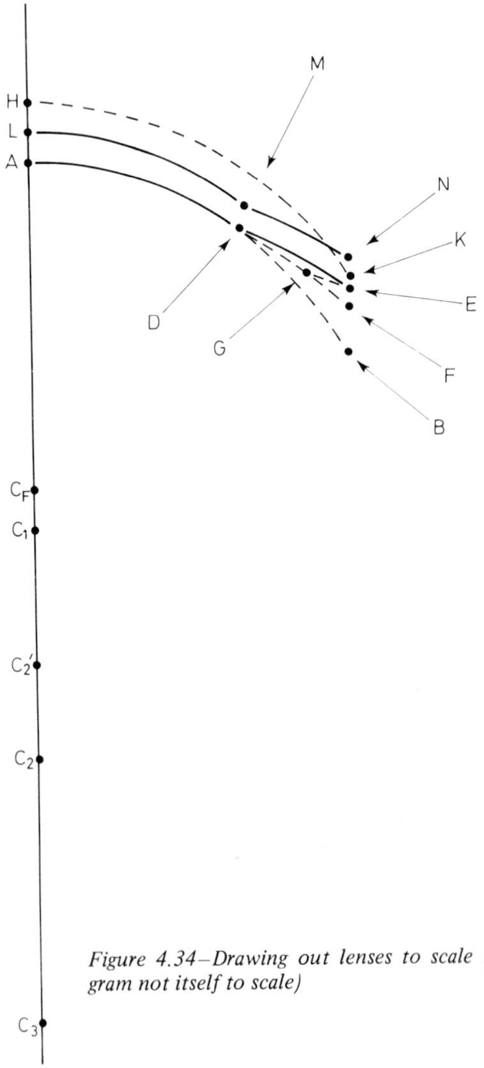

Figure 4.34–Drawing out lenses to scale (diagram not itself to scale)

The front surface of the lens may be drawn, having first determined its radius according to the BVP required, by estimating centre thickness as described on page 129. The centre thickness is marked off from A to point H. The centre for the front surface radius is then found by measuring off its radius from H to C_F. The FCOR (C_FH) is then drawn in from H to K, the latter point being the edge of the front surface. Thus, the edge thickness EK may be determined, and if too great or small an edge thickness results then the centre thickness can be adjusted appropriately (after checking by calculation or slide rule that this does not alter the FCOR required to give the correct BVP). If necessary a lenticular can be designed as shown in *Figure 4.34* where the centre thickness has been reduced from AH to AL. The edge of the FCOD is marked off as required at, say, M, and a suitable curve MN (which could be parallel to DE) constructed for the FPOR, so as to give a satisfactory junction thickness at MD and edge thickness at NE.

For negative lenses of high power a front junction radius similar to that shown in *Figure 4.32* can easily be constructed.

Drawing out to scale in this manner can be done for any type of lens and it has the advantage of permitting the designer to specify something which it is feasible for the manufacturer to make. It is also useful in that it allows the complete front and back surface to be specified, which encourages accurate reproduction of a lens on future occasions if duplicates are required.

EXAMINATION QUESTIONS AND ANSWERS

The following questions have all been taken from past papers in Visual Optics of the Advanced Contact Lens Examination set by the British Optical Association, and are reproduced by their kind permission. The date of the questions and their answers are given in brackets after each question. Only the numerical type of questions have been included. It is hoped that these will be helpful to those people preparing for such examinations.

(1) An aphakic eye is 25 mm long and has a cornea (assumed infinitely thin) of 8 mm radius of curvature in front of the pupil area. The refractive index of the aqueous and vitreous may be assumed as 1.336. What is the ocular refraction?

What would be the percentage reduction in retinal image size in this eye, given by an infinitely thin contact lens as compared to an infinitely thin spectacle lens worn 12 mm in front of the cornea? (*September, 1968; +11.44 D, 12.1%*)

(2) Describe in detail:
  (a) the error in back vertex power recorded by a focimeter having an aperture stop of 6 mm diameter when used for measuring a lens of back surface specification C2/8.00: 7.00/8.50: 9.00 and true back vertex power of +16 D.
(*September, 1968; +0.15 D*)

(3) Calculate the required back vertex power of the toroidal contact lens fitted to match the cornea of an eye having spectacle refraction of −5.00/−1.00 X 180 (vertex distance 12 mm) and keratometer readings: 7.55 mm along 90
                                    8.00 mm along 180.
How much of the cylindrical correction would be incorporated on the front surface of the lens (assumed thin), which has back central optic radii the same as the keratometer readings? The cornea may be assumed as a single refracting surface of the same refractive index as the tears, 1.336. The contact lens refractive index is 1.49.
(*November, 1968; −4.72/−0.88 X 180, +2.77 X 180*)

(4) For the practitioner one of the greatest problems in verifying the characteristics of a corneal lens is that of back surface peripheral radii of curvature. Discuss methods that have been used to verify these radii and the limitations of such methods.

The following corneal lens has been ordered from a laboratory:

C2. 7.80: 6.50/8.00: 9.50/−6.00 D. (Refractive index 1.490).

On checking the following values were obtained:
  Centre thickness   0.10 mm
  Back vertex power   −6.00 D
  BCOR   7.80 mm
  Back vertex power of
    peripheral zone   −5.00 D
  Thickness at centre of
    peripheral zone   0.20 mm

Does the peripheral radius of curvature conform to specification?
(*July, 1970; No − 7.90 mm*)

(5) A patient with the following refractive details is to be fitted with minimum clearance haptic lenses in order to provide a satisfactory level of vision binocularly. Calculate the necessary back vertex powers of the lenses if the back central optic radii of the contact lenses are R and L 8.30 mm.
RX   R. +4.00 D/−2.00 D. Cyl. axis 180.
       Vertex distance 15 mm
       L. +5.00 D Sph

Keratometer readings R and L   along 90°
                                          7.64 mm
                                  along 180°
                                          8.00 mm
(*January, 1971; R + 5.78/−0.22 X 180, say +5.75 D.S. L +6.93/+1.98 X 180, say +7.00 with +2.00 D.C. X 180 on front surface*)

(6) A patient is fitted with an aircell underwater haptic contact lens. Calculate the radius of curvature of the front optic surface of the haptic component from the following details:

R eye   Spectacle Rx   +5.00 D.S.
                         −2.00 D. Cyl. axis 180
                         Vertex distance 15 mm

Keratometer readings 90° 7.80 mm 180° 8.20 mm

BCOR 8.60 mm. Centre thickness 0.4 mm. Refractive index 1.490.
(*July, 1971; 7.76 mm assuming contact lens BVP of +7.25 D*)

(7) Discuss the relative merits and usefulness of the following instruments for checking contact lenses: keratometer, radiuscope, focimeter and slit-lamp.

A focimeter may be used to check the BCOR of a corneal lens if a lens of known characteristics is available. Given a lens of known characteristics (BCOR 8.2 mm, BVP +6.00 D) calculate the BCOR of an unknown lens given the following details:

BVP of known and unknown lens +4.00 D
BVP of known and unknown lens +3.00 D
with water (n.c. 1.336) between lenses.
Centre thickness of unknown lens 0.2 mm,
lens material refractive index 1.49.
(*January, 1972; 7.68 mm*)

(8) Although spectacle/contact lens systems have been used as subnormal vision aids, they have severe limitations. If a system to be used with an emmetropic patient consists of a spectacle lens power +12.00 D vertex distance 15 mm and a contact lens, calculate the magnification produced by such a system for a distant object, and also the ocular accommodation exerted to view an object one metre from the spectacle lens (assume the system remains in normal adjustment).
(*January, 1972; X1.22, +1.46 D*)

(9) A preformed haptic (scleral) trial lens is placed on an eye and gives a satisfactory minimum clearance fit. The supplementary refraction is:

+2.50 DS/+2.00 DC X 90 vertex distance 12 mm.

The trial lens has a front surface radius of 8.25 mm and refractive index of 1.49.

What will be the front surface radii of the final contact lens if it has the same rear surface construction, thickness and refractive index?

What can you deduce about the possible origins of the astigmatism if it is known that the patient normally wears spectacles with the following correction?

−6.00 DS/−2.00 DC X 90 vertex distance 12 mm.
(*July, 1972; 7.64 mm 180, 7.91 mm 90, crystalline lens astigmatism*)

(10) A patient with a PD of 60 mm wears a spectacle correction of −8.00 sph R and L in plano-concave form at a vertex distance of 13 mm. Subsequently a corneal lens correction is provided. Calculate the demands on accommodation and convergence when fixation is changed from a distant object to one at 32 cm from the spectacle plane using the two forms of correction.

What are the clinical implications of this calculation?
(*July, 1972; Spectacles: accommodation +2.47 D, convergence 7.34 prism dioptres each eye. Contact lenses: accommodation +3.00 D, convergence 8.70 prism dioptres each eye*)

(11) A contact lens having a BCOR of 8 mm and a thickness of 0.15 mm has a front vertex power of −20.00 D. It is used in combination with a plano-convex spectacle lens of back vertex power +16.00 DS and 10 mm thick to provide magnification for an emmetropic eye of low visual acuity. Assume that the material of both lenses has a refractive index of 1.49. Neglect the liquid lens. Calculate:

(a) front surface radius of contact lens;
(b) lens separation for normal adjustment;
(c) the magnification.
(*July, 1972; (a) 11.99 mm, (b) 12.5 mm, (c) X1.25 not allowing for shape factor*)

(12) A myope having a spectacle correction of −12 D, right and left, worn at a vertex distance of 12 mm and 25 mm from the centres of rotation of the eyes, is fitted with contact lenses. So, too, is a bilateral aphakic of spectacle refraction +12 D worn at the same vertex distance and the same distance from the eyes' centres of rotation as the myope. Each has a distance CD for the spectacles of 60 mm.

Determine in each case: (a) the difference in convergence required for an object 25 cm in front of the spectacle plane, when wearing spectacles and contact lenses; (b) the alteration in the clear field of view (assuming that, in both cases, lenticular spectacle lenses with a circular aperture of 30 mm diameter are used) between contact lens wear and spectacle lens wear.

(January, 1973; (a) Myope in spectacles, 17.14 prism dioptres. In contact lenses, 21.82 prism dioptres. Hypermetrope in spectacles; 30.00 prism dioptres. In contact lenses, 21.82 prism dioptres. (b) Myope: 76° in spectacles, unlimited in contact lenses but 62° if spectacle frame present. Hypermetrope: 45.5° in spectacles, unlimited in contact lenses but 62° if spectacle frame present.)

(13) Two solid concentric bifocal contact lenses of polymethylmethacrylate of refractive index 1.49 are made up so as to give the patient a near addition of +2.00 D. One has a front surface addition and the other a back surface addition. In each case the distance portion is in the centre and is of −2.00 D BVP and 0.20 mm centre thickness. The BCOR of the front surface addition lens is 7.60 mm, and the same radius is used on the portion of the back surface used for the near addition of the other lens. Assuming a refractive index of 1.336 for tears, calculate the two front surface radii of the front surface addition lens, and the BCOR and FCOR for the back surface addition lens.

(January, 1973; FCOR, DP 7.91 mm; FCOR, NP 7.67 mm; BCOR 6.92 mm, FCOR 7.19 mm)

(14) A parallel bitoric corneal lens has a back vertex power in air of −2.00/−5.00 X 180. It is fitted so that the back central optic surface exactly matches the with-the-rule corneal contour, and there is an afocal liquid lens. The contact lens also exactly corrects the eye's ocular refraction.

The back central optic radii of the lens are 7.25 and 8.00 mm. What is the power and axis direction of the positive cylinder which has been worked on the front surface? (Assume an infinitely thin contact lens and, for ease of calculation, refractive indices of: lens material, 1.5; tears and cornea, 1.333.) How much of the ocular astigmatism is corneal and how much is due to the crystalline lens?

(July, 1973; +1.47 X 180, corneal astigmatism +4.31 X 180, crystalline lens astigmatism +0.69 X 180)

(15) A young emmetropic patient has an alternating esotropia of 15°, and uses the R.E. for distance and the L.E. for near (assumed as 25 cm from the spectacle plane). Following an accident his macular areas undergo degenerative changes and his accommodation is considerably reduced. He requires a telescopic aid for the R.E. and a 'microscopic' aid for the L.E. Corneal lenses are to be used for the eyepieces and spectacles worn at a vertex distance of 16 mm for the objectives of these aids. As his corneae are identical, two similar corneal lenses are made up, of BCOR 7.50 mm and FCOR 12.00 mm. (Assume an infinitely thin contact lens of refractive index 1.5.) If the L.E. continues to use the same working distance, what back vertex powers must the two spectacle lenses have and what magnification would they afford?

(July, 1973; R.E. +17.86 D, X1.40; L.E. +21.86 D, X1.40)

(16) A soft contact lens, when fully hydrated, has a back optic radius of 8.00 mm, a refractive index of 1.35, centre thickness of 0.30 mm and back vertex power of −3.00 D.

It is allowed to become partially dehydrated and its refractive index goes up to 1.40. Calculate the change in back vertex power on the basis of the refractive index change alone.

What other factors associated with dehydration would also contribute to a change in BVP?

(January, 1975; −0.40 D; curvature and thickness changes)

(17) A fused bifocal corneal lens has a segment of refractive index 1.58 in the lower part of the back central optic portion and coming into contact with the tears layer of refractive index 1.336. The lens has a back central optic radius of 7.00 mm. The main part of the lens has a refractive index of 1.49. Calculate the interface radius necessary to give the lens a near addition, on the eye, of +3.00 D. (Assume thin lens theory.)

Explain what different factors would be taken into consideration in determining the interface radius, had the segment been on the front surface.

(January, 1975; 5.67 mm)

ACKNOWLEDGEMENTS

We are indebted to the following people for help in the preparation of this chapter; Mr Roger Phillips for programming the computer and producing the figures on which Appendix D is based; Mrs Rita Watts for help in the calculations for Appendices A and B; and Mr R. G. Stone for drawing many of the diagrams.

REFERENCES

Baron, H. (1975). 'Some remarks on the correction of astigmatic eyes by means of soft contact lenses.' *Contacto* 19(6), 4–8

Bennett, A. G. (1966). *Optics of Contact Lenses*, 4th ed. London: Association of Dispensing Opticians

Bennett A. G. (1967). 'Personal communication cited in later reference by Stone, J. (1967)

Bennett, A. G. (1968). 'The corrected aphakic eye: a study of retinal image sizes.' *Optician* 155, 106–111 and 132–135

Bennett, A. G. (1972). 'Retinal image sizes in the aphakic eye.' *Contact Lens* 3(7), 2–6; also in *Contact Lens* 4(2), 24–28 (1973) with publisher's errors corrected

Bennett, A. G. (1976). 'Power changes in soft contact lenses due to bending.' *Ophthal. Optician* 16, 939–945

Capelli, Q. A. (1964). 'Determining final power of bitoric lenses.' *Br. J. physiol. Optics* 21, 256–263

Carney, L. G. (1975). 'The basis for corneal shape change during contact lens wear.' *Am. J. Optom.* 52, 445–454; reproduced in *Optician* 171(4415), 11, 15–16, 20–22 (1976)

Clark, B. A. J. (1970). 'Sagitta nomograms for contact lens calculation.' *Contact Lens* 2(7), 3–6

Creighton, C. P. (1964). *Contact Lenses Fabrication Tables*. New York: Creighton

Emsley, H. H. (1955). *Visual Optics*, Vol. 1 – Optics of Vision, 5th ed. London: Hatton Press

Fletcher, R. J. (1965). 'Haptic Lenses.' In *Contact Lens Practice: Basic and Advanced*, ed by R. B. Mandell. Springfield, Ill.: Thomas

Ford, M. W. (1974). 'Changes in hydrophilic lenses when placed on an eye.' Paper read at the joint International Congress of The Contact Lens Society and The National Eye Research Foundation, Montreux, Switzerland

Ford, M. W. (1976). 'Computation of the back vertex powers of hydrophilic lenses.' Paper read at the Interdisciplinary Conference on Contact Lenses, Department of Ophthalmic Optics and Visual Science, The City University, London

Francis, J. L. (1968). *Optical Tables for Contact Lens Work*. London: Hatton Press (these are now incorporated in the present book)

Gordon, S. (1965). 'Contact lens hydration: a study of the wetting-drying cycle.' *Optom. Wkly* 56, 55–62

Harris, M. G. and Chu, C. S. (1972). 'The effect of contact lens thickness and corneal toricity on flexure and residual astigmatism.' *Am. J. Optom.* 49, 304–307

Kerns, R. L. (1974). 'Clinical evaluation of the merits of an aspheric front surface contact lens for patients manifesting residual astigmatism.' *Am. J. Optom.* 51, 750–757

Mackie, I. A. (1973). 'Design compensation in corneal lens fitting.' In *Symposium on Contact Lenses*, Transactions of the New Orleans Academy of Ophthalmology. St. Louis: Mosby

Mandell, R. B. (1975). 'Corneal oedema from hydrogel lenses.' *Int. Contact Lens Clinic* 2(1), 88–98

Mandell, R. B. and Polse, K. A. (1969). 'Corneal thickness changes as a contact lens fitting index – experimental results and a proposed model.' *Am. J. Optom.* 46, 479–491

Obstfeld, H. (1978). *Optics in Vision*. London: Butterworths

Polse, K. A. (1972). 'Changes in corneal hydration after discontinuing contact lens wear.' *Am. J. Optom.* 49, 511–516

Rabbetts, R. B. (1976). 'Large corneal lenses with constant axial edge lift.' *Ophthal. Optician* 16, 236, 239

Rengstorff, R. H. and Arner, R. S. (1971). 'Refractive changes in the cornea: mathematical considerations.' *Am. J. Optom.* 48, 913–918

Sarver, M. D. (1963). 'The effect of contact lens tilt upon residual astigmatism.' *Am. J. Optom.* 40, 730–744

Sarver, M. D., Ashley, D. and Van Every, J. (1974). 'Supplemental power effect of Bausch and Lomb Soflens contact lenses.' *Int. Contact Lens Clinic* 1(1), 100–109

Sarver, M. D., Harris, M. G. and Polse, K. A. (1975). 'Corneal curvature and supplemental power effect of the Bausch and Lomb Soflens contact lens.' *Am. J. Optom.* 52, 470–473

Sorsby, A., Leary, G. A. and Richards, M. J. (1962). 'The optical components in anisometropia.' *Vision Res.* 3, 43–51

Stone, Janet (1959). 'Factors governing the back central optic diameter of a microlens.' *Optician* 138, 20–22

Stone, Janet (1966). 'The use of contact lenses in the correction of astigmatism.' *Optica Internat.* 3, 6–23

Stone, Janet (1967). 'Near vision difficulties in non-presbyopic corneal lens wearers.' *Contact Lens* 1(2), 14–25

Stone, Janet (1973). 'Contact lens wear in the young myope.' *Br. J. physiol. Optics* 28, 90–134

Stone, Janet (1975). 'Corneal lenses with constant axial edge lift.' *Ophthal. Optician* 15, 818–824

Strachan, J. P. F. (1973). 'Some principles of the optics of hydrophilic lenses and geometrical optics applied to flexible lenses.' *Aust. J. Optom.* 56, 25–33

Swaine, W. (1956). 'Optics of contact lenses and their prescription.' *Br. J. physiol. Optics* 13, 147–163

Voerste, K. (1976). 'Analysing the clinical results of fitting a type of soft contact lens.' *Optician* 171(4414), 15–18 and 23

Westerhout, D. (1969). 'Clinical observations in fitting bitoric and toric forms of corneal lenses.' *Contact Lens* 2(3), 5–21 and 36

Westheimer, G. (1962). 'The visual world of the new contact lens wearer.' *J. Am. optom. Ass.* 34, 135–140

Wichterle, O. (1967). 'Changes of refracting power of a soft lens caused by its flattening.' In *Corneal and Scleral Contact Lenses*, The Proceedings of the International Congress, March 1966, ed. by L. J. Girard. Paper 29, pp. 247–256. St. Louis: Mosby

Chapter 5

Keratometry and Slit Lamp Biomicroscopy

Michael Sheridan

A keratometer and slit lamp biomicroscope are the two major instruments used in contact lens practice. The first provides information which is helpful in deciding on the initial fitting lens and in monitoring corneal changes during the adaptation and after-care period; the second is indispensable for effective investigation of the condition of the cornea and the fit of the contact lens at every stage of fitting and after-care.

KERATOMETRY

The main function of a keratometer is the measurement of the radius of curvature of the central portion of the front surface of the cornea, usually referred to as the optic cap (*see* Chapter 11). This result is obtained indirectly by measuring the angular size of the reflected image, formed by the cornea, of an object of known angular size. In most instruments, this is an object, the linear size of which is fixed or measurable, at a predetermined distance from the image plane.

The technique is usually attributed to von Helmholtz, though Mandell (1960) has argued that Jesse Ramsden was, in fact, the inventor. Its subsequent development has been discussed by Emsley (1955), and the development of the allied technique of keratoscopy has been discussed by Levene (1965).

The derivation of the radius is shown in *Figure 5.1*, where B and Q represent the limits of an object of size h. The images B' and Q', formed by reflection at the front surface of the cornea, are the limits of an image of size h' formed slightly in front of the focal plane of the cornea (which intersects the axis at F, the principal focus) and at a distance d from the object plane BQ. A is the pole of the cornea and C its centre of curvature. Thus, the radius $r = AC$ and $r/2 = AF$.

Figure 5.2 illustrates the doubling principle by which the measurement of image size is made. If a prism of power P prism dioptres is interposed in half the observation aperture, an image of size h' will be seen doubled, and the doubled images will only be positioned exactly adjacent to one another at the distance a, such that $h'/a = P/100$.

In practice, the extremities of the object are represented by a pair of internally illuminated mires, the corneal images of which are observed and seen magnified through a short-focus telescope (or long-focus microscope). This incorporates a doubling device which gives rise to the four images seen in the telescope field, the two central ones being brought into contact or superimposed as shown in *Figures 5.3* and *5.4*. To obtain adjacent or superimposed images, either h' (*Figure 5.1*) may be varied by altering the mire separation h while the power and position of the doubling device are fixed (fixed doubling); or the image size h' and mire separation h may be fixed while the power of the doubling device P or its distance a from the image plane is varied (variable doubling). In most modern instruments employing variable doubling, it is the distance a which is varied, the doubling prism travelling along the axis of the instrument between the objective and eyepiece.

In most keratometers, doubling takes place in one meridian only − along the line joining the mires. Such an instrument must be rotated about its optical axis in order to align it with each of the principal meridians of the cornea in turn and it is therefore known as a two position keratometer. A one position keratometer is an instrument in which variable doubling of mutually perpendicular pairs of mires is produced by two doubling devices

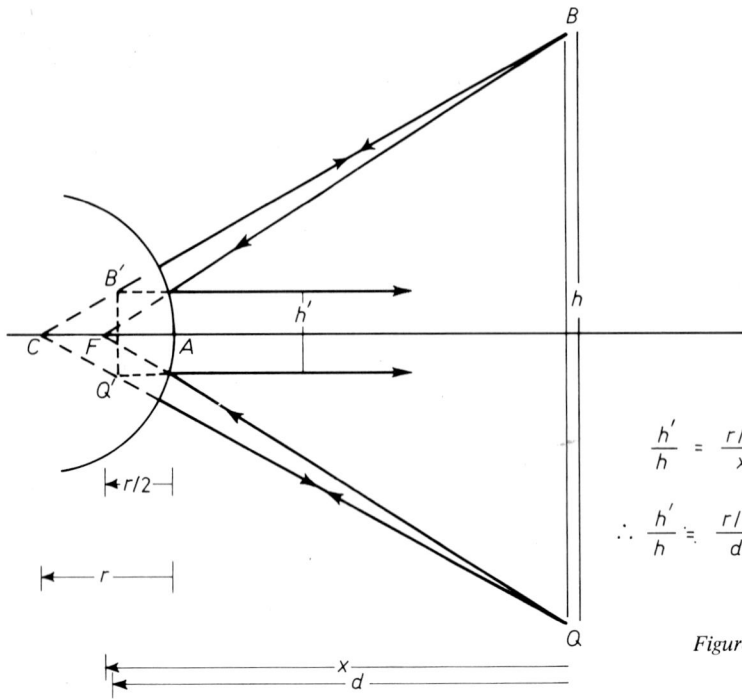

$$\frac{h'}{h} = \frac{r/2}{x} \qquad \text{But } d \doteq x$$

$$\therefore \ \frac{h'}{h} \doteq \frac{r/2}{d} \qquad \therefore \ r \doteq \frac{2\,d\,h'}{h}$$

Figure 5.1–Optical principle of keratometry

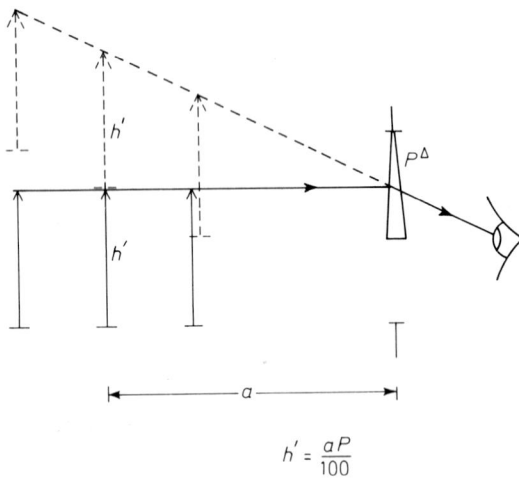

Figure 5.3–Javal Schiötz mires as used in the Haag-Streit keratometer

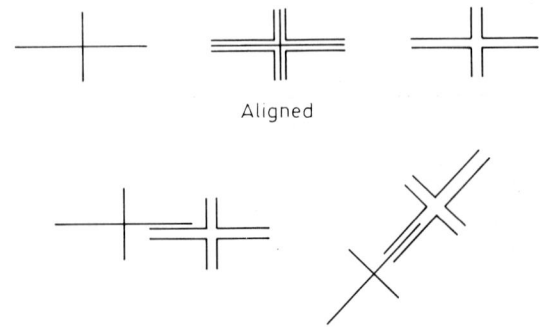

$$h' = \frac{aP}{100}$$

Figure 5.2–The doubling principle

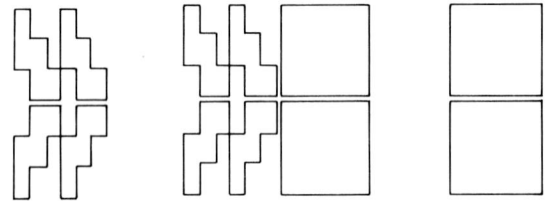

Not along principal meridian   Along principal meridian

Figure 5.4–Mires used in the Zeiss ophthalmometer

in the corresponding meridians. The instrument is rotated about its axis to align the mires with both principal meridians of the cornea (which are assumed to be at right-angles to each other) and the images in each can then be brought into contact without further rotation. A skilled observer operating both doubling devices can therefore make almost simultaneous measurements. If, however, the cornea is very toroidal, a focus adjustment must also be made as the pairs of mire reflections are formed in different planes for each meridian (Stone, 1962). The Bausch and Lomb keratometer is probably the best known instrument of this type. *Figure 5.5* shows the appearance of its mire images when out of focus and at the end point of the measurement. Topcon produces a similar instrument. The American Optical Company's CLC Ophthalmometer is a more recent one position design, but its mire pattern is almost identical in appearance to that of the Bausch and Lomb instrument. The American Optical Company also produces a hybrid instrument in which mire images in both principal meridians are viewed simultaneously, but a single variable doubling device is used and rotated through 90° to measure each principal meridian in turn.

SOURCES OF ERROR

Some of the factors which influence the accuracy of a keratometer measurement are not under the control of the observer but are functions of the design of the instrument. The relationships derived in *Figure 5.1* are based on paraxial optical theory, which has been shown by Emsley (1960 and 1963) and Bennett (1966) to oversimplify the situation. The corneal areas from which the mire images are reflected are too far from the axis of the system to be considered as being in the paraxial zone of a surface with a reflecting power of about -260 D. The resulting third order aberrations are too large to permit a keratometer to be calibrated by paraxial theory. Bennett (*op. cit.*) has shown that the difference in the aberrations of convex and concave surfaces can account for the corrections which have to be applied when a keratometer is used to measure the back central optic radius of a contact lens (*see* Chapter 12), whereas the paraxial formulae apply equally to concave and convex surfaces.

The second of the equations derived in *Figure 5.1* ($r = 2dh'/h$) is an approximation in which d, the separation of object and image, is assumed to be the same as x, the distance of the object from the focal point. This assumption is used in the design of most keratometers, the mires being

mounted relatively close to the eye. The error thus introduced is small because of the high reflecting power of the cornea. Emsley (1955) calculates that for a cornea of 8 mm radius it amounts to 0.10 D (0.02 mm) with the Bausch and Lomb keratometer in which d is 72 mm, and that if d is increased to 150 mm the error is reduced to 0.02 D (0.003 mm). It can be completely eliminated by making the mires the targets of a collimating system. This course is adopted in the Zeiss, the Gambs and the Guilbert Routit Topographic instruments.

Figure 5.1 also shows that the light from the mires is reflected, not from the keratometric pole towards which the telescope is directed but from two small areas on either side of it. The instrument is calibrated on the assumption that these two areas are on a spherical surface and the resulting radius is attributed to the keratometric pole. If the areas from which the mire images are reflected have a curvature different from that of the pole, or from each other, the measurement will be incorrect. This error is more likely to be serious if the two reflection areas are large or widely separated, or if the keratometric pole is markedly decentred within the optic cap. It can be reduced by reducing the size and separation of the mires (Noble, 1962; Mandell, 1962a and 1965). *Figure 5.6* shows the separations of the mire reflection areas in some current instruments, and *Table 5.1* shows the diameters of the corneal reflection areas for a single mire as determined by Lehmann (1967).

Table 5.1

Keratometer	Diameter in mm of corneal area in which each mire is reflected when the corneal radius is:		
	7.00 mm	9.00 mm	10.00 mm
Bausch and Lomb	0.1	0.1	
Zeiss	0.2		0.4
Gambs	0.2		0.4
Guilbert Routit Topographic	0.5		0.8
Haag-Streit	0.4		0.3

The main source of error which is under the control of the observer is focusing. If the mire images formed by the objective are not accurately focused in the intended primary image plane, the radius measurement will be incorrect since the object—image separation is then incorrect, and the out-of-focus mire images have a different separation from sharply focused ones. These out-of-focus images may not appear to be blurred if the observer accommodates. Collimated mires and a fully

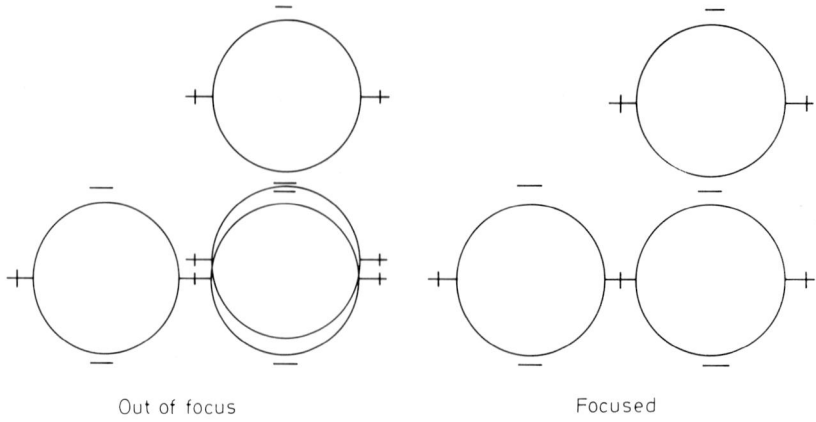

Figure 5.5 – The Bausch and Lomb keratometer mires

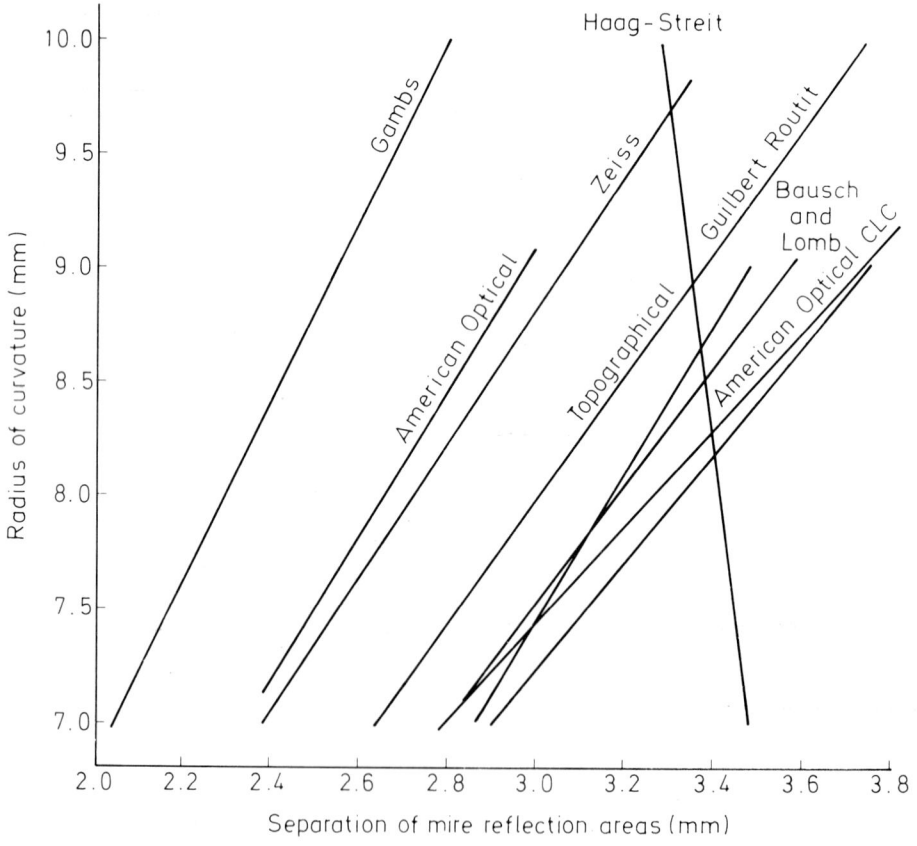

Figure 5.6 – Graphs showing the separation of the mire reflection areas on the corneal cap for radii of curvature from 7 to 10 mm for various modern keratometers (after Mandell and Lehmann)

telecentric viewing system, as in the Zeiss or Guilbert Routit Topographic instruments, eliminate this source of error; or the observer's judgment of focus can be assisted by including a Scheiner disc in the viewing system as in the American Optical Company CLC, the Topcon and the Bausch and Lomb keratometers, where the central mire image is seen double if it is not accurately focused (*Figure 5.5*). In instruments with a fixed graticule in the primary image plane, there should be no parallax between the mire images and the graticule when the observer moves his eye from side to side; this test is valid whether or not the observer is accommodating.

The commonest cause of focusing error is proximal accommodation by the observer. The following precautions should reduce this to a minimum by avoiding unnecessary stimulation of accommodation. The observer should keep both eyes open and suppress the image in the disengaged eye. If the instrument has an adjustable eyepiece, it should be carefully focused on the graticule by turning it as far as possible in the positive direction (outwards) and then resetting it until the graticule is just clear. To ensure that convergent light emerges from the eyepiece when the instrument is out of focus, thereby encouraging the observer's accommodation to remain relaxed, the instrument should be moved as far as possible from the patient and then slowly moved forward until the mire images are just clear. By keeping errors to a minimum, readings should be repeatable to 0.02 mm, but the scales of some instruments are difficult to interpolate to this degree of accuracy (Stone, 1962).

USES OF THE KERATOMETER

A standard keratometer may be used by a contact lens practitioner for three purposes: to decide on an appropriate back central optic radius during fitting; to monitor changes in central corneal and soft lens front surface curvature during after-care; and to check the radii of finished contact lenses.

As an Aid to Fitting

The value of a keratometer in fitting contact lenses depends on the fitting technique employed. If, as is usual, the specification of the prescription lens is derived by examining the fit of a number of trial lenses, the function of the keratometer is limited to indicating a starting point and providing a base record with which the measurements made in the after-care period may be compared and from which

the power of the tears lens may be calculated (*see* Chapter 4). This assists in computation of the correct back vertex power. In soft lens fitting, keratometry can be carried out with the lens in place; the quality of the mire images and the stability (or instability) of the radius reading indicating whether the lens is flat or steep (*see* Chapter 14, Volume 2). If a keratometer is available, it is usually possible to arrive at a final specification with about half the number of trial lens insertions that would be required if it were not. This materially speeds up the fitting procedure and reduces discomfort to the patient.

In After-care

In the after-care period, comparison of keratometer readings made on successive visits provides a valuable means of detecting corneal changes produced by contact lens wear. During the adaptation period, the radius of the cornea changes in an unpredictable way even with an apparently well-fitting lens. Bier (1957) suggests that a lens which is flatter than the cornea will lead to corneal flattening and vice versa, but this view has not been confirmed by subsequent investigators (Sabell, 1962; Hodd, 1962; Rengstorff, 1965a and b, 1967 and 1969b; Spurrett, 1973). Regular increases or decreases in radius of up to 0.1 mm are usually tolerable during the first six weeks of wear, provided that spectacle blur is not persistent.

There may also be irregular changes of curvature. These are revealed by distortion of the mire images, sometimes to such an extent that no satisfactory reading can be obtained. Appearances of this kind, which show that the contact lens is deforming the cornea, are common with badly fitting lenses, but slight distortion of the mire images may occur during the adaptation period even with a lens which is a good fit. It is most likely to occur with a lens whose apex clears the cornea, since the transition or peripheral zones may bear on the cornea close to the zones from which the mire images are reflected.

In order that there should be a minimum apparent variation in corneal radius due to experimental error, follow-up measurements should be made by the same observer, using the same instrument and, in view of the diurnal variations in radius reported by Reynolds (1959) and Noble and Sheridan (1962), at the same time of day.

If the front surface of a soft lens becomes coated or dirty the mire images appear indistinct, and they appear distorted if the fit is poor. Steepening of curvature indicates probable dehydration of the lens.

In the Checking of Contact Lens Radii

Since the optic radii of a contact lens are similar to those of the cornea, a keratometer may be used to check them. Keratometers are calibrated to measure convex surfaces and require re-calibration when used for concave ones. The principles of re-calibration have been investigated by Emsley (1963) and Bennett (1966), and a conversion scale for concave surfaces is available for the Bausch and Lomb, Topcon and American Optical Company CLC keratometers. The practical aspects of this use of keratometry are discussed in Chapter 12.

It sometimes happens that the surface to be measured has a radius which lies outside the range for which the keratometer is calibrated. The haptic surface of a scleral contact lens or the apex of a conical cornea are examples. The range may be extended by fitting an auxiliary lens (such as a spectacle trial case lens) in front of the objective of the keratometer to change the working distance of the instrument: a positive auxiliary lens enables shorter radii to be measured; a negative lens extends the range to allow measurement of longer radii. The instrument must be re-calibrated with the auxiliary lens in place (Sampson and Soper, 1970). Steel ball-bearings of known radii and guaranteed accuracy are ideal for this purpose. For each auxiliary lens, a graph may be drawn showing the actual radius of the balls against keratometer readings and, provided that the same auxiliary lenses are employed, these graphs may be used for future measurements (cf Chapter 12, page 286).

KERATOMETRY AND KERATOSCOPY OF THE PERIPHERAL CORNEA

Contact lenses usually extend well beyond the optic cap and, since their use became widespread, interest in the contour of the peripheral cornea has been intensified. This has resulted in the design of a number of new keratometers and the modification of existing designs to give more accurate measurements of the peripheral portion of the cornea. Mandell (1962a and b, and 1965) modified a Bausch and Lomb keratometer so as to reduce the mire separation from 64 mm to 26 mm. With the addition of a series of off-axis fixation points, he was able to make measurements of the periphery of the cornea. Noble (1962) and Noble and Sheridan (1962) achieved a small mire separation by mounting small slit mires above an aperture in the telescope tube and reflecting the light along the axis of the system with a semi-silvered mirror.

Bennett (1964) has described the design of a keratometer based on Drysdale's principle and intended for measurement of both central and peripheral cornea.

The system employed by Bonnet and Cochet (1960) and Bonnet (1964) and incorporated in the Guilbert Routit Topographic keratometer makes use of only one mire for the peripheral readings, which are obtained from a corneal area of only 0.5 mm in diameter. The central radius is determined by 'classical' keratometry, using two mires over a much larger chord (*Figure 5.7*). The Zeiss keratometer also provides facilities for single

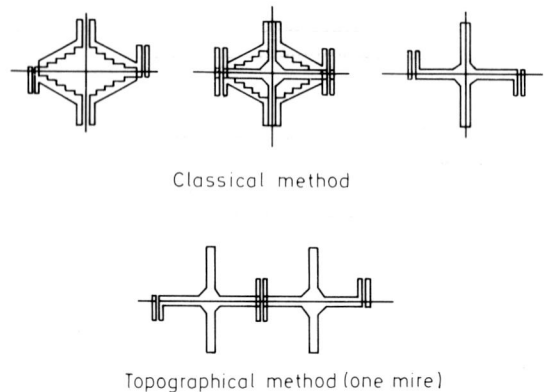

Classical method

Topographical method (one mire)

Figure 5.7 – The mires used in the Guilbert Routit topographical ophthalmometer

mire keratometry and the movable fixation point and extended radius scale which are necessary for peripheral readings.

The Topogometer (Soper, Sampson and Girard, 1962; Sampson, Soper and Girard, 1965; Sampson and Soper, 1970) is a movable fixation device designed to fit the Bausch and Lomb keratometer. As the full mire separation is used, measurement of peripheral radii is not accurate: it is used to find the position, radii and diameters of the optic cap. A similar device is available for the American Optical Company CLC ophthalmometer.

The corneal contour has also been investigated by various photokeratoscopic techniques by Reynolds (1959), Reynolds and Kratt (1959), Blair (1960), Knoll (1961), Stone (1962), Ludlam and Wittenberg (1966), Ludlam et al. (1967) and Mandell and York (1969a and b). Further information is given on page 163 in Chapter 6, and page 174 in Chapter 7. Stereophotogrammetry – a method of stereophotography used for determining surface contour – has been employed by Bertotto (1948), Rzymkowski (1954), and Bonnet (1959 and 1964). Bier (1956 and 1957) used specially constructed peripheral fitting lenses and

Collignon-Brach, Papritz and Prijot (1966) employed profile photography.

This activity has produced many results of scientific interest but few developments of practical clinical value, with the exception of Dunn's (1959) independent curve fitting technique – a development of Bier's method – and photoelectronic keratoscopy (PEK). All the other methods are much more time consuming than using a fitting set, and the order of accuracy obtainable with photokeratoscopy is low (Stone, 1962), though improvements have been reported by more recent workers (Cochet and Amiard, 1966 and 1969; Ludlam *et al.*, 1967; Mandell and York, 1969*a*). In a contact lens context, the desire to make precise measurements of the contour of an individual cornea implies that if this information were available it would be possible, without any trial fitting, to specify the back surface of a contact lens which would fit that cornea perfectly. As the fit of a contact lens depends on factors other than the relationship of its back surface to the cornea, this implication seems unlikely to be true although the PEK system attempts to take some of these factors into account in designing the lens. At present, use of a fitting set is the most reliable way of arriving at the specification for a prescription lens, though keratometry – as already described – can play a useful auxiliary part.

SLIT LAMP BIOMICROSCOPY

The slit lamp biomicroscope is an essential tool for the contact lens practitioner. No other method permits such a detailed examination of the anterior segment of the eye or reveals possible pathological changes at such an early stage. These advantages are obtained because a slit lamp gives a stereoscopic view, at magnifications of up to ×60, of a field of view which can be illuminated in many different ways and at high intensity. Most modern slit lamps can be operated with one hand, leaving the other free to manipulate the patient's lids if necessary. The clinical aspects of the use of this instrument are discussed in Chapter 7, as part of the initial examination, and in Chapter 16, Volume 2 in relation to after-care. The entire anterior segment of the globe, the tears film, the canthi and the lids may be examined in detail, using suitable techniques and stains such as fluorescein and bengal rose (Norn, 1974). With suitable attachments, the apparent thickness of the cornea and depth of the anterior chamber can be measured with great accuracy.

The illuminating system, which gives the instrument its name, is essentially a projection system of short throw, in which the slide is replaced by a slit of variable width, the image of which is focused on the patient's eye. In most instruments it is possible to use a circular aperture if desired and to vary the colour and intensity of the illumination. The slit image is usually vertical, but in some instruments it may be arranged in any desired meridian. It is now common practice to mount the illuminating system vertically, with a narrow reflecting prism or mirror to direct the beam on to the eye. This makes it easy for the illuminating system and microscope to be arranged co-axially for gonioscopy or fundus examination (*see* Chapter 24, Volume 2); but in routine examination of the anterior segment, it is rare to arrange the instrument in this way or to orientate the slit image in any meridian but the vertical.

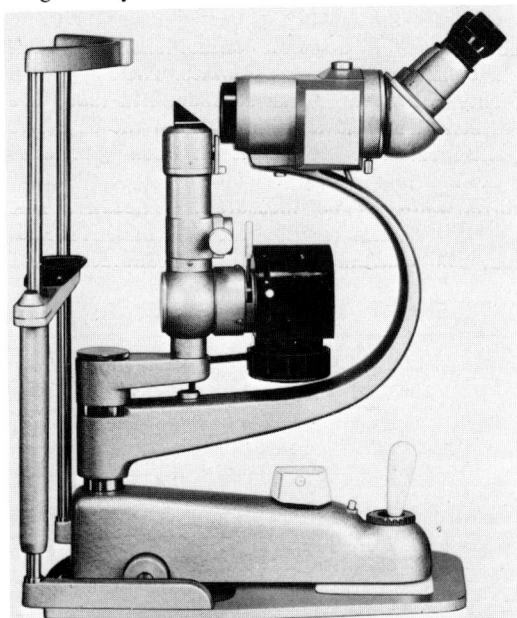

Figure 5.8–The Zeiss slit lamp biomicroscope 100/16 (reproduced by kind permission of Carl Zeiss, Oberkochen)

The slit lamp and binocular microscope are usually mounted on a common pivot and both are focused at a point above the centre of rotation unless deliberately uncoupled. This arrangement means that both may be focused at the same time, using a joystick control, since the part of the eye illuminated by the slit focus will be in focus in the centre of the microscope field. The routine of focusing the slit accurately has been described by Stone (1966 and 1979); if the lamp is oscillated about its pivot, the slit image will remain stationary if accurately focused. A 'with' movement shows that the focus is behind the illuminated surface and an 'against' movement shows that it is in front. *Figure 5.8* shows a typical modern slit lamp.

TYPES OF ILLUMINATION

It is conventional to describe five or six methods of illuminating the eye with a slit lamp (Doggart, 1949; Goodlaw, 1961). These are direct and indirect illumination, oscillating illumination, examination of the zone of specular reflection, retro-illumination and illumination by sclerotic scatter. To this list should be added diffuse illumination, since some modern instruments now have a diffuser which can be placed in front of the reflecting mirror or prism. This is useful for general observation of the anterior eye and adnexa with low magnification. However, the first three methods mentioned are carried out simultaneously by the experienced observer, who continually varies the angle between the lamp and microscope while observing the whole of the microscope field, part of which is directly illuminated and the remainder indirectly illuminated by the slit. These methods of illumination are illustrated diagrammatically in *Figure 5.9*; they are particularly useful for general examination of the anterior segment at the first visit. Direct illumination with a narrow slit and a large angle between the lamp and microscope provides the best means of assessing the depth of an opacity

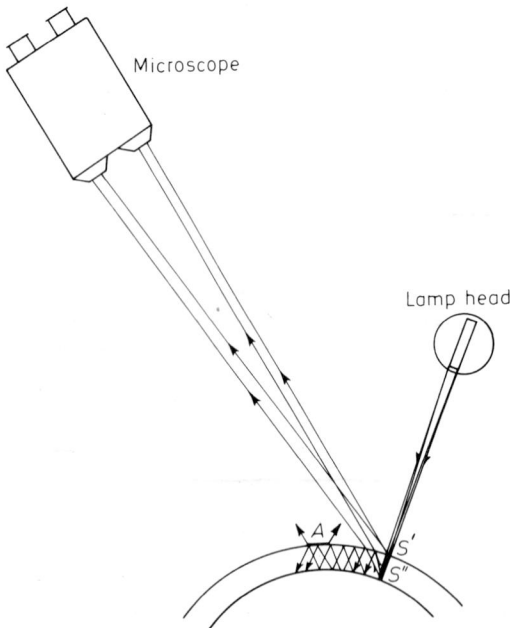

Figure 5.10—Specular reflection. The slit beam is focused at S'. NS' is the normal to the cornea. By arranging the microscope and illuminating system at equal angles on either side of this, any irregularities of the focused surface are seen against a brilliantly lit background

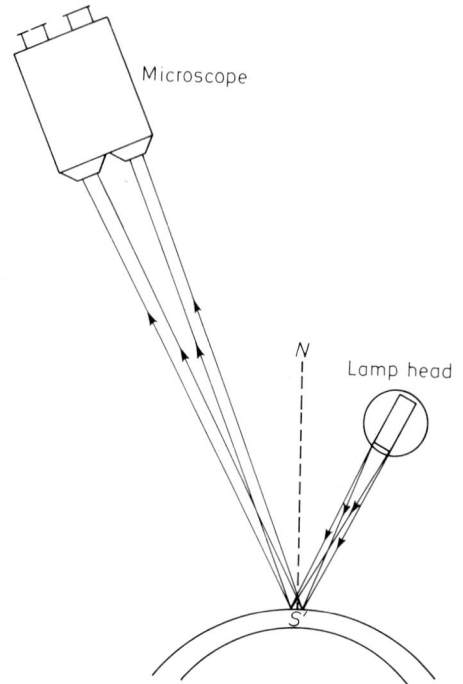

Figure 5.9—Direct and indirect illumination. The slit and microscope are focused at S', and the section of cornea S'S" is seen by direct illumination. Due to some light being reflected and scattered within the cornea an irregularity at A, well outside the beam, is also seen in the microscope field by indirect illumination

or the corneal clearance of a contact lens (Marriott and Woodward, 1964). A larger width of slit allows a parallelepiped of cornea to be viewed; and by varying the depth of focus, the front surface, intermediate area and back surface may be examined. In this way may be observed the vertical striae at the back of the cornea, associated with corneal oedema following soft lens wear.

Examination of the zone of specular reflection requires, as shown in *Figure 5.10*, an appropriate adjustment of the angle between slit beam and microscope. It reveals minute surface defects very clearly. These appear as dark areas on a brilliant background. The discovery of corneal dimples by this method of illumination may provide the first indication that a corneal lens is damaging the surface.

Retro-illumination and sclerotic scatter are shown in *Figures 5.11* and *5.12*. They are most easily carried out with the slit lamp and microscope uncoupled so that the microscope can be focused in front of the slit. Sclerotic scatter — in

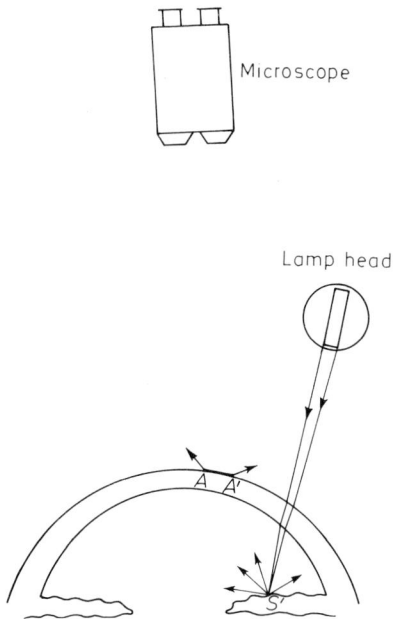

Figure 5.11–Retro-illumination. The slit beam and microscope may be uncoupled. An irregularity at AA', focused in the microscope field, is seen against the light background of the iris where the slit is focused at S'

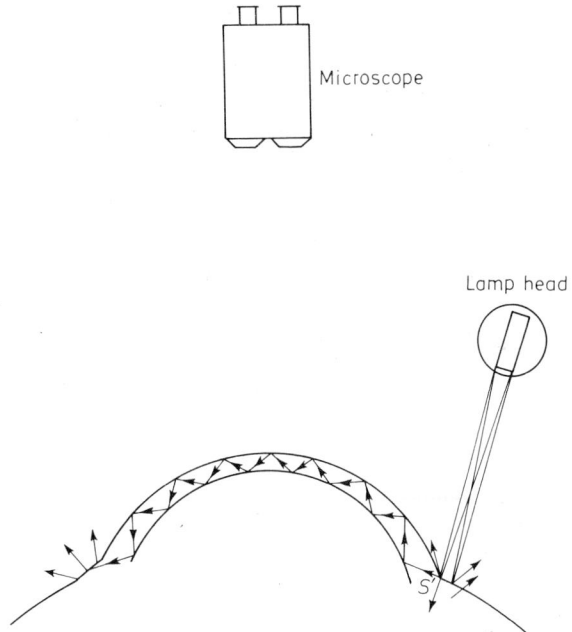

Figure 5.12–Sclerotic scatter. The slit beam is focused at the limbus at S'. Light is totally internally reflected by the corneal surfaces as shown and emerges at the opposite limbus where it is scattered by the scleral tissue and shows up as a glow of light. Any corneal irregularity would similarly scatter the light which would then be seen either with or without the microscope

which the slit is focused at the limbus and opacities or oedema revealed as luminous areas on an otherwise dark cornea — is a particularly useful technique for the contact lens practitioner, who is concerned during after-care not with gross corneal defects but with subtle signs of interference with corneal metabolism. The ease with which slight oedema of the cornea is revealed by sclerotic scatter is illustrated in *Figure 5.13*. The central circular cloudy patch, which is the manifestation of oedema following corneal lens wear, is most easily seen without the aid of a microscope. It is comparable to a newsprint picture, the form of which is difficult to determine if seen magnified. However, detail, such as micro-cysts and epithelial cell oedema, may be seen with the microscope focused on the corneal surface and uncoupled from the beam.

The slit lamp may also be used for the examination of contact lenses, both on and off the eye. Besides the estimation of corneal clearance already mentioned, the behaviour of the lens on the eye may be studied in great detail — especially its effect on the flow of tears and the behaviour of the pre-corneal film. The effect of a sharp transition

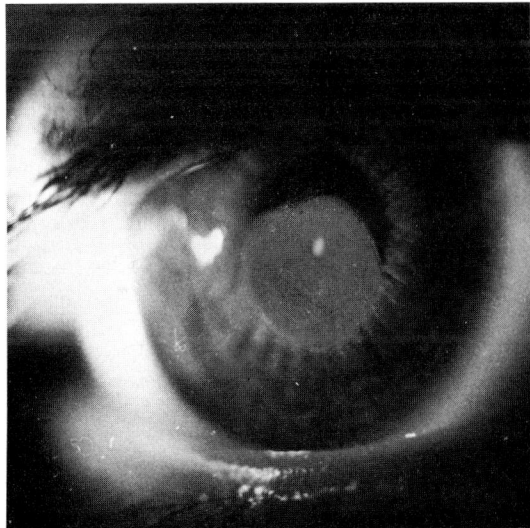

Figure 5.13–Central corneal epithelial oedema shown up by scleral scatter

or the edge of a fenestration hole in converting a bubble into froth can be clearly seen by this method of examination, as can the formation of dimple veil when small bubbles are pressed into the corneal surface by the lens. Slit lamp examination also reveals the presence of unsuspected small bubbles under a corneal lens. Stone (1967) has discussed these appearances fully.

When the slit lamp is used as an illuminated binocular microscope for examining the surface quality and edge form of contact lenses (*see* Chapter 12), the lens is either mounted in a suitable holder and observed directly or by reflection in a mirror arranged at 45 degrees to the axis of the illuminating system, or viewed directly by mounting in Plasticine. Surfaces, fenestrations and edges may be readily examined in this manner. However, the front surface of a contact lens is best studied when on the eye. The effects of scratches on the wettability of the surface may then be judged and the adherence to the surface of sebaceous matter from the back surface of the lids can more easily be seen in this way.

MEASUREMENT OF CORNEAL THICKNESS

Measurement of corneal thickness (pachymetry or pachometry) has been carried out for many years as a special technique. Langham and Taylor (1956) reported that corneal thickness increased during contact lens wear, while Hedbys and Mishima (1966) demonstrated a linear relationship between stromal hydration and thickness. The popularity of the technique as a means of monitoring the fit of contact lenses has increased rapidly since Miller (1968) found corneal curvature and thickness changes to be well correlated. This finding was not confirmed by Mandell and his co-workers (Mandell and Polse, 1969 and 1971; Mandell, Polse and Fatt, 1970). They did, however, find a positive association between central corneal clouding and thickness change. They also found that hard lenses which were a good fit produced an initial corneal thickening which gradually subsided during adaptation, but that poorly fitting lenses produced a persistent increase in thickness. This effect was especially marked with steep lenses. They suggest that increased thickness may be a better indicator of fit than corneal curvature changes since a central swelling may be confined to an area within the keratometer reflection points.

Polse and Mandell (1970) showed that the corneal thickness increased on reduction of the oxygen tension at the epithelial surface, and Polse (1972) has shown that fluctuations of corneal thickness occur on discontinuing contact lens

wear; these are accompanied by curvature changes similar to those described by Rengstorff (1967 and 1969*a*).

Since 1970 there has been a rapid increase in the number of soft lenses fitted and this has further increased the popularity of pachymetry as a means of monitoring lens-induced corneal changes, because a poorly fitting soft lens may produce a generalized corneal oedema which is much more difficult to detect by scleral scatter than the central oedema produced by a badly fitting hard lens (Stone, 1974).

Figure 5.14 shows the principle of pachymetry. If a narrow slit beam is directed normally at the corneal surface, the apparent thickness of the cornea can be found by measuring the width of the optical section seen through the microscope. This is now the usual technique. An alternative method in which the axis of the microscope is normal to the corneal surface was used by Donaldson (1966) and Mandell and Polse (1969). The true thickness can be found if the radius of curvature of the front surface and the refractive index of the cornea are known. For clinical purposes, measurement of the apparent thickness is sufficient, since the object is to detect changes in thickness rather than absolute values.

The measurement of optical section width is made by means of a doubling device in the viewing system. The doubling is varied until (as in a keratometer) the doubled images are juxtaposed, the front surface of one image being aligned with the back surface of the other. To facilitate this adjustment, the slit lamp microscope is usually fitted with a special eyepiece so that the observer sees the top half of one image and the bottom half of the other, as shown in *Figure 5.15*. Provided the angle between the slit lamp and the microscope is kept constant, the instrument can be calibrated to read apparent depth directly.

SOURCES OF ERROR IN PACHYMETRY

It will be apparent from *Figure 5.14* that the measurement of apparent thickness depends on the slit beam being normal to the corneal surface. If the beam is not kept normal to the surface, an error of measurement will result. Mishima and Hedbys (1968) used two small lights mounted at the same angle to the slit beam as the microscope, but on the opposite side of it. The images of these lights appeared on the front surface of the corneal image, one in the upper and one in the lower half of the field, only when the slit beam was normal to the cornea. A similar device, but with the lights mounted above and below the microscope objective, was used by Donaldson (1966) and Mandell

$$BQ' = \frac{BE}{\sin\theta}$$

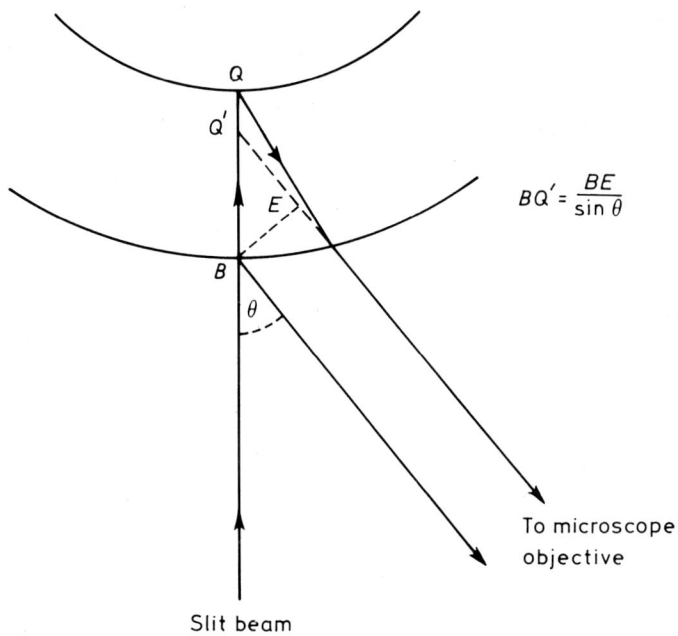

Figure 5.14–Optical principle of pachymetry

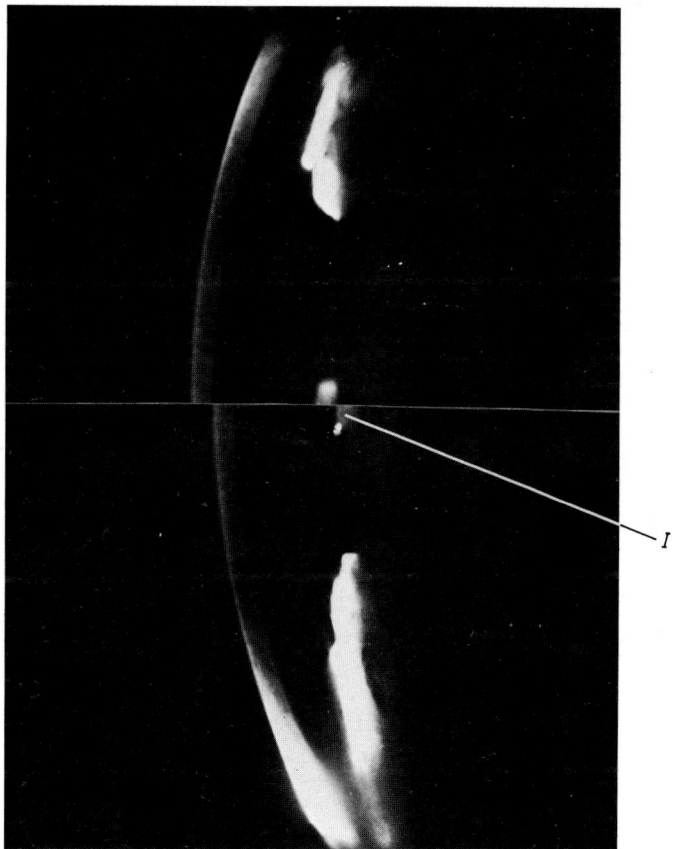

To microscope
objective

Slit beam

Figure 5.15–Appearance of slit section at end-point of measurement (Stone, 1974). Note vertical bisection of 1st Purkinje image, I

and Polse (1969) to ensure that the microscope axis was normal to the corneal surface.

When measuring the thickness of the central cornea, normal incidence can be more simply maintained by asking the patient to look at the centre of the slit and checking that the reflected beam from the cornea returns to the slit aperture. A piece of translucent paper may be mounted above the slit aperture to receive the reflected beam. Vertical alignment can be checked by ensuring that the first Purkinje image of the slit, which is visible at the front surface of the crystalline lens, is bisected by the dividing line between the upper and lower halves of the field, as shown in *Figure 5.15* (Stone, 1974).

Peripheral corneal thickness measurements will be of value only if the patient's head is restrained and the slit lamp fitted with a fixation device which can be accurately and repeatably positioned so that the section measured is the same on each occasion.

It is easier to set the doubled images in co-incidence if the slit beam is narrow. Norn (1974) pointed out that if a corneal parallelepiped is visible, it is possible to include the width of the slit in the corneal thickness measurement. A narrow beam, however, makes it difficult to judge the focus on the cornea and an out-of-focus image will also give an inaccurate reading. In setting up the instrument, it is essential to ensure that the slit beam and microscope are accurately focused on the corneal section. The highest magnification available should be used for this purpose. Once accurate focus has been achieved, the slit beam can be narrowed until there is just enough light to make the measurement, using the highest possible light output from the bulb.

Another possible source of error in comparative measurements arises from the fact that there is a diurnal variation in corneal thickness. Mandell and Fatt (1965) and Gerstmann (1972) found that the cornea is thicker on waking and thins, rapidly at first, then more gradually, throughout the waking day. Errors from this source can be minimized by ensuring that measurements on any particular patient are always made at the same time of day.

Kruse Hansen (1971), using the Haag-Streit instrument, found a systematic difference between the results obtained for the right eyes of his sample and those for the left, the thickness measured for the left eyes being significantly greater than those found in the right eye at the 1 per cent level of probability. Ehlers and Kruse Hansen (1971) attribute this variation to the fact that in the Haag-Streit instrument, the microscope is always on the right side of the slit lamp during pachymetry; this means that the observation is made through a nasal portion of the cornea in the right eye and a temporal portion in the left. As the visual axis does not pass through the apex of the cornea, measurements made with the patient fixing the centre of the slit will be made at different inclinations to the optical axis in the right and left eyes. The differences reported by Kruse Hansen are small (0.004 mm between the sample means for the right and left eyes) but in the light of these findings and those of Spurrett (1973), who found a systematic difference between right and left eyes in a group of contact lens wearers, the thickness of the right cornea apparently increasing more than that of the left, it is evident that apparent differences between the right and left eyes should be treated with caution.

REFERENCES

Bennett, A. G. (1964). 'A new keratometer and its application to corneal topography.' *Br. J. physiol. Optics* **21**, 234–235

Bennett, A. G. (1966). 'The calibration of keratometers.' *Optician* **151**, 317–322

Bertotto, E. V. (1948). 'The stereophotogrammetric study of the anterior segment of the eye.' *Am. J. Ophthal.* **31**, 573–579

Bier, N. (1956). 'A study of the cornea.' *Br. J. physiol. Optics* **13**, 79–92

Bier, N. (1957). *Contact Lens Routine and Practice*, 2nd ed. London: Butterworths

Blair, W. A. (1960). 'Photo-electronic keratoscopy testing.' *Contacto* **4**, 217–227

Bonnet, R. (1959). 'Stéréophotogrammetrie de la cornée humaine.' *Revue Opt. théor. instrum.* **38**, 447–462

Bonnet, R. (1964). *La Topographie Cornéenne*. Paris: Desroches

Bonnet, R. and Cochet, P. (1960). 'Nouvelle méthode d'ophtalmometrie topographique.' *Bull. Mém. Soc. Fr. Ophthal.* **73**, 687–716 (translated by E. Eagle (1962). *Am. J. Optom.* **39**, 227–251)

Cochet, P. and Amiard, H. (1966). 'La photokeratoscopie, élément de biométrie cornéenne.' *Bull. ds. Soc. d'ophthal. Franç.* **66**, 1094–1104

Cochet, P. and Amiard, H. (1969). 'Photography and contact lens fitting.' *Contacto* **13**(2), 3–9

Collignon-Brach, J., Papritz, F. and Prijot, E. (1966). 'Etude de l'applatissement périphérique de la cornée au moyen d'une technique photographique.' *Bull. Soc. belge Ophtal.* **144**, 971–982

Doggart, J. H. (1949). *Ocular Signs in Slit Lamp Microscopy*. London: Kimpton

Donaldson, D. D. (1966). 'A new instrument for the measurement of corneal thickness.' *Archs Ophthal.* **76**, 25–31

Dunn, G. M. (1959). 'Independent curve corneal fitting.' *Optician* **138**, 501–503

Ehlers, N. and Kruse Hansen, F. (1971). 'On the optical measurement of corneal thickness.' *Acta Ophthal. (Kbh.)* **49**, 65–81

Emsley, H. H. (1955). *Visual Optics, Vol. 1,* 5th ed., pp.301–331. London: Butterworths

Emsley, H. H. (1960). 'Revival of the keratometer.' *Optician* **139**, 585–589

Emsley, H. H. (1963). 'The keratometer: measurement of concave surfaces.' *Optician* **146**, 161–168

Gerstmann, D. R. (1972). 'The biomicroscope and Vickers image splitting eyepiece applied to the diurnal variation in human central corneal thickness.' *J. Microscopy* **96**, 385–388

Goodlaw, E. I. (1961). 'The use of slit lamp biomicroscopy in the fitting of contact lenses.' In *Encyclopaedia of Contact Lens Practice,* Vol. 3, ed. by P. R. Haynes. South Bend, Indiana: International Optics Publishing Corporation

Hedbys, B. O. and Mishima, S. (1966). 'The thickness– hydration relationship of the cornea.' *Exp. Eye Res.* **5**, 221–228

Hodd, F. A. B. (1962). 'Contact lenses in general ophthalmic practice.' *Ophthal. Optician* **2**, 852–861

Knoll, H. A. (1961). 'Corneal contours in the general population as revealed by the photokeratoscope.' *Am. J. Optom.* **38**, 389–397

Kruse Hansen, F. (1971). 'A clinical study of the normal human central corneal thickness.' *Acta Ophthal. (Kbh.)* **49**, 82–89

Langham, M. E. and Taylor, I. S. (1956). 'Factors affecting the hydration of the cornea in the excised eye and in the living animal.' *Br. J. Ophthal.* **40**, 321–340

Lehmann, S. P. (1967). 'Corneal areas utilised in keratometry.' *Optician* **154**, 261–264

Levene, J. R. (1965). 'The true inventors of the keratoscope.' *Br. J. History Science* **2**, 324–342

Ludlam, W. M. and Wittenberg, S. (1966). 'Measurements of the ocular dioptric elements utilizing photographic methods. Part II. Cornea – theoretical considerations.' *Am. J. Optom.* **43**, 249–267

Ludlam, W. M., Wittenberg, S., Rosenthal, J. and Harris, G. (1967). 'Photographic analysis of the ocular dioptric components. Part III. The acquisition, storage, retrieval and utilization of primary data in photokeratoscopy.' *Am. J. Optom.* **44**, 276–293

Mandell, R. B. (1960). 'Jesse Ramsden – inventor of the ophthalmometer.' *Am. J. Optom.* **37**, 633–638

Mandell, R. B. (1962a). 'Small mire ophthalmometry.' Paper read before annual meeting of American Academy of Optometry, Miami, December, 1962

Mandell, R. B. (1962b). 'Methods to measure the peripheral corneal curvature. Part 3: Ophthalmometry.' *J. Am. optom. Ass.* **33**, 889–892

Mandell, R. B. (1965). *Contact Lens Practice Basic and Advanced.* Springfield, Ill: Thomas

Mandell, R. B. and Fatt, I. (1965). 'Thinning of the human cornea on awakening.' *Nature* **208**, 292–293

Mandell, R. B. and Polse, K. A. (1969). 'Corneal thickness changes as a contact lens fitting index.' *Am. J. Optom.* **46**, 479–491

Mandell, R. B. and Polse, K. A. (1971). 'Corneal thickness and central clouding.' *Am. J. Optom.* **48**, 129–132

Mandell, R. B., Polse, K. A. and Fatt, I. (1970). 'Corneal swelling caused by contact lens wear.' *Archs Ophthal.* **83**, 3–9

Mandell, R. B. and York, M. A. (1969a). 'A new calibration system for photokeratoscopy.' *Am. J. Optom.* **46**, 410–417

Mandell, R. B. and York, M. A. (1969b). 'Corneal contour from birth to five years – a cross-sectional study. Part II – corneal contour measurements.' *Am. J. Optom.* **46**, 818–825

Marriott, P. J. and Woodward, E. G. (1964). 'A method of measuring the corneal clearance of a haptic lens.' *Br. J. physiol. Optics* **21**, 61–83

Miller, D. (1968). 'Contact lens induced curvature and thickness changes.' *Archs Ophthal.* **80**, 430–432

Mishima, S. and Hedbys, B. O. (1968). 'Measurement of corneal thickness with the Haag-Streit pachometer.' *Archs Ophthal.* **80**, 710–713

Noble, D. (1962). 'The corneal contour and its measurement.' Paper read to The Yorkshire Optical Society, Bradford, January, 1962

Noble, D. and Sheridan, M. (1962). 'The normal cornea, its variations and measurement.' Paper read to the Contact Lens Society, Bradford, July, 1962

Norn, M. S. (1974). *External Eye, Methods of Examination,* 1st ed. Copenhagen: Scriptor

Polse, K. A. (1972). 'Changes in the corneal hydration after discontinuing contact lens wear.' *Am. J. Optom.* **49**, 511–516

Polse, K. A. and Mandell, R. B. (1970). 'Critical O_2 tension at the corneal surface.' *Archs Ophthal.* **84**, 505–508

Rengstorff, R. H. (1965a). 'The Fort Dix report.' *Am. J. Optom.* **42**, 156–163

Rengstorff, R. H. (1965b). 'Corneal curvature and astigmatic changes subsequent to contact lens wear.' *J. Am. optom. Ass.* **36**, 996–1000

Rengstorff, R. H. (1967). 'Variations in myopia measurements.' *Am. J. Optom.* **44**, 149–161

Rengstorff, R. H. (1969a). 'Variations in corneal curvature measurements.' *Am. J. Optom.* **46**, 45–51

Rengstorff, R. H. (1969b). 'Relationship between myopia and corneal curvature changes after wearing contact lenses.' *Am. J. Optom.* **46**, 357–362

Reynolds, A. E. (1959). 'Corneal topography as found by photo-electronic keratoscopy.' *Contacto* **3**, 229–233

Reynolds, A. E. and Kratt, H. J. (1959). 'The photo-electronic keratoscope.' *Contacto* **3**, 53–59

Rzymkowsky, J. (1954). 'Stereophotographic and stereophotogrammetric reproduction of the cornea and sclera of the living eye.' (Translated by W. P. Schumann.) *Am. J. Optom.* **31**, 416–422

Sabell, A. G. (1962). 'Surface distortions of the cornea from contact lenses.' In *Transactions of the International Ophthalmic Optical Congress,* 1961. London: Crosby Lockwood

Sampson, W. G. and Soper, G. W. (1970). 'Keratometry.' In *Corneal Contact Lenses,* 2nd ed. Ed. by L. J. Girard. St. Louis: Mosby

Sampson, W. G., Soper, J. W. and Girard, L. J. (1965).

'Topographical keratometry and contact lenses.' *Trans. Am. Acad. Ophthal. Otolaryngol.* **69**, 959–969

Soper, J. W., Sampson, W. G. and Girard, L. J. (1962). 'Corneal topography, keratometry and contact lenses.' *Archs Ophthal.* **67**, 753–760

Spurrett, A. J. (1973). *Corneal Contact Lens Design and Corneal Change.* M.Sc. Thesis, University of Bradford

Stone, Janet (1962). 'The validity of some existing methods of measuring corneal contour compared with suggested new methods.' *Br. J. physiol. Optics* **19**, 205–230

Stone, Janet (1966). 'The use of the slit lamp in ophthalmic practice.' *Ophthal Optician,* **6**, 637–640, 645, 646

Stone, Janet (1967). 'The use of the slit lamp in contact lens practice.' *Contact Lens Practitioner,* June 1967

Stone, Janet (1979). 'The slit lamp biomicroscope in ophthalmic practice.' *Ophthal. Optician* **19**, 439–455

Stone, Janet (1974). 'The measurement of corneal thickness.' *Contact Lens J.* **5**(2), 14–19

Chapter 6

External Eye Photography

D. C. Burns

It is not intended, in a book of this nature, to attempt coverage of the whole field of ocular photography, let alone the realm of medical photography. Nor was it felt necessary in a book intended for such a specialized readership to include the usual glossary of optical definitions and terms. The purpose of this chapter is to provide that basic data which will enable the practitioner to employ routine photography in his contact lens work. The bibliography gives references for further study in special areas.

The aim must be a speedy and accurate recording of features of clinical interest, such results to be obtained with the minimum of disturbance to the practitioner's routine and the least possible inconvenience and discomfort to the patient. In this context the author must make clear his dislike of camera stands, head rests, bellows and other such items which serve to impede the swift and convenient use of the camera. This must be a personal preference as much excellent work has been done with these devices, but it can only be said that first class results are possible without such aids. Apart from the use of copy stand, bellows and transillumination stage for higher magnification photography of contact lens defects, all of the clinical work to be described here can be undertaken with the camera and flash hand-held.

Many practitioners feel that their most valuable photographic record is that of the external eye, life-size, taken before fitting is commenced (*Colour Plate I*). Features such as lid position and conjunctival vascularization can be very clearly recorded and reference back to this photograph can be most useful.

THE CAMERA

By far the most suitable camera is the single lens reflex, normally referred to as an SLR (*Figure 6.1*). The particular advantage of this type is the complete absence of parallax, so important to close-up work. All except the very cheapest SLRs have automatic diaphragm control which permits framing and focusing to be done with the lens at full aperture. The diaphragm is then automatically stopped down to the chosen aperture just before the shutter releases. It is rare to find an SLR camera where the lens is not interchangeable. This facility permits the use of extension tubes, bellows and lenses of different focal lengths, all of which are important in close-up photography. Examples of such accessories are shown in *Figure 6.2*.

The focusing screen fitted as standard equipment to most cameras has a circular central microprism, surrounded by ground glass and/or a Fresnel lens to improve edge brightness. Although this arrangement is excellent for general photography, it is generally agreed that a plain ground glass or fine Fresnel screen is more satisfactory for telephoto and close-up work. A few cameras, such as the Nikon F, Olympus OM1 and Contax RTS feature interchangeable screens, allowing a flexible approach. Another most important, though insufficiently considered, point is that the photographer should find the camera comfortable to hold (*Figure 6.3*). This does not necessarily mean the smallest, lightest camera, as someone with large hands may find small cameras — such as the Olympus OM1 or the latest Pentax M — difficult to operate, whilst a lady with small hands may find

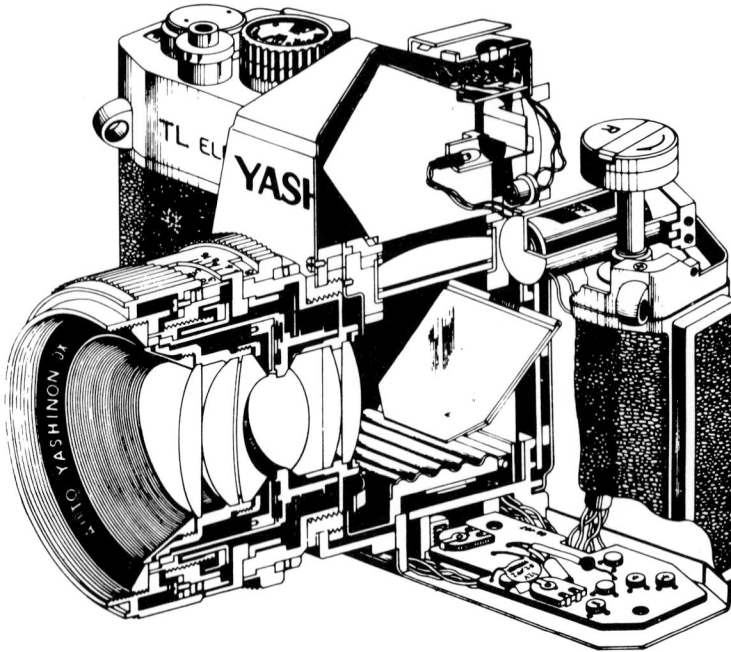

Figure 6.1–Section through a single lens reflex camera. The 45° mirror, allowing through-the-lens viewing, can be seen. This springs out of the way when the shutter is released (reproduced by kind permission of Yashica)

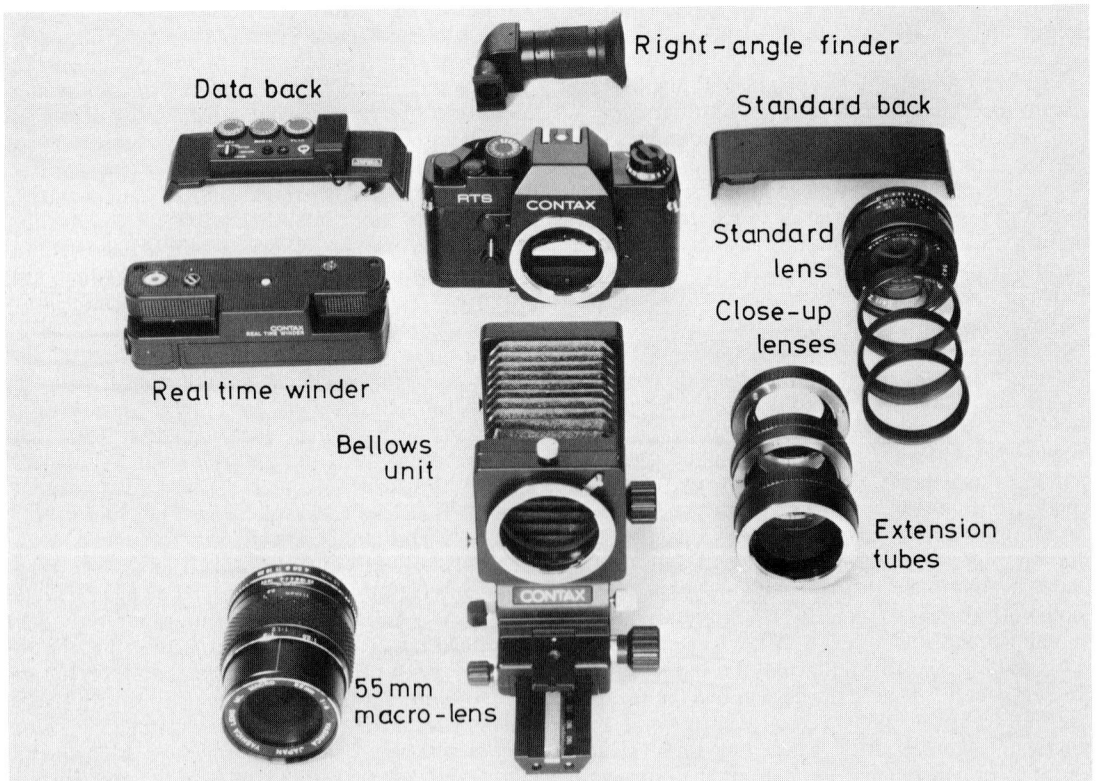

Figure 6.2–Accessories for macro-photography using the Contax system

it suits her perfectly. Zeiss even went to the lengths of retaining the Porsche car design department to develop the body and control layout of the new Contax RTS for near-perfect ergonomic efficiency. The practitioner should try holding and firing the complete equipment; that is, the camera, the flash and the close-up equipment of choice, with one hand, as the other hand is frequently required for steadying oneself against the patient's brow or manipulating the lids.

Among the camera systems which meet all or most of the above requirements are those by Practika, Pentax, Topcon, Olympus, Minolta, Canon, Nikon, Contax and Leicaflex. The smallest and lightest is probably the Pentax M, the largest and heaviest the Leicaflex. Possibly the most widely used are the Pentax, Olympus and Nikon instruments.

It is necessary to warn against the ordering of eyepiece correction lenses by direct reference to the user's spectacle prescription; many cameras do not have the viewing screen image at infinity, but have a built-in 'refractive error' of their own! The only way to ensure accurate correction is to interpose trial lenses between the eye and the viewfinder lens until the best result is found by trial and error.

Special cameras for clinical photography have been developed by Polaroid and the Dine Company in the United States. Lester Dine has cleverly adapted the Kodak Instamatic Cameras for use at close range. The various magnifications are set by different close-up lenses in conjunction with a variable distance device which fixes the correct separation between the camera and the patient's cheek.

THE LENS

Most SLR cameras, as mentioned in the previous section, have interchangeable lenses with automatic diaphragm control. The camera is normally supplied with a so-called 'standard' lens having a nominal focal length of 50 mm and a maximum aperture of around f2. This lens is likely to focus down to about 2 ft, and for closer work either supplementary lenses, bellows, extension tubes or a specially designed macro-lens must be employed (*Figure 6.2*). The best known macro-lenses are the Micro-Nikkor (Nikon), the Macro-Takumar (Pentax) and the Macro-Zuiko (Olympus). These special lenses have a longer focal length than standard lenses (for example, 55 mm), and are computed to give best results at much closer working distances than standard lenses. They allow a slightly longer working distance than bellows or extension tubes with standard lenses, thereby lessening illumination problems. They may also be used quite satisfactorily for general photography. The Micro-Nikkor macro-lens, for example, focuses from infinity down to 1:2 (half life size) without interruption and, with the addition of an automatic extension ring, right down to 1:1.

However, it is convenient to use a lens of normal focal length for clinical photography up to

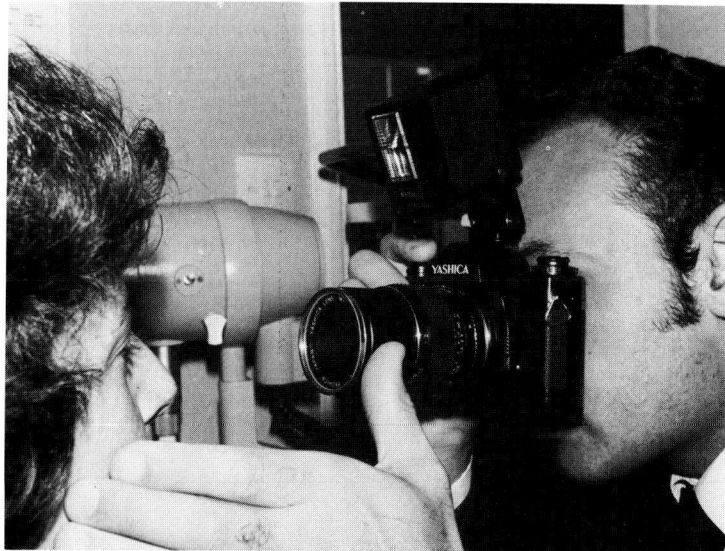

Figure 6.3–Single lens reflex system in use, showing one hand steadying the camera against the patient's face and the other hand holding the camera with forefinger ready to operate the shutter release

1:1 (life size) as the working distance with this lens enables the photographer to steady himself against the patient's brow with the finger tips of his left hand (if normally right-handed) while the thumb is rested on the lens mount (*Figure 6.3*). A longer focal length makes lighting rather easier, but may increase the working distance too much for the above steadying technique to be employed. It must be emphasized that there is no advantage in using either longer or shorter focal length lenses in so far as depth or field is concerned, as this is a function of magnification and aperture and is independent of focal length.

CLOSE-UP LENSES

Although these are normally sold in powers of +1, +2 or +3 dioptres, for closer ranges very satisfactory results have been obtained with lenses of +10, or even +15 dioptres. These lenses should, of course, be anti-reflection coated. Since it is essential in ocular photography to work at small apertures in order to yield adequate depth of field, the aberrations which would normally preclude the use of such powerful supplementary lenses, are adequately controlled. Examples of focusing distances for lenses of +3 and +6 dioptres are shown in *Table 6.1*.

EXTENSION TUBES

Extension tubes are fitted between the camera lens and the camera body. As they do not contain any optical elements they do not affect the optical performance of the lens, except that the lens used may be operating in a magnification range for which it was not designed. Tubes are normally sold in sets of three and may be used either singly or in combination to give the required magnification (*Table 6.2*).

BELLOWS

Bellows may be regarded as continuously variable extension tubes, but although it is possible to obtain them for some cameras with automatic diaphragm coupling, they are not as convenient in use as tubes.

THE FILM

The choice of films can be broken down in two ways. Are slides or prints required? Should the film be fast (for use in fluorescein photography), or slow for general external photography? (Colour film is assumed to be a necessity.)

Prints

Although prints may be more convenient, slides are cheaper and give much better contrast and detail. If, however, prints are preferred, suitable negative films are Kodacolor II, Agfacolor CNS 2 or Fujicolor FII, although if accustomed to other brands the practitioner can be assured that there are far more likely to be marked variations between

Table 6.1—Close-up Lens Chart for +3D and +6D

| Scale setting on camera (m) | Close-up lens strength | |
| | +3D | +6D |
	Focusing distance from lens to subject (mm)	
infinity	333	167
20	328	165
15	326	165
10	322	164
5	312	161
3	300	158
2	286	154
1.5	273	150
1	250	143
0.7	226	135
0.5	200	125

Table 6.2—Increase in Magnification with Extension (Macro-Takumar 50 mm f4 lens with distance scale set at 0.234 m)

Magnification	Tubes to be used	Area to be photographed (mm)	Film-to-subject distance (mm)	Exposure factor
0.50	Not used	48 × 72	234	× 2.3
0.73	1 (12 mm)	33 × 49	213	× 3.2
0.86	2 (19 mm)	28 × 42	209	× 3.7
1.00	3 (26 mm)	24 × 36	208	× 4.3

the En Print type processing of one firm compared with another, than between the performances of different films. Until very recently there has not been a freely available colour negative film which was ideal for ultra-violet illuminated work, but with the arrival of Fuji 400 and Kodacolor 400 this is now a possibility.

Transparencies

For general clinical photography Kodachrome 25 is widely considered to offer the best combination of sharpness, colour quality and processing reliability. Ektachrome X, Agfacolor CT18 and Kodachrome 64 can also be recommended. Where extra film speed is called for, Ektachrome 200 is a most

carefully balanced, consistent light output and is cheap to buy and run. The flash duration is very short, typically less than 1/1000 of a second, eliminating any danger of subject movement.

The flashgun should, ideally, have a light source with a small aperture as this will produce a correspondingly small reflex when photographing subjects such as the cornea.

TECHNIQUE

The flashgun is best fitted to a tilting flash adaptor and both mounted on the camera accessory shoe. It must be remembered that this will normally render the 'hot shoe' (direct contact) feature

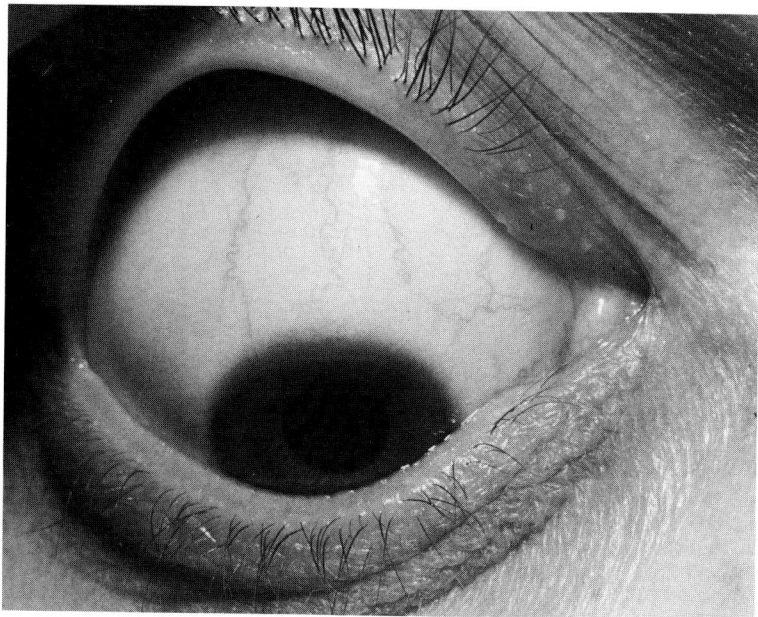

Figure 6.4 – The external eye photographed at 1:1 magnification on the negative, and utilizing the technique shown in Figure 6.3. The photographs in Figures 6.5 and 6.6 were also taken in the same way

versatile material as it can, by varying its development times, be rated at speeds from its normal 200 ASA up to an astonishing 2,000 ASA! Naturally, quality suffers when the film is 'pushed' to this degree, but very acceptable results are obtained by rating it up to 1½ stops faster, that is, up to about 500 ASA.

ILLUMINATION

The modern, compact electronic flashgun combines all of the requirements for a light source in clinical photography. It is light in weight, powerful, has

inoperative so that the flash unit must be connected to the X synchronization contact on the camera. The flashgun is then tilted downwards so as to point directly at the subject; if this angle is carefully adjusted it is possible to produce perfectly illuminated photographs even as close as for life size (that is, 1:1) shots (*see Figures 6.3 – 6.6*). Although, in theory, the ring flash seems more suitable, in practice it produces a most inconvenient reflex right in the centre of the cornea. The light output of the smallest flash units has been found to be quite adequate even with such slow films as Kodachrome 25, producing excellent results at apertures as small as f16.

Larger flashguns, whilst useful in ultra-violet photography, are of no help in normal colour work as they are too powerful and many camera lenses (for example, Nikon) cannot cope with the extra illumination as they do not stop down further than f16.

Most cameras must be set to a speed of around 1/60 of a second or slower as their focal plane shutters will otherwise produce partially exposed frames. It is of no advantage to set the shutter speed at a value slower than that required for flash photography as the result may well show blurring due to the effect of the ambient illumination, even though the flash duration is so short. The lighting used for focusing must be very carefully controlled; if it is too dim it is impossible to see properly to focus, and if too bright, particularly with ultra-violet work, the colour rendering is affected.

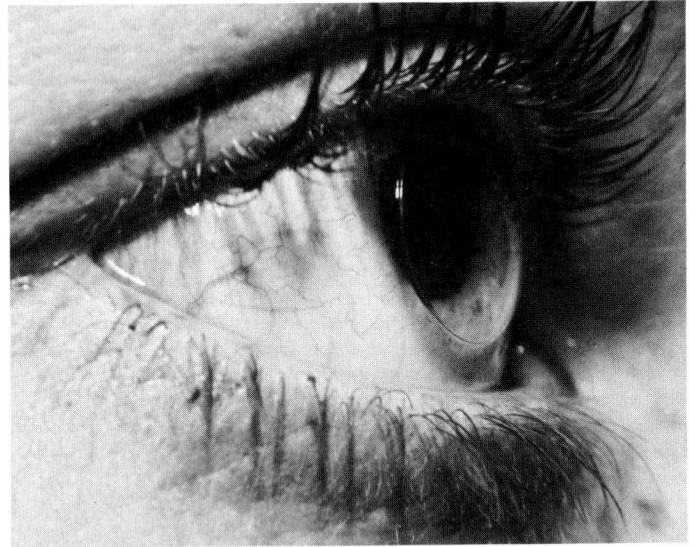

Figure 6.5–Photographs showing the position taken up by a corneal lens. (a) From the side. (b) From in front. Notable also is the low lower lid position and in (b) the shadow cast on the iris by the edge of the lens

(a)

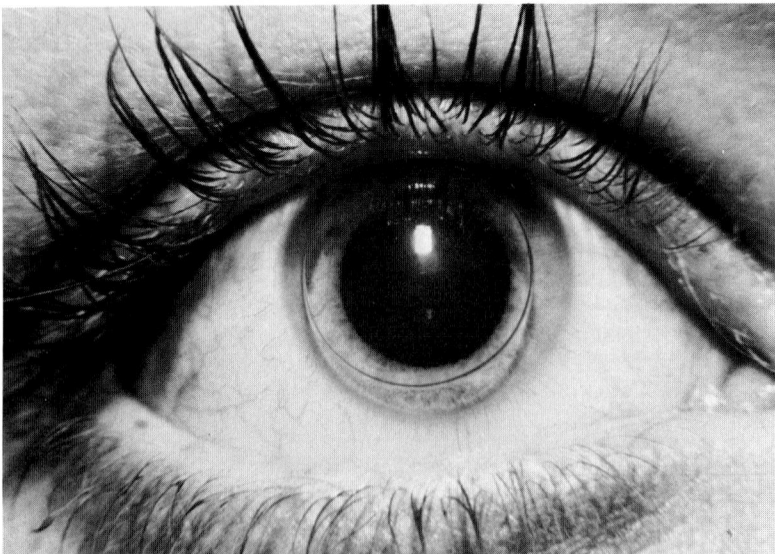

(b)

ULTRA-VIOLET PHOTOGRAPHY

The recording of corneal staining or of the fit of a contact lens requires some adaptation to the above technique (*see Colour Plate II*). It is most convenient if a second camera body is available, permanently loaded with the faster film required (for example, Ektachrome 200 or 400, or Kodacolor 400). With only one camera body it is inevitable that it is loaded with the wrong film when required!

A small electronic flashgun covered with Kodak Wratten 47B Gelatin Filter, which is blue, should be mounted on a tilting flash shoe (for example, Kaiser) and angled sharply downwards. In order to increase the blue/yellow-green contrast of the photograph a pale yellow (*2X*) filter must be fitted over the camera lens.

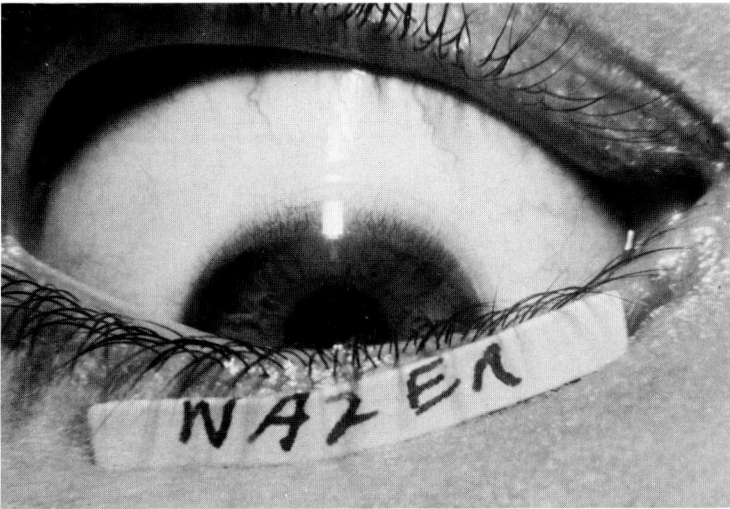

(a)

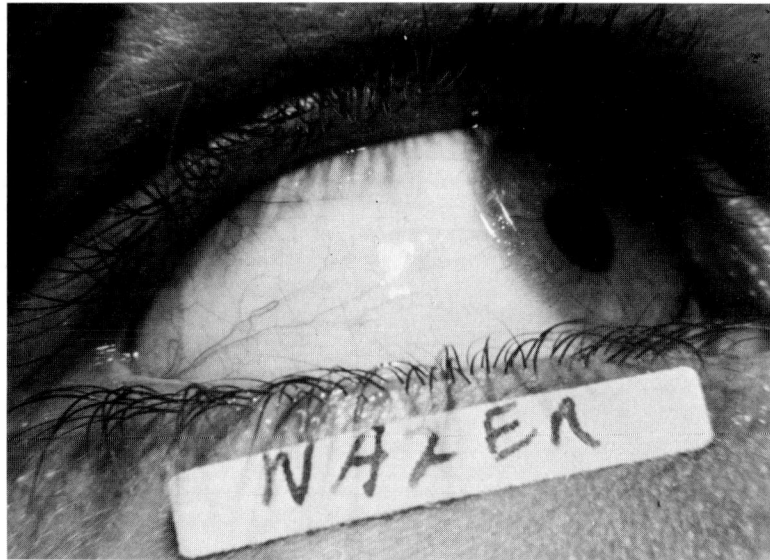

(b)

Figure 6.6–Photographs showing the positioning of a soft lens on the eye. (a) With gaze depressed and upper lid raised. (b) Looking nasally

SLIT LAMP PHOTOGRAPHY

If photographs of the external eye are required, the results obtained with a conventional camera system are superior (and very much cheaper) to those obtained with a photo slit lamp. When slit section photographs are called for, such as that in *Figure 6.7*, there is no substitute for a specially designed photo slit lamp such as those made by Zeiss (West Germany), Zeiss Jena or Gambs (*Figure 6.8*). The special procedures required when using these instruments are, of course, very fully described in the appropriate instruction books.

EXPOSURE

Although it is theoretically possible to calculate the correct exposure from the flash factor and the film speed, in practice the result is usually unreliable due to the very short distances involved. A much simpler method is to make an 'exposure gradient' test. The chosen film/flashgun/magnification combination is used to produce a series of test exposures from maximum to minimum aperture of the lens used. When the slides (or prints) are returned they should be viewed by whichever method will subsequently be employed, that is, projection, viewer

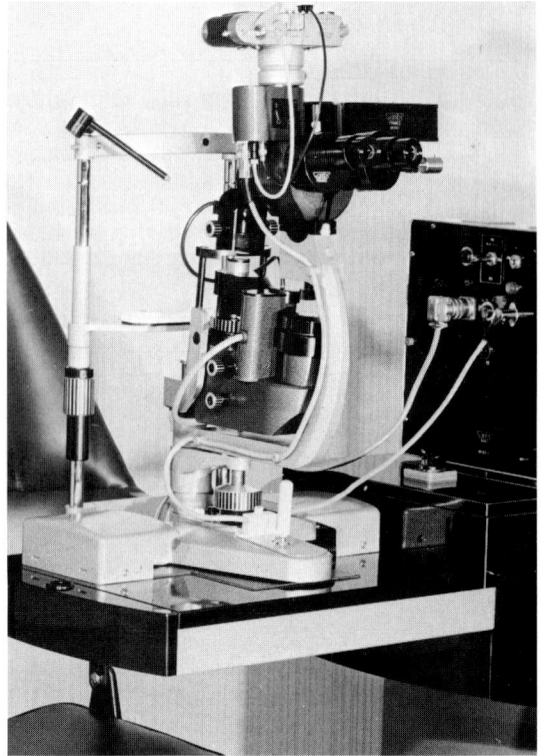

Figure 6.8–The Gambs photo slit lamp

or lightbox for slides, and the exposure of the best slide (or print) chosen. It is sometimes possible to refine this result still further by selecting an intermediate aperture, although not all lenses have 'click' settings at half stop intervals. This information should then be recorded on a label stuck to the camera or flashgun (for example, K25/1:1/ f16). This will, of course, have to be repeated for different film/filter combinations, although it has been found that reasonable changes in magnification, for example, between 3:1–1:1½ make little difference. The reason for this is that the inverse square laws relating to the increase in illumination versus the extra exposure required with greater extension, cancel each other out.

FUNDUS CAMERAS

Besides the equipment already described, fundus cameras, such as the Zeiss (Jena) model, may be used for external eye photography, yielding high quality transparencies. Magnification can be varied from about twice life size (2:1) down to one-third life size (1:3).

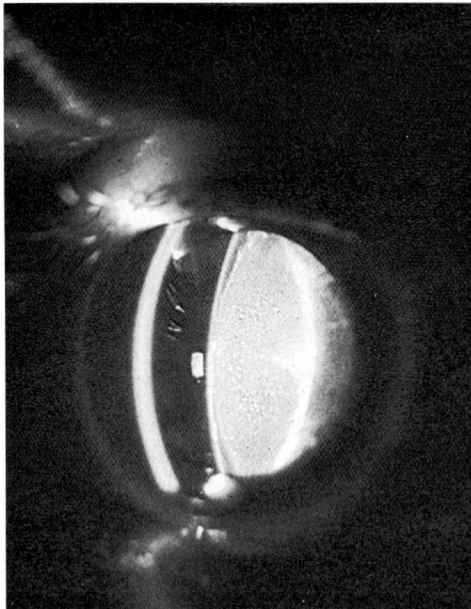

Figure 6.7–Section of cornea and crystalline lens taken with a Zeiss (Oberkochen) photo slit lamp

Table 6.3–Typical Exposure Data

Film	K.25*	E200*	E400*
Magnification	1:2	1:2	1:2
Lens	50 mm	50 mm	50 mm
Filter (camera)	None	2X yellow	2X yellow
Filter (flash)	None	47B	47B
Flashgun	– –	Vivitar 121	– –
Aperture	f16	f2.8	f5.6

* K.25 is Kodachrome 25, that is, film speed 25 ASA.
 E200 is Ektachrome 200, that is, film speed 200 ASA.
 E400 is Ektachrome 400, that is, film speed 400 ASA.
 (All three films are made by Kodak.)

PHOTOKERATOSCOPY

This is a technique for photographing the regularity of the corneal front surface or the front surface of a soft contact lens by means of Placido disc-type rings. Examples can be seen in *Figures 14.6, 14.9, 14.13, 14.22* and *14.35* in Chapter 14, Volume 2. The technique is also used for measuring the corneal contour and in one system black and white Polaroid photographs of the corneal image are automatically scanned to give corneal curvature and eccentricity values in the two principal meridians. Corneal lenses are then designed by computer from this information (*see* page 174, Chapter 7). Other references to photokeratoscopy are given on page 147, Chapter 5.

BIBLIOGRAPHY

Bishop, C. (1976). 'Basic aspects of ophthalmic photography.' *Ophthal. Optician* **16**, 719–720, 729–731, 762–764, 769, 817–820, 845–848, 853–854

Eastman Kodak Data Book, Publication N-3. (1972). *Clinical Photography*

Eastman Kodak Medical Publication N-18. (1973). *Medical Photography (Clinical, Ultra-Violet and Infrared)*

Hall, J. (1973). 'Ophthalmic optics and the visual sciences.' *Ind. comml. Photogr.* **13**, March, 1973, 84–91

Horder, A. (1956). *The Ilford Manual of Photography*, 4th ed. Ilford, Essex: Greenwood

Kodak Information Sheet (AM-900(H)). (1977). *An Introduction to Infrared Photography*

Littman, G. (1965). 'Slit image photography.' *Zeiss Inf.* No. 56, 3–11

Lang, M. M. (1971). 'Fluorescence colour photography of the eye with the polaroid CU5 camera.' *Aust. J. Optom.* **54**, 7, 242–248

Maude, N. (1976). 'Developments of ophthalmic photography in the field.' *Br. J. Photogr.* **123**, 298–299

Pearce, N. (1974). 'Slit lamp photography of the eye.' *Med. biol. Illust.* **24**(1), 21–27

Rosen, E. (1976). 'Recent advances in retinal photography.' *Med. biol. Illust.* **26**(1), 27–31

Stein, H. A. and Slatt, B. J. (1971). 'Eye photography.' In *The Ophthalmic Assistant*, Chapt. 23, 2nd ed. St. Louis: Mosby

Wagstaff, D. F. (1970). 'External eye photography in ophthalmic practice.' *Ophthal. Optician* **10**, 17–28

Wilmot, F. R. H. (1966). 'An integrated system for contact lens photography.' *Ophthal. Optician* **6**, 924–926

Chapter 7

Indications and Contra-Indications for Contact Lens Wear

Janet Stone

INTRODUCTION

Many people would like to wear contact lenses. For various reasons, only some of these ever visit a contact lens practitioner. The contact lens practitioner must select for fitting only those deemed to be suitable. Careful selection benefits both the patient and the practitioner by avoiding time wasted in attempting to fit unsuitable patients.

As far as ocular contour is concerned, it is now possible to fit any eye with a contact lens — but successful wearing depends on adequate patient motivation and absence of contra-indications. Patient selection depends on adequate recognition of these factors by the practitioner.

Certain pathological and abnormal conditions of the eye and adnexa are a definite *indication* for contact lenses.

INDICATIONS AND CONTRA-INDICATIONS FOR CONTACT LENS WEARING

These may be considered broadly under three headings: (1) psychological influences; (2) pathological, anatomical and physiological factors; and (3) personal and external factors. Some overlap between the three is inevitable.

PSYCHOLOGICAL INFLUENCES

Patients should be made aware of the essential differences between the fitting and wearing of spectacles and of contact lenses. This is necessary to avoid subsequent disillusionment on the part of the patient. From the legal standpoint, it is as well to issue the patient with a printed booklet in which certain general facts about contact lenses are emphasized. This is also helpful because many patients are not fully attentive at the initial interview and may forget what is said by the practitioner, who may himself omit to mention or emphasize certain points.

Prior to embarking on the actual fitting of contact lenses, the practitioner should draw the patient's attention to the following special aspects of contact lens fitting and wear, so that the patient has the opportunity to reject them before being placed under any obligation.

Time Taken for Fitting

Since this varies from patient to patient, and depends on the skill of the practitioner and the type of lens to be fitted, it is up to each practitioner to say how long the entire fitting is likely to take. Including tuition of lens handling some 3 hours is an average for corneal lenses, as long as 10 hours for scleral lenses because of modifications which may have to be made, and up to 4 hours for soft lenses. Numerous visits to the practitioner may be necessary; and if the fitting proves complicated, a longer time may be involved.

Tolerance trials add to the time spent by both patient and practitioner. Some practitioners like to arrange for a two-week trial of contact lenses. Four hours is about the desirable minimum length for a corneal lens tolerance trial. With scleral lenses these trial wearing periods are difficult to arrange unless spare lenses of a reasonable fit are available. Again, a minimum length of 4 hours is desirable. For potential soft lens wearers the desirable length of tolerance trial depends on the water content of the lens. For example, if fitting extended or continuous wear lenses (usually of high water content) it is advisable to arrange a 24-hour tolerance trial commencing early in the day, and to see the patient again at the end of the day, as well as the following morning after the lenses have been worn all night. For slightly lower water content lenses (55–70 per cent) a tolerance trial is desirable of a minimum duration of 6 hours. The lower water content lenses (approximately 40 per cent) should ideally be tried out for at least 4 hours. All this adds up to another hour or so of 'chair-side' time to the fitting, and if more than one tolerance trial is necessary the time involved with the patient during fitting may extend to 12 hours or more, and the patient may be involved for much longer.

Fitting children with contact lenses can be very time consuming and parents should be advised of this. It is especially important with children that they be dealt with in an unhurried but reassuringly firm fashion. If under the age of 12 years, ideally the child should be fitted in the presence of one of the parents, both to give the child reassurance and to demonstrate lens handling to the parent who may subsequently be required to insert and remove the lenses, particularly if the child is under the age of 7 years. At the first visit, besides the preliminary examination and measurements it is often enough just to insert one lens and leave proper fitting for a further visit. Several hours practise are often needed for a child to perfect insertion and removal techniques, although children whose parents wear contact lenses may accomplish insertion and removal very quickly, and can be less troublesome and time consuming than adults.

Patients should also be made aware of the importance of adequate after-care and the need to allow sufficient time for this to be carried out.

Initial Discomfort – Physical and Visual

Patients used to wearing spectacles are sometimes totally unprepared for the initial difficulties with contact lenses and should be warned of the likelihood of corneal and lid sensation, photophobia, flare, after-wear blur with spectacles, and so on, as appropriate. These difficulties are less noticeable with soft lenses, but are still liable to occur. Also, soft lenses may give rise to fluctuations of vision during wear.

Gradual Wearing Procedure

The advisability of building up wearing time slowly, particularly with corneal lenses, is well recognized. Patients must be made fully aware of this, otherwise they may think that changing to contact lenses is as simple as changing their spectacle prescription. Only extended and continuous wear soft lenses do not always require a build-up time. Instead, several visits to the contact lens practitioner are necessary in the first 2 weeks of wear.

Special Storage

Owing to their effective cost, and the softness of the plastics material from which they are made, contact lenses deserve to be handled and stored very carefully. Because of their wetting and hydration properties and the danger of transferring harmful organisms on to the eye, they must be kept in sterile conditions and certain solutions must be employed during their handling and storage. This aspect is of extreme importance with soft lenses, and patients must be informed early on that on no account must any solution intended for use with hard lenses, ever come into contact with a soft lens.

Extra Hygiene

Spectacle wearers may spend one minute or less each day cleaning their spectacles, whereas contact lenses must be thoroughly cleansed with an antiseptic or other suitable solution appropriate to the type of lens material. During handling the hands should be kept clean and free of grease and nicotine. Contamination of the lenses with face or eye make-up preparations must also be avoided, and special make-up creams may be necessary (Cordrey, 1972). Eye cosmetics are known to be a source of potentially serious infection (Bruch, 1973; Wilson et al., 1973), and cases of conjunctival-embedded pigment from mascara and eye-liner causing long-term discomfort and excessive lacrimation have been reported by Stewart (1973). It is helpful to issue patients with a leaflet explaining the safest methods of using eye and other make-up with contact lenses, such as that issued by the Department of Optometry and Visual Science, The City University, London (1974), which is based on articles by McConnell (1967) and Gustafson (1967). Patients should also examine their lenses daily to avoid wearing badly scratched, cracked or chipped lenses. These aspects add to the 'nuisance value' of the lenses and patients who are not prepared to take the necessary time and trouble to keep their lenses clean should preferably not be fitted. This is particularly so with soft lenses which are more easily contaminated than hard lenses. Some types of soft lens require disinfection by boiling and this, unfortunately, adds to the time and the initial cost of keeping the lenses clean, although in the long term the use of solutions is more costly than boiling.

Stringent After-care at Regular Intervals

Abrasions of the cornea are easily caused by contact lenses, especially hard lenses; and corneal sensitivity is lowered during hard contact lens wear (Boberg-Ans, 1955; Millodot, 1976). Examination of the eyes and lenses at intervals of not greater than one year is advisable so that the practitioner may detect any changes which may have taken place and advise the patient accordingly. This routine after-care check is, of necessity, longer and more detailed than that given to a normal spectacle wearer. Some patients require more frequent after-care checks because of recurrent symptoms or pathology. Also, if continuous or extended wear soft lenses are fitted, more frequent after-care checks should be made.

Need for and Cost of Insurance

Corneal lenses are easily lost; scleral lenses less so. Soft lenses are easily damaged, particularly ultra-thin and high water content lenses. Loss or damage is most likely to occur during the initial wearing period before complete adaptation to the lenses takes place, and before facility of handling has been mastered. It is therefore essential for patients to insure lenses for their replacement value plus the estimated cost of the practitioner's fee at the time of replacement. The insurance premium may be as much as 20 per cent of the original fee plus the cost of the lenses. This is the rate normal for soft lenses, although usually it is about 5–10 per cent for hard lenses. Some of the lens manufacturers run insurance or replacement schemes of their own, which can be helpful to both patient and practitioner.

Lack of Protection from Foreign Bodies

Spectacle wearers who transfer to contact lenses always, at first, miss the protection afforded by their spectacles and should be warned of initial troubles in windy and dusty atmospheres. *Colour Plates II* and *XIII* show the effect of foreign bodies on the cornea. Scleral lenses and soft lenses provide more protection from foreign bodies than hard corneal lenses – the degree of protection being related to the size of the lens.

Cost of Lenses, Examination Fees and Accessories

Conscientious practitioners usually include up to one or two years after-care in the initial fitting fee, which must therefore be adequate to cover the practitioner for the time likely to be spent with the average patient during that time. It is only fair to warn patients of other costs they are likely to incur, such as travelling expenses, and the costs of soaking and wetting solutions and boiling units for soft lenses.

Fear of Lenses

Another barrier that has to be overcome is the patient's fear of having anything put on the eye. Patient handling is dealt with in Chapter 8, and it is sufficient here to say that a practitioner who inspires confidence is usually able to help a patient overcome this fear very quickly. Children (and the parents who accompany them) often require a very special approach.

Apart from these possible 'psychological' disadvantages, there are many definite indications for contact lenses which have a psychological background, as will be seen from the following.

Safety

Fear of damage to the eyes from broken spectacle lenses in sports such as football, rugby and cricket is removed. There are many cases of contact lenses having afforded definite protection to the eyes, where otherwise a blow to the eye might have resulted in both external and internal ocular damage (Rengstorff and Black, 1974).

Security

A feeling of safety is engendered by wearing contact lenses as opposed to spectacles when worn for horse riding, cycling (especially in the rain), shooting in rough country, skiing and bob-sleighing.

Clarity of Vision

The removal of the nuisance value of spectacles which steam up when playing badminton, tennis, squash and table tennis is a distinct advantage; also, spectacles become coated with spray when sailing.

Cosmetic reasons

Intense dislike of spectacles, particularly if very thick lenses are worn, has often meant that contact lenses bring about a marked cosmetic improvement. This can and does result in a beneficial personality change from introvert to extrovert. To some patients spectacles are an advertisement of a personal disability which is relieved by wearing contact lenses.

Restoration of Normal Appearance

Similar psychological benefits have been afforded to people (especially children) with disfigured eyes which are fitted with prosthetic lenses to give a normal appearance; for example, in albinism, aniridia, microphthalmos or an ugly eye due to injury or disease. *Colour Plate III* shows such an example.

Children

Unfortunately, children who wear spectacles, still sometimes suffer taunts from their classmates. If children are of fairly placid disposition they may adapt very readily to contact lenses and thereby avoid the mental suffering which wearing spectacles occasionally entails.

However, it is definitely not desirable to force children to wear contact lenses because of some whim on the part of the parents. To a child, the fitting of contact lenses can be a very traumatic experience and if it is carried out entirely against the will of the child it can lead to considerable upset and possible long-lasting psychological disturbance to the child. For this reason, if contact lenses are essential for some pathological or serious visual condition, it may be desirable for them to be fitted under general anaesthesia in a hospital environment, if the child is very young.

PATHOLOGICAL, ANATOMICAL AND PHYSIOLOGICAL FACTORS

Some patients are selected for contact lens wear because no other form of visual correction is suitable. Others may be rejected due to the presence of an abnormal anatomical feature or because of the existence of a pathological condition. These aspects will now be dealt with in more detail.

Cases where Contact Lenses are indicated for Pathological Reasons

In these cases the patient is frequently referred to the contact lens practitioner by his medical adviser. If not, before fitting is undertaken, medical co-operation should be sought (*see* Chapter 8). Chapters 20 and 21, Volume 2 deal with fitting these cases.

Keratoconus

Early cases may be suitable for corneal lenses as may be some medium keratoconic corneas, but most medium and advanced cases are best corrected with scleral lenses. Soft lenses with a hard corneal lens fitted steep on the front surface have been tried successfully in keratoconus. In one or two cases a soft lens has been used underneath a scleral lens (Westerhout, 1973).

Corneal Irregularities and Scars

Unless these are small and near the limbus (when a small, carefully centred corneal lens may be fitted), soft or scleral lenses are advisable. If the irregularity is great, flush fitting of the cornea with a scleral lens may yield best results.

Soft lenses are definitely recommended where sterile superficial corneal ulcers are present as they assist corneal healing. However, they should not be used if any infection exists, as the presence of the lens only exacerbates the condition (Leibowitz and Rosenthal, 1971). Soft lenses, either with or without the use of hypertonic saline solution every two hours, are also recommended for bullous keratopathy and greatly alleviate discomfort (Takahashi and Leibowitz, 1971). The results of their wear may be spectacular, sometimes obviating the need for enucleation and often giving considerable visual improvement. Soft lenses are also of assistance as a form of splint to assist corneal healing following penetrating corneal wounds when they prevent leakage of aqueous and collapse of the anterior chamber (Leibowitz, 1972). Both hard and soft lenses have been put to similar use as splints following operations for cataract extraction and to hold corneal grafts in place following keratoplasty.

Protection Against Radiation

During irradiation of malignant tumours on or near the eye, a special lead contact shell is used for protection (*see* Chapter 24, Volume 2).

Protection Against Drying and Foreign Bodies

There are a number of conditions in which tears output is reduced. If these lead to drying of the eye, corneal opacification and infection may occur. An alternative to tarsorrhaphy (stitching the lids together) is the wearing of a protective scleral or soft lens with a suitable solution of artificial tears (*see* Chapter 3). A protective lens may also be required if there is lagophthalmos or marked ectropion. Trichiasis and entropion can lead to damage of the cornea and here a protective scleral lens may be indicated rather than epilation and surgery. Soft lenses are worth trying in such cases but a scleral lens affords protection to a greater area of the eye's front surface and the choice of lens must depend on the eye's actual condition.

Protection Against Light

Contact lenses can be tinted and can have an artificial iris portion incorporated, the latter being most effectively done in scleral lenses, the extra thickness of which permits the effect of an anterior chamber to be achieved. However, corneal lenses with an iris pattern are being fitted more frequently now that manufacturing techniques have improved. Tinted and prosthetic soft lenses are also available. People with aniridia or albinism are still usually helped best with scleral lenses. In albinism, an opaque haptic portion prevents scattering of light within the eye by the sclera. The resulting improvement in acuity usually reduces the nystagmus commonly found in albinos, provided that the fitting is undertaken early in life, preferably before the age of 2 years. Fitting has been undertaken before the age of 1 year, but this type of fitting must be done under general anaesthesia. Patients suffering visual difficulties due to iridectomy or polycoria experience similar advantages to the albino when fitted with a lens incorporating an artificial iris. Where an upper iridectomy has been performed during cataract extraction, it is usually covered by the upper lid and there is no need for an artificial iris.

Corneal lenses are the easier method of prescribing a tint – and tints are essential where there is photophobia, such as immediately following cataract extraction. Manufacturers can supply details of the transmission curves of tinted corneal lenses. Tinted soft lenses are available but they are not cosmetically satisfactory if larger than the size of the iris. In some cases a non-toxic vegetable dye can be applied daily to the lens, but as these dyes leach out of the material the tint lightens towards the end of the day. Their use has been over too short a time to know if any eye irritation results from the prolonged application of these dyes. Other possible dangers of tinted lenses are dealt with in Chapter 24, Volume 2.

Prosthetic Contact Lenses and Shells

In addition to the type of eye mentioned in the preceding section, prosthetic contact shells may be fitted as prostheses where an eye has become blind or shrunken. For squinting or pronouncedly disfigured eyes – as in the case of severe burns – a sighted artificial pupil may be incorporated at an appropriate location, if useful vision can thereby be obtained. A tinted corneal lens may be sufficient to mask a corneal opacity or disfigurement of the pupil or iris. However, a prosthetic corneal or soft lens incorporating an iris pattern is even better if the cornea is sufficiently regular to be fitted with one. Corneal cosmetic shells can be surprisingly successful, even on grossly scarred corneas. In such cases the psychological benefit to the patient is often often remarkable, provided that a normal appearance is restored; but the effect may be detrimental if, for example, a squinting eye is fitted with a scleral shell having a displaced iris which then rotates! Obviously, great care in fitting must be exercised for the patient to derive maximum benefit.

Aphakia

Unilateral aphakics usually obtain some form of binocular vision, and even some stereopsis, with a contact lens for the aphakic eye. Other than an intraocular implant a corneal lens is likely to give the smallest possible retinal image size in this eye (*see* Shape Factor, Chapter 4) and may therefore be optically slightly better than a scleral lens, but soft lenses are as good as corneals, for they are usually only a little thicker and are usually much more stable. An opaque shell (scleral or corneal or soft) may help if a unilateral aphakic experiences disturbing binocular diplopia, and it may be fitted to the eye with the poorer visual acuity. Of course, any patient suffering from binocular diplopia may be helped in the same way, provided that the underlying cause has been medically investigated to rule out active pathology.

Young aphakics usually accept contact lenses more readily than the elderly, because elderly people may find the psychological disturbance of being fitted as great as the disturbance caused by a high positive spectacle correction. However, the optical advantages of contact lenses are so pronounced (especially in unilateral aphakia) that their use is to be recommended if the patient is likely to co-operate. The weight of the lenses may be reduced by using a lenticular construction, but with corneals this may lead to disturbing reflections as the lens moves on the cornea, if the pupil is large. Even this may be overcome to a large extent by modern lens designs, where the peripheral carrier portion of the lens is designed to attach to the upper lid and move with it (*see* Chapters 4 and 11). A well-fitting, thin scleral lens is easier for the aphakic to see (and find, if lost); is often easier to handle; and the optical result is, if at all, only very slightly inferior to that of a corneal lens. In the unlikely event that residual astigmatism is present, a scleral lens is the more reliable type for its correction. If the patient has a fairly spherical cornea or is prepared to wear additional spectacles to correct astigmatism and provide a near addition, soft lenses are highly satisfactory and are also often found to be easier to handle than corneals.

Considerable success has been reported with continuous wear soft lenses fitted at the time of operation for cataract extraction (Kersley, 1975).

High Myopia

A definite improvement of visual acuity is usually obtained with contact lenses, although this may be partially offset by difficulties with convergence and accommodation (*see* Chapter 4). Here, consideration must be given to the looseness of the lids and to the state of exophthalmos. Scleral lenses are less satisfactory cosmetically, particularly if the eyes protrude slightly. However, thick edges on corneal lenses make corneals difficult to tolerate by myopes with tight lids. Also, the thick edge of a high negative corneal lens is often gripped by the upper lid, and corneal lenses may therefore ride so high on the cornea as to cause visual disturbance due to the peripheral zone or even the edge of the lens intersecting the pupil area. However, lens constructions are available (*see* page 131 and *Figure 4.32*, Chapter 4) which overcome these difficulties (Mandell, 1974), but the problem then becomes one of manufacture rather than fitting (*see* Chapters 11 and 22, Volume 2). Soft lenses, unless otherwise contra-indicated, are ideal, although there are still the problems of high positioning with corneal sized

lenses, due to lid traction, and if a lenticular semi-scleral lens is used the upper lid may push the lens downwards due to pressure on the thick transition between the lenticular portion and the carrier zone.

Microphthalmos

Scleral lenses yield good results both optically and cosmetically, and are easier for the patient to handle. It may be necessary to construct a specially small impression tray in order to do the fitting, as most impression trays and most preformed trial lenses are far too large. Corneal lenses are not ruled out, but being of high positive power are liable to drop and ride low unless made lenticular with a suitable carrier portion which will attach to the upper lid. Soft lenses are satisfactory if they can be manufactured sufficiently accurately to the high positive prescription required. The very steep front optic surface of scleral and soft lenses in particular, are apt to make the patient look keratoconic when the contact lens is *in situ* and spherical aberration is a problem as the lenses move (*Figure 4.22*).

Non-tolerance of Spectacles

Occasionally, spectacles are not tolerated owing to trauma, skin disease, nervous troubles or even absence of one or both external ears. Scleral, corneal or soft lenses may then be suitable, but some skin diseases may be made worse by the wearing of contact lenses and appropriate medical advice should be sought. People who 'cannot bear' spectacles may well not be able to put up with the trials and tribulations of getting used to contact lenses and should not be led to believe that they are essential when a lighter-weight spectacle frame may be all that is required. However, because soft lenses are so easy to adapt to, they may be a great help in such cases, if the patient is otherwise suitable.

Partial Sight

Young people with partial sight may be helped by wearing a telescopic aid to give magnification. A scleral, soft, or corneal lens can form the eyepiece of such a system, with a spectacle lens as the objective (*see* Chapter 24, Volume 2). Generally speaking, corneal lenses perform least well because their mobility makes them a poorer eyepiece for such a system, than is afforded by a soft or scleral lens. Whilst, in theory, such systems can be used to assist any person with low visual acuity, elderly people find it extremely difficult to adapt to the contact lenses as well as to the magnification of the telescopic-type system.

Ocular Conditions Needing Medication

Special scleral lenses are sometimes used in hospitals for keeping medicaments in contact with the eye to promote healing and treat infection (*see* Chapter 24, Volume 2). Particularly for the treatment of glaucoma with miotics, soft lenses hydrated in pilocarpine which is slowly released on to the eye, are now being used very satisfactorily (Hillman, 1976). Soft lenses obviously have considerable potential in the field of medication for those cases where it is desirable to keep a drug in contact with the eye for an extended period of time (*see* Chapter 24, Volume 2).

Pathological Defects Found During the Examination of the Eye for Contact Lenses

If any previously unsuspected pathological condition is found during the course of the preliminary examination, or if the history reveals the existence of a pathological condition, contact lenses should not be fitted until medical advice has been sought. Both general and ocular conditions indicating referral will be considered below.

General Conditions

General debility. Tolerance of contact lenses is likely to be poor unless general health is good.

Diabetes. Unless refraction is stable, contact lenses are not practicable. The low rate of epithelial healing is an additional disadvantage. Soft lenses are therefore advised if contact lenses must be fitted.

Hyperthyroidism.* The disturbed metabolism which results in exophthalmos and lack of blinking can make contact lens wear difficult as there is liable to be an insufficient tears flow to the cornea, with all its attendant problems.

Chronic catarrh and sinusitis. The risk of ocular infection is increased if corneal abrasions from contact lenses occur. The associated mucus in the tears also causes visual problems most noticeable with scleral lenses but still very trouble-

---

* Loewi's adrenaline eye test for the detection of hyper-excitability of the sympathetic nervous system should not be confused with the dilatation of the pupil when adrenaline, 0.1 per cent, is instilled following a local anaesthetic prior to the taking of eye impressions.

some with soft and corneal lenses. Frequently the naso–lacrimal drainage channels become blocked, leading to epiphora which is exacerbated by contact lens wear (*see* page 173).

Herpes simplex of the mouth. There is a danger of corneal infection from 'cold sores' when contact lenses are worn. Contact lenses should not be licked. Even so, the virus may be transferred by hand from the mouth to the eye.

Skin conditions and allergic reactions. There is a slight risk of some patients being hypersensitive to certain plastics (or the residual monomer therein) and to the contents of some contact lens solutions. Careful questioning about allergies is advisable before fitting. Backman and Bolte (1974) have shown that desensitization treatment for chronic allergic conjunctivitis, although lengthy, is successful in most cases and useful for contact lens patients. If there is any doubt a medical investigation is desirable to establish whether or not the patient is allergic to the plastics material which it is intended to use. For hard lenses the polymethyl methacrylate used should preferably be the clinical quality (CQ) which is available through contact lens manufacturers, although the standard of purity of ordinary polymethyl methacrylate is also very high and allergic reaction to the material is very rare indeed.

Where there are infections of the eye or its adnexa, soft lenses should not be fitted except under medical supervision, because the lens material is liable to become contaminated, with the risk of extending the infection.

Norn (1964), Mackie (1967) and others have shown that instillation into the conjunctival sac of one drop of rose bengal 1 per cent will show up desquamated conjunctival and corneal epithelium and mucus, indicative of active or sub-clinical conditions likely to be irritated by contact lenses. Typical of such conditions are the following, in which very special care should be taken during the fitting, with prolonged tolerance trials – despite which the contact lenses may have to be abandoned if the skin condition worsens or the eye becomes involved.

Atopic eczema is associated with asthma and hay fever. When contact lenses are fitted, they may cause an urticarial reaction. This should be minimized with soft lenses but the lens surfaces may degrade rapidly due to excessive protein deposits. If hard lenses are used sclerals or small corneals have been found to give the best results.

Kerato-conjunctivitis sicca (Sjögren's syndrome) is associated with rheumatoid arthritis; there is a lack of tears secretion, and filamentary keratitis is common. Hard corneal lenses should not be fitted. Soft lenses may be fitted if saline solution or artificial tears drops are instilled at regular intervals throughout the day. Even so, the lenses may dehydrate and be unwearable. Sealed scleral lenses used with a suitable artificial tears solution (*see* pages 67 and 81, Chapter 3) are most likely to prove satisfactory and are a good way of protecting the cornea. Fenestrated scleral lenses may be equally good or better, and generally allow a longer wearing time, but are only satisfactory if there are sufficient tears to supplement the artificial tears which tend to evaporate or drain away because of the fenestration hole. Sometimes channelled scleral lens provides the best compromise.

Xerophthalmia (vitamin A deficiency), congenital ichthyosis (dry skin) and sarcoidosis are three conditions in which scleral lenses may prove satisfactory but corneal lenses may lead to persistent corneal abrasions. Soft lenses are best but the material is likely to deteriorate quickly.

Several other skin conditions, such as the following, may flare up when contact lenses are worn.

Seborrhoeic eczema manifests itself as dandruff, blepharitis, and otitis externa. Only scleral or very small corneal lenses are usually tolerated as they give rise to minimal lid irritation. Soft lenses are contra-indicated in the presence of blepharitis, but if this can be resolved, they can be ideal as they cause less irritation to the eye and lids than any other type of lens. However, the patient should be advised to discontinue soft lens wear during recurrences of the condition. An effective treatment for blepharitis (Mackie, 1977) is a half-dose of tetracycline, taken orally; 250 mg twice daily for 6 weeks. This must not be taken in milk, which inactivates it. It may be prescribed by arrangement with the patient's general medical practitioner, but should not be given to young children or pregnant women as it can cause side-effects such as discoloration of growing teeth.

Acne vulgaris, which occurs around the age of puberty, is not markedly aggravated by contact lens wear, but greasing and frothing of the tears may prevent satisfactory wear of any type of lens. Prolonged tolerance trials are useful to establish whether or not this is likely to occur. If hard lenses are worn astringent lotions may give temporary relief (*see* Chapter 3), and wetting and soaking solutions containing polyvinyl alcohol minimize greasing of hard lenses. Thin, well-fitting scleral lenses or corneals fitted within the palpebral aperture give fairly good results since there is no massaging effect on the lids to increase the output of sebum. Soft lenses may be satisfactory but rapid deterioration of the lens surfaces is liable to occur due to contamination by sebum from the eyelids.

Acne rosacea is accentuated as the foreign body reaction to contact lenses increases the blood vessel dilatation of the skin of the face and conjunctiva. Punctate keratitis is associated with the condition and may be exacerbated by contact lens wear. In the absence of keratitis, soft lenses or small corneal lenses may be tolerated — otherwise, if contact lenses are essential, sclerals are the lens of choice provided they are fitted to avoid any corneal touch.

Psoriasis is not directly aggravated by the wearing of contact lenses, but the generally associated nervous disposition may lead to a worsening of the condition during the initial difficult period of adaptation to contact lenses. For this reason soft lenses are likely to perform best.

Other indications of general or ocular pathology. These should be referred for medical advice whether or not they are specific contra-indications to contact lens wear.

Ocular Conditions

A number of different techniques must be employed to examine the eyes for suitability for contact lenses. Norn (1974) has compiled an exhaustive list of techniques used in the external examination of the eye, with an excellent description of each technique. Some of these techniques are routinely used by ophthalmic opticians and optometrists in the examination of the eye. These will not be further elaborated; but those specific to contact lens fitting will be mentioned in more detail. Reference should also be made to Chapter 5 for a description of some of the equipment used. Any evidence of pathology found should indicate the need for referral.

Slit Lamp Examination in Ocular Conditions

The anterior segment of the eye and its adnexa should be examined. $X20$ magnification is recommended for routine use, with $X40$ for examination of detail. Fluorescein should be instilled and, if necessary, the excess removed by irrigation to prevent masking of small stained areas by fluorescein in the tears film. Bengal rose, 1 per cent may also usefully be instilled. The use of these stains is discussed further on page 173.

Normal signs, using a broad beam from the side. The eye should be viewed from in front, and both white light and blue light (cobalt filter) should be used.

Cornea and limbus. Dust particles are apparent in the tears film and move with blinking. The cornea appears to have a granular structure owing to the presence of cell bodies. Several very fine nerve fibres may extend across to the centre of the cornea. Limbal blood vessel loops normally encroach into the cornea about 1 mm, but a little more than this at the upper limbus. The radial arrangement of myelinated nerve fibres around the limbus should show that the myelin ceases about 1 mm in from the limbus. Aqueous veins (usually in the horizontal meridian) may be seen. A ring or crescent of more opaque corneal tissue separated from the limbus by a narrow, normally transparent, band is frequently seen. It is normally associated with advancing age and is then known as arcus senilis, but is often seen from the early teens onwards and is usually situated near the upper and lower limbus, and is thought to be cholesterol deposits. Posterior embryotoxin may be evident as a semi-opaque, linear structure, about the width of a blood vessel, situated at the posterior corneal surface, near the limbus, and usually in the horizontal meridian where it runs parallel to the limbus (Becker, 1972). It appears to be more common than is indicated in textbooks of ophthalmology. Usually the termination of the endothelium at the anterior chamber angle is not visible except by gonioscopy when it is known as Schwalbe's line, but if tags of endothelium extend into the anterior chamber or the endothelium is raised at that point, then it becomes visible by normal direct illumination with the slit lamp. Its significance, when visible like this, is that the anterior chamber angle is likely to become blocked more easily; hence, care should be exercised when fitting soft or scleral lenses to avoid corneal oedema near the limbus. The rest of the endothelium should be carefully scanned to rule out the presence of any abnormalities or striate lines, which might later, subsequent to soft lens wear, be attributed to corneal oedema (*see* Chapter 16, Volume 2).

Bulbar conjunctiva and sclera. Conjunctival blood vessels appear to move with respect to the deeper scleral vessels during blinking and eye movements. Most conjunctival blood vessels are normally almost empty and the transparency of the conjunctiva is apparent with the slit lamp. The presence of pigment, mainly near the limbus region, is normal in Asians and Negroes, but not in white-skinned races. With age, fat is deposited in the conjunctiva within the region of the palpebral aperture and appears as thickened yellow irregularities. The incidence of pingueculae also increases with age, as does the irregularity of the conjunctiva and its looseness at the limbus. Whilst

these findings are normal, irregularities of the conjunctiva such as those described, may encourage xerosis of the conjunctiva during corneal and soft lens wear and contribute to limbal dessication of the corneal epithelium at the three and nine o'clock positions during corneal lens wear. It is thought that these irregularities, combined with the presence of the lens, prevent the upper eyelid from massaging the mucoid layer into the surface conjunctival and corneal epithelium which normally permits these tissues to remain wetted.

Plica semilunaris and caruncle. Fine hairs are normally visible on the caruncle. The blood vessels should not appear unduly engorged. Both tissues should appear smooth and not granular.

Iris and pupil. Small pigment deposits of normal chromatophores and xanthophores are frequently visible, as are pupillary remnants arising from the region of the collarette. The pupil shape and reactions may be checked.

Anterior lens surface. Epicapsular pigment stars, often associated with pupillary remnants, may be seen. The 'orange peel' effect of the anterior capsular epithelium should be visible.

Lid margins. By slightly everting the lids, their margins may be seen under magnification. Any abnormalities, such as blocking of the orifices of the Meibomian glands, can be detected and appropriate action taken. Small marginal cysts, which disappear after a few days, are often visible. They give rise to discomfort when corneal lenses are worn.

Normal signs, using a narrow beam from in front. The microscope should be moved round to one side.

Cornea. When normally transparent, this shows as a slightly granular tissue in cross-section, with a brighter reflex from both the front surface (lacrimal layer and epithelium) and back surface. With age, a few pigment spots become deposited on the back surface of the cornea due to disintegration of the iris pigment epithelium. Hassal Henle endothelial warts appear in old age.

Anterior chamber. This should appear optically empty except for normal pupillary remnants and, with age, a few pigment granules. Its depth can be assessed and the chamber angle estimated (van Herick, Shaffer and Schwartz, 1969). It is important to rule out those patients with shallow anterior chamber angles if soft lenses which may cause corneal oedema are to be fitted, for in soft lens wear the cornea is thought to swell backwards slightly, into the anterior chamber. In this connection, it is wise to refer for medical advice before fitting, any patient in whom the depth of the chamber at the limbus appears to be equal to a quarter of the thickness of the cornea, or less, as seen by optical section. (The microscope should be used from directly in front of the patient with the narrow slit beam at 60 degrees to one side.) Such narrow angles are potentially capable of closure.

Staining

Several stains may be employed to detect abnormality. Fluorescein is the most common.

Fluorescein. A drop of 1 or 2 per cent sterile sodium fluorescein solution should be instilled into the conjunctival sac or applied from a sterile impregnated paper strip moistened with sterile saline solution. The excess may be rinsed out with sterile normal saline solution if necessary. The cornea should be examined under magnification with suitable long wavelength ultraviolet light. (Short wavelength ultra-violet rays are dangerous.) This is followed by slit lamp examination using $X20$ magnification. Any staining of the cornea prior to contact lens fitting, except if caused by a foreign body (the prior presence of which may usually be elucidated by questioning the patient) is abnormal, although Norn (1970) states that a few punctate dots of stain, increasing in number with age, are normal in about 20 per cent of the population. Extensive staining indicates the probable need for referral. (Following an illness or head cold, the corneal permeability is increased and the cornea absorbs some fluorescein; but this gives only a slight green haze, unlike the bright green stain of an abraded area. When the corneal permeability is grossly increased, some fluorescein may enter the anterior chamber.)

The patency of the puncta and lacrimal drainage channels may be demonstrated by asking the patient to blow his nose on to a paper tissue, which should stain green. Each side should be checked separately. It is unwise to proceed with fitting contact lenses if the naso-lacrimal passages are blocked, for the conjunctival sac is less likely to be sterile. Also the presence of contact lenses, causing excess tears production, is bound to lead to epiphora in such a case. Referral is indicated for the use of decongestant eye and/or nasal drops*, or if necessary, irrigation of the naso-lacrimal passages, to clear them. Blockage is common in catarrh and hay fever sufferers, and in those with dry eyes when the passages may easily get blocked with epithelial debris.

Bengal rose. The instillation of a drop of 1 per cent solution should not cause any marked corneal

* Otrivine-Antistin (*CIBA*).

or conjunctival staining. If such staining is seen, the tears output may be reduced or an abnormal skin condition may exist and further advice should be obtained before fitting. The mucus strip along the lid margins normally stains red and thus becomes apparent. It often detaches from the lid margin during contact lens wear and if it adheres to the lens or floats in the pre-corneal film it may interfere with vision. (Bengal rose should be instilled after the use of fluorescein, for it occasionally causes the appearance of punctate staining with fluorescein.)

Alcian blue and trypan blue. Norn (1964) and Kemmettmüller (1962) have described the use of these dyes for the detection of abnormality. Since their action is liable to be prolonged, their use in normal contact lens practice is not appropriate.

Sensitivity

An anaesthetic cornea is an abnormal cornea. Before contact lenses are fitted to an eye with an insensitive cornea, medical advice should be obtained. Great care is needed in fitting such an eye as abrasions caused by poorly fitting lenses do not give rise to the normal discomfort symptoms and injury to the eye can occur without the wearer's realization. For this reason soft lenses are the most appropriate in such cases. People with insensitive corneas readily accept contact lenses and it is essential to give them strict advice concerning wearing schedules and after-care, and to warn them of the dangers of ignoring this advice. Sensitivity may be quickly checked by gently holding the lids apart and touching a wisp of sterile cotton wool on to the cornea from one side, so that its approach is not seen by the patient. Touching the lashes should be avoided. A normal blink reflex response should result from both apical and limbal touch. More refined methods whereby measurements of sensitivity can be obtained are useful if there is any doubt as to whether or not sensitivity is normal. Suitable instruments are the aesthesiometer and sensitometer; and air puff methods are also available (*see* Chapter 2). Schirmer and Mellor (1961) have shown that reduced sensitivity is to be expected following cataract extraction in the sector of the cornea corresponding to the incision. Lowered sensitivity also follows interstitial keratitis and past ulceration of the cornea (as well as hard and soft contact lens wear, the latter causing the least loss in sensitivity, with recovery in both cases being rapid (Millodot, 1976).

Pachometry

The use of the slit lamp to observe the thickness of the cornea is aided by the use of a pachometer (pachymeter) or other doubling device for actual measurement of corneal thickness (*see* Chapter 5). A very thin or irregular cornea, as in keratoconus, indicates the need for referral prior to fitting. Many surgeons prefer to carry out keratoplasty while the cornea is still reasonably thick. As a thickened cornea is an indication of oedema, it is desirable to measure corneal thickness prior to contact lens fitting, as a reference for future measurements. It is also useful to know the normal values found in pachometry – the apparent central thickness of the majority of normal corneas falling between 0.50 mm and 0.60 mm.

Classical keratometry. This allows measurement of the curvature of the central cornea. Most corneas have central radii within the range 7.2– 8.6 mm. Radii outside this range may indicate abnormalities such as keratoconus (steep radii) and megalocornea or cornea plana (flat radii).

The amount of corneal astigmatism present is also measured. A very toric cornea may give rise to difficulties in fitting, and it is as well to anticipate these in order to warn the patient of extra time required for fitting. A big difference between ocular and corneal astigmatism should lead the practitioner to expect a large amount of residual astigmatism with a hard spherical lens, probably requiring a cylindrical correction. Again, this should indicate a more lengthy fitting procedure, and fair warning can be given to the patient at an early stage. Some manufacturers of spherical soft lenses recommend that they are not fitted to corneas having more than 1.5 D of astigmatism.

The keratometer also reveals surface irregularities of the cornea, some so small as to be invisible with the slit lamp. Any irregularity should be further investigated prior to fitting.

Peripheral keratometry. Bonnet and Cochet (1962) developed a topographical keratometer which enabled the periphery of the cornea to be measured and the rate of flattening from apex to limbus to be determined. This was of considerable help when fitting irregular corneas, where the lens design was based on the measurements found. Similar results are obtainable (some, with less accuracy) using special attachments to a classical keratometer (*see* Chapter 5). Such measurements have the inherent disadvantage that the value found for the curvature is not the true corneal curvature at that point, because its centre of curvature does not lie on the visual axis, *see Figure 11.4* (Chapter 11).

Photokeratoscopy

The keratoscope, of which the most simple variety is the Placido disc, provides useful information regarding regularity and curvature of the anterior corneal surface, the amount and type of corneal astigmatism, displacement of the corneal apex and variations in the amount of peripheral flattening from one sector of the cornea to another. Any abnormalities indicate further examination before fitting. If a photokeratoscope is used, records of unusual cases may be kept for further reference. The photographs printed by some photokeratoscopes can be scanned by an electronic computer, enabling a suitable lens design for the patient to be computed, and allowing any corneal curvature changes after contact lens wear to be monitored (Bibby, 1976).

Tears Output

Both insufficient and excessive tears output may indicate some abnormality of the lacrimal or conjunctival glands or of their nerve supply. Tears output is also affected by certain drugs (*see* pages 179 and 180). To fit corneal lenses to a dry cornea could be harmful, whereas excessive tears would prevent a corneal lens being worn satisfactorily. Soft or scleral lenses could be beneficial in either case, but the abnormality should be medically investigated before fitting. It should be borne in mind that soft lenses may alter curvature considerably on dry eyes and can only be fitted if saline solution or artificial tears are repeatedly instilled.

The usual test for the measurement of tears flow is that described by Schirmer (*see* Chapter 2), but because the test papers may irritate the eye, it is really only adequate for the detection of gross abnormality. Nevertheless, it is very useful in revealing those very dry eyes in which even the irritation from the Schirmer test paper fails to produce any tears. It is therefore a test recommended for use before fitting any type of contact lens.

Norn's test (Norn, 1965) is more accurate than Schirmer's test, for it involves judging the dilution of the tears in the lacrimal rivus over the central part of the lower lid exactly 5 minutes after 10 μl of a mixture of rose bengal, 1 per cent, and fluorescein, 1 per cent, is instilled into the lower fornix. Using the slit lamp a comparison is made with known dilutions of the mixture in capillary tubes. Ford (1974) has interpreted Norn's work very carefully, and is able to predict the amount of refractive change likely to take place due to dehydration of soft lenses on the eye, on the basis of the tears output measured by this test. He advocates the use of the test but points out the difficulty of instilling the correct amount of the fluorescein and rose bengal mixture in the first place.

The break-up time (BUT test) of the pre-corneal film is another very useful test (*see* pages 175–176, Pre-corneal film).

General External Examination of the Eye

This may be carried out with a suitable white light and loupe, as well as using the slit lamp (*see* page 171).

Abnormalities of the sclera and bulbar conjunctiva, such as pterygium or old operation scars, may make scleral lenses difficult to fit and may distort a semi-scleral soft lens. Loose conjunctival tissue at the limbus can block the fenestration hole of a scleral lens or prevent tears flow through a channelled scleral lens, and can prevent tears from being pumped under a semi-scleral soft lens by forming a seal. When large corneal lenses which bump into the limbus region are worn, any loose conjunctival tissue becomes easily injected, inviting new blood vessel growth.

Pingueculae are apt to be irritated by any sort of contact lens and it is only fair to warn patients of the conjunctival hyperaemia which is likely to detract from their cosmetic appearance when contact lenses are worn. Contact lenses of any sort are contra-indicated where there is a limbal growth due to spring catarrh.

Lids. The lids should be everted; and if concretions or other elevations are seen, the patient should be referred for treatment before fitting. Folliculosis of the palpebral conjunctiva makes contact lens wearing very difficult. The recovery period is protracted and treatment may be of very little help. Contact lenses are best abandoned until the tissue returns to normal.

If ectropion, entropion or trichiasis is evident contact lenses are advisable to protect the cornea as described under the heading *Protection Against Drying and Foreign Bodies* on page 168. Incomplete lid closure (usually due to lagophthalmos following VIIth nerve paralysis) again indicates the need for a protective contact lens (*see* page 168).

Special scleral lenses can be fitted where there is ptosis of the upper lid (*see* Chapters 20 and 24, Volume 2).

Blepharospasm, if it is persistent, can be a nuisance to corneal lens wearers as considerable discomfort ensues. In such cases scleral lenses are advisable. Soft lenses may be satisfactory but the excessive lid pressure usually distorts the lens. In any case the cause of the blepharospasm should be investigated before fitting. It should be borne in mind that those people who are somewhat apprehensive about wearing contact lenses may exhibit an unusual amount of blepharospasm at an initial interview, simply due to nervousness, and this subsequently disappears.

Soft lenses should not be fitted in the presence of blepharitis. Corneal lenses are also difficult to fit satisfactorily to eyes with blepharitis, or where the lid margins are highly sensitive. (Lid margin sensitivity may be checked with a wisp of cotton wool or an aesthesiometer.) Recurrent styes are a contra-indication to either soft or corneal lenses, so are any lid margin growths. Where there is absence of lashes — a sign of eczema and/or alopecia — fitting should proceed with great care: the patient (and practitioner) may have difficulty in gripping the lids during insertion and removal of lenses.

The depth of the fornices should be checked before fitting scleral lenses. Past injury or surgery may restrict the limits of the conjunctival sac, making sclerals unsuitable or difficult to fit, and if very restricted, semi-scleral soft lenses may also be contra-indicated. Conversely, in certain inflammatory conditions such as the Stevens–Johnson syndrome and ocular pemphigus, scleral lenses may be necessary to maintain the depth of the fornices and prevent the adherence of palpebral and bulbar conjunctiva.

The palpebral aperture size is a useful guide to the size of lens to fit. However, as shown by Hill and Leighton (1965), a vertical palpebral aperture of less than 6 mm is likely to rule out hard contact lenses since the temperature increase behind the contact lens in an eye with a small palpebral aperture may be too great to allow normal corneal metabolism to continue. In spite of this, small fenestrated corneal lenses may be satisfactory as the fenestrations facilitate tears flow in the retro-lens area by preventing negative pressure under the lens. For similar reasons, the same type of lens is often successful where lids are tight and exert heavy pressure on the lens, which would otherwise restrict retro-lens tears flow. Lens materials of increased oxygen permeability and wettability should also help.

If a tolerance trial with corneal lenses induces the formation of a white deposit at the canthi within half an hour of insertion, the implication is that there is an excessive temperature rise and that corneal lenses should probably be rejected unless lengthy tolerance trials with different types of lens can be arranged. Soft lenses are often more successful however, and ultra-thin lenses and those of high water content are least likely to upset corneal metabolism.

The presence of foam at the outer canthus is fairly normal (Norn, 1963), but its production is increased by blinking and the presence of foreign bodies such as contact lenses. The production of excessive mucus during a tolerance trial is also a contra-indication to fitting, as is excessive Meibomian activity which may give rise to subsequent greasing problems.

Lacrimal gland. This should be checked for normality — for size, position and colour. If it is large and prominent and scleral lenses are to be fitted, the temporal portion of the lens must be made sufficiently thin to slide under the gland without bumping it.

Pre-corneal film. A number of qualitative tests may be used to assess the normality of the pre-corneal film prior to fitting contact lenses. These have been described by McDonald (1969) and their relevance to contact lens fitting elaborated by Hill (1973).

The wettability of the tears layer is a function of the mucoid layer, and its efficiency may be judged by observing through the biomicroscope the reflection of an ordinary movable lamp in the lacrimal rivus or prism at the lower lid margin. This prism has three zones: an upper convex one against the lower cornea, a middle concave one at the centre of the rivus, and another convex one at the limit of the tears layer on the rear of the lower lid. As the lamp is slowly moved up and down, three smoothly moving bright reflections should be seen in the prism — the upper and lower ones giving a 'with' movement and the centre an 'against' movement. It may be necessary to ask the patient to look downwards to see all three, but if all or parts of these reflections are missing, the wettability of the tears is abnormal.

The quality of the surface oily layer which controls the rate of evaporation of the aqueous layer behind it, can be judged by looking in the same way at the corneal surface reflection of the lamp. The patient should blink normally about once every four seconds, and the reflection of the lamp should remain bright all the while. If streaks of interference colours appear the tears layer is too thin (or there is too great an evaporation rate). If the reflection is irregular and pocked, the surface is very dry.

A test of viscosity may be made by watching the movement of bubbles or debris in the lower tears prism. Surface particles should move more slowly than deeper ones. If the movement is simultaneous and rapid, insufficient viscosity is indicated and not enough tears will be retained on the eye. Simultaneous but slow movement indicates tears which are too viscous, and contact lenses would tend to become greasy and dirty if worn.

Other phenomena indicating tears which are too viscous are the 'pleated drape' and 'rolled scum' phenomena. The former is seen by reflection of a lamp in the upper tears prism at the start of each blink, when waves, like pleats, form interference colours which close together as the lid comes down and then open out as the lid goes up. The 'rolled scum' effect is left on the lower third of the cornea after each blink, where the two lids have parted and left an oily deposit. This is visible with a wide slit beam and is more noticeable after a high cholesterol intake. It is therefore felt that tears chemistry is related to diet (Lowther, Miller and Hill, 1970; Young and Hill, 1973).

Normal phenomena are the 'crumple' effect seen with a broad vertical slit at about $15°$ to the microscope axis, when the surface oil molecules undergo lateral pressure from the lids at the start of each blink and cause a diffuse (instead of uniform) reflection rather like wet silk; the epithelial drying effect, when the tears layer can be seen to evaporate after about 20 seconds without blinking which causes a reduction in acuity; and the epithelial touch effect, when a foreign body such as an eyelash or a bubble of carbon dioxide or air under a contact lens forms a furrow in the epithelium. In the latter case, after the foreign body is washed away, the furrow — visible by its oily margins — gradually widens for up to 5 minutes and then slowly narrows as the normal tears layer reforms. Such furrows retain fluorescein and, in the case of contact lens wearers, are called dimples. The speed with which the furrow disappears may well be a measure of epithelial fragility. *Colour Plate IV* shows dimples and furrows under a corneal lens.

Another test of the epithelial drying effect has been described by Polse (1975). He has stated that a deficiency of mucus production results in corneal dry spots which show up when the tears film is seen to break up into droplets. The test is known as the BUT (break-up-time) test. It is best seen by applying fluorescein below the cornea and observing with the slit lamp, with blue light and the largest possible circular aperture to illuminate the entire cornea. The patient is instructed to make one complete blink and then hold the eyes wide open. In normal individuals dry spots, which show up as black areas within the fluorescein-covered corneal surface, usually only appear if the lids are held apart for 20 seconds or more after a complete blink; whereas they appear within 10 seconds after a complete blink in certain pathological and dry-eye conditions (*see Colour Plate XXV b*, Volume 2) and if there is a mucus deficiency (Lemp *et al.,* 1970, 1971; Koetting, 1976). Polse feels that the appearance of such abnormal dry spots on the cornea is a contra-indication to successful contact lens fitting, and this is confirmed by Koetting who has shown a correlation between the surface contamination/coating of hydrophilic lenses and a low tears film break-up-time. However, Vanley, Leopold and Gregg (1977) have cast doubts on the usefulness of the BUT test as they found considerable variation in individual eyes from one patient visit to the next. Before rejecting a patient for contact lenses on the grounds of poor tears output, several different tests should be carried out and repeated at intervals in order to get a true picture.

Most of these tests and phenomena may be observed with a corneal lens in place. The tears prism at the temporal edge of the lens may be used for checking wettability and viscosity, and the lens surface for rate of evaporation; although the surface of a contact lens dries more quickly than the surface of the cornea.

Lowther, Bailey and Hill (1971) have also found that a normally wetted bulbar conjunctiva which appears smooth may become dry and irregular following corneal lens wear, due to the mechanical effect of the lids being held off the conjunctiva (especially in the three and nine o'clock positions) by the lens edge, so that the conjunctiva is not properly wetted. This can occur when the tears chemistry is normal: so that the remedy is one of lens design (thinner edges and less peripheral clearance) rather than patient rejection. *Colour Plate V* shows '3 and 9 o'clock' staining.

Puncta. Their presence and apposition to the globe should be checked.

Pupil size and reactions. Reactions should be normal. Large pupils create difficulties for some corneal lens wearers, particularly motorists who do a lot of night driving, and also for bifocal contact lens wearers. The deeper the anterior chamber the larger should be the central optic portion of the lens for a given pupil diameter (Stone, 1959). The transition between the central optic portion and the peripheral optic zone should be made as gradual as possible to minimize flare. (At the initial interview a patient's pupils may appear more dilated than normal, due to apprehension.) The maximum pupil size is readily judged by ultra-violet illumination in a dark room when the fluorescence of the crystalline lens shows up the pupil size.

Iris. Normality should be established. Special lenses may be fitted if the iris is wholly or partially absent, to occlude the unwanted iris apertures. This can result in a considerable improvement in vision. Scleral, corneal or soft lenses may be used depending on the severity of the condition.

Exophthalmos or enophthalmos. Abnormalities such as Horner's syndrome should be looked for and pathological conditions ruled out. Iris-sized soft lenses or corneal lenses are cosmetically better for exophthalmos, although they may have to be fitted slightly steep in order to be retained on the cornea. In exophthalmos there is a risk of reduced tears flow behind the lens. For enophthalmos, sclerals look better but need to be made small to facilitate insertion and removal.

Ophthalmoscopy

This is carried out to check the media and fundi to establish absence of abnormalities. Any disturbance of the normal reflex fundus glow — for example, due to lid pressure on the cornea — should be noted in case it is later mistaken for the after-effects of contact lens wear.

Visual Fields

These should be checked if there are any doubts about their normality.

Tonometry

This is usually carried out if raised intraocular tension is suspected. Cases have been encountered where a scleral lens has been thought to cause a rise of tension in an already abnormal eye. Khoo (1974) found that during the first hour of soft lens wear intraocular pressure rises slightly, but then returns to normal. Because of the possible risk of contact lenses increasing intraocular tension by pressure on the anterior ciliary veins, or in the case of soft lens wear when corneal oedema could result in a narrowing of the anterior chamber angle, it is wisest to carry out tonometry both before and after fitting, whenever there is the slightest suspicion of high intraocular pressure.

Visual Acuity and Refraction

A consideration of the optical effects of contact lenses (*see* Chapter 4) shows that, in theory, contact lenses should give a better visual acuity than spectacles as there are no oblique aberrations or distortion with contact lenses.

In *myopes*, contact lenses give bigger retinal images than spectacles, in proportion to the strength of the correction. This can lead to initial disorientation with contact lenses but should give better visual acuity. More ocular accommodation is needed, and the convergence required is greater than with spectacles, owing to the absence of the prism base-in effect. Thus, myopes tend to experience near-vision difficulties not encountered with spectacles, although the accommodation-convergence relationship should remain the same (Stone, 1967). They also have to move their eyes about more. From the point of view of others, the myope's eyes look bigger in contact lenses, as the reduced magnification of spectacles has been removed. All these effects are proportional to the power of the lenses.

In *hypermetropes*, the effects of contact lenses are the opposite to those for myopes. Smaller retinal images are obtained than with spectacles, and the eyes look smaller than in spectacles. Accommodation needed is less, convergence required is reduced and the eyes have to move less than with spectacles.

Astigmats. Spectacle wearers learn to compensate for the distortion of the retinal image afforded by an astigmatic spectacle correction. This compensation by the brain is continued when contact lenses are first worn, and it gives rise to a false experience of distortion which usually soon disappears. A comparison of ocular astigmatism with that measured by the keratometer allows prediction of the approximate amount of residual astigmatism with a hard spherical contact lens. A suitable lens construction may be chosen in advance if residual astigmatism is likely to cause a reduction in visual acuity. If soft lenses are being considered, any excess of ocular astigmatism over corneal astigmatism greater than 1 D suggests that a toric lens is necessary or else hard lenses capable of incorporating a cylindrical correction should be used. Where ocular astigmatism is negligible but corneal astigmatism is present, which neutralizes any crystalline lens astigmatism, soft lenses are optically ideal, provided the corneal astigmatism is not so great as to disrupt the fit.

Anisometropes. In most cases, contact lenses should not be used for axial anisometropia, as aniseikonia is thought to be induced. Sorsby, Leary and Richards (1962) have shown that most naturally occurring anisometropia is axial. Thus, in high anisometropia where a spectacle correction affords good binocular vision, contact lenses are probably ruled out. Even if the anisometropia is known to be re-

fractive, if spectacles give satisfactory binocular vision, contact lenses may induce a state of pseudo-aniseikonia owing to the relative difference between the two eyes of the change in retinal image size. An investigation of the binocular state in contact lenses is advisable before proceeding to supply final lenses. This is well worth while since a number of highly successful cases have been reported (Hodd, 1970). Where the eye with the higher refractive error is also amblyopic the author has often found that contact lens wear slowly improves the visual acuity in that eye. Part-time occlusion of the other eye, while very fine visual tasks are undertaken, has been found to help.

It may be found that non-comitant heterophorias are recorded at first with contact lenses, as the brain still continues to compensate for the ocular movements made with the anisometropic spectacle correction.

Monocular aphakia is an example in which a contact lens correction may give binocular vision where spectacles will not. However, a contact lens is worn some distance in front of the entrance pupil of the eye and it is by no means certain that contact lenses will give satisfactory binocular vision in this condition because of the residual aniseikonia. The patient may well prefer monocular vision to disturbed binocularity, giving rise to asthenopic symptoms.

Binocular Vision

Heterotropias. In general, contact lenses perform as well as spectacles in the treatment and correction of squints. Very often, all that is required to correct a squint is a full spectacle correction determined with the aid of a cycloplegic. However, this may mean the patient wearing a heavy and/or unsightly pair of spectacle lenses which tend to be abandoned to the detriment of the squint. In such cases contact lenses are invaluable. The author has had some success in cases of anisometropic esotropia by fitting the more hypermetropic eye with a contact lens of power equal to the difference between the two eyes. A balanced spectacle correction is then worn in addition to the one contact lens, but it is usually easier to fit contact lenses to both eyes. However, a combination of spectacles and contact lenses permits variations in negative additions for exotropes to be made on the spectacle lenses, and where bifocals would be prescribed for either esotropia or exotropia, contact lenses can be worn for general purposes with additional spectacles to be worn for close work. Difficulties arise where there is a residual high heterophoria requiring prismatic correction or where there is a vertical element needing prism to correct it (*see* below). As most patients requiring refractive corrections for heterotropias are children, soft lenses are particularly useful as they are quicker to adapt to and cause less discomfort in fitting. Also, if they are to be used in combination with spectacles, the latter can be used to provide any necessary cylindrical or prism correction.

High heterophorias are difficult to prescribe for, using contact lenses, as only about 4 prism dioptres can be satisfactorily incorporated into a contact lens. With scleral lenses, the prism base can be put in any direction, as long as the haptic portion is a good fit and the lens does not rotate. This allows a maximum of 8 prism dioptres difference between the two eyes. However, with soft and corneal lenses, the base always rotates downwards due to gravity, which limits any prismatic correction to 4 prism dioptres base-down. In fact, 2 prism dioptres is a more reasonable figure as all the prism must be put on one lens. Discomfort is likely with a very thick lower edge; also the prism base usually takes up a slightly nasal position due to lid action.

Myopes often require less prism in contact lenses than in spectacles, presumably because the bigger retinal image size with contact lenses affords a better binocular lock. However, the mobility of the retinal image, in corneal lens wear, may necessitate greater prism. There is no general rule, but the minimum prism to get rid of any fixation disparity and/or symptoms should be prescribed.

Amblyopia. Care must be taken to see that any improved visual acuity given by contact lenses does not give rise to an insuperable diplopia. As visual acuity improves, orthoptic exercises may be needed to help consolidate binocular vision.

Eye movements. Pareses of extraocular muscles give rise to diplopia with contact lenses as with spectacles. As already stated, contact lenses can affect the amount of eye movement required because they remove the prismatic effects of spectacle lenses, so that both version and vergence movements may be affected.

Aniseikonia. A combination of spectacles and contact lenses can be used to create size differences to relieve symptoms due to aniseikonia. The principles are those of a Galilean telescope system, similar to the type used as an aid to the partially sighted (*see* Chapter 24, Volume 2).

Uniocularity. Contact lenses are a hazard – even if only a very slight one – and it may be in the best interests of a uniocular person, or one with intractable amblyopia in one eye, not to fit him with contact lenses unless this considerably improves vision as compared with spectacles, or is otherwise necessary. In any case the patient should be warned of the risk, however small. If spectacles are prescribed these should have plastics or toughened lenses.

PERSONAL AND EXTERNAL FACTORS

Age and Sex

Incentive, enthusiasm and handling ability are generally better in younger people, although there are remarkable exceptions. Presbyopic contact lens wearers need to use spectacles for near work unless bifocal contact lenses are fitted – and even when it is possible to fit these, they have certain limitations in use.

Women undergoing the menopause may experience difficulties with their lenses. Xerosis sometimes occurs during the menopause. Occasionally hormonal changes lead to psychological disturbances and consequent loss of motivation to wear contact lenses. Such changes are most likely to take place at the time of a pregnancy or during the menopause. Pregnancy also frequently disturbs contact lens wearing, presumably due to metabolic changes in the cornea. The change in hormone balance alters the water content of all tissues, including the cornea and lids – which may result in a corneal thickness or curvature change and a consequent alteration in lens fit. The fit of corneal lenses can become dramatically tighter, with very little peripheral clearance where plenty existed before; and if modifications are made to alleviate the ensuing discomfort the lenses can be made wearable again until the termination of the pregnancy. Then, the cornea returns to its original state and the modified lenses become loose and uncomfortable, and must either be made smaller or replaced. In this respect soft lenses are less likely to cause problems than hard lenses, although tears output is often reduced during periods of water retention, and this coupled with corneal curvature and thickness changes can make even soft lens wearing difficult.

Similar effects have been recorded in women taking oral contraceptives (Koetting, 1966), although improvements in these drugs have now reduced the effects to a minimal amount. Difficulties in wearing contact lenses associated with premenstrual tension have also been reported (Dalton, 1970). Dalton, a gynaecologist, states . . . 'Difficulty with contact lenses may occur before or during menstruation and I usually advise patients when first starting to use contact lenses, to practise first, after menstruation. During the premenstruum, ocular symptoms are common; non-infective conjunctivitis related to menstruation was noted as early as 1521 (Roy, 1961), and raised intraocular pressure also occurs. Landesman *et al.* (1953) studied the menstrual changes of the peripheral vascular bed of the bulbar conjunctiva and demonstrated changes during the premenstruum when the blood flow is diminished, the vessels become dilated and engorged and the arterioles constricted.'

'My own experience suggests that women who manage contact lenses will only have problems if they are on an unsuitable contraceptive pill and are getting other side-effects, for example, headaches, bloatedness or nausea. By changing the contraceptive pill and eliminating other side-effects, the ocular symptoms also disappear.'

'Similarly, women suffering from toxaemic symptoms of pregnancy (vomiting, headache, depression, lethargy) are also likely to have difficulty with contact lenses, but the ocular symptoms are eased as soon as the pregnancy symptoms are eased by treatment or the passage of time.'

'I have always assumed that in women with premenstrual exacerbations, or those taking the contraceptive pill, and during pregnancy, that it was the deficient progesterone and/or oestrogen excess which was responsible for their symptoms. In my experience, it is rare for women to complain of difficulty with contact lenses while on progesterone for premenstrual migraine, depression and irritability.'

Farrall (1976) has shown that a reduction in tears output with associated drop in lysozyme and relative increase in globulin-type protein is to be expected when women first take the oral contraceptive pill, or change to another type, or cease to take it. The effects of increased corneal oedema, reduced lacrimal secretion and increased mucus and lipid content of the tears film may last a few weeks but gradually subside. In a contact lens wearer, though, they may be sufficient to cause abandonment of hard lens wear.

Ability to Handle Lenses

Contact lenses should not be supplied unless they can be handled properly by the patient, who should be able to see both the lenses and any engraving on them. A light (neutral) tint may help. In cases such as aphakia, a spectacle frame can be supplied, glazed to a suitable prescription on one side only, the other 'eye' being left empty and the lower rim removed. The first contact lens is then inserted through the empty 'eye' of the frame, which enables the patient to see it with the other eye. The frame is then removed as the patient is able to see the second contact lens with the first in place.

People with very clumsy or shaky hands are usually able to handle scleral lenses better than corneals, but may too easily damage soft lenses.

In the case of very young children or elderly people who must wear contact lenses but are unable to handle them, a relative or someone close to the patient should be taught the various insertion and removal techniques and be given all the necessary information.

Working and Living Conditions

Corneal lenses and soft lenses (and, to a much lesser extent, scleral lenses) can be difficult to wear in a number of conditions: dusty and smokey atmospheres, very hot or cold temperatures, windy weather, and very dry and very humid atmospheres.

If the light is poor, the pupil may dilate to greater than the central optic diameter so that diplopia (ghost images) or peripheral blur is seen.

If excessive light is likely, a tint may be necessary. Choice of tint must depend on the absorption required and the colour rendering. A neutral tint is preferable for most purposes because, as Fletcher and Nisted (1963) have shown, some tints can be dangerous if used under a monochromatic illumination the wavelength of which is not transmitted by the tint. The effects of tints on dark adaptation should also be remembered.

Certain head postures do cause difficulty with corneal lenses, and the bubble in a fenestrated scleral lens can be a nuisance in some head positions.

Small palpebral apertures, when continually looking downwards as when reading, may give rise to veiling due to an upset in metabolism. This may be caused by covering the fenestration in a scleral lens, or — with any type of lens — due to too great a rise in temperature with the reduction in palpebral aperture size.

Continuous rapid eye movements (as, for example, those eye excursions made by a copy typist) can cause considerable limbal bumping and associated limbal injection, when hard lenses are worn.

Soft lenses have been found to be very beneficial in hot climates. They are more liable to dry out in very windy or dry atmospheres, and instillations of saline solution may be needed. Soft lenses are absolutely contra-indicated for people coming into contact with any noxious fumes such as workers in the chemical industry.

Drugs

Drug-taking can influence metabolism, which in turn may influence contact lens wear. Tolerance trials extended over 4 weeks if necessary (as, for example, in the case of women under hormone treatment) may be advisable before prescribing contact lenses for some patients, as the corneal curvature, especially peripherally, may alter quite dramatically. The effects of oral contraceptives on tears output and corneal oedema have been dealt with under the heading Age and Sex, page 179.

Thyroxine treatment has been reported to cause intolerance to contact lenses (Marsh, 1975). Mackie, Seal and Pescod (1977) have shown that beta-adrenergic blocking drugs such as practolol and tolamolol, as used for certain heart conditions, may reduce tears output and lysozyme concentration, although very low doses of the latter drug may increase lysozyme concentration. Contact lenses may therefore be contra-indicated for patients on prolonged courses of these drugs.

Habits

Hygiene is essential in the handling of contact lenses. People who rub their eyes a lot and who blink excessively should not be given corneal lenses unless they can cease these habits. Smoking may be a disadvantage to the wearer of contact lenses.

Hobbies

Bearing in mind the high cost of insurance premiums for contact lenses, people who intend to use them only for sports and swimming are still likely to be best satisfied with scleral lenses, although special lenses for sports purposes, have been designed (Levey, 1965). Corneal lenses fitted steeply are frequently satisfactory, but they may be too steep to give all day wear — and they are still more easily lost than a scleral-type lens. Soft lenses are more likely to stay in place than corneals, but have been known to wash out of the eye during swimming. Also they are likely to become contaminated by the chlorine in swimming pool water. Despite their difficulties, however, corneal lenses or soft lenses have become the contact lenses of choice for the majority of contact-lens-wearing sports enthusiasts.

For those who need contact lenses for the stage and films, arc lights make photophobia a difficulty. Various tints are available, as are lenses having artificial irides. For effects purposes,

contact lenses in the form of prosthetic lenses can be used to alter the appearance and colour of the eyes.

If contact lenses are required for only occasional wear, as for social events, soft lenses are by far the best lens to fit. With hard lenses difficulties are likely to be encountered as a satisfactory tolerance must always be built up beforehand, especially with corneals; and with fenestrated sclerals a varying amount of settling may take place so that bubble trouble may occur on one occasion whilst corneal touch symptoms are experienced on another.

Special Occupations

In the United Kingdom there are certain restrictions regarding the wearing of contact lenses whilst driving, or piloting an aircraft, and in certain other occupations. Similar restrictions may apply in other countries and regulations regarding such use of contact lenses are normally available from the appropriate vehicle or driver/pilot licensing authority in that country or from the prospective employer. At the time of writing the following regulations apply in the United Kingdom.

Drivers

As far as drivers are concerned, The Department of the Environment Driver and Vehicle Licensing Centre at Swansea has stated the following in a personal communication (September, 1975) to the author.

'For ordinary car drivers who normally wear contact lenses and will have to remove them and change to spectacles for any reason, they should wait for two to three hours before driving, in order to allow time for adaptation in the new form of correction.'

'Drivers of heavy goods vehicles and public service vehicles and other professional drivers should not wear contact lenses.'

The Department of the Environment has elaborated on the second paragraph above, as follows.

'There are no prescribed eyesight requirements for applicants for heavy goods vehicle drivers' licences other than that which applies generally to holders of 'ordinary' driving licences: the ability to read (with glasses, if worn) a clean number plate at a distance of 75 feet for letters and figures $3\frac{1}{2}$ inches high or at 67 feet for letters and figures $3\frac{1}{8}$ inches high.'

'The medical standards for heavy goods vehicle drivers which guide the statutorily independent Licensing Authorities and doctors carrying out

Room T211
Civil Aviation Authority
CAA House
45–59 Kingsway
(main entrance Kemble Street)
London WC2B 6TE
Telephone 01-379 7311   2799

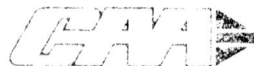

CAA

Medical Department

CONTACT LENSES – PROFESSIONAL PILOTS, LICENSED AIRCREW AND STUDENT AND PRIVATE PILOT LICENCES (S/PPL)

APPLICANTS FOR AND HOLDERS OF THE ABOVE LICENCES MAY WEAR CONTACT LENSES FOR THE CORRECTION OF VISION BUT THE FOLLOWING REQUIREMENTS MUST BE FULFILLED

A   The fields of vision must be normal.

B   The unaided vision in each eye should be correctable in the case of the professional pilot to 6/9 and in the case of licensed aircrew and S/PPL correctable to 6/12.

C   Reports in connection with the wearing of contact lenses should contain the following details:

    a) Record of the <u>unaided</u> visual acuity in each eye.

    b) The corrected vision in each eye with i) spectacles and ii) contact lenses.

    c) Prescriptions for both contact lenses and spectacles should be included in the report.

    d) There should be written confirmation that contact lenses have been worn constantly and successfully for several hours every day over a period of at least six months.

If these requirements are met and provided the medical examination report is in other respects satisfactory contact lenses may be approved to be worn while exercising the privileges of the licence subject to carrying a pair of spectacles which when worn correct the vision immediately after removal of the contact lenses.

Should the contact lenses be changed or if this form of correction is abandoned further ophthalmic reports should be provided.

Any expense incurred in obtaining information is the responsibility of the applicant.

Figure 7.1–Copy of the Civil Aviation Authority regulations governing the wearing of contact lenses by applicants for professional pilots licences as well as for student and private pilots licences and by licensed aircrew (reproduced by kind permission of the CAA)

examinations for licensing purposes are those recommended by the Medical Commission on Accident Prevention in the booklet *Medical Aspects of Fitness to Drive*. The Commission recommends, in the case of vision, that these drivers much reach a Snellen standard of 6/12 in one eye and 6/36 in the other, with glasses, if necessary; and that they (and other professional drivers) should not wear contact lenses. The Commission considers that although contact lenses may give drivers visual acuity as good as that achieved with the aid of spectacles, they have certain disadvantages when worn continuously. The most limiting of these are eye irritation, blurring of vision, and inflammation which often occur after they have been worn for long periods. They may also be easily ejected by coughing or sneezing.'

It is hoped that these regulations will be reviewed in the light of modern types of contact lenses and todays high standards of contact lens fitting.

Civil Pilots

The Medical Department of the Civil Aviation Authority in London, also in a personal communication to the author, dated February 1980, has stated:

'The rules and regulations regarding the wearing of contact lenses by pilots have recently been amended as outlined in the enclosed regulations.'

These regulations are reproduced in *Figure 7.1* and cover the licensing of aircrew, student and private pilots, as well as professional pilots.

Royal Air Force Personnel

A personal letter from the consultant adviser in ophthalmology, dated October 1976 and confirmed in February 1980, states:

'There are no regulations, as such, about the wearing of these lenses, other than that all potential wearers must be referred to me; also the Civil Aviation Authority require referral of civilian aircrew to their consultant adviser.'

'The reason for this rule is that although contact lenses, in many cases, may give good visual acuity at ground level, they may not, under certain conditions of flight, give as good a correction as a properly fitted pair of corrected flying spectacles.'

'So far as hard lenses are concerned, low flight deck humidity, which in a Boeing 707 may fall as low as 7 per cent, and kinetic heating in high-speed, low-level flight can give problems with corneal epithelial hydration behind the lens.'

'Also exposure to low ambient atmospheric pressure, either very high altitude flight or accidental exposure to an altitude of over approximately 23,000 ft can give rise to bubble formation behind the lens. These bubbles certainly degrade vision and, if the lenses are not removed, can produce staining abrasions of the corneal epithelium. De Vries and Hoogerheide, *Aeromedica Acta* (1958). **VI**, pp. 141–153 describe an experiment to confirm this finding, and as a result of this, and other incidents, we prefer not to take the risk with our aircrew.'

'With regard to soft lenses, we do not yet know the pros and cons, and I am at present carrying out a trial of various lenses with Mr Ruben. It is possible that low oxygen transmission and kinetic heating might introduce problems, as might the absorption of toxic fumes and chemicals by the lenses and slow release to the globe.'

'We have had some success with the fitting of hard lenses to non-pilot aircrew, this solely to retain very experienced crewmen in some form of flying role, but at present this is not a general practice. However, we are still keeping an open mind on this subject.'

Royal Navy Personnel

A letter to the author from the Medical Directorate (Navy) branch of the Ministry of Defence dated November 1976, and confirmed in February 1980, states:

'Whilst there is in general no restriction to the wearing of contact lenses to improve visual efficiency the nature of the task in some branches of the Service requires a certain level of unaided vision. If this is not achieved, personnel may not be admitted to that particular branch of the Service regardless of whether or not they wear contact lenses.'

Applicants to the Royal Navy would obviously have to find out whether or not their particular task would permit the wearing of contact lenses.

Army Personnel

The Army informed the author that there are no regulations regarding the wearing of contact lenses and that they are acceptable as long as a visual acuity of 6/12 or better in each eye is achieved.

Police

The Metropolitan Police provided the following information.

'Contact lenses are permitted provided that the aided visual acuity is 6/6 and the unaided vision is 6/18.'

This applies to the Essex Police and presumably to other police forces throughout the United Kingdom.

London Transport

Bus and tube train drivers are not allowed to wear contact lenses.

British Rail

Locomotive drivers are not allowed to wear contact lenses.

Legislative Control of Contact Lenses and Solutions

The availability of some contact lenses and solutions is limited in certain countries by government regulations. Thus, at the time of writing, citizens of the United States of America are unable to obtain contact lenses for continuous or extended wear unless they are necessary for a pathological condition or have been asked to wear them as part of an investigational procedure and are prepared to submit to strict after-care examinations as set out by the Food and Drugs Administration (FDA), which is part of the United States Department of Health, Education and Welfare, Public Health Service.

A brief outline of the current (1980) situation is appropriate here.

In the United Kingdom, since 1975, all contact lens solutions and preparations have been subject to licensing under the Medicines Act. The Department of Health and Social Security (DHSS) were approached in 1973 by the Faculty of Ophthalmologists, to bring preparations used in association with contact lenses under the control of the Medicines Act. This was because justifiable doubts had been cast on the efficacy of some solutions to kill harmful microorganisms in a suitable length of time. Also, it was felt that the toxicity of these solutions should be investigated. The DHSS, after due consideration, then set up a Working Party to consider guidelines which might be used in judging these preparations in the light of their mode of use. Then, in late 1975, contact lenses and associated preparations were brought under the control of the newly established Committee on Dental and

Surgical Materials which was set up by Statutory Instrument to advise the Licensing Authority on various aspects of such materials.

This Committee set up a sub-committee in 1977 to advise it on 'the safety, quality and efficacy of contact lenses, contact lens blanks, contact lens fluids, such other substances or articles to which any provision of the Medicines Act 1968 is applicable and which are for administration to the human eye or which are for preventing, diagnosing, or treating adverse conditions of the human eye.' The DHSS Working Party has made recommendations to this Committee and it is evident that contact lens materials and cases, as well as solutions and their containers, and sizes of the latter will become subject to Statutory control in due course.

In the United Kingdom licensing of contact lens solutions became obligatory on 1st January 1980, but contact lenses and materials are still under consideration. It is understood that guidelines for their licensing have already been prepared and that such licensing will shortly come into effect.

Some idea of what is involved may be obtained from the experience of practitioners in the United States of America where all new contact lens materials (that is, other than PMMA) are considered as drugs. Prior to approval for general use they are subjected to clinical trials on rabbits and humans, and microbiological, toxicological and allergy tests are carried out with both lenses and solutions as well as tests on the associated use of their respective containers. Thus, several years may elapse between the original application to permit testing of the new lens/solution/system and its final approval. As far as extended wear contact lenses are concerned the FDA requires the clinical trials to include at least 200 patients using the lenses for daily wear first, for at least 100 days. Pachometry, checks of the corneal endothelium (by specular microscopy), slit lamp examination of the upper tarsal plate, and other observations are all to be included in the clinical trials, as well as oxygen permeability studies on the lenses and their uptake of solution preservatives. If they pass these stringent daily wear trials they may then be used for similar extended wear trials lasting 6 months, at least.

Regulations also exist in certain European countries, but are less stringent than those of the United States. In Japan, the Ministry of Health and Welfare insists on independent testing of contact lens materials, methods of manufacture, and on contact lens solutions. University departments normally carry out the tests over a 3–5 year period which includes clinical trials. At present only a few companies are licensed to produce soft lenses. Even PMMA for hard lenses is subject to testing, and firms wishing to set up as hard lens manufacturers are rigorously controlled. As far as contact lens solutions are concerned, most mercurial compounds, such as thiomersalate, are banned.

Thus, in future, it may be that the practitioner's choice of lenses, solutions and containers will become much more limited, though it is to be hoped that bureaucratic intervention will not hamper genuine advances in the field of contact lenses.

Sufficient has now been said about indications, contra-indications and selection of patients and contact lenses, as well as the factors to be considered in the choice of the best type of lens to fit. The reader must realize that both frustration and satisfaction are to be the lot of the contact lens practitioner at different times and with different patients.

REFERENCES

Backman, H. and Bolte, C. (1974). 'Chronic allergic conjunctivitis and its effect on contact lenses.' *Optom. Wkly* **65**(31), 26–30

Becker, S. C. (1972). *Clinical Gonioscopy: A Text and Stereoscopic Atlas,* pp. 165–167. St. Louis: Mosby

Bibby, M. M. (1976). 'Computer-assisted photokeratoscopy and contact lens design.' Part 1, *Optician* **171**(4423), 37, 39, 41, 43; Part 2, *Optician* **171**(4424), 11, 14–15, 17; Part 3, *Optician* **171**(4425), 22–23; Part 4, *Optician* **171**(4426), 15, 17

Boberg-Ans, J. (1955). 'Experience in clinical examination of corneal sensitivity.' *Br. J. Ophthal.* **39**, 705–726

Bonnet, R. and Cochet, P. (1962). 'New method of topographical ophthalmometry – its theoretical and clinical applications.' *Am. J. Optom.* **39**, 227–251

Bruch, C. W. (1973). 'Eye products: handle with care.' *Optician* **166**(4297), 22, 27

Cordrey, P. (1972). *Cosmetics and the Eye/Contact Lens System.* London: Cordrey

Dalton, K. (1970). Personal communication

Department of Optometry and Visual Science, The City University, London (1974). 'Eye beauty should be safe: eye make-up and contact lenses.' *Optician* **168**(4355), 9, 13

Farrell, H. (1976). 'Some effects of oral contraceptive steroids on the eye, related to corneal lens wear.' *Optician* **171**(4423), 8–9, 13

Fletcher, R. J. and Nisted, M. (1963). 'A study of coloured contact lenses and their performance.' *Ophthal. Optician* **3**, 1151–1154, 1161–1163, 1203–1206, 1212–1213

Ford, M. W. (1974). 'Changes in hydrophilic lenses when placed on an eye.' Paper read at the joint International Congress of The Contact Lens Society and The National Eye Research Foundation, Montreux, Switzerland

Gustafson, J. C. (1967). 'Patient symptoms resulting from cosmetics and their correction.' *Contacto* **11**(1), 16–19

Hill, R. M. (1973). 'Tears: the missing link.' *Ophthal. Optician* **13**, 792, 797–798, 800

Hill, R. M. and Leighton, A. J. (1965). 'Temperature changes of human cornea and tears under a contact lens. Part II: Effects of intermediate lid apertures and gaze.' *Am. J. Optom.* **42**, 71–77

Hillman, J. S. (1976). 'The use of hydrophilic contact lenses.' *Optician* **172**(4458), 9–11

Hodd, F. A. B. (1970). Personal communication

Kemmettmüller, H. (1962). 'Corneal lenses and keratoconus.' *Contacto* **6**, 188–193

Kersley, H. J. (1975). 'Continuous wear lenses after aphakic operation.' *Optician* **170**(4393), 12–13, 15–16, 18

Khoo, F. B. H. (1974). Paper read at National Optical Congress, University of Lancaster, September, 1974

Koetting, R. A. (1966). 'The influence of oral contraceptives on contact lens wear.' *Am. J. Optom.* **43**, 268–274

Koetting, R. A. (1976). 'Tear film break-up time as a factor in hydrogel lens coating – a preliminary study.' *Contacto* **20**(3), 20–23

Landesman, R., Douglas, R. G., Dreishpoon, G. and Holze, E. (1953). 'The vascular bed of the bulbar conjunctiva in the normal menstrual cycle.' *Am. J. Obstet. Gynec.* **66**, 988–998

Leibowitz, H. M. (1972). 'Hydrophilic contact lenses in corneal disease. IV. Penetrating corneal wounds.' *A.M.A. Archs Ophthal.* **88**, 602–606

Leibowitz, H. M. and Rosenthal, P. (1971). 'Hydrophilic contact lenses in corneal disease. I. Superficial, sterile, indolent ulcers.' *A.M.A. Archs Ophthal.* **85**, 163–166

Lemp, M. A., Dohlman, C. H. and Holly, F. J. (1970). 'Corneal dessication despite normal tear volume.' *Ann. Ophthal.* **2**, 258–261 and 284

Lemp, M. A., Dohlman, C. H., Kuwabara, T., Holly, F. J. and Carroll, J. M. (1971). 'Dry eye secondary to mucus deficiency.' *Trans. Am Acad. Ophthal. Otolaryngol.* **75**, 1223–1227

Levey, E. M. (1965). 'The sports wearer of contact lenses.' *Am. J. Optom.* **42**, 21–23

Lowther, G. E., Bailey, N. J. and Hill, R. M. (1971). 'Conjunctival xerosis associated with contact lenses.' *Am. J. Optom.* **48**, 754–758

Lowther, G. E., Miller, R. B. and Hill, R. M. (1970). 'Tear concentrations of sodium and potassium during adaptation to contact lenses. 1. Sodium observations.' *Am. J. Optom.* **47**, 266–275

Mackie, I. A. (1967). 'Lesions at the corneal limbus at 3 o'clock and 9 o'clock in association with the wearing of contact lenses.' pp.66–73. In *Contact Lenses, XXth International Congress of Ophthalmology Symposium,* Munich-Feldafing, August 13th 1966, ed. by O. H. Dabezies, H. Laue, A. Schlossman and G. P. Halberg. Basel and New York: Karger

Mackie, I. A. (1977). Personal communication

Mackie, I. A., Seal, D. V. and Pescod, J. M. (1977). 'Beta-adrenergic receptor blocking drugs: tear lysozyme and immunological screening for adverse reaction.' *Br. J. Ophthal.* **61**, 354–359

Mandell, R. B. (1974). 'What is the gravity lens?' *Int. C.L. Clin.* **1**(4), 29–35

Marsh, R. (1975). 'Thyroxine and contact lenses.' In 'Points from Letters', *Br. med. J.* **2**, 689

McConnell, J. (1967). 'Cosmetics and contact lenses.' *Contacto* **11**(1), 40–43

McDonald, J. E. (1969). 'Surface phenomena of the tear film.' *Am. J. Ophthal.* **67**, 56–64

Millodot, M. (1976). 'Effect of the length of wear of contact lenses on corneal sensitivity.' *Acta Ophthal.* **54**, 721–730

Norn, M. S. (1963). 'Foam at outer palpebral canthus.' *Acta Ophthal. (Kbh.)* **41**, 531–537

Norn, M. S. (1964). 'Vital staining in practice using a mixed stain and alcian blue.' *Br. J. physiol. Optics* **21**, 293–298

Norn, M. S. (1965). 'Lacrimal apparatus tests: A new method (lacrimal streak dilution test) compared with previous methods.' *Acta Ophthal. (Kbh.)* **43**, 557–566

Norn, M. S. (1970). 'Micropunctate fluorescein vital staining of the cornea.' *Acta Ophthal. (Kbh.)* **48**, 108–118

Norn, M. S. (1974). *External Eye: Methods of Examination.* Copenhagen: Scriptor

Polse, K. A. (1975). 'Observation of corneal dry spots.' *Optom. Wkly* **66**(18), 20–21

Rengstorff, R. H. and Black, C. J. (1974). 'Eye protection from contact lenses.' *J. Am. optom. Ass.* **45**, 270–276

Roy, A. M. (1961). 'Menstrual red eye.' Letter in *Br. med. J.* **1**, 590

Schirmer, K. E. and Mellor, L. D. (1961). 'Corneal sensitivity after cataract extraction.' *A.M.A. Archs Ophthal.* **65**, 433–436

Sorsby, A., Leary, G. and Richards, M. J. (1962). 'The optical components in anisometropia.' *Vision Res.* **2**, 43–51

Stewart, C. R. (1973). 'Conjunctival absorption of pigment from eye make-up.' *Am. J. Optom.* **50**, 571–574

Stone, J. (1959). 'Factors governing the back central optic diameter of a micro-lens.' *Optician* **138**, 20–22

Stone, J. (1967). 'Near vision difficulties in non-presbyopic corneal lens wearers.' *Contact Lens* **1**(2), 14–16, 24–25

Takahashi, G. H. and Leibowitz, H. M. (1971). 'Hydrophilic contact lenses in corneal disease. III. Topical hypertonic saline therapy in bullous keratopathy.' *A.M.A. Archs Ophthal.* **86**, 133–137

van Herick, W., Shaffer, R. N. and Schwartz, A. (1969). 'Estimation of width of angle of anterior chamber.' *Am. J. Ophthal.* **68**, 626–629

Vanley, G. T., Leopold, I. H. and Gregg, T. H. (1977). 'Interpretation of tear film breakup.' *A.M.A. Archs Ophthal.* **95**, 445–448

Westerhout, D. (1973). 'The combination lens and therapeutic uses of soft lenses.' *Contact Lens* **4**(5), 3–12, 16–18, 20 and 22

Wilson, L. A., Kuehne, J. W., Hall, S. W. and Ahearn, D. G. (1973). 'Microbial contamination in ocular cosmetics.' *Optician* **166**(4298), 4, 6 and 12

Young, W. and Hill, R. M. (1973). 'Cholesterol levels of human tears: case reports.' *J. Am. optom. Ass.* **45**, 424–428

Chapter 8

Patient Management and Instruction

K. W. Atkinson and M. J. A. Port

Some of the psychological factors likely to influence a patient have already been mentioned in Chapter 7. Many of these are worth repeating because the way in which a patient is managed is as important as pure technical ability and can make the difference between success and failure.

It is necessary for the patient to have confidence in the practitioner. This is essential in order that the patient commences to wear contact lenses, continues to wear them in spite of occasional difficulties and accurately follows any instructions given.

Simple terms should be used in explanations. Before examining a patient's eyes, it is wise to discuss the general characteristics of contact lenses and correct any mistaken ideas the patient has acquired. This is especially true since the advent of hydrophilic lenses. They have received a great deal of publicity — much of which is often over-optimistic. The practitioner should beware of making extravagant claims which may lead to loss of patient confidence or even legal proceedings if they are not met. A full explanation and discussion must cover any points on which the patient may require information.

The reason given by the patient for wanting contact lenses is important. It has a considerable effect on the successful outcome of contact lens wearing, assuming that the practitioner is fully competent to deal with any fitting difficulties. Prime motivations may be rationalized to other reasons on enquiry by the practitioner, but cosmetic results are the usual consideration in general practice. Intelligence, dexterity, environment, motivation and the needs of the patient all have a bearing on the type of lens selected.

A demonstration of corneal, scleral and hydrophilic lenses by the practitioner on his own eyes is useful. If lens insertion and removal can be shown to be smooth, simple, and painless procedures, confidence in the practitioner is enhanced and at the same time the patient's apprehension is reduced regarding his own ability to tolerate a contact lens.

Discussion tends to relax patients. They are normally tense and worried at the first visit. This discussion should include the advantages and disadvantages of contact lenses together with a brief résumé of adaptive difficulties. Reasons for using different types of contact lens can be given. It is important to anticipate a particular patient's visual expectations wherever possible, especially if the practitioner is considering fitting soft lenses. Current hydrophilic materials give wide variation in terms of 'quality of vision' and 'visual performance'. The practitioner should explain how much time is involved in fitting and what this entails. At this stage, the cost of the lenses and professional fees may be mentioned. The patient should be informed of the annual cost of wearing contact lenses; this normally consists of a fee for an after-care examination, an insurance premium to cover accidental loss of lenses, and the cost of any wetting, soaking or cleaning solutions. Most patients wish to know how long their lenses are going to last them. With careful handling and storage hard lenses should last 5–15 years. The useful life of a soft lens is difficult to quantify due to the difference in materials. Five years for a poly-HEMA lens is fairly common. However, taking loss or breakage of a lens into account there may well be little difference between the average life of a hard and a soft lens.

The practitioner must lay great emphasis on the need for regular after-care visits after the initial supervised period. These may be carried out at 9 or 12 month intervals. After the first year of wear a fee is normally charged.

ROUTINE EXAMINATION

Routine examination helps to determine the limitations that the patient himself may impose on the possibility of successful contact lens wear. It also helps to determine which type of lens will be most suitable. The patient's history is most important and should cover all the contra-indications mentioned in Chapter 7, with particular reference to general systemic conditions, systemic medication, previous ocular pathology and general ocular history (squint, amblyopia, eye operations and diseases).

The refractive condition of the patient should be considered as follows.

(1) Degree and type of ametropia, and whether or not corrected. Differences between the corneal astigmatism and the spectacle astigmatism are worth noting.

(2) Length of time spectacles have been worn. The patient may feel incomplete without spectacles if these have been worn for a considerable number of years. Conversely, the ability to see clearly without spectacles may be a strong motive.

(3) Whether the prescription is worn continually or only intermittently. A patient who wears a spectacle correction intermittently may not have sufficient motivation to persevere with contact lenses.

(4) The best visual acuity with the spectacle correction worn, the best visual acuity obtainable, and whether or not the patient has been fully corrected previously.

(5) Vocation and corrected acuity. It may well be that a gardener or housewife will accept a lower level of acuity with contact lenses than, say, a surveyor or printer.

(6) The need of a correction for near vision. Motivation may be lessened when the patient realizes that a near correction is still necessary with contact lenses, be this in the form of bifocal contact lenses (*see* Chapter 19, Volume 2) or supplementary reading spectacles. Myopes invariably find that presbyopia appears a few years earlier if they are wearing contact lenses rather than spectacles.

(7) Tints. Corneal lenses are available in a variety of tints and a light tint may be incorporated in every pair of corneal lenses. Neutral tints help those who are photophobic; different densities of the same colour tint are normally available. Tinted lenses are used to change the apparent iris colour. These lenses may have a uniform tint throughout the lens or a clear centre with a tinted periphery. A tinted lens helps the patient to locate the lens if it is displaced on to the bulbar conjunctiva or if the lens is dropped

(*see* Chapter 11). Although not as common as tinted corneal lenses, soft lenses are available with the central portion tinted — the portion over the sclera being left clear. Scleral lenses can also be supplied with a tinted optic portion.

If the patient knows other contact lens wearers, their success or failure may affect his attitude and it may be worthwhile to mention individual variations in contact lens tolerance; for example, hours worn, degree of adaptation, lens comfort.

GENERAL OCULAR EXAMINATION

Some parts of this examination assume added importance in contact lens work, but the following is a guide to the necessary tests (Chapter 7 gives an expansion of this information).

(1) External examination.

(2) Motility.

(3) Measurement of heterophorias at distance and at near. (Vertical prism can be included in both corneal and scleral lenses but horizontal prisms can only be incorporated in scleral lenses and then only up to 3Δ in each lens.) Cover test for squint. Speed of recovery of heterophoria. Measurement of near point of convergence. Fixation disparity tests.

(4) Visual acuity with spectacles.

(5) Ophthalmoscopy.

(6) Retinoscopy: a swirling movement may be indicative of keratoconus.

(7) Refraction. If the best acuity obtainable with trial lenses, of one or both eyes, comes below 6/6, the practitioner should endeavour to find a reason for this. Checking with a pin-hole disc may be useful.

EXTERNAL OCULAR CHARACTERISTICS RELATED TO CONTACT LENSES

(1) General considerations.

(*a*) Vertical and horizontal measurement of palpebral apertures.

(*b*) Vertical and horizontal visible iris diameters.

(*c*) Pupil diameters in average illumination and the maximum diameter in low illumination.

(*d*) Any irregularity of the pupil shape and any difference in size between the two.

(*e*) The profile of the cornea should be observed against the lower lid margin for Munson's sign (this is visible in keratoconus when the ectatic cornea distorts the outline of the lower lid margin). The anterior chamber depth, the central corneal radius and the nature of the limbal junction may be estimated at the same time.

(f) When fitting scleral lenses, the size of the globes should be noted — that is, large or small — and the general shape of the sclera.

(g) Lid tension, texture and thickness.

(h) Conjunctival texture, thickness and vascularity. Abnormalities are recorded; for example, pingueculae, limbal injection, blebs.

(2) A drawing may be made of the normal lid position relative to the cornea, as this affects the centration of a hard corneal lens or a hydrophilic lens.

(3) Active corneal and conjunctival conditions can be detected by instilling staining agents such as fluorescein and rose bengal (see Chapter 3).

(4) Corneal sensitivity can be established grossly with a wisp of tissue. Correct use of a corneal aesthesiometer will give more accurate information.

(5) Keratometry (see Chapter 5).

(6) A thorough slit lamp examination (see Chapters 5, 7, and 16 in Volume 2). Where possible this should include pachometry, to measure at least the central corneal thickness (Stone, 1974).

(7) A Placido disc, Klein keratoscope or photo-electric keratoscope (PEK) should be used if prior examination has led the practitioner to suspect the presence of keratoconus or corneal irregularity. Keratometry, slit lamp examination, refraction and visual acuity also give clues.

(8) A test for lacrimal output. Only gross differences from the norm are detectable as the test itself usually involves the reflex production of extra tears. Schirmer test paper strips are widely used for this test (see Chapters 2 and 7).

(9) Tears film integrity (see Chapter 7). Assessment of time for dry spots to appear in the tears film of the open eye. Lemp, Dohlman and Holly (1970) found that a time of less than 10 seconds was critical.

(10) Photography of the external eye with both white light and ultra-violet light (see Chapter 6).

Not all the above tests are necessary for every patient. Tests 7, 8, 9 and 10 may be carried out at the discretion of the practitioner, although it may be valuable to do them for every patient.

If the history or ocular examination yields evidence that an active pathological process is present, then it is necessary by statute to refer the patient to his doctor. If the patient is receiving treatment for a general condition it is prudent to contact the general medical practitioner concerned and ask his opinion as to the advisability of fitting contact lenses. Those who refuse to consult a medical person should be asked to provide a letter stating their reasons for refusal, and careful records should be kept.

The practitioner must be very careful to examine the eyes for active or passive pathological conditions before proceeding to place a contact lens on the eye. As stated above, with any active condition, referral is imperative before fitting is started. In the case of a passive condition, careful notes and diagrams should be entered on the patient's record card. Such conditions may not prevent successful contact lens wear, but the patient should be made aware of their presence.

If, for example, an early case of endothelial dystrophy had been discovered and it is decided not to proceed with fitting, it would be wise to inform the patient and provide him with a covering note to this effect. The practitioner should obviously keep a copy for his own protection. This same patient might well consult someone else with a view to having contact lenses fitted. Such a subtle condition could well be overlooked and contact lenses might be supplied to the detriment of the patient's cornea, unless the patient has already been told why he was rejected for contact lenses. Where conditions exist that are 'abnormal' but may not fit precisely into an 'active' or 'passive' category the opinion of an ophthalmologist should be sought, who may also be able to give opinions as to whether such conditions would be aggravated by the wearing of contact lenses.

Changes in the condition of the eyes in subsequent years may be blamed on contact lenses. These changes may be old or may have arisen concurrently with contact lens wear. Accurate records monitoring the condition of the eyes over the years are therefore of paramount importance.

At this stage it is necessary to decide whether to proceed with fitting, bearing in mind the contraindications which might have been discovered. Some conditions may impose restrictions on the performance of contact lenses and the patient should be made aware of these limitations.

If the practitioner decides to proceed with the fitting, he must also decide whether to fit hard (scleral or corneal) or soft lenses, taking all considerations into account.

INSERTION OF THE FIRST LENS

The methods of lens insertion and removal by the practitioner and by the patient are very similar — though, of course, the patient may occupy a different position, either sitting or reclining backwards when the lens is being inserted by the practitioner, and leaning over some flat surface or over a mirror when doing it himself. The methods described in detail are only some of those which can be used, and variations can be left to the ingenuity of the individual.

It is better to use finger methods as these are much less likely to cause trauma. And when it comes to handling lenses, confidence is more easily achieved when a minimum of artificial aids is necessary.

The patient who has lost his suction holder and is dependent on it to remove his lenses can be in a real dilemma. For this reason suction holders should only be supplied for removing lenses from the cornea as a last resort after all other methods have been tried in vain. To eliminate this danger, the safe keeping of the suction holder must be emphasized to this group of patients. Recommending spare suction holders to be kept safely at work and at home is expedient.

INSERTION AND REMOVAL OF CORNEAL LENSES

Insertion is more easily managed by working from the same side as the eye on to which the lens is to be placed, so that the facial contours do not interfere with lens manipulation.

FINGER METHOD OF INSERTION

The lens is placed on the forefinger of one hand. The second finger of this hand is used to hold the bottom lid down and also to steady the inserting hand. The other hand is used to hold up the top lid, and while some fixation point is regarded with the other eye, the lens is gently placed on to the cornea. If the lids are held apart for a moment after the lens has been placed on the cornea, then the lens is less likely to be dislodged on the first strong blink. The patient should then look down. Best lid control is obtained if the lids are held near to but not actually over the lashes (*Figure 8.1*).

By the Practitioner

Standing beside the patient, ideally the practitioner should work on the same side as the eye being fitted, for best lens control. It needs a little practice to become equally adept with either hand, but the ease of doing it this way makes the practice worth while. The patient is instructed to look at a suitable object so that the line of sight is depressed, and the lens is gently placed on to the upper part of the cornea and allowed to move into place before the lids are released.

By the Patient

This may be done over a horizontally placed mirror. Fixation is maintained by the eye which is not receiving the lens. This reduces the avoidance reflex causing eye deviation if the lens is watched as it approaches the cornea. When the lens insertion technique has been mastered efficiently with the mirror the patient should try to insert the lens without the mirror. The eye receiving the lens has to fixate the lens, or, better still, looks at some object directly ahead so that the cornea remains centred within the palpebral aperture. Many patients prefer to learn this way as they find it upsetting to watch themselves in a mirror.

Some patients prefer to use a vertical mirror. They should be warned that the lens is more likely to slip off the finger and get lost with this method.

The patient learning to insert corneal lenses has to remember a number of points and they are not always co-ordinated immediately. Three main points are worth underlining when instructing the patient: (1) keep a very firm grip on the lid margins; (2) only let the lids go when the lens is definitely felt to have settled on the cornea; (3) keep fixation stationary until both lids have been gently released.

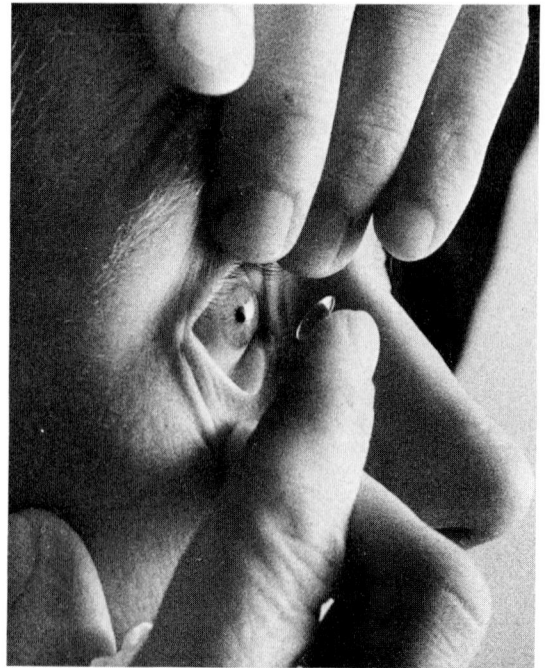

Figure 8.1–Insertion of a corneal lens

INSERTION BY THE SUCTION HOLDER METHOD

Instead of being placed on the forefinger, the lens is lightly pressed on to the end of a moistened suction holder and transferred from this to the eye by the technique set out above. This is a less satisfactory method than placing the lens on the forefinger as it is more likely to cause damage when inexpertly used and generally causes a larger avoidance eye movement. It also relies on the patient always having a suction holder to hand.

Variations of the suction holder technique are sometimes employed and usually incorporate a fixation target such as a light seen through the hollow handle. High hyperopes, presbyopes, and aphakics may have to resort to such methods of lens insertion if they cannot see to manipulate the lens at short distances. They may also find it useful to have a spectacle frame, glazed on one side only with a prescription for near work. The lower part of the front on the other side is removed from the frame and the first contact lens is inserted through the empty half of the frame. It should then be possible to see to insert the other lens.

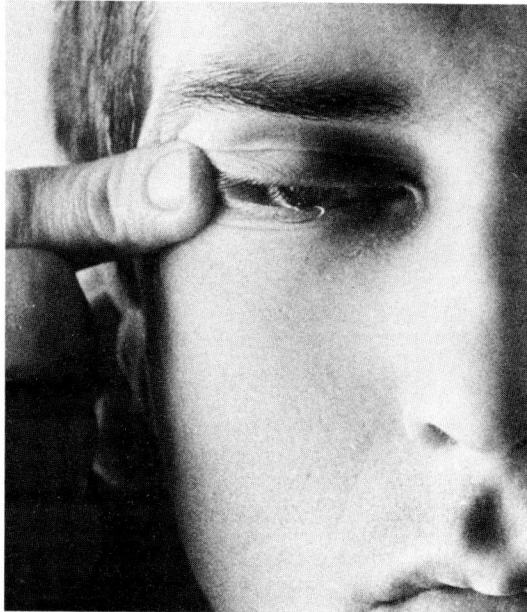

Figure 8.2–Lid removal of a corneal lens using one finger

ONE-HANDED INSERTION

This method is occasionally necessary when a patient has only one hand which can be used. In this case, the lids are held apart with the first and third fingers while the second finger is used to place the lens on the eye. Some patients can inhibit the blink reflex so well that they only need hold the bottom lid down with the middle finger and place the lens on the cornea with the forefinger.

INSERTION TECHNIQUE VARIATIONS

Patients often develop ingenious and sometimes awkward-looking methods for inserting and removing contact lenses. As long as the method is unlikely to damage their eyes or lenses there is no reason for change.

REMOVAL BY BOTH THE PRACTITIONER AND THE PATIENT

With the cornea central in the palpebral aperture, the lids are opened as wide as possible. To keep the lids taut the patient should be told to keep his eyebrows raised and stare wide all the time until the lens is expelled. The forefinger, middle finger or thumb is placed at the outer canthus. The lids are then pulled outwards in the direction of the top of the ear so that both lids are tensioned equally at the top and bottom of the lens. An extra pull with the finger or a strong blink will then lift the lens off the eye as shown in *Figure 8.2*. Some patients find that a slight head turn to position the cornea just in the nasal part of the aperture is a useful posture to adopt prior to starting the removal technique. As the lens comes off the cornea it may drop, in which case it may be caught with a free hand. Alternatively it may stick on the lashes. In this case the patient closes his eyes and then the lens is removed with the fingers.

'SCISSORS' METHOD OF REMOVAL

Using One Hand

The cornea is again positioned centrally or slightly nasally in the palpebral aperture. The middle finger is placed on the upper lid margin and the third finger on the lower lid margin as shown in *Figure 8.3*. The two fingers can control the upper and lower lids independently. It is important that the margins are in contact with the globe; an 'ectropion' lid posture cannot result in successful lens removal. When correctly positioned, the lids are pulled towards the ear as described above.

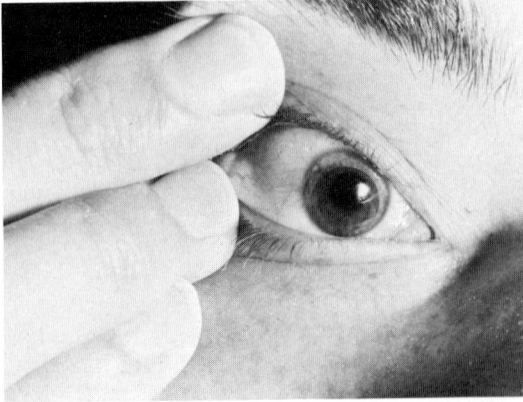

Figure 8.3—Lid removal of a corneal lens using two fingers

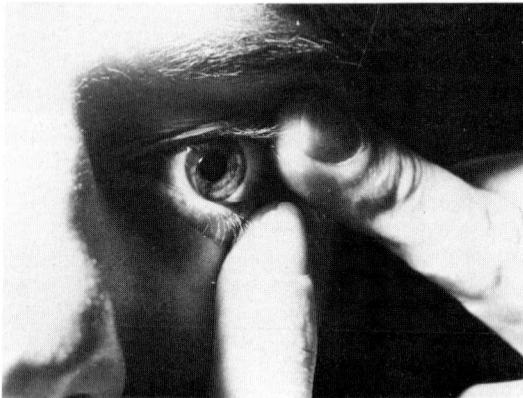

Figure 8.4—Lid removal of a corneal lens using one finger of each hand

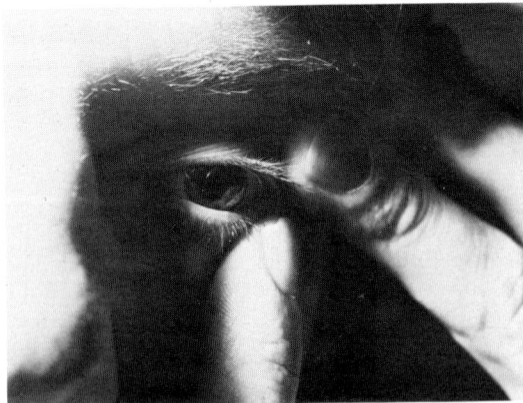

Figure 8.5—Later stage of removal. The lens is just coming away from the cornea. Temporal movement of the lens is almost inevitable

Using Two Hands

The forefingers of each hand are positioned on the top and bottom lids as shown in *Figures 8.4 and 8.5*. The method is essentially the same as in using one hand only.

The scissors method is normally used when the conventional method is inadequate; the usual reason for failure being the top lid descending over the lens while the pulling action occurs. Before trying the scissors method it may be worth positioning the single finger more on the top lid rather than exactly at the outer canthus.

SUCTION HOLDER REMOVAL OF LENS

The lids are held apart in the same way as that used for inserting a lens. With the top lid held up by the free hand and the lower lid held down by the hand using the moistened suction holder, the thumb and forefinger hold the suction holder bulb, which is squeezed before the flat end is pressed gently against the lens. When the thumb and forefinger are eased apart, the lens is sucked on to the holder and can be removed from the eye. Sometimes a small twist as the lens comes off the cornea helps to break the suction between lens and cornea (*Figure 8.6*). This method is often useful when dealing with a tense patient.

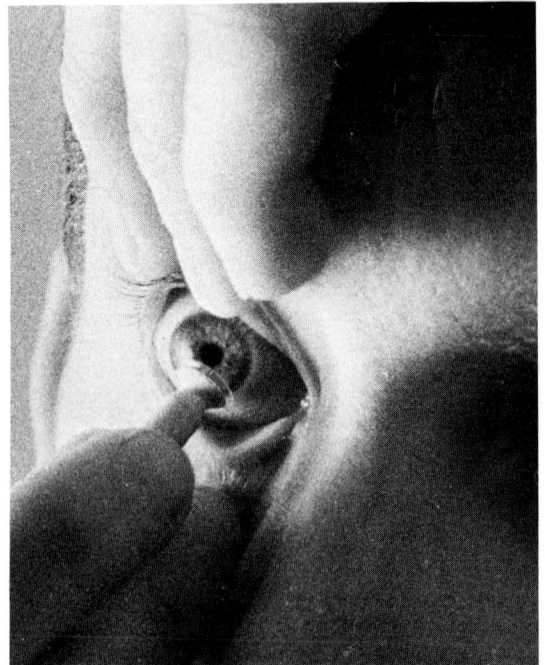

Figure 8.6—Using a suction holder to remove a corneal lens

A large amount of suction is not required in most cases. The common fault is not getting the cup end of the suction holder central and parallel to the lens. Patients having to use this method as a last resort usually have narrow apertures and/or enophthalmic eyes.

Before any repeated attempts are made at lens removal by this method, the patient should be instructed to check that the lens is still on the cornea in order to prevent possible corneal insult by the suction holder.

With all the above methods of lens removal the practitioner must be willing and able to help the patient by demonstrating on himself. It is also useful for him to remove a lens from the patient's eye to demonstrate a particular aspect; for example, the force used by the fingers when pulling the lids. When using the fingers in conjunction with a mirror the practitioner must emphasize that pulling on the lids after the top lid has passed over the lens edge can have no effect except to keep the lens in and make the eye sore. Similarly, it is difficult to remove a corneal lens if there is excessive lacrimation. Tears should be allowed to subside before attempting removal. The lid margins can then grip and pass under the lens edges more effectively.

LENS ON THE BULBAR CONJUNCTIVA

Some corneal lens wearers habitually place the lens on to the conjunctiva and then centre it. Occasionally, the practitioner may place the lens on to the conjunctiva of a nervous patient and then move it carefully on to the cornea. More frequently a corneal lens locates itself on the conjunctiva from faulty insertion or removal technique. The patient must be able to find the lens if this happens, and it must be emphasized that the lens cannot get lost behind the eye. The position of the lens can usually be located because it can be felt as the eye moves, except when in the upper fornix. To expose the lens maximally it is usually easier to use a vertical mirror. The patient can expose various sections of the bulbar conjunctiva by appropriate head movements; for example, tilting the head down and looking up, if the lens is displaced downwards. Pulling the lids away from the globe can also help in the search for a misplaced lens. Having found the lens it can be removed with a suction holder or recentred on to the cornea.

The lens can be centred by using the lid margin to push the lens into the required position or back on to the cornea. *Figure 8.7* shows a lens being moved from the lower conjunctival sac towards

the cornea. The lid is pulled down as necessary, so that the margin is beyond the furthest edge of the lens. Then, using two fingers to prevent the lens moving sideways, the lid margin is used to push the lens back on to the cornea. It is useful to press down gently on the edge of the lens furthest from the cornea. This will lift the lens edge closest to the cornea and minimize the risk of abrasion when the lens is centred. From the patient's point of view the lens is most easily centred when it is on the upper or lower sectors of the conjunctiva.

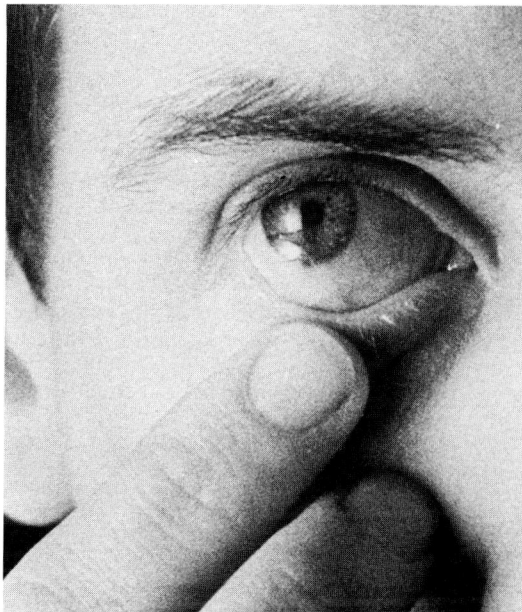

Figure 8.7–Centring a corneal lens with the lower lid

It is often simpler to move the lens into one of these areas before attempting to centre it. Again, the lid margin can be used to move the lens across the conjunctiva to the desired area. When using the lower lid to manipulate the lens, it is best to tell the patient to hold the upper eyelid up, out of the way, and vice versa.

Alternatively, the lens can sometimes be located by closing the eye and feeling through the lids with one or two fingers. The lens may be centred by forming the fingertips of one hand into a circle and, with the eye still closed, massaging through the lids to centralize the lens. This is a haphazard approach and is often unsuccessful. It can be useful if the lens has moved into the superior fornix and may be occluded by the orbital margin.

INSERTION AND REMOVAL OF SCLERAL LENSES

INSERTION

The insertion methods are the same whether done by the practitioner or by the patient. The lens is best inserted into the superior fornix. With the eye looking down, the upper lid is lifted by the opposite hand. The lens is grasped at or slightly below its horizontal meridian on each side by the thumb and second finger (*Figure 8.8*). If the lens is fenestrated, then the fenestration should be orientated before the lens is inserted on to the eye. The first finger is positioned against the lower front optic portion and serves to support the lens. The top edge of the lens is gently touched on to the superior portion of the bulbar conjunctiva and allowed to follow the contour of the eye into the superior fornix. While it is held in this position by the fingers, the forefinger of the other hand is used to manipulate the top lid down over the lens, which holds the lens in position. The patient then looks up and the lower lid is simultaneously pulled down so that the lower portion of the lens moves on to the inferior bulbar conjunctiva and the lens is then in position. During this procedure, blinking or closing the eyes must be resisted as a really hard blink may trap the lower lid under the lower edge of the lens and it is then necessary to pull the lid free so that it moves comfortably over the lens.

REMOVAL

Removal is accomplished by looking downwards, which exposes the upper edge of the lens when the upper lid is raised. The tip of the forefinger is used to hold the top lid at its nasal margin close against the eye above the lens, and pulling it taut up across the superior aspect of the eye causes the lid margin to move under the top edge of the lens and lever it away from the eye. By looking upwards and pulling the lower lid away from the eye, the lens is finally expelled (*Figure 8.9*).

Alternatively, a small suction holder placed on to the superior haptic portion of the lens may be used to pull the top of the lens away from the eye, if the lid method is not successful. A slight twist of the suction holder helps to break any suction between lens and eye.

Care should be taken to supervise patients habitually using the lid removal method to make sure that a fingernail is not used to lever the top of the lens from the eye as this could lead to trauma and, possibly, infection.

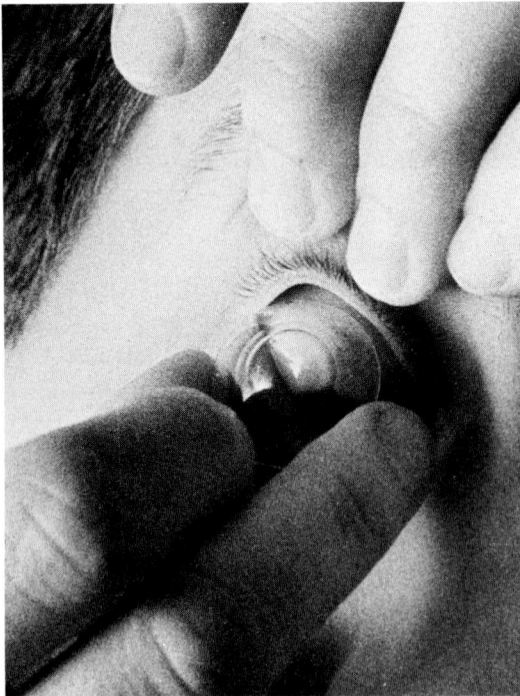

Figure 8.8–Inserting a scleral lens

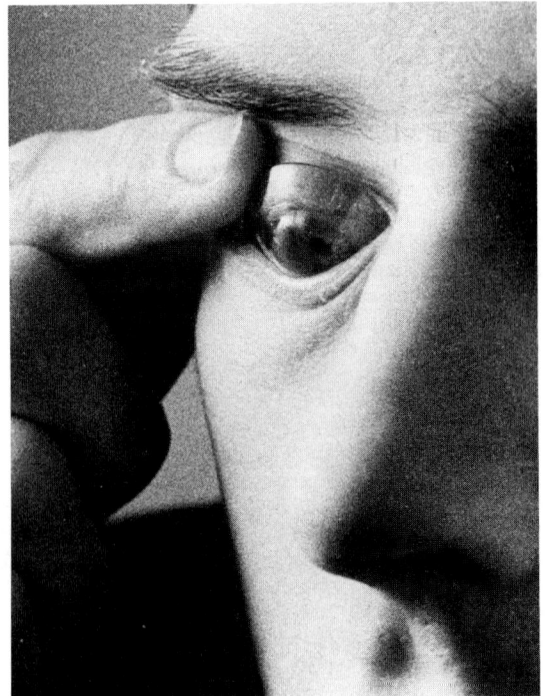

Figure 8.9–Lid removal of a scleral lens

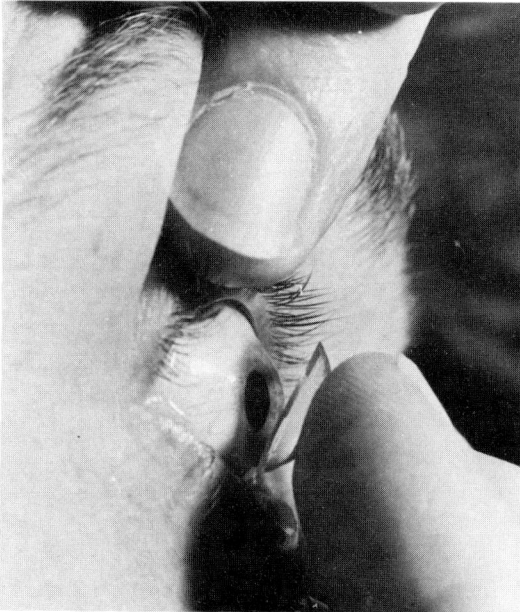

Figure 8.10–Practitioner insertion of a semi-scleral hydrophilic lens

INSERTION AND REMOVAL OF
HYDROPHILIC LENSES

INSERTION

If the lids are loose and the palpebral aperture is
large compared with the overall size, a soft lens
can be inserted exactly as described above for
insertion of hard corneal lenses. The greater bulk
of the hydrophilic lens means that it can more
easily fall off the finger during insertion and it is
more likely to catch on the lashes. *Figure 8.10*
shows a practitioner inserting a soft lens and
Figure 8.11 shows patient insertion of a lens
using a horizontal mirror. Insertion with the
head held horizontally minimizes the risk of the
lens falling off the finger. Ultra-thin lenses must be
allowed to dry for a few moments before insertion
otherwise they turn inside out on the finger.

If the above method is unsatisfactory the lens
can be placed on the temporal, inferior or superior
conjunctiva and then if it does not centre itself it
can be gently manipulated by means of the lid or a
finger on to the cornea – *Figure 8.12* shows this
operation. Care must be taken that fingernails
do not damage the lens. If the patient makes large
avoidance eye movements when a lens approaches
the cornea, thus precluding the use of the first
method, this indirect method of insertion is
normally successful.

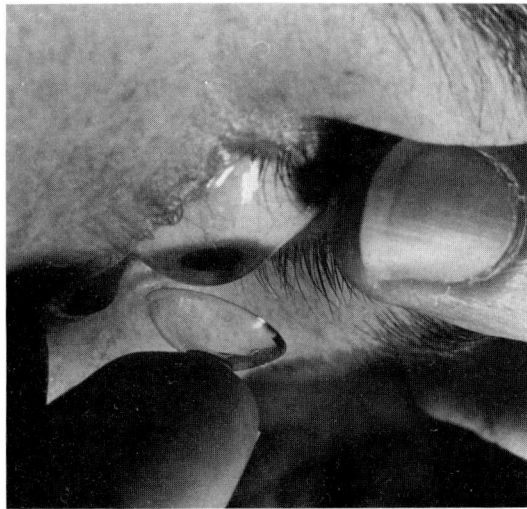

Figure 8.11–Patient inserting a hydrophilic lens

Another method is to fold the lens in half
vertically between thumb and forefinger, and with
the patient looking down and the upper lid raised
the lens is tucked under the upper lid and allowed
to unfold on to the eye. It may then be centred
if necessary, but it usually centres itself.

Before hydrophilic lenses are inserted it is wise
to check that the lens is not inside out. Classically
the profile of the lens should indicate if this has
happened. *Figures 8.13* and *8.14* show a lens the
correct way round and the same lens inside out.
With very thin lenses the difference is not so
obvious. A further check can be made by folding
the lens inwards gently between thumb and
forefinger. If the edges move inwards the lens
is the right way round, if they bend outwards it
is inside out.

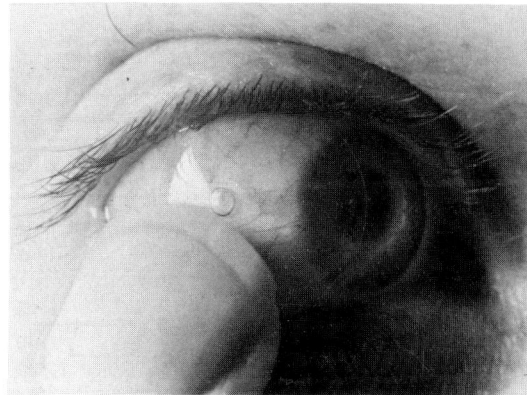

Figure 8.12–A hydrophilic lens being moved from the
temporal conjunctiva to the cornea

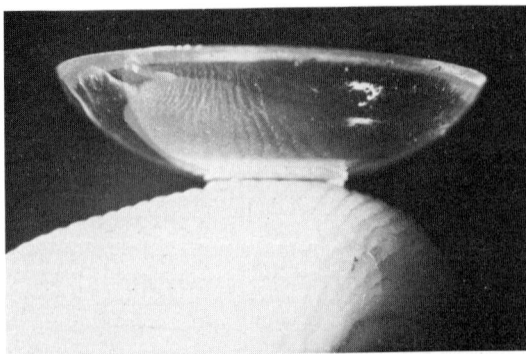

Figure 8.13–A hydrophilic lens the right way round

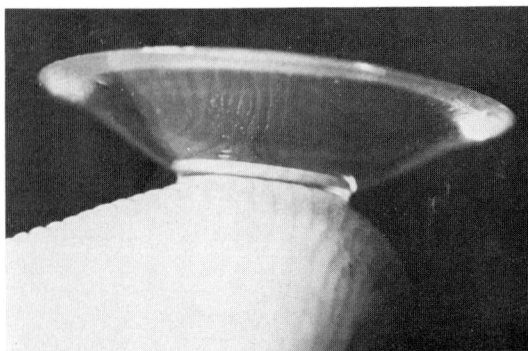

Figure 8.14–The same lens as shown in Figure 8.13, but inside out

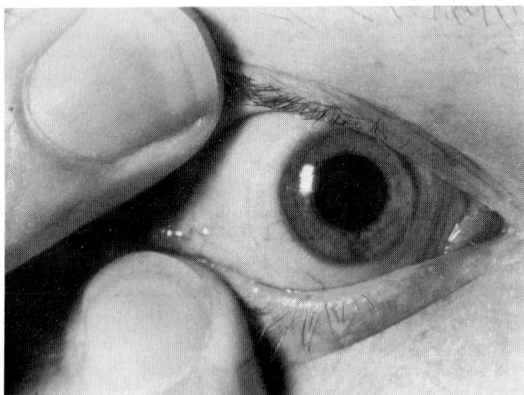

(a)

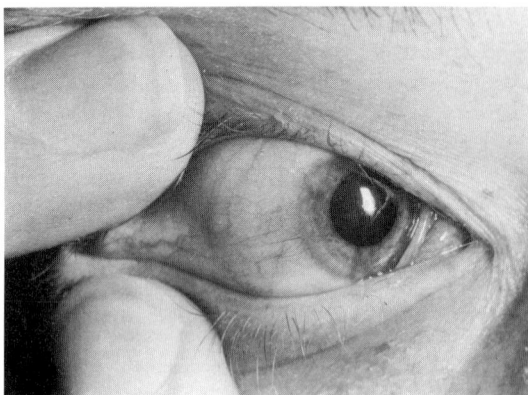

(b)

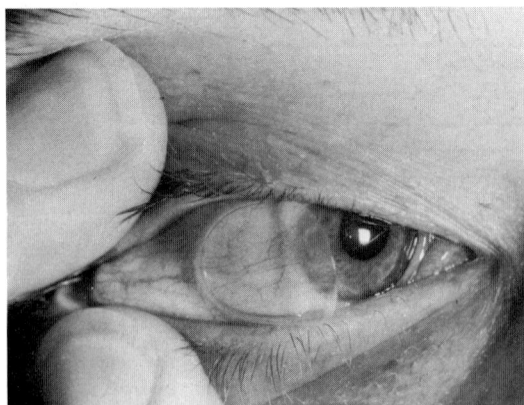

(c)

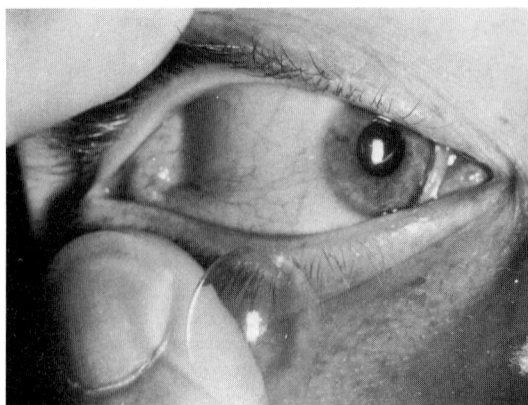

(d)

Figure 8.15–(a)–(d). Removal sequence of a hydrophilic lens using one finger of each hand

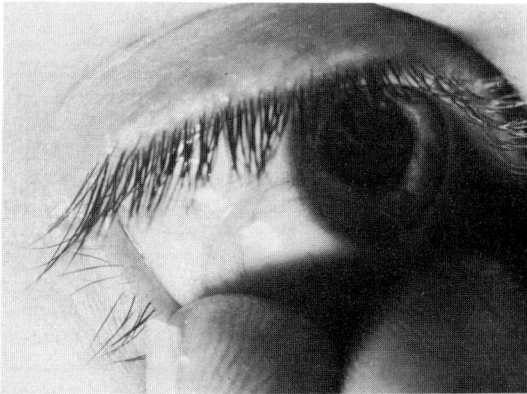
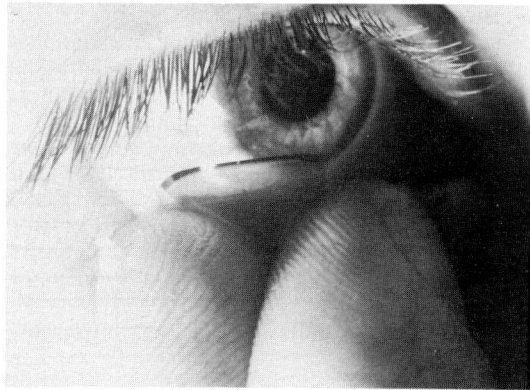

(a)   *(b)*

Figure 8.16—(a) and (b). Pinching a hydrophilic lens between finger and thumb of one hand to remove the lens from the lower fornix

REMOVAL

The method chosen to remove a soft lens will depend on dexterity, size of lens, lid and palpebral aperture characteristics as well as factors such as lens thickness and lens material. It is worthwhile consulting the manufacturer's literature regarding lens removal.

The first method is essentially the same as the 'scissors' method described for removing hard corneal lenses although the lids must be held slightly further apart to allow for the larger lens size. The forefinger of each hand is used on the lid margins. *Figure 8.15a–d* shows the removal sequence. If the patient glances nasally towards the end of the operation, this often facilitates removal.

The second method involves moving the lens from the cornea to the inferior or temporal conjunctiva. With the lens in this position the patient or practitioner can gently pinch the lens between forefinger and thumb and remove the lens from the eye. Again, great care must be taken to avoid damaging the lens or eye with the fingernails. This method causes considerable lens flexure and if the finger pressure is too great the material may be affected adversely over a long period. *Figure 8.16a and b* shows a soft lens being pinched off the eye.

The third method utilizes a suction holder. The lens is moved on to the inferior or temporal conjunctiva with a finger. (The importance of this should be stressed to the patient.) With a small amount of suction the lens can then be removed in the same way as a hard corneal lens is removed from the conjunctiva. *Figure 8.17* shows removal with a suction holder.

REACTIONS TO THE FIRST LENS

Cleanliness is important in all aspects of contact lens practice. The patient should be made aware of this both by instruction as well as by the practitioner's own example of hygiene.

The patient must be prepared physically and psychologically for the insertion of the first lens. It should be stated that some initial discomfort (use of the word 'pain' is deprecated) and lacrimation is quite normal. It is explained that these initial symptoms usually subside quickly and the lens becomes more tolerable. Most patients admit that the first lens feels much better than expected and there is no harm in telling a new patient this before the lens is inserted.

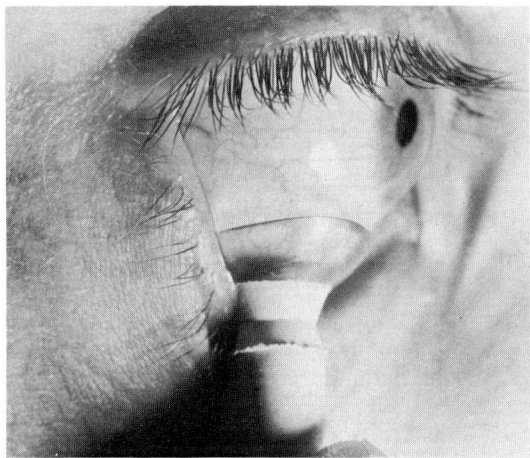

Figure 8.17—Removal of a hydrophilic lens from the lower fornix using a suction holder

There may well be some irritation for the first minute or two. The new patient has no experience in deciding what may be the cause of this irritation. The practitioner should bear in mind such factors as pH, tonicity, solutions and foreign bodies. A small piece of dust or fluff behind a lens can be very irritating. Removing the lens, cleaning it appropriately and re-inserting it can often give a dramatic improvement. With a soft lens it is often sufficient to move the lens on to the conjunctiva for a few seconds and then centre it back on the cornea.

The patient should always be sitting comfortably with his head supported. He should be given a tissue to wipe his cheeks if tears overflow.

If a hard lens is selected this should be first cleaned in a suitable antiseptic solution and then thoroughly rinsed in cold water. This minimizes the adhesion of fluorescein to the front surface. A lens with a greasy front surface can cause fluorescein adhesion and the true assessment of the fluorescein pattern becomes difficult. Hard lenses coated with wetting solution may also give confusing fluorescein patterns.

A soothing explanation of what is taking place helps to calm the patient. It should be treated as a matter of course if the lens should fall before being inserted, or if the first attempt is not successful. It is essential not to panic at any stage.

Excess lacrimation, blepharospasm, engorgement of conjunctival vessels or extreme sensitivity may contra-indicate the use of contact lenses, if these symptoms do not subside in a reasonable time.

Unless a scleral lens is fitting very poorly the patient does not experience much discomfort relative to that felt with a hard corneal lens. If the lens is too large there may be localized sensation at the edges. It is often reported that the eye feels full and hot.

With a hard corneal lens most of the sensation comes from the top lid moving over the lens edge, because the lid margins are very sensitive. The lids being somewhat tense will cause some pressure effects on the lens. These points can easily be demonstrated by the practitioner moving the lids well away from the lens; the patient then admits that the sensation virtually disappears completely. It may be worthwhile for the practitioner to assess the edge fit; if too tight it can produce discomfort. Assuming no foreign bodies and a reasonable fit, the symptoms from a corneal lens soon pass. Patient relaxation and reduction in corneal sensitivity obviously assist this process. The patient can be told this will occur.

Most people react very favourably to hydrophilic lenses. There is often significantly less reaction than with a hard lens, and although the

reaction of the patient is of consequence the practitioner must not choose a lens type on this basis. Other significant factors must be taken into account before this very important decision is taken.

A patient who sweats profusely, sways about in the chair, complains of a 'stuffy atmosphere', or turns pale, may be in the early stages of fainting or vomiting. It is useful to be prepared for this after the insertion of the first lens. If in doubt, the patient should be asked if he feels well, and if necessary his head may be held down. The patient should not be left alone in this state as he may fall from the chair and injure himself. The contact lens should be removed as soon as it is practicable to do so and the patient given adequate time to recover. It is usually of no use to continue the fitting as the patient may faint again if another lens is inserted. It is useful to be able to obtain assistance easily in any emergency so that a glass of water or smelling salts can be handed to the patient. The presence of another person may be desirable for the practitioner's own protection and be reassuring to the patient.

After the initial symptoms have passed — and this may take 5 or 10 minutes — the fit and performance of the first lens is observed. Some patients are very apprehensive about the instillation of fluorescein to check the fit. If they look down and in, or up and in, while a minimal quantity is applied to the bulbar conjunctiva from an impregnated strip, they are usually soon reassured by the lack of discomfort. After assessing all aspects of the fit of the first lens, it is then removed. Excess lacrimation and renewed tension at this prospect often make removal difficult. It is essential, therefore, that the practitioner is proficient at this. He must have several methods at his disposal, and he should be able to vary them according to the circumstances so that the lens is quickly removed with minimum discomfort.

The basic fitting methods for hard corneal lenses, scleral lenses, and hydrophilic lenses are dealt with in Chapters 11, 9, 10, and 14 in Volume 2 respectively.

REFRACTION WITH CONTACT LENSES

HARD LENSES

The special technique of refraction using FLOM lenses is dealt with in Chapter 10.

With corneal lenses, excess lacrimation, mucus production and lens movement make patient observation difficult. Hence, a satisfactory endpoint in subjective refraction is not always easy. If the lens does not centre well or the patient blinks at a high rate, then again refraction is variable. The duochrome chart may help. The maximum positive power acceptable should be given and the Humphriss balancing technique is useful in helping to keep accommodation relaxed.

Although in most cases only a spherical correction is necessary, the astigmatism manifested with a contact lens in place should still be measured. This may be done most easily with a retinoscope – but if good acuity is not obtainable with a spherical correction, or if the patient is hypercritical, a subjective measurement should be made. The methods and criteria for correcting residual astigmatism are set out in Chapter 18, Volume 2. It is generally found that up to 0.75 D of astigmatism may be left uncorrected without reducing visual acuity, though individual acceptance varies.

It is important to check for any vertical heterophoria when the patient has a lens in each eye. The spectacle correction gives a clue as to whether correcting prism may have to be incorporated.

It is often useful to order the power of a lens +0.25 D more than the power deduced from the refraction. The excess lacrimation with the trial lens provides a temporary increase in negative power and the discomfort of a contact lens can cause the patient to accommodate slightly. In addition, most practitioners find – if it is necessary later to modify a lens – that it is relatively easy to add negative power or reduce positive power but more difficult to reduce negative power or increase positive power (see Chapter 23, Volume 2).

If power changes are necessary, they can be carried out once the patient is fully adapted. It is then easier for the patient to concentrate and make accurate judgments in subjective testing. For this reason, binocular balancing is best left until this time.

HYDROPHILIC LENSES

Many of the points mentioned above in relation to hard lenses still apply to soft lenses. It is important to remember that neither the practitioner nor the soft lens laboratory can satisfactorily modify the power of finished lenses.

To ensure accurate refraction with hydrophilic lenses a stable lens fit is required. 'Vaulting' by a steep lens proves particularly troublesome. A trial lens with power and other parameters as close as possible to the patient's intended prescription is helpful, as well as behaving more nearly like the final lens.

Most corneal astigmatism is transmitted by a soft lens. Residual astigmatism is sometimes less and sometimes more than expected. It should be measured, recorded, and its effects anticipated in every case.

Lenses should be well settled before a refraction is performed. It is preferable and convenient to do this after a tolerance trial, but 20 minutes wear would be a minimum before a final assessment is made. If vision checks are performed during fitting a shorter time for the lens to settle has to be allowed even though this is not ideal.

Vision which cannot be stabilized to a satisfactory level is a contra-indication for fitting soft lenses. If it is stable and the quality is poor the practitioner should think of alternative lens designs (soft and hard). The quality of vision may be judged by asking the patient to look at a small spotlight in the dark. If it does not appear round and well-defined, but instead looks distorted, or streaky, then the quality of vision is poor. The use of toric hydrophilic lenses may be helpful if poor quality is related to residual astigmatism that is quantitatively constant (see Chapter 4, pages 109–111 and 115–118, also Chapter 18, Volume 2).

TOLERANCE TRIALS

A tolerance trial should be carried out routinely. Whether this is a short term trial of an hour or two, or an extended trial depends on the practitioner and the individual patient.

From the patient's point of view a tolerance trial gives him an opportunity of wearing contact lenses for a period and assessing his own reaction to the experience. Gross causes of intolerance; for example, acne rosacea, can show up. The cornea is put under 'stress' for a short time. The practitioner can then assess the corneal reaction with the slit lamp. Corneal changes may indicate the desirability of an extended tolerance trial, that is, a period greater than 2 hours.

There are several reasons why a short tolerance trial may be of little use. The practitioner may not be able to find a pair of lenses near the required specification in terms of fit and power. The patient may well show worse results from poor fitting lenses than from those of the correct specification. Long-term effects may not show up; for example, 3 o'clock and 9 o'clock staining, spectacle blur, effects of oedema and poor motivation. The practitioner must also consider the time factor in administering the tolerance trials.

If, at this stage, the practitioner considers the patient to have a good chance of being a successful contact lens wearer he may order a pair of lenses of the required specification. The patient then has an extended tolerance trial of up to a month, following a full instruction session. Most practitioners can quote examples of patients who perform badly on short tolerance trials and in the long term turn out to be very successful. Conversely, there are people who do well with a short trial but eventually cannot wear their lenses for longer than about 6 hours. If the patient progresses well the ordered lenses can be retained by the patient. Most patients seem prepared to pay a fee for an extended trial of this nature and have their case reviewed at the end of the period. If both the patient and the practitioner are quite happy with progress then the balance in fees can be paid. On the other hand, it may be quite obvious that to continue would be a waste of the patient's money as well as wasted time for both parties.

If the practitioner does not order lenses specially for the tolerance trial he will have to draw on his own stock of lenses. Lenses with back vertex powers close to the correct prescription should give a fair impression of the visual acuity expected with contact lenses. Otherwise, low power lenses can be used and the patient wears his own spectacles in conjunction with the contact lenses to obtain reasonable visual acuity. If the back surface specification of the lenses differs from the correct values the patient should be so informed. The practitioner must also take this into account when assessing the results of the trial. Hard corneal lenses used for tolerance trials should be kept in soak in a storage solution for 24 hours beforehand so that they are fully hydrated (Phillips, 1969).

At the end of the tolerance trial the following points should be checked and compared with similar observations made at the commencement of the trial.

Hard Corneal Lenses

(1) Lens comfort and patient's reactions. State of eyelids and margins. Condition of conjunctivas.

(2) Refraction and visual acuity with lenses *in situ.*

(3) Lens position and movement.

(4) Lens fit with fluorescein. If the fit has flattened, especially centrally, the possibility of central corneal epithelial oedema should be borne in mind. Pachometry may be useful.

(5) Slit lamp biomicroscopy. Epithelial oedema and its sequelae, corneal drying, staining and abrasions (other than those due to foreign bodies) must be carefully investigated. *Colour Plates II, IV* and *V* illustrate some of the appearances which may be seen. If abnormalities are discovered a further tolerance trial may be required using lenses of different specifications.

Epithelial oedema may be relieved by fenestration (single or multiple) with holes 0.25—0.50 mm diameter in the central portion (*see*

Colour Plate VI), or by making the lens smaller and/or flatter (*see* Chapter 16, Volume 2). The central and peripheral portions of the lens must be considered. Alterations to the back central optic diameter, width of peripheral bands and blending of curves all need thought when considering changing specifications. Corneal drying and staining in the 3 o'clock and 9 o'clock positions is normally only seen after an extended trial. It may be remedied by thinner lenses, using a closer fitting periphery, changing the lens mobility by altering the overall size of the lens or possibly by teaching the patient to blink properly. Stains due to transitions and edges can be remedied by blending and reshaping respectively. Central corneal abrasions may be due to flat fitting or oedema.

(6) Keratometry. An alteration in curvature of more than 0.2 mm suggests that a modification in the lens design is required. Oedema is often accompanied by corneal steepening and thickening.

(7) Spectacle refraction and visual acuity. Ideally, this should be unchanged. No more than 1.00 D of spectacle blur is normally acceptable.

Scleral Lenses

Similar observations should be made with scleral lens wearers provided that suitable (fenestrated) tolerance trial lenses are available. Usually, the final lenses must be ordered for tolerance trials and these are then modified according to the results of the trial. Particular attention should be paid to ensuring mobility of limbal bubbles under the lens, as a cornea which dries due to a stagnant bubble often subsequently vascularizes. *Colour Plate VII* shows neo-vascularization of the cornea.

Hydrophilic Lenses

The changes induced by soft lenses are normally less than those seen with hard lenses. There is rarely any spectacle blur, keratometer readings from the cornea vary only by very small amounts, pachometry and aesthesiometry both reveal little change. Corneal staining is normally small in degree and area. It is useful to assess the residual refraction and visual acuity with the lenses *in situ*. The amount of residual astigmatism may bear little relation to the best sphere visual acuity. Stable visual acuity should be established and the quality of vision ascertained. The patient's observations are useful especially if blurred vision is noticed before or after a blink. Retinoscopy can be useful in assessing optical stability as can keratometry from the front surface of the soft lens. Mire clarity before and after blinking can help to assess the lens fit.

It is very important to inspect the conjunctiva for edge indentation by semi-scleral soft lenses. Positive indentation necessitates a change of lens specification, a different type of soft lens or a different water content material.

Obviously the fit of the lens needs careful observation. The criteria vary from one design to another and the practitioner must be aware of these.

Inspection of the front surface of the lens for accumulated debris and deposits is useful. Similarly, material trapped between the back of the lens and the cornea may be indicative of future problems.

Early signs of oedema caused by soft lenses are usually more difficult to detect than the oedematous changes caused by hard lenses. Correct illumination and observation of the cornea with the slit lamp are essential (*see* Chapters 5, 7, and 16 in Volume 2). Vertical striae of the posterior cornea are visible by direct illumination, and generalized oedema is noticeable as an increase in translucence of the cornea by indirect illumination. All practitioners fitting hydrophilic contact lenses should ensure that they can recognize these subtle changes.

Post-wear changes are discussed in more detail in Chapter 16, Volume 2.

LENS INSERTION AND REMOVAL BY THE PATIENT

During the initial examination, some practitioners like to give patients some experience in inserting and removing lenses themselves. This can help the patient's confidence in his ability to wear and handle lenses. Whether this is done depends on time available, but it is useful to have some idea of the patient's ability to handle lenses before proceeding further. Inability to insert and remove lenses is as important a contra-indication to contact lens wear as any of the others. However, with a very tense patient, further instruction may solve any difficulty of lens handling; and the use of an eyebath between consultations may aid relaxation. It has been found very useful with children to instruct them to spend 5 or 10 minutes daily practising the techniques of lens placement and removal. They should do this in front of a mirror and are told to get a drop of water on the insertion finger and imagine that it is the lens. This not only helps them to relax, but also gives them confidence in handling their eyes, so that by the time they collect their lenses they are usually adept at

controlling their eyelids and eye movements. Adults can, of course, benefit similarly from such practice.

ORDERING

The practitioner has now amassed the information needed to decide if the lenses are to be ordered and, if so, the necessary specification. He must be sure that the patient stands a reasonable chance of successfully adapting to contact lenses and wishes to continue. If the patient is likely to have any particular difficulty, then he should be told of this before the practitioner continues. If the patient still desires lenses and there are no disqualifying contra-indications, then an appointment is made to collect the finished lenses.

Before the patient leaves, a careful examination of the cornea is essential. A prophylactic, for example, sulphacetamide 10 per cent may be administered if any abrasions are present. If the conjunctiva is injected, a vasoconstrictor may be instilled for cosmetic reasons.

COLLECTION OF LENSES

From the moment a patient starts to wear the lenses prescribed for him, the practitioner is responsible for the continued well-being of the patient's eyes. This can only be achieved with painstaking care.

The lenses should be checked for accuracy and rejected, or modified to correct them, if necessary (*see* Chapters 12 and 15 and 23 in Volume 2). Hard corneal lenses should be stored in a sterile soaking solution for at least 24 hours before issue, to ensure that hydration is complete and that the lenses have attained a constant dimension. A further check of the hydrated BCOR serves to ensure that only the expected alteration has taken place (Phillips, 1969).

When the patient arrives, he should be informed as to the sequence of events at this consultation. A great deal of information is imparted on this occasion and it is very useful to have a printed sheet, covering the main points, which can be given to the patient for future reference. Addenda I and II, pages 203 and 207, give examples of information sheets for wearers of hard and soft lenses respectively. This is reassuring from the patient's point of view, as it provides an available source of information and guidance. It is also a source of protection to the practitioner if he should forget to mention anything, and is desirable from a legal standpoint.

CARE AND HYGIENE OF LENSES

Identification marks on the lenses and lens container should be shown. The patient should be instructed in how to remove the lenses from the container and how to insert the lenses for storage. Preferred methods of cleaning contact lenses should be explained and in the case of hydrophilic lenses a clear account of the ascepticizing regimen must be given. Details of, and applications of, any solutions handed to the patient must be clear. Future purchases of solutions must be applicable to the type of lens in use; the dangers of using the wrong solutions must be stressed. The patient must be made aware of the reasons for hygiene and must be educated in all aspects related to contact lenses and their usage.

The lenses can be inserted and as the patient adjusts to them further information can be given. Points which should be dealt with are: the methods of handling lenses; the adaptive difficulties that may be encountered; the fact that lenses cannot get lost behind the eye; the wearing schedule and consequences of over-wear; what to do if a foreign body enters the eye; the advantages of contact lens insurance. The patient is told to attend wearing his lenses at first and subsequent aftercare visits, having worn them for the maximum time indicated for that date by the wearing schedule. This enables the practitioner to assess the effects of several hours of wear.

When the practitioner is satisfied that the patient has adapted as much as possible to his lenses, an assessment of the fit may then be made. All the usual characteristics of the lens fit should be recorded, together with visual acuities. It is usually unwise to alter the power of the lenses at this stage unless the acuity is very poor. Scleral lenses may well need some small modifications before they are issued.

INSTRUCTION OF INSERTION AND REMOVAL

The patient should insert and remove his lenses several times before being allowed to leave with them. If this is not done efficiently at the first visit, he should return for further instruction before the lenses are issued.

When teaching insertion and removal, the practitioner must have several methods at hand and be able to vary them according to the needs of the patient. Failure of a particular method must be analysed for reasons of failure, and a new approach must be introduced. Failure often arises from lack of dexterity, lid characteristics and poor fixation.

The patient must be taught to retrieve a lens which has become displaced on to the bulbar conjunctiva, as discussed earlier.

ADAPTIVE AND OTHER DIFFICULTIES

It must be emphasized that adaptive symptoms do not arise with all patients, but they are expected and normal and should disappear within a few weeks. The reason for mentioning this is to prevent the patient from panicking if the unexpected occurs. The reaction when a foreign body gets under the lens, and the remedy, should be explained. Holding the lids apart may help to eject a foreign body, but often it is necessary to either remove the lenses or use the lids to move the lens off the cornea on to the bulbar conjunctiva to obtain relief. A foreign body which is ignored may cause a severe abrasion of the corneal epithelium. Other points which should be covered are the effects on lens wear of different atmospheric and environmental conditions; the effects of reflected light, for example, with night driving; photophobia; lacrimation and excessive lens movement; spectacle blur; the effects of poor health and of physical or emotional states on lens comfort; and the need for gradual re-adaptation if wearing has been suspended.

WEARING SCHEDULES

A daily wearing programme should be given to the patient. With hard lenses the first day may start with anything from half an hour to three hours depending on the patient. Half an hour extra per day is added to this time if it is comfortable to do so. The wearing period may be split into two daily periods. Using this schedule patients can attain all-day wear within a month. It should be stressed that a longer period of adaptation does not constitute failure on their part it merely underlines individual variation. Quicker rates of progress are possible, but a conservative approach is wise. A description of the 'over-wear syndrome' may be beneficial to those patients who are likely to exceed a safe rate of progress. The possibility of suffering severe ocular pain, accompanied by photophobia and lacrimation, as well as reduced vision is usually sufficient warning to prevent over-wear, especially if it is pointed out that these symptoms usually occur in the early hours of the morning, a few hours after removing the lenses. It may also be worth mentioning that the pain and discomfort may be considerably relieved by taking soluble aspirin, if over-wear symptoms do occur. A balance has to be struck between building up too slowly, when the patient may lose interest, and building up too quickly when the cornea may suffer.

The eyelid margins take between 7 and 14 days to adapt to corneal lens wear (Lowther and Hill, 1968). During this time, the lids may become oedematous, causing excess pressure on the contact lens and thence on the cornea, interrupting normal tears flow and disturbing corneal metabolism. The result is usually corneal epithelial oedema, and in its presence the fit of the lens may alter and abrasion of the oedematous area may result. If the corneal sensitivity has become lowered due to pressure on the nerve endings, it is possible for such an abrasion to remain unnoticed by the patient until some hours after lens removal, when the corneal sensitivity returns to normal. To assist adaptation and encourage adequate tears flow beneath the contact lens, the patient should be taught regular, relaxed blinking with complete eyelid closure at each blink (Wilson, 1970).

Patients wearing soft lenses encounter fewer adaptive difficulties than their hard lens counterparts. Most hard lens wearers who give up often do so because of discomfort from the lenses. With soft lenses this is rarely a cause of failure; it is more likely to be poor vision. The wearing schedule for the soft lens wearer can normally permit a quicker time increase than for the wearer of hard lenses. All-day wear achieved in a week or two is not uncommon. Most manufacturers offer advice on wearing schedules for their own lenses and it is as well to consult their literature on the subject.

If it is possible for the patient to keep a record of his contact lens wearing times, this can be of great help to the practitioner and to the patient in monitoring progress. Such a diary may be made out as follows.

Date	Wearing time	Any special reasons for lens removal, etc.
3/4/80	2½ hr	None
4/4/80	3 hr	Slight soreness of left eye

The patient should be made aware that if his eyes are in real need of attention he should contact his own practitioner if possible or, if the circumstances do not allow this, any other contact lens practitioner, ophthalmic optician, doctor or hospital casualty department.

With all the advice and tuition he has received, the patient should now be able to commence his period of adaptation to contact lenses.

The lenses, accessories and instructions should be presented and any arrangements made for insuring the lenses and paying the fees relating to the supply of the lenses. An appointment should be made for the first after-care visit and the patient is then, for the first time, able to wear his contact lenses without the direct supervision of the practitioner.

The practitioner can only exert his responsibility for the ocular well-being of the contact lens wearer by careful fitting, complete instruction and tuition, and continuing after-care.

FITTING CHILDREN WITH CONTACT LENSES

There is nothing particularly unusual about childrens' eyes. Teenagers are usually very good patients if they are well motivated. Most of this group are myopic girls. Maturing earlier, girls usually have a more responsible attitude towards contact lenses than boys of the same age. If the parents are paying for the lenses good communication and co-operation is absolutely essential.

Fitting children under the age of 10 years presents a few more problems. They often cannot see the point of it, they get bored quickly and communication can be minimal or unreliable. The practitioner requires greater patience than for older age-groups. Very young children and babies are best fitted in hospital departments. Scleral lenses are often prescribed and a general anaesthetic is used for impression taking. Parents have to be taught how to insert and remove the lenses if the child himself is not old enough to do it efficiently. Extended wear lenses will almost certainly be used more in the future for young children. Reliable toric soft lenses will be needed as a high percentage of potential wearers will need astigmatic corrections.

ADDENDUM I

Every practitioner must issue written instructions to each patient to supplement those given verbally. These should cover such information as lens handling and hygiene, insertion and removal methods with illustrative pictures or diagrams if possible, care of the eyes and normal symptoms and the wearing programme advised. Terminology used should be simple enough for the patient to comprehend. Minor variations may be made by each individual practitioner and the type of hard lens material may govern the solutions recommended.

The following section is taken from the Instruction Booklet used by one of the Editors in his practice and that used by the London Refraction Hospital.

INSTRUCTIONS TO PATIENTS WEARING HARD CONTACT LENSES

Most contact lenses are made of hard plastic material. They are ground and polished to very fine limits of accuracy using expensive equipment, so that when fitted they rest on your eye but still allow a film of tears to flow between the eye and the lens. Both they and your eyes deserve special care and attention.

HANDLING THE LENSES

(1) Hands must be clean and free of creams and nicotine. All traces of soap must be rinsed off. Avoid contamination of the lenses with perfumes and when using hair lacquer keep the eyes closed until the air has cleared.

(2) Whilst handling the lenses, always work over a smooth, soft surface such as a paper handkerchief spread over a table. This avoids scratching or losing a lens on the floor.

(3) If a lens is dropped, do not move until the lens is located. Always lift a dropped lens by wetting a fingertip or suction holder and gently touching the surface. Lenses must not be slid across table surfaces.

(4) Never wipe your lenses with a handkerchief or other material. When wiping is necessary, use only the softest of paper tissues.

(5) To avoid distorting the lenses, never leave them near heat, and handle very gently. Avoid holding the lenses by the edges.

(6) Fingernails should be clean and kept reasonably short to avoid scratching the eyes or contact lenses.

HYGIENE AND LENS STORAGE

Absolute cleanliness is essential in the handling and storage of contact lenses. In order to prevent dirt or any harmful organisms being transferred to the eye, the following rules must be observed.

(1) The lenses should be stored in the container provided, in one of the recommended soaking solutions.

(2) The level of soaking solution should be maintained in the container so that each lens is completely immersed in the solution. At least once a week the container should be emptied out and cleaned by being filled with I.C.I. 'Savlon'.* This is left for a period of at least half an hour (for instance, while the lenses are being worn) and then rinsed out with running tap water (or, ideally, boiled water that has been allowed to

---

* It is not advisable to recommend this solution if hard lenses are made from materials other than PMMA.

cool). The container is then refilled with fresh solution. (Never use bleach or other antiseptic solutions as they may be absorbed by the plastic of the container and then contaminate the lenses.)

(3) The lenses must *never* be stored dry as this allows the growth of bacteria and affects the curvature of the lens and the wetting ability of its surface.

(4) Before inserting your lenses, rinse off the soaking solution with cold water and apply one drop of recommended wetting solution to each lens, spreading it on to both surfaces of the lens with the fingers. The wetting solution maintains lens sterility, helps the surface wet more easily and forms a protective cushion in the event of a lens being inserted too quickly.

(5) On the removal of your lenses, clean with Savlon* (diluted with an equal quantity of water for this purpose), and rinse off the cleaning solution with fresh tap water before replacing the lenses in their container. Be sure to put the plug in the hand basin before rinsing lenses under running tap water.

(6) Never lick your lenses as harmful organisms can be transferred from the mouth to the eye.

(7) Keep hair clean and free of dandruff as this may lead to eye discomfort with contact lenses.

(8) Examine the lenses regularly for scratches and chips and to ensure that each lens is being worn in the correct eye. One or both lenses may be engraved with dots or R and L to identify them.

(9) You are strongly advised to insure your lenses against loss.

CORNEAL LENSES

INSERTION OF LENSES

Place the wetted lens on the tip of the forefinger of one hand, where it will be retained. Look downwards and, using two fingers of the other hand, hold the upper lid and eyelashes well up clear of the cornea. Now use the middle finger of the hand holding the lens to pull down the lower lid by the very edge. Keep the head and eyes pointing in the same direction and place the lens gently on to the cornea. Remove the forefinger, release the lower lid and *finally* the upper lid. The whole procedure is repeated for the other eye. The very tip of the second finger may be used as an alternative, with the third finger holding down the lower lid, if any difficulty is experienced using the forefinger.

If the lens slips on to the white of the eye, it may be replaced by lifting one lid beyond the lens and pushing it back on to the cornea with the lid margin, using a finger on either side of the lens as a guide. A mirror will aid lens location, and this should be held so that the eye is looking in the *opposite* direction from where the lens is positioned. Alternatively, a suction holder may be used if one is available.

If you cannot remove it from the white of the eye — **do not panic** — it is quite safe to leave it there, overnight if necessary, until you can obtain assistance. It cannot disappear behind the back of the eye as a fold of tissue prevents this. Nevertheless, in the case of an apparently lost lens, remember to check that it has not moved well under the lids.

REMOVAL

Although the first method described below is the simplest and most commonly used, you are strongly advised to practise all three techniques so that should one not work an alternative method may be used.

(1) Again, work over a table or hold the free hand cupped to catch the lens. Bend the head slightly and tilt it so that the eye is turned slightly towards the nose. Open the eyes as wide as possible, so that both lids are beyond the edges of the lens. Stare straight in front of you and place a finger at the outer corner of the eye, separating the lids slightly. Pull the lids towards the direction of the top of the ear and give a single blink, when the lens should be ejected from the eye. At first it may often stick to the lashes, from where it is easily removed. A quick glance in the opposite direction to the pull of the fingers at the same instant as the blink may aid lens ejection.

(2) The second method is to place the forefinger of each hand on the very edge of the upper and lower lid at the inner corner of the eye. Each lid is then slowly stretched around the lens and then together. Working over a mirror may be helpful at first, though this should be discarded as soon as possible as such artificial aids may not be available in an emergency. This also applies to the use of a suction holder as suggested in the third method of removal described below and a suction holder should not be used except where there is any initial difficulty with either of the above methods.

(3) The free hand should hold the upper lid away from the lens. Squeeze the bulb of the moistened suction holder firmly and place the end gently against the dome of the lens. Release the pressure on the bulb and slowly withdraw both holder and lens.

SCLERAL LENSES

INSERTION

Hold the lens by its edges with the middle finger and thumb of the right hand and with the forefinger resting on the optic portion (or dome of the lens) so that the wide part of the haptic rim of the lens will fit on the temporal side of the eye and the narrow part on the nasal side. Raise the upper lid with a finger of the left hand, placed over the lashes and edge of the lid. Pull the lid right up and look down at the chin. Gently place the upper edge of the lens on the white of the eye, and slide it up under the upper lid as far as it will go. Remember — **keep looking down all the time.** Release the upper lid but keep the lens pushed well up all the time. With the left hand, now pull down the lower lid from behind the lens, still gently pushing up the lens with the right forefinger. At the same time, look slowly and steadily upwards until the lens is settled under the lids. The vision may be blurred for a few minutes until the lens has filled with tears.

REMOVAL

The lens is removed by sliding the upper lid margin behind the lens. Look down towards the chin. Place a fingertip firmly on the edge of the upper lid, near the nose. Pull the edge of the lid up and back, at the same time sliding the finger along the edge and stretching the lid tightly behind the top edge of the lens. The lid should ease the lens off the eye and pass underneath the lens. Now look slowly upwards, and as the lens comes out catch it with a free hand.

A suction holder may be used instead. Squeeze the bulb of the holder and apply it firmly to the upper central part of the lens, avoiding the fenestration hole (if one is present). Leave the holder in position and look right down. Raise the upper lid as high as possible. Tilt the suction holder downwards and twisting it slightly, ease the top edge of the lens away from the eye. Now look slowly upwards and remove the lens from the eye.

CARE OF THE EYES

(1) Insert and remove lenses gently and slowly to avoid scratching the eyes.

(2) In the event of a foreign body becoming trapped behind the lens, the following procedure should be carried out.

If initial blinking does not move the particle, look downwards and hold the upper lid away from the eye for a few seconds. Repeat several times if necessary. If the particle is still present, remove the lens, clean and replace. The lens must *not* be left on the eye if there is a foreign body beneath it. If there is any discomfort when the lens is removed, the lens should not be re-inserted until the following day. If the discomfort persists until the following day, report to your practitioner for examination.

(3) Always seek advice if: (*a*) your eyes remain red or painful during or after wear; (*b*) you continually see coloured haloes around lights or if your vision becomes misty; (*c*) you notice white spots on the cornea which do not move on blinking.

(4) Always report for an examination of your eyes and lenses when advised to do so. An after-care examination is advised at least once a year after the first twelve months.

(5) Do not wear your lenses if you are ill or have a bad cold; or at least reduce your wearing period. Female patients may occasionally experience slight lens discomfort during the menstrual period, and possibly in the first month or two of taking the contraceptive pill or in the later stages of pregnancy. Advice should be requested where necessary.

NORMAL SYMPTOMS

Some symptoms, such as the following, are normal during the adaptation period and should not cause anxiety.

(1) Excessive blinking and watering of the eyes.

(2) Discomfort in bright lights, high winds, dusty atmospheres and on looking upwards. Use sun-spectacles if helpful.

(3) Discomfort when reading and in a stuffy atmosphere. Avoid both where possible in the first few weeks during lens wear.

(4) Comfort is greater out of doors than indoors.

(5) Moments of blurred vision and temporary double vision.

(6) Blurred vision with spectacles after wearing contact lenses. This is due to the gentle massaging effect of the lenses. The slightly blurred vision it produces is normally expected to last between 10 minutes and 3 hours. Report any great difference between the two eyes.

(7) Displacement of lenses on the eye. Usually due to poor insertion or removal.

(8) Annoying reflections from lights due to the increased lens movement present over the first few weeks.

(9) Headaches and tension in the face and forehead. Often found where the wearer is not relaxing the muscles in the brow.

If you are in any doubt about symptoms, please ask for advice.

WEARING PROGRAMME

The speed of adaptation varies greatly from individual to individual. The following gives a good guide, though it may be necessary to adapt slightly more slowly or quickly depending on individual tolerance.

On the first day, wear the lenses for from ½ to 2½ hours, depending on comfort. Increase by ½ an hour every day until 5 hours have been attained. Now add ¾ of an hour every day until 10 hours have been achieved, when 1 hour may be added each day until maximum tolerance is achieved. The final daily increase should never be greater than 1¼ hours.

Wear your lenses every day. This is very important during the adaptation period.

Never wear your lenses longer than the recommended period no matter how comfortable they may be. Severe discomfort may be experienced several hours after lens removal if there has been gross over-wear. If the lenses have been left out for several days, for example, due to illness, re-adapt over several days. In cases of prolonged illness, special advice should be requested.

Slight discomfort of both lenses towards the end of the wearing schedule may be ignored, but the lenses should be removed if there is any marked discomfort of one or both lenses. If any discomfort occurs every day, mention this to the practitioner as occasionally a small modification to the lens becomes necessary as it settles on the eye.

Never leave your lenses in all night. You may rub the eyes during sleep and have sore eyes on waking. Also the presence of the lens deprives the cornea of its oxygen supply.

Do not drive with contact lenses in until you are fully adapted to them and have comfortable vision. This is particularly so at night when you may notice haloes or streamers around lights. Remember to keep a pair of spectacles in the car in case emergency removal of your contact lenses is necessary; for example, you may lose a lens or get something in your eye. These spectacles should provide good vision – do no rely on an old pair. Cyclists and motor cyclists should wear protective goggles or glasses. In daytime, sun-glasses can give protection from both light and dust, but **never** wear tinted glasses at night or at dusk even though glare from headlights may be troublesome with contact lenses, for the tint could then cause you to miss seeing poorly lit cars and pedestrians.

Where possible, wear your lenses outdoors at first and try to do something which will take your mind off your lenses. For instance, do not sit watching television or reading a book.

Make a note in your diary that in the event of an accident your contact lenses should be removed.

When you report for your first re-examination, usually after one to two weeks, **you must be wearing your lenses** and have been wearing them for the maximum period of tolerance that you have achieved; that is, if you have achieved a wearing time of 6½ hours, then you must have been wearing your lenses for this time when you come for your appointment.

ADDENDUM II

The following is based very largely on the Instruction Booklet used by one of the Editors (A. J. Phillips) in his practice.

INSTRUCTIONS FOR THE CARE AND HANDLING OF SOFT CONTACT LENSES

Patient's name . . . .

Date lenses issued . . . .

Hydrophilic (soft) contact lenses are designed to cover the entire cornea. Some lenses may overlap on to the 'white' of the eye. Virtually all soft lenses will tear or 'crack' and it is therefore essential that they are handled with great care. As the lenses contain a high proportion of fluid, daily disinfection of lenses worn for all waking hours is necessary. Lenses which are not clean greatly increase the risk of eye infection and ulceration. There are several methods of lens disinfection depending on the lenses you have been prescribed.

For 'daily wear' lenses you are advised to:

(1) Boil the lenses daily *only*.

or

(2) Disinfectant them using special solutions *only*.

or

(3) Use either of the above methods depending on convenience and the practitioner's recommendations.

For 'continuous wear' lenses you are advised to clean and disinfect your lenses every ..... weeks or as advised by the practitioner.

BOILING METHOD OF LENS DISINFECTION

Since tears contain a proportion of salt, it is important for comfort that the lenses are stored in a normal saline solution. This is conveniently obtained from a pharmacist in the transparent flexible containers (normally one litre) used as saline drips in hospitals. Alternatively, it can be prepared as follows.

(1) Fill the small squeeze bottle provided with purified water to the fill line.

(2) Add one salt tablet (prepared by the same laboratory as the squeeze bottle). Shake until the tablet is dissolved. It is probably better to do this a few hours before the lenses are removed from the eyes. Saline solution made up in this way is not sterile, but to prevent the growth of harmful organisms it is sensible to keep the solution in the refrigerator when not in use.

On removal, place the lens in the palm of the hand, concave side up. Wet it with saline solution (or preferably cleaning solution — *see* below) and rub gently but thoroughly with the fingertip. Take great care not to touch the lens with the fingernail. Alternatively, the lens may be cleaned by rubbing it between thumb and index finger. After cleaning, rinse thoroughly with saline solution. This should be done over a hand basin with the plug in place.

Having filled your container with fresh saline solution, place each lens in the appropriate compartment as instructed, and close the caps tightly.

Using distilled, purified or boiled water, fill the boiling unit (aseptor) to the correct level (usually indicated by a mark or line).

The lens container and aseptor lid are placed in position. The activating lever is then pressed. If the mains supply is on and the unit is functioning, a red light will come on. After about 15 minutes the light will go out and the water in the aseptor will have evaporated. After cooling to room temperature, the lenses are ready for wear. If the lenses are disinfected last thing at night the cooling period causes no inconvenience.

If the aseptor should not be functioning, or if you are away from home, then simply place the lens container (with lenses inside) into a saucepan of boiling water for 15 minutes, taking care that all the water in the saucepan does not evaporate. Alternatively, place the lens container (with lenses inside) into a vacuum flask of boiling water. Cap the flask normally and leave overnight. Ensure that the container has cooled before removing the lenses and inserting them in your eyes. This may be speeded up, if necessary, by holding the lens container under running cold tap water.

When the lens container is opened the lens may not be on its convex mount (if this is the type of container supplied). If this is so, empty the case and catch the lens in the palm of your hand.

If the solution has escaped from the container and the lens is adhering to the mount, fill the container full with saline (or storage solution), replace the cap and tighten. Then shake the container. Let the lens soak until it moves freely. Ideally, the lenses should then be boiled again to make sure they are properly disinfected.

If the lens *always* stings slightly on insertion try filling the squeeze bottle to a maximum of ¼ inch above or ¼ inch below the fill line.* Advise your practitioner if you do this.

STERILIZATION BY SPECIAL SOLUTIONS

Solutions have been developed exclusively for the disinfection of soft contact lenses. As soft lenses have the effect of concentrating some antiseptics on the lens surfaces (and hence causing eye irritation) it is of vital importance that all solutions specifically state that they are for use with hydrophilic or soft lenses (gel lenses or hydrogel lenses are other terms which are used). Under no circumstances should the lenses be stored in tap water, purified or distilled water, or hard lens solutions of any sort.

The storage routine is as follows.

(1) Any solution already in the container should be emptied out and the container filled with fresh solution direct from the bottle. It is important that this is done *daily* as the low antiseptic concentration is unlikely to maintain lens sterility beyond 24 hours when the lenses are in use.

(2) Your lenses *should/should not* then be cleaned by the following method. On removal, place the lens in the palm of the hand, concave side up. Wet it with storage solution (or preferably cleaning solution – *see* later) and rub gently but thoroughly with the fingertip. Take great care not to touch the lens with the fingernail. Alternatively, the lens may be cleaned by rubbing it between the thumb and index finger. After cleaning, rinse the lens thoroughly with the storage solution. All this should be carried out over a hand basin with the plug in place.

(3) The clean lenses are then placed in the container as instructed.

(4) The lenses may be inserted direct from the container the next morning.

* Practitioners should bear in mind that this may cause very slight changes in lens parameters.

COMBINATION OF DISINFECTION METHODS

Disinfection by boiling has the advantage that it is less expensive in the long term, it is an efficient method of disinfection of the lenses, and there is no risk of the remote possibility of the patient becoming allergic to the preservatives used in chemical disinfecting solutions. It has the disadvantage of some inconvenience when travelling (travelling cases are now available) although the lenses may be boiled in their container in a saucepan of water or kept in a vacuum flask of boiling water overnight (*see* above). Disinfection using special solutions has the advantage of simplicity, portability and greater likelihood of maintaining lens sterility if the lenses are not worn for several days.

In practice, of course, a combination of both methods may be ideal and possibly desirable. Most lenses may be disinfected by either technique and you will be advised if this is not so. Some manufacturers recommend one particular technique although the lens material allows either method to be used. In such cases, if boiling is recommended, the lenses may be disinfected using hydrophilic storage solutions, for example, during holidays. Some practitioners recommend weekly boiling in saline solution, with the special storage solution used for the rest of the week. If storage solutions are recommended, the lenses may still be boiled in saline solution (if the lens material is suitable) in their container, once a week if time and facilities permit, as an added precaution to ensure lens sterility. *Always discuss with your practitioner the advisability of changing from one method to another.*

PROTEIN BUILD-UP ON LENSES

Unless lenses are thoroughly cleaned before soaking or boiling (asepticizing), proteins from the tears accumulate on the lens, and the soaking or boiling then alters the state of the protein so that it adheres to the lens and can irritate the eye. You may then notice any or all of the following symptoms to a small degree.

(1) A drop in the standard of vision; (2) loss of comfort; (3) lens discoloration; and (4) a red eye.

One manufacturer makes a lubricating solution* which is gently rubbed on to the lens before insertion and which is stated to reduce protein and mucus build-up on the lens. Other manufacturers produce cleaning solutions† which you are strongly recommended to use daily after removing your lenses to get rid of surface deposits prior to

* Hydrosol – *Contactasol.*

sterilization. Also produced are enzyme tablets*
which remove any protein deposits which may
have built up on the lens. The latter method should
be used once a week or as often as necessary.
Maintenance of surface cleanliness will not only
improve lens comfort but also contributes to lens
life and significantly improves the efficiency of
the disinfection method†.

LENS INSERTION

To prevent the right and left lenses being interchanged accidentally, they should be removed
from their soaking container and inserted one at a
time. The following procedure is carried out for
the right eye (and reversed for the left eye) after
ensuring that the lens is not inside out (*see* below).

(1) Support the lens on the ball of the forefinger
(or middle finger) of the right hand. Work over a
large, smooth, flat surface if possible. A mirror is
sometimes helpful at first. Allow ultra-thin lenses
to dry out for a few seconds.

(2) Bring the left hand down over the forehead,
look right down, and grasp the upper right lid
firmly with the middle finger. Now look straight
ahead (at your eye in the mirror).

(3) Pull down the lower lid with the middle
finger (or fourth finger) of the right hand, keeping
the lens away from the eye.

(4) Bend the head well forward over the mirror
or the flat surface, and holding the lids well apart
gently place the lens on the cornea. Obviously,
the distance between the lids must be greater than
the lens diameter; the lashes must be kept well out
of the way.

(5) Slowly release both lids.

There may be very slight irritation for the first
minute or so. In the case of marked irritation, a
particle of dust or fluff may have become trapped
behind the lens; it should be removed, rinsed with
sterile saline or storage solution, and re-inserted.
Sometimes a small foreign body behind the lens
can be removed by moving the lens on to the white
of the eye (the side nearest the ear is most convenient), massaging it there for a few seconds and
then sliding it back on to the cornea.

Rather than insert the lens directly on to the
cornea some patients may prefer to look in the
mirror, turn the head to the right, and place
the lens on the white of the eye, then use a finger
on the lens to gently move it on to the cornea.
When inserting the left lens the head is turned to

the left, or you can look up and place it below the
cornea.

Before placing the lens on the eye always
ensure that it has not accidentally become turned
inside out. There are two simple methods of
checking that this is not the case.

(1) Place the lens on the tip of the forefinger,
concave side upwards, and hold it up to a light or
a window. Look at the shape of the lens from the
side in silhouette. If the lens is the correct way
round the edges will point almost vertically. If the
lens is inside out the edges will turn slightly
outwards.

(2) Balance the lens on the tips of the thumb
and forefinger, concave side upwards. Gently fold
the lens inward slightly. If the edges bend inwards
then the lens is the right way round and vice versa.

Also, some lenses are marked and this can be
checked to ensure it is the right way round.

LENS REMOVAL

Method 1

(*a*) Hold the upper and lower lids apart as described
in Insertion above. This time the mirror may be
used in either a vertical or horizontal position.

(*b*) Turn your head so that you are looking
across your nose into the mirror, that is, for the
right eye, turn your head to the right so that you
are then looking to the left to see in the mirror.

(*c*) Using the index finger slide the lens off the
cornea (towards the ear) on to the white of the
eye.

(*d*) Keep hold of the upper lid but take away
the right hand and turn so that the side of the
thumb and forefinger are facing the eye.

(*e*) Keeping the head position constant, hold
the lids at the corner of the eye apart with the side
of the thumb and forefinger and *gently* pinch the
lens off the eye, with the thumb and forefinger.

Method 2

Bend the chin into the neck so that you look
upwards to see the eye in the mirror. Slide the
lens below the cornea and pinch off using thumb
and forefinger (or middle finger) as before. If you
have long fingernails, deep set eyes or a smaller
than average distance between the lids, Methods
1 and 2 may prove difficult.

Method 3

(*a*) Raise the eyebrows and keep staring wide.

(*b*) Use one finger of each hand. Put one fingertip on the edge of the top lid and the other on the
edge of the bottom lid. Both lids should be held
about half way along.

---

* Cleaner No. 4 or Softmate (*Barnes-Hind*), Pliagel (*Alcon*);
  Preflex (*Burton, Parsons*); Sterisolv (*Sauflon*); Softgel
  (*Hydron*).
† Hydrocare or Hydron or Soflens Cleaning tablets
  (*Allergan*); Amiclair tablets (*Abatron*); and Clean-O-Gel
  (*Burton, Parsons*) for lipid removal.

(*c*) Pull the lids towards the ear keeping the edges of the lids in close contact with the white of the eye.

(*d*) Look towards your nose almost at the same time as (*c*). The lens should be expelled from the eye.

Method 4

Proceed as in Method 1 or 2 but instead of pinching the lens off the white of the eye between finger and thumb use a rubber suction holder.

WEARING SCHEDULE

Unless otherwise advised, start at 3 or 4 hours on the first day and increase by 1 or 2 hours each day if it is comfortable to do so. Endeavour to wear your lenses every day during the adaptation period. The lenses may need changing in both fitting and power as they settle.

An alternative wearing schedule may be advised as follows.

1st day	5th day ....
2nd day	6th day ....
3rd day	7th day ....
4th day	8th day ....

GENERAL NOTES

(1) Always wash your hands thoroughly before handling soft lenses to ensure they are free from all traces of creams, make-up, nicotine, etc. Dry them on a lint-free, well-washed towel.

(2) If your lenses accidentally dry out (becoming smaller and losing their flexibility) handle them with extreme care. Preferably drop saline solution on to them and let them soften for half an hour before touching them. Then place them loosely in the container and soak in saline or storage solution for *at least* 2 hours. Ideally, they should then be re-disinfected by your usual method before wear. *Never put a partly dry lens on an eye.*

(3) As most lenses are not marked right and left, great care must be taken not to get them confused.

(4) There is very little chance of dust getting beneath a lens during wear. *See* under Lens Insertion in case this happens. If discomfort persists, consult your contact lens practitioner or doctor.

(5) There is little risk of lens loss from the eye, even when swimming, though they may be displaced on to the white of the eye if the eyes are rubbed. Swimming in highly chlorinated water should be avoided as the chlorine may be absorbed by the lens causing marked subsequent irritation. Swimming goggles may, of course, be worn.

(6) Take great care to keep the eyes closed when using aerosol or other sprays. Remember that the droplets may persist in the room for several minutes. Such foreign chemicals may again cause subsequent irritation and often ruin the lens permanently.

(7) If the lens is irritating your eye and you suspect that it may be contaminated with make-up, etc., clean the lens very carefully. Boil the lens for at least an hour in distilled water and return the lens to normal saline or storage solution for at least one additional hour. If this procedure is ineffective go through the recommended routine with an enzyme cleaner. If discomfort persists, stop wearing the lens and get in touch with your practitioner.

(8) Unless your lenses are designed for continuous or extended wear *never sleep in your lenses* for more than very short periods of time. If you should forget, however, check immediately on waking to see if the lenses will move on the eyes. If they do not move readily, do not attempt to remove them. Place several drops of saline solution in the eyes every few minutes and try moving them again. If, after several applications, the lenses will still not move you must consult your contact lens practitioner.

(9) If after placing a lens on the eye you do not see clearly through it, massage the closed lid gently to centre the lens and express any air bubbles from beneath it. If vision is still not clear, check to see if you have put in the wrong lens or if the lens is inside out.

(10) You are strongly advised to insure your lenses.

(11) The lenses should not be worn if you are using medicated eyedrops of any sort.

(12) Make a note in your diary that you are a soft contact lens wearer and that in the event of an accident the lenses should be removed within a few hours.

(13) After-care check-ups will be advised at periodic intervals until complete integrity of the eyes has been ascertained. Further appointments at longer intervals, but never less than once a year, are essential to ensure that no abnormal corneal changes are taking place, as often these may cause you no symptoms. If you are in any doubt about the state of your eyes or lenses, always seek advice.

(14) Always bring your spectacles to every after-care appointment. These should be worn for at least 3–4 hours after every visit as the drops used to check the integrity of the eye may permanently stain the lens.

ACKNOWLEDGEMENTS

The authors are indebted to Mr R. Taylor for preparing photographs for *Figures 8.1, 8.2* and *8.6—8.9* and to Mr E. G. Woodward for *Figures 8.3—8.5* and *8.10—8.17.*

REFERENCES

Lowther, G. E. and Hill, R. M. (1968). 'Sensitivity threshold of the lower lid margin in the course of adaptation to contact lenses.' *Am. J. Optom.* **45**, 587—594

Lemp, M. A., Dohlman, C. H. and Holly, F. J. (1970). 'Corneal dessication despite normal tear volume.' *Ann. Ophthal.* **2**, 258—261, 284

Phillips, A. J. (1969). 'Alterations in curvature of the finished corneal lens.' *Ophthal. Optician* **9**, 980—986, 1043—1054, 1100—1110

Stone, J. (1974). 'The measurement of corneal thickness.' *Contact Lens J.* **5**(2), 14—19

Wilson, M. S. (1970). 'Instruction of contact lens patients with particular reference to hospital practice.' Paper read at the summer Clinical Conference of The Contact Lens Society, Bradford, 1970

BIBLIOGRAPHY

Anon (1974). 'Why we do not find keratometer changes and spectacle blur in gel lens wearers.' *Internat. cont. Lens Clin.* **1**(1), 34

Bailey, I. L. and Carney, L. G. (1973). 'Corneal changes from hydrophilic contact lenses.' *Am. J. Optom.* **50**, 299—304

Barradell, M. J. (1975). 'Future requirements of soft lenses.' *Optician* **169**(4363), 14—16

Berman, M. R. (1972). 'Central corneal curvature and wearing time during contact lens adaptation.' *Optom. Wkly* **63**, 132—135

Bier, N. (1957). *Contact Lens Routine and Practice,* 2nd ed. London: Butterworths

Black, C. J. (1972). 'Experiences with soft lenses.' *Contacto* **16**(1), 57—58

Brundgardt, T. F. and Potter, C. E. (1972). 'Adaptation to corneal lenses: profile of clinical tests.' *Am. J. Optom.* **49**, 41—49

Enoch, J. M. (1972). 'The fitting of hydrophilic (soft) contact lenses to infants and young children.' *Cont. Lens med. Bull.* **5**(3—4), 41—49

Filderman, I. P. and White, P. F. (1968). *Contact Lens Practice and Management.* Philadelphia: Chilton

Finnemore, V. (1973). 'Common factors in contact lens failure.' *Am. J. Optom.* **50**, 50—55

Fletcher, R. J. (1961). 'Routine and records in contact lens practice.' *Ophthal. Optician* **1**, 429—431

Fletcher, R. J. and Nisted, M. (1963). 'A study of coloured contact lenses and their performance.' *Ophthal. Optician* **3**, 1203—1213, 1259—1262, 1269

Grosvenor, T. (1963). *Contact Lens Theory and Practice.* Chicago: Professional Press

Grosvenor, T. (1972). 'Visual acuity, astigmatism, and soft contact lenses.' *Am. J. Optom.* **49**, 407—412

Grosvenor, T. (1972). 'Soft lens patient selection and criteria for success.' *J. Am. optom. Ass.* **43**, 330—333

Harris, M. G. (1972). 'Identifying potentially unsuccessful contact lens patients.' *Contacto* **16**(3), 50—58

Harris, M. G. and Sarver, M. D. (1971). 'Health history and failure in wearing contact lenses.' *J. Am. optom. Ass.* **42**, 550—553

Harris, M. G. and Sarver, M. D. (1972). 'The prefitting eye examination and failure in wearing contact lenses.' *Am. J. Optom.* **49**, 565—568

Harris, M. G. and Messinger, J. H. (1973). 'Personality traits and failures in wearing contact lenses.' *Am. J. Optom.* **50**, 641—646

Harris, M. G., Blevins, R. J. and Heiden, S. (1973). 'Evaluation of procedures for the management of spectacle blur.' *Am. J. Optom.* **50**, 293—298

Hill, J. (1973). 'Tear analysis for successful contact lens wear.' *Optom. Wkly* **64**, 943—946

Hill, J. (1973). 'Physical and physiological differences in fitting soft contact lenses.' *Optom. Wkly* **64**, 621—623

Hill, J. (1975). 'A comparison of refractive and kerato-metric changes during adaptation to flexible and non-flexible contact lenses.' *J. Am. optom. Ass.* **46**, 290—294

Hill, R. M. (1970). 'Comments on contact lens adaptation: osmotic pressure of the tears.' *Cont. Lens Soc. Am. J.* **4**(4), 36—39

Hill, R. M. (1971). 'Apertures and contact lens control.' *J. Am. optom. Ass.* **42**, 749—750

Holden, B. (1973). 'The present and future of contact lenses.' *Austr. J. Optom.* **56**, 429—442

Koetting, R. A. (1973). 'Keratometric reflexes on flexible lens surfaces.' *Am. J. Optom.* **50**, 722—726

Koetting, R. A. and Mueller, R. C. (1961). 'A routine for examination of contact lens patients.' *Am. J. Optom.* **38**, 211—220

Larke, J. R. and Sabell, A. G. (1971). 'A comparative study of the ocular response of two forms of contact lens.' *Optician,* **162**(4187), 8—12 (Part 1); **162**(4188), 10—14 (Part 2)

Lemp, M. A. and Hamill, J. R. (1973). 'Factors affecting tear break-up time in normal eyes.' *Archs Ophthal.* **89**, 103

Mackie, I. A. (1970). 'Blinking mechanisms in relation to 3 o'clock and 9 o'clock limbal lesions associated with contact lens wear.' *Cont. Lens med. Bull.* **3**(2), 16—20

Mandell, R. B. (1971). 'Contact lens adaptation.' *J. Am. optom. Ass.* **42**, 45—50

Mandell, R. B. (1974). 'Lathe cut hydrogel lenses.' *Internat. Cont. Lens Clin.* **1**(1), 54

Mandell, R. B. (1974). *Contact Lens Practice: Hard and Flexible Lenses,* 2nd ed. Springfield, Ill: Thomas

McMonnies, C. W. (1972). 'Predicting residual astigmatism with flexible hydrophilic contact lenses.' *Austr. J. Optom.* **55**, 106—111

Morrison, R. J. (1973). 'Comparative studies in visual acuity with spectacles and flexible lenses: ophthal-mometer readings with and without flexible lenses.' *Am. J. Optom.* **50**, 807—809

Moss, H. L. and Polishuk, A. (1972). 'Oral contraceptives and contact lenses.' *J. Am. optom. Ass.* **43**, 654—656

Phillips, A. J. (1969). 'Contact lens plastics, solutions and storage — some implications.' *Ophthal. Optician*

8, 1058, 1075–1076, 1134–1136, 1143, 1190–1192, 1203–1205, 1234–1238, 1312–1315, 1405–1408; **9**, 19–20, 25–27, 65–66, 75–79

Polse, K. A. and Mandell, R. B. (1971). 'Contact lens adaptation.' *J. Am. optom. Ass.* **42**, 45–50

Racusen, F. R. *et al.* (1964). 'An explanatory investigation of factors associated with success or failure in contact lens wearing.' *Am. J. Optom.* **41**, 232–240

Rocher, P. (1972). 'Optical and metabolic problems with hydrophilic contact lenses.' *Optician* **162**(4209), 6–8

Sabell, A. G. (1970). 'Oral contraceptives and the contact lens wearer.' *Br. J. physiol. Optics* **25**, 127–137

Sarver, M. D. (1972). 'Vision with hydrophilic contact lenses.' *J. Am. optom. Ass.* **43**, 330–333

Schoessler, J. P. and Lowther, G. E. (1971). 'Slit lamp observations of corneal oedema.' *Am. J. Optom.* **48**, 666–671

Schmidt, P. P. *et al.* (1974). 'Adaptation: "hard" vs "soft" contact lenses.' *J. Am. optom. Ass.* **45**, 282–284

Stein, H. A. and Slatt, B. J. (1973). 'Clinical impressions of hydrophilic contact lenses.' *Canad. J. Ophthal.* **8**, 83–91

Stewart, C. R. (1968). 'Functional blinking and contact lenses.' *Am. J. Optom.* **45**, 687–691

Stevens, A. V. (1972). 'A simple device for the removal of contact lenses.' *Br. J. Ophthal.* **56**, 442

Tabak, S. (1972). 'A short Schirmer test.' *Contacto* **16**(2), 38–42

Watts, G. (1973). 'Soft lens wearers: how are they doing?' *Optician* **165**(4282), 25–26, 30

Wilson, M. S. (1970). 'Corneal oedema from contact lens wear, its causes and treatment.' *Trans. U.K. Soc. Ophthal.* **90**, 31–45

York, M. *et al.* (1971). 'Variation in blink rate associated with contact lens wear and task difficulty.' *Am. J. Optom.* **48**, 418–425

Chapter 9

Ocular Impressions and Scleral Lens Fitting

P. J. Marriott

The successful fitting of a scleral contact lens depends entirely on obtaining a final result which interferes as little as possible with the physiology and metabolism of the eye. The ideal lens must be considered to be that lens which does not alter the metabolism of the eye at all − a lens which leaves a normal and uninterrupted flow of tears over the cornea and does not interfere with their normal disposal by evaporation or via the lacrimal apparatus. This is impossible to achieve; but it is possible to fit the lens so that the interference is minimal and not beyond the adaptability of the eye.

The scleral contact lens must fulfil the three following basic criteria in order to achieve, as nearly as possible, these physiological requirements.

(1) The haptic portion must be in apposition to the globe. If the weight and pressure of the haptic portion is spread evenly over the scleral surface, it is then possible to support the optic portion accurately and its correct position. A correctly fitting haptic portion does not, in itself, cause a tight 'glove' fit.

(2) The corneal clearance must be such as to allow an even and correct flow of tears over the cornea. This clearance is critical (Marriott and Woodward, 1964). In a fully settled lens, it must be between 0.04 mm and 0.08 mm.

(3) Adequate clearance at the limbus in order not to interfere with the limbal circulations.

The technique of constructing and fitting a scleral lens by means of making an impression of the eye requires a knowledge of the contours of the tissues on which the haptic portion of the lens rests, the corneal contours which must be accurately cleared, and the shape and position of the limbus.

The positions of the muscle insertions, the position of the globe in the orbit, and the configuration of the orbit are extremely important features which affect the final fit of the lens. A résumé therefore follows.

The classical description of the positions of the insertions of the rectus muscles is shown in *Figure 9.1*. The insertion of the medial rectus approaches to between 4 mm and 5 mm from the corneal margin, followed by the inferior rectus (6.5 mm), the lateral rectus (7.0 mm) and the superior rectus (7.5 mm).

The position of the globe in the orbit, and the configuration of the orbit, is shown diagrammatically in *Figure 9.2*.

The temporal wall of the orbit is inclined to the nasal wall at an angle of approximately 45 degrees. The primary axis of the globe is approximately parallel to the nasal wall, and at an angle of 22½ degrees with the midline of the orbit.

An analysis of the anterior global contours (Marriott, 1966) showed certain constants which must be considered when constructing the lens. These constants are as follows.

(1) The temporal portion of the sclera is spherical, and remains so during most eye movements − steepening slightly on convergence and flattening slightly in divergence.

(2) The nasal portion is very flat − even conical when the eye is converged more than 6−8 degrees from the primary position − and becomes increasingly spherical as the eye diverges from this position.

(3) The centres of curvature of the corneal and scleral curves do not lie on the same axis. They are off-set in relation to each other. In general, the flatter the scleral radius the greater the angle of off-set (*Figure 9.3*).

(4) The limbal area, in the vast majority of cases, is a horizontal oval, and the 'anatomical' limbus is about 1 mm beyond the 'visible' limbus.

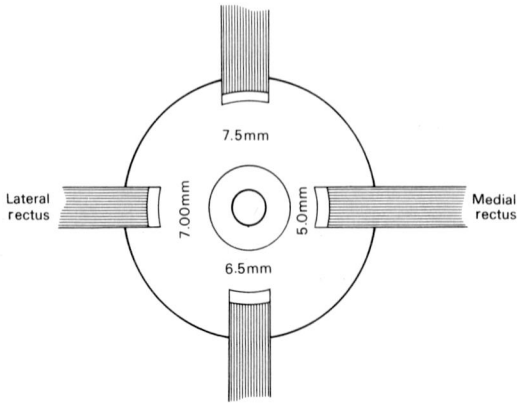

Figure 9.1–Insertions of rectus muscles relative to the limbus (diagrammatic)

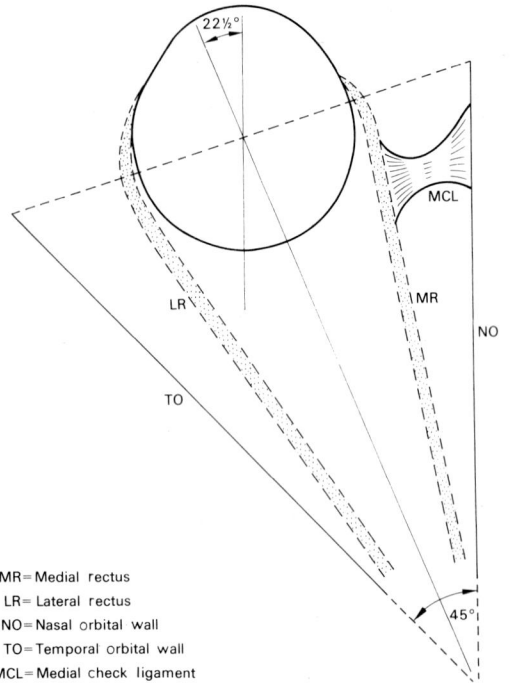

MR = Medial rectus
LR = Lateral rectus
NO = Nasal orbital wall
TO = Temporal orbital wall
MCL = Medial check ligament

Figure 9.2–Configuration of the globe and medial and lateral rectus muscles in the orbit (left eye seen from above)

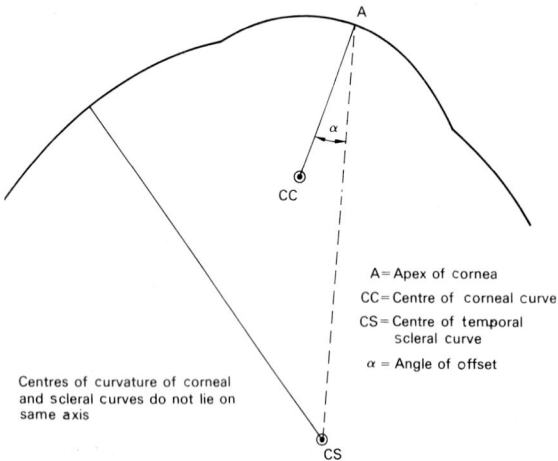

A = Apex of cornea
CC = Centre of corneal curve
CS = Centre of temporal scleral curve
α = Angle of offset

Centres of curvature of corneal and scleral curves do not lie on same axis

Figure 9.3–Diagrammatic representation of the angle of offset of the cornea with respect to the temporal sclera

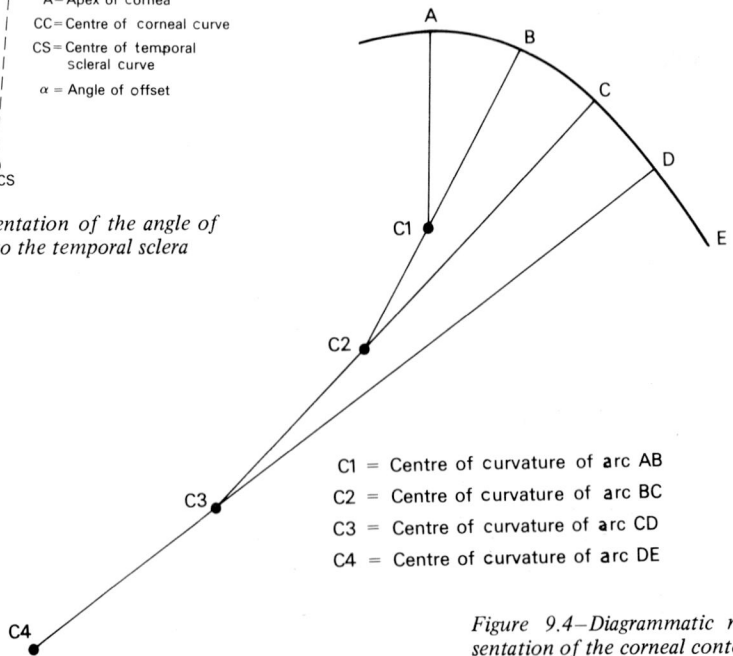

C1 = Centre of curvature of arc AB
C2 = Centre of curvature of arc BC
C3 = Centre of curvature of arc CD
C4 = Centre of curvature of arc DE

Figure 9.4–Diagrammatic representation of the corneal contour

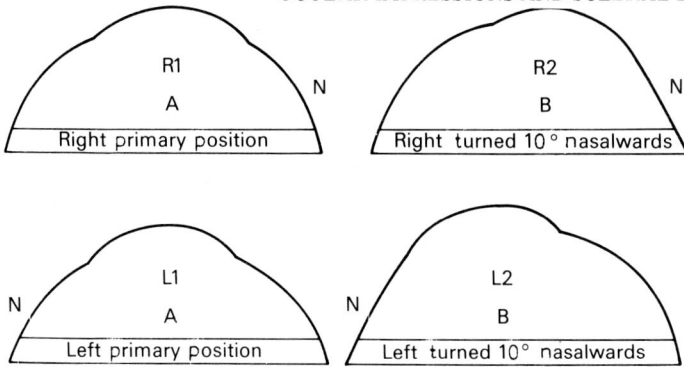

Figure 9.5–Drawings of casts showing change of global contours in convergence – horizontal sections viewed from below

(5) The cornea is very seldom spherical, even at its so-called 'central cap'. It is generally paraboloidal in shape. An analysis of casts of corneal impressions showed the shape as. illustrated in *Figure 9.4* (Marriott, 1966). Mandell (1965) also showed this to be so by using a keratometric technique.

The change in shape of the global contours on version movements is illustrated by the following tracings of casts of impressions made of eyes when they were (a) in the primary position, and (b) turned approximately 10 degrees nasalwards. Note that the nasal portions of the casts in *Figure 9.5*A are spherical, and in *9.5*B they are almost straight lines or conical. The change in shape of the temporal contour is not nearly so marked.

Reference to the anatomy of the globe and its configuration in the orbit (*Figure 9.2*) provides the explanation for this. The origins of the medial and lateral recti, at the apex of the orbit, cause the muscles to leave the globe approximately parallel to their respective orbital walls. Thus, there is a tendency for the lateral rectus to wrap around the globe to the equator, whilst the medial rectus leaves the globe soon after its insertion. These conditions are accentuated when the eye turns nasalwards.

When a scleral lens is fitted on to an eye, it fits over these muscle insertions and parts of the medial and lateral rectus muscles. This is shown diagrammatically in *Figure 9.6*. The temporal haptic portion rests over the insertion of the lateral rectus (IL) and part of the muscle (LR). As the lateral rectus adheres closely to the globe, the contour is almost a regular sphere. The nasal haptic portion fits over the insertion (IM) and part of the medial rectus muscle (MR). Although when the eye is in the primary position the medial rectus tends to leave the globe before the lateral rectus, the nasal side is still spherical but of a longer radius than that of the temporal side.

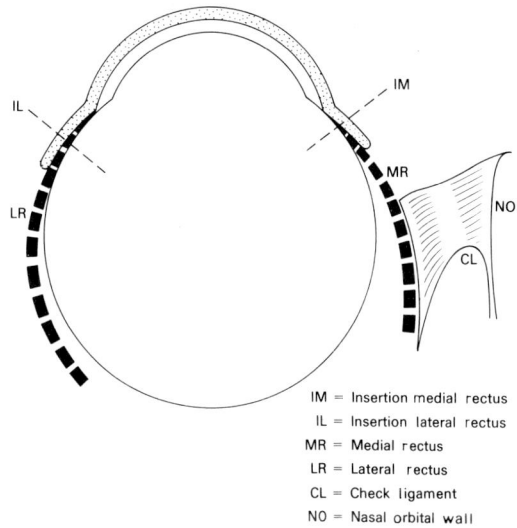

IM = Insertion medial rectus
IL = Insertion lateral rectus
MR = Medial rectus
LR = Lateral rectus
CL = Check ligament
NO = Nasal orbital wall

Figure 9.6–Scleral lens fitted to the globe in the primary position

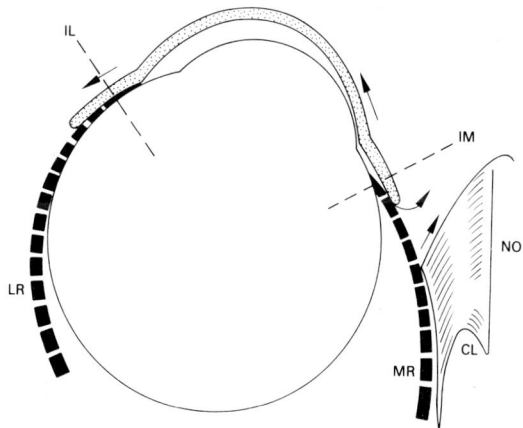

Figure 9.7–Effect on the fit of the lens shown in Figure 9.6 when the eye converges 10 degrees

When the eye turns nasalwards approximately 8–10 degrees, the lateral rectus muscle tends to wrap further round the globe, and its contour remains relatively unaltered. The medial rectus muscle, however, tends to stand further away from the globe, and its contour becomes straight or conical. This change in contour is increased by the pull of the medial check ligament, a thickening of the muscle itself and a 'bunching' of the conjunctiva. This is illustrated in *Figure 9.7* and the effect on the lens also shown in the same Figure.

during all normal ocular movements. Certainly there should be no suspicion of corneal touch when the eyes are converged to the reading position. These conditions obtain if the impression is made when the eye is turned inwards at an angle of approximately 6–8 degrees, when most of the flattening of the nasal contour of the globe has taken place. Thus, the direction of fixation of the eye is critical when an impression is made. If it is incorrect, there is very little chance of the final lens fitting correctly.

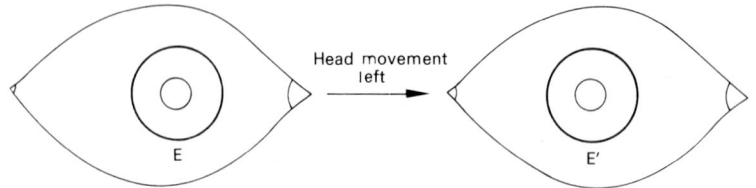

Figure 9.8—Effect of head movement on the position of the eye in the palpebral aperture even though fixation of a target is accurately maintained

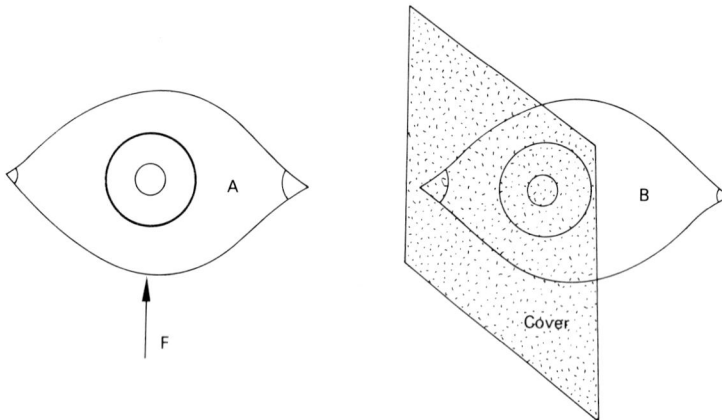

Figure 9.9—Arranging correct fixation which will maintain the eye in its correct position irrespective of head movements

The nasal edge of the lens is lifted in the direction of the arrow. As the temporal contour of the globe remains relatively unchanged, the temporal haptic still fits correctly, and the lens slides temporalwards in the direction of the arrow, causing heavy nasal corneal touch.

It is obvious that even an impression lens can give only a compromise fit. The contour of the temporal globe alters very little on version movements but does become slightly steeper when the eye turns nasalwards, and slightly flatter when the eye turns temporalwards. Generally, a good fit of the temporal globe is maintained for all except extreme version movements. As has been shown, the nasal contour of the globe alters considerably. It is essential that the correct fit be obtained when the lens is in such a position that there is no nasal corneal touch except on extreme inward rotation of the eye, giving complete corneal clearance

THE IMPRESSION TECHNIQUE – INTRODUCTION

METHOD OF FIXATION

The usual method of using a stationary fixation target does not necessarily ensure that the eye is fixating correctly. Even though the patient's head is firmly pressed into a headrest, there is always the possibility of a slight lateral movement of the head. Then, although the patient is still accurately fixating the target, the eye is not correctly positioned in the orbit (*Figure 9.8*). If an eye, E (*Figure 9.8*), is fixating a target and the head is then turned slightly in the direction of the arrow, when the eye continues to fixate the target, it will be positioned in the palpebral aperture as E'.

A more accurate method dispenses with a stationary fixation target, is quite independent of head movements, and compensates for heterophorias and heterotropias. The position of the fixating eye in its palpebral aperture is noted, when the 'impression' eye, under cover, is in its correct position for the impression. A mark is then made with a grease pencil on the lower lid of the fixating eye directly below the centre of the pupil. In *Figure 9.9*, *B* is the eye on which the impression is to be made, and *A* is the free or fixating eye. Eye *A* fixates the practitioner's finger, whilst eye *B* is screened by a cover and cannot see the finger, although the practitioner can observe eye *B* behind the cover. The practitioner then moves his finger until eye *B* is in the correct position for the impression. A mark, *F*, is then made on the lower lid of eye *A* directly below the centre of the pupil. When the impression material has been injected into the shell of eye *B* (or the shell inserted if the insertion method is being used), the practitioner instructs the patient to fixate his finger, which he moves until eye *A* is in its correct position with the centre of the pupil directly above the mark *F* on the lower lid. This then ensures that eye *B* is correctly positioned regardless of any lateral head movement of the patient.

IMPRESSION MATERIALS

The three impression materials in most common use today are listed below. These materials are used for dental impressions and are suitable for ophthalmic work, in some cases after slight modification. Those impression materials used in contact lens work are all alginates which are derived from seaweed.

Ophthalmic Zelex*

This substance produces good impressions because it can be spatulated into a very smooth free-flowing cream, which may be varied by using less or more water, depending on whether a stiff or thin mix is required. The normal ratio is 5 g of Zelex to 6.5 cc of water. If the powder is kept for a month or two, it produces a lumpy paste instead of a smooth cream. The gelling time appears to be rather gradual, commencing quite early during the spatulation period, while the setting time is long – two to three minutes.

Tissutex†

This dental material makes excellent impressions. It can be mixed into a rather thicker cream than Zelex, but it appears to have a longer free-flow period. Earlier, it was rather uncomfortable on the eye as it contained a peppermint flavouring. There was, however, some advantage in this as it caused slight lacrimation, which prevented suction between the impression and the eye and so made removal of the impression easier. Tissutex is now being manufactured without the peppermint, specially for ophthalmic work. The mixing proportions are very important – equal parts of water and powder (volume) or 2 g of Tissutex to 7 cc of water. Spatulation time must not exceed one minute.

Kromopan‡

This dental alginate offers a mixing technique which eliminates the necessity of timing the spatulation period. It changes colour twice during manipulation, each change denoting a stage in its preparation. Initially, the mixture is violet in colour. This changes to pink, indicating the end of the spatulation period, when the syringe or shell should be loaded. The final change is from pink to white. This is the stage for insertion for dental work. It is still very free-flowing at this stage, but for ocular work it is better to commence injection as soon as the syringe is loaded. Usually, therefore, the mixture is still a pale pink colour when injection is commenced, and is very free-flowing. It turns white just before, or at the end of, the injection. The material gels fairly rapidly – 20 to 30 seconds after turning white – and the impression may be removed after 1 or 1½ minutes in the eye.

The mixture is best made with equal parts (volume) of loosely packed powder and water, or 2 g of Kromopan to 7 cc of water, but the proportion is not as vital as with other impression materials. Spatulation must be carried out rapidly if a smooth mixture is to be obtained by the time it changes colour from violet to pink; and it is best done with a thin stainless steel spatula, mixing the material in a thin flexible rubber bowl. The mixture can then be 'stropped' easily against the side of the bowl.

The resulting impression is often not as smooth as with Tissutex or Zelex but, owing to its longer 'free-flow' period, there is less chance of creating conjunctival folds and 'ruckings' and of distorting the cornea and limbal region.

---

* Ophthalmic Zelex (*Amalgamated Dental Co. Ltd.*)

† Tissutex (*Dental Manufacturing Co. Ltd.*)
‡ Kromopan (*F. H. Wright Dental Co. Ltd.*)

There are other impression materials. The practitioner should use them all, and choose the one which gives the best results with his own personal methods (Frost, 1973).

SUPPORT OF IMPRESSIONS

No impression material keeps its shape without support, and this support is provided by impression shells or trays.

There are two main types of impression shell (or tray) — those used for the injection method, and those used for the insertion method. The injection-type shell has a hollow handle fixed over the corneal portion, through which the

holes are shown in *Figure 9.10*A and the shape of the holes is shown in *Figure 9.10*B. The reason for the shape of the hole is obvious. The large wedge-shaped countersink at the front end of the hole allows a relatively large wedge of impression material to gel and firmly lock the impression on to the shell. The back of the hole is only slightly countersunk, to avoid corneal damage during the insertion of the shell and to allow an easy start to the flow of the cream through the hole.

Size of Shell

The largest size of shell which can be reasonably inserted and removed should be used. A larger

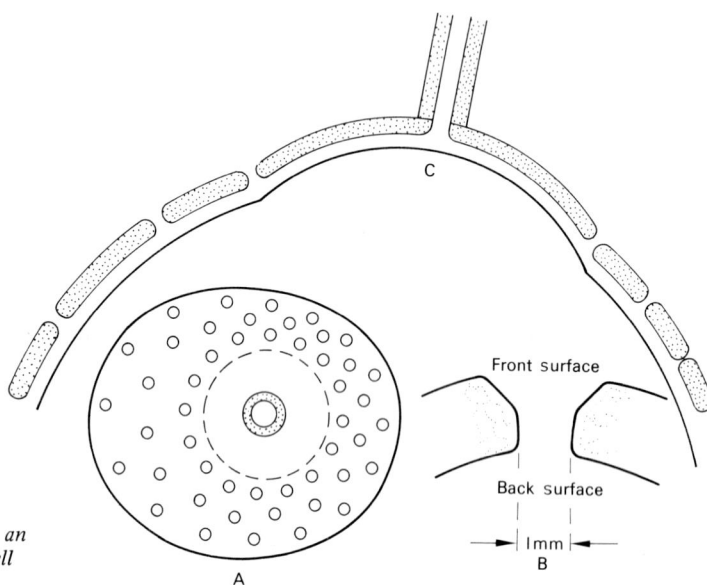

Figure 9.10–Construction of an injection impression tray or shell

impression material is injected with a syringe. The insertion-type shell may have a solid or hollow handle, or no handle at all; in the latter case, it is manipulated with a rubber suction holder.

Both types of shell fulfil the same function — that of supporting the impression when on the eye and, later, during the casting of the impression. The impression must adhere firmly to the shell during removal from the eye. As the impression material is not sticky, holes are drilled in the shell, through which the material extrudes to set on the shell's front surface, thus locking the impression to the shell. The size, position, shape and number of holes in the shell are very important. The best size of hole is approximately 1.00 mm in diameter. The position and number of

shell can be used for the injection method than is used for the insertion method. The shells should be oval in shape and up to 29 × 27 mm in overall size. The most usual sizes for the injection method are 29 × 27 mm and 27 × 25 mm. Even the latter overall size would be large for use with the insertion method.

Thickness of Shell

The thinner the shell — consistent with safety — the better. The thinner the shell the larger the size that can be used, and the less pressure exerted by the lids on the shell and on the impression material. The shell should not be more than

0.6 mm thick. This is thick enough to prevent flexing and possible distortion of the impression, and it allows a large shell to be used. The thinness certainly facilitates the insertion of the shell when using the insertion method.

Shape of Back Surface of Shell

The impression shell, or tray, should rest on the eye only at its extremities, and there should be an even clearance elsewhere between it and the eye in order to obtain an impression of even thickness (*Figure 9.10C*). This clearance is not so important when using the injection method as the shell is held away from the eye during the injection of the material. As long as the shell clears the cornea adequately, and is a generally a 'steep' fit, the fact that the impression is thicker over the cornea than elsewhere is of no importance.

When using the insertion method, it is important that the shell more nearly matches the contour of the globe. A large range of shells, both steep and flat, is therefore desirable. Conical-shaped shells are useful in order to obtain corneal clearance in cases of advanced keratoconus.

IMPRESSION TECHNIQUES

There are two techniques for ocular impressions, as follows.

INJECTION TECHNIQUE

An impression shell with a hollow handle is inserted under the lids. Impression material is injected from a syringe through the hollow handle of the shell to fill the space between the eye and the shell.

INSERTION TECHNIQUE

An impression tray, held with either a small handle or a rubber suction holder, is first filled with impression material and then inserted under the lids on to the eye.

SUITABILITY OF TECHNIQUE

Both techniques have advantages and disadvantages, although these are relative to the practitioner concerned. Most practitioners become more skilled at one technique than the other and are consequently less affected by its disadvantages – which may not appear to them to be disadvantages. With this reservation, the advantages and disadvantages are listed below.

INJECTION METHOD

Advantages

(1) In general, and certainly for most beginners, this is the easier technique of the two.

(2) There is a longer working time as the shell is already on the eye.

(3) It is easier to use when the patient has 'tight' lids or a small palpebral aperture.

(4) As larger shells can be used, a larger supported area of impression is obtained.

Disadvantages

(1) Care is needed to ensure that the impression material covers the whole of the anterior globe. It is relatively easy to 'miss' a quadrant by inadvertently pressing the shell against one section of the globe.

(2) Owing to the larger shell, the impression is sometimes more difficult to remove.

(3) The larger impression may cause more suction between it and the eye and also cause removal to be slightly more difficult.

INSERTION METHOD

Advantages

(1) There is more time, after insertion of the shell, to position it and arrange fixation.

(2) Removal may be easier as the shell and impression are smaller and there may not be so much suction.

Disadvantages

(1) Smaller supported impressions are obtained as smaller shells are used.

(2) It is sometimes difficult to insert the shell with patients who have tight lids and/or small palpebral apertures.

(3) It may be difficult to control the position of the impression in the shell, thus obtaining an impression that is extended too much at the top with too little at the bottom, and vice versa.

MATERIAL AND APPARATUS REQUIRED

The following is a list of the drugs, materials and apparatus which may be needed for taking an impression of an eye.

Drugs

Novesine 0.4 per cent (or other local anaesthetic — *see* Chapter 3)
Fluorescein Sod. 2 per cent or Fluorets
Sodium Bicarb. 2 per cent
Sodium Chloride 1 per cent
Sulphacetamide Sod. 10 per cent (or other chemo-therapeutic agent — *see* Chapter 3)
Cetavlon 1 per cent
Adrenaline Hydrochloride 0.1 per cent (or other decongestant — *see* Chapter 3)

Materials

Dental impression powder
Dental stone
Distilled water

Apparatus

Two measuring glasses
Two undines
Two spatulas (preferably thin, stainless steel)
Four thin rubber bowls
Kidney bowl
Two glass dishes or beakers
Tissues
Selection of impression trays for both insertion and injection methods
Stands for holding shells when making casts
Grease pencil or waterproof fibre pen for marking shells (if necessary) and lower lid for fixation purposes. A thin lipstick sharpened to a fine point is ideal for this purpose.

IMPRESSION TAKING

PREPARATION OF PATIENT

The taking of an eye impression must be presented to the patient as a simple and straightforward fitting process — which, in fact, it is. It is absolutely essential that the procedure be explained to the patient in simple terms, impressing upon him that the process involves no more than inserting a contact lens containing an impression material or one to be filled with an impression material after insertion. The patient must previously have had a scleral lens inserted, and it must be explained to him that he should feel even less during the impression-taking than he did during the insertion of the first contact lens — which is quite true if the eye has been correctly anaesthetized. The majority of patients suffer no discomfort at all, either during or after the taking of an impression. If there is any resultant soreness of the eyes, it is usually less than that encountered after a session of preformed lens fitting. The more relaxed the patient the easier to obtain a good impression.

An explanation to the patient of what is being done at all stages of the procedure generally arouses his interest and allays any fears or misgivings. For example, the practitioner knows that the impression material and water must be mixed in accurate quantities and automatically proceeds with this preparation; but to the patient seeing the quantities being meticulously measured out — especially if stainless steel instruments are used — it may appear that this is the preparation for a surgical operation. If, however, it is explained to him that it is essential to have the exact mixture for success, he should not worry. Patients like to co-operate and think they are helping the practitioner in other ways than by just obeying instructions. If the practitioner is working without an assistant, then the patient may be given the syringe to hold while the impression material is being spatulated; and he may be asked to pull down his own lower lid when the insertion method is being used, etc. The patient should be seated normally and comfortably as for a normal refraction. If the method of fixation already described is used, it is unnecessary to have the patient sitting rigidly still with his head against a head-rest.

(1) An external examination should have been carried out during the initial examination of the patient, when assessing his suitability for contact lenses. But it is wise to check again for recent abrasions and corneal staining, using fluorescein. The cornea should be carefully examined, using the slit lamp.

(2) The following should also be noted.

(*a*) Any irregularities of the sclera or bulbar conjunctiva such as scars, pingueculae, and thickened muscle insertions. Later, these can be related to any irregularities on the cast.

(*b*) Prominent lateral check ligaments, and size and position of the plica semilunaris. These may affect the position of the impression shell. If a lateral check ligament is trapped under the shell, it causes a groove in the impression.

(*c*) Protruding lacrimal gland tissue.

(3) The fixation position of the eye (as already described) should be checked.

(4) One drop of local anaesthetic is then instilled and, after half a minute, corneal anaesthesia checked by lightly touching the cornea with a wisp of cotton wool. The anaesthetic is instilled into both lower conjunctival sacs as this helps to lessen blinking.

(5) The correct-sized shell is selected, cleaned, inserted and checked. The shell should be as large as can conveniently be inserted. This may be up to 29 × 27 mm — a size frequently used — or even larger for the injection method. A check should be made to ensure that the shell can be manipulated to fit snugly behind the caruncle, and that it does not trap folds of conjunctiva from the lower fornix under its lower edge.

If the insertion method is to be used, it is useful at this stage to do a 'dummy-run' with an empty shell and show the patient how to pull down his lower lid, etc., (*see* right-hand column, last paragraph).

(6) The shell is then removed.

(7) The correct quantities of impression material and water are measured out ready for mixing.

(8) One drop of adrenaline hydrochloride 0.1 per cent or one drop of Otrivine-Antistin* may then be instilled to constrict the conjunctival vessels which may have become injected. This is very seldom needed in present-day practice, as the use of anaesthetics of weaker strengths rarely causes any significant injection.

(9) After one minute, a second drop of local anaesthetic is instilled in the upper conjunctival sac of the eye on which the impression is to be made.

To this stage, the procedure is the same for both the insertion and injection methods; but it is subsequently different for each method.

INSERTION TECHNIQUE

(10) The impression material is mixed with water in a thin rubber bowl and spatulated for the correct time — or, if using a colour change material, until it has changed to the correct colour. Although this may seem a simple operation, it is one of the most frequent causes of failure and needs considerable skill and practice. There are several factors to which the practitioner must pay particular attention:

Mixture

The proportions of powder and water are very critical with some alginates. Trial mixes should be

* Otrivine-Antistin (*CIBA*)

made by the practitioner to ascertain the proportions which result in a thin free-flowing cream. This is usually equal parts alginate and water (volume), but Zelex and Tissutex, for instance, need to be tapped down into the measure. If Kromopan is tapped down, it gives too stiff a mixture. The most accurate method is to weigh the material: Zelex — 5 g to 6.5 cc of water; Tissutex and Kromopan — 2 g to 7 cc of water (Frost, 1973).

Spatulation

This operation also needs considerable practice. It is not sufficient just to stir the mixture. It must be stropped rapidly against the side of the bowl, preferably with a thin stainless steel spatula, until all the powder has been mixed and the resultant mixture is a thin, smooth, free-flowing cream that just runs off the spatula and contains no lumps. This must be achieved in a short space of time as the more it is spatulated the stiffer it becomes. Zelex and Tissutex should not be spatulated for more than one minute, and Kromopan until just before it turns white.

Temperature

The room and water temperatures influence the setting time. A room temperature of 21°C (70°F) greatly accelerates the rate of gelling. In these conditions, it is wise to have the water as cold as possible and, if necessary, syringes, shells and spatulas should be left soaking in cold water until they are required.

(11) The impression material is then placed in the impression tray.

(12) The tray is inserted. This procedure should have been rehearsed with the patient when selecting the correct shell. The patient, holding a tissue in his free hand, bends his head forward until the plane of his face is parallel with the floor. He looks down towards his chin and, at the same time, pulls down his lower lid. The practitioner then pulls up the patient's upper lid as far as possible, holding it away from the globe. The shell is then inserted under the upper lid and gently pushed upwards as far as possible. The practitioner must maintain a slight outward pull on the shell in order to keep it against the lid and away from the globe as much as possible. The patient is now instructed to look upwards as far as possible, at the same time raising his head but still keeping his lower lid pulled downwards. As he looks upwards, the practitioner maintains the upward pressure on

the shell and manipulates the lower edge of the shell under the lower lid. At this stage, having raised his head, when the lower edge of the shell is inserted the patient is sitting upright and looking straight in front of him. This makes it easier for the practitioner to ensure that the shell is, in fact, inserted and that the lower lid has not been trapped under the shell. This may be difficult to ascertain as the lower lid is frequently hidden by excess impression material. The practitioner may now take the tissue from the patient and wipe away some of the excess material and, if necessary, using the tissue to grip it, pull out the lower lid from beneath the shell. It is practically impossible to do this without a tissue as the impression material makes the skin of the lower lid too slippery to pull down with the ball of the finger. Instead, the lower lid may be pulled and held down by previously sticking one end of a small strip of adhesive tape to the lid and pulling down on the other end.

(13) The shell is allowed to sink back on to the eye. It is possible that during insertion the shell may have become twisted. This is not serious; but if the material has not commenced to gel, the shell may be rotated to its correct position. If there is not time, the new horizontal axis must be marked on the shell, with grease-pencil, before removal.

(14) The patient's other eye is directed to its correct fixation position, which should be maintained until the impression has set. This takes approximately one-and-a-half to two minutes.

INJECTION TECHNIQUE

(10) The impression shell is inserted and checked to see that it is placed neatly behind the caruncle, that the conjunctiva from the lower fornix is not folded into the lower half of the shell, and that the lateral check ligament is not under the temporal edge of the shell. The shell is most easily settled by easing it gently away from the globe after insertion, rotating it gently a few degrees in both directions and then allowing it to settle back.

(11) The impression material is mixed and spatulated.

(12) The syringe is filled and checked to ensure that no air bubbles are present.

(13) The patient is instructed to look straight in front of him while the impression material is being injected. The exact fixation position is taken up immediately the shell is filled.

(14) The impression material is injected through the hollow stem of the impression shell. This is the most critical stage of the technique. The practitioner must ensure that the impression material flows evenly over all of the anterior surface of the globe.

This can only occur if there is sufficient space between the impression shell and the globe. Before commencing the injection, the practitioner should hold the stem of the shell between his thumb and forefinger and rest the remaining fingers on the patient's forehead. The shell is then eased forward away from the globe, the pressure being adjusted by means of the fingers on the patient's forehead. The nozzle of the syringe is inserted into the stem of the shell, and the material is injected slowly and steadily, without pause, until sufficient has been injected. It is better to inject too much than too little. Care must be taken not to push the shell on to the eye with the syringe. In order to ensure that the impression material covers all of the globe, the handle may be tilted nasally, temporally, upwards and downwards during the injection – although this is often not necessary if the shell is held away from but parallel to the globe. As soon as the injection is finished, the shell is allowed to sink gently back on to the globe. It needs no pushing; the lid pressure is quite sufficient. The handle of the shell must be supported while the material is gelling.

(15) The patient's other eye is directed to its correct fixation position.

REMOVAL OF IMPRESSION (both techniques)

If sufficient material has been used and it has extruded through the holes in the shells and formed an efficient 'key', and if the impression is removed correctly, there is no possibility of it becoming separated from the shell. The worst that can happen is for a small portion which is beyond the shell to become detached. This is unimportant as it would not, in any case, be used. The only possible way in which the impression can become separated from the shell is if the practitioner attempts to *pull* the impression directly off the eye or uses a shell with an insufficient number of holes, or with incorrectly placed or incorrectly countersunk holes.

(1) The patient is reassured. The procedure is explained and he is told not to be alarmed if the removal seems to take a long time. Although removal takes probably less than a minute, to the patient a minute may seem a very long time, and he may become alarmed and think it is becoming impossible to remove the impression.

(2) Excess material is removed from the patient's lids (and lower cheek if necessary), and the position of the shell is checked. If it has turned, the new horizontal axis is marked with a grease pencil.

(3) The patient is asked to look downwards and his upper lid is pulled up to free his lashes from

the material. A muscle hook is used, if necessary, to pull long eyelashes out of the impression.

(4) The patient is then instructed to look upwards as far as he possibly can. At the same time, the lower lid is pulled down until the lower lid margin is below the edge of the impression. The lid margin is gently pushed against the sclera. Air is admitted, and any suction between the impression and the eye is thereby relieved. The handle of the shell is held and the patient is instructed to look very slowly downwards, when the impression should slide out over the lower lid. Very occasionally, a strong suction is produced between the eye and the impression. This is felt as soon as the patient looks downwards. The impression does not slide out. The patient must be instructed to look upwards again while more pressure is exerted on the lower sclera until, quite suddenly, the impression comes free.

There is therefore no pulling of the impression away from the eye. It is allowed to slide out, thus avoiding any possibility of the impression being separated from the shell.

(5) The impression is inspected and its quality is assessed. First, the position of the corneal portion is noted. It should be displaced nasally. Flaws such as small air bubbles or torn or broken edges are looked for. Small flaws are unimportant as they may easily be removed from the final cast. Experience soon enables the practitioner to tell whether it is worth making a cast from the impression or whether it is necessary to take another impression.

(6) The shell is placed in a suitable holder in readiness for making a dental-stone cast, which should be done as soon as possible.

INSPECTION OF THE EYE AND CLEANING

The eye must be thoroughly inspected for any loose bits of impression material which may have become detached. With modern materials, small pieces are rarely left. Any pieces which remain are usually large thin pieces which 'overflowed' from the edges of the shell. These are easily seen and removed. Any small pieces are very soft and work their way into the inner canthus without causing any discomfort. As irrigation of the eyes is an uncomfortable process for the patient, it is better not to irrigate unless large pieces cannot otherwise be dislodged. In most cases, it is quite unnecessary and is only extra punishment to an eye that has already been subjected to pressure, and whose corneal epithelium has been softened by the use of an anaesthetic. Where irrigation is necessary, warm normal saline solution or sodium bicarbonate

solution may be used from an undine and the overflow collected in a kidney dish held against the patient's face. The patient's clothing must be protected.

The cornea must be inspected – using fluorescein and ultra-violet light – and given a thorough examination using the slit lamp. A diffuse, general dull staining of the cornea is almost invariably seen after impression taking. This is due to a softening of the corneal epithelium, caused by the anaesthetic and pressure. This staining is quite different from the brilliant green colour seen in the staining of an abrasion, and it should cause no alarm.

PROPHYLAXIS

Instillation of one or two drops of sulphacetamide 10 per cent (Albucid) or other chemotherapeutic drops, is a wise precaution. A very small number of patients experience some discomfort when the effect of the anaesthetic wears off. This is quite distinctive. They experience the sensation of the sudden appearance of a foreign body on the centre of the cornea. The eye lacrimates copiously for a few minutes, and then the sensation disappears. It is as well to warn all patients that this may happen as it may save them considerable anxiety.

If the eye continues to be painful and sore for more than 3–4 hours, the patient must contact the practitioner as soon as possible. As the epithelium is soft, the patient must be warned not to rub his eyes until the effect of the anaesthetic has worn off as this may cause an abrasion. The patient should also be warned to wear his spectacles out of doors until the anaesthetic has worn off as he would not feel a foreign body enter the eye, and spectacles afford some protection.

MAKING AND PREPARATION OF CAST

The making of a positive dental-stone cast of the impression is a very simple procedure, but it must be done very carefully. It is well worth while taking trouble with this as a perfectly good impression may be rendered useless if it is spoiled by careless casting.

(1) The shell and impression are mounted in a suitable and stable holder.

(2) The dental-stone powder is slowly added to cold water, stirring all the while until the mixture begins to stiffen but still runs easily off the spatula. The mixture is then spatulated until evenly mixed and of a smooth creamy texture. One of the best

materials for this is Caléstone*, which is hard and does not shrink.

(3) The mixing bowl must be vigorously tapped on a hard surface for several minutes to bring all the air bubbles to the surface. This is very important as any air bubbles left in the mixture may spoil the cast.

(4) A little of the mixture is poured into the impression and tapped down gently with the end of the spatula, taking care not to go through the mixture and damage the impression. More mixture is added to the centre and is tapped down from the centre to make it creep up the sides of the impression and so faithfully copy it contour. This also helps to free any remaining air bubbles.

(5) This is left for at least 1½−2 hours to ensure complete setting.

(6) When the cast has set, before removing it from the impression, the horizontal meridian is marked along the base of the cast. The nasal and temporal edges and the top of the cast are also marked and the patient's name is written on it.

(7) The cast is gently removed from the impression and inspected carefully. The cast must be of a high quality as it is the basis of the whole fitting procedure of an impression lens. Without this good foundation, a well-fitting lens cannot be produced. The following points should be noted.

(a) The position of the cornea. This should be well to the nasal side of the cast.

(b) The contours of the nasal and temporal portions. The nasal portion should be almost conical and the temporal portion spherical, and the cornea should have the appearance of being tilted nasalwards.

(c) The limbal region should be clearly marked. Without this, it is difficult to accurately locate the position of the transition and the centre of the back optic portion of the lens.

PREPARATION OF THE CAST

Generally, little alteration should be made to the cast except for cutting to shape and overall size with a sharp knife. It is better to leave the cast as large as possible and cut the lens to size when it has been made. Any small bumps or irregularities and small conjunctival wrinkles may be scraped off, keeping the general contour of the cast. The less the cast is adulterated the better. Reference back to the cast can always be made if there is any fault with the final lens fitting; but if the cast has been drastically reshaped, it is impossible to decide whether any fault in the fitting of the

* Caléstone (*Amalgamated Dental Co. Ltd.*)

final lens is due to the alteration of the cast or to incorrect manufacture. Certainly a cast should never be polished, as is done by some laboratories. If the practitioner wishes to experiment with or alter a cast, it is wise to leave the original untouched and make a copy of it with which to experiment. A copy is easily made by making a cast of a shell pressed from the original cast.

The corneo-scleral junction, which should be clearly delineated on the cast, must be accurately pencilled in, using an ordinary pencil. This is best done under magnification to ensure accuracy. A binocular loupe is excellent. This ensures the exact positioning of the transition.

THE CONSTRUCTION OF IMPRESSION LENSES

If a scleral lens — either an impression lens or a preformed lens — is to give long, comfortable and trouble-free wearing time, it must be constructed so as to give a correct physical fit and a correct physiological fit. The physical fit is the matching of the haptic portion to the anterior contours of the globe. The physiological fit is the arranging of the correct clearance of the lens from the cornea and the limbal region so as to cause as little interference as possible with the physiology of the anterior segment of the eye. Correct corneal clearance allows an almost uninterrupted normal flow of tears over the cornea, and the correct limbal clearance ensures that there is no constriction of any of the limbal circulations.

There are three criteria which, when satisfied, ensure a correct physical and physiological fit; these are as follows.

(1) The haptic portion in apposition to the globe (physical fit).

(2) Correct corneal clearance and alignment
(3) Correct limbal clearance } (physiological fit).

These are shown in *Figure 9.11*. The haptic portion, *H*, is in apposition to the globe. The optic portion clears the cornea centrally at *A*. This central corneal clearance is very critical and must be between 0.04 and 0.08 mm. Less than 0.04 mm may cause discomfort; and if more than 0.08 mm, the lens may not fill or it may have an excessively large bubble. This clearance should increase gradually to reach its maximum over the limbal area, *B*, and extend to approximately 2 mm beyond the visible corneo-scleral margin. This gives a fluorescein picture of pale green centrally, increasing to a deeper green over the limbus (*Figure 9.12*).

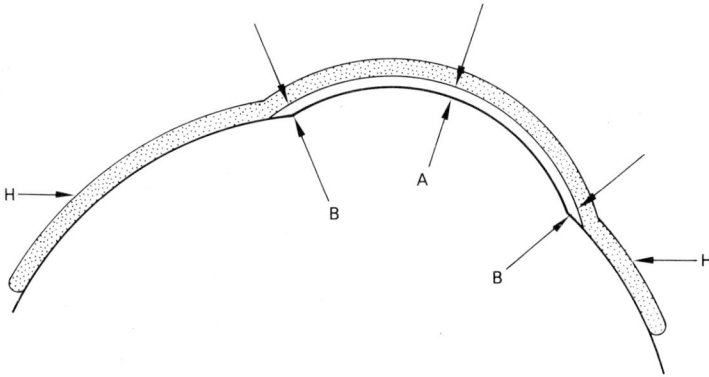

Figure 9.11–Criteria of a correctly fitting scleral lens

When a lens is made from a cast, the haptic fit is already produced and needs no construction. The lens would, however, also conform to the limbus and cornea. Thus, these portions of the lens have to be ground out to give the correct clearances. The back optic or corneal portion is ground out to a depth of approximately 0.15– 0.20 mm evenly over the whole cornea, whatever its shape or contour. This allows for the lens to

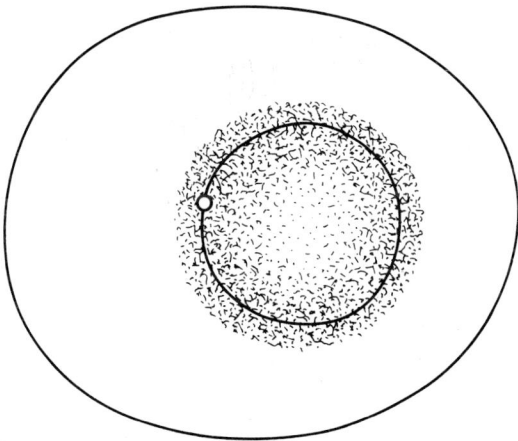

Figure 9.12–Fluorescein picture of a fully settled scleral lens. Shaded area indicates depth of fluorescein when viewed under ultra-violet light

settle, leaving a final central clearance of 0.06 mm.

The radius of the back optic portion is usually 0.2 mm flatter than the flattest keratometer reading. This contrasts with the back optic radius of preformed lenses, which is approximately 0.70–1.00 mm flatter than the flattest keratometer reading.

FACTORS AFFECTING THE CONSTRUCTION OF IMPRESSION LENSES

An analysis of casts of impressions of eyes (Marriott, 1966) has shown that several critical factors must be taken into account when constructing a lens from the cast. The casts were consistently found to have the following features, with varying measurements (*see Figure 9.3*).

(1) Fairly regular spherical temporal curves which were generally considerably flatter than was once thought to be the case. They ranged from 12.25 to 28.75 mm, with 57 per cent within the range 14.00–18.00 mm.

(2) The nasal curves were very flat, or conical, with some even exhibiting a negative curve.

(3) The vertical curves were fairly regular and spherical but flat, ranging from 15.3 mm to conical, measured on a section vertically through the 'cornea'.

(4) The centres of curvature of the temporal portion and the corneal portion did not lie on the same axis. This angle of 'offset' (angle α, *Figure 9.3*), the angle made at the corneal apex between the lines drawn from the respective centres of curvature, varied from 3½ degrees temporally to 27 degrees nasally. The majority (75 per cent) were within the range of 5–18 degrees nasally. In general, the longer the temporal radius the greater was the angle of offset.

(5) The vast majority of eyes had a limbus that was a horizontal oval in outline. A great many, too, had corneal astigmatism 'with-the-rule'.

If the impression, and consequently the cast, is correct and a shell is pressed accurately over the cast, then the temporal, nasal and vertical curves of the global contours are accurately reproduced. As these have only to be polished during lens manufacture, they need not be considered further.

One of the fitting variables − the fit of the haptic portion − is eliminated and no modifications to the haptic portion should ever be necessary.

It is necessary, however, to grind out the corneal and limbal portions to give correct central corneal clearance and correct limbal clearance, which must be maintained during all but extreme rotations of the eye. It is during these operations that the angle of offset can be altered and an incorrectly shaped transition portion produced.

ANGLE OF OFFSET

The angle of offset is very critical. An alteration in the optic axis, and therefore the angle of offset, by as little as 5 degrees may easily cause peripheral corneal touch, or touch on only small version movements of the eye. This is illustrated in *Figure 9.13*. In *Figure 9.13*, DE is the back optic curve giving correct clearance of the cornea. Its centre of curvature, C', is on the optic axis BAC. A is the apex of the cornea and C its centre of curvature.

If the back optic curve had been ground with its centre of curvature at C_2, lying on the axis BC_2, which makes an angle of 5 degrees with the correct axis BAC, the resultant back optic curve would be the dotted line, FG. This comes much closer to the cornea nasally than the correctly aligned curve, and would cause nasal touch after only a slight inward version movement of the eye. Note that the 'centre' B, of both curves gives almost the same apical clearance, AB.

The usual method of grinding out the back optic curve is by mounting the lens on a holder and allowing it to spin on a diamond-impregnated grinding tool of the desired radius (*Figure 9.14*). The grinding tool spins about the axis DC, and the lens, held slightly off vertical, is either allowed to spin or is revolved manually and oscillated to and fro across the tool. For the purpose of illustration, the lens is kept still and the tool oscillates, giving the same effect (*Figure 9.15*). In this illustration, the lens remains on a vertical axis but the tool oscillates about its centre of curvature as well as spinning around its axis DC. From this figure it can be seen that if the lens is allowed to take up its position freely it is self-centring, and the primary axis of the back optic passes through the centre of curvature of the tool. If, however, the curve on the shell is irregular, the lens tends to be ground out off-axis (*Figure 9.16*). In *Figure 9.16*, B is an irregularity on the surface of the back optic curve. When the lens is placed on the tool, it tends to take up a position, on each revolution of the lens, as at D, and the curve is ground out along the dotted line FG, with its centre of curva-

ture at C' instead of C. Although it is still ground with its optical centre at A, its primary axis is AC' instead of AC, and the offset is incorrect by the angle α. This is very difficult to control, and it is not usually possible to correct it after the grind-out has been finished. However, if a final impression lens shows peripheral corneal touch, this almost certainly is the reason and generally a new lens has to be made.

SHAPE OF BACK OPTIC AND TRANSITION

A large number of eyes fitted with contact lenses have some corneal astigmatism 'with-the-rule', and an even larger number have a cornea that is horizontally oval in shape. Thus, the transition on the lens must generally be a horizontal oval shape to give correct clearance at all points of the limbus.

When a shell is pressed over a cast, it reflects the corneal astigmatism and so usually has a steeper curve vertically than horizontally. When this is ground out with a spherical tool, the resulting back optic is a vertical oval − the opposite to that which is required. This gives too much corneal clearance in the vertical meridian. If the transition is then blended in between the back optic and the haptic, it too becomes a vertical instead of a horizontal oval.

The shape of the limbal area varies in different meridians, and the type of transition − that is, curved or conical − should also vary. Generally, it needs to be a curve, sometimes almost a deep channel, especially at the upper limbus, then flatter at the temporal and lower limbus and approximately conical at the nasal limbus. This generally happens automatically as the grinding of the transition is carried out, but it frequently needs local adjustment in the final lens.

MANUFACTURE OF IMPRESSION LENSES

It has been stated by many contact lens practitioners that the impression method of fitting scleral lenses does not produce a higher percentage of well-fitting results than the preformed method, and that equally as many adjustments need to be made to both types of lens to obtain a satisfactory fit. Obviously, if the impression is good, an impression lens should fit perfectly and need adjustments only to the clearances over the cornea and limbus. Any other faults must be due entirely to incorrect manufacture of the lens. Unfortunately, laboratory methods of manufacture frequently do not produce the desired result. The

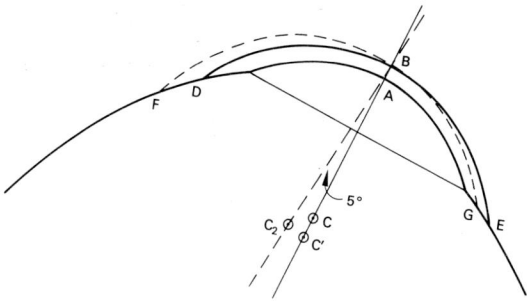

Figure 9.13–Effect on alignment of the back optic curve when it is ground out along an incorrect axis

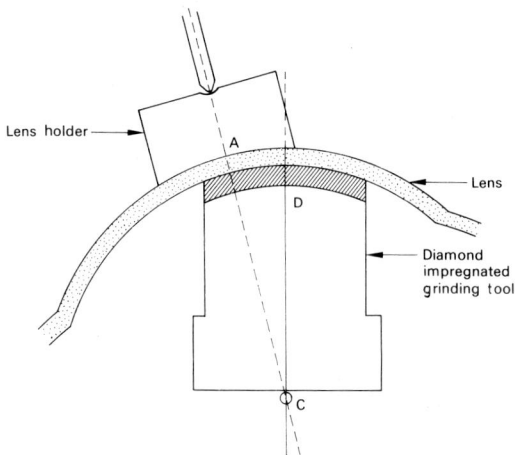

Figure 9.14–Grinding out the back optic curve

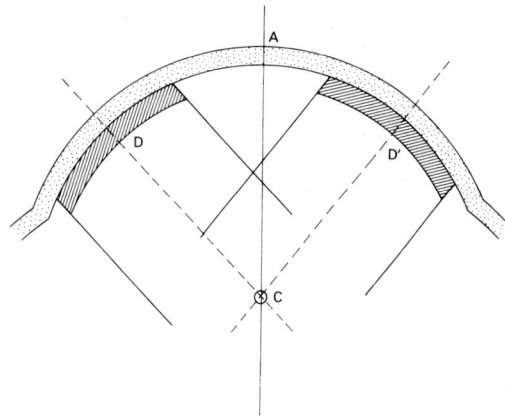

Figure 9.15–Tool oscillating and spinning on its axis with the lens remaining stationary (theoretical – to illustrate how the back optic curve is ground out on the correct axis)

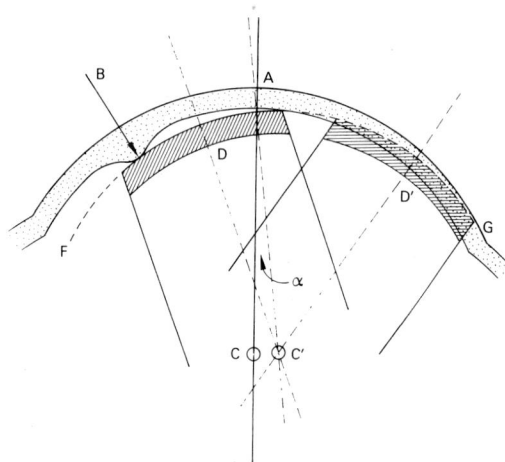

Figure 9.16–Irregularity on the back surface of the shell causing the back optic surface to be 'tilted' and ground out on an incorrect axis

usual laboratory process comprises three stages, as follows.

(1) Pressing of the shell over the cast.

(2) Grinding the back central optic to the radius and clearance specified by the practitioner. The radius usually selected is approximately 0.7 mm flatter than the flattest corneal radius found by keratometry.

(3) Blending of the junction of the optic curve with the haptic.

This method, as previously explained, frequently produces a vertically oval back central optic and transition. This shaped back central optic gives too much corneal clearance in the vertical meridian, and the transition, as such, cannot be accurately located over the limbus at any point. Theoretically, this method of manufacture can only produce a correctly fitting lens for an eye whose cornea is nearly spherical and whose limbus is round and not oval.

A different sequence of manufacture must be used to produce consistently the correct physical and physiological fit as illustrated in *Figure 9.11*.

The pressing of the shell over the cast produces a correctly fitting haptic portion which should need no adjustment at all. The second stage commences with the marking of the limbus on the shell and is followed by grinding out the transition. This sequence ensures that the transition is accurately located over the limbus and is of the correct shape. Some local or general adjustment may be required in the final lens to increase the limbal clearance locally or all round.

Grinding of the back central optic to the correct radius and clearance follows, after the transition has been formed.

In order to obtain consistently perfect fitting, the practitioner who does not manufacture his own lenses needs to become skilled at certain processes of manufacture. He must make the necessary adjustments to the transition and back central optic. These operations need considerable practice. It is extremely difficult, if not impossible, to communicate to the laboratory just what is required and to expect a third person to effect this without seeing the lens on the patient. There follows, therefore, a description of suitable manufacture by the practitioner and the tools required.

THE SHELL

A very simple but accurate method is used. The cast, with the extremities of the limbus marked on it in pencil, is mounted on a block B (*Figure 9.17*)

accurately over the edges of the cast. As one end is sealed, a build-up of air pressure in the tube helps to press the Perspex accurately over the cast. The pencil lines drawn on the cast are visible on the shell and may be used as a check on the accuracy of the pressing. When cool, the tube is removed and the edges of the cast are marked round with a grease pencil. The shell is tapped smartly on a hard surface to remove the cast.

The following description of constructing the lens involves the use of a flexible drive handpiece and a suitable selection of tools. This needs practice, but when proficiency has been achieved it is generally the quickest and most accurate method. Other methods may be used, such as mounting the tools on a vertical or horizontal spindle.

The shell is cut off, using a side burr mounted in the flexible drive. The edges are shaped and rounded, using a hard conical grinding stone — first by bringing to a V edge (A in *Figure 9.18*) and then rounding it off (B in *Figure 9.18*). The

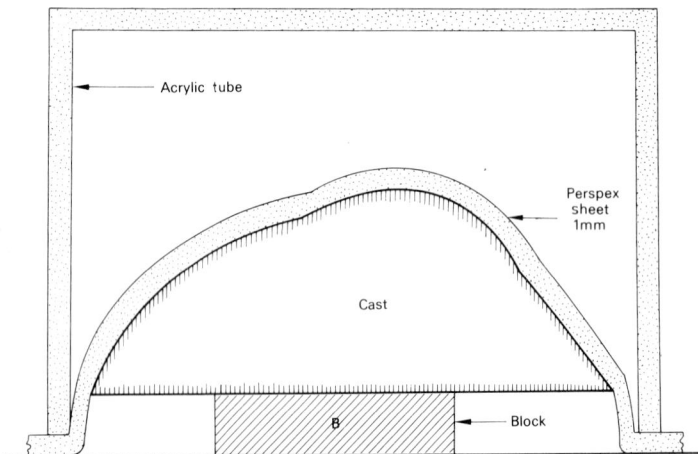

Figure 9.17–Pressing the shell over the cast (cross-section)

and is adjusted to the correct level by sticking it on to the block with Plasticine. A square of Perspex*, 1 mm thick, is mounted in a metal clamp, placed over an infra-red spectacle frame heater and heated for approximately two minutes, until it is suitably soft. It is then placed on the cast, and pressed, and 'pulled down' over the cast by means of an acrylic tube, one end of which is sealed and whose internal diameter is only slightly larger than the cast and thickness of Perspex. Using an acrylic tube has the advantage that it sticks slightly to the Perspex and drags it down

* Perspex (*I.C.I. Ltd.*)

edge is then polished, using a hard felt buff and Tripoli or Lustre wax polish, to remove all the grinding stone marks. The final polish is obtained by polishing at high speed with a linen mop. The edge must then be examined with a binocular loupe to ensure that it is well-rounded, with no ridges, and well polished.

THE TRANSITION

The limbus should have been already pencilled-in on the cast. The shell is then placed on the cast, and with a grease pencil or waterproof fibre pen

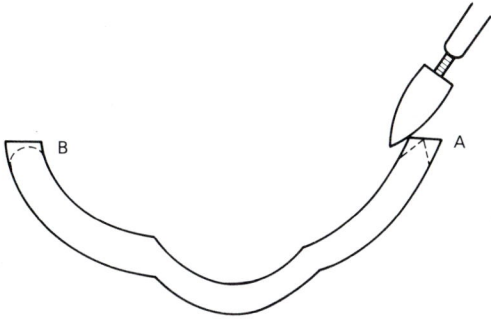

Figure 9.18–Edging the shell using a conical stone mounted in the handpiece of a flexible drive (cross-section)

placed on the eye and fluorescein is instilled. This is to check that a good impression and a faithful copy of the anterior global surfaces has been obtained. If the shell is good, inspection with ultra-violet light will show that all the fluorescein has been displaced, and that the shell is a complete matching fit all over the sclera and cornea (see (1) physical fit on page 224). The shell must have been fenestrated in order to check this. If not, it may well rest on a layer of tears trapped underneath, and will exhibit a false corneal clearance.

Before removing the shell, the centre of the pupil is marked. For want of a better reference, this locates the apex of the cornea and the centre of the back optic.

the limbus is marked on the front surface of the shell. The shell is then placed on the eye to check that the marking does, in fact, coincide with the limbus. Any small adjustments to the alignment with the limbus are then made with the shell *in situ*. The position of the fenestration is also marked (see Chapter 10, page 252).

The shell is then removed, and fenestrated, as described in Chapter 23, Volume 2. It is again

The shell is then removed and, before the pupil-centre mark gets rubbed off, a tiny pip is made with a small drill over the centre marking. A line is then drawn with the grease pencil approximately 2 mm beyond the limbus line to mark the extremity of the limbal clearance. Another circle, of approximately 6–8 mm in diameter, is drawn round the centre mark (*Figure 9.19*). The shaded area is then ground out by hand to a depth of approximately

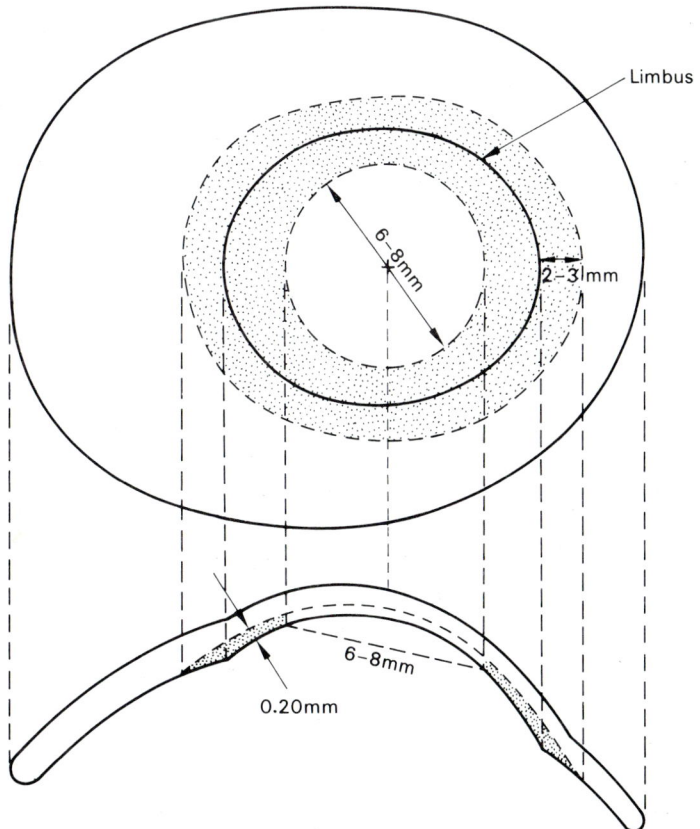

Figure 9.19–Plan and elevation of first grind-out (by hand) to give correct limbal clearance

0.2 mm, the greatest depth being over the limbus (*Figure 9.19*). This grind-out should taper off towards the haptic but leave a step in the optic portion, which is blended off when the back optic is ground out.

The grind-out of the transition and peripheral optic portion may be done with a dental rose burr or a 10 mm diameter grinding ball used in a handpiece. It may seem an impossible task to do this accurately by hand and match the corneal contours, but it is relatively easy with practice. It must be remembered that the tools do not cut very rapidly and that it is not necessary to take out all the material in one go. Several attempts may be made; and the shell may be tried on the eye after each attempt, to ascertain whether enough material has been removed.

When it is estimated that the correct clearance has been obtained, this ground-out area must be polished. It is first ground to a fine matt finish with a grit-impregnated rubber wheel, used wet. At the same time, the back haptic portion is also ground to a fine matt finish. This must be done at this stage. If it is left until after the correct corneal clearance has been obtained, the lens would then settle and be brought too close to the cornea.

The back surface is then polished, using a hard felt wheel impregnated with Tripoli. A final polish is later put on, using a linen buff impregnated with Silvo*, but this is not necessary until the fitting has been completed.

The shell is then placed on the eye, fluorescein instilled, and examined with ultra-violet light. If enough substance has been removed evenly all round, the fluorescein picture should be that of heavy central touch over the central 6–8 mm (from which no material has been removed) and full and even clearance of the peripheral cornea and limbus to about 2 mm beyond the limbus (*Figure 9.27*). It may at this stage appear that too much material has been removed, and there may be some fairly large bubbles in the limbal area. These disappear once the correct central clearance is given; but before this, the lens rests heavily on the corneal apex. However, the lens settles when this central portion is ground out to give the correct central clearance.

When the correct peripheral corneal and limbal clearance is obtained, it should be remembered that this is a fairly true matching clearance, whatever the corneal curves may be and no matter how much they varied towards the periphery, and that the limbus has been cleared no matter what its shape. It would in many cases be quite impossible to have achieved this by grinding out with spherical curves.

* Silvo (*Reckitt and Colman*)

CHOICE OF BACK CENTRAL OPTIC RADIUS

Before removing the shell from the eye, the limit of the area of central touch should be carefully marked with a grease pencil. The shell is then removed and the back optic radius is ground on, using a diamond impregnated grinding tool that just 'takes up' over the area marked (central area, *Figure 9.27*). This is best done by trial and error, starting with a tool that is about 0.2 mm flatter than the flattest keratometer reading. If the shell is held with its centre over the centre of the tool and the tool is used dry, it can be ascertained just where the tool is taking up. If it starts evenly all round the limits of the area of touch, it is of the correct radius. The centre thickness of the shell is measured. It is then mounted on a runner and spun and oscillated across the diamond tool until 0.2 mm of substance has been removed. The optic is then polished, using a wax polishing tool cut to the correct radius and well soaked with Silvo. If the correct radius has been selected, the back central optic blends in with the hand grinding, leaving an almost 'continuous curve' back optic surface to the lens with no transitions. If there are any transitions, they must be blended out.

There are reasons for leaving such a small back central optic as 6–8 mm. First, it lessens the risk of altering the angle of offset when grinding it out (and this is also helped by making sure the tool takes up correctly before spinning the lens freely on it); and secondly, in cases of high astigmatism, the oval shape produced is very much less than if the whole back optic surface had been ground out with a single spherical curve or multiple spherical curves.

It has been advocated that FLOM lenses may be used to determine the back central optic radius to be used on an impression lens. This is not so, and the use of these can be very misleading. It must be remembered that a FLOM lens has a round back central optic, and it is being fitted to clear a limbus that is nearly always horizontally oval in shape. Though the FLOM may appear to give a good corneal fit, it is impossible to reproduce this round back central optic on an impression shell that already incorporates the ocular astigmatism.

ASSESSMENT OF FIT AND MODIFICATIONS

If the impression has been done correctly, with the eye in the correct fixation position and the shell accurately pressed over the cast, no haptic adjustments should be necessary.

The lens is inserted to observe the rate of filling. In 15 minutes, or when the bubble has become very small or is non-existent, a drop of fluorescein 2 per cent is introduced through the fenestration hole and the lens is inspected, using ultra-violet light.

POSITION OF OPTIC

The optic portion should be accurately centred over the cornea. If there is any corneal touch, it should be central and should remain so on all but extreme version movements. If the lens is not centred correctly, corneal touch is evident nasally or temporally.

Corneal Touch Nasally

This is usually caused by the impression having been taken with the eye turned insufficiently nasalwards. To check, the nasal haptic curve should be observed; if it is spherical and similar to the temporal curve, then the cause is confirmed. Rarely can it be corrected. It is usually quicker and easier to take another impression. The second cause is an incorrect 'offset', the tool having 'taken up' and ground out along an incorrect axis. If more substance is needed to be removed from the back optic, it is sometimes possible to alter the angle of offset during regrinding by holding the lens slightly off axis until the tool 'takes up' along the correct axis. Other causes are the provision of insufficient clearance when the back central optic is ground and/or a back central optic radius which is too steep. This is easily rectified by giving additional clearance and/or altering the radius.

Corneal Touch Temporally

The causes are the same as for nasal touch but in opposite directions. Correction is frequently possible by grinding out locally. Otherwise, procedures as for nasal touch must be adopted.

CENTRAL CORNEAL CLEARANCE

If 0.15 mm substance has been removed from the back central optic, the lens usually shows central corneal touch after settling. This touch is corrected by the grinding out process, in steps of not more than 0.05 mm.

LIMBAL CLEARANCE

The back surface transition frequently needs local or general modification. Where extra clearance is needed, the area of touch must be very carefully and accurately marked on the front of the lens with a grease pencil before removing the lens. The area is then ground out with a small carborundum ball and repolished. Very little substance should be removed. It is better to make several adjustments than to remove too much substance as, obviously, it cannot be replaced and this may mean starting again. It is a wise precaution to make a cast of the lens at this stage before commencing adjustments. If the lens is then over-adjusted and ruined, a new lens can be made from the cast instead of starting again from the very beginning.

Obtaining a good and accurate fit of an impression scleral lens requires a considerable amount of skill and manual dexterity on the part of the practitioner, and it can be time consuming. However, these skills, and perhaps more, are required to make a preformed lens fit — frequently with not nearly such good results.

ALTERNATIVE METHOD OF LENS CONSTRUCTION

A more accurate and less tedious method of obtaining the correct corneal clearance and alignment — and one requiring less skill — is to build up the corneal portion of the cast to a known amount before pressing the shell. This automatically gives the correct clearance and alignment without any hand grinding.

This may be done using acrylic laminates of a known thickness and form, as described in a paper read in 1969 at the World Contact Lens Congress at Eastbourne (Marriott, 1970).

Acrylic laminates may be lathe-cut to any desired thickness or combination of thicknesses. The most usual is 0.24 mm thick with a thinner central area 0.20 mm thick over a diameter of 6—8 mm (*Figures 9.20* and *9.28*). The central thinner portion produces less clearance on the shell over this area, leaving slight central touch — just enough to allow for working on the back central optic. This is exactly the same principle as for hand grinding.

MARKING THE POSITION OF THE LAMINATE ON THE CAST

For the successful use of laminates, the original impression must be of high quality and must have caused little or no deformation of the cornea, although this is sometimes unavoidable in cases of advanced keratoconus. Allowances can, however, be made for this.

As it may be necessary to make shells with different corneal clearances, it is preferable to make duplicate casts on which to mount the laminates rather than using the original. If a laminate of incorrect thickness is stuck on the original cast or is wrongly centred, it cannot be removed and the cast is ruined. Duplicate casts can be made quite easily by making a shell from the original cast and making as many casts of that shell as may be required.

In most cases, there is no doubt as to the position of the limbus, but it is a wise precaution to check this. The shell that was used for making the duplicate casts is edged, fenestrated and placed on the eye. The limbus is then drawn on the shell, when *in situ*, and the centre of the pupil is marked with a grease pencil. Before removing the shell from the eye, fluorescein is instilled to check that it is a good matching fit. If there is already some corneal or limbal clearance, allowance must be made for this by using a thinner laminate. The shell is removed, and another line is drawn 2–3 mm beyond the limbus to mark the extent of the laminate, exactly as previously described for hand grinding (*Figure 9.19*). If these markings are then

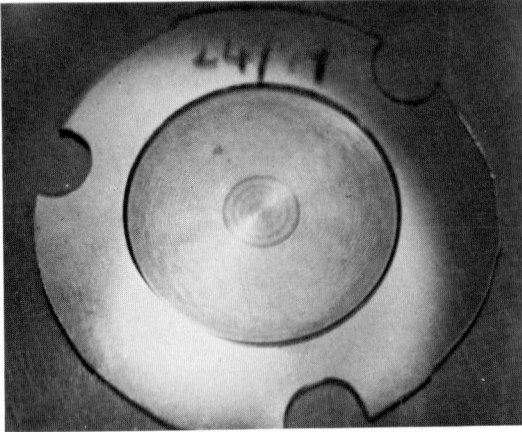

Figure 9.20–Acrylic laminate, 0.24 mm thick, with a central portion of 8 mm diameter, which is 0.20 mm thick

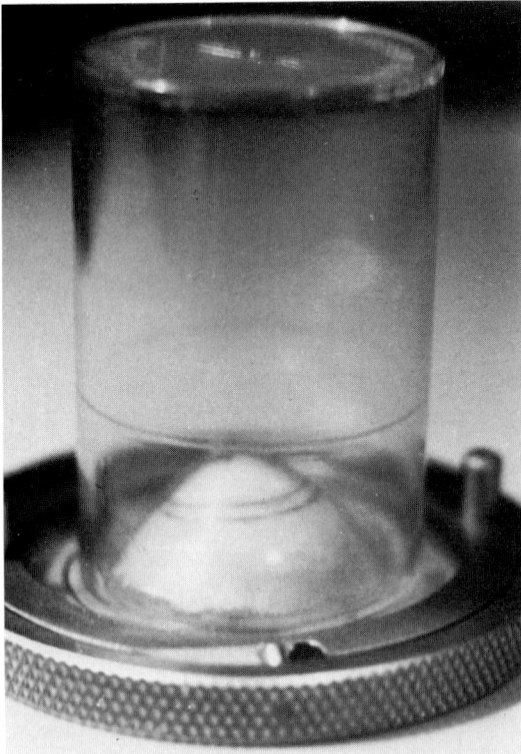

Figure 9.22–Backing sheet marked before removing from the cast. After removal this must be marked over again on the back surface of the laminate

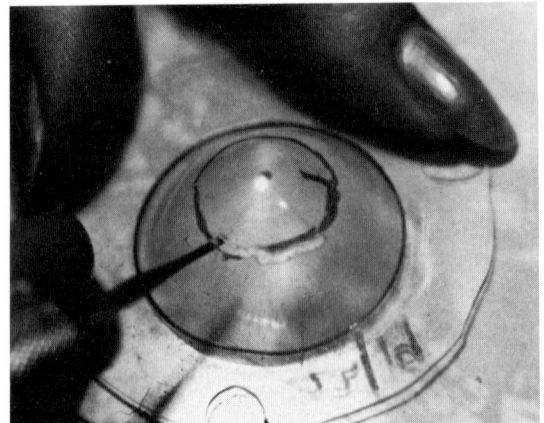

Figure 9.21–Laminate and backing sheet being pressed over the cast

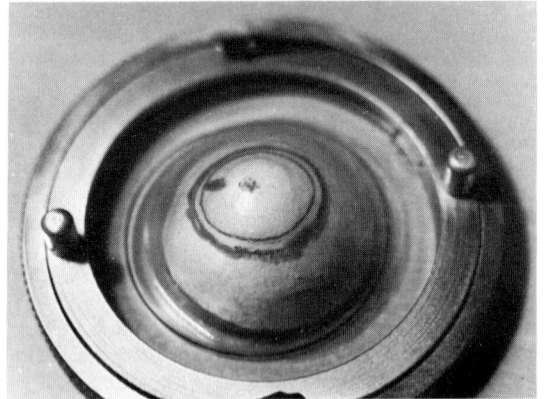

Figure 9.23–Cutting off the laminate

drawn over on the *back surface* of the shell with a grease pencil, when a cast is made the grease pencil marks are left on the cast showing accurately the limbal area and the centre of the optic portion.

FORMING THE LAMINATE

The laminate is placed in a ring clamp, lathe-side downwards, and its upper surface is smeared with a thin oil. Another disc of 1 mm Perspex is placed on top of it, and the two are firmly clamped together. The centre of the laminate is marked with a grease pencil so that it can be accurately centred on the cast. The clamp is then placed over an infra-red heater and heated for approximately two minutes. The correct temperature is obtained when the film of oil between the two sheets of Perspex begins to form fine bubbles. The two sheets are then pressed over the cast, the laminate in contact with the cast (*Figures 9.21* and *9.29*).

When the Perspex has cooled, before removing it from the cast, the extremities of the laminate must be marked. This must be done on the backing sheet of Perspex, and when both laminate and backing sheet have been removed from the cast the marking must be transferred to the back surface of the laminate before separating them (*Figure 9.22*). The laminate is easily separated from the backing sheet as the oil prevents them from sticking together. The laminate is then checked for accuracy and even thickness over the area to be used. There is a fairly consistent loss of thickness of 0.02 mm in the peripheral portion and 0.01 mm at the centre. Thus, a laminate of 0.24 mm at the periphery and 0.20 mm at the centre, after pressing, generally measures 0.22 mm and 0.19 mm respectively, with a variation over the surface of ±0.01 mm. Thus, the exact clearance over the cornea and limbus is known; and should this prove to be incorrect, other laminates, thinner or thicker, may be used.

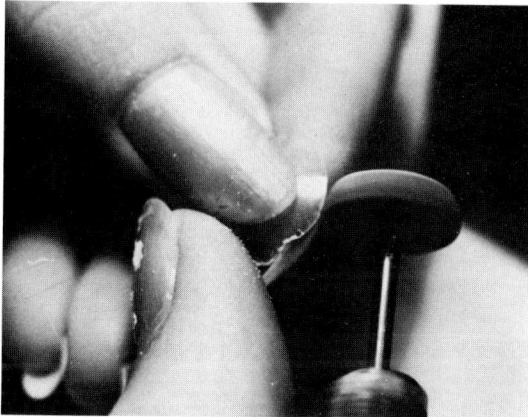

Figure 9.24–Trimming the laminate to size

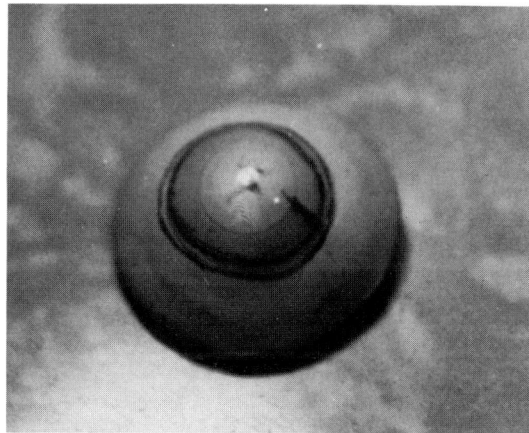

Figure 9.26–Laminate stuck on the cast

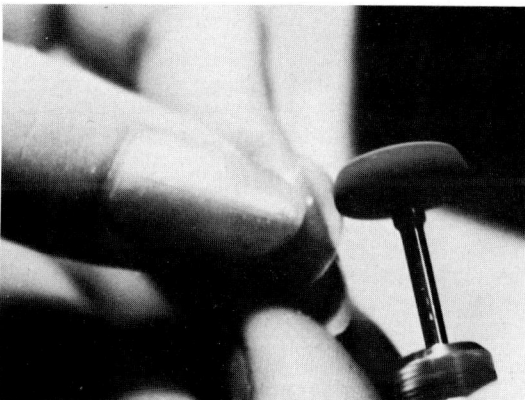

Figure 9.25–Chamfering the laminate to a knife edge

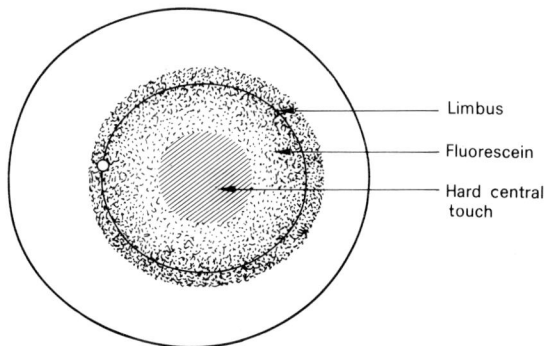

Figure 9.27–Fluorescein picture after the first grind-out showing correct limbal clearance but hard central touch

The laminate is then cut off approximately to size (that is, cutting outside the grease pencil marks), using a very fine dental side-burr mounted in a flexible drive (*Figure 9.23*).

When cut off, it is trimmed to the correct size and shape, using an impregnated rubber grinding wheel (*Figure 9.24*). When the correct size is obtained, the edge is chamfered off to a knife-edge, using the same rubber wheel (*Figure 9.25*).

The laminate, accurately centred, is then stuck on the cast using Durofix* or some similar adhesive

* Durofix (*The Rawlplug Co. Ltd.*)

(*Figures 9.26* and *9.30*). When the adhesive is dry and the laminate is firmly stuck to the cast, a shell is pressed over in the usual way.

FINISHING AND POLISHING THE SHELL

A shell pressed over the combination of cast and laminate has a fairly smooth back surface, especially over the area covered by the laminate. It does, however, need to be polished as even the lathe marks from the laminate are reflected on to the shell. The central 8 mm over which the back optic

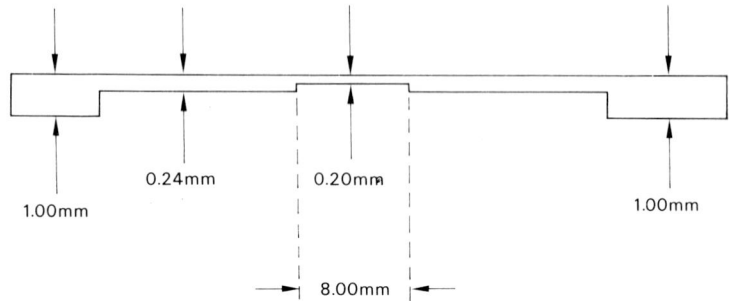

Figure 9.28–Cross-section of Perspex laminate

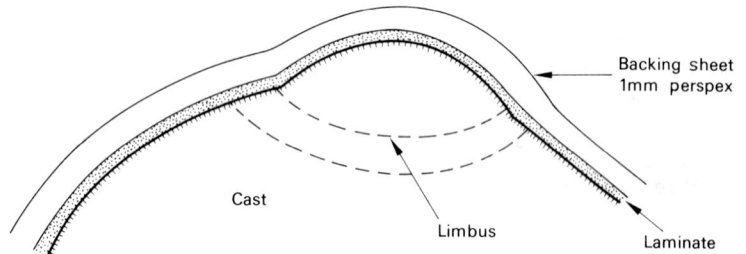

Figure 9.29–Laminate and backing sheet pressed over the cast

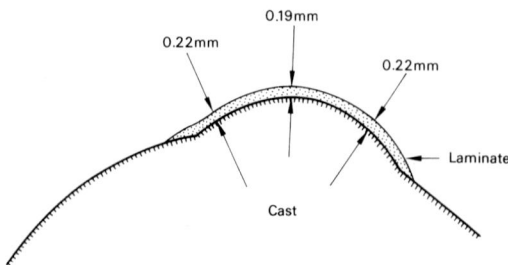

Figure 9.30–Cross-section of the laminate cut, trimmed, and chamfered to a knife edge and stuck on to the cast

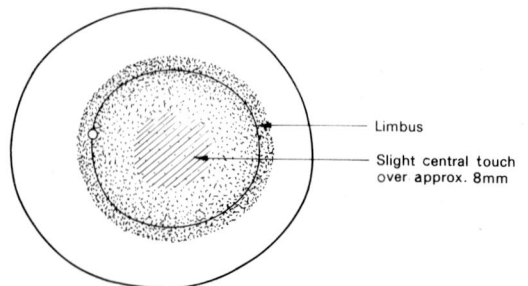

Figure 9.31–Fluorescein picture of the shell pressed over the combination of cast and laminate of Figure 9.30. The slight central touch allows for the back central optic to be worked

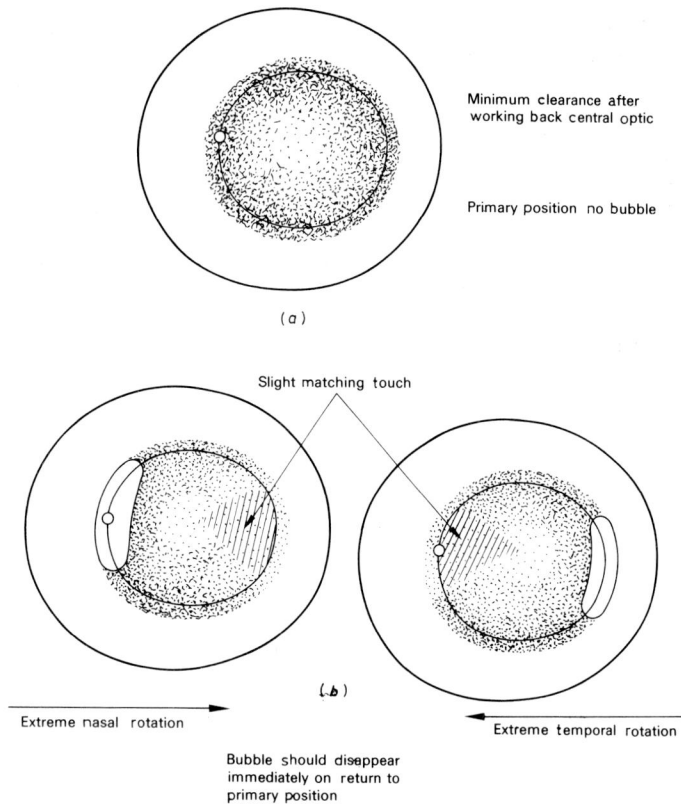

Minimum clearance after
working back central optic

Primary position no bubble

(a)

Slight matching touch

(b)

Extreme nasal rotation

Extreme temporal rotation

Bubble should disappear
immediately on return to
primary position

*Figure 9.32–Fluorescein pictures when
back central optic has been worked
showing, (a) no bubble in primary position, and (b) bubble appearing only on
large version movements*

is to be worked is always clearly visible. This is
marked round with a grease pencil, and the rest
of the back surface of the shell is finely ground
and polished.

At this stage, the shell may be fenestrated and
tried on the eye. The fit should be correct everywhere except for a slight matching central touch
over the central 8 mm (*Figure 9.31*). If this is so,
the back central optic may be worked on. The
radius of the tool used should match the radius of
the shell, which is usually about 0.2 mm flatter
than the flattest keratometer reading, that is,
flatter by the thickness of the laminate.

The final fluorescein picture should be that of
even capillary clearance all over the cornea,
extending to 2–3 mm beyond the limbus, with no
bubble. A bubble should appear only on version
movements, and it should disappear immediately
the eye returns to the primary position (*Figure
9.32*). *Colour Plates VIII* and *IX* show fluorescein
pictures of this type of fit. A rapid exchange of
tears liquid may be observed, and there should be
a good liquid balance.

A more rapid exchange of liquid may be
obtained by the inclusion of a fairly deep (0.25 mm
deep and 1.5 mm wide) superior-temporal channel
in the shell, as well as fenestrating. This occasionally
assists in eliminating frothing as small bubbles
tend to escape up the channel, provided that the
channel is deep enough to remain as an 'air channel'
rather than a 'liquid channel', that is, the bulbar
conjunctiva does not herniate into it and block it.

CHOICE OF LAMINATE

For most non-pathological cases of hypermetropia
and medium myopia, the most used thickness of
laminate is 0.24 mm, with a thinner central portion
of 0.20 mm over a diameter of 8 mm (*Figure 9.28*),
which reduces by 0.02 or 0.03 to 0.22 (0.21)/0.19
(0.18) mm after pressing. This usually gives correct
mid-corneal and limbal clearance with just enough
central touch to allow for working the back central
optic.

High myopic and aphakic eyes, which are
frequently 'soft', need thicker laminates as these

eyes are often more compressed during impression taking; also the lens has a tendency to settle more. A laminate of 0.26/0.22 mm may be necessary.

In cases of advanced keratoconus with a very steep cone, the cone is invariably compressed when taking the impression, and a laminate of equal thickness all over is necessary to allow for this. A laminate of 0.25/0.24 mm may be used, which achieves an even thickness of 0.23 mm when pressed. Occasionally, it is necessary, in these cases, to use a laminate that is thicker in the centre than at the periphery (*see* Chapter 20, Volume 2).

ORDERING OF IMPRESSION LENSES

Impression lenses may be ordered according to British Standard 3521: 1979.

This states that the cast should be marked on the back with R or L and a line indicating the horizontal, its nasal and temporal ends being marked N and T respectively. The patient's name or reference may be added. On the front of the cast, the peripheral limit of the haptic portion should be outlined. Alternatively, the overall size or back haptic size and the displacement of optic should be specified.

This cast should be sent to a laboratory requesting a lens and giving the following specifications.

(*i*) Eye and impression scleral lens.

(*ii*) Back central optic radius.

(*iii*) Back central optic diameter, if appropriate.

(*iv*) Back peripheral optic radius, where one is to be worked.

(*v*) External diameter of peripheral optic zone, if appropriate.

(*vi*) Detail of transition(s).

(*vii*) Clearance between cast and back central optic portion at its geometrical centre.

(*viii*) Back haptic size, and long and short axes, with orientation of long axis in standard notation.

(*ix*) Back vertex power or an adequate alternative, and any prism decentration or addition.

(*x*) Centre thickness.

(*xi*) Any front surface requirements.

(*xii*) Any other requirements such as tint, truncations, edge form, fenestrations, channels, distinguishing marks and haptic thickness.

Note: The dimensions given in items (ii) to (v) above are interrelated to the back haptic form. Since the latter is not geometrical, the peripheral zone(s) cannot be exactly specified.

Thus, the order accompanying the cast might be:

Right impressions scleral lens, BCOR 8.25, well blended transition, 0.2 clearance, BHS 25 H X 23 V (or as marked on cast), BVP −4.00 D, 0.7 haptic thickness.

This may be abbreviated to: R Imp S/8.25/ well blended transition/vertex clearance 0.2/ B 25.00 X 23.00 or as marked on cast/L 180/ −4.00/0.7 etc.

As has been previously stated, this frequently produces a very unsatisfactory lens. It is much better for the practitioner to become acquainted with a laboratory and make sure that the staff of the laboratory know how he requires his lenses to be constructed. Thus, a plain unworked shell may be ordered and the lens constructed by the practitioner by the methods already described, or by a laboratory if there is a good understanding with the practitioner, after the shell has been correctly marked up.

REFERENCES

British Standard 3521 (1979). *Glossary of Terms Relating to Ophthalmic Lenses and Spectacle Frames – BS 3521: 1979. Part 3. Glossary of terms relating to contact lenses.* London: British Standards Institution

Frost, C. J. (1973). 'Alginates.' *Ophthal. Optician* **13**, 1027–1032

Mandell, R. B. (1965). *Contact Lens Practice, Basic and Advanced.* Springfield, Ill.: Thomas

Marriott, P. J. and Woodward, E. G. (1964). 'A method of measuring the corneal clearance of a haptic lens.' *Br. J. physiol. Optics* **21**, 61–83

Marriott, P. J. (1966). 'An analysis of the global contours and haptic lens fitting.' *Br. J. physiol. Optics* **23**, 3–40

Marriott, P. J. (1970). 'The use of acrylic laminates in fitting haptic lenses.' *Br. J. physiol. Optics* **25**, 29–43

Chapter 10

Preformed Scleral Lens Fitting Techniques

E. G. Woodward

The preformed method of fitting scleral contact lenses is one which is difficult to justify in theoretical terms, particularly in a country where the use of local anaesthetics by those who are not medical practitioners is legal. This might be expected to make the impression technique the method of choice. The basic assumptions on which most of the preformed fitting sets were designed no longer appear to be valid, and a prerequisite of this method is a financial outlay for fitting sets which is probably higher than in any other fitting method.

The method has some theoretical advantages and one very great practical advantage; namely, it works. Many thousands of lenses have been successfully fitted this way, possibly more than by any other method of fitting scleral lenses. The relative success of this method may be explained by two factors.

(1) Assumptions which have since proved to be incorrect have virtually all related to the contour of the sclera and hence to the shape of the haptic portion of the lens. Paradoxically, in a scleral lens the fit of the portion which rests on the sclera is relatively unimportant. Quite large departures from a 'glove fit' in the haptic portion cause no trouble whatsoever provided that the optic portion is well balanced in relation to the cornea, both geometrically and hydraulically. The degree of this departure has not been appreciated as distortion and compression of the conjunctiva conceal quite large variations in the haptic fit.

(2) Impression techniques were highly developed several years ago, but the weak link in the chain has always been the actual preparation of the lens from the cast — particularly in regard to the formation of the transition which clears the limbus, and choice of axis for the optic portion.

Bearing in mind these factors which concern the theoretical basis of the whole method, the detailed advantages and limitations of fitting by the preformed method now follow.

ADVANTAGES

(1) Before ordering any lenses specifically for the patient, the practitioner can put on the patient's eye a lens which, even at its worst, is an approximate fit for the eye. Thus, the patient is given the 'feel' of a scleral lens — a most useful experience at the preliminary investigation. This is vital for tolerance trials.

(2) Whatever method of fitting is used, a scleral lens is needed to carry out a contact lens refraction. This lens is preformed in so far as the characteristics of the optic portion are known. Use of a corneal lens, or resort to inexact calculations using ocular refraction and keratometer readings, is a poor alternative.

(3) Specifications having been decided upon, the lens can be ordered by telephone or mail. There is no need to send or preserve casts at this stage.

(4) A preformed scleral lens allows the most accurate interpretation of the practitioner's instructions. Even more important, in most cases, the way in which instructions have been obeyed by the manufacturer can be checked.

(5) The specification of a preformed lens is a set of figures. If optic grind-outs or other adjustments have to be made, appropriate alterations can be made to the original specification. Thus, theoretically, it should be possible to reproduce a lens exactly when a replacement lens is necessary. But in actual practice, few if any manufacturers

can produce two lenses which have identical specifications and have the same corneal clearance on the eye. Even so, replacement lenses are a comparatively simple proposition.

(6) Some preformed scleral lenses can be turned from solid material, which can give a thinner lens than one moulded over a cast.

(7) In certain cases, such as patients with one blind eye, fitting by the impression technique may become very difficult due to visual fixation problems. The preformed method avoids this. Cases of nystagmus may give better results with preformed lenses, and the taking of impressions on high myopes carries a small but definite risk of retinal detachment.

LIMITATIONS

The limitations of the preformed method are mainly financial and organizational. If unlimited funds were available, preformed lenses of every possible combination of parameters could be made in the form of a huge trial case. This would allow selection of the one correct trial lens, amongst many thousands, for each eye fitted. In practice, enough trial lenses must be available to make the method feasible without having a prohibitively large number of lenses. With a basic fitting set of eight haptic portion fitting lenses and twenty-eight fenestrated lenses for optic measurement (FLOM), practically any eye worth fitting with preformed lenses can be fitted. If preformed scleral lens fitting is the only method in use, a much larger fitting set is required. Irregular eyes cannot be fitted with preformed lenses unless the latter are subsequently modified so much that they cease to be preformed.

TYPES OF PREFORMED LENS

A preformed scleral lens is a contact lens, not an impression lens, whose back surface is of some predetermined form. The latter is a mathematical form, thus excluding from consideration the Dallos 'type shells', which are shells based on impressions of different sizes and shapes of eye (Dallos, 1937). The appropriate 'type' lens is selected on the basis of the type of eye being fitted (see Chapter 1, and Chapter 24 in Volume 2).

'True' preformed scleral lenses, fall broadly into two main groups, as follows.

(1) Those in which the haptic fitting and optic fitting are done with the same lenses.

(2) Those in which the haptic portion is fitted with one set of lenses and the optic portion fitted with an entirely different type of optic measuring lens.

GROUP I

Conical Lenses

These were developed by William Feinbloom (1936) from 1936 onwards. Each consists of a spherical optic portion, a haptic portion of which the major part is conical, and a crescent on the temporal side which has a spherical curve (*Figure 10.1*).

In the original 'Tangent Cone' series of lenses there were three variables:

(1) The angle of the cone.
(2) The radius of the temporal crescent.
(3) The back haptic size.

The choice of cone angles was restricted to 86, 92 and 98 degrees, and the radius of the temporal portion varied from 20 to 38 mm. Later, the range was extended to give a choice of basic optic diameters, and 'double cones' were included to fit toroidal eyes.

These lenses are not usually very comfortable as the lens only rests on the sclera where this is tangential to the conical section — and except on a very flat scleral curve, this is not a very large area.

Some of these lenses are still being fitted, but they are no longer widely used.

Wide Angle Lenses

These lenses were introduced by G. Nissel in 1947 and an introductory paper was written by Cowan in 1948 (Jenkin and Tyler-Jones, 1964). The design is a composite one based on the ground spherical lens and the Feinbloom cone lens, the aim being to combine the 'firm haptic fit' of a spherical lens with the good limbal clearance of Feinbloom's cone lens (*Figure 10.2*).

As can be seen in *Figure 10.2*, the optic and haptic are spherical but the transition is conical. The 'corneal chord' (BCOD) is standardized at 11.5 mm and the 'limbal chord' at 16 mm. The terms 'corneal' and 'limbal' chord are used rather than the normal nomenclature because as the lens is usually pressed out over a master tool the more usual measurement of the primary optic diameter cannot readily be made. If the lens is produced by cutting from solid, the terms 'back optic diameter' and 'peripheral diameter of cone' may be substituted for 'corneal chord' and 'limbal chord' respectively.

The variables in this lens are the back optic radius, the back haptic radius and the cone angle of the transition. The cone angles vary from 90 to 108 degrees in 3 degree steps for each 0.25 mm change in back optic radius from 7.50 to 9.00 mm.

Based on the assumption that the best transitional form is one in which the transition is tangential to the back optic curve, an attempt has been made to pair each angle with a particular back optic radius. For example, a 7.50 mm back optic radius is joined by a transition of cone angle 90 degrees, and a 7.75 mm radius with 93 degrees and so on. The selection of these relationships is empirical. The lenses are pressed from master tools with a predetermined haptic form and interchangeable optic portions whose primary sags can be varied. Unless the lens is specially made, there is no choice of the transition cone angle. Another disadvantage with this method of manufacture – the usual one for wide angle lenses – is that after the lens is pressed it is then mounted and the optic portion first ground with a diamond impregnated tool and then polished with a wax polisher. The amount of material removed in this process is an unknown quantity and could vary considerably with the skill of the operator. Thus, lenses with apparently identical specifications could have varying primary sags.

Wide Angle Hapticon Lenses

This lens, developed by S. M. Braff (1965), may be considered as a more sophisticated version of the original wide angle lens. In its production, the die

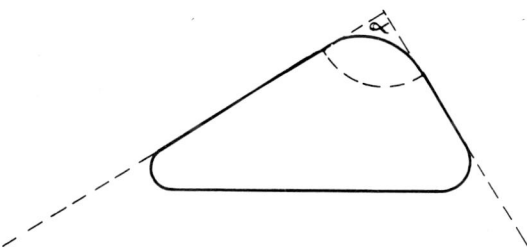

Figure 10.1–Feinbloom conical lens (cone angle α)

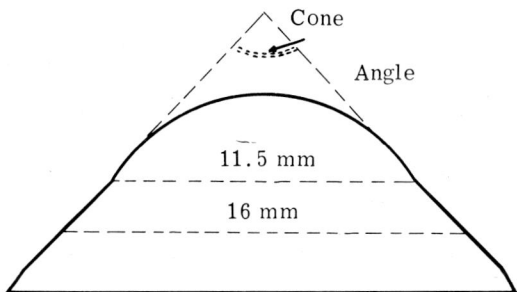

Figure 10.2–Wide angle lens

is made up of three parts instead of only two as in the wide angle lens. The extra part is the transitional portion, which in the original version is allowed to free form by suspension over a void. This extra part gives better control over the form of the transition. In the later version of this lens, the transition is no longer a flat angled section but is a spherically arched section. The optic and limbal chords are still kept the same as in the original wide angle series.

In the manufacture of this lens, after the die and plastics blank have been pre-heated, the blank is moulded to the die under air pressure. This is claimed to give much greater accuracy than the type of hand-operated press and infra-red heater lamps commonly used in England to manufacture wide angle lenses.

GROUP II

Spherical Preformed Lenses

This type of lens is a direct descendant of the original Zeiss ground lens, developed in 1912–13 (von Rohr and Boegehold, 1934). The lens, in its present form, is based on Bier's Transcurve Lens (Bier and Cole, 1948), and both back optic and haptic curves are spherical and are joined by a spherical transition whose radius of curvature is the mean of the back optic and haptic radii and of 2 mm width. The great advantage of this type of lens construction is that it lends itself to the method of cutting from solid material. These

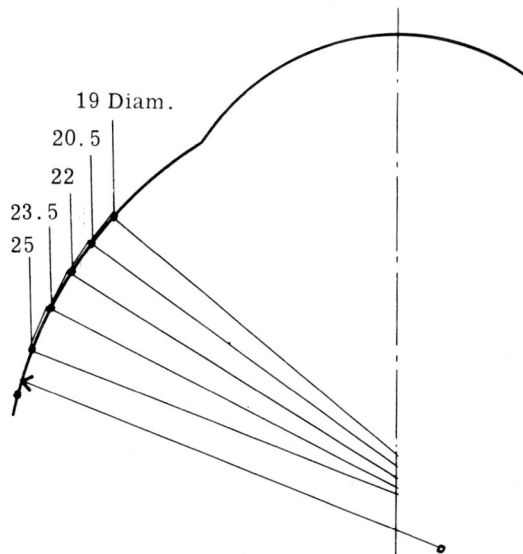

Figure 10.3–'Forknall' offset lens design

lenses can probably be made more accurately than any others. Once made, they can also be checked with greater certainty than those which have been pressed out over a die. When fitted, however, they do seem to need more adjustment in the transitional region than some of the other types of lens.

The fit of the optic portion is measured with FLOM lenses as described on page 246.

Offset Lenses

These very interesting lenses, developed by the late A. J. Forknall between 1947 and 1951, were first described in a paper given to the Contact Lens Society in December, 1951 (Forknall, 1953). The basis of their design was the so-called 'Spherical Rule' connecting the back haptic size with haptic curvature. This rule states that, to maintain the same fit, any increase in back haptic size must be accompanied by a corresponding increase in back haptic radius and the converse. Approximately 1.5 mm increase in back haptic size requires 0.25 mm extra on the back haptic radius. Forknall drew, on a larger scale, a series of curves following this rule and joined them together with a single curve (*Figure 10.3*).

He found that the resultant curve needed a larger radius than the component radii, and also that its centre of curvature had to be 'offset' to the distal side of the axis of symmetry. This was the nature of the curve used in the design of these lenses. There have been two sets of offset lenses: the original ones were used for several years and then Forknall decided that they tended to give slightly too much stand off on the temporal edge and, using slightly different data, he designed the 'x Offsets', which he claimed were more satisfactory in this respect.

Like spherical preformed scleral lenses, the offset lenses are used in conjunction with a FLOM fitting set, but with more possibility of a discrepancy in the process of manufacture. As in the wide angle lenses, the shells were originally pressed out over a die with interchangeable (protruding) steel balls to form the optic portion. A back central optic diameter is specified, but the primary sag may vary somewhat according to the allowance made by the operator in adjusting the height of the steel ball to allow for subsequent 'take-up' of the polishing tool.

BSD Lenses (Bi-Sphériques Décentrés)

These comparatively new lenses have been developed by Henri Biri (1968) and, although as yet few have been fitted, they appear to hold much promise. Their general principle is not unlike that of the Forknall offset lens, but the haptic portion consists of two spherical curves of which only the second one has its centre of curvature decentred nasally with respect to the axis of symmetry of the lens (*Figure 10.4*).

The variables in these lenses are the first haptic radius (RS_1), the second haptic radius (RS_2), the displacement of the centre of curvature of the second haptic radius from the axis of symmetry (D). The second haptic radius is flatter than the first by 0.50–1.00 mm, the greater difference being on the flatter lenses. For example, the trial lens equivalents to spherical lenses of 12.50 mm, 13.75 mm and 14.25 mm back haptic radii would be 12.25/12.75 mm, 13.50/14.25 mm and 14.00/15.00 mm respectively.

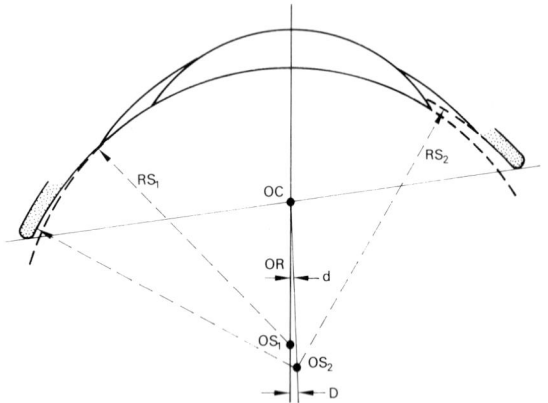

Figure 10.4 – BSD lens (reproduced from Les Cahiers des Verres de Contact by kind permission of H. Biri, les Fréres Lissac, Paris)

The displacement of the centre of curvature of the second haptic radius from the axis of symmetry varies between 0.20 and 0.40 mm. The transition is spherical and of radius equal to the mean of the first haptic radius and back optic radius, plus 0.75 mm. The centre of curvature of the transition is displaced by approximately half the displacement of the second haptic radius from the axis of symmetry. The lenses are usually made horizontal oval with 1 mm difference in back haptic size between the major and minor axes. All trial lenses have back haptic sizes of 23.50 × 22.50 mm or 24.50 × 23.50 mm.

Variation of the displacement of the centre of curvature of the second haptic radius from the axis of symmetry is used when, although the haptic fit appears good, there is excessive clearance at the temporal limbus with nasal limbal tightness on the slightest convergence. This very familiar picture with spherical preformed lenses can be radically altered by this extra variable available with BSD lenses.

Although FLOM lenses are used in conjunction with this lens, the back central optic radius and primary optic diameter so obtained are not used directly in the final lens characteristics. The designer of this lens has prepared a table (*Table 10.5*) which gives the optic characteristics for the final lens for a given FLOM fitting, and the final lens has a steeper back optic radius than that of the FLOM lens, usually by about 0.25 mm. *Table 10.5* is at the end of section on FLOM fitting (page 251).

FITTING SETS

The absolute prerequisite for fitting preformed scleral contact lenses is a fitting set. In Great Britain, at the time of writing, most preformed lenses are wide angle, spherical or offset. There follows a discussion of the fitting sets for these three types of lens.

WIDE ANGLE FITTING SETS

The optic portion is fitted simultaneously with the haptic portion, and a fairly large fitting set is obviously necessary. The minimum desirable set is shown in *Table 10.1*.

Table 10.1–Minimum Wide Angle Fitting Set

Back haptic radius (mm)	Back optic radius (mm)				
12.50	8.00	8.25	8.50		
12.75	8.00	8.25	8.50		
13.00	8.00	8.25	8.50	8.75	
13.25	8.00	8.25	8.50	8.75	9.00
13.50	8.00	8.25	8.50	8.75	9.00
13.75		8.25	8.50	8.75	9.00
14.00			8.50	8.75	9.00
14.25			8.50	8.75	9.00

(30 lenses)

It is known that making a lens round or oval does not make such a great difference to the fit as was once thought. Most practitioners eventually fit oval lenses because they find them more stable in wear, and it is probably best to order horizontal oval lenses. If a 2 mm difference is used between principal meridians, the horizontal back haptic

size can be 23 mm in the steeper part of the range and up to 24.5 mm in the flatter lenses.

SPHERICAL PREFORMED FITTING SETS

The lenses used for obtaining the haptic fit in this set have a very steep back optic radius (8.00 or 8.25 mm) to avoid resting on the cornea, thereby creating a pseudo haptic fit. Virtually all cases that can be fitted with preformed scleral lenses are within the range of estimation of eight fitting lenses (*Table 10.2*).

Table 10.2–Minimum Spherical Fitting Set

Back haptic size (mm)	Back haptic radius (mm)				
22.50	12.50	13.00	13.50	14.00	
24.00		13.00	13.50	14.00	14.50

Steps of 0.25 mm are not essential since it is a fairly easy matter to estimate when an intermediate lens is needed from the flatter and steeper lenses. Round or oval lenses can be used with spherical preformed lenses as with wide angle lenses. Most stock fitting sets sold by manufacturers contain too many lenses in the steeper range and not enough in the flatter range. In the type of patient usually fitted with scleral lenses, a back haptic radius of 14.25 and 14.50 mm is quite a common requirement, yet not many fitting sets contain such lenses.

OFFSET FITTING SETS

The basic offset fitting set originally consisted of thirteen lenses marked with two letters. The first letter gave the 'equivalent' conventional spherical back haptic radius. It must be emphasized that it

Table 10.3–Offset Trial Set Markings

First code letter and equivalent back haptic radius (mm)	(mm)	Second code letter, back haptic size and displacement of optic (mm)
A 11.00	H 12.75	
B 11.25	J 13.00	
C 11.50	K 13.25	E = 22 D 1.5
D 11.75	L 13.50	L = 23.5 × 22.5 D 2
E 12.00	M 13.75	T = 24.5 × 23.5 D 1.5
F 12.25	N 14.00	
G 12.50		

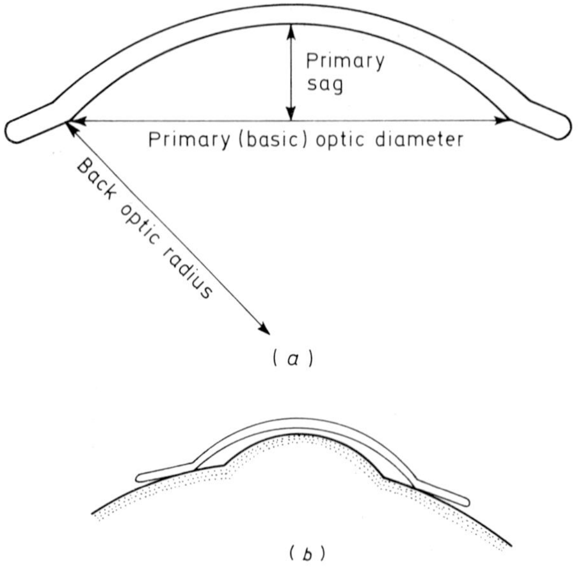

Figure 10.5—(a) Cross-section of a fenestrated lens for optic measurement (FLOM). (b) Diagrammatic representation showing how a FLOM transition rests on the sclera and avoids creating a pseudo fit

no possibility of the haptic rim influencing the corneal fit. This avoids a false impression of corneal clearance being given. The lens is designed to rest on the eye at the transition between the back optic surface and the haptic rim. This transition is deliberately left sharp, although this makes these lenses somewhat uncomfortable *(Figure 10.5)*.

The FLOM is identified by the back optic radius and the primary (basic) optic diameter. If all or some lenses of each back optic radius are optically worked, these lenses can be used for refraction purposes. This avoids having to find for refraction a scleral lens which fills properly with tears to provide a liquid lens. It also eliminates the calculations involved when such a lens does not have the same back optic radius as the one to be ordered. Twenty-eight FLOM lenses, as shown in *Table 10.4*, are usually adequate.

A large (1.5 mm) fenestration hole is provided in each lens, and the front transition should be smooth to permit handling with a suction holder.

was an equivalent because the curve of the haptic portion, although spherical, is a much flatter one with an 'offset' centre of curvature. The second letter designated the back haptic size *(Table 10.3)*.

These lenses have a steep optic portion and are used with separate FLOM lenses.

FLOM LENSES

These lenses were first described by Bier (1948), using the term 'Corneal Ventilated Trial Lenses'. They consist of an optic portion with a narrow haptic rim of approximately 2 mm width. This haptic portion is usually of approximately 13 mm radius, which is almost invariably flatter than the sclera in the limbal region, so that there should be

GENERAL CONSIDERATIONS IN HAPTIC FITTING

The haptic portion of the lens is only there to hold the optic portion in the correct position. Provided that the haptic portion keeps the optic portion reasonably centred during ocular excursions of up to 30 degrees, with an apical corneal clearance of approximately 0.07 mm, and is neither uncomfortable nor cosmetically ugly, the means and reasons whereby this is achieved are relatively unimportant. Much has been written on the fitting and adjustment of the haptic portion, but less attention has been paid to the optic and transitional fits which, somewhat paradoxically, are the most important aspects of scleral lens fitting.

The easily compressed bulbar conjunctiva absorbs minor imperfections in the haptic fit and,

Table 10.4—FLOM Fitting Set

Back optic radius (mm)	Primary optic diameter (mm)								
8.00	13.00								
8.25		13.00	13.25	13.50	13.75	14.00			
8.50			13.25	13.50	13.75	14.00	14.25		
8.75				13.50	13.75	14.00	14.25	14.50	
9.00				13.50	13.75	14.00	14.25	14.75	14.75
9.25					13.75	14.00	14.25	14.50	14.75
9.50									14.75

provided that the optic portion centres well, the basic principles are as follows.

(1) The lens should be comfortable, with the weight, as far as possible, evenly distributed. To achieve this, the maximum possible surface area should rest on the bulbar conjunctiva, as long as the lower haptic portion is not so large as to cause the lens edge to be supported by the inferior fornix.

(2) The lens should not move on the globe any more than necessary. Excessive lateral movements can cause the bubble under the optic portion to move excessively and disturb vision. Undue rotation of the lens can cause the fenestration to be covered by one of the lids for far too long, thereby upsetting corneal metabolism.

(3) The lens should be as large as possible without bumping on either the caruncle or the lateral check ligaments on version movements. This is cosmetically desirable and distributes the weight of the lens over as large an area as possible.

THE TECHNIQUE OF FITTING THE HAPTIC PORTION

It is important to emphasize that the fitting of this portion of the lens is very simple. If the third or fourth trial lens inserted is not the correct one, the practitioner should be in a position to say that the patient is not suitable for preformed scleral lenses. An impression should then be taken. The so-called 'spherical rule' has tended to complicate the fitting of this portion. It suggests that the sclera is hyperbolic in shape, not spherical; and thus, to maintain the same fit, the back haptic radius must be varied as the back haptic size is altered. The relationship is that for an increase of 1.5 mm in back haptic size the radius must be lengthened by 0.25 mm (although some practitioners make a 0.25 mm increase in back haptic radius for each 1 mm increase in back haptic size, which appears to be more realistic).

Marriott (1966) indicates that the temporal anterior sclera is, in fact, roughly spherical but with a much larger radius than previously thought and with a centre of curvature not necessarily on the axis of symmetry of the cornea. When the back haptic size is increased by 0.75 mm, the increase in back haptic radius, for example, from 13.50 to 13.62 mm is less than 1 per cent, suggesting an insignificant amount which in fact appears to make no difference. In recent years, some practitioners have ignored this rule completely. Its only application might be when ordering a lens considerably larger than the largest trial lens available or when fitting an oval spherical lens to a toroidal eye, as explained below. It also applies only to spherical lenses and not to any of the offset types.

As Marriott states (*see* page 225), the sclera is much flatter than the back haptic radii fitted to it. There may therefore be some justification for using the rule. Any increase in back haptic size must introduce extra clearance of the lens from the eye unless the back haptic radius is flattened at the same time. The theory is similar to that of FLOM fitting. *Figure 10.12* illustrates the increase in clearance given by an increase in size, and *Figure 10.11* illustrates the reduction in clearance obtained by using a flatter radius. Thus, one alteration can be used to counteract the other, or each may be used separately to improve the fit of the haptic portion.

Theoretically, in fitting a spherical lens to a toroidal eye, a steeper back haptic radius than that which aligns the flatter meridian of the sclera may be used providing the back haptic size is reduced along this flatter meridian. The reduction in size along the flatter meridian allows the lens to rest close to the eye and the steeper back haptic radius allows a compromise fit between the two meridians.

In practice, horizontal, oval, preformed, spherical lenses do give a slightly better fit on eyes with 'against-the-rule' toricity, but vertical, oval, preformed, spherical lenses do not usually locate correctly on eyes having 'with-the-rule' toricity. As the latter is the more common state of affairs, the possibility of fitting toroidal eyes with spherical lenses by varying their shape is so remote as to be rarely worth considering.

The sequence of events in fitting the haptic portion follows.

The object is to determine the back haptic radius, back haptic size and the optic displacement. Provided there is no corneal touch (giving a pseudo haptic fit), the optic portion is of little interest at this stage. A lens with a steep back optic radius should therefore be chosen in order to give corneal clearance.

Patient Preparation

The patient should be told what is about to happen, and that his cornea is very sensitive and his sclera relatively insensitive. If he follows instructions and looks in the direction indicated, corneal touch can be avoided. It often helps at this stage to touch the bulbar conjunctiva lightly with the edge of a scleral lens, after assuring the patient that the lens is not going to be inserted. The fact that he can hardly feel this usually boosts the patient's morale.

Local anaesthetics are contra-indicated at this stage of the fitting. They are not needed, and the patient's subjective reactions are a useful guide.

Choice of First Lens

The eye to be fitted should be examined and an estimate made of its relative flatness or steepness; a lens is chosen accordingly. A surprisingly good estimate of radius can be made with very little practice. Eyes having steep corneas also tend to have steep scleras, etc., so that keratometry may give a guide to the relative steepness or flatness of the eye.

Insertion of Lens First Chosen

At this stage, only two dimensions — back haptic size and back haptic radius — need be considered. If the back haptic size is too small, it has little effect on the radius. If it is too big, the lens may be lifted by the caruncle and/or the lateral check ligament, giving an erroneous picture. It is important to watch for any such fitting. Too large a lens tends to remain stationary as the eye moves behind it. The lens should be large enough for the edges to remain invisible in the palpebral aperture during normal eye movements.

If the eye can be fitted with spherical preformed scleral lenses, the radius may be too steep, too flat or correct (*Figure 10.6*). Following

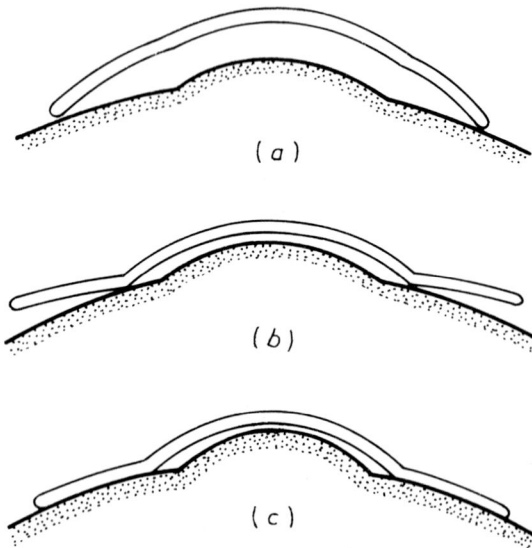

Figure 10.6—Cross-section of a scleral lens. (a) Haptic fit too steep. (b) Haptic fit too flat. (c) Correct

the instillation of fluorescein, the fit may be observed with white light and ultra-violet illumination, having made sure that there is no corneal touch which would invalidate the fit of the haptic portion.

(1) If the back haptic radius is too steep, the lens is tight at the edges and may cause blanching of the conjunctival blood vessels, and fluorescein or air extends from the optic too far towards the periphery of the lens, that is, well past the transition.

(2) If the back haptic radius is too flat, the edges stand off the eye, there is mid-haptic blanching of the bulbar conjunctival vessels, and fluorescein is restricted to within the limbal region.

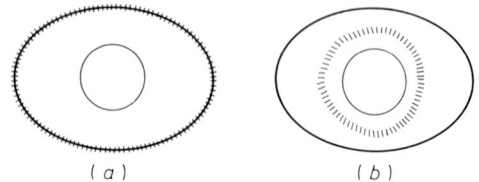

Figure 10.7—Blanching (indicated by lines) in (a) steep, and (b) flat haptic fits (cf. Figure 10.6)

The lens is first examined with white light and the following noted.

(3) Overall size and back haptic size of lens: the lens should be as large as possible. If it is ordered too large, the back haptic size can be reduced — but the converse does not apply.

(4) Blanching: where local pressure is exerted by the lens upon the conjunctiva and the episclera, the blood columns in smaller vessels are squeezed, producing blanching or whiteness in excess of normal (*Figure 10.7*).

Peripheral blanching indicates too steep a lens. Mid-haptic blanching usually accompanies an edge which 'stands off', indicating too flat a lens.

(5) Frothing: a collection of fine bubbles usually indicates a channel.

(6) Edge 'stand-off': looseness or stand-off at the edge of the haptic portion may admit a bubble locally, or trap a pocket or annulus of tears liquid.

Fluorescein Picture

The lens is then examined, using fluorescein and an ultra-violet source. The insertion of fluorescein demonstrates that a preformed scleral lens fit is never a 'text-book' picture, which should not be expected. If the lens fits well over three-quarters of the haptic, this is usually adequate. Pooling in the lower nasal quadrant occurs frequently and can initially be ignored if the haptic fits elsewhere.

Fluorescein pictures indicate steepness or flatness of the lens, as shown in *Figure 10.8*.

If the lens is too steep, there is a large central pool (*Figure 10.8a*).

If the lens is too flat, there is a small central pool, and perhaps pooling round the edges (depending on how the lens tilts on its supporting annulus of sclera) associated with mid-haptic blanching (*Figure 10.8b*).

In an ideal fit, the pool extends evenly just beyond the optic portion (*Figure 10.8c*).

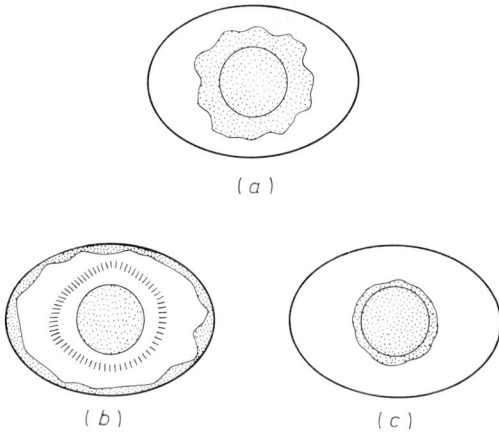

Figure 10.8–Fluorescein pictures with (a) steep, (b) flat and (c) correct haptic fittings respectively. Blanching is indicated by line shading and fluorescein by dot shading

It cannot be emphasized too strongly that during the determination of the haptic fit (with the optic portion clearing the cornea) the depth of the central fluorescein pool is of no interest; only its size is of importance.

Displacement of Optic

The required optic displacement is estimated by putting a suitable lens of known displacement on the eye. Normal displacements fall within the range 0.5–2.5 mm. The lens is inserted, bearing in mind possible alterations of optic displacement and their effects on the disposition of the haptic on either side of the cornea. The trial of alternative lenses with different displacements serves well. For example, too large a nasal haptic portion may cause nasal corneal touch which disappears when a lens of the same back haptic size but bigger displacement of optic is used.

If the ideal fit described above is not obtainable, the eye is rather irregular or toroidal.

An irregular eye requires an impression lens. Toroidal fitting sets are available for preformed spherical, conical, wide angle and offset scleral lenses. The impression method is also suitable for these cases and, consequently, there appears to be no advantage in using toroidal preformed lenses. For satisfactory results, a large and expensive fitting set is needed — hardly justifiable on economic grounds.

It is possible to estimate and order a toroidal lens by estimation from the spherical lens which aligns with the flattest meridian.

Forknall (1959) claimed that nearly all toroidal eyes could be fitted with either 0.50 mm or 0.75 mm difference in back haptic radius between the principal meridians. It is often possible, therefore, to align the flattest meridian and order a lens such that the meridian in which the edge stands off most is 0.50 mm steeper and obtain a satisfactory final lens. Low degrees of toricity can be dealt with by lens adjustment. For example, a spherical lens on an eye having with-the-rule scleral and corneal toricity may give the best fit when the lens aligns the horizontal meridian of the eye but allows a large vertical oval-shaped fluorescein pool extending well beyond the upper and lower cornea accompanied by slight stand-off of the upper and lower edges. This additional limbal space may encourage air bubbles to collect and remain at the 6 and 12 o'clock positions of the limbal region. As such immobile bubbles may cause corneal dessication, such a lens (*Figure 10.9*) would then need a localized back haptic grind-out on either side of the fluorescein pool horizontally followed possibly by slight grinding out of the back haptic near the upper and lower 'mid-rim' portions of the lens. As these back haptic grind-outs permit the lens to settle back on to the eye,

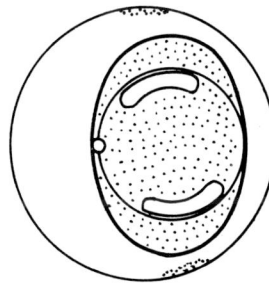

Figure 10.9–Static bubbles in the upper and lower limbal region when an eye having fairly marked corneal astigmatism (with-the-rule) is fitted with a spherical lens. The fluorescein picture is a typical vertical oval with slight vertical edge stand-off (shown by dot shading). In more marked astigmatism the fluorescein pool would break through to the edge

localized transitional grind-outs at 3 and 9 o'clock may also then be needed to relieve limbal touch, followed by a possible back optic grind-out to relieve subsequent central corneal touch.

This demonstrates why large amounts of toricity are best fitted with toroidal lenses or impressions taken.

Haptic fitting determines the dimensions of the back haptic radius, back haptic size and optic displacement. The next step is the determination of the optic specifications. As explained earlier, some types of preformed trial lens are arranged in sets in which both the optic and haptic specifications vary, so that the same lenses are used for fitting both haptic and optic portions. In which case a lens with the correct back haptic radius but with a flatter back optic radius than used during haptic fitting, is selected, until the correct optic and haptic fit is achieved — *see Figures 10.8c and 10.15*. This is the procedure adopted in fitting wide angle lenses. Otherwise, the optic fitting is continued with FLOM lenses.

THE TECHNIQUE OF OBTAINING OPTIC SPECIFICATIONS WITH FLOM LENSES

Fenestrated lenses for optic measurement are not fitted in the sense that they represent a lens to be worn. They simulate the optic portion of a complete scleral lens. The FLOM is simply a measuring device and it may be legitimate to instil a local anaesthetic with a sensitive patient, for the following reasons.

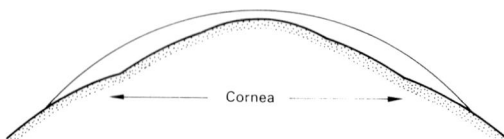

Figure 10.10—Cross-section of the desired corneal clearance

First, these lenses are not comfortable to wear and the patient's subjective response is of no particular value. Secondly, the FLOM giving the desired corneal clearance is not necessarily any more comfortable than any other FLOM. Thirdly, a lens permits a more accurate refraction, with less chance of ciliary spasm, if it is not too uncomfortable. Finally, corneal abrasions caused whilst inserting and removing the trial lenses are less likely if the patient is relaxed and not apprehensive.

The purpose of FLOM fitting is as follows. It is required to arrive at a curve (or series of curves) which clear the centre of the cornea by

an amount between 0.04 and 0.08 mm, with adequate clearance in the limbal region (Marriott and Woodward, 1964).

A suitable optic radius must be considerably flatter than the mean corneal radius (*Figure 10.10*). The difference in radius between the back optic of the lens and the keratometer reading is usually in the region of 0.50–0.70 mm, which dictates the back optic radius of the first trial lens to be inserted. Corneal clearance is achieved in two ways. A lens with a single back optic radius has two variables — the radius of curvature and the primary optic diameter — both of which affect the clearance of the lens from the cornea.

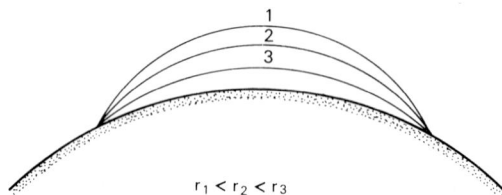

Figure 10.11—The effect on clearance of alterations in back optic (or haptic) radius when primary optic diameter (or back haptic size) is kept constant

Decreasing the back optic radius without altering the primary optic diameter increases the corneal clearance and vice versa (*Figure 10.11*).

Decreasing the primary optic diameter without altering the optic radius reduces the corneal clearance and vice versa (*Figure 10.12*).

Alteration of both variables at once produces either an additive or a subtractive result, or preserves the status quo. In practice, often, a given apical corneal clearance must be maintained while

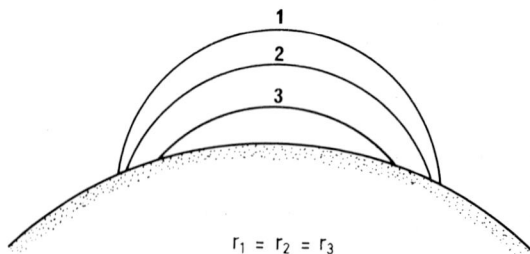

Figure 10.12—The effect on clearance of increasing and decreasing diameter keeping radius constant

the variables are altered for other reasons — for example, to increase or decrease limbal clearance. Usually, there is a simple relationship (*Figure 10.13*) which allows variation of radius and diameter to give the required apical and limbal clearance.

A FLOM lens (*a*) laying on a flat surface has a certain primary sag. If the radius of curvature is increased (*b*) to maintain the same primary sag, its diameter must be increased. The sagitta formula dictates that, for the typical values encountered in FLOM fitting, if the back optic radius is increased by 0.50 mm the primary optic diameter must be increased by the same amount to give approximately the same primary sag. This relationship, although not exact, works well in general.

However, a lens fitted to an eye is not resting on a flat surface but on a curved surface, flatter than the lens itself. *Figure 10.13* shows that if the back optic radius is flattened, an even greater

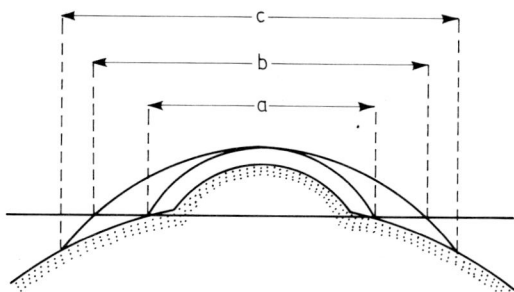

Figure 10.13—The relationship between radius and diameter for a given clearance

diameter (*c*) is needed than on a flat surface to preserve the same corneal clearance. Clinically, it is found that if the back optic radius is increased by a certain amount, then the primary optic diameter must be increased by *twice* that amount to preserve the same corneal clearance. For example, FLOMS 8.00/13.00, 8.25/13.50 and 8.75/14.50 all give the same apical corneal clearance on a certain eye. Because of this, such lenses are known as *clinical equivalents* (although they give different limbal clearances).

The best method of inserting the FLOM is for the patient to look straight ahead while the practitioner gently parts the lids and places the lens symmetrically on the cornea and limbus as if inserting a large corneal lens. If a local anaesthetic has been used, this is perfectly straightforward; otherwise, it is sometimes necessary to place the lens in the upper fornix and then slide it down, with a much greater risk of corneal abrasion. The use of a suction holder allows easier manipulation of the lens during its placement on the eye.

FIRST TRIAL LENS

To choose the back optic radius of this first lens, 0.50–0.70 mm is added to the mean keratometer reading and a lens of the nearest radius is used. If,

for example, the mean keratometer reading is 8.00 mm, an 8.50 mm or 8.75 radius is indicated. In a FLOM fitting set there are usually five lenses of each radius, with diameters, in this example, from 13.25 to 14.50 mm. A lens in the middle of this diameter range (probably an 8.75/14.00) is the first FLOM to insert. It has been suggested that the visible iris diameter is a guide to primary optic diameter, but as this is not a measurement which can be determined accurately and the primary optic diameter range of FLOMs of a given radius only extends over 1 mm there is little or no help from this measurement.

The first FLOM, after cleaning, is inserted without solution and left for up to five minutes to see whether it fills with tears liquid, at what rate it fills, and with what shaped bubble. If the radius is too steep, the bubble tends to cross the pupil; if the radius is too flat, a ring bubble extends a considerable way round the limbus region; if the fit is correct, a small sausage-shaped bubble forms with its concave surface inwards. The bubble shape is an indication of the relationship between the back optic radius and the corneal radius — a round bubble indicating too steep a lens and an annular bubble too flat a lens. The size of the bubble is an indication of the amount of clearance (*Figure 10.14*). Colour Plate X shows a FLOM with excessive apical clearance and insufficient limbal clearance.

If the bubble shape indicates that the radius is too steep, the primary optic diameter is maintained but the radius is flattened by one step (0.25 mm).

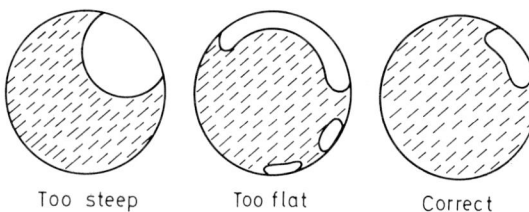

Too steep   Too flat   Correct

Figure 10.14—Bubble shapes in FLOM fitting

A bubble shape indicating that the radius is too flat must be confirmed with fluorescein. If the lens does not fill at all, the primary optic diameter is reduced until the lens does fill or, if this does not have the desired effect, the radius is flattened. At this stage, one variable at a time should be altered — otherwise, it may not be clear which is having the greater effect. In theory, a flattening of 0.25 mm in radius has twice the effect of a 0.25 mm reduction in diameter in reducing the apical corneal clearance (*Figure 10.13*).

White light inspection takes the fitting to the stage where a lens has been selected which fills with tears liquid within two or three minutes and has a satisfactory bubble. Fluorescein is then instilled and the fit is observed under ultra-violet light, enabling two factors to be checked which are not easily observed with any other method: (1) the presence or absence of corneal touch; (2) limbal clearance.

These two factors must be considered in relation to each other. There are now four possible situations in the typical case, as follows.

(1) Central corneal touch with limbal tightness (*Figure 10.15i*). The same radius is maintained and the primary optic diameter is increased to give more clearance until both the touch and tightness are eased.

(2) Central corneal touch with adequate limbal clearance, requiring a shorter radius with the same primary optic diameter (*Figure 10.15ii*).

(3) Limbal tightness with correct central corneal clearance (*Figure 10.15iii*). This requires an increase in primary optic diameter with a compensatory increase in the radius of curvature to

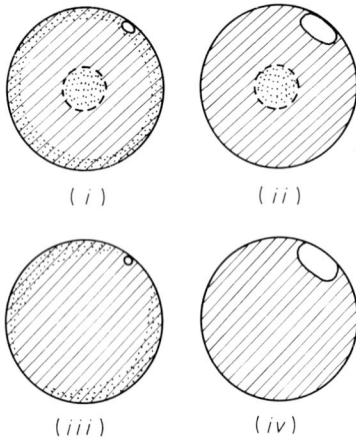

Figure 10.15—Fluorescein pictures in FLOM fitting (see text). Line shading indicates fluorescence, and dot shading corneal touch

preserve the same central corneal clearance. Thus, if the lens which gives limbal tightness with correct apical corneal clearance is 8.50/13.50, the diameter may be increased to 14.00 mm while altering the radius to 8.75 mm to preserve the same apical corneal clearance.

(4) The correct lens shows neither signs of limbal tightness nor apical corneal touch (*Figure 10.15iv*). The bubble circulates freely around the limbus on eye movements, bubble position being opposite to the direction of gaze.

Gentle pressure, for example, with a glass rod, on the apex of the correctly fitting FLOM should demonstrate minimal apical corneal touch while limbal clearance is still maintained.

Figure 10.16 shows diagrammatically the possible sequence of events and the action to take.

The desired optic fit is now represented by two measurements towards the final specification. The only value these figures have in isolation is possibly when FLOM lenses are used to determine the required radius of curvature for the back optic surface of an impression lens.

MULTIPLE CURVE OPTICS

Occasionally, there occurs an eye on which it is impossible to achieve the required fit and reach the desired final specification with ordinary FLOM lenses. There is perhaps the correct shaped bubble and good limbal clearance, but it is impossible to avoid central touch no matter how the radius and basic optic diameter are varied. These are the cases in which multiple back surface radii are needed (*Figure 10.17*).

Multiple curve fitting sets are available, but they are difficult to check and are needed fairly infrequently. A method of fitting which avoids recourse to these fitting sets and is adequate for the average practice is as follows.

The eye is fitted with single curve FLOMs, in the normal way, to find the lens which gives adequate limbal clearance with correct bubble size and shape but which still touches centrally. The diameter of the touch area is then measured and 2 mm is added to determine the diameter of the new back central optic, whose radius is 0.50 mm steeper.

If, for example, the first lens is 9.00/14.50, giving a touch area of 6 mm in diameter, an optic with 8.50 mm radius and a back central optic diameter of 8.00 mm is ordered with a 9.00 mm peripheral optic radius and back peripheral optic diameter of 14.50 mm. (For refraction purposes, an 8.50 mm radius lens must be used or the appropriate power allowance made.)

This method works well in practice and avoids using a double curve fitting set of doubtful veracity.

INTERPRETATION OF RESULTS

A lens may then be ordered. There are normally no allowances to be made in the specification of the haptic portion. The back haptic radius is the one that was chosen as the best fit — or, if the exact trial lens required was not available, the one deduced by interpolation.

Lens inserted

Lens does not fill:
(1) Reduce diameter
until lens fills.
(2) If lens still
does not fill flatten
radius until lens
does fill

Lens fills

Observe bubble size and shape

If large bubble
impinging on
central area,

If bubble correct
shape but too large,
keep radius same,
reduce diameter
until correct size

flatten radius
until correct
shape bubble

If bubble correct
size and shape
insert fluorescein
and check no
touch and limbal
clearance

If no bubble insert
fluorescein and look
for central touch

No central touch:
increase diameter
and check limbal
clearance

If central touch:

If plenty of room in
limbus region, same
diameter, shorten radius
until no touch

If tight on limbus
region: same radius
and increase diameter
until no touch

Lens should have correct shaped
bubble. Lens with same radius
but 0.25 mm greater diameter
should give too large a bubble.
With 0.25 mm less diameter, there
should be central touch. There
should be adequate limbal clearance

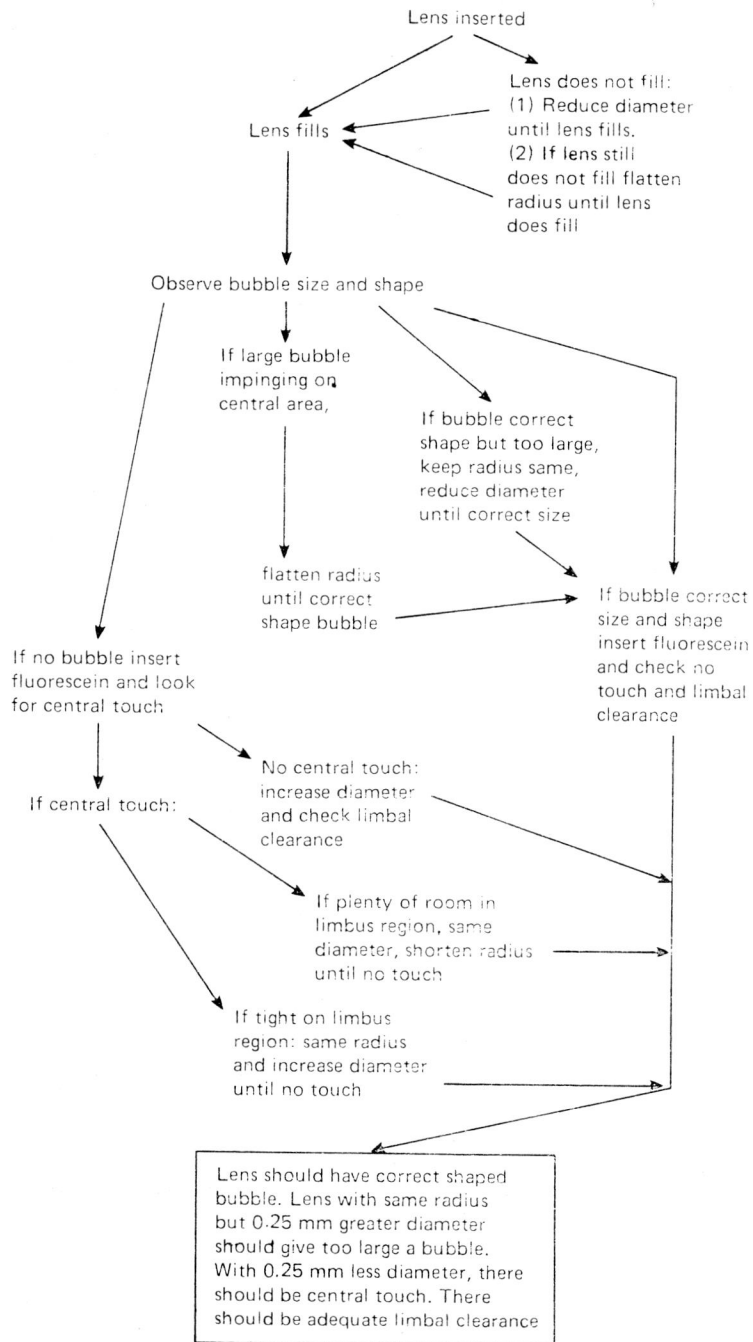

Figure 10.16—FLOM fitting schema

If composite fitting lenses were used, it may be necessary to order the final lens with a primary optic sag varied by ±0.05–0.10 mm because the range of lenses giving the correct haptic fit may not give the correct central corneal clearance. Estimation based on the apical touch and other factors such as bubble size may be required.

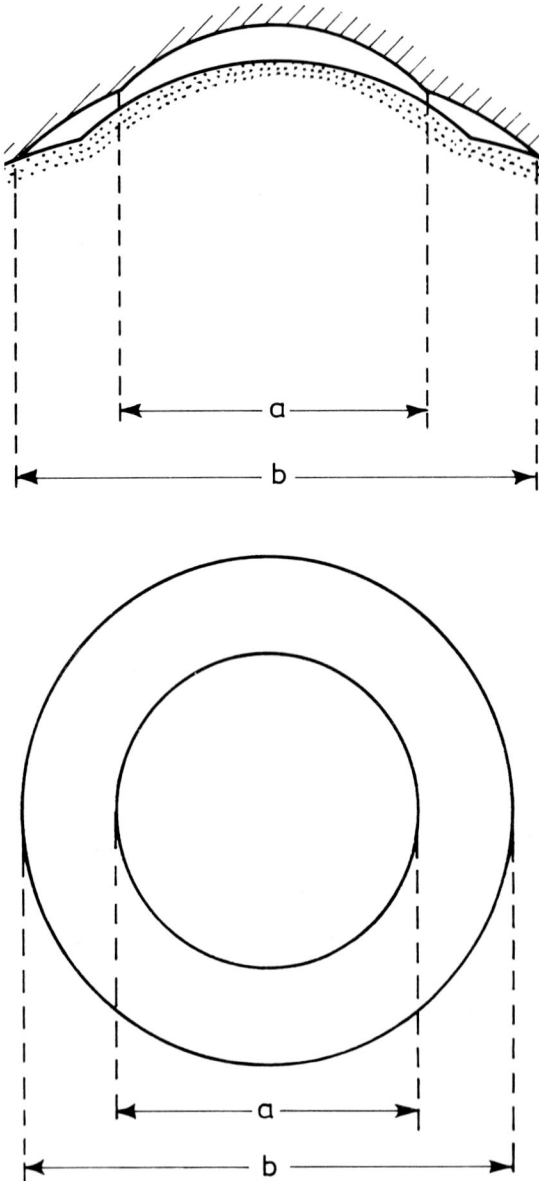

Figure 10.17–Cross-section and plan view of a multiple curve optic. (a) is the back central optic diameter, and (b) the back peripheral optic diameter

Possibly because of the relatively imperfect fit on the sclera, preformed scleral lenses settle closer to the eye after a period of time. More corneal clearance is required initially than may be acceptable in the finally fitted lenses in order to allow for settling to take place. The amount of settling varies considerably from patient to patient, being most on big, soft eyes often found in high myopes.

Settling is compensated for by ordering a primary optic diameter larger than that of the correctly fitting FLOM lens. Elaborate guides have been given (for example, Bier, 1957) for the allowances to be made in a particular case, but an addition of 0.25 mm suffices in most cases. For example, if the final FLOM is 8.75/13.75, then the optic specification 8.75/14.00 should be ordered. If a greater allowance is made, the patient is likely to be bothered by excessively large bubbles in the first few weeks of wear. It is no great comfort for the patient to be told that these bubbles should diminish in a few weeks if they are at that moment interfering with his daily life. Most patients have to earn a living, and they find it difficult to wear such lenses enough for them to settle sufficiently. The extra 0.25 mm may not give sufficient extra clearance – in which case, the lens may give apical corneal touch after some weeks of wear. It is then a relatively simple matter to grind 0.05 or 0.10 mm from the back optic portion with modern modification tools (*see* Chapter 23, Volume 2).

An ideally fitting fully settled scleral lens has a central corneal clearance between 0.04 and 0.08 mm with no bubble when the eye is in the primary position. Bubbles appear on version movements but should rotate freely around the limbus and then disappear when the eye has returned to the primary position for a few seconds. This is shown in *Colour Plates VIII* and *IX*.

As mentioned previously, when fitting BSD lenses the optic characteristics are obtained from a table prepared by the designer, and not as in the method just described (*see Table 10.5*).

REFRACTION

Refraction is best carried out using a FLOM which has a known back vertex power. The lens used fulfil the following four requirements.

(1) It should have the same back central optic radius as the prescription lens. Alternatively, the nearest radius available is used and the necessary calculations are made (*see* Chapter 4, page 113).

(2) The lens must fill adequately.

(3) There must be adequate, and, as near as possible, correct corneal clearance. Excessive corneal touch may flatten and distort the cornea,

Table 10.5—Suggested Back Central Optic Radii and Primary Optic Diameters to be Ordered in Relation to the Ideal Fitting Set Lens Parameters when Fitting BSD Lenses

FLOM fitting set BOR (mm)	FLOM fitting set POD (mm)						
	12.75	13.00	13.25	13.50	13.75	14.00	14.25
8.00	7.75/13.00	7.75/13.50 −0.02	7.80/13.50	7.80/13.75 −0.02	7.87/14.00 +0.02	7.87/14.25 +0.02	7.87/14.50
8.25	8.00/13.00 +0.02	8.00/13.25	8.00/13.50	8.00/13.75 −0.02	8.05/14.00	8.05/14.25 −0.02	8.12/14.50
8.50	8.25/13.00 +0.02	8.20/13.25	8.25/13.50 +0.02	8.25/13.75	8.25/14.00	8.50/14.25 −0.02	8.50/14.50
8.75	8.37/13.00	8.37/13.25 −0.02	8.45/13.50 +0.02	8.50/13.75 +0.02	8.50/14.00	8.50/14.25	8.50/14.50
9.00	8.62/13.00 +0.02	8.62/13.50	8.62/13.50 −0.02	8.70/13.75	8.75/14.00 −0.02	8.75/14.25	8.75/14.50

It will be seen from the table that the final lens invariably has a steeper BOR than the FLOM lens fitting indicated, and the degree of steepening is greater on the smaller primary optic diameters.

When figures such as +0.02 or −0.02 are seen, these are instructions to the manufacturer to give this much more or less primary sag, the amount being measured in millimetres.

giving a false refraction. Too much clearance introduces too large a bubble or at least provides another source of error, the thicker tears layer having an optical effect different from that which is required.

(4) The front surface of the lens must stay wet, wetting solutions being used if necessary.

Ideally the lens should also be as near as possible to the final back vertex power required (*see* Chapter 4).

Any favoured refractive technique may be used, and if two suitable powered lenses are available the refraction should be binocular.

Residual astigmatism should be measured but, at this stage, only the best sphere ordered. Residual astigmatism may vary or even disappear when the lenses have been worn for a while. If it does not disappear, it is still necessary for the lenses to assume their final resting position before the axis may be marked with the lens *in situ*, as even horizontal, oval, preformed, scleral lenses rarely lay with the major axis exactly along the horizontal meridian.

The vertex distance of the supplementary trial lens from the eye must be measured and its effective power at the cornea calculated (*see* Appendix A, page 304). With a knowledge of the keratometric findings, the approximate power of the liquid lens can be calculated and, thus, the contact lens power compared with the spectacle prescription. Any large discrepancies found must be investigated. On the higher positive powers, the thickness of the trial contact lens used must also be taken into account. This part of the procedure of fitting preformed scleral lenses is the part where there is the least excuse for error.

FENESTRATION AND LOCAL ADJUSTMENTS

At this stage, the lenses have arrived from the laboratory and been checked, and the patient has returned for final fitting.

Insertion of the lenses is preceded by an explanation that, until the lenses are fenestrated, vision is likely to be unclear. If necessary, the lenses can be inserted filled with liquid to avoid this.

The fit of the lenses is then checked with white light and with fluorescein to detect gross errors of fitting. Minor areas of tightness and leaks may safely be left until after fenestration since they may then alter or disappear. Fenestration helps to equalize the pressure in front of and behind the lens, allowing it to settle back on the eye. The back haptic size must be corrected before fenestration, particularly if it is too large. Also, if the back haptic size is too great in any one meridian this must be remedied before fenestration, otherwise the fenestration may come to rest in the wrong place with respect to the lids. If the lens is too small, there is no remedy and the lens should be re-ordered.

The back haptic size can be reduced on a grindstone or grinding ball, or with a file — the latter method being slower but safer. The edge is then reshaped with a narrow file, or fine carborundum ball, and smoothed with fine sandpaper. Final polishing is carried out on a soft buff (see Chapter 23, Volume 2).

Assuming that the size is now correct, the lens is re-inserted, after a grease pencil or waterproof line has been drawn along the proposed horizontal meridian. A lens with grease pencil on the outer surface may feel gritty, and the patient should be warned of this. (Waterproof fibre pens are more satisfactory, but paraffin has to be used to remove the marking.) The patient is then instructed to look in every direction in turn and execute some rapid eye movements. It does not matter if the lens rotates a little, provided that it always returns promptly to the same position. If it does not do this, the back haptic size is probably still too big. Alternatively, corneal touch may be present, causing the lens to spin on the cornea; or there may be an area of heavy haptic touch acting as a pivot for the lens. This must be remedied. When the lens is stable, it is ready for fenestration.

The fenestration should be positioned on the optic portion on the temporal side in the shadow of the upper lid when the eye is in the primary position. If it is placed too far towards the centre of the cornea, it may subsequently cause a localized area of dimpling. If it overlies the sclera, it becomes too readily visible. With a small hole of 0.50–0.70 mm correctly positioned just in front of the iris pattern, the fenestration should be visible only to the trained observer. This size appears optimum as a larger diameter gives a poor cosmetic effect and a smaller diameter tends to clog with mucus fairly easily.

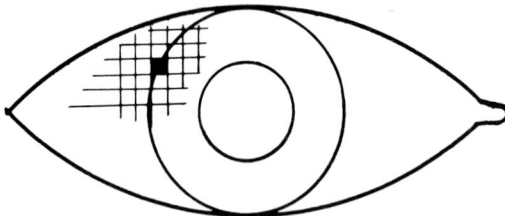

Figure 10.18–Cross-hatching drawn on a scleral lens to mark the fenestration position (upper lid slightly retracted)

Marking the fenestration position may be done while the patient looks straight ahead — a cross being made with a grease pencil or waterproof fibre pen to indicate the correct position. An alternative method is to draw a squared grid in the appropriate limbal area before the lens is inserted. When the lens is inserted, it is simply a

matter of making a mental note in which square of the grid the hole should be drilled. In *Figure 10.18*, the hole would be correctly positioned in the centre square of the centre row.

The hole is best made by hand, using a 0.50 mm or 0.70 mm drill mounted in a pin-vice. It is better to make a slight mark on the front surface first with a sharply pointed tool to stop the drill

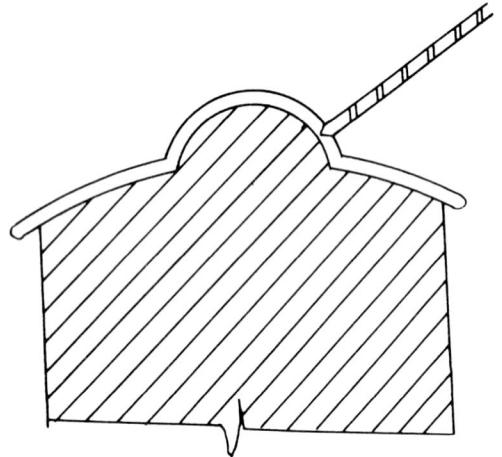

Figure 10.19–Drilling a fenestration with the lens mounted on a cast

slipping sideways. With thinner lenses and smaller holes, the angle of the hole is of little significance and it is drilled at right-angles to the front surface. If the lens is hand-held, the hole can be drilled from the back, but by mounting the lens on a plaster mount, good contact is obtained by boring from the front (*Figure 10.19*).

The hole is countersunk at both ends with a small dental ball tool and then polished, as described in greater detail in Chapter 23, Volume 2.

The lens and fenestration hole are thoroughly cleaned and the lens is placed without solution on the patient's eye. Minor tight and loose areas should not be modified at this stage because they may alter after a few hours' wear. Initially the patient may notice a clicking noise as air is expressed or enters via the fenestration hole during eye movements and blinking. This usually goes as the lens settles. The lens should only be adjusted under the circumstances listed below.

(1) The lens does not fill. It must be settled by evenly grinding out the back haptic portion until it fills well enough to give reasonable visual acuity.

(2) There is corneal touch. As this is likely to increase after a few hours' wear, a back optic grind-out must be performed immediately.

(3) There is limbal tightness. This must be relieved before the patient wears the lens.

(4) The back haptic size is still too large. The size must be reduced, particularly if it causes heavy nasal bumping on the limbus region on convergence.

(5) The power is more than ±0.75 DS incorrect. A correction is then necessary before the lens is worn.

All other adjustments should be carried out at subsequent visits – probably on the first visit at which the patient arrives having worn the lenses for a few hours. It is important that all transitions are smooth and well-blended, the fenestration hole well polished, and that the final corneal and limbal clearance are correct, otherwise frothing of the bubble may occur with resultant dimpling of the corneal epithelium, and dimple 'veil' occur after lens removal (*see* Chapter 16, Volume 2).

INSERTION AND REMOVAL

The only acceptable method of insertion is by the use of the fingers. Suction holders are generally unnecessary and unaesthetic. The only acceptable method of removal is by using the upper lid. Methods involving hooking the lens out with the fingernails are dangerous.

Insertion and removal is best taught by the practitioner, who first demonstrates with his own lenses. It is made clear to the patient that, in both insertion and removal, he should keep his sensitive cornea out of harm's way. With regard to positioning of the lens, the patient is told that the fenestration hole goes on the side towards the ear (*see* Chapter 8).

LENS ORDERING

The result of a preformed scleral lens fitting being simply a set of figures, and not a cast as in impression fitting, it is very important that these figures are conveyed to the prescription laboratory (or anyone else) in a form which is unambigious and universally accepted.

At the time of writing, the only British Standards relating to preformed scleral lenses are BS 5562: 1978 and BS 3521:1979. Their terms are applicable to spherical preformed scleral lenses.

The essentials of its recommendations regarding back surface specification are as follows:

Dimensions (in millimetres) and orientations are invariably to be given in the following order:

(*i*) Eye and preformed scleral lens (S denotes scleral).

(*ii*) Back central optic radius.

(*iii*) Back central optic diameter.

(*iv*) Back peripheral optic radius, if present.

(*v*) External diameter of back peripheral optic zone (if applicable).

(*vi*) Back haptic radius.

(*vii*) Back haptic size or overall size and long and short axes. (*Note:* Where BHS is specified it should be preceded by a letter B, otherwise the dimension is assumed to be the OS).

(*viii*) Orientation of long axis in standard axis notation.

(*ix*) Displacement of optic and direction.

(*x*) Details of transitions.

Example:

LS/8.50: 11.50/11.00: 13.50/13.50:
(*i*) (*ii*)   (*iii*)   (*iv*)   (*v*)   (*vi*)

B24.00 *X* 22.00/L 10/D 1.00 in/ sharp transitions
 (*vii*)   (*viii*) (*ix*)   (*x*)

The previous British Standard recommendation was written in 1962 and then the back surface specification was written in the sequence required by a technician cutting the lens from solid material, namely:

(*i*) Radius of back haptic surface.

(*ii*) Radius of back central optic surface.

(*iii*) Primary optic diameter.

(*iv*) (Subsidiary optic dimensions)

(*v*) Back haptic size or overall size.

(*vi*) Orientation of long axis.

(*vii*) Displacement of optic.

Example:
(*i*)   (*ii*)   (*iii*)   (*v*) (*vii*)
14.00/8.50/13.50/B24 D1 in.

At the current time (1979) most fitting sets have lenses labelled in this old sequence. Great care is therefore necessary to avoid confusion, particularly where parameters of similar dimensions such as back haptic radius and basic optic diameter could be inadvertently interchanged.

(1) Radius of back central optic surface.

(2) Primary optic diameter.

(3) Radius of back haptic surface.

(4) Back haptic size.

(5) Displacement of optic.

The example previously written would then become:

8.50/13.50/14.00/B 24 D1 in.

It can be seen that the 1962 Standard presents a technician cutting a preformed lens from solid with the dimensions in the order that he needs to know them, and this may have been the original reason for this particular scheme. If the latest suggested method is adopted, care will have to be taken when using fitting sets marked with the original system as the back haptic radius and basic optic diameter are usually of similar dimensions and could be confused.

WIDE ANGLE LENSES

The corneal and limbal chords being standardized on these lenses, the specifications to be given are as follows.
  (1) Back optic radius.
  (2) Back haptic radius.
  (3) Back haptic size.
  (4) Displacement of optic.
In the old system back haptic radius was written first followed by back optic radius and most fitting sets available are labelled using the old system.

As this is a 'composite' type of lens, where the haptic and optic specifications are obtained with the same lens, the final lens required is often not in the fitting set. The nearest lens is usually ordered, together with the instructions 'raise (or lower) optic by x-tenths of a mm' according to whether greater or less corneal clearance is required.

OFFSET LENSES

These lenses are ordered in the following way.
  (1) Back optic radius.
  (2) Primary optic diameter.
  (3) The first letter on the fitting set lens (that is, the 'equivalent' back haptic radius).
  (4) The 'size' letter (*see Table 10.3*).

Example:

(1) (2) (3) (4)
8 / 13 / K / T

whereas the old system was to give 'K / 8 / 13 / T' which is still used on these fitting sets.

BSD LENSES

These lenses are ordered in a similar way to spherical preformed lenses but, in addition, the displacement of the centre of curvature of the second haptic radius from the axis of symmetry must be specified.

With all types of preformed lens the power of the lens is to be given in the back vertex form. Lens thickness is easily controlled with preformed lenses and this can be ordered as desired. 0.50– 0.60 mm is a good thickness to aim for after doing any necessary modifications.

SUMMARY

The fitting of scleral lenses by the preformed method is a matter of applying simple rules and accepting the limitations of each lens type. Complex formulae are of no help when attempting to fit an eye with a lens whose design is intrinsically wrong for the contours of the eye being fitted. Over the last few years, there seems to have been a renewed interest in fitting preformed lenses and several promising designs have emerged. More attention is now being paid to the transitional form and allowance is being made for the differing axes of symmetry of the scleral and corneal curves. Hours spent on local adjustments to remedy basic defects of fit due to unsatisfactory lens design are no longer acceptable.

The familiar appearance of a large bubble at the temporal limbus may become a thing of the past. Although the preformed spherical lens still serves well in demonstrating steep and flat fits, and FLOM fitting is an exercise in logical thinking, it is increasingly recognized that a lens with more variables in its design is needed for satisfactory preformed scleral lens fitting.

For sports purposes and swimming, for short periods of wear up to four hours, a minimum clearance, sealed (non-fenestrated) scleral lens is ideal as it gives such stable vision and cannot fall out of the eye. Such lenses must be inserted filled with a suitable solution (*see* Chapter 3, page 81); and this may present a little difficulty as the head must be held down during insertion so that the solution is not spilled.

The advent of gas permeable hard lens materials together with better wetting materials could well increase the number of scleral lenses fitted. There is no doubt that in the higher power ranges, both positive and negative, a lathe-cut scleral lens can give the best vision of any type of contact lens. The larger front optic that can be worked, combined with the lens stability gives steady vision unequalled by other lenses. Residual astigmatism can be most satisfactorily corrected with scleral lenses and in all these types of case the scleral lens may well again become the lens of choice.

REFERENCES

Bier, N. (1948). 'The practice of ventilated contact lenses.' *Optician* **116**, 497–501

Bier, N. and Cole, P. J. (1948). 'The transcurve contact lens fitting shell.' *Optician* **115**, 605–606, 610

Bier, N. (1957). *Contact Lens Routine and Practice,* 2nd ed. London: Butterworths

Biri, H. (1968). 'Le B.S.D. nouveau verre scléral de form géométrique.' *Cah. Verres Contact* **16**, 8–16

Braff, S. (1965). 'The design and development of a scleral lens.' *J. Am. optom. Ass.* **36**, 217–223

British Standard 3521 (1979). *Glossary of Terms Relating to Ophthalmic Lenses and Spectacle Frames.* BS 3521: 1979. *Part 3. Glossary of terms relating to contact lenses.* London: British Standards Institution

Cowan, J. M. (1948). 'The wide angle contact lens.' *Optician* **115**, 359

Dallos, J. (1937). 'The individual fitting of contact glasses.' *Trans. Ophthal. Soc. U.K.* **57**, 509–520

Feinbloom, W. (1936). 'A plastic contact lens.' *Trans. 15th Congress Am. Acad. Optom.* **10**, 44

Forknall, A. J. (1953). 'Pre-formed lenses, corneal fit, with a note on the slit lamp.' *Br. J. physiol. Optics* **10**, 15–22, 49

Forknall, A. J. (1959). 'Some notes on haptic lenses.' *Br. J. physiol. Optics* **16**, 96–115

Jenkin, L. and Tyler-Jones, R. (1964). *Theory and Practice of Contact Lens Fitting,* pp. 15–16. London: Hatton Press

Marriott, P. J. and Woodward, E. G. (1964). 'A method of measuring the corneal clearance of a haptic lens.' *Br. J. physiol. Optics* **21**, 61–83

Marriott, P. J. (1966). 'An analysis of global contours and haptic lens fitting.' *Br. J. physiol. Optics* **23**, 3–40

von Rohr, M. and Boegehold, H. (1934). *Das Brillenglass als Optisches Instrument,* p. 17. Berlin: Springer

Chapter 11

Corneal Lens Fitting

A. J. Phillips

BASIC REQUIREMENTS

The student new to contact lens practice is often confused by the multitude of different fitting techniques and lens types available, each claiming its own special advantages. The basic requirements of a good fitting contact lens are often forgotten and should be stressed from the outset. These are simply:

(1) Maintenance of corneal integrity (including integrity of the related ocular and extraocular tissues).

(2) Adequate vision.

(3) Patient comfort.

(4) Invisibility.

It follows, therefore, that the best fitting technique or lens construction to use in any one particular instance is the one which most readily satisfies these criteria. For many patients, several different techniques may all perform adequately; in others, the use of a specific technique may give improved results.

CORNEAL CONTOUR

In the fitting of corneal lenses, a knowledge of corneal contours is essential. To review the enormous volume of research on this single topic would be impossible in this chapter. Nevertheless, for fitting purposes, a basic knowledge will suffice.

In the late 1940s and early 1950s, the main instrument available for measurement of corneal curvature was the keratometer. This gave an accurate value for the central corneal curvature; but a single curve lens made to this curvature and an overall size of 9.0–10.0 mm showed a fluorescein picture (*see* page 260) of central and peripheral touch with intermediate corneal clearance (*Figure 11.1*).

Observations such as this led Bier (1956) to conceive the idea of a triple zone cornea (*Figure 11.2*). Bier believed there to be a central, regular and positively curved zone; outside this a less curved or *relatively* negative zone; and beyond this a further zone of steeper curvature. From this general idea arose the concept of a 'corneal cap'. This commonly used term in contact lens practice was meant to indicate the central, regular corneal area. Bier stated that in the average case the corneal cap was decentred 0.2–0.6 mm nasally and 0.2 mm superiorly.

Modifications to the keratometer confirmed the peripheral flattening of the cornea but representations of this flattening were often incorrectly shown, as in *Figure 11.3*.

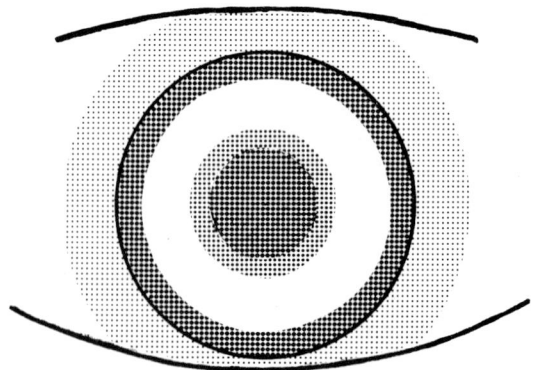

Figure 11.1—Fluorescein picture obtained when fitting a monocurve corneal lens of approximately the same curvature as the central cornea. Shading within the lens circumference indicates corneal bearing and the unshaded ring indicates corneal clearance

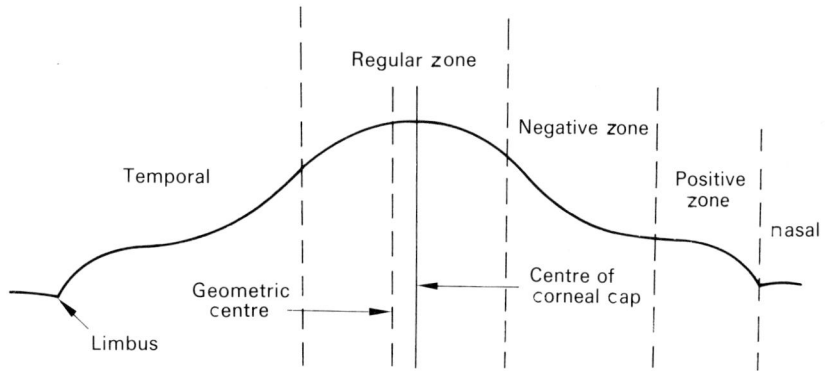

*Figure 11.2–Diagrammatic repre-
sentation of the corneal contour
(after Bier, 1956)*

Cap decentred $^1/5 - ^3/5$ mm nasally
and approximately $^1/5$ mm superiorly.

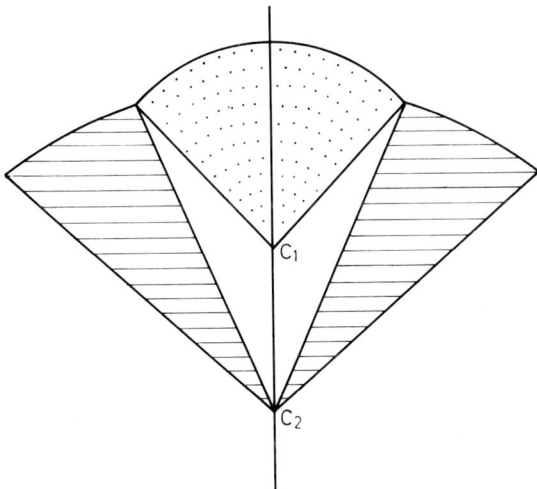

*Figure 11.3–Incorrect representation of peripheral corneal
flattening as measured by a keratometer*

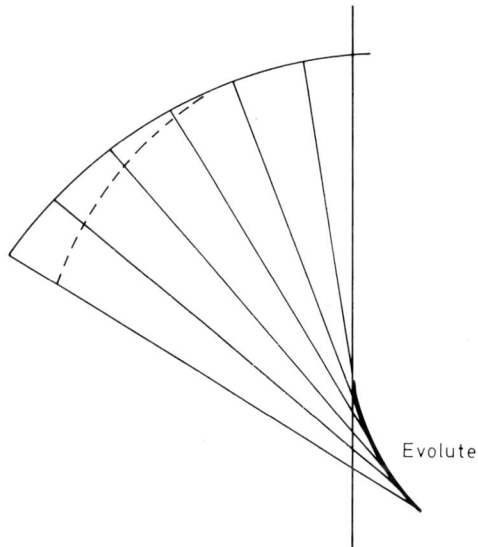

Figure 11.4–General appearance of a corneal evolute

The centre of curvature for the central region lies at C_1, and at C_2 for the peripheral portion. The construction so produced supported the concept of a central corneal cap, a secondary negative zone and a tertiary positive zone.

The introduction of more accurate methods of assessing corneal contour — such as single mire keratometry, photokeratoscopy and other photographic methods — have shown that the cornea has a constantly varying radius of curvature; also, that the centre of curvature is constantly changing to a new position, the centres of curvature forming a locus of points which extends from the centre of curvature of the central point to an off-axis

position. The locus of centres of curvature for a constantly varying curve is known as an *evolute*. The general appearance of a corneal evolute is shown in *Figure 11.4*.

It is now possible to see why the original single curve lens made to the same curvature as the central keratometer reading gave the fluorescein picture shown in *Figure 11.1*, and how this led to the concept of a triple zone corneal configuration as described by Bier. However, although the conception of a 'corneal cap' is not strictly correct, for clinical purposes it is often convenient to assume that one does exist, for the following reasons.

(1) The flattening close to the centre of the cornea is so small that the central region may be assumed close to spherical, in each principal meridian, for clinical purposes.

(2) The keratometer reading obtained for fitting purposes is not the curvature value at the geometric centre of the cornea but of two points some 1.2–1.8 mm each side of the centre (*see* Chapter 5). For a typical back central optic diameter (BCOD – *see* page 259) of 6.00–7.00 mm, the keratometer

(3) Where it is attempted to align too large a central area of the cornea with one single curve of a lens, the peripheral corneal flattening shows a circle of non-alignment of the fluorescein pattern in the mid-periphery of the curve, similar to that shown in *Figure 11.1*. Earlier writers on corneal lens fitting claimed that this was because the back central optic diameter was larger than the corneal cap, and they recommended that a smaller BCOD be used. While it has been shown that the corneal

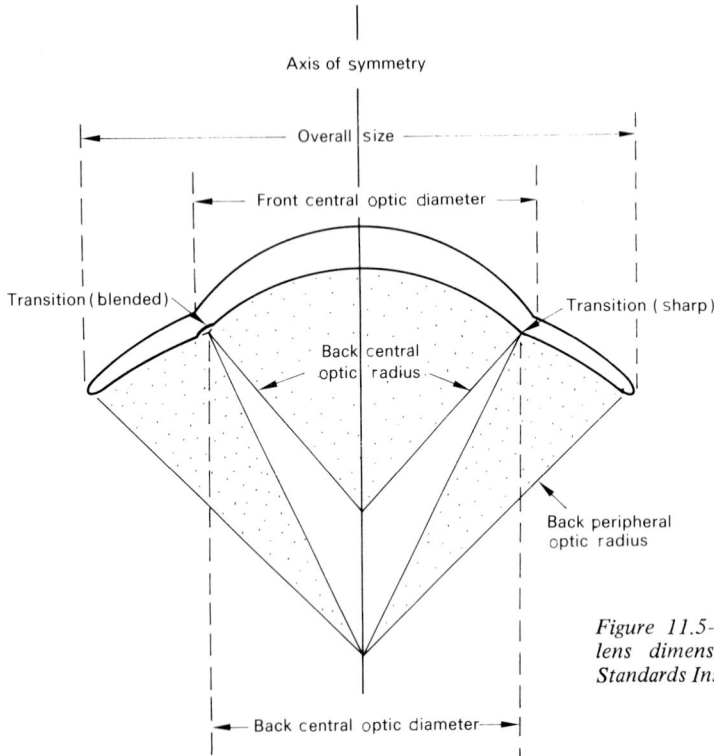

Figure 11.5–Diagrammatic representation of corneal lens dimensions as recommended by the British Standards Institution

reading is therefore approximately the mean value of the curvature at the geometric centre* and that at the edge of the back central optic portion. A curvature value is therefore obtained which should closely approach the cornea over this diameter.

* Arias (1960) has pointed out that, since the visual and geometric centres of the cornea do not normally coincide, when the patient fixates the keratometer target he is looking along the visual axis and a slightly flat value of central curvature is obtained. The curvature at the geometric centre may be 0.02–0.05 mm steeper than the keratometer reading. This has been confirmed for emmetropes by Sheridan (1970) though in myopes the visual axis appears to pass through the steepest part of the cornea.

cap is a misconception, the clinical remedy of improving the area of alignment by reduction of the BCOD still holds good as an attempt to align a spherical contact lens with a non-spherical cornea.

TERMS RELATING TO CORNEAL LENSES

Before proceeding further, it is necessary to define the terms used to describe the form and dimensions of corneal lenses. It became apparent several years ago that workers in different countries were using varying terms to describe the same dimension of a lens and that ambiguity in the terms used could give rise to confusion. Accordingly, British Standards BS 5562:1978 and BS 3521:1979 were published to define terms used to describe the power, form, dimension and specification of corneal, scleral and soft lenses. It is only possible in this chapter to define some of the more commonly used terms, and the student is strongly urged to obtain copies of both these Standards.

DEFINITIONS

(1) *Corneal lens:* A contact lens designed to be worn in front of the cornea only.

(2) *Central optic portion* (COP): The central region of the optic portion (of specified diameter and radius of curvature) a term applicable only when there is a peripheral optic zone. (Back central optic radius – BCOR – is the radius of this portion.)

(3) *Peripheral optic zone* (POZ): An annulus of specified dimensions surrounding the central optic portion. (In practice, there may be several curves in this peripheral zone which are usually termed first back peripheral optic radius – BP_1OR, second back peripheral optic radius – BP_2OR, etc.)

(4) *Overall size* (OS): The maximum external dimension(s) of the finished lens or shell. In non-circular shapes, the long axis (LA) is first determined as the maximum dimension. The short axis (SA) is the perpendicular distance between tangents to the lens periphery on either side of, and parallel to, the long axis.

(5) *Optic diameter(s)*: The diameter of any specified optic portion, measured to the surrounding junction. If the latter is not circular the major and minor diameters define the size. The term may be qualified, for example, back central optic diameter (BCOD) which is the optic diameter of the back central optic portion. In practice the presence of blending may make this dimension uncertain.

(6) *Back vertex power* (BVP): Back vertex power of the (central) optic portion of the lens, measured in air, that is, the reciprocal of the back vertex focal length measured in metres.

(7) *Centre thickness* (t_c): The thickness of the (central) optic portion measured at its geometrical centre.

FORCES AFFECTING THE LENS ON THE EYE

For a correctly fitting lens, a balance is necessary between those forces acting to hold the lens against the cornea and those acting to move the lens or eject it from the eye. The most important of these forces are reviewed as follows.

Capillary Attraction

The force of attraction between the lens and the cornea varies inversely with the distance between the two surfaces (Wray, 1963). In other words, the more nearly a lens surface matches the corneal contour the greater is the force of attraction. If the lens curvature is made slightly flatter than that of the cornea, the capillary attraction is lessened and the lens moves more easily. Since the cornea is not spherical, it should be impossible to achieve exact alignment with a spherical corneal lens. However, since the cornea is compressible, lenses which closely approximate the corneal curvature can 'mould' the cornea to the shape of the lens and appear as a good alignment fitting. With lenses fitted steeper than the corneal curvature, although capillary attraction is lessened, the compressibility of the cornea allows the edge of the lens to press into the cornea during blinking, and lens movement is reduced by reason of the suction effect so produced.

In practice, while it is desirable to achieve a reasonable area of corneal alignment with the lens to prevent corneal insult, a lens which *exactly* conforms to the corneal contour over the *whole* of its surface cannot be comfortably tolerated. In this instance the capillary attraction would be so great that lens movement would be minimal and adequate tears circulation beneath the lens would be prevented.

Gravity

The effects of gravity on the lens are most easily envisaged by the use of the concept of the centre of gravity. This has the property that the object acts as though all of its weight were concentrated at that one point. For a corneal lens, the position of the centre of gravity is near the back surface or actually behind the lens. The further the centre of gravity moves behind the lens the greater the area of support above the centre of gravity. As the centre of gravity moves towards the front surface of the lens, there is less support for the lens and it tends to drop or 'lag' more readily under the effect of gravity.

The position of the centre of gravity is affected by the lens overall size, back vertex power, thickness and BCOR (*Figure 11.6*). Thus, the effect of gravity is less for a negative lens, minimal centre thickness and steep corneal curvature.

Related to and affected by gravity is the lens mass or weight. Augsburger and Hill (1971) have published the five following 'rules of thumb' for relating alterations in the parameters of negative corneal lenses to changes in their mass.

(1) A change of 0.01 mm in t_c can change lens mass by 3–12 per cent.

(2) A change of 0.1 mm in OS can change lens mass by as much as 4 per cent for a −5.00 D lens of OS 8.00 mm, or as little as 2 per cent for a −1.00 D lens of OS 10.00 mm.

(3) A change of 1.00 D in BVP can change lens mass by 2–6 per cent.

(4) A change of 0.1 in the BCOD/OS ratio can change lens mass by 3–4.5 per cent over the BVP range −1.00 to −5.00 D.

(5) A change of 0.1 mm in BCOR changes lens mass by only 0.3–1.5 per cent.

It is thus apparent that changes in lens thickness, overall size and power are most likely to affect lens position on the eye.

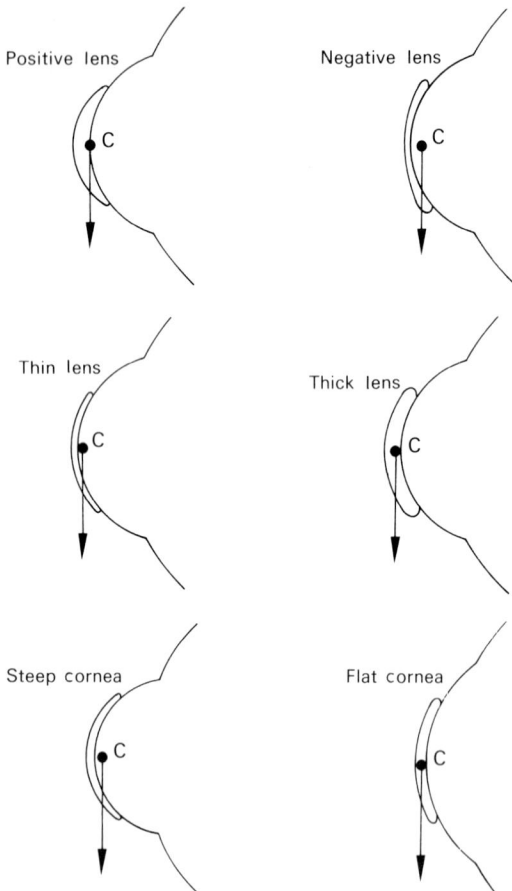

Positive lens   Negative lens

Thin lens   Thick lens

Steep cornea   Flat cornea

Figure 11.6—Diagrammatic representations of the centre of gravity (C) with lenses of differing power, thickness and BCOR

Tears Meniscus

The existence of a tears meniscus under the edge of a corneal lens is essential for its centration (Mackie, Mason and Perry, 1970; Mackie, 1973). For any given lens, the greater the circumference of the meniscus, the better the lens centration. Fenestration holes which permit the formation of a tears meniscus between lens and cornea, also therefore aid in lens centration, as they add to the effective 'length' of the tears meniscus between lens and cornea.

Lid Force and Position

Many corneal lenses ride in such a position that the upper lid covers a small portion of the lens. The lens is thus held between the cornea and lid. This force contributes to but is not necessary for holding the lens on the eye.

In many cases, the lower lid is sufficiently high for the lens to rest on it between blinking.

Frictional Forces

A corneal lens tends to remain stationary on the eye because of frictional forces. This is largely due to the viscosity of the pre-corneal film. If the pre-corneal layer is thin, friction may also occur directly between the surface of the lens and the corneal epithelium.

Variations in the viscosity of the pre-corneal film affect the frictional forces and so affect the position of the lens on the cornea. Thus, the foreign body reaction produced by a lens when first worn, or by a lens with a misshapen or damaged edge, causes an increase in lacrimal production. This serous liquid is less viscous than the normal pre-corneal liquid and lowers its frictional effect, allowing greater lens movement. Since the pre-corneal film thickness is also increased, the capillary attraction is lessened and, again, lens movement is increased.

FLUORESCEIN PATTERNS

Fluorescein patterns (*see Colour Plates XI to XVIII*) are the pictures obtained when one drop of 2 per cent sodium fluorescein is instilled into the lower fornix or on to the bulbar conjunctiva above the lens in order to give colour to the tears. The lens fit is then viewed under ultra-violet light, which renders the tears fluorescent. A different pattern is obtained as the lens moves upwards and downwards following each blink and as the fluorescein gradually drains from behind the lens. It is thus a dynamic picture and not easily represented pictorially. The following diagrams and cross-sectional representations can only serve as a useful guide and must be complementary to clinical study (*Figure 11.7*).

FITTING TECHNIQUES

In the following review, the student should not forget that the fitting technique is but a means to the end of achieving the desiderata listed at the beginning of this chapter. The fitting technique selected should be that which most easily allows the fulfilment of these desiderata. However, whilst considering the following techniques the reader should bear in mind the accumulated experience of many contact lens practitioners over the past three decades. This is that the fitting technique least likely to upset corneal integrity is the so-called 'alignment' technique, whereby the central optic portion of the corneal lens follows as closely as possible the central corneal contour. It is obviously difficult to align a toroidal cornea with the spherical back surface of a lens, but *Table 11.3* on page 271 gives an idea of the BCOR likely to give the best possible approximation to alignment in such cases, as well as indicating when a lens with a toroidal back surface should be considered. Although a spherical lens fitted to a markedly toroidal cornea is often optically satisfactory and encourages tears flow beneath the lens, it may mould the cornea so much as to cause a considerable alteration in the spectacle refraction with a resultant severe drop in V.A. if the original spectacle prescription is worn. Thus, alignment fitting using a toroidal surface becomes necessary provided that adequate tears flow can be maintained. A careful balance must always be achieved between the need for tears flow and minimizing the moulding effect on the cornea. As a general guide when fitting a spherical BCOR to a toroidal cornea the BCOR chosen should be slightly steeper than the flattest corneal meridian by approximately one-third of the astigmatic difference of the cornea. In all cases the fit should be checked with fluorescein to confirm its adequacy. With spherical and almost spherical corneas it may be necessary at times to choose a BCOR slightly flatter (up to 0.10 mm) than the keratometer reading, especially if a large BCOD (7.00–8.00 mm) is chosen. This is because the cornea flattens beyond the region measured by the keratometer, and in order to achieve an overall alignment it is necessary to fit flatter than the flattest radius measured by keratometry.

Many techniques and lens constructions are available, each claiming its own especial advantages. Many are very similar and may be divided into two main groups:

EXTRA-PALPEBRAL APERTURE FITTING TECHNIQUES

This group of techniques utilizes lenses larger than the vertical inter-palpebral aperture (though smaller than the vertical visible iris diameter). Three main examples follow.

Contour Technique

This technique was one of the first which attempted to follow more closely the contour of the cornea, from which it derived its name. It arose from the observations of Bier (1957), who attempted to improve on the fitting of the monocurve 'micro-lens'. As it had proved impossible to align a single curve lens with the cornea over the whole of its surface when made to the same curvature as the keratometer reading, the micro-lens was generally fitted about 0.3 mm flatter than the central corneal curvature (Dickinson, 1954). This resulted in heavy central bearing, excessive lens movement, alteration in corneal curvature, and usually eventual corneal insult and lens rejection.

Bier suggested a back central optic diameter of around 7.00 mm over which it should be possible to align closely to the cornea. The peripheral curve is fitted flatter than the cornea in order to prevent the lens edge from pressing into the cornea. The clearance given must also be sufficient to prevent the edge from digging in on lens movement to the flatter corneal periphery. The fluorescein picture is that shown in *Figure 11.7a*, so that a reservoir of tears collects beneath the peripheral zone. As the lens is moved up and down by the action of the lids, the tears pass under the back central optic portion, thereby maintaining normal corneal metabolism.

In cases of corneal astigmatism, the lens is fitted to align with the flattest corneal meridian or may be fitted slightly steeper than this meridian since the flatter meridian often becomes more steep with lens wear (*see* page 271).

Further details of this technique are discussed under Fitting Routine, page 270.

Advantages

(1) The back surface of the lens parallels the cornea closely enough to distribute the lens

262

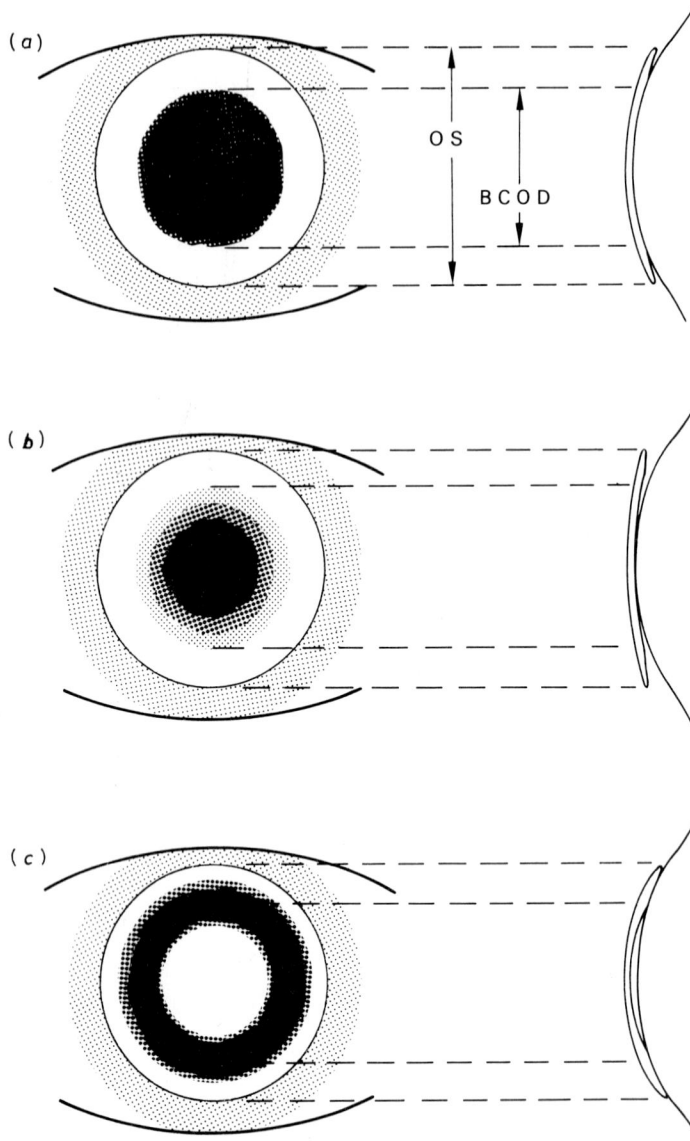

Figure 11.7–Typical fluorescein patterns of corneal lenses with the lens centred and lids slightly separated. The cross-section of the lens fit is shown on the right-hand side. Shading within the lens circumference indicates corneal bearing and the unshaded area indicates corneal clearance. (a) Alignment of the back central optic portion and clearance of the peripheral optic zone (a 'contour' fit). The fluorescein pattern appears as a dark area of alignment over the BCOD and a bright fluorescein band beyond (cf. Colour Plate II). (b) Flat back central optic portion and peripheral optic zone. The fluorescein pattern appears as a dark area of contact towards the centre of the back central optic portion and shows increasing fluorescence towards the lens periphery (cf. Colour Plate XII). (c) A lens with BCOR steeper than the cornea showing central clearance and bearing on the transition between the back central and peripheral curves (an example of a 'tight' lens fit). The fluorescein pattern appears as a central trace of fluorescein, the amount depending on the relative steepness of the lens, a dark ring of bearing in the transition region, and a bright ring of fluorescein towards the lens edge where the lens is flatter than the cornea (cont.)

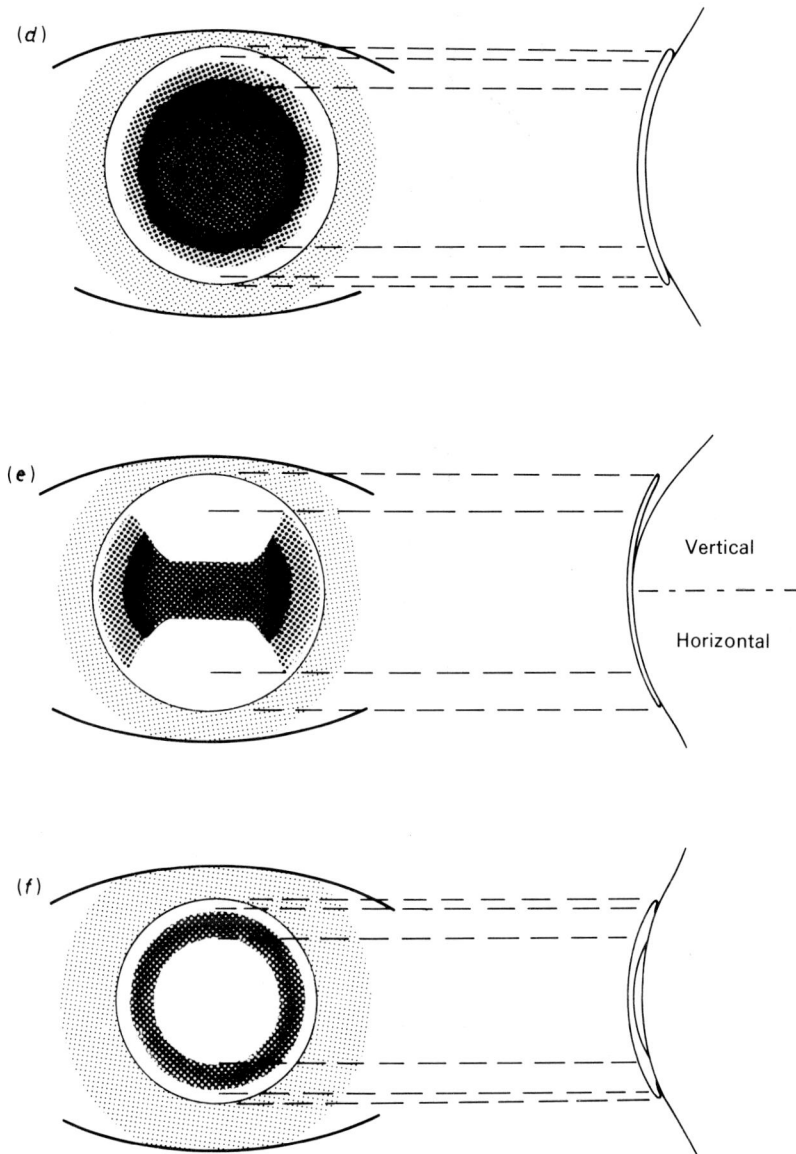

Figure 11.7 (cont.)–(d) Alignment or slight clearance of the back central optic portion, near alignment of the first peripheral curve moving towards shallow clearance, and complete clearance of the narrow second peripheral curve (a 'modified contour' fit) (cf. Colour Plate XI). The fluorescein pattern appears as a dark area of central alignment gradually merging into a bright ring of fluorescein towards the lens edge. (A similar appearance is given by the correct fitting of a 'tapered' and an 'all-aspheric' continuous curve lens) (cf. Colour Plates XIII and XIV). (e) A 'contour' lens on a 'with-the-rule' astigmatic cornea. In the horizontal meridian the lens shows alignment of the back central optic curve and has been fitted with near alignment of the peripheral curve in this meridian to reduce excessive edge clearance in the vertical meridian (see split cross-sectional diagram) (cf. Colour Plate XVII). (f) A small lens showing central clearance, alignment of the first peripheral curve and clearance of the narrow second peripheral curve ('Bayshore' technique). The fluorescein pattern appears as a bright circle of fluorescein over the back central optic portion, a dark area of alignment over the first peripheral curve and a bright ring of fluorescein over the second peripheral curve

weight evenly and yet differs enough from the true corneal curvature to allow tears circulation beneath the lens.

(2) The even distribution of the lens weight gives rise to a minimum of spectacle blur (*see* Chapter 16, Volume 2) or corneal distortion.

(3) The success of this method is shown by the fact that it was the most commonly used fitting technique for many years. and that all modern fitting methods are extensions of the same technique.

Disadvantages

(1) Occasional poor centring. Once the lens moves to the peripheral cornea, it often stays there due to alignment of the peripheral zone with the cornea.

(2) Lenses often 'ride high', due to the top of the lens being held by the upper lid.

(3) Moderately large lens movement. This very commonly shows as a ring or part ring of indentation around the limbus, which collects fluorescein where the lens edge has indented the bulbar conjunctiva in this region.

(4) A small amount of corneal steepening (for example, due to oedema) or slight lens flattening gives rise to a flat fitting lens with the accompanying disadvantages mentioned above.

(5) Nearly all possible modifications to the lens effectively make the fit flatter (*see* Effect of Variations in the BCOD, page 275).

Summary of Typical Specifications

$$BCOR = K_F \pm 0.10 \text{ mm}*$$
$$BPOR = BCOR + (0.40 \to 0.80) \text{ mm}$$
$$BCOD = 6.50 \to 7.50 \text{ mm}$$
$$OS = 8.50 \to 10.00 \text{ mm}$$

Modified Contour Technique

This technique (*see Colour Plate XI*) is similar to the contour technique but attempts to eliminate some of the disadvantages associated with that method. The first peripheral curve is made to approach the cornea more closely and there is usually a small, flat, second peripheral curve at the very edge to act as a tears reservoir and to prevent the edge digging in on lens movement (*Figure 11.7d*). The junction between the BCOR and BP$_1$OR must be well blended since both curves are close to corneal alignment. The BCOR may be

---

* K_F = flattest corneal meridian in mm as measured by the keratometer.

fitted slightly steeper than the flattest corneal meridian to aid lens centration in certain cases (*see* pages 267 and 271).

Advantages over Contour Technique

(1) Better centration and less lens movement.

(2) High-riding lenses are less common since the lens adheres more to the cornea than the upper lid, due to the greater area of corneal alignment with this technique.

(3) The lens is more amenable to modification and there is less likelihood of a flat fit.

(4) There is less edge sensation since the edge lies closer to the cornea.

Disadvantages

(1) Greater accuracy is required in fitting, especially of the first peripheral curve.

(2) Many laboratories have difficulty in manufacturing an accurate first peripheral curve, which greatly affects the efficacy of this method.

(3) Following from (1) and (2) above, it is relatively easy to obtain a 'tight' lens, that is, a fitting where the lens weight is concentrated on to a narrow band, usually at a transition or near the lens edge, causing a restriction in tears flow under the lens.

Summary of Typical Specifications

$$BCOR = (K_F - 0.05) \pm 0.05 \text{ mm}$$
$$BP_1OR = BCOR + (0.30 \to 1.00) \text{ mm}$$
$$BP_2OR = 9.50 \to 12.50 \text{ mm}, 0.20 \to 0.40 \text{ mm wide}$$
$$BCOD = 6.00 \to 7.50 \text{ mm}$$
$$OS = 8.50 \to 9.50 \text{ mm}$$

Multi-curve or Tapered Lenses

A further attempt to match the corneal contour more closely and to eliminate some of the disadvantages associated with the two foregoing techniques is the multi-curve lens (Hodd, 1958) (*see Colour Plates XII, XIII* and *XV*). Typically, these lenses have four or five back surface curves, usually well blended with a similar number of curves. The edge clearance is not as excessive as may be imagined (*see* discussion and table of examples of edge lifts on page 271), and there is less likelihood of edge or transition indentation. The main disadvantage is the difficulty of checking the narrow peripheral curves (*see* Chapter 12). Either the central alignment or minimal apical clearance methods of fitting may be used and the

Table 11.1–Fitting Set Designed by J. Stone with a Constant Axial Edge Lift of 0.15 mm at the OS of 9.00 mm

| | | | | | | | | Edge lift | | | Ratio |
| | | | | | | | | Axial (AEL) | | Radial (REL) | $\frac{REL}{AEL}$ |
BCOR	BCOD	BP$_1$OR	BP$_1$OD	BP$_2$OR	BP$_2$OD	BP$_3$OR	OS	at 7.8	at 8.6	at 9.0	at 9.0	at 9.0
7.00	7.0	7.40	7.8	8.40	8.6	10.00	9.00	0.018	0.083	0.147	0.113	0.77
7.10	,,	7.55	,,	8.60	,,	10.20	,,	0.019	0.085	0.148	0.115	0.78
7.20	,,	7.70	,,	8.80	,,	10.40	,,	0.020	0.086	0.148	0.116	0.78
7.30	,,	7.85	,,	9.10	,,	10.40	,,	0.021	0.091	0.149	0.118	0.79
7.40	,,	8.10	,,	9.30	,,	10.50	,,	0.025	0.095	0.150	0.120	0.80
7.50	,,	8.30	,,	9.50	,,	10.60	,,	0.028	0.097	0.150	0.121	0.80
7.60	,,	8.40	,,	9.70	,,	10.80	,,	0.027	0.097	0.150	0.122	0.81
7.70	,,	8.55	,,	9.90	,,	11.00	,,	0.028	0.098	0.149	0.121	0.81
7.75	,,	8.65	,,	10.00	,,	11.10	,,	0.029	0.098	0.150	0.123	0.82
7.80	,,	8.75	,,	10.10	,,	11.30	,,	0.029	0.098	0.150	0.123	0.82
7.85	,,	8.80	,,	10.20	,,	11.40	,,	0.029	0.098	0.150	0.123	0.82
7.90	,,	8.85	,,	10.40	,,	11.50	,,	0.028	0.099	0.150	0.124	0.82
8.00	,,	9.00	,,	10.60	,,	11.70	,,	0.028	0.100	0.151	0.125	0.83
8.10	,,	9.20	,,	10.80	,,	11.90	,,	0.030	0.101	0.150	0.125	0.83
8.20	,,	9.30	,,	11.00	,,	12.10	,,	0.030	0.101	0.150	0.126	0.84
8.30	,,	9.45	,,	11.30	,,	12.40	,,	0.029	0.101	0.150	0.126	0.84
8.40	,,	9.60	,,	11.60	,,	12.60	,,	0.029	0.102	0.150	0.127	0.85
8.50	,,	9.80	,,	11.70	,,	12.90	,,	0.031	0.101	0.150	0.128	0.85
8.60	,,	10.00	,,	11.90	,,	13.10	,,	0.032	0.102	0.150	0.128	0.86
8.70	,,	10.40	,,	12.00	,,	13.20	,,	0.036	0.104	0.150	0.129	0.86

peripheral flattening varied to allow adequate tears flow and prevent indentation by this zone on lens movement.

Summary of Three Typical Specifications

BCOR $= (K_F - 0.05) \pm 0.05$ mm

Three possible variations of the peripheral zone curves follow

(1) BP$_1$OR = BCOR + 0.50 mm
BP$_2$OR = BCOR + 1.00 mm
BP$_3$OR = BCOR + 1.50 mm
BP$_4$OR = 12.25 mm

(2) BP$_1$OR = BCOR + 0.50 mm
BP$_2$OR = BCOR + 1.25 mm
BP$_3$OR = BCOR + 2.25 mm
BP$_4$OR = 12.25 mm

(3) BP$_1$OR = BCOR + 0.50 mm
BP$_2$OR = BCOR + 1.50 mm
BP$_3$OR = BCOR + 2.70 mm
BP$_4$OR = 12.25 mm

BCOD = 7.00 mm
BP$_1$OD = 7.60 mm
BP$_2$OD = 8.20 mm
BP$_3$OD = 8.80 mm
OS = 9.20 mm

The range for BCOD and OS, which has been omitted to avoid over-complication, is the same as for the modified contour technique.

Constant Axial Edge Lift Lenses

Stone (1975a) and Rabbetts (1976) have designed multi-curve lenses of various overall sizes so that throughout each fitting set the lenses all have the same axial edge lift (see page 268 and Chapter 4, pages 133–136). These lenses are a much more logical approach to fitting, since if the axial edge lift is constant throughout the set, all lenses are equally likely to have similar peripheral clearances on the eyes to which they are fitted; whereas with a standard flattening in radius of the first and second peripheral curves throughout the fitting set, the flat lenses have a much smaller edge lift than the steep lenses (see page 271). The flat lenses therefore give less peripheral clearance to the eyes on which they are fitted, than do the steep lenses.

Lenses with constant edge lift are fitted by the modified contour technique. Full specifications are given in Chapter 4, pages 135–136 but a typical example of a fitting set with an axial edge lift of 0.15 at the OS of 9.0 is as shown in *Table 11.1*.

Other types of lens having constant edge lift are dealt with later (see page 268).

Lens—Lid Attachment (Parallel-Surfaced Peripheral Zone Lenses)

Corneal lens intolerance has been related, amongst other reasons, to the development of corneal oedema under the lens and corneal dessication in areas that the lens does not cover. Oedema can be avoided (assuming the lens is fitted correctly) provided a smaller area of cornea is covered or, alternatively, the movement of the lens on the cornea is increased. The small lens, which satisfies both these criteria, has the disadvantage of sometimes inducing abnormal blinking because it is often unstable after each blink. According to Korb and Korb (1974), the ideal contact lens should simulate the actions and movements of the tears layer in order to prevent this oedema occurring.

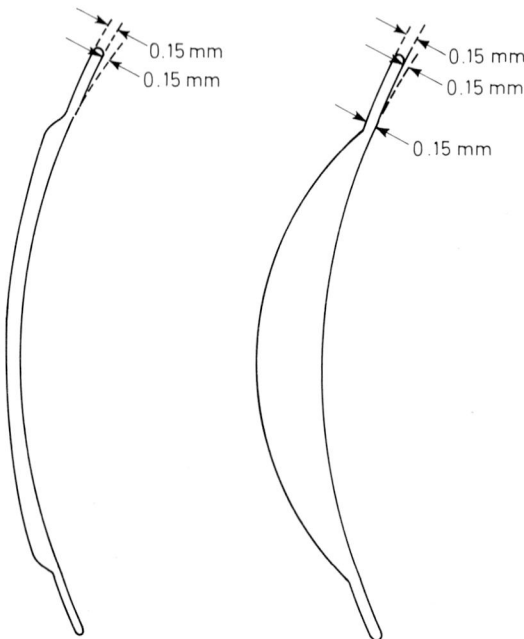

Figure 11.8—Cross-sections of parallel-surfaced peripheral zone lenses: negative (left) and positive (right). The carrier zone is held by the upper lid

Since almost all pre-corneal film movement is the result of upper lid action, and since the pre-corneal film may in effect be considered as attached to the upper lid, Korb and Korb argue that the ideal contact lens should therefore be effectively attached to the upper lid. This concept of lens performance, in which the lens remains immobile without upper lid action or eye version movements, but moves during blinking as if the corneal lens were attached to the upper lid, facilitates the movement of tears during the acts of blinking and eye movement, and permits the successful training of blinking.

The main technique of 'lid attachment' is achieved by arranging that 0.75–1.00 mm of the most peripheral portion of the lens has parallel front and back surfaces or is even slightly negative in cross-section (that is, slightly thicker at the very edge). This may be done by simply requesting it from the laboratory; by tables (Korb and Korb, 1974); by drawing to x40 magnification (Mackie, 1973), or by calculation (Stone, 1975b). The latter two methods are dealt with in Chapter 4, pages 130–137.

Unlike all other techniques, Korb and Korb recommend that the lens is fitted flatter than the central cornea to give an approximate alignment fit when riding superiorly on the cornea and actually moving some 3 mm onto the inferior sclera during blinking. The lens edge is made more blunt and rounded than normal to increase the tears meniscus. This is acceptable since the upper lid does not have to pass over the lens edge. Lens mass is kept to an absolute minimum.

Summary of Typical Specifications

BCOR $= K_F + (0.40 \rightarrow 0.50)$ mm
BPOR $=$ fitted to give satisfactory clearance with the lens in the superior position
FPOR $=$ arranged to be parallel with the back surface over $0.75 \rightarrow 1.00$ mm. A lenticulated lens is usually necessary
BCOD $=$ typically 7.00 mm
OS $\quad = 8.20 \rightarrow 9.40$ mm, typically 9.00 mm
t_c $\quad =$ minimum possible to allow lens manufacture and to keep edge thickness to around 0.06 mm for plano lenses, with a range of $0.05 \rightarrow 0.12$ mm

In spite of the Korbs' recommendation to fit flat, Stone (1975b) has found the technique of using parallel-surfaced peripheral zones very successful using a modified contour technique and an axial edge lift of approximately 0.15 mm. Lenses are drawn out to scale or calculated to give edge thickness of approximately 0.15 mm and are made lenticular with the FCOD equal to the BCOD. This technique is particularly successful for making positive lenses and low-power negative lenses (up to −2.0 D) ride high. For lenses of −7.0 D and upwards the technique is also helpful as it minimizes edge thickness. For very high-power negative lenses an extra front surface junction curve must be worked on and the appearance then is similar to the Gravity Lens described by Mandell (1974) (*see Figures 4.32 and 11.8*).

Whereas Stone uses peripheral thicknesses of 0.15 mm and axial edge lifts of 0.15 mm, Mackie uses peripheral thicknesses of 0.10 mm and radial edge lifts of 0.10 mm. Both report considerable success with this modification of Korb's technique.

For drawing out lenses to scale at $x40$ magnification large sheets of graph paper, a drawing board and a beam compass are required. The drawing itself is simple and is done by normal geometrical principles.

If lens curvatures are determined by calculation, sag tables (Appendix C) and an electronic calculator are ideal (Stone, 1975b) – see Aspects of Lens Design, Chapter 4, page 128.

Another technique for assisting the upper eyelid to hold up a corneal lens has been described by Hersh (1974). This involves making a groove, some 0.05 mm deep and 0.08 mm in width, in the front peripheral portion of the lens, about 0.4–0.8 mm in from the edge depending on lens overall size. The inner margin of the upper eyelid aligns and penetrates the groove at the upper part of the lens thereby holding it up. It is essential that the groove is well polished, otherwise the patient suffers considerable lid sensation.

INTERPALPEBRAL APERTURE FITTING TECHNIQUES

This group of techniques utilizes lenses smaller than the vertical interpalpebral aperture. Lester and Braff (1963) list the following conditions as particularly suitable for these small lenses.
(1) When the lid aperture is narrow.
(2) When the lids are more sensitive than average.
(3) When large lenses do not centre.
(4) When the peripheral cornea is highly irregular.
(5) When the cornea abrades easily.
(6) When the lenses are worn in hot or humid climates.
(7) When very large lenses of high positive power would otherwise be necessary.
(8) When the patient has a backward head tilt with conventional lenses.

To which may be added

(9) In cases of moderate corneal astigmatism where the fitting of a small lens may obviate the need for a lens with a toroidal back surface.
(10) When the wearer spends most of his time doing close work.
(11) When the lower lid margin is situated below the lower limbus.
(12) Some cases of 3 and 9 o'clock staining (although often a larger lens works better).
(13) Persistent corneal oedema.

Small Bi-curve and Tri-curve Lenses

The fitting technique is basically that of the contour or modified contour philosophy except that the overall size of the lens is made smaller than the interpalpebral aperture but should be at least 2.00 mm larger than the maximum pupillary diameter. Jessen (1961) suggests overall sizes in the range of 7.50–8.40 mm, Morrison (1967) an average of 7.80 mm, Davis (1964) from 7.30 to 8.20 mm, and Moore (1974) from 8.00 to 8.30 mm.

The BCOR necessary to give an alignment fitting may be slightly steeper than the keratometer reading since the cornea steepens towards its apex, and this becomes more apparent with the generally smaller BCOD (see page 258). The central thickness of the smaller lenses is often less than that of the extrapalpebral aperture lenses. Various other modifications to small lens fitting have been suggested. Morrison (1967), for example, utilizes a narrow peripheral zone width of 0.30–0.40 mm and a relatively large BCOD.

Summary of Typical Specifications

BCOR = K_F – (0 → 0.15) mm
BPOR = BCOR + (0.30 → 1.00) mm
BCOD = 5.00 → 6.50 mm
OS = 7.30 → 8.40 mm

Bayshore Technique

Probably the most well known of the interpalpebral aperture fitting techniques (although not now fitted so frequently), this method (see Colour Plate XVI) reverses the bearing surfaces of the contour technique to give central clearance, first peripheral curve alignment and a small, flat second peripheral curve (Figure 11.7f). The overall size is normally determined by the vertical lid aperture less 0.20 mm, with a minimum of 7.00 mm and a maximum of 8.80 mm (Bayshore, 1963).

The main advantage of this method is the excellent lens centration. This arises from the fact that it is possible to achieve much better alignment of the non-spherical cornea with a narrow first peripheral curve than with the wider back central optic portion. Thus, the cornea is steeper on one side of the bearing surface and flatter on the other, giving the lens a strong tendency to move to the position of first peripheral curve alignment. It is therefore important to stress the accuracy with which this curve must be fitted. The disadvantages of this method are mainly those that apply to the modified contour technique, also the corneal oedema and surface irregularity which often arise unless fitted extremely carefully.

The Bayshore technique may also be applied as an extrapalpebral technique in certain cases, though some of the advantages of the smaller lens may be lost. In this instance, the recommendation of subtracting 0.30 mm from the radius of the flattest corneal meridian to give the BCOR (Bayshore, 1962 and 1963) would give rise to excessive central clearance from the cornea with the use of a wider BCOD. Approximately half this amount gives the same central clearance as the smaller lens.

Summary of Typical Specifications

BCOR	$= K_F - 0.30$ mm
BP$_1$OR	= Generally $1.00 \rightarrow 1.50$ mm flatter than BCOR to give alignment
BP$_2$OR	= 17.00 mm radius*, $0.10 \rightarrow 0.30$ mm wide
BCOD	$= 5.60 \rightarrow 6.60$ mm, generally governed by subtraction of the first peripheral curve width (ideally $0.80 \rightarrow 0.90$ mm) and second peripheral curve width, from the overall size
OS	$= 7.00 \rightarrow 8.80$ mm (interpalpebral aperture less 0.20 mm)
Fenestration	A central fenestration, $0.20 \rightarrow 0.25$ mm in diameter is recommended if a restriction of lacrimal interchange should cause objective symptoms or subjective signs of oedema.

Lester and Braff (1963) list some of the dis-advantages of interpalpebral fitting lenses as follows.

(1) They are more difficult to handle and are more easily lost.

(2) The lens edges need more precise finishing.

(3) There is less variation possible for a good fit.

(4) If the corneal apex is decentred, the small lens is also usually decentred.

(5) There is often a problem with flare.

(6) Modification of small lenses usually requires greater care.

(7) They tend to lose their dimensional stability more than larger lenses.

---

* In practice, if this curve is polished, using a soft felt tool which tends to take up the shape of the lens, it is unlikely that the curve will remain as flat as this after polishing. The writer would not recommend such a flat curve if harder tools (for example, those made of wax or hard felt) are to be used.

CONTINUOUS CURVE LENSES

These more recent types of lens construction (*see Colour Plate XIV*) may be used for either inter-palpebral or extrapalpebral aperture fitting techniques. As their name would suggest, these types of lens eliminate transitions, so that the back surface of the lens is apparently of one continuous curve. In practice, the back surface may be made with a single aspherical curve or the peripheral zone may follow on from the edge of the back central optic portion without a sharp junction. The accurate use of terminology used to describe them is therefore most important. The advantages claimed for this lens-type are as follows.

(1) It is possible to align more accurately the gradually flattening cornea with a non-spherical lens construction.

(2) There is no risk of corneal abrasion from a transitional area.

(3) There is less likelihood of flare.

(4) The precise lens construction is, in theory, easier to reproduce.

(5) Due to fewer parameters, they are generally simpler to fit.

The main disadvantage is that the practitioner is at the mercy of the laboratory in as much as it is impossible at the present time to check accurately all such peripheral zone constructions. Stone (1975a), however, has described methods of checking radial and axial edge lifts.

There are three basic types of lens construction, as follows.

Offset Peripheral Curve Lenses

The back peripheral curve is cut on a conventional lathe but the centre of curvature is offset so that its radius passes through the centre of curvature of the back central optic portion at the transition between the two curves (*Figure 11.9*). This eliminates a sharp transition between the two curves which, at that point, both have a common tangent. As the centre of the peripheral curve is offset to the opposite side of the centre of curvature of the central portion, as in *Figure 11.9*, it is known as a 'contra-lateral offset continuous curve' lens. Bennett (1968) has termed this type of lens construction a 'continuous bi-curve' lens.

The amount of flattening is usually specified by the distance, at the lens edge, between the back central optic curve (extrapolated to this point) and the peripheral curve(s). The distance, in milli-metres, is normally measured along a line parallel to the axis of symmetry (*Figure 11.9*) and is known as the axial edge lift – previously known as

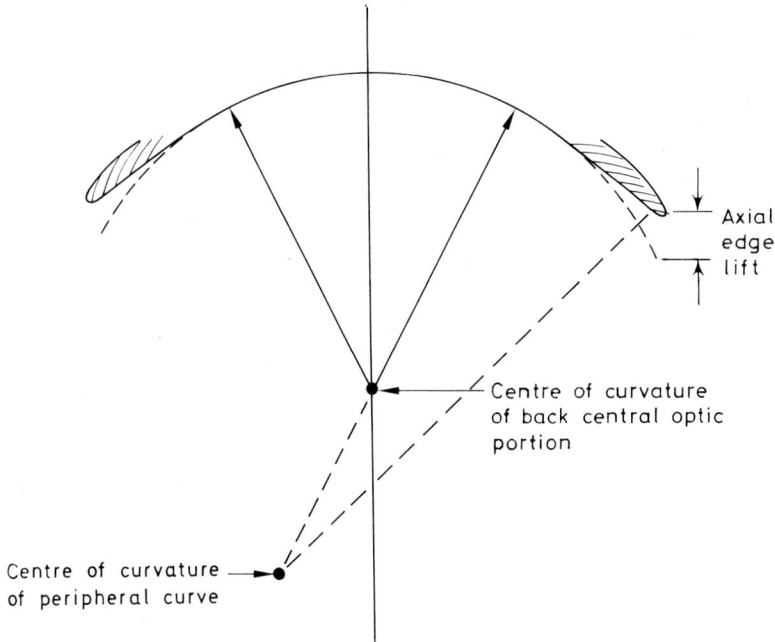

Figure 11.9–Contralateral offset or continuous bi-curve lens

the 'flattening factor' or 'Z value' (Bennett, 1968). Some writers prefer to measure the radial edge lift along the radius of curvature of the back peripheral optic portion at the lens edge – previously known as the 'Z factor' (Ruben, 1966; Hodd, 1966). When comparing peripheral lens flattening, it is important to check if axial or radial edge lifts are being referred to.

The centre of curvature of the peripheral curve may also be displaced to some homolateral point, though this does not give a 'continuous curve' lens when a flatter peripheral curve is used.

Conical Peripheral Zone Lenses

With this type of lens, it can be readily appreciated that for each BCOR at a certain BCOD there is one tangent to the lens at this point. A tangent rotated around the axis of symmetry gives a conical peripheral zone with no visible transition. The cone angle is expressed in degrees as the included (apical) angle of the conical surface (*Figure 11.10*).

In the 'Conoid'* type of construction (Thomas, 1967), the lens rests on the conical peripheral region and shows central optic clearance. Centration is extremely good with this type of fitting, as with the Bayshore technique, and the same degree of

* Conoid – *Focus Laboratories Ltd.* under licence from Corneal Lens Corporation Pty. Ltd., Australia.

central steepness of BCOR is recommended for both techniques ($K_F - 0.30$ mm). It is argued that the gradually increasing and decreasing bearing across the contact band in the conical periphery gives rise to less corneal discomfort and distortion than that of the conventional spherical lens on the aspheric cornea. In the optimum fitting of this technique there is a bright glow of fluorescein over the central area, surrounded by a dark band of contact which should circle the apical clearance. The apical pool may be circular or elliptical in shape, depending on the degree of corneal astigmatism present. Around the edge of the lens there should be a band of fluorescein 0.30 mm wide at the narrowest part of the band. A 0.25 mm

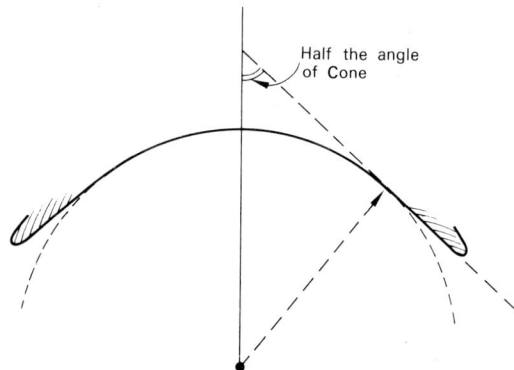

Figure 11.10–Conical periphery continuous curve lens

diameter fenestration, 2.00 mm in from the lens edge (with a lens of overall size 9.00 mm), aids lacrimal interchange. Comparison with the fenestration diameter during fitting aids selection of the cone angle to give the correct width of peripheral clearance. Toroidal back central optic portions with elliptical conoidal peripheries are available where the corneal astigmatism does not permit a complete ring of corneal bearing with a standard lens. Conoid lenses are generated with a lathe working on the pantograph system and the cone angles are claimed to be accurate to within 0.1 degree. A new instrument is currently undergoing evaluation which should enable the practitioner to check the accuracy of the conical peripheral zone.

In the 'Conic'* construction (Stek, 1975), the back central optic portion is fitted to align the cornea, while the conical peripheral zone is adjusted (normally by the laboratory) to give a constant radial edge lift of 0.10 mm (considered to be the ideal). Where there is excessive peripheral corneal flattening this may be increased. The cone angle is always within 2 degrees of being an exact tangent so that, while it may not be a true 'continuous curve' lens, the transition is virtually eliminated. It is argued by the originators of the technique that the constant radial edge lift in conjunction with almost complete lack of transition permits a more normal corneal metabolism and causes less corneal distortion than with other lens designs. Conic lenses appear to be suitable in cases of up to 3.00 D of corneal astigmatism and Conic peripheries in conjunction with toroidal back central optic portions are available for use where the corneal astigmatism is in excess of this value.

Complete Aspheric (or Conicoid) Lenses

The third type of lens construction has a complete single aspheric back surface curve from lens centre to edge and may therefore be correctly termed a 'continuous curve' lens. Over a central 1.00 mm diameter area, the curvature is extremely close to spherical and this serves as the nominal central curvature of the lens.

Nissel (Steele, 1969) has produced three aspheric fitting sets, each set having the same axial edge lifts for every lens. Thus:

Set 1 –   Known as the 12/18 set has an axial lift of 0.12 mm at a diameter of 8.00 mm and of 0.18 mm at a diameter of 9.50 mm.

Set 2 –   Known as the 7/11 set has an axial lift of 0.07 mm at a diameter of 8.00 mm and of 0.11 mm at a diameter of 9.50 mm.

Set 3 –   Known as the 5/8 set has an axial lift of 0.05 mm at a diameter of 8.00 mm and of 0.08 mm at a diameter of 9.50 mm.

Each set can be made with any desired overall size. The addition of a small, flat 0.50 mm wide well-blended curve at the lens margin has been found to prevent indentation of the lens edge at the corneal periphery (Gegg, 1969).

In the fitting of this type of lens, the aim is to match the aspherical surface of the cornea with the continuous aspheric back surface of the lens. Since the keratometer gives the corneal curvature approximately 1.5 mm each side of the geometric centre, the correctly fitting lens is generally some 0.10 mm steeper than this value since the nominal lens curvature is taken at the lens centre (Steele, 1969). This may be varied by individual practitioners, however, according to their own fitting philosophy.

A similarly constructed lens has been produced by Focus Contact Lens Laboratory Ltd., and is known as the 'Uni A' lens.

Examples of Axial Edge Lifts

It is of interest to compare edge lifts for various types of lens construction (*Table 11.2*). It should be emphasized that the values given are axial edge lifts (measured along a line parallel to the axis of symmetry) and not radial edge lifts (measured along a line normal to the lens edge).

The significance of the edge lift must be considered in relation to the different types of lens construction and the ways in which these bear upon the cornea. Thus, two lenses having the same edge lift and the same OS may give different edge clearances as well as different widths of peripheral corneal clearance.

FITTING ROUTINE

The following are required before fitting commences.

(1) General discussion with the patient on advantages and disadvantages of contact lenses, patient suitability, etc., as discussed in Chapters 7 and 8.

(2) Corneal, as well as lid and limbal, integrity should be established with a slit lamp (*see* Chapters 5 and 7).

_____

* Conic – *Optimedic Ltd.*

Table 11.2–Back Surface Specifications and Edge Lift Values of Comparable Corneal Lenses

	Axial edge lift (mm)
Bi-curve lenses	
C2/7.20:7.00/7.70:9.00	= 0.06
C2/7.80:7.00/8.30:9.00	= 0.05
C2/8.40:7.00/8.90:9.00	= 0.04
Tri-curve lenses	
C3/7.20:7.00/7.70:8.40/10.00:9.00	= 0.12
C3/7.80:7.00/8.30:8.40/10.00:9.00	= 0.09
C3/8.40:7.00/8.90:8.40/10.00:9.00	= 0.06
Multi-curve lenses	
C4/7.20:7.00/7.70:7.80/8.20:8.60/10.50:9.00	= 0.13
C4/7.80:7.00/8.30:7.80/8.80:8.60/11.00:9.00	= 0.10
C4/8.40:7.00/8.90:7.80/9.40:8.60/12.00:9.00	= 0.09

Conoid lenses
Not applicable since these lenses are fitted with apical clearance and use the peripheral curve as the bearing surface.

Conic lenses
Constant for every BCOR and OS (BCOD = 6.80 mm) at: 0.10

Kelvin Continuous Curve lenses
Impression moulded lenses with a spherical back central optic portion surrounded by an annulus whose curvature constantly changes from the edge of the central optic portion. Toroidal continuous curve lenses are also available. Various radial edge lifts are possible and each is held constant for every BCOR. Thus a lens with a *constant* radial edge lift of 0.10 mm at 9.00 mm OS will give the following axial edge lifts (AEL) for:

BCOD = 7.00 mm
	BCOR = 7.20, AEL	= 0.14
	„ = 7.80, „	= 0.13
	„ = 8.40, „	= 0.12

Nissel Continuous Offset lenses

Set. 1 (Ref. 3/4/2).
BCOD = 6.50 mm
OS = 9.50 mm
	BCOR = 7.40 mm	= 0.09
	„ = 7.80 mm	= 0.08
	„ = 8.40 mm	= 0.06

Set 2 (Ref. 146/0914).
BCOD = 6.50 mm
OS = 9.50 mm
	BCOR = 7.30 mm	= 0.15
	„ = 7.80 mm	= 0.12
	„ = 8.35 mm	= 0.09

Set 3 (Ref. 5/2/51/2).
BCOD = 6.50 mm
OS = 9.50 mm
	BCOR = 7.20 mm	= 0.19
	„ = 7.80 mm	= 0.16
	„ = 8.40 mm	= 0.12

Nissel Aspheric (Conocoid) lenses

Set 1 (Ref. 12/18).
All nominal BCOR
	At 8.00 mm diam.	= 0.12
	At 9.50 mm diam.	= 0.18

Set 2 (Ref. 7/11).
All nominal BCOR
	At 8.00 mm diam.	= 0.07
	At 9.50 mm diam.	= 0.11

Set 3 (Ref. 5/8).
All nominal BCOR
	At 8.00 mm diam.	= 0.05
	At 9.50 mm diam.	= 0.08

(3) Accurate keratometer readings. These govern the choice of the BCOR of the first trial lens (*see* Chapters 4 and 5).

(4) Horizontal and vertical visible iris diameters (which approximately equal the corneal diameters). These partly govern the choice of overall size.

(5) Interpalpebral aperture size. Again, this partly governs the choice of overall size.

(6) Pupil size in average and low illuminations. This largely governs the choice of BCOD.

(7) Accurate spectacle refraction and calculation of ocular refraction. This enables a subsequent check on the liquid lens power to be made, which should be zero in a true alignment fit.

(8) Decision of lens type to be used – corneal, hydrophilic or scleral.

SELECTION OF THE FIRST TRIAL LENS

For simplicity it will be assumed that the fitting of a bicurve contour lens is being carried out. The basic routine varies only with the lens dimensions, as discussed under the different fitting techniques.

BCOR

It is best to approach alignment from the steep side rather than the flat side as a central fluorescein pool is easier to see than fluorescein just inside the transition. For this reason, lenses as much as 0.20 mm flatter than correct alignment may *appear* to give an alignment picture. The student new to contact lens practice is well advised to select a BCOR approximately 0.15 mm steeper than the flatter keratometer reading for the first trial lens so that a definite central fluorescein pool is obtained. The BCOR may then be flattened in steps of 0.05 mm until central alignment is obtained.

Table 11.3

Astigmatism (by keratometer)	Approximate BCOR
Under 0.75 D	Flattest keratometer reading to 0.05 mm steeper
0.50–1.00 D	0.05–0.10 mm steeper than the flattest keratometer reading
1.00–2.00 D	Steeper than the flattest keratometer reading by approximately one-third of the difference between the principal meridians (consider a toroidal back central optic portion)
Over 2.00 D	As above, but a toroidal back central optic portion is recommended (*see* Chapter 18, Volume 2)

The majority of contact lens patients have some degree of corneal astigmatism. Keratometry indicates the corneal radii and amount of corneal astigmatism. *Table 11.3* indicates the optimum value of BCOR found from clinical experience in the majority of cases.

BCOD

This should be at least 1.00 mm bigger than the pupil diameter in average room illumination, and larger if the lenses are to be used in the dark (for example, for night-driving).

It has been found from clinical experience that if a given BCOR over a certain BCOD gives a satisfactory central alignment, then 0.05 mm should be added to the BCOR for each 0.50 mm increase in BCOD in order to maintain a satisfactory fit (*see* page 275).

BPOR

To give adequate peripheral clearance, this must be approximately 0.50 mm flatter than the BCOR, more for flat corneas (8.20 mm and above) and less for steep corneas (7.60 mm and below). Toroidal peripheral curves may be considered for corneal astigmatism of about 3.00 D and over (*see* Chapter 18, Volume 2).

In assessing the fit of the peripheral curve, it must be ensured that this curve shows adequate clearance when centred on the cornea but not such excessive clearance that the lens can pass over the limbal region. Conversely, if inadequate clearance is given, the lens may dig into the peripheral cornea on lens movement, necessitating a flatter peripheral curve or the addition of an even flatter second peripheral curve. In general, several peripheral curves are preferable to one, in order to give the desired peripheral clearance.

Overall Size

This should be at least 1.40 mm smaller than the largest visible iris diameter, and often 2.00 mm smaller. If the lids are tight, or if there is a narrow vertical palpebral aperture or a lot of corneal astigmatism, a smaller overall size may be selected.

ASSESSMENT OF THE FIT

At least five minutes should be allowed after insertion of the first lens for lacrimation to subside. This is not normally necessary with subsequent lenses. Patients usually comment that the lens is more comfortable than expected and the practitioner should maintain conversation to reassure patients and to take their minds off any irritation produced by the lens. While adapting to the lens, the patient should be instructed to look downwards (where the lids are at their most relaxed) and blink normally.

White Light Assessment

(1) Lids in the normal position: as the eye moves, the lens should remain within the limbal area.

(2) Lids separated: the lens should drop slowly when pushed to the top of the cornea. A flat fitting lens falls more quickly and often drops in a curved path as it pivots around the apex of the cornea. A steep fitting lens falls more slowly and often remains at the corneal apex.

Ultra-Violet Light Assessment

One drop of 2 per cent fluorescein is applied from a wetted impregnated paper strip, or with a sterile glass rod, on to the conjunctiva above the cornea with the patient looking down and the lids retracted.

Lens Centred

Table 11.4 supplements the fluorescein patterns represented pictorially in *Figure 11.7*.

Table 11.4

Fit		Fluorescein picture
Central	Peripheral	
Ideal align- ment	–	Even dark blue over BCOD with a 0.5–1.0 mm wide green band at edge of lens. A central trace of fluorescein is acceptable
–	Flat	Bright green under the entire peripheral zone
Flat	–	Green encroaching under periphery of central portion
–	Steep	Narrow blue touch band at extreme edge, green within this. Possible blue transition touch with wide peripheral curves
Steep	–	Blue transition with green under central portion and bubble if very steep

Lens Displaced Upwards

Fluorescein should disappear from under the upper periphery of the lens, except at the extreme edge, and should collect under the lower periphery and lower part of the central portion. Care should be taken to ensure that the extreme edge of the lens does not indent the peripheral cornea.

Movement

With fluorescein present, the movement of the lens is observed with the lids in the normal position, during blinking and normal eye rotations (*Table 11.5*). The BCOD is checked relative to the pupil

Table 11.5

Lens position	Possible cause*
Continually high, not dropping after blinks	Flat peripheral zone; too large a lens; too wide a peripheral zone; lens too thin; thick edges; (lens slightly steep, occasionally); lens too light in weight due to small overall size, or too thin, or both; negative lens
Continually low, with rapid dropping after blinks	Too small a lens; too thick a lens; (prism) ballasted lens; too heavy a lens due to large overall size or thickness, or both; positive lens
Continually to one side	Apex of cornea displaced; lens too small or too flat; spherical lens on an 'against-the-rule' cornea
Hardly any movement from the centre	Lens too steep
Lens moving about too much and beyond limbus	Profuse lacrimation due to foreign body or poor lens edge; lens too flat, allowing excessive movement; lens too flat or too steep, causing irritation and lacrimation; spherical lens on a toric cornea

* Reference should also be made to *Figure 11.6* for the effects of centre of gravity on lens position.

size as the lens moves. The lens should centre itself after each blink and eye movement. Whenever a lens consistently takes up an incorrect position, areas where the transition or edge may be bearing on the cornea should be looked for and blended.

Fitting Astigmatic Corneas

When fitting a spherical lens to an astigmatic cornea, a compromise fit is called for as dealt with in under BCOR on page 271. If a 'with-the-rule' astigmatic cornea is assumed fitted with a lens showing central alignment of the flattest meridian and a peripheral zone also showing near alignment in this meridian, then the fluorescein picture should show:

Centrally – an elongated H or dumb-bell-shaped blue touch area as wide as the BCOD (*see Colour Plate XVII*).

Peripherally – blue touch in the horizontal meridian and green stand-off in the vertical. The peripheral alignment should not occupy more than one-third of the lens circumference. Vertical stand-off is liable to cause discomfort when blinking. This can be minimized by making the lens as small as possible and the peripheral zone narrow (*see Colour Plates XVII and XVIII*).

Refraction

This should be performed with the patient wearing the lens whose BCOR is the nearest to the correct fitting. The contact lens refraction is a means of checking the fit, as in exact alignment the liquid lens power should be zero and the contact lens refraction (plus any power of the trial contact lens) equal to the ocular refraction. If the contact lens refraction shows less negative or more positive power than the ocular refraction, then a slightly flat fitting should be suspected, and vice versa.

TOLERANCE TRIALS

Once the desired fitting information has been obtained, the practitioner should order the lenses in the manner described later. Following an instruction session (*see* Chapter 8) and once the practitioner is satisfied with his ability to handle the lenses, the patient is then issued with his lenses for a tolerance trial of usually 1–2 weeks. Because of the curvature change with hydration, lenses should ideally be soaked for 24 hours before being worn (*Figure 11.11*). It should be explained to the patient that he is being *loaned* his lenses for an assessment period. It should also be stressed that the patient is free to consult the practitioner should any problems arise or if he should decide not to have contact lenses (when an appropriate fee will be charged). Similarly, the practitioner must reserve the right to reject any patient he considers as being unsuitable for corneal lenses.

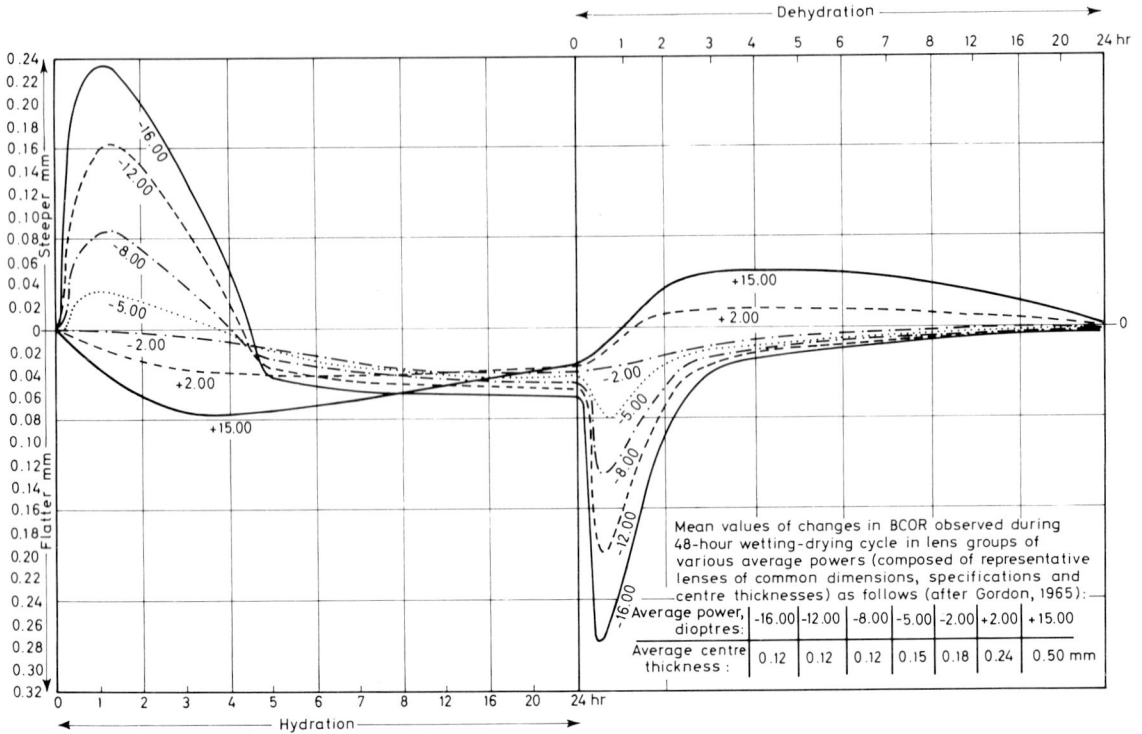

Figure 11.11 – The wetting-drying cycle of polymethyl methacrylate corneal lenses

At the end of the tolerance trial, the fitting of the lenses is noted (and any necessary modifications carried out), the patients objective and subjective reactions noted, and the corneas examined for oedema or any abrasion which may indicate epithelial fragility. Tolerance trials are discussed fully in Chapter 8.

FITTING SETS

Ideally, a large number of trial sets of varying dimensions and powers is desirable. In most average-sized practices this is unrealistic although a small but growing number of practitioners are now fitting from (a large) stock covering the most commonly used parameters. The student may begin with one or two sets and aim at extending these as soon as possible.

A tri-curve back surface and a fairly sharp transition between the three curves allows an accurate assessment of the fit of both back central and peripheral regions. Further transitional or

peripheral curves may then be ordered on the final lens if found to be needed. Trial lenses may be ordered with slightly greater central thickness than prescription lenses to aid maintenance of lens curvature with handling. Since most contact lens patients are myopic, many trial sets are made with low to moderate negative power. Lenses which are approximately afocal have the advantage that, in many cases, the patient may wear his spectacle correction over the contact lenses during a short tolerance trial but the effect of the correct lens power on lens position and movement is thereby sacrificed.

Table 11.6 gives the minimum requirements for an initial fitting set. Those in lighter type show additional lenses which may be obtained later. Additional fitting sets are shown in *Tables 11.7* and *11.8*.

Further fitting sets may be acquired as the practitioner develops his own techniques. Sets of high positive and negative lenses are useful for fitting aphakics and high myopes. The thickness variations cause such lenses to behave differently

Table 11.6–Initial Nineteen Lens Fitting Set (Heavy Type) Extending to Twenty-seven Lenses

BCOR	BCOR	BCOR	
7.20	7.70	8.15	
7.30	7.75	8.20	
7.35	7.80	8.25	BCOD 7.00 mm
7.40	7.85	8.30	
7.45	7.90	8.35	BVP approximately afocal.
7.50	7.95	8.40	
7.55	8.00	8.45	BPOR 0.50 mm flatter than
7.60	8.05	8.50	BCOR, 0.70 mm after
7.65	8.10	8.60	BCOR 8.00 mm
			t_c 0.23–0.25 mm
			OS 9.00 mm

Table 11.7–Second Fitting Set

Specifications as for the initial set but with:

BCOD 6.50 mm and OS 8.50 mm
BVP −3.00 D t_c 0.19–0.22 mm

Table 11.8–Third Fitting Set

Specifications as for the initial set but with:

BCOD 7.25 mm and OS 9.50

on the eye from low-powered lenses of otherwise similar specifications, although when made in lenticular form, as is usual, high positive lenses with parallel-surfaced or negative carrier zones, behave like low-powered negative lenses. Even when high-powered negative lenses are made lenticular it is difficult to stop them from riding high on the cornea, due to upper lid traction, but the 'Gravity Lens' type of construction (*see* page 266) helps, particularly if the edge is made like that of a positive lens.

Becoming increasingly popular are fitting sets with a constant axial edge lift as discussed earlier (*see* pages 133 and 265).

All trial lens specifications should be checked at frequent intervals as these may alter with age, handling, etc. All curvatures should be noted to the nearest 0.01 mm and each lens engraved with some suitable identification engraving. Lenses may be lightly tinted in some colour sequence to help prevent confusion of the trial set order.

ORDERING

During the fitting routine, it is unlikely that a single lens will be available which will be correct in all its specifications. It may be necessary to combine specifications from several lenses or to extrapolate a dimension from the nearest available trial lens. The following notes indicate those allowances necessary.

BCOR

Effect of Variations in the BCOD

As mentioned earlier, since the cornea flattens towards its periphery, as the BCOD is increased, the BCOR must be flattened to maintain the nearest to an alignment fit. The opposite applies on reducing the BCOD. It has been found from clinical experience that for every 0.50 mm increase in BCOD the BCOR must be flattened by approximately 0.05 mm, and vice versa.

Effect of Hydration

Due to plastics expansion, all lenses flatten with hydration. Thus, since lenses flatten during storage and wear, an allowance should be made for this at the time of ordering (Phillips, 1969). A table of average hydration flattening has been given by Gordon (1965) and is reproduced in *Table 11.9*. Generally, as the lens is made thinner so the flattening with hydration is increased. *Figure 11.11* shows the effects of hydration and dehydration on the BCOR of PMMA lenses of different powers. Lenses made of other materials, such as cellulose acetate butyrate, show fairly similar hydration and dehydration changes. CAB, however, is generally less stable than PMMA and the changes are much more marked (Stone, 1978).

BPOR

The same allowances apply as for the BCOR, both for alterations in the overall size and hydration flattening (usually taken to the nearest 0.05 mm owing to the difficulty of accurately manufacturing and checking peripheral curves).

BCOD AND OS

See notes under BCOR and BPOR.

Table 11.9–Flattening of Back Central Optic Radius with Maximum Hydration of PMMA Lenses

Range of powers of lenses (dioptres)	Lens centre thickness (mm)	Flattening at maximum hydration	
		Group flattening range (mm)	Mean value of lens flattening (mm)
+10.00 to +20.00	0.40 to 0.60	0.020 to 0.035	0.028
+5.00 to +9.00	0.25 to 0.40	0.020 to 0.035	0.030
+1.00 to +3.00	0.20 to 0.28	0.025 to 0.040	0.033
−1.00 to −3.00	0.12 to 0.22	0.030 to 0.045	0.038
−4.00 to −6.00	0.10 to 0.20	0.030 to 0.050	0.042
−7.00 to −9.00	0.08 to 0.18	0.035 to 0.060	0.047
−10.00 to −13.00	0.08 to 0.17	0.035 to 0.065	0.052
−14.00 to −18.00	0.08 to 0.16	0.040 to 0.070	0.058
−19.00 to −22.00	0.07 to 0.15	0.045 to 0.080	0.065

As measured by Gordon (1965). Each group contained 20 lenses and 90 per cent of the findings fell within the group flattening range.

BVP

Comparison of Spectacle and Contact Lens Correction

The initial spectacle refraction is best written in negative cylinder form since the tears lens acts as a negative cylinder in a lens aligning the flattest corneal meridian and corrects most of the corneal astigmatism (see Chapter 4). Thus, the power of these two negative cylinders can be compared, and where the spectacle astigmatism and keratometer astigmatism are approximately the same, the astigmatism should be corrected by the tears lens and then the cylinder in the spectacle correction may be ignored. The spherical component of the spectacle refraction referred to the corneal plane should then equal the liquid lens power along the flattest corneal meridian, plus the BVP of the contact lens. If there is more than 0.50–0.75 D difference between spectacle and keratometer astigmatism, depending on individual patient acuity and tolerance, it may be necessary to incorporate a front surface cylindrical correction. To maintain lens orientation in these cases, a prism-ballasted lens or double truncation may be used where the cornea is close to spherical; alternatively a toroidal back surface lens may be fitted where possible (see Chapter 18, Volume 2).

Vertex Distance

A refraction is carried out with the trial contact lens in place, and provided adequate visual acuity is achieved the 'best sphere' power is used.

The BVP of the trial contact lens is then added to the power of the spectacle addition, having made due allowance for the vertex distance, to give the BVP of the lens to be ordered.

A table of vertex distance allowances is given in Appendix A, page 304. It can be seen that for spectacle corrections of less than 4.00 D the effects of vertex distance may generally be ignored, provided that the latter lies within normal limits.

Effect of Variations in the BCOR

It may be necessary to carry out the refraction with a trial contact lens whose BCOR is not the same as that to be ordered on the final lens. As any alteration of the BCOR alters the power of the tears liquid lens, an allowance must be made to the BVP of the lens to be ordered. It can be calculated that, for small amounts and for corneas of average curvature, an alteration of 0.05 mm in the BCOR requires an alteration in BVP of 0.25 D.

Thus, if the trial lens used is of BCOR 8.00 mm and BVP −3.00 D, and the lens ordered has a BCOR of 8.05 mm, then the liquid lens becomes more negative powered and the BVP of the lens must be ordered as −2.75 D to compensate for this.

No alteration to the BVP should be made where the BCOR is altered to compensate for flattening with hydration. This allowance normally disappears when the lens becomes fully hydrated.

CENTRE THICKNESS

Although the centre thickness of a lens is normally specified, the edge thickness is just as important clinically. An edge which is either too thick or too thin gives rise to lid irritation. An edge thickness of around 0.14–0.18 mm appears to be the ideal. A lens which is too thin flattens excessively with hydration and often becomes distorted if handled incorrectly. Conversely, a lens which is too thick is relatively heavy and constantly positions low on the cornea.

A list of suggested centre thicknesses for variations in BVP and OS is given in Table 11.10.

Table 11.10–Corneal Lens Thickness Chart

Negative powered lenses

BVP (D)	Overall size (mm)					
	8.50 to 8.80	8.90 to 9.20	9.30 to 9.60	9.70 to 10.00	10.10 to 10.30	10.40 and over
Afocal to −0.50	0.215	0.210	0.210	0.210	0.200	0.180
−0.75 to −1.00	0.215	0.210	0.200	0.190	0.190	0.170
−1.25 to −1.50	0.210	0.200	0.190	0.190	0.175	0.160
−1.75 to −2.00	0.200	0.200	0.190	0.180	0.165	0.155
−2.25 to −2.75	0.190	0.190	0.175	0.170	0.155	0.150
−3.00 to −3.25	0.180	0.180	0.160	0.155	0.150	0.145
−3.50 to −4.25	0.170	0.160	0.150	0.145	0.140	0.130
−4.50 to −5.00	0.160	0.155	0.140	0.135	0.125	0.115
−5.25 to −5.50	0.150	0.145	0.130	0.120	0.110	0.105
−5.75 to −6.00	0.140	0.135	0.120	0.105	0.100	0.100
−6.25 to −7.00	0.130	0.120	0.110	0.105	0.100	0.100
−7.00 and over	0.100	0.100	Make in lenticular form			

Positive powered lenses

BVP (D)	Overall size (mm)					
	8.40 to 8.70	8.80 to 9.20	9.30 to 9.70	9.80 to 10.00	10.50 (approx.)	11.00 (approx.)
Afocal to +1.00	0.210	0.220	0.230	0.235	0.240	0.245
+1.25 to +2.00	0.230	0.240	0.250	0.255	0.265	0.270
+2.25 to +3.00	0.260	0.270	0.280	0.290	0.310	0.330
+3.25 to +4.00	0.280	0.295	0.310	0.325	0.350	0.370
+4.25 to +5.00	0.305	0.315	0.330	0.360	0.395	0.450
+5.25 to +6.00	0.330	0.345	0.365	0.385	0.420	0.470
+6.25 to +7.00	0.350	0.370	0.395	0.440	0.470	0.520
+7.00 and over	Make in lenticular form					

The figures given above for centre thickness (mm) are the average for the power and overall size groups and generally give an edge thickness of about 0.14−0.18 mm for an average tri-curve lens (Bryant, 1975). Lens thicknesses should be ordered to two decimal places only.

Note: Lenses with a BVP of about ±5.00 D may be made in lenticular form. Lenses with a BVP of ±7.00 D or more should be made in lenticular form. To reduce the incidence of oedema, centre thickness of greater than 0.40 should be avoided where possible by the use of lenticulation. Some practitioners advocate lenticular construction for all positive lenses to minimize centre thickness but give adequate edge thickness.

It is suggested that the higher powers are made in lenticular form since this provides a great reduction in lens weight, thereby aiding lens centration and giving easier control of edge thickness. When a lens is ordered in lenticular form, it is necessary to specify a front central optic diameter (FCOD), and the desired final edge thickness. The FCOD is generally around 0.50 mm larger than the BCOD. Junction thickness may also be specified (*see* page 130, Chapter 4).

TRANSITIONS

These may be left sharp or blended lightly, moderately or heavily. Although a heavily blended transition lessens any risk· of corneal abrasion caused by this area, there are two possible disadvantages. First, it is difficult to check if the BCOD has been made correctly: if incorrect, it effectively alters the fit of the central portion. Secondly, the transition, if polished well into the BCOD, reduces its effective diameter, often causing flare under conditions of low illumination. Ideally, the transition should be ordered lightly blended and the blending increased later by the practitioner as necessary.

If blending is carried out, a tool should be chosen whose radius lies one-third to mid-way between the BPOR and BCOR so that most of the lens substance is removed from the peripheral curve.

DISTINGUISHING MARKS FOR RIGHT AND LEFT LENSES

Right and left lenses should be distinguished by the letters R and L or by small dots — one for the right lens and two for the left (British Standard, BS 5562:1978). Although used mainly for scleral lenses, if dots are used for identification marks, often only the right lens is so marked since the drilling of two small holes into the lens surface may weaken the lens. A hole filled with black pigment shows less against the iris background, in most cases. A dot is more easily visible to presbyopes even without their near correction. All marks are positioned near the lens edge so that there is no risk of visual interference and, ideally, both lenses should be engraved. A disadvantage of lens engraving marks is that they are sometimes inadvertently removed when power alterations are carried out.

LENS TINT

The use of tinted plastics material enables the contact lens practitioner to prescribe a tinted lens for his patient either for photophobia or to alter or enhance the iris colour within certain limits. Surface-dyed lenses are no longer used since the tint is not permanent and it has been suggested that certain of the pigments used in the dyeing process may be carcinogenic.

The arguments used by Giles (1960) to deprecate the over-prescribing of tinted spectacle lenses also apply to tinted contact lenses. However, the use of very light neutral tints in contact lenses, for example, code numbers 911 (very light grey) and 912 (light grey), is often beneficial in practice for two reasons. First, location of a clear lens on the sclera or in a bowl of water is extremely difficult, whereas even a lightly tinted lens can be easily observed. Secondly, the contact lens wearer is often more light sensitive than when wearing spectacles and the use of a lightly tinted lens may help to relieve this. The reasons for this photophobia have been suggested as three in number (Phillips, 1968), as follows.

(1) The increased light transmission of the contact lens since there is only one air-lens surface, which causes the greatest light loss by reflection. (However, the wearing of plano spectacle lenses over the contact lenses does not relieve the photophobia — Bergevin and Millodot, 1967.)

(2) The small amount of corneal oedema usually present in new wearers whilst adapting to their lenses, which causes increased scattering of light.

(3) The foreign-body sensation of the lens edges, again present in new wearers, which probably causes reflex iris blood vessel dilatation, iris congestion, and pain on sphincter constriction.

Since both (2) and (3) above are normally temporary in nature, the temptation to prescribe a deeper tint should be avoided. However, in the case of a badly fitting lens causing increased corneal oedema, or a poor lens edge exaggerating the foreign-body reflex, the photophobia may well be excessive and prolonged. In these instances, the answer lies in improving the lens design or construction and not in prescribing a deeper tint.

Tinted lenses are discussed further in Chapter 24, Volume 2. Where available, the use of CQ (clinical quality) material is recommended.

FENESTRATION

While some practitioners utilize fenestrations initially in every case the majority of practitioners fenestrate lenses only as a subsequent modification, usually to eliminate corneal oedema or staining due to inadequate tears flow under the lens. Fenestrations should only be used in those central areas which are definitely clear of the cornea, otherwise an additional tears meniscus is formed between lens and cornea which tends to reduce lens movement. In addition there is a greater risk of epithelial trauma from the edge of the fenestration.

Atkinson and Phillips (1971) have listed the proposed advantages of fenestrations in corneal lenses.

(1) To relieve oedema and corneal staining not alleviated by other methods (Friedberg, 1961; Korb, 1961, 1962a,b; Sellers, 1964; Boyd, 1965).

(2) To allow larger than normal lenses or back central optic diameters to be fitted, for example, in the case of large pupils or high-riding lenses, where the large lens would cause oedema (Haynes, 1960; Korb and Filderman, 1961; Korb, 1962a,b; Boyd, 1965; Neill, 1967).

(3) For non-blinkers, where there is constant oedema (Boyd, 1965).

(4) To remove small bubbles under the lenses not removed by other modifications (Korb and Filderman, 1961; Boyd, 1965).

(5) For patients who have difficulties in hot, stuffy atmospheres (Korb, 1961, 1962a,b; de Carle, 1965, 1967).

(6) To reduce or remove photophobia caused by an interference with normal corneal physiology (Korb, 1962a,b).

(7) To allow normal tears flow with lenses that have to be fitted steeper than the flattest corneal meridian and/or with less than normal lens movement (Sellers, 1960, 1964; Korb and Filderman, 1961; Bayshore, 1962; Korb, 1962a,b; Neill, 1967).

(8) To lighten heavy hyperopic lenses by making eight to ten fenestrations (Boyd, 1965).

(9) In high plus corrections where the thickness of the lens induces physiological problems (Korb and Filderman, 1961; Korb, 1962a,b).

(10) To improve tears circulation in toric back surface and truncated lenses which do not rotate and therefore have a poor tears flow beneath them (Friedberg, 1961; Korb, 1961, 1962b).

(11) To allow quicker lens settling and to improve the patient's speed and regularity of adaptation (Sellers, 1960, 1964).

(12) To prevent 'corneal exhaustion' where this has arisen by a minimal but prolonged interference with normal corneal metabolism (Korb, 1961, 1962b).

(13) To aid in reducing spectacle blur in certain cases (Friedberg, 1961).

(14) To improve normal corneal physiology in high-riding lenses with superior pooling (Friedberg, 1961).

The suggested size of fenestrations fall into three main groups: (1) around 0.10 mm diameter, often positioned centrally; (2) the most com-monly suggested group, around 0.25 mm diameter, and positioned near the edge of the back central optic portion; and (3) a larger fenestration of around 0.50 mm.

Hill and Uniacke (1968) have shown that there is little oxygen movement (via the tears) through the fenestration itself but that any physiological improvement is more likely to be due to the prevention of negative pressure under the lens.

A method of lens fenestration by the practitioner is described in Chapter 23, Volume 2. Lenses fenestrated by a laser beam permit multiple well-finished fenestration holes of 0.10 mm diameter. These are reported by Brucker (1975) to be very successful.

THE WRITTEN PRESCRIPTION

The form of the written prescription has been recommended by British Standard BS 3521:1979.

The radius of each portion is given in turn from the centre outwards, immediately followed by its external diameter. Dimensions are invariably to be given in the following order:

(i) The letter C followed by the figure 1 for a single curve, 2 for a double curve, 3 for a triple curve lens, etc.

(ii) Radius of the back central optic surface followed by its diameter or the overall size, whichever applies.

(iii) Radius of each surrounding back optic surface followed by its external diameter or the overall size, whichever applies.

(iv) Displacement of the optic (where applicable).

Examples

(1) Please supply one corneal lens

$\quad$ (i) $\qquad$ (ii) $\qquad$ (iii) $\qquad$ (iii) $\quad$ (iv)

R. C3/7.70:6.50/8.15:8.00/10.00:8.80/D1

BVP − 6.00 D

t_c 0.14 mm

Transitions left sharp.

Mark one dot (black).

Clear tint.

(2) Please supply one pair corneal lenses

R. C2/8.00:7.00/8.50:9.30

BVP − 3.25 D

t_c 0.17 mm

L. C2/8.05:7.00/8.55:9.30

BVP − 1.00 D

t_c 0.20 mm

Transitions light blended.

Engrave R & L.

912 CQ tint.

(3) Please supply one corneal lens

R. C3/8.15:7.00/8.70:8.20/9.50:9.40

BVP − 7.00 D

Front surface lenticular, FCOD 8.00 mm, to give edge t = 0.20 ± 0.02 mm

Transitions moderately well blended.

Engrave R.

911 tint.

Other Examples

The following example indicates the importance of knowing the accurate parameters of the trial set in use and the final lens to be fitted. At the same time it illustrates the importance of the various allowances discussed earlier.

Supposing a trial lens is engraved as	7.80 mm BCOR and 7.00 mm BCOD
but actually measures	7.77 mm BCOR and 7.20 mm BCOD
A lens is ordered to the same parameters as the trial lens but comes as	7.82 mm BCOR and 6.80 mm BCOD
that is, net effect on the lens fit is	≡ 0.05 mm flat ≡ 0.04 mm flat

Now the lens is also a −10.00 D and the flattening with hydration has been ignored. This will average 0.06 mm.

The total effect of the fit will therefore be

≡ 0.05 + 0.04 + 0.06 mm flat

≡ 0.15 mm flat.

The lens will therefore appear grossly flat in this instance.

Whilst the use of trial lenses, over-refraction, etc., is considered essential by most authorities it may be instructive to consider the following example of 'theoretical' fitting:

Keratometry, right eye 7.80 at 180, 7.71 at 90

Spectacle R_x − 6.00/− 0.75 X 180

Horizontal cornea diameter: 11 mm

Maximum pupil size   :   6 mm

First, applying the rule-of-thumb that 0.05 mm change in radius ≡ 0.25 D change in power, we can see by comparing the K readings that there is approximately 0.50 D corneal astigmatism, that is, 0.25 D less than the spectacle astigmatism, indicating that theoretically there should be approximately 0.25 D of residual astigmatism.

The lens ordered may be typically:

C4/7.73:7.00/8.25:8.00/10.00:8.40/12.25:8.80

BVP −5.75 D

t_c 0.10 mm

t_e 0.16−0.18 mm

Transitions moderately blended.

912 tint.

Engrave R.

The BCOR is derived from a compromise of the K readings, as explained earlier, of 7.77 mm + (−0.04 mm) hydration allowance for this BVP.

The BVP is derived from −5.50 D (after allowing 0.50 D for the vertex distance) + (−0.25 D) to compensate for the positive powered liquid lens which will be introduced as the BCOR is 0.04 mm steeper than the flattest K reading, that is, 7.81− 7.77 mm (the hydration allowance can be ignored, as explained earlier).

THE FINAL LENS

The final lens is first checked as described in Chapter 12. Ideally, the transitions are blended to facilitate tears flow under the lens and prevent bubble entrapment and corneal abrasion. The lenses are fully hydrated before being checked on the eye — carried out in the same manner as in the fitting routine. A gradual transition across the lens from touch to clearance is the ideal for most fitting philosophies. If any hard blue arcuate bearing areas (possibly indicative of a relatively sharp transition or too steep a peripheral curve) are apparent, either with the lens centred or as it moves on the cornea, these should be blended.

The patient is instructed in the wear and handling of his lenses, as described in Chapter 8, and the period of after-care then begins.

REFERENCES

Arias, C. M. (1960). 'Are we measuring the true apex of the cornea with the keratometer?' *Contacto* **4**, 195−198

Atkinson, K. W. and Phillips, A. J. (1971). 'Fenestrations in corneal lenses.' *Br. J. physiol. Optics* **26**, 1−14

Augsburger, A. R. and Hill, R. M. (1971). 'Contact lens mass: the most elusive feature.' *J. Am. optom. Ass.* **42**, 78−82

Bayshore, C. A. (1962). 'Report on 276 patients fitted with micro-corneal lenses, apical clearance and central ventilation.' *Am. J. Optom.* **39**, 552–553

Bayshore, C. A. (1963). 'Report on 600 cases of micro-corneal lenses fitted with apical clearance.' *Am. J. Optom.* **40**, 351–353

Bennett, A. G. (1968). 'Aspherical contact lens surfaces.' *Ophthal. Optician* **8**, 1037–1040, 1297–1300, 1311; **9**, 222–230

Bergevin, J. and Millodot, M. (1967). 'Glare with ophthalmic and corneal lenses.' *Am. J. Optom.* **44**, 213–221

Bier, N. (1956). 'A study of the cornea in relation to contact lens practice.' *Am. J. Optom.* **33**, 291–304

Bier, N. (1957). 'The Contour lens.' *J. Am. optom. Ass.* **28**, 394–396

Boyd, H. H. (1965). 'Perforation of contact lenses.' *Am. J. Ophthal.* **60**, 726–728

British Standard 5562 (1978). *Specification for Contact Lenses.* London: British Standards Institution

British Standard 3521 (1979). *Glossary of Terms Relating to Ophthalmic Lenses and Spectacle Frames – BS 3521: 1979. Part 3. Glossary of Terms Relating to Contact Lenses.* London: British Standards Institution

Brucker, D. (1975). 'Laser fenestrated lenses.' Chapter 20 in *Micro-Corneal and Soft Contact Lenses* by S. K. Dastoor. Bombay: Popular Prakashan

Bryant, P. (1975). Personal communication

Carle, J. de (1965). 'A comparison of materials used in the manufacture of contact lenses.' *Contact Lens Practnr* **6**, 29–32

Carle, J. de (1967). 'Small lenses.' *Contact Lens Practnr.* **8**, 9–11

Davis, H. E. (1964). 'Why the small contact lens?' *Br. J. physiol. Optics* **21**, 215–218

Dickinson, F. (1954). 'Report on a new corneal lens.' *Optician* **128**(3303), 3–6

Friedberg, M. A. (1961). 'Contact lens apertures and toric curve designs.' *J. Am. optom Ass.* **32**, 642–644

Gegg, B. R. (1969). 'Aspherical contact lenses – developments and doubts.' *Contact Lens* **2**(5), 20–24, 31

Giles, G. H. (1960). *The Principles and Practice of Refraction,* London: Hammond, Hammond

Gordon, S. (1965). 'Contact lens hydration: a study of the wetting-drying cycle.' *Optom. Wkly* **56**, 55–62

Haynes, P. R. (1960). 'Aperture venting techniques in corneal contact lenses.' In *Encyclopedia of Contact Lens Practice.* Ed. by Haynes, P. R. South Bend, Indiana: International Optics Publishing Corporation

Hersh, D. (1974). 'The Hersh palpebral traction lens.' *Internat. Contact Lens Clin.* **1**(4), 65–71

Hill, R. M. and Uniacke, N. P. (1968). 'Lacrimal fluid and lens design.' *Contacto* **12**, 59–61

Hodd, F. A. B. (1958). 'Clinical experience in fitting micro-lenses.' *Br. J. physiol. Optics* **15**, 205–226

Hodd, F. A. B. (1966). 'A design study of the back surface of corneal contact lenses.' *Ophthal. Optician* **6**, 1175–1178, 1187–1190, 1203, 1229–1232, 1235–1238; **7**, 14–16, 19–21, 39

Jessen, G. N. (1961). 'New bifocal technique results in more comfortable single vision lenses.' *Contacto* **5**, 237–243

Korb, D. R. (1961). 'Contact lens news and views: application of multiple micro-holes.' *J. Am. optom. Ass.* **32**, 11, 891–892

Korb, D. R. (1962*a*). 'The evolution of fenestrated corneal lenses.' *Pennsylvania Optom.* **22**(3), 23–28

Korb, D. R. (1962*b*). 'Recent advances in corneal lens fenestration.' In *Encyclopedia of Contact Lens Practice.* Vol. 3, Suppl. 14, pp. 58–66. Ed. by Haynes, P. R. Sound Bend, Indiana: International Optics Publishing Corporation

Korb, D. R. and Filderman, I. P. (1961). 'A new approach to contact lens ventilation.' *Optom. Wkly* **52**, 2375

Korb, D. R. and Korb, J. E. (1974). 'Fitting to achieve a normal blinking and lid action.' *Internat. Contact Lens Clin.* **1**(3), 57–70

Lester, R. and Braff, S. (1963). 'The management of small corneal contact lenses.' Calcon Comment, El Monte, California. Cited by R. B. Mandell in *Contact Lens Practice, Basic and Advanced.* Springfield, Ill.: Thomas

Mackie, I. A., Mason, D. and Perry, B. J. (1970). 'Factors influencing corneal contact lens centration.' *Br. J. physiol. Optics* **25**, 87–103

Mackie, I. A. (1973). 'Design compensation in corneal lens fitting.' In *Symposium on Contact Lenses: Transactions of the New Orleans Academy of Ophthalmology.* St. Louis: Mosby

Mandell, R. B. (1974). 'What is the gravity lens?' *Internat. Contact Lens Clin.* **1**(4), 29–35

Moore, C. (1974). 'A new concept for fitting ultrathin lenses.' *Internat. Contact Lens Clin.* **1**(3), 47–54

Morrison, R. J. (1967). 'Minalens technique.' *Refractionist* January/March, 35–44

Neill, J. C. (1967). 'Electronic venting of corneal contact lenses.' *Contacto* **11**, 9–11

Phillips, A. J. (1968). 'Filters used by drivers at night.' *Ophthal. Optician* **8**, 707–713, 756–763

Phillips, A. J. (1969). 'Alterations in curvature of the finished corneal lens.' *Ophthal. Optician* **9**, 980–986, 1043–1054, 1100–1110

Rabbetts, R. B. (1976). 'Large corneal lenses with constant axial edge lift.' *Ophthal. Optician* **16**, 236, 239

Ruben, M. (1966). 'Use of conoidal curves in corneal contact lenses.' *Br. J. Ophthal.* **50**, 642–645

Sellers, F. J. E. (1960). 'The adjustment of multi-curved corneal lenses.' *Contact Lens Practnr* **1**, 26–32

Sellers, F. J. E. (1964). 'Fenestrations first – not last.' *Contacto* **8**, (2), 17–30

Sheridan, M. (1970). 'The investigation of corneal form.' *Ophthal. Optician* **10**, 892–894

Steele, E. (1969). 'The fitting of aspheric contact lenses.' *Contacto* **4**, 55–58

Stek, A. W. (1975). 'Conic contact lens – design and fitting technique.' *Optician* **169**(4378), 30–35

Stone, J. (1975*a*). 'Corneal lenses with constant axial edge lift.' *Ophthal. Optician* **15**, 818–824

Stone, J. (1975*b*). Personal communication

Stone, J. (1978). 'Changes in curvature of cellulose acetate butyrate lenses during hydration and dehydration.' *J. Br. Contact Lens Ass.* **1**, 22–35

Thomas, P. F. (1967). *Conoid Contact Lenses.* Australia: Corneal Lens Corporation

Wray, L. (1963). 'An elementary analysis of the forces retaining a corneal contact lens on the eye.' *Optician* **146**, 239–241, 373–376

Chapter 12

Hard Lens Verification Procedures

Rita Dickins

Contact lenses should be checked for quality and physical characteristics whether they are for prescription use, contact lens sets or research purposes. Contact lens manufacturers are not bound by any statutory regulations, but many laboratories publish details of the accuracy to which their lenses are made, and the British Standards Institution has issued guidance on tolerances for use by practitioner and laboratory (*see* Addenda I and II, pages 299 and 300).

This chapter is divided into the following sections: parameters to be checked; and verification procedures.

PARAMETERS TO BE CHECKED

Table 12.1 shows the various parameters which may need checking in each group for corneal and scleral lenses, they are: (1) radii; (2) diameters and linear parameters; (3) thickness; (4) the optic; and (5) quality, tint, etc.

A pair of lenses should match for tint, transition and edge forms. Diameters and zone widths should not differ by more than a certain tolerance. The maximum difference in thickness for a pair of lenses of relatively equal power should not exceed a specified tolerance unless this is specifically requested to facilitate lens checking.

VERIFICATION PROCEDURES

RADII

Various methods are available for verifying contact lens radii.

Radiuscopes

There are several instruments available (*Figure 12.1*) which differ in construction, but all use Drysdale's method for the measurement of small radii (Drysdale, 1900). This method is based on the principle that for a curved mirror an image is formed in the same plane as the object when the object is at the centre of curvature of the surface. This is because the reflected light returns along its incident path. An image may also be formed on the surface, and the distance between the two images — which is equal to the radius of the surface — is measured (*Figure 12.2*).

A radiuscope consists essentially of a microscope with a dial gauge attached (calibrated to 0.01 mm) to read the position of the microscope body or microscope stage. Light from an illuminated target (consisting of a ring of dots or radial lines) attached to the microscope is imaged by the microscope objective after being reflected through a right-angle by a semi-transparent mirror.

Some modern radiuscopes (*Figure 12.3*) have dispensed with the external dial gauge shown in *Figure 12.1*, and the radius reading is shown on a scale at one side of the field of view in the microscope. The knurled knob on the left-hand side of the instrument in *Figure 12.3*, just above its nameplate, is used to set a pointer to zero on this scale when the surface image of a concave surface is in focus. To focus the centre of curvature image, the coarse and fine focusing wheels at the lower back of the instrument are used to raise the microscope objective and at the same time this movement is recorded by the pointer on the scale — so giving the radius reading directly. The use of instruments with dial gauges is outlined below.

Table 12.1–Contact Lens Parameters which may need Verifying

Group	Corneal lenses	Scleral lenses
Radii	Back central optic radius Back peripheral radii Front optic radii (spherical and/or toroidal)	Back haptic radius Back optic radius/radii Transition radii Front optic radii (spherical and/or toroidal)
Diameters and linear parameters	Back central optic diameter Back intermediate diameters Overall size Displacement of optic Lenticular, front central optic diameter Bifocal segment size and position Axial and/or radial edge lift	Back central optic diameter Back intermediate diameters Back peripheral optic diameter Primary optic diameter Lenticular, front central optic diameter Back haptic size Overall size Displacement of optic Transition widths
Thickness	Central Edge Lenticular junction	Central optic Average haptic Edge
Optic – lens prescription	Back vertex power Front vertex power Near addition Prism Cylinder Aberration	As for corneal lenses
Quality, etc.	Finish and quality Polish Edge Form Transitions Tint	As for corneal lenses

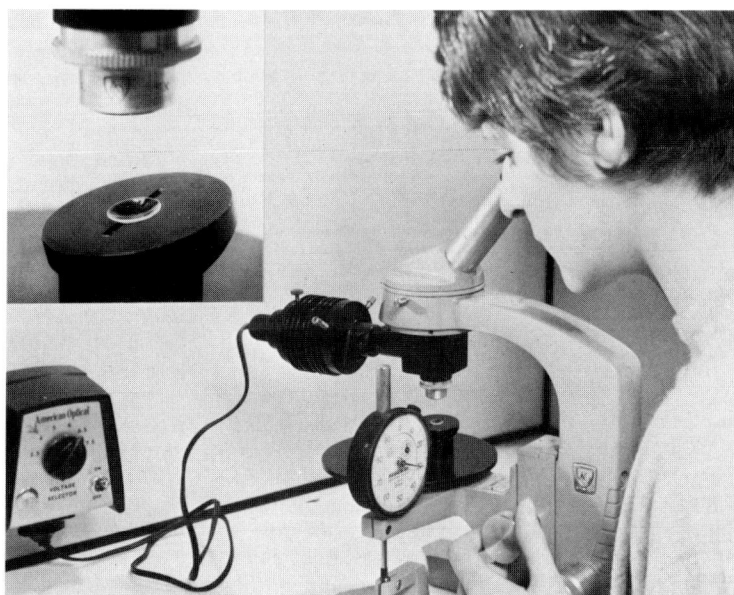

Figure 12.1–American Optical Company Monocular Radiuscope with corneal lens in place for measurement of back central optic radius. Inset: Close-up of lens in place, holder tilted to measure back peripheral radius

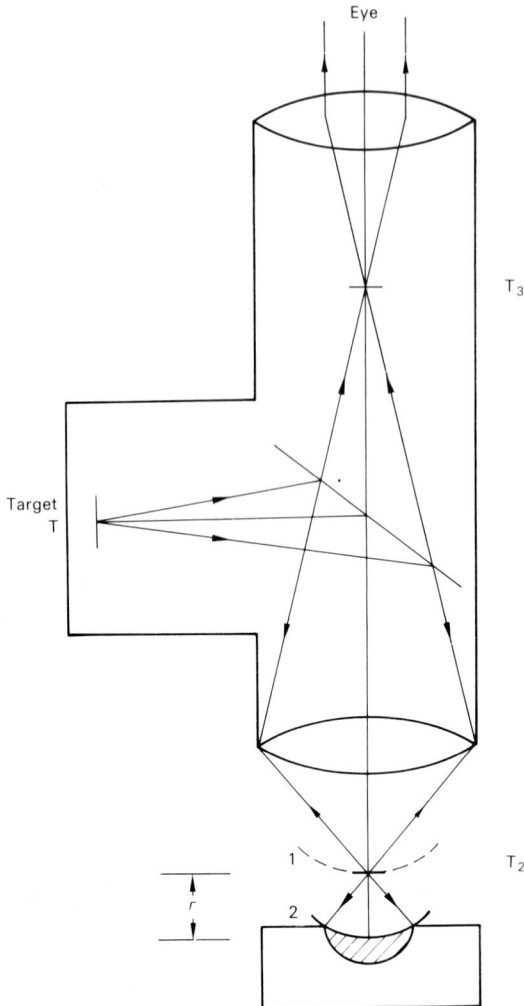

Figure 12.2–Diagram to show Drysdale's principle. 1 – First position of lens, image focused on lens surface. 2 – Second position of lens, image is now at centre of curvature of surface. r = lens radius

Procedure for Using a Radiuscope, Concave Surfaces

(1) A suitable lens holder is filled with water.

(2) The clean lens is placed centrally on the holder, convex surface in complete contact with the water. The water minimizes reflections from the front surface of the lens since its refractive index is very similar to that of the lens material. (Without the water present, the images formed by reflection at the front surface are as bright as the images formed by the back surface, and it then becomes difficult to tell quickly which image is required.) Only a small quantity of water should be used, otherwise the lens floats and may move during measurements.

(3) The holder is placed on the microscope stage and centred.

(4) The microscope eyepiece is correctly adjusted, and then by observation through the microscope the target is imaged on the surface of the lens by moving either the microscope and target or the microscope stage, depending on the type of instrument used.

(5) The dial gauge reading is recorded (or the dial gauge is set to zero).

(6) A second focus, at the centre of curvature of the surface, is obtained by racking the microscope up or the stage down.

(7) The second reading is recorded.

(8) The difference between the two dial gauge readings gives the radius of curvature of the surface.

(9) This procedure should be repeated twice and the average of the three readings taken. To minimize user errors, the fine focusing drum should be racked in the same direction when making each setting. The radius should also be measured at different points on the lens as it may vary (Tannehill and Sampson, 1966).

The focused target must be central. Usually, it is possible to move the microscope stage horizontally to centralize the image. A diaphragm and/or rheostat is incorporated in most instruments to reduce brightness.

The target image will appear distorted if the surface is irregular. If any water is left on the surface being measured, it can result in distorted surface images. On toroidal surfaces, two measurements for the principal radii must be made. When a radial line target is being used, the lens must be rotated so that its principal meridians coincide with one pair of perpendicular radial lines.

On some instruments it is necessary to use a special holder (*Figure 12.4*) when measuring back haptic radius. By using the holder, the travel of the microscope is increased to cope with the larger radii encountered.

Measurement of Back Peripheral Radii

A similar procedure is followed but the lens holder is tilted and the microscope stage moved across so that the target is focused in the peripheral band of the lens. Care is needed to centre the surface image in this band. Provided that the band is 1 mm wide, it is possible to measure its radius. It is therefore possible to measure any

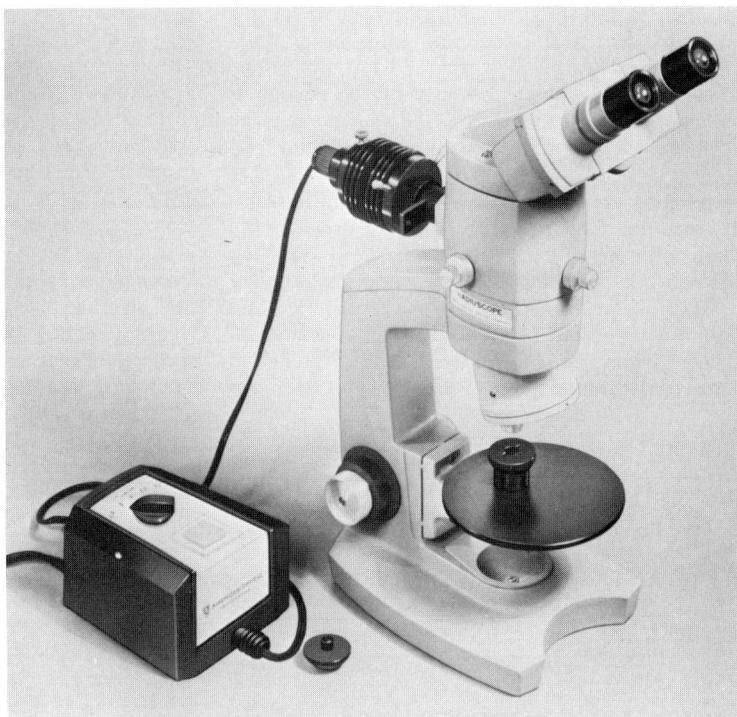

Figure 12.3–American Optical Company Binocular Radiuscope with internal scale. (Photograph kindly provided by British American Optical Company)

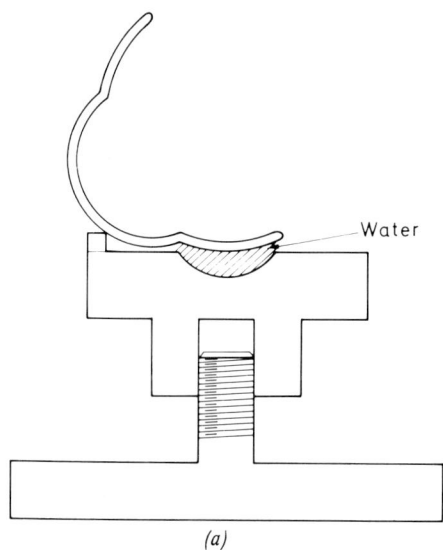

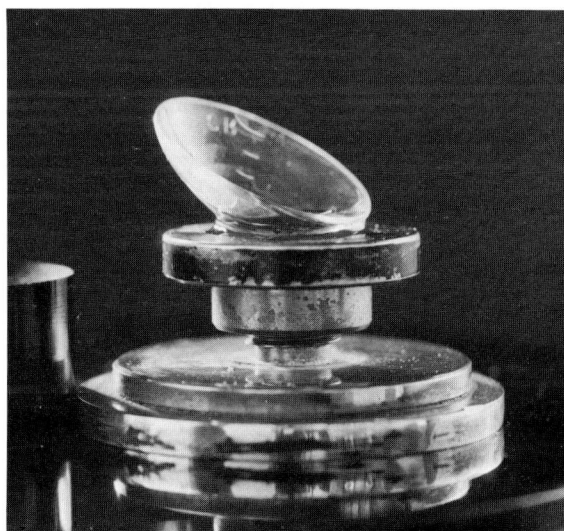

(a)

(b)

Figure 12.4–Scleral lens holder for use with Drysdale's method. (a) Diagram of section through holder with lens in place. Note screw section by means of which a greater distance may be obtained between the lens surface and microscope objective. (b) Holder in use, back haptic radius being measured

intermediate radii on the lens which occur over a wide enough band. (Attempts have been made (Brungardt, 1962) to measure back peripheral radii using a focimeter. Because of the change in back surface radius between the centre and the periphery, it may be possible to obtain two power readings on the focimeter. Provided that the front surface is one single curve, the difference between the two power readings is due to the radius difference on the back surface. If the back central optic radius is known, its corresponding negative surface power may be obtained from radius/power tables* and the back peripheral surface power found by adding the difference in focimeter readings (the periphery has the less

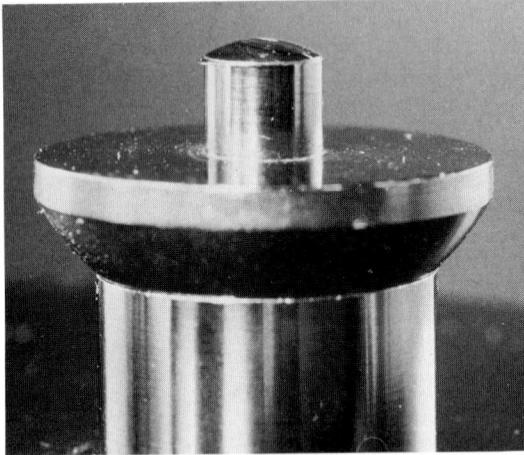

Figure 12.5–Holder for measuring convex surfaces on the radiuscope. The lens has been displaced slightly in order to make it visible

negative value). By further using radius/power tables, the back peripheral radius may be determined. This method is inaccurate with multicurve lenses. The thickness difference between centre and periphery contributes to the inaccuracy for all lenses.)

Measurement of Convex Surfaces

The concave surface is mounted on water, if possible, or blacked out with a soft grease pencil or felt-tip pen. The convex surface is placed uppermost on a special holder (*Figure 12.5*) on a radiuscope. A similar procedure to that outlined above for concave surfaces is followed, but the surface and centre of curvature images are reversed.

---

* Tables for radius to power conversion – *see* Appendix B, *Table II*, page 310.

Keratometers

The keratometer is used with a special contact lens holder (*Figure 12.6*) which utilizes a front surface silvered mirror and a lens support. The lens rests on water in a small depression on a horizontal support. The mirror is set at 45 degrees to the optical axis of the instrument and reflects light from the instrument on to the surface to be measured.

Another type of holder (*Figure 12.7*) requires that the lens be attached to a depression, which lies in a vertical plane, by some adhesive substance such as Plasticine or double-sided sticky tape. There is a possibility that the lens may be distorted using this procedure.

The keratometer can be used to measure central optic radii of corneal lenses and optic radii of scleral lenses. Since an area of approximately 3 mm in diameter is needed to check a particular radius using conventional keratometers (Lehmann, 1967), it is not possible to measure intermediate and peripheral radii on corneal lenses by this method. Using a single mire of the topographic ophthalmometer (*see* Chapter 5), which utilizes a very small area of reflecting surface, such readings may be possible, however.

Because the keratometer mires are reflected from regions of the surface outside the paraxial zone, an allowance is made during calibration for the aberrations thus introduced. As keratometers are calibrated for convex surfaces, and when used to measure back optic radii of contact lenses, concave surfaces are involved, an error is introduced. This is because the aberrations produced by a concave surface are different from those produced by a convex surface. As stated in Chapter 5, page 146, Bausch and Lomb and other keratometer manufacturers have produced conversion tables for converting convex to concave radii and these show the error to range from 0.02 mm for steep radii (of the order of 6.50 mm) up to 0.04 mm for flat radii (of about 9.50 mm). In all cases the radii for concave surfaces are greater than for convex surfaces. Thus, for most of the back central optic radii encountered in contact lens work it is sufficient to add 0.03 mm to the radius reading given by the keratometer.

To measure back haptic radii the range of the keratometer needs extending. This may be done by recalibrating the keratometer using a −1.00 D or −2.00 D trial case lens taped in front of the objective as mentioned on page 146. Three steel balls are used for recalibration having accurately known radii of say 9.00 mm, 12.00 mm and 15.00 mm. A graph is then drawn of measured radius (ordinate) against actual radius (abscissa).

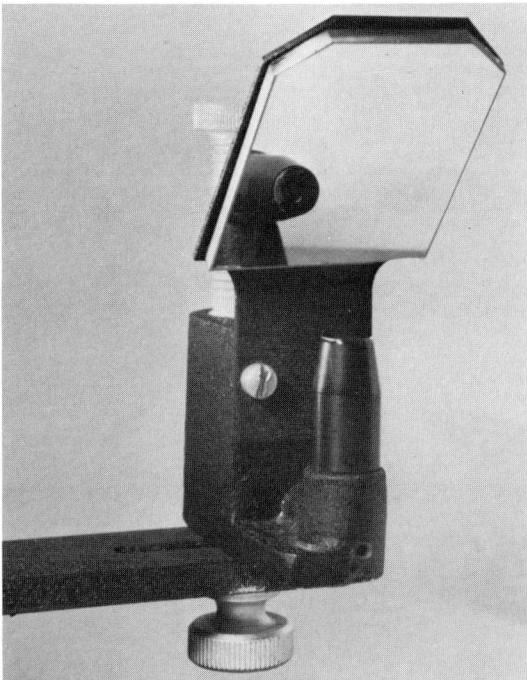

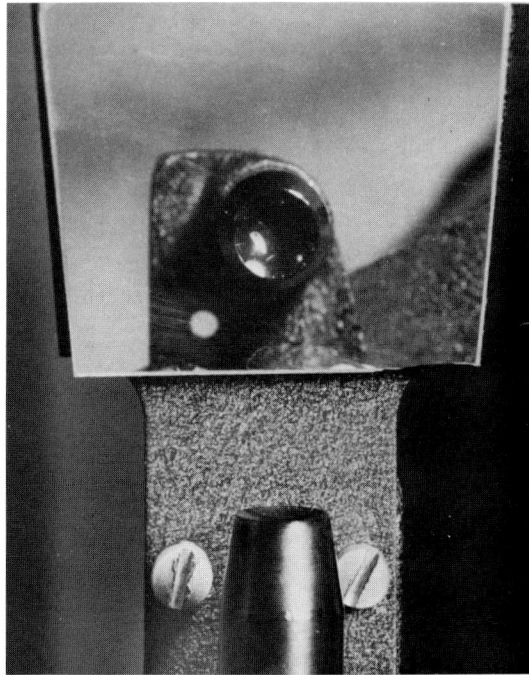

(a)   (b)

Figure 12.6–Mirror-type contact lens holder for use with a keratometer. (a) On the keratometer. (b) Close-up. The lens, which is resting on the concave depression of the support, can be seen reflected in the mirror

Provided the same trial case lens is always employed, the same graph may then be used for determining longer radii than the keratometer was designed to measure. Steep radii may be determined similarly, by taping a positive trial case lens, of about +1.50 D, in front of the keratometer objective

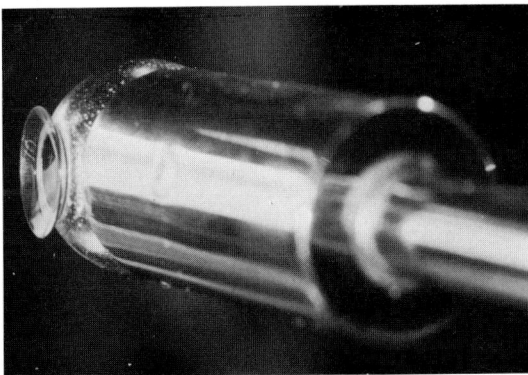

Figure 12.7–Contact lens holder for use with keratometer. The holder is screwed to the head-rest arm, and the lens is held in the depression by an adhesive substance

and recalibrating with steep steel balls and drawing another graph. (This is useful for measuring the radii of keratoconic corneas, if sufficiently undistorted readings can be obtained.)

The Radius Checking Device

This device (*Figure 12.8*), developed by Sarver and Kerr (1964), is used in conjunction with a focimeter. The device is made of plastics, refractive index 1.49, and has a depression on one surface which is flatter than the front surface radius of most corneal contact lenses. The other surface has a convex portion, radius 8.87 mm, designed to rest in the plane of the focimeter stop. A small amount of liquid of refractive index 1.49 is placed in the depression and the lens to be measured is placed with its convex surface in contact with the liquid. The device with lens in place can be considered as a thick lens since all the components — device, liquid and lens — have the same refractive index.

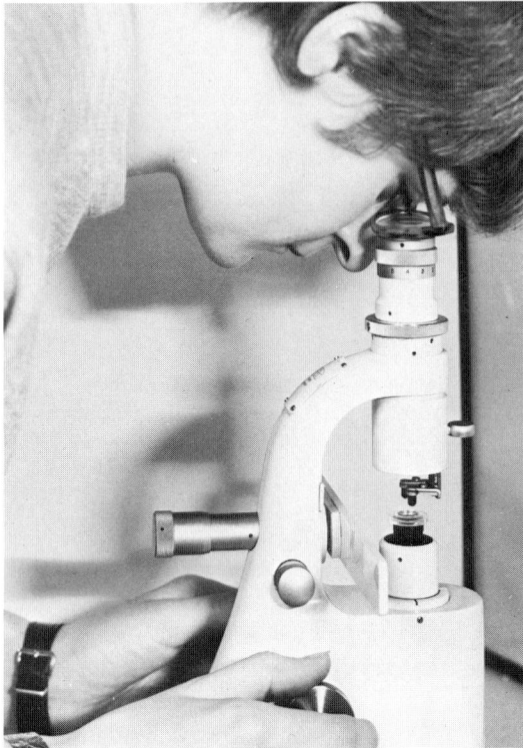

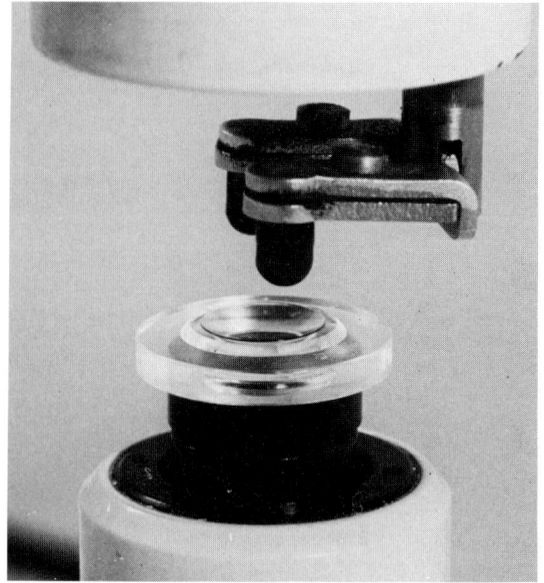

(b)

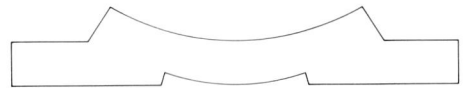

(a)   (c)

Figure 12.8 – The radius checking device. (a) On the focimeter. (b) Close-up of device on the focimeter. (c) Diagram of cross-section of device. Note design of the convex side. The outer flat section rests on the focimeter stop, and the convex part is in the same plane

Thus if,

front surface of device	$= F_1$ D $= +55.24$ D
thickness of device	$= t_1$ mm
thickness of contact lens	$= t_2$ mm
back surface power of contact lens	$= F_2$ D
back surface radius of contact lens	$= r_2$ mm
front vertex power of the system	$= F_v$ D

then

$$F_v = \frac{F_2}{1 - \left(\frac{t_1 + t_2}{1000n}\right) F_2} + F_1$$

from the formula for front vertex power.

From the above

$$r_2 = \underbrace{\frac{(1-n)1000}{F_v - F_1}}_{(a)} + \underbrace{\frac{(t_1 + t_2)(1-n)}{n}}_{(b)}$$

The front vertex power of the system is found using the focimeter. The thickness of the liquid between lens and device is negligible. The thickness of the contact lens is determined by a suitable method. Tables have been prepared and published (Dickins, 1968) for use with the device. Thus, once F_v and $(t_1 + t_2)$ have been determined, two figures are obtained from the appropriate tables for the two parts of the formula (*a*) and (*b*). This device can only be used to measure the back central optic radius of a corneal lens. It is possible that a separate device could be designed for use with scleral lenses.

Templates

Plastics rings of various radii, with chamfered edges, have been used to measure back haptic radii (Stone, 1964).

Other Methods

There are various other methods for measuring contact lens radii which are in the main only laboratory techniques. It is possible that other instrumentation may be developed using these techniques.

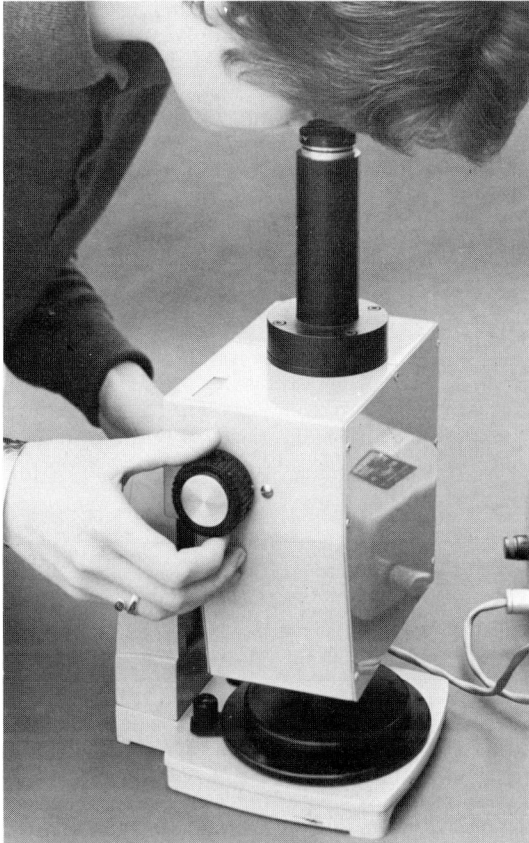

Figure 12.9–The Toposcope

Interference Patterns

Interference patterns, which may be parallel fringes or rings, can be produced in a number of ways. Interference fringes are the basis of many lens testing techniques. Moiré fringes are utilized in the Toposcope (*Figure 12.9*). It is used for measuring radii and diameters of corneal lenses. The target, which consists of a series of straight lines, is viewed through a screen with similar lines. The shape and orientation of the fringes formed are a function of the relationship between the two sets of lines. Straight parallel fringes indicate a spherical surface, curved fringes indicate an elliptical surface. Any warpage or dimples in the surface are indicated by irregularly shaped fringes.

The lens to be measured is placed on a holder with the convex surface in contact with a small amount of water. The instrument is adjusted until horizontal fringes are formed parallel to the horizontal index in the eyepiece. The radius is then read from a scale which has 0.01 mm divisions. At the extremities of the field of view, a second band of fringes aligned in a different direction may be seen. The back peripheral radius (and similarly any intermediate radii) can be measured by aligning these fringes to the horizontal index (*Figure 12.10*).

Aspheric central and peripheral curves can be measured with this instrument by noting those points of the curved fringes which are parallel to the horizontal index.

Garner (1970), undertook an investigation concerning the measurement of contact lens radii using Newton's rings. Although his apparatus was too complicated to form the basis for an instrument for use by practitioners, it made use of test plates and was accurate to 0.003 mm in radius determination. With it he showed that hydration of hard lenses maintains the spherical nature of their

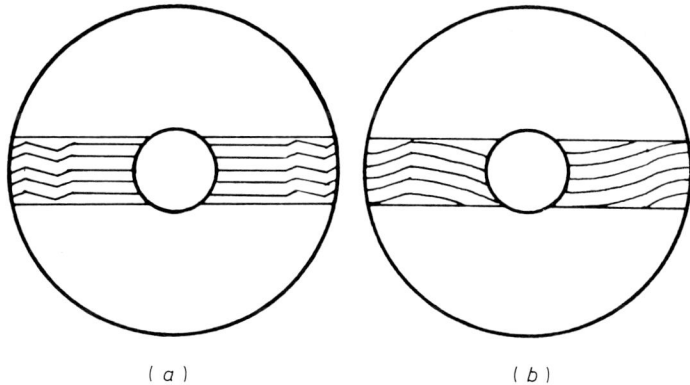

Figure 12.10–Fringes as seen with the toposcope. (a) Straight parallel fringes indicate spherical curves; central fringes correspond to the back central optic radius, peripheral fringes the back peripheral radius. A transition zone and edge bevel are apparent. (b) Curved fringes indicating an elliptical surface

(a)   (b)

surfaces (if spherical to start with), and that surface polishing with wax tools can lead to flattening of the periphery of a spherical surface with effective steepening at the centre due to distortion.

Pneumatic Gauging

This method uses an air jet as part of a direct reading spherometer (Smith, 1966), the pressure from a small air jet being proportional to the sagitta of surfaces to which it is applied.

Focimeter and Trial Lenses

Linnell Fearn (1970), suggested taking a focimeter reading with the front surface of a trial lens resting on the back surface of a test lens of unknown dimensions. A second reading is taken with water between the contact surfaces. The difference between the readings gives the liquid lens power. Knowing the front surface radius of the trial lens and assuming a negligible liquid lens thickness, and refractive index of 1.336, the back central optic radius of the test lens can be determined. The fluid lens power must be kept to a minimum. This requires the use of about three trial lenses with different known front surface radii depending on the BCOR of the lens to be tested.

Accuracy of Methods

Of the methods described for determining contact lens radii, the radiuscope appears to be the most accurate and versatile (Dickins and Fletcher, 1964). The keratometer is limited since a large area is usually needed on which to take measurements. Most keratometers are not calibrated with a sufficiently small scale to measure to 0.01 mm positively. Since a keratometer utilizes reflections from outside the paraxial zone, it is calibrated to allow for the aberrations introduced by convex surfaces. When used for measuring concave surfaces the radius is slightly underestimated by approximately 0.02–0.04 mm (Bennett, 1966) (see page 286).

The accuracy of the radius checking device has been investigated (Dickins, 1966a and b) and found to be reasonable. Measurements can be made to an accuracy of 0.02 mm provided that the constants of the device are accurately known.

Templates provide only an approximate value for the back haptic radius. Sources of error are the pliability of the lens and the difficulty of rotating the template about the axis of symmetry of the lens.

In an investigation into the accuracy of the Toposcope, Storey (1969) found it to be poor, particularly for peripheral radii, and most errors were negative. However, a more recent study by Janoff (1977) has shown that with an experienced observer the Toposcope proved quicker to use and gave less variable readings than the radiuscope. Also the Toposcope utilizes fringes formed over the whole back central optic and is capable of detecting and measuring aspheric surfaces to a limited degree of accuracy.

Methods of measuring radii using fringes may be needed more in the future with the developments in aspheric and continuous curve surfaces.

It should be remembered when checking contact lens radii that finished corneal lenses alter in curvature with hydration and with release of any stresses in the lens material (Phillips, 1969).

DIAMETERS AND LINEAR PARAMETERS

Several devices are available for measuring the different linear parameters. With some methods the problem of parallax occurs as the measuring scale is not in the same plane as the parameter being measured.

Measuring Magnifier

The measuring magnifier (*Figure 12.11*) has an adjustable eyepiece through which an engraved scale is viewed. The lens is held with the concave surface towards the scale. The overall size of the lens may be checked with this device. The back central optic diameter and any intermediate optic diameters may also be checked in this way provided that the transitions are reasonably sharp. The lens should be rotated and several readings taken to check overall and central optic roundness. Any displacement of the optic may be checked with this instrument. Since the scale is usually only 20 mm long, the device is only used with corneal lenses.

V Gauge

V gauges (*Figure 12.12*) are made of metal or plastics and have a V-shaped channel cut into the material. The channel may vary in width from 6.00 to 12.50 mm. The corneal lens to be measured is placed at the widest end of the channel, concave side downwards, and then allowed to slide down under gravity until it is stopped by the sides of the gauge. The overall size is then read from a scale

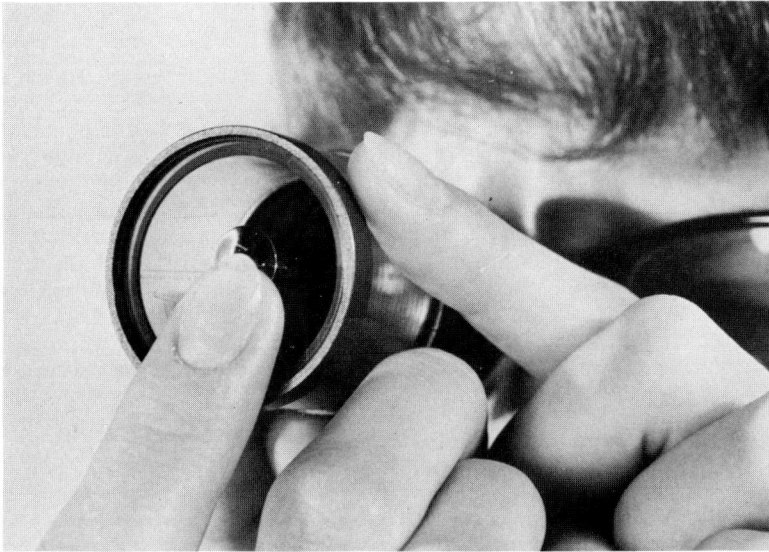

(a)

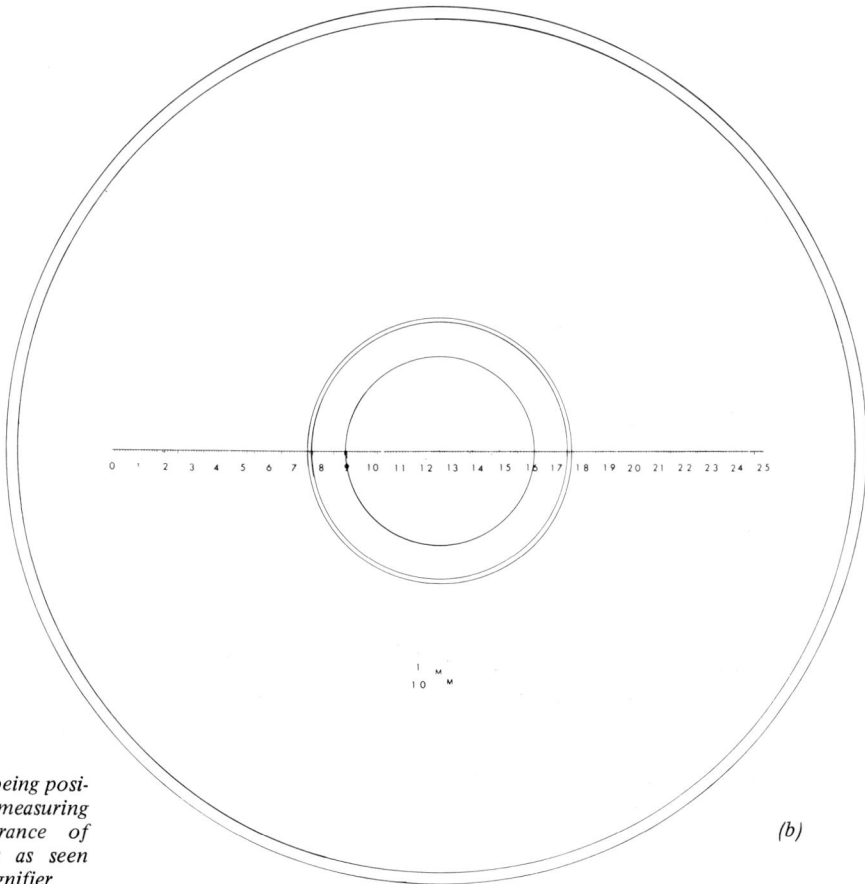

(b)

Figure 12.11—(a) Lens being positioned against scale of measuring magnifier. (b) Appearance of zones of corneal lens as seen through a measuring magnifier

beside the channel. The lens must be clean and dry or it will not slide freely. The lens must not be forced along the channel as this can result in compression and even breakage.

The Toposcope

The Toposcope has a reticule within the eyepiece which is used for measuring back central optic diameter, overall size, intermediate diameters, size and location of distorted areas, all on corneal lenses. Prior to measurement the instrument is set to give a constant magnification.

Cast, Dividers, Transparent Rule

Most scleral lens parameters are measured on a cast of the lens (*Figure 12.13*). The cast is made from dental stone mixed with a small amount of water to a smooth paste. The lens is supported horizontally on Plasticine. After ensuring that all air bubbles have escaped from the dental stone by tapping the sides of the mixing bowl, the dental stone is poured into the lens until it is completely full. When the dental stone is set, the cast is removed from the lens, using a fingernail. Care must be taken that an excess of dental stone does not drip over the sides of the lens and so cause

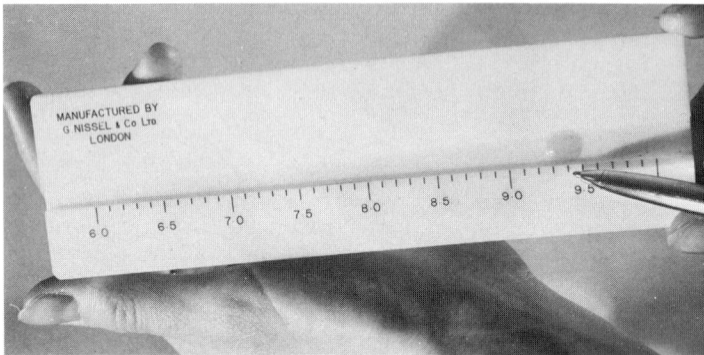

Figure 12.12 – V gauge in use. Pen indicates position, to read lens overall size of 9.40 mm to nearest 0.10 mm

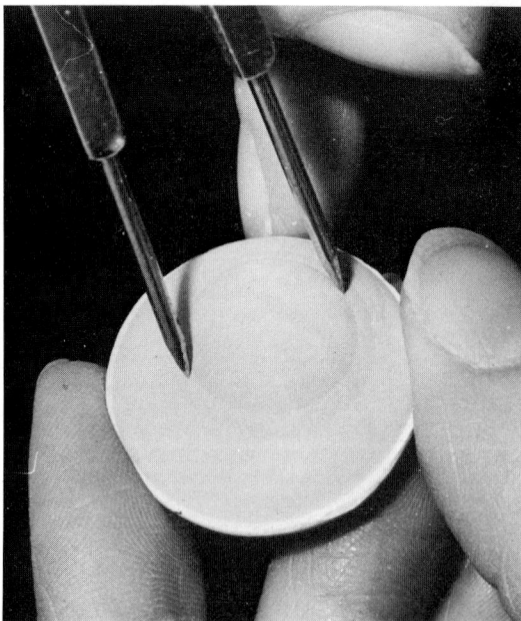

(a)

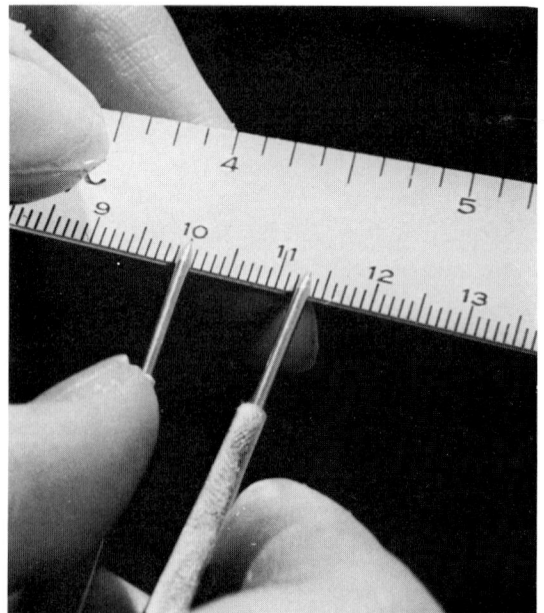

(b)

Figure 12.13 – (a) Cast of scleral lens with dividers placed to measure back central optic diameter. (b) Dividers placed against scale giving measurement of 13.0 mm

Micrometer and Spheres

A special problem arises in checking the primary optic diameter of a scleral lens since the sharp demarcation between back optic and haptic surfaces is usually removed by the transition. It is possible to measure this diameter by finding the difference between optic and haptic sags (Stone, 1964).

A sphere with radius equal to the back haptic radius of the lens to be measured is placed on the base plate of a vertical micrometer (*Figure 12.14*) with the lens on top. The maximum measurement x (*Figure 12.15*) is determined. From this is subtracted the thickness of the optic, t, and $2h$, the diameter of the sphere, to find the difference between the sags, a.

Tables are now referred to*. The value a is found in the appropriate table indicated by the back haptic radius and back optic radius, and the primary optic diameter can then be read off. Values of a have been computed for back central optic radii from 7.00 to 10.50 mm in 0.125 mm steps, back haptic radii from 11.50 to 15.50 mm in 0.25 mm steps, and primary optic diameters from 12.00 to 15.50 mm in 0.125 mm steps.

* Tables used when measuring primary optic diameter with a micrometer (Stone, 1964).

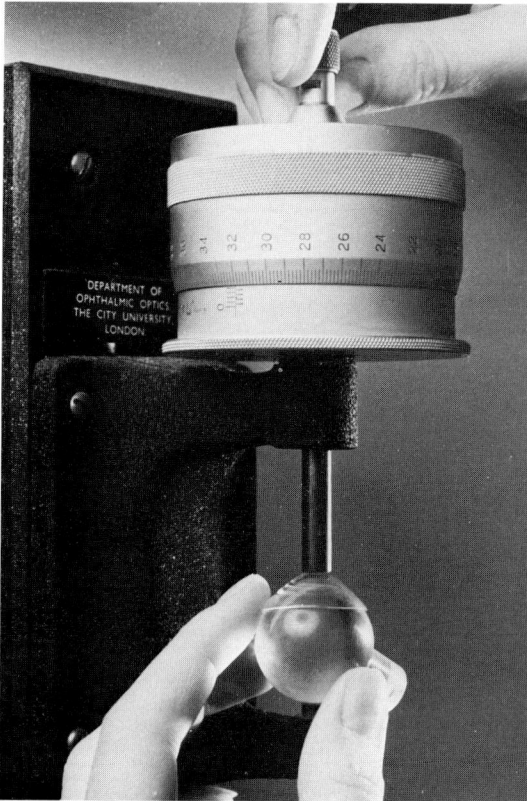

Figure 12.14–Micrometer method of measuring primary optic diameter. The lens is placed on a sphere. When the vertical plunger is in contact with the front surface of the lens the scale reading gives the distance x (Figure 12.15)

difficulty in the removal of the cast. The cast has all the lens features clearly marked on it. The transition width, back central optic diameter and optic displacement can be measured from the cast by placing the dividers at the appropriate points and measuring the distance apart of the dividers with a rule. The primary optic diameter of a preformed scleral lens may be deduced by adding the transition width to the back optic diameter, measured on a cast at the point where the transition curve intersects the optic curve. Displacement of optic is found by measuring on the cast, the major and minor haptic chords (usually on the temporal and nasal sides respectively) and taking half the difference between the two. A haptic chord is measured from the outer edge of the transition to the edge of the cast.

The overall size and back haptic size of a scleral lens are determined by direct measurement with a transparent rule.

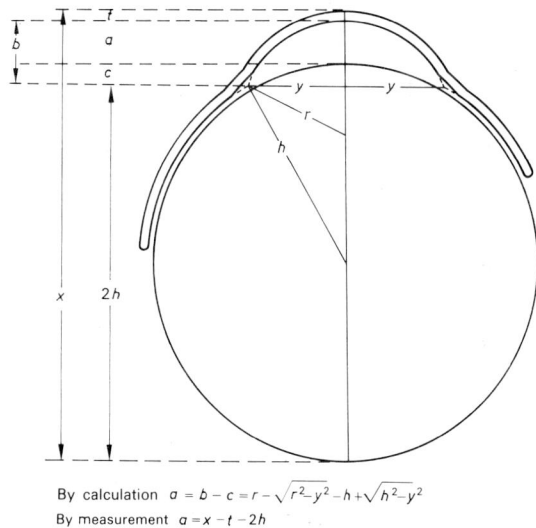

By calculation $a = b - c = r - \sqrt{r^2 - y^2} - h + \sqrt{h^2 - y^2}$

By measurement $a = x - t - 2h$

Figure 12.15–Principle of micrometer method of measuring primary optic diameter. h = back haptic radius; r = back optic radius; 2y = primary optic diameter; b and c are determined from the exact sag formula

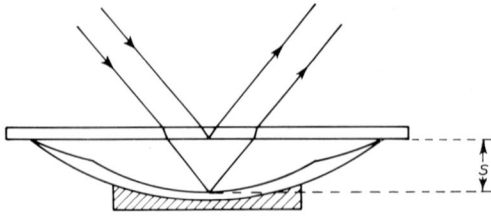

Figure 12.16–Axial edge lift measurement. A cover slide on the lens (which is placed in the radiuscope holder) permits s to be measured

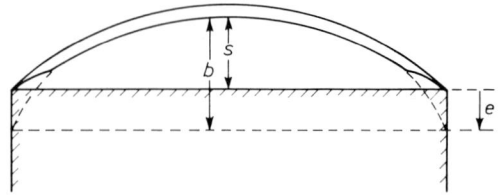

Figure 12.17–Axial edge lift e = b − s. Here the lens is placed on a holder having a stem diameter equal to its overall size. Other stem diameters may be used

Axial Edge Lift Measurement

Stone (1975) has described two methods, as follows.

Method 1

The lens is placed on the radiuscope holder in the usual manner, and a microscope cover slide placed on top (*Figure 12.16*). Central readings are taken successively on the underside of the cover slide and then the back surface of the lens. The difference between these readings gives the lens primary sag. From sag tables (*see* Appendix C, page 332) the sag *b*, corresponding to the back central optic radius of the lens under test at a diameter corresponding to the overall size of the lens, is found. The axial edge lift $e = b − s$ (*Figure 12.17*). This does not allow for edge rounding.

Method 2

The radiuscope is first focused on the flat uppermost surface of a holder or stem of known diameter such as that shown in *Figure 12.17*. The test lens is then placed on this, convex surface upwards, and the radiuscope is re-focused at the apex of the convex surface. The difference between these readings gives the sag *s* plus the lens thickness. From sag tables (*see* Appendix C) the sag *b* corresponding to the back central optic radius of the lens under test at a diameter equal to that of the stem is found. The axial 'edge' lift $e = b − s$. This gives the true axial edge lift at the known diameter of the stem.

Radial Edge Lift

As described by Newlove (1974) and Stone (1975), and shown in *Figure 12.18*, the radial edge lift also may be found by placing the lens concave surface down on a holder of known diameter. It can be seen from the right-angled triangle in *Figure 12.18*, that by Pythagoras' theorem:

$$(\text{Radial edge lift} + \text{BCOR})^2$$

$$= \left(\frac{\text{Stem diameter}}{2}\right)^2 + (\text{BCOR} − \text{sag})^2$$

If stem diameter = $2y$ and sag = s, then

$$\text{Radial edge lift} = \sqrt{y^2 + (\text{BCOR} − s)^2} − \text{BCOR}$$

s is found as described above, by focusing the radiuscope first on the upper flat surface of the

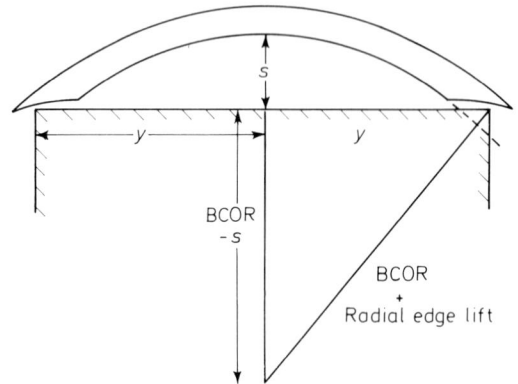

Figure 12.18–Determination of radial edge lift (after Newlove)

stem and then at the apex of the front surface of the lens, and subtracting the centre thickness of the lens from the measurement obtained.

Note: If the stem diameter is the same as the overall size of the lens, the sag value, *s*, obtained is that of the primary sag of the lens.

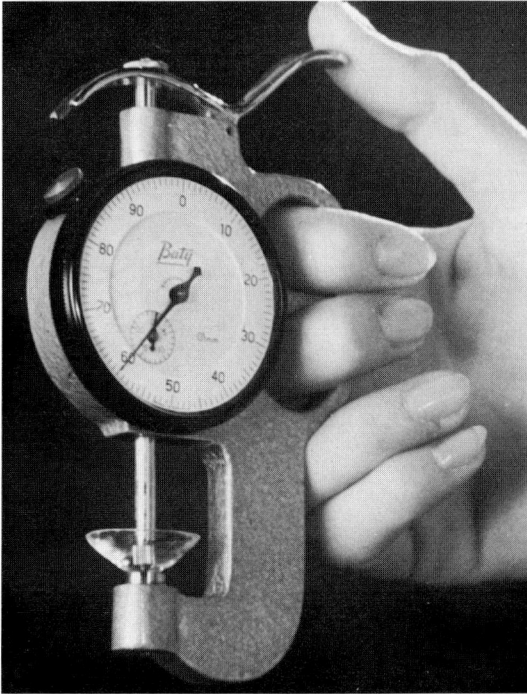

Figure 12.19–Measurement of the optic thickness of a scleral lens. Scale reading 0.60 mm

THICKNESS

The thickness of the centre and edge or any other part of a corneal lens, as well as the optic and haptic of a scleral lens, may be determined with a suitable thickness gauge. Thickness gauges usually incorporate a dial gauge calibrated to 0.01 mm (*Figure 12.19*).

Alternatively, a lens measure may be used; but this method is deprecated because the lens surface may be damaged by the points on the legs of the lens measure. One newer lens measure does, however, have spherical tips to the legs and would therefore be safer.

Another method is to use the radiuscope. Water is not used in the lens holder when the thickness of a lens is being determined. The target is focused on each lens surface in turn. The distance between the two foci multiplied by the refractive index of the material gives the lens thickness. Or a flat plate may be put on the radiuscope holder, on which surface the radiuscope is first focused and set at zero. The lens is then placed, convex side down, on the plate and the radiuscope focused at the centre of its back surface. This gives a direct reading of the lens centre thickness.

OPTIC – LENS PRESCRIPTION

The back vertex power of a contact lens may be measured using a focimeter. If the focimeter is mounted vertically, the lens can rest freely on the stop. A corneal lens, if held against the stop, may

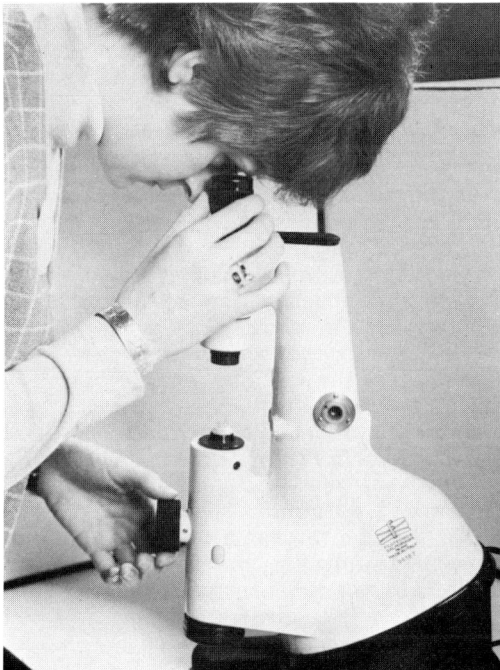

(a)

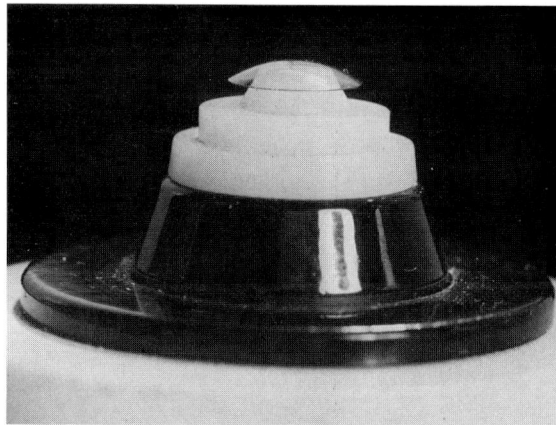

(b)

Figure 12.20–(a) Measurement of back vertex power on a focimeter. (b) Close-up of lens in place against stop. It can be seen that the back vertex of the lens is not in the plane of the stop

be distorted by the pressure of the fingers. Unless its construction permits angling to a vertical position, it is possible to arrange for a focimeter to be mounted vertically by means of a special stage (*Figure 12.20*). The focimeter is used in the normal way to determine the prescription. Care is needed in centring the lens to determine any prism.

One problem in determining the back vertex power of a contact lens is that the back surface of the lens may not be in the plane of the focimeter stop. This is because contact lenses have highly curved surfaces. With scleral lenses, the haptic portion may prevent the back surface of the lens

may then be determined by calculation or from tables (Appendix D, page 336) if the central optic thickness and back central optic radius are known.

SURFACE QUALITY AND POLISH, EDGE FORM, TINT

A binocular microscope (*Figure 12.22*), radiuscope, toposcope or measuring magnifier may be used to examine the surface of a contact lens. Alternatively, the lens is observed against a uniformly

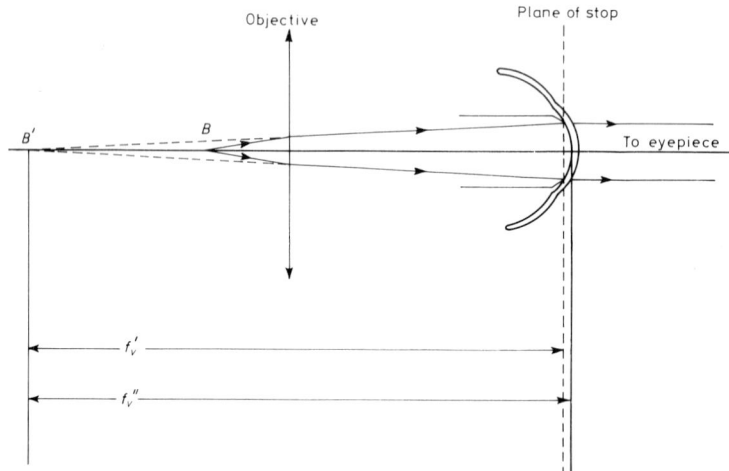

Figure 12.21–Error in measuring back vertex power. f'_v = back vertex focal length of lens under test as measured on the instrument; f''_v = true back vertex focal length; B = target; B' = image of target formed by objective

from lying in the correct plane. The back vertex power may therefore be recorded as being a greater positive or smaller negative value than it actually is. This is because the back vertex focal length of a lens is measured from the plane of the stop to the target position (*Figure 12.21*). Since the back surface of the lens is not in the plane of the stop the true back vertex focal length is actually greater. This error can be minimized either by using a smaller stop or removing the stop collar, if possible, so that the back surface of the lens is in approximately the correct position. (Rodenstock make a special attachment to their focimeter, for measuring corneal lenses. The stop may be screwed up or down depending on the BCOR of the lens which is indicated on a scale.)

Alternatively, instead of back vertex power, front vertex power may be measured by resting the front surface of the contact lens on an optical flat placed in the focimeter's stop. The former

illuminated background with or without magnification. The blending of the transition may be observed at the same time.

Any distortion of the optic or unwanted cylinder may be found using a crossline chart and the lateral and rotational tests, or by using a focimeter, radiuscope or toposcope.

The shape of the edge of a contact lens may be examined by observation with a binocular microscope with the lens mounted on a suitable rotating holder as shown in *Figure 12.22*. Casting the edge in dental stone or pressing the lens edge into Plasticine may be utilized and in each case the impression left on the material is examined under magnification with a binocular microscope, for example, on a slit lamp. The edge is cast by inserting the edge of the lens into a small pool of dental stone on top of a rubber band on a square of plastics material (*Figure 12.23*). The lens is placed at right-angles to the rubber band. When the dental

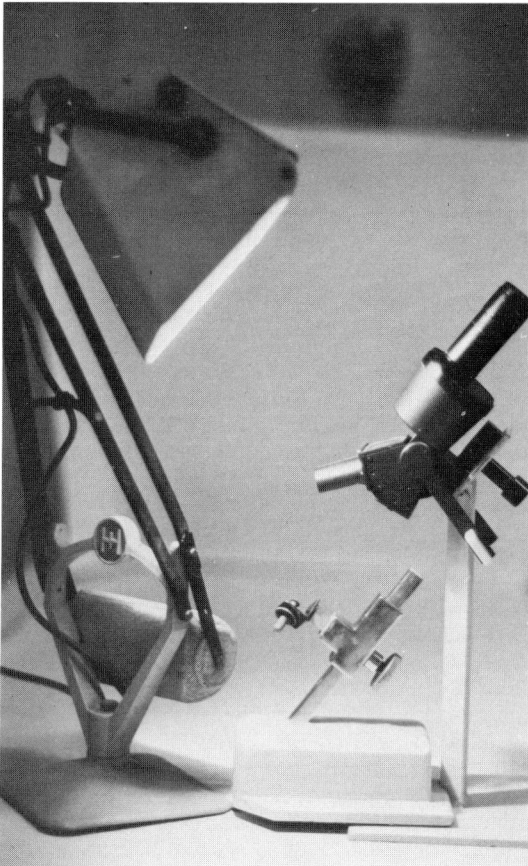

(a)

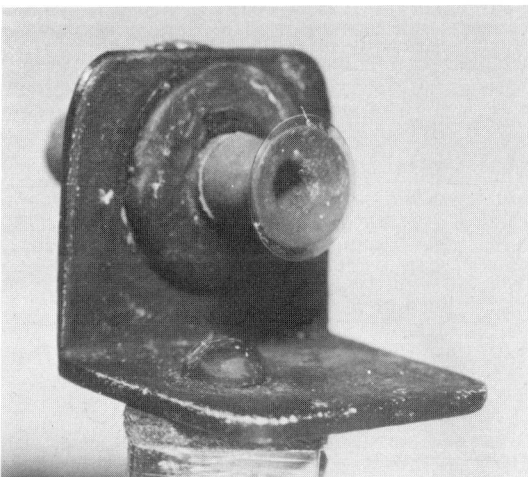

(b)

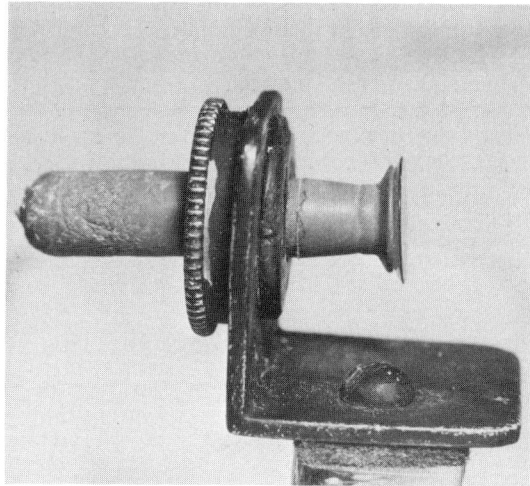

(c)

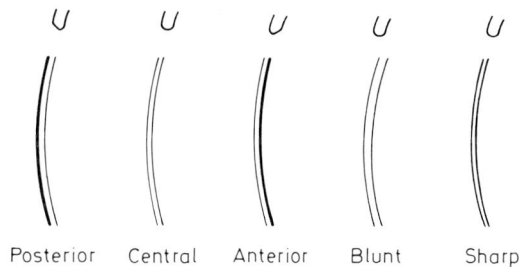

| Posterior | Central | Anterior | Blunt | Sharp |

(d)

Figure 12.22–(a) Binocular microscope used to inspect lens surfaces and edges. An external light source is used. The lens is held on the suction holder which can be rotated about its own axis and about the plane of the lens, the rotating holder being movable along its angled support to permit accurate focusing. Thus, the entire edge can be quickly scrutinized. (b) Close-up of lens surface which is seen to be dirty. (c) Close-up of lens edge as seen through the microscope. The width of the central bright reflection can be used to judge the edge shape as shown in (d). (d) The position and width of the bright edge reflection (shown as the gap between the lines) from several corneal lens edges whose profiles are shown above, and with the position of the peak of the edge given below. (The rotating lens holder was built by Ronald B. Rabbetts ((Rabbetts, 1978)) for the London Refraction Hospital, and (d) is reproduced by kind permission)

stone is set, the lens is removed and the dental stone is pulled off the rubber band. The dental stone is scored on the back by the rubber band so that it is easy to break in half and the edge cast can be examined in cross-section.

Plasticine provides a quick and easy means to examine the edge, but the cast tends to loose shape. If the lens is left in the Plasticine, the edge shape can be seen in profile against the Plasticine when examined with the binocular microscope.

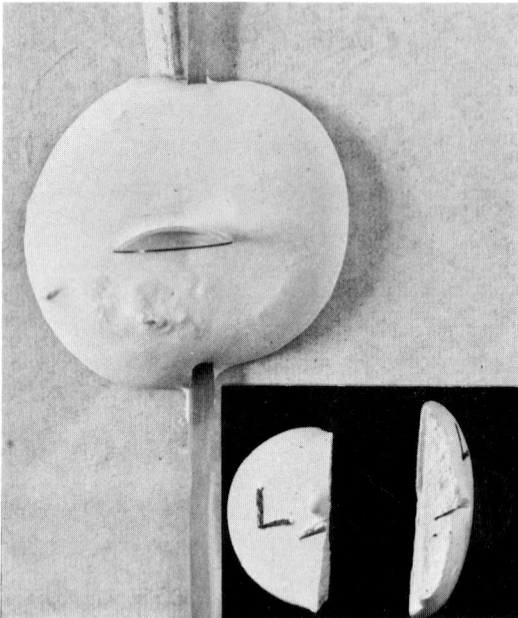

(a)

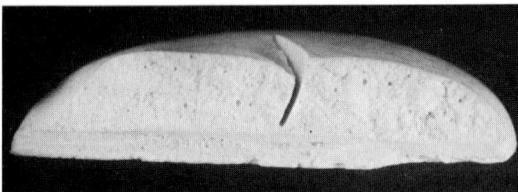

(b)

Figure 12.23—(a) Lens edge being cast in dental stone: Inset – cast broken in half. (b) Magnified view of section through cast. A square-shaped edge is seen

The edge should be examined at a number of different points by one of the above methods.

The entire circumference of the lens edge should also be rotated before a binocular microscope to check for any localized distortions (*see Figure 12.22*).

The colour of a contact lens may be observed against a white background.

STRESS

Stress may be checked by placing the lens between crossed polarized filters. If stress is present a strain pattern is seen, otherwise the appearance is devoid of any pattern.

Surface and undersurface stresses can lead to subsequent flaking of the surface layers, in final lens working, polishing or in later use (Cordrey, 1973).

TORIC LENSES

When a radiuscope is used to check toroidal surfaces, the target image formed on the lens surface appears uniformly focused as seen through the microscope, but as a toroidal surface has two centres of curvature corresponding to the two principal meridians there is not a uniformly focused target image formed at the two centre of curvature positions. Instead, only one of the target lines will appear sharply focused and the lens must be rotated so that each principal meridian coincides with one of the target lines. Then the centre of curvature of each principal meridian is located by focusing the two perpendicular target lines in turn. If the target consists of a ring of dots there is no need to rotate the lens to locate the principal meridians.

If a keratometer is used, the procedure is the same as for carrying out keratometry on a toroidal cornea, the usual small allowances being made for the measurement of a concave surface instead of a convex one.

The back central optic diameter of a corneal lens may be oval, depending on the method of manufacture, so maximum amd minimum values should be found.

For checking the power of toric lenses, *see* Chapter 18, Volume 2.

BIFOCAL LENSES

The addition may be checked using a focimeter. For solid bifocals, where the addition is on the back surface, its value in air is 3.18 times that on the eye (*see* Chapter 4, page 123). The diameter and position of the near vision zone may be checked using a measuring magnifier.

ACKNOWLEDGEMENTS

The author is indebted to Mr C. Wilson, formerly of the Department of Optometry and Visual Science, The City University, London, and now at Bath University, for preparing photographs for all the figures; and to Mr G. Nissel for the loan of the toposcope for photography.

Addendum I

Dimensional Tolerances For Hard Contact Lenses

All dimensions are in millimetres

	Corneal	Scleral	Method of test
Back central optic radius	±0.02	±0.05	(a) Keratometer (calibrated for concave surfaces) (b) Radiuscope (c) Interferometry techniques
Back central optic diameter	±0.20	±0.20	10 × measuring magnifier
Back haptic radius (of preformed lenses)	–	±0.10	(a) Keratometer (calibrated for concave surfaces) (b) Radiuscope (c) Interferometry techniques
Basic or primary optic diameter	–	±0.10	Sagitta method
Peripheral optic radius	±0.10	±0.10	(a) Keratometer (calibrated for concave surfaces) (b) Radiuscope (c) Interferometry techniques
Back peripheral optic diameter	±0.20	±0.20 (for preformed lenses)	10 × measuring magnifier
Axial edge lift	±0.02	for all lenses	(a) Radiuscope (b) Sagitta method*
Radial edge lift	±0.02	for all lenses	(a) Radiuscope (b) Sagitta method*
Overall size	±0.10	±0.25	(a) V-channel gauge (b) 10 × measuring magnifier (c) Projection magnifier with scale
Front central optic diameter	±0.20	±0.20	10 × measuring magnifier
Bifocal segment height	±0.10	–	10 × measuring magnifier
Centre thickness	±0.02	±0.03	(a) Measuring dial gauge† (b) Radiuscope (c) Projection magnifier with scale
Edge thickness	±0.02	–	Hard: Measuring dial gauge†
Vertex clearance (from cast)	–	±0.02	Measuring dial gauge†
Fenestration Truncation Displacement Haptic thickness	10% allowance on specification		

* Sagitta method – see Stone, Janet (1975). 'Corneal lenses with constant axial edge lift.' *Ophthal. Optician* 15, 818–824
† Measuring dial gauge calibrated in units of 0.01 mm in accordance with BS 2795: Part 1

(Reproduced by kind permission of the British Standards Institution from *BS 5562:1978 Specification for Contact Lenses*)

Addendum II

Optical Tolerances for Hard Contact Lenses

	Corneal	*Scleral*	*Method of test*
Back vertex power (in the weaker meridian):			
+10.00 D to −10.00 D	±0.12 D	±0.12 D	Focimeter with an aperture of not
Over ±10.00 D	±0.25 D	±0.25 D	less than 4 mm
Prism (measured at geometrical centre of optic portion)	±0.50 △	±0.50 △	Focimeter with an aperture of not less than 4 mm
Optical centration (maximum error)	0.50 mm	0.50 mm	Focimeter with an aperture of not less than 4 mm
Cylinder power:			
Up to 2.00 D	±0.25 D	±0.25 D	Focimeter with an aperture of not
2.00 D to 4.00 D	±0.37 D	±0.37 D	less than 4 mm
Over 4.00 D	±0.50 D	±0.50 D	
Cylinder axis	±5°	±5°	For a prism ballast front surface toric lens, the resultant cylinder axis is measured with the prism base down, that is, the base-apex line at 90°. For a bitoric lens the resultant cylinder axis is measured with respect to the orientation of the flattest meridian of the back toroidal surface

(Reproduced by kind permission of the British Standards Institution from *BS 5562:1978 Specification for Contact Lenses*)

REFERENCES

Bennett, A. G. (1966). 'The calibration of keratometers.' *Optician* **151**, 317–322

Brungardt, T. F. (1962). 'A fast, accurate and practical measurement of the secondary curve radius.' *J. Am. optom. Ass.* **34**, 131–134

Cordrey, P. (1973). 'Technical and economic effects of contact lens production methods.' *Ophthal. Optician* **13**, 230–236

Dickins, R. (1966a). 'An investigation into the accuracy of the radius checking device.' *Optician* **151**, 265–269

Dickins, R. (1966b). 'Further results using the radius checking device.' *Optician* **152**, 135–137

Dickins, R. (1968). 'Tables for use with the radius checking device.' *Optician* **155**, 292–294

Dickins, R. and Fletcher, R. J. (1964). 'Contact lens measurement, a comparison of several devices.' *Br. J. physiol. Optics.* **21**, 107–115

Drysdale, C. V. (1900). 'On a simple direct method of measuring the curvature of small lenses.' *Trans. opt. Soc.* **2**, 1–12

Garner, L. (1970). Personal communication. 'The design and measurement of the back surface of contact lenses.' Ph.D. Thesis, The City University, London

Janoff, L. E. (1977). 'A pilot study of the comparison of validity and reliability between the radiuscope and toposcope.' *Int. Contact Lens Clinic,* **4**(2), 68–73

Lehmann, S. (1967). 'Corneal areas utilised in keratometry.' *Optician* **154**, 261–264

Linnell Fearn, W. W. (1970). 'The use of the focimeter for measuring the central radii of contact lenses.' *Contact Lens* **2**(6), 20–22

Newlove, D. B. (1974). 'Development of a new hard lens material.' *Optician* **169**(4368), 16–23

Phillips, A. J. (1969). 'Alterations in curvature of the finished corneal lens.' *Ophthal. Optician* **9**, 980–982, 985, 986, 1043–1046, 1051–1054, 1100–1104, 1109, 1110

Rabbetts, R. B. (1978). 'Corneal lens edge checking device.' *Ophthal. Optician* **18**, 202

Sarver, M. D. and Kerr, K. (1964). 'A radius of curvature measuring device for contact lenses.' *Am. J. Optom.* **41**, 481–489

Smith, I. C. P. (1966). 'Pneumatic gauging applied to contact lenses.' *Br. J. physiol. Optics.* **23**, 161–167

Stone, J. (1964). 'Checking preformed contact lenses.' *Br. J. physiol. Optics,* **21**, 264–286

Stone, J. (1975). 'Corneal lenses with constant axial edge lift.' *Ophthal. Optician,* **15**, 818–824

Storey, S. (1969). 'An assessment of the O.M.I. Topo-scope.' Student project, The City University, London

Tannehill, J. C. and Sampson, W. G. (1966). 'Extended use of the radiuscope in contact lens inspection.' *Am. J. Ophthal.* **62**, 538–540

BIBLIOGRAPHY

Anon (1963). 'What's new – B.A.O. Radiuscope.' *Ophthal. Optician* **3**, 76

Bailey, N. J. (1959). 'The examination and verification of a contact lens.' *J. Am. optom. Ass.* **30**, 557–560

Bennett, A. G. (1958). 'On accuracy in contact lens manufacture.' *Optician* **135**, 357–358

Bennett, A. G. (1966). *Optics of Contact Lenses,* 4th edn. London: Association of Dispensing Opticians

Blackstone, D. (1961). 'A new instrument.' *Ophthal. Optician* **1**, 614–615

Blackstone, M. (1966). 'The toposcope examined.' *Optician* **152**, 38–39

Charman, W. N. (1972). 'Diffraction and the precision of measurement of corneal and other small radii.' *Am. J. Optom.* **49**, 672–680

Emsley, H. H. (1963). 'The keratometer – measurement of concave surfaces.' *Optician* **146**, 161–168

Fletcher, R. J. and Nisted, M. (1961). 'The accuracy of corneal contact lenses.' *Ophthal. Optician* **1**, 217–219

Forst, G. (1971). 'Optical homogeneity and contour of contact lenses and tests.' *Ophthal. Optician* **11**, 739–744

Freeman, M. H. (1965). 'The measurement of contact lens curvature.' *Am. J. Optom.* **42**, 693–701

Goldberg, J. B. (1961). 'Lens evaluation inadequacies.' *Contacto* **5**, 357–358

Haynes, P. R. (1960). 'Quality control and inspection of contact lenses.' In *Encyclopaedia of Contact Lens Practice,* **1**, Ch. 23, 8–63. South Bend, Indiana: International Optics

Laycock, D. E. (1957). 'A microlens measuring aid.' *Am. J. Optom.* **34**, 538–539

Mandell, R. B. (1965). *Contact Lens Practice: Basic and Advanced.* Springfield, Illinois: Thomas

Nissel, G. (1962). 'Measuring instruments used in the manufacture and checking of contact lenses.' *Optician* **144**, 58–64

Sarver, M. D. (1963). 'Verification of contact lens power.' *J. Am. optom. Ass.* **34**, 1304–1306

Appendices

APPENDIX A

SPECTACLE AND OCULAR REFRACTION, OR EFFECTIVE POWER OF SPECTACLE LENSES IN AIR AT VARIOUS VERTEX DISTANCES: POSITIVE LENSES

(Body of Table shows effective power at stated vertex distance)

Ocular refraction in dioptres for vertex distances in mm of:

Spectacle refraction or spectacle lens power (BVP) in dioptres	6	7	8	9	10	11	12	13	14	15	16	17	18	19	20
+0.25	0.25	0.25	0.25	0.25	0.25	0.25	0.25	0.25	0.25	0.25	0.25	0.25	0.25	0.25	0.25
.50	0.50	0.50	0.50	0.50	0.50	0.50	0.50	0.50	0.50	0.50	0.50	0.50	0.50	0.50	0.51
.75	0.75	0.75	0.75	0.76	0.76	0.76	0.76	0.76	0.76	0.76	0.76	0.76	0.76	0.76	0.76
+1.00	1.01	1.01	1.01	1.01	1.01	1.01	1.01	1.01	1.01	1.02	1.02	1.02	1.01	1.02	1.02
.25	1.26	1.26	1.26	1.26	1.27	1.27	1.27	1.27	1.27	1.27	1.28	1.28	1.28	1.28	1.28
.50	1.51	1.52	1.52	1.52	1.52	1.52	1.53	1.53	1.53	1.53	1.54	1.54	1.54	1.54	1.55
.75	1.77	1.77	1.78	1.78	1.78	1.79	1.79	1.79	1.80	1.80	1.80	1.81	1.81	1.81	1.81
+2.00	2.02	2.03	2.03	2.04	2.04	2.04	2.05	2.05	2.06	2.06	2.07	2.07	2.07	2.08	2.08
.25	2.28	2.29	2.29	2.30	2.30	2.31	2.31	2.32	2.33	2.33	2.34	2.34	2.35	2.35	2.36
.50	2.54	2.54	2.55	2.56	2.56	2.57	2.58	2.58	2.59	2.60	2.60	2.61	2.62	2.62	2.63
.75	2.79	2.80	2.81	2.82	2.82	2.83	2.84	2.85	2.86	2.87	2.87	2.88	2.89	2.90	2.91
+3.00	3.06	3.06	3.07	3.08	3.09	3.10	3.11	3.12	3.13	3.14	3.15	3.16	3.17	3.18	3.19
.25	3.31	3.33	3.34	3.35	3.36	3.37	3.38	3.39	3.40	3.42	3.43	3.44	3.45	3.46	3.48
.50	3.58	3.59	3.60	3.61	3.63	3.64	3.65	3.67	3.68	3.69	3.71	3.72	3.74	3.75	3.76
.75	3.84	3.85	3.87	3.88	3.90	3.91	3.93	3.94	3.96	3.97	3.99	4.00	4.02	4.04	4.05
+4.00	4.10	4.12	4.13	4.15	4.17	4.18	4.20	4.22	4.24	4.26	4.27	4.29	4.31	4.33	4.35
.25	4.36	4.38	4.40	4.42	4.44	4.46	4.48	4.50	4.52	4.54	4.56	4.58	4.60	4.62	4.64
.50	4.63	4.65	4.67	4.69	4.71	4.73	4.76	4.78	4.80	4.83	4.85	4.87	4.90	4.92	4.95
.75	4.89	4.91	4.94	4.96	4.99	5.01	5.04	5.06	5.09	5.12	5.14	5.17	5.19	5.22	5.25
+5.00	5.15	5.18	5.21	5.24	5.26	5.29	5.32	5.35	5.38	5.41	5.43	5.46	5.49	5.52	5.56
.25	5.42	5.45	5.48	5.51	5.54	5.57	5.60	5.63	5.67	5.70	5.73	5.76	5.80	5.83	5.87
.50	5.69	5.72	5.75	5.79	5.82	5.85	5.89	5.92	5.96	6.00	6.03	6.07	6.11	6.14	6.18
.75	5.96	5.99	6.03	6.06	6.10	6.14	6.18	6.22	6.25	6.29	6.33	6.37	6.41	6.46	6.50
+6.00	6.22	6.26	6.30	6.34	6.38	6.42	6.46	6.51	6.55	6.59	6.64	6.68	6.72	6.77	6.82
.25	6.49	6.54	6.58	6.62	6.67	6.71	6.76	6.80	6.85	6.90	6.94	6.99	7.04	7.09	7.14
.50	6.77	6.81	6.86	6.91	6.95	7.00	7.05	7.10	7.15	7.20	7.26	7.31	7.36	7.42	7.47
.75	7.04	7.09	7.14	7.19	7.24	7.29	7.35	7.40	7.46	7.51	7.57	7.63	7.69	7.75	7.82
+7.00	7.30	7.36	7.41	7.47	7.52	7.58	7.64	7.70	7.76	7.82	7.88	7.94	8.01	8.07	8.14
.25	7.58	7.64	7.70	7.76	7.82	7.88	7.94	8.01	8.07	8.14	8.20	8.27	8.34	8.41	8.48
.50	7.86	7.92	7.98	8.05	8.11	8.18	8.24	8.31	8.38	8.45	8.53	8.60	8.67	8.75	8.83
.75	8.13	8.20	8.26	8.33	8.40	8.47	8.55	8.62	8.70	8.77	8.85	8.93	9.01	9.09	9.17

	6	7	8	9	10	11	12	13	14	15	16	17	18	19	20
+8.00	8.40	8.47	8.55	8.62	8.70	8.77	8.85	8.93	9.01	9.09	9.17	9.26	9.35	9.43	9.52
.25	8.68	8.76	8.83	8.91	8.99	9.07	9.16	9.24	9.33	9.42	9.51	9.60	9.69	9.78	9.88
.50	8.96	9.04	9.12	9.21	9.29	9.38	9.47	9.56	9.65	9.75	9.84	9.94	10.04	10.14	10.25
.75	9.23	9.32	9.41	9.50	9.59	9.68	9.78	9.87	9.97	10.07	10.17	10.28	10.38	10.49	10.60
+9.00	9.51	9.61	9.70	9.79	9.89	9.98	10.09	10.19	10.30	10.41	10.52	10.63	10.74	10.86	10.98
.25	9.79	9.89	9.99	10.09	10.19	10.30	10.41	10.52	10.63	10.74	10.86	10.98	11.10	11.22	11.35
.50	10.07	10.17	10.28	10.38	10.49	10.60	10.72	10.83	10.95	11.07	11.20	11.33	11.45	11.59	11.72
.75	10.35	10.46	10.57	10.68	10.80	10.92	11.04	11.16	11.29	11.42	11.55	11.68	11.82	11.96	12.11
+10.00	10.64	10.75	10.87	10.99	11.11	11.24	11.36	11.49	11.63	11.76	11.90	12.05	12.20	12.35	12.50
.25	10.92	11.04	11.17	11.29	11.42	11.55	11.69	11.83	11.97	12.11	12.26	12.41	12.57	12.73	12.89
.50	11.21	11.33	11.46	11.60	11.73	11.87	12.01	12.16	12.31	12.46	12.62	12.78	12.95	13.12	13.29
.75	11.49	11.63	11.76	11.90	12.05	12.19	12.34	12.50	12.66	12.82	12.98	13.15	13.33	13.51	13.69
+11.00	11.78	11.92	12.06	12.21	12.36	12.51	12.67	12.84	13.00	13.17	13.35	13.53	13.72	13.91	14.10
.25	12.06	12.21	12.36	12.52	12.68	12.84	13.01	13.18	13.35	13.53	13.72	13.91	14.11	14.31	14.52
.50	12.35	12.51	12.66	12.83	12.99	13.16	13.34	13.52	13.71	13.90	14.09	14.29	14.50	14.71	14.93
.75	12.64	12.80	12.97	13.14	13.31	13.49	13.68	13.87	14.06	14.26	14.47	14.68	14.90	15.13	15.36
+12.00	12.93	13.10	13.27	13.45	13.64	13.83	14.02	14.22	14.42	14.63	14.85	15.08	15.31	15.54	15.79
.25	13.22	13.40	13.58	13.77	13.96	14.16	14.36	14.57	14.79	15.01	15.24	15.47	15.72	15.97	16.23
.50	13.51	13.70	13.89	14.08	14.29	14.49	14.71	14.93	15.15	15.38	15.62	15.87	16.13	16.39	16.67
.75	13.81	14.00	14.20	14.40	14.61	14.83	15.05	15.28	15.52	15.77	16.02	16.28	16.55	16.83	17.11
+13.00	14.10	14.30	14.51	14.72	14.94	15.17	15.40	15.64	15.89	16.15	16.41	16.69	16.97	17.27	17.57
.25	14.39	14.60	14.82	15.04	15.27	15.51	15.76	16.01	16.27	16.54	16.82	17.10	17.40	17.71	18.03
.50	14.69	14.91	15.14	15.37	15.61	15.86	16.11	16.37	16.65	16.93	17.22	17.52	17.83	18.16	18.49
.75	14.99	15.21	15.45	15.69	15.94	16.20	16.47	16.74	17.03	17.32	17.63	17.94	18.27	18.61	18.96
+14.00	15.28	15.52	15.77	16.02	16.28	16.55	16.83	17.11	17.41	17.72	18.04	18.37	18.72	19.07	19.44
.25	15.58	15.83	16.08	16.35	16.62	16.90	17.19	17.49	17.80	18.12	18.46	18.80	19.16	19.54	19.93
.50	15.88	16.14	16.40	16.68	16.96	17.25	17.55	17.87	18.19	18.53	18.88	19.24	19.62	20.01	20.42
.75	16.18	16.45	16.72	17.01	17.30	17.61	17.92	18.25	18.59	18.94	19.31	19.69	20.08	20.49	20.92
+15.00	16.48	16.76	17.04	17.34	17.65	17.96	18.29	18.63	18.99	19.35	19.74	20.13	20.55	20.98	21.43
.25	16.79	17.07	17.37	17.68	18.00	18.33	18.67	19.02	19.39	19.77	20.17	20.59	21.02	21.47	21.94
.50	17.09	17.39	17.69	18.01	18.34	18.68	19.04	19.41	19.79	20.19	20.61	21.04	21.50	21.97	22.46
.75	17.39	17.70	18.02	18.35	18.70	19.05	19.42	19.81	20.21	20.62	21.06	21.51	21.98	22.48	22.99
+16.00	17.70	18.02	18.35	18.69	19.05	19.42	19.80	20.20	20.62	21.05	21.51	21.98	22.47	22.99	23.53
.25	18.01	18.34	18.68	19.03	19.40	19.79	20.19	20.60	21.04	21.49	21.96	22.45	22.97	23.51	24.07
.50	18.31	18.65	19.01	19.38	19.76	20.16	20.57	21.01	21.46	21.93	22.42	22.93	23.47	24.03	24.63
.75	18.62	18.97	19.34	19.72	20.12	20.53	20.96	21.41	21.88	22.37	22.88	23.42	23.98	24.57	25.19
+17.00	18.93	19.30	19.68	20.07	20.48	20.91	21.36	21.82	22.31	22.82	22.35	23.91	24.50	25.11	25.76
.25	19.24	19.62	20.01	20.42	20.85	21.29	21.75	22.24	22.74	23.27	23.83	24.41	25.02	25.66	26.34
.50	19.55	19.94	20.35	20.77	21.21	21.67	22.15	22.65	23.18	23.73	24.31	24.91	25.55	26.22	26.92
.75	19.87	20.27	20.69	21.12	21.58	22.06	22.55	23.07	23.62	24.19	24.79	25.42	26.08	26.78	27.52
+18.00	20.18	20.59	21.03	21.48	21.95	22.44	22.96	23.50	24.06	24.66	25.28	25.94	26.63	27.36	28.12
.25	20.49	20.92	21.37	21.84	22.32	22.83	23.37	23.93	24.51	25.13	25.78	26.46	27.18	27.94	28.74
.50	20.81	21.25	21.71	22.20	22.70	23.23	23.78	24.36	24.97	25.61	26.28	26.99	27.74	28.53	29.37
.75	21.13	21.58	22.06	22.56	23.08	23.62	24.19	24.79	25.42	26.09	26.79	27.52	28.30	29.13	30.00
+19.00	21.44	21.91	22.41	22.92	23.46	24.02	24.61	25.23	25.89	26.57	27.30	28.06	28.88	29.73	30.65
.25	21.76	22.25	22.75	23.28	23.84	24.42	25.03	25.68	26.35	27.07	27.82	28.61	29.46	30.35	31.30
.50	22.08	22.58	23.10	23.65	24.22	24.82	25.46	26.12	26.82	27.56	28.34	29.17	30.05	30.98	31.97
.75	22.40	22.92	23.46	24.02	24.61	25.23	25.88	26.57	27.30	28.06	28.87	29.73	30.64	31.61	32.64
+20.00	22.73	23.26	23.81	24.39	25.00	25.64	26.32	27.03	27.78	28.57	29.41	30.30	31.25	32.26	33.33

SPECTACLE AND OCULAR REFRACTION, OR EFFECTIVE POWER OF SPECTACLE LENSES IN AIR AT VARIOUS VERTEX DISTANCES: NEGATIVE LENSES

(Body of Table shows effective power at stated vertex distance)

Ocular refraction in dioptres for vertex distances in mm of:

Spectacle refraction or spectacle lens power (BVP) in dioptres	6	7	8	9	10	11	12	13	14	15	16	17	18	19	20
−0.25	0.25	0.25	0.25	0.25	0.25	0.25	0.25	0.25	0.25	0.25	0.25	0.25	0.25	0.25	0.25
−0.50	0.50	0.50	0.50	0.50	0.50	0.50	0.50	0.50	0.50	0.50	0.50	0.50	0.50	0.50	0.50
0.75	0.75	0.75	0.75	0.75	0.74	0.74	0.74	0.74	0.74	0.74	0.74	0.74	0.74	0.74	0.74
−1.00	0.99	0.99	0.99	0.99	0.99	0.99	0.99	0.99	0.99	0.99	0.98	0.98	0.98	0.98	0.98
.25	1.24	1.24	1.24	1.24	1.23	1.23	1.23	1.23	1.23	1.23	1.23	1.22	1.22	1.22	1.22
.50	1.49	1.48	1.48	1.48	1.48	1.48	1.47	1.47	1.47	1.47	1.46	1.46	1.46	1.46	1.46
.75	1.73	1.73	1.73	1.72	1.72	1.72	1.71	1.71	1.71	1.71	1.70	1.70	1.70	1.69	1.69
−2.00	1.98	1.97	1.97	1.96	1.96	1.96	1.95	1.95	1.95	1.94	1.94	1.93	1.93	1.93	1.92
.25	2.22	2.22	2.21	2.21	2.20	2.20	2.19	2.19	2.18	2.18	2.17	2.17	2.16	2.16	2.15
.50	2.46	2.46	2.45	2.44	2.44	2.43	2.43	2.42	2.42	2.41	2.40	2.40	2.39	2.39	2.38
.75	2.71	2.70	2.69	2.68	2.68	2.67	2.66	2.66	2.65	2.64	2.63	2.63	2.62	2.61	2.61
−3.00	2.95	2.94	2.93	2.92	2.91	2.90	2.90	2.89	2.88	2.87	2.86	2.85	2.85	2.84	2.83
.25	3.19	3.18	3.17	3.16	3.15	3.14	3.13	3.12	3.11	3.10	3.09	3.08	3.07	3.06	3.05
.50	3.43	3.42	3.40	3.39	3.38	3.37	3.36	3.35	3.34	3.33	3.31	3.30	3.29	3.28	3.27
.75	3.67	3.65	3.64	3.63	3.61	3.60	3.59	3.58	3.56	3.55	3.54	3.52	3.51	3.50	3.49
−4.00	3.91	3.89	3.88	3.86	3.85	3.83	3.82	3.80	3.79	3.77	3.76	3.75	3.73	3.72	3.70
.25	4.14	4.13	4.11	4.09	4.08	4.06	4.04	4.03	4.01	4.00	3.98	3.96	3.95	3.93	3.92
.50	4.38	4.36	4.34	4.33	4.31	4.29	4.27	4.25	4.23	4.22	4.20	4.18	4.16	4.15	4.13
.75	4.62	4.60	4.58	4.56	4.54	4.51	4.49	4.47	4.45	4.43	4.42	4.40	4.38	4.36	4.34
−5.00	4.85	4.83	4.81	4.78	4.76	4.74	4.72	4.69	4.67	4.65	4.63	4.61	4.59	4.57	4.55
.25	5.09	5.06	5.04	5.01	4.99	4.96	4.94	4.91	4.89	4.87	4.84	4.82	4.80	4.77	4.75
.50	5.32	5.30	5.27	5.24	5.21	5.19	5.16	5.13	5.11	5.08	5.06	5.03	5.01	4.98	4.96
.75	5.56	5.53	5.50	5.47	5.44	5.41	5.38	5.35	5.32	5.29	5.27	5.24	5.21	5.18	5.16
−6.00	5.79	5.76	5.72	5.69	5.66	5.63	5.60	5.56	5.53	5.50	5.47	5.44	5.41	5.39	5.36
.25	6.02	5.99	5.95	5.92	5.88	5.85	5.81	5.78	5.75	5.71	5.68	5.65	5.62	5.59	5.56
.50	6.26	6.22	6.18	6.14	6.11	6.07	6.03	6.00	5.96	5.92	5.89	5.85	5.82	5.79	5.75
.75	6.49	6.45	6.41	6.37	6.33	6.29	6.25	6.21	6.17	6.13	6.09	6.06	6.02	5.98	5.95
−7.00	6.72	6.67	6.63	6.58	6.54	6.50	6.46	6.41	6.37	6.33	6.29	6.25	6.22	6.18	6.14
.25	6.94	6.90	6.85	6.81	6.76	6.72	6.67	6.63	6.58	6.54	6.50	6.46	6.41	6.37	6.33
.50	7.18	7.13	7.08	7.03	6.98	6.93	6.88	6.84	6.79	6.74	6.70	6.65	6.61	6.57	6.52
.75	7.41	7.35	7.30	7.25	7.19	7.14	7.09	7.04	6.99	6.94	6.90	6.85	6.80	6.76	6.71
−8.00	7.63	7.58	7.52	7.46	7.41	7.35	7.30	7.25	7.19	7.14	7.09	7.04	6.99	6.94	6.90
.25	7.86	7.80	7.74	7.68	7.62	7.56	7.51	7.45	7.40	7.34	7.29	7.24	7.18	7.13	7.08

	6	7	8	9	10	11	12	13	14	15	16	17	18	19	20
.50	8.09	8.03	7.96	7.90	7.84	7.78	7.72	7.66	7.60	7.54	7.49	7.43	7.37	7.32	7.27
.75	8.31	8.24	8.18	8.11	8.05	7.98	**7.92**	7.86	7.79	7.73	7.67	7.62	7.56	7.50	7.45
−9.00	8.54	8.47	8.40	8.33	8.26	8.19	8.12	8.06	7.99	7.93	7.87	7.81	7.75	7.69	7.63
.25	8.76	8.69	8.61	8.54	8.47	8.40	8.33	8.26	8.19	8.12	8.06	7.99	7.93	7.87	7.81
.50	8.98	8.90	8.83	8.75	8.67	8.60	8.53	8.45	8.38	8.31	8.24	8.18	8.11	8.05	7.98
.75	9.21	9.12	9.04	8.96	8.88	8.80	8.73	8.65	8.58	8.50	8.43	8.36	8.29	8.22	8.16
−10.00	9.43	9.35+	9.26	9.17	9.09	9.01	8.93	8.85	8.77	8.70	8.62	8.55	8.47	8.40	8.33
.25	9.65+	9.56	9.47	9.38	9.29	9.21	9.12	9.04	8.96	8.88	8.80	8.73	8.65+	8.58	8.50
.50	9.88	9.78	9.69	9.59	9.50	9.41	9.32	9.24	9.15+	9.07	8.99	8.91	8.83	8.75+	8.68
.75	10.10	10.00	9.90	9.80	9.71	9.61	9.52	9.43	9.34	9.26	9.17	9.09	9.01	8.93	**8.85**
−11.00	10.32	10.21	10.11	10.01	9.91	9.81	9.72	9.62	9.53	9.44	9.35+	9.27	9.18	9.10	9.02
.25	10.54	10.43	10.32	10.22	10.11	10.01	9.91	9.81	9.72	9.63	9.53	9.44	9.36	9.27	9.18
.50	10.76	10.64	10.53	10.42	10.31	10.21	10.11	10.00	9.90	9.81	9.71	9.62	9.53	9.44	9.35
.75	10.98	10.86	10.74	10.63	10.51	10.40	10.30	10.19	10.09	9.99	9.89	9.79	9.70	9.61	9.51
−12.00	11.19	11.07	10.95−	10.83	10.71	10.60	10.49	10.38	10.27	10.17	10.07	9.97	9.87	9.77	9.68
.25	11.41	11.28	11.16	11.03	10.91	10.80	10.68	10.57	10.46	10.35	10.24	10.14	10.04	9.94	9.84
.50	11.63	11.49	11.36	11.24	11.11	10.99	10.87	10.75+	10.64	10.53	10.42	10.31	10.20	10.10	10.00
.75	11.84	11.71	11.57	11.44	11.31	11.18	11.06	10.94	10.82	10.70	10.59	10.48	10.37	10.26	10.16
−13.00	12.06	11.92	11.78	11.64	11.50	11.37	11.25	11.12	11.00	10.88	10.76	10.65	10.54	10.43	10.32
.25	12.27	12.13	11.98	11.84	11.70	11.56	11.43	11.30	11.18	11.05+	10.93	10.81	10.70	10.59	10.47
.50	12.49	12.34	12.18	12.04	11.89	11.76	11.62	11.49	11.35+	11.23	11.10	10.98	10.86	10.74	10.63
.75	12.70	12.54	12.39	12.24	12.09	11.94	11.80	11.66	11.53	11.40	11.27	11.14	11.02	10.90	10.78
−14.00	12.91	12.75+	12.59	12.43	12.28	12.13	11.99	11.84	11.71	11.57	11.44	11.31	11.18	11.06	10.94
.25	13.13	12.96	12.79	12.63	12.47	12.32	12.17	12.02	11.88	11.74	11.60	11.47	11.34	11.21	11.09
.50	13.34	13.16	12.99	12.83	12.66	12.50	12.35+	12.20	12.05+	11.91	11.77	11.63	11.50	11.37	11.24
.75	13.55+	13.37	13.19	13.02	12.85+	12.69	12.53	12.38	12.22	12.08	11.93	11.79	11.66	11.52	11.39
−15.00	13.76	13.57	13.39	13.22	13.04	12.87	12.71	12.55+	12.40	12.24	12.10	11.95+	11.81	11.67	11.54
.25	13.97	13.78	13.59	13.41	13.23	13.06	12.89	12.73	12.57	12.41	12.26	12.11	11.97	11.82	11.69
.50	14.18	13.98	13.79	13.60	13.42	13.24	13.07	12.90	12.74	12.58	12.42	12.27	12.12	11.97	11.83
.75	14.39	14.19	13.99	13.80	13.61	13.42	13.25	13.07	12.90	12.74	12.58	12.42	12.27	12.12	11.98
−16.00	14.60	14.39	14.18	13.99	13.79	13.61	13.42	13.25	13.07	12.90	12.74	12.58	12.42	12.27	12.12
.25	14.81	14.59	14.38	14.18	13.98	13.79	13.60	13.42	13.24	13.07	12.90	12.73	12.57	12.42	12.26
.50	15.01	14.79	14.58	14.37	14.16	13.96	13.77	13.59	13.40	13.23	13.05+	12.88	12.72	12.56	12.41
.75	15.22	14.99	14.77	14.56	14.35−	14.14	13.95−	13.76	13.57	13.39	13.21	13.04	12.87	12.71	12.55
−17.00	15.43	15.19	14.97	14.74	14.53	14.32	14.12	13.92	13.73	13.55	13.37	13.19	13.02	12.85+	12.69
.25	15.63	15.39	15.16	14.93	14.71	14.50	14.29	14.09	13.89	13.70	13.52	13.34	13.16	12.99	12.83
.50	15.84	15.59	15.35+	15.12	14.89	14.68	14.46	14.26	14.06	13.86	13.67	13.49	13.31	13.13	12.96
.75	16.04	15.79	15.54	15.30	15.07	14.85+	14.63	14.42	14.22	14.02	13.82	13.64	13.45+	13.27	13.10
−18.00	16.24	15.98	15.73	15.49	15.25+	15.02	14.80	14.59	14.38	14.17	13.97	13.78	13.59	13.41	13.23
.25	16.45+	16.18	15.93	15.68	15.43	15.20	14.97	14.75+	14.54	14.33	14.13	13.93	13.74	13.55+	13.37
.50	16.65+	16.38	16.12	15.86	15.61	15.37	15.14	14.91	14.70	14.48	14.28	14.07	13.88	13.69	13.50
.75	16.85+	16.58	16.31	16.04	15.79	15.54	15.31	15.08	14.85+	14.63	14.42	14.22	14.02	13.83	13.64
−19.00	17.06	16.77	16.49	16.23	15.97	15.72	15.47	15.24	15.01	14.79	14.57	14.36	14.16	13.96	13.77
.25	17.26	16.96	16.68	16.41	16.14	15.89	15.64	15.40	15.16	14.94	14.72	14.50	14.30	14.09	13.90
.50	17.46	17.16	16.87	16.59	16.32	16.06	15.80	15.56	15.32	15.09	14.86	14.65−	14.43	14.23	14.03
.75	17.66	17.35+	17.06	16.77	16.49	16.23	15.97	15.72	15.47	15.24	15.01	14.79	14.57	14.36	14.16
−20.00	17.86	17.54	17.24	16.95−	16.67	16.39	16.13	15.87	15.62	15.38	15.15+	14.93	14.71	14.49	14.29
.25	18.06	17.74	17.43	17.13	16.84	16.56	16.29	16.03	15.78	15.53	15.29	15.06	14.84	14.62	14.41
.50	18.25	17.93	17.61	17.31	17.01	16.73	16.45	16.19	15.93	15.68	15.44	15.20	14.97	14.75+	14.54
.75	18.45+	18.12	17.80	17.49	17.19	16.89	16.61	16.34	16.08	15.83	15.58	15.34	15.11	14.88	14.66

Ocular refraction in dioptres for vertex distances in mm of:

Spectacle refraction or spectacle lens power (BVP) in dioptres	6	7	8	9	10	11	12	13	14	15	16	17	18	19	20
−21.00	18.65−	18.31−	17.98	17.66−	17.36−	17.06	16.77	16.50	16.23	15.97	15.72	15.48	15.24	15.01	14.79
.25	18.85−	18.50−	18.16	17.84	17.53	17.22	16.93	16.65−	16.38	16.11	15.86	15.61	15.37	15.14	14.91
.50	19.04	18.69	18.35−	18.01	17.70	17.39	17.09	16.80	16.53	16.26	16.00	15.75−	15.50	15.26	15.04
.75	19.24	18.88	18.53	18.19	17.86	17.55+	17.25−	16.95+	16.67	16.40	16.13	15.88	15.63	15.39	15.16
−22.00	19.43	19.05+	18.71	18.36	18.03	17.71	17.40	17.11	16.82	16.54	16.27	16.01	15.76	15.51	15.28
.25	19.63	19.25+	18.89	18.54	18.20	17.88	17.56	17.26	16.97	16.68	16.41	16.14	15.89	15.64	15.40
.50	19.82	19.44	19.07	18.71	18.37	18.04	17.72	17.41	17.11	16.82	16.54	16.30	16.01	15.76	15.52
.75	20.02	19.62	19.25+	18.88	18.53	18.20	17.87	17.56	17.25−	16.96	16.68	16.40	16.14	15.88	15.63
−23.00	20.21	19.81	19.43	19.05+	18.70	18.36	18.02	17.71	17.40	17.10	16.81	16.53	16.27	16.01	15.75+
.25	20.40	20.00	19.60	19.23	18.86	18.52	18.18	17.85+	17.54	17.24	16.95−	16.66	16.39	16.13	15.87
.50	20.60	20.18	19.78	19.40	19.03	18.67	18.33	18.00	17.68	17.38	17.08	16.79	16.52	16.25−	15.99
.75	20.79	20.36	19.96	19.57	19.19	18.83	18.48	18.15−	17.82	17.51	17.21	16.92	16.64	16.37	16.10
−24.00	20.98	20.55−	20.13	19.74	19.35+	18.99	18.63	18.29	17.96	17.65−	17.34	17.04	16.76	16.48	16.22
.25	21.17	20.73	20.31	19.90	19.52	19.14	18.78	18.44	18.10	17.78	17.47	17.17	16.88	16.60	16.33
.50	21.36	20.91	20.48	20.07	19.68	19.30	18.93	18.58	18.24	17.91	17.60	17.30	17.00	16.72	16.44
.75	21.55−	21.10	20.66	20.24	19.84	19.45+	19.08	18.73	18.38	18.05−	17.73	17.42	17.12	16.83	16.56
−25.00	21.74	21.28	20.83	20.41	20.00	19.61	19.23	18.87	18.52	18.18	17.86	17.54	17.24	16.95−	16.67
.25	21.93	21.46	21.01	20.58	20.16	19.76	19.38	19.01	18.66	18.32	17.99	17.67	17.36	17.06	16.78
.50	22.12	21.64	21.18	20.74	20.32	19.91	19.52	19.15−	18.79	18.44	18.11	17.79	17.48	17.18	16.89
.75	22.31	21.82	21.35+	20.91	20.48	20.07	19.67	19.29	18.93	18.58	18.24	**17.79**	17.60	17.29	**17.00**
−26.00	22.49	22.00	21.52	21.07	20.64	20.22	19.82	19.43	19.06	18.71	18.36	18.03	17.71	17.40	17.11
.25	22.68	22.17	21.69	21.23	20.79	20.37	19.96	19.57	19.19	18.83	18.48	18.15	17.83	17.51	17.21
.50	22.86	22.35+	21.86	21.39	20.95	20.52	20.10	19.71	19.33	18.96	18.61	18.27	17.94	17.62	17.32
.75	23.05+	22.53	22.04	21.56	21.11	20.67	20.25−	19.85−	19.46	19.09	18.73	18.39	18.06	17.74	17.43
−27.00	23.23	22.71	22.20	21.72	21.26	20.82	20.39	19.98	19.59	19.22	18.85+	18.50	18.17	17.84	17.53
.25	23.42	22.88	22.37	21.88	21.41	20.96	20.53	20.12	19.72	19.34	18.98	18.62	18.28	17.95+	17.64
.50	23.61	23.06	22.54	22.05−	21.57	21.11	20.68	20.26	19.86	19.47	19.10	18.74	18.40	18.06	17.74
.75	23.79	23.23	22.71	22.20	21.72	21.26	20.82	20.39	19.98	19.59	19.22	18.85+	18.50	18.17	17.84
−28.00	23.97	23.41	22.88	22.36	21.87	21.41	20.96	20.53	20.11	19.72	19.34	18.97	18.62	18.28	17.95−
.25	24.15+	23.58	23.04	22.52	22.03	21.55+	21.10	20.66	20.24	**19.84**	**19.46**	19.08	18.73	18.38	18.05+
.50	24.34	23.76	23.21	22.68	22.18	21.70	21.24	20.79	20.37	19.96	19.57	19.20	18.84	18.49	18.15+
.75	24.52	23.93	23.38	22.84	22.33	21.84	21.38	20.93	20.50	20.09	19.69	19.31	18.95−	18.59	18.25+
−29.00	24.70	24.11	23.54	23.00	22.48	21.99	21.51	21.06	20.63	20.21	19.81	19.43	19.05+	18.70	18.36
.25	24.88	24.28	23.70	23.15	22.63	22.13	21.65−	21.19	20.75	20.33	19.92	19.54	19.16	18.80	18.45+
.50	25.06	24.45−	23.87	23.31	22.78	22.27	21.79	21.32	20.88	20.45−	20.04	19.65−	19.27	**18.90**	18.55+
.75	25.25−	24.62	24.03	23.47	22.93	22.42	21.93	21.45+	21.00	20.57	20.16	19.76	19.38	19.01	18.65+
−30.00	25.42	24.79	24.19	23.62	23.08	22.56	22.06	21.58	21.13	20.69	20.27	**19.87**	**19.48**	19.11	18.75

APPENDIX B

TABLE I. Surface Powers in Dioptres for Various Radii and Refractive Index Differences

Radii, r in mm	1.568−1	1.376−1	1.3375−1	1.490−1.336	radii, r in mm	1.586−1	1.376−1	1.3375−1	1.490−1.336
5.00	113.600	75.200	67.500	30.800	8.55	66.433	43.977	39.474	18.012
5.10	111.373	73.725	66.176	30.196	8.60	66.047	43.721	39.244	17.907
5.20	109.231	72.308	64.904	29.615	8.65	65.665	43.468	39.017	17.803
5.30	107.170	70.943	63.679	29.057	8.70	65.287	43.218	38.793	17.701
5.40	105.185	69.630	62.500	28.519	8.75	64.914	42.971	38.571	17.600
5.50	103.273	68.364	61.364	28.000	8.80	64.545	42.727	38.352	17.500
5.60	101.429	67.143	60.268	27.500	8.85	64.181	42.486	38.136	17.401
5.70	99.649	65.965	59.211	27.018	8.90	63.820	42.247	37.921	17.303
5.80	97.931	64.828	58.190	26.552	8.95	63.464	42.011	37.709	17.207
5.90	96.271	63.729	57.203	26.102	9.00	63.111	41.778	37.500	17.111
6.00	94.667	62.667	56.250	25.667	9.10	62.418	41.319	37.088	16.923
6.10	93.115	61.639	55.328	25.246	9.20	61.739	40.870	36.685	16.739
6.20	91.613	60.645	54.435	24.839	9.30	61.075	40.430	36.290	16.559
6.30	90.159	59.683	53.571	24.444	9.40	60.426	40.000	35.904	16.382
6.40	88.750	58.750	52.734	24.063	9.50	59.789	39.579	35.526	16.211
6.50	87.385	57.846	51.923	23.692	9.60	59.167	39.167	35.156	16.042
6.60	86.061	56.970	51.136	23.333	9.70	58.557	38.763	34.794	15.876
6.70	84.776	56.119	50.373	22.985	9.80	57.959	38.367	34.438	15.714
6.80	83.529	55.294	49.632	22.647	9.90	57.374	37.980	34.091	15.556
6.90	82.319	54.493	48.913	22.319	10.00	56.800	37.600	33.750	15.400
7.00	81.143	53.714	48.214	22.000	10.10	56.238	37.228	33.416	15.248
7.05	80.567	53.333	47.872	21.844	10.20	55.686	36.863	33.088	15.098
7.10	80.000	52.958	47.535	21.690	10.30	55.146	36.505	32.767	14.951
7.15	79.441	52.587	47.203	21.538	10.40	54.615	36.154	32.452	14.808
7.20	78.889	52.222	46.875	21.389	10.50	54.095	35.810	32.143	14.667
7.25	78.345	51.862	46.552	21.241	10.60	53.585	35.472	31.840	14.528
7.30	77.808	51.507	46.233	21.096	10.70	53.084	35.140	31.542	14.393
7.35	77.279	51.156	45.918	20.952	10.80	52.593	34.815	31.250	14.259
7.40	76.757	50.811	45.608	20.811	10.90	52.110	34.495	30.963	14.128
7.45	76.242	50.470	45.302	20.671	11.00	51.636	34.182	30.682	14.000
7.50	75.733	50.133	45.000	20.533	11.10	51.171	33.874	30.405	13.874
7.55	75.232	49.801	44.702	20.397	11.20	50.714	33.571	30.134	13.750
7.60	74.737	49.474	44.408	20.263	11.30	50.265	33.274	29.867	13.628
7.65	74.248	49.150	44.118	20.131	11.40	49.825	32.982	29.605	13.509
7.70	73.766	48.831	43.831	20.000	11.50	49.391	32.696	29.348	13.391
7.75	73.290	48.516	43.548	19.871	11.60	48.966	32.414	29.095	13.276
7.80	72.821	48.205	43.269	19.744	11.70	48.547	32.137	28.846	13.162
7.85	72.357	47.898	42.994	19.618	11.80	48.136	31.864	28.602	13.051
7.90	71.899	47.595	42.722	19.494	11.90	47.731	31.597	28.361	12.941
7.95	71.447	47.296	42.453	19.371	12.00	47.333	31.333	28.125	12.833
8.00	71.000	47.000	42.188	19.250					
8.05	70.559	46.708	41.925	19.130					
8.10	70.123	46.420	41.667	19.012					
8.15	69.693	46.135	41.411	18.896					
8.20	69.268	45.854	41.159	18.780					
8.25	68.848	45.576	40.909	18.667					
8.30	68.434	45.301	40.663	18.554					
8.35	68.024	45.030	40.419	18.443					
8.40	67.619	44.762	40.179	18.333					
8.45	67.219	44.497	39.941	18.225					
8.50	66.824	44.235	39.706	18.118					

The Refractive Indices given pertain to the following materials:

1.568	Hyfrax
1.490	Polymethyl methacrylate
1.376	Cornea
1.3375	Most keratometers
1.336	Tears

APPENDIX B

TABLE II. Surface Powers in Air for n = 1.49 (PMMA), r = radius of curvature, F = surface power

r mm	F Dioptres	r mm	F Dioptres	r mm	F Dioptres	r mm	F Dioptres	r mm	F Dioptres	r mm	F Dioptres	r mm	F Dioptres
4.90	100.00	5.30	92.45	5.70	85.96	6.10	80.33	6.50	75.38	6.90	71.01	7.30	67.12
.91	99.80	.31	92.28	.71	85.81	.11	80.20	.51	75.27	.91	70.91	.31	67.03
.92	99.59	.32	92.11	.72	85.66	.12	80.07	.52	75.15	.92	70.81	.32	66.94
.93	99.39	.33	91.93	.73	85.51	.13	79.93	.53	75.04	.93	70.71	.33	66.85
.94	99.19	.34	91.76	.74	85.37	.14	79.80	.54	74.92	.94	70.60	.34	66.76
.95	98.99	.35	91.59	.75	85.22	.15	79.67	.55	74.81	.95	70.50	.35	66.67
.96	98.79	.36	91.42	.76	85.07	.16	79.55	.56	74.70	.96	70.40	.36	66.58
.97	98.59	.37	91.25	.77	84.92	.17	79.42	.57	74.58	.97	70.30	.37	66.49
.98	98.39	.38	91.08	.78	84.78	.18	79.29	.58	74.47	.98	70.20	.38	66.40
.99	98.20	.39	90.91	.79	84.63	.19	79.16	.59	74.36	.99	70.10	.39	66.31
5.00	98.00	5.40	90.74	5.80	84.48	6.20	79.03	6.60	74.24	7.00	70.00	7.40	66.22
.01	97.80	.41	90.57	.81	84.34	.21	78.90	.61	74.13	.01	69.90	.41	66.13
.02	97.61	.42	90.41	.82	84.19	.22	78.78	.62	74.02	.02	69.80	.42	66.04
.03	97.42	.43	90.24	.83	84.05	.23	78.65	.63	73.91	.03	69.70	.43	65.95
.04	97.22	.44	90.07	.84	83.90	.24	78.53	.64	73.80	.04	69.60	.44	65.86
.05	97.03	.45	89.91	.85	83.76	.25	78.40	.65	73.68	.05	69.50	.45	65.77
.06	96.84	.46	89.74	.86	83.62	.26	78.27	.66	73.57	.06	69.41	.46	65.68
.07	96.65	.47	89.58	.87	83.48	.27	78.15	.67	73.46	.07	69.31	.47	65.60
.08	96.46	.48	89.42	.88	83.33	.28	78.03	.68	73.35	.08	69.21	.48	65.51
.09	96.27	.49	89.25	.89	83.19	.29	77.90	.69	73.24	.09	69.11	.49	65.42
5.10	96.08	5.50	89.09	5.90	83.05	6.30	77.78	6.70	73.13	7.10	69.01	7.50	65.33
.11	95.89	.51	88.93	.91	82.91	.31	77.65	.71	73.03	.11	68.92	.51	65.25
.12	95.70	.52	88.77	.92	82.77	.32	77.53	.72	72.92	.12	68.82	.52	65.16
.13	95.52	.53	88.61	.93	82.63	.33	77.41	.73	72.81	.13	68.72	.53	65.07
.14	95.33	.54	88.45	.94	82.49	.34	77.29	.74	72.70	.14	68.63	.54	64.99
.15	95.15	.55	88.29	.95	82.35	.35	77.17	.75	72.59	.15	68.53	.55	64.90
.16	94.96	.56	88.13	.96	82.21	.36	77.04	.76	72.49	.16	68.44	.56	64.81
.17	94.78	.57	87.97	.97	82.08	.37	76.92	.77	72.38	.17	68.34	.57	64.73
.18	94.59	.58	87.81	.98	81.94	.38	76.80	.78	72.27	.18	68.25	.58	64.64
.19	94.41	.59	87.66	.99	81.80	.39	76.68	.79	72.16	.19	68.15	.59	64.56
5.20	94.23	5.60	87.50	6.00	81.67	6.40	76.56	6.80	72.06	7.20	68.06	7.60	64.47
.21	94.05	.61	87.34	.01	81.53	.41	76.44	.81	71.95	.21	67.96	.61	64.39
.22	93.87	.62	87.19	.02	81.40	.42	76.32	.82	71.85	.22	67.87	.62	64.30
.23	93.69	.63	87.03	.03	81.26	.43	76.21	.83	71.74	.23	67.77	.63	64.22
.24	93.51	.64	86.88	.04	81.13	.44	76.09	.84	71.64	.24	67.68	.64	64.14
.25	93.33	.65	86.73	.05	80.99	.45	75.97	.85	71.53	.25	67.59	.65	64.05
.26	93.16	.66	86.57	.06	80.86	.46	75.85	.86	71.43	.26	67.49	.66	63.97
.27	92.98	.67	86.42	.07	80.72	.47	75.73	.87	71.32	.27	67.40	.67	63.89
.28	92.80	.68	86.27	.08	80.59	.48	75.62	.88	71.22	.28	67.31	.68	63.80
.29	92.63	.69	86.12	.09	80.46	.49	75.50	.89	71.12	.29	67.22	.69	63.72

r mm	F Dioptres
7.70	63.64
.71	63.55
.72	63.47
.73	63.39
.74	63.31
.75	63.23
.76	63.14
.77	63.06
.78	62.98
.79	62.90
7.80	62.82
.81	62.74
.82	62.66
.83	62.58
.84	62.50
.85	62.42
.86	62.34
.87	62.26
.88	62.18
.89	62.10
7.90	62.03
.91	61.95
.92	61.87
.93	61.79
.94	61.71
.95	61.64
.96	61.56
.97	61.48
.98	61.40
.99	61.33
8.00	61.25
.01	61.17
.02	61.10
.03	61.02
.04	60.95
.05	60.87
.06	60.79
.07	60.72
.08	60.64
.09	60.57
8.10	60.49
.11	60.42
.12	60.34
.13	60.27
.14	60.20
.15	60.12
.16	60.05
.17	59.98
.18	59.90
.19	59.83
8.20	59.76
.21	59.68
.22	59.61
.23	59.54
.24	59.47
.25	59.39
.26	59.32
.27	59.25
.28	59.18
.29	59.11
8.30	59.04
.31	58.97
.32	58.89
.33	58.82
.34	58.75
.35	58.68
.36	58.61
.37	58.54
.38	58.47
.39	58.40
8.40	58.33
.41	58.26
.42	58.19
.43	58.13
.44	58.06
.45	57.99
.46	57.92
.47	57.85
.48	57.78
.49	57.72
8.50	57.65
.51	57.58
.52	57.51
.53	57.44
.54	57.38
.55	57.31
.56	57.24
.57	57.18
.58	57.11
.59	57.04
8.60	56.98
.61	56.91
.62	56.84
.63	56.78
.64	56.71
.65	56.65
.66	56.58
.67	56.52
.68	56.45
.69	56.39
8.70	56.32
.71	56.26
.72	56.19
.73	56.13
.74	56.06
.75	56.00
.76	55.94
.77	55.87
.78	55.81
.79	55.75
8.80	55.68
.81	55.62
.82	55.56
.83	55.49
.84	55.43
.85	55.37
.86	55.30
.87	55.24
.88	55.18
.89	55.12
8.90	55.06
.91	54.99
.92	54.93
.93	54.87
.94	54.81
.95	54.75
.96	54.69
.97	54.63
.98	54.57
.99	54.51
9.00	54.44
.01	54.38
.02	54.32
.03	54.26
.04	54.20
.05	54.14
.06	54.08
.07	54.02
.08	53.96
.09	53.91
9.10	53.85
.11	53.79
.12	53.73
.13	53.67
.14	53.61
.15	53.55
.16	53.49
.17	53.43
.18	53.38
.19	53.32
9.20	53.26
.21	53.20
.22	53.15
.23	53.09
.24	53.03
.25	52.97
.26	52.92
.27	52.86
.28	52.80
.29	52.75
9.30	52.69
.31	52.63
.32	52.58
.33	52.52
.34	52.46
.35	52.41
.36	52.35
.37	52.29
.38	52.24
.39	52.18
9.40	52.13
.41	52.07
.42	52.02
.43	51.96
.44	51.91
.45	51.85
.46	51.80
.47	51.74
.48	51.69
.49	51.63
9.50	51.58
.51	51.52
.52	51.47
.53	51.42
.54	51.36
.55	51.31
.56	51.25
.57	51.20
.58	51.15
.59	51.09
9.60	51.04
.61	50.99
.62	50.94
.63	50.88
.64	50.83
.65	50.78
.66	50.72
.67	50.67
.68	50.62
.69	50.57
9.70	50.52
.71	50.46
.72	50.41
.73	50.36
.74	50.31
.75	50.26
.76	50.20
.77	50.15
.78	50.10
.79	50.05
9.80	50.00
.81	49.95
.82	49.90
.83	49.85
.84	49.80
.85	49.75
.86	49.70
.87	49.65
.88	49.60
.89	49.54
9.90	49.49
.91	49.45
.92	49.40
.93	49.35
.94	49.30
.95	49.25
.96	49.20
.97	49.15
.98	49.10
.99	49.05
10.00	49.00
.01	48.95
.02	48.90
.03	48.85
.04	48.80
.05	48.76
.06	48.71
.07	48.66
.08	48.61
.09	48.56
10.10	48.51
.11	48.47
.12	48.42
.13	48.37
.14	48.32
.15	48.28
.16	48.23
.17	48.18
.18	48.13
.19	48.09
10.20	48.04
.21	47.99
.22	47.95
.23	47.90
.24	47.85
.25	47.81
.26	47.76
.27	47.71
.28	47.67
.29	47.62
10.30	47.57
.31	47.53
.32	47.48
.33	47.44
.34	47.39
.35	47.34
.36	47.30
.37	47.25
.38	47.21
.39	47.16
10.40	47.12
.41	47.07
.42	47.03
.43	46.98
.44	46.94
.45	46.89
.46	46.85
.47	46.80
.48	46.76
.49	46.71

r mm	F Dioptres	r mm	F Dioptres	r mm	F Dioptres	r mm	F Dioptres	r mm	F Dioptres	r mm	F Dioptres
10.50	46.67	10.90	44.95	11.30	43.36	11.70	41.88	12.10	40.50	12.50	39.20
.51	46.62	.91	44.91	.31	43.32	.71	41.84	.11	40.46	.51	39.17
.52	46.58	.92	44.87	.32	43.29	.72	41.81	.12	40.43	.52	39.14
.53	46.53	.93	44.83	.33	43.25	.73	41.77	.13	40.40	.53	39.11
.54	46.49	.94	44.79	.34	43.21	.74	41.74	.14	40.36	.54	39.08
.55	46.45	.95	44.75	.35	43.17	.75	41.70	.15	40.33	.55	39.04
.56	46.40	.96	44.71	.36	43.13	.76	41.67	.16	40.30	.56	39.01
.57	46.36	.97	44.67	.37	43.10	.77	41.63	.17	40.26	.57	38.98
.58	46.31	.98	44.63	.38	43.06	.78	41.60	.18	40.23	.58	38.95
.59	46.27	.99	44.59	.39	43.02	.79	41.56	.19	40.20	.59	38.92
10.60	46.23	11.00	44.55	11.40	42.98	11.80	41.53	12.20	40.16	12.60	38.89
.61	46.18	.01	44.51	.41	42.95	.81	41.49	.21	40.13		
.62	46.14	.02	44.47	.42	42.91	.82	41.46	.22	40.10		
.63	46.10	.03	44.43	.43	42.87	.83	41.42	.23	40.07		
.64	46.05	.04	44.38	.44	42.83	.84	41.39	.24	40.03		
.65	46.01	.05	44.34	.45	42.80	.85	41.35	.25	40.00		
.66	45.97	.06	44.30	.46	42.76	.86	41.32	.26	39.97		
.67	45.92	.07	44.26	.47	42.72	.87	41.28	.27	39.94		
.68	45.88	.08	44.22	.48	42.68	.88	41.25	.28	39.90		
.69	45.84	.09	44.18	.49	42.65	.89	41.21	.29	39.87		
10.70	45.79	11.10	44.14	11.50	42.61	11.90	41.18	12.30	39.84		
.71	45.75	.11	44.10	.51	42.57	.91	41.14	.31	39.81		
.72	45.71	.12	44.07	.52	42.54	.92	41.11	.32	39.77		
.73	45.67	.13	44.03	.53	42.50	.93	41.07	.33	39.74		
.74	45.62	.14	43.99	.54	42.46	.94	41.04	.34	39.71		
.75	45.58	.15	43.95	.55	42.43	.95	41.00	.35	39.68		
.76	45.54	.16	43.91	.56	42.39	.96	40.97	.36	39.64		
.77	45.50	.17	43.87	.57	42.35	.97	40.94	.37	39.61		
.78	45.46	.18	43.83	.58	42.31	.98	40.90	.38	39.58		
.79	45.41	.19	43.79	.59	42.28	.99	40.87	.39	39.55		
10.80	45.37	11.20	43.75	11.60	42.24	12.00	40.83	12.40	39.52		
.81	45.33	.21	43.71	.61	42.21	.01	40.80	.41	39.48		
.82	45.29	.22	43.67	.62	42.17	.02	40.77	.42	39.45		
.83	45.25	.23	43.63	.63	42.13	.03	40.73	.43	39.42		
.84	45.20	.24	43.60	.64	42.10	.04	40.70	.44	39.39		
.85	45.16	.25	43.56	.65	42.06	.05	40.66	.45	39.36		
.86	45.12	.26	43.52	.66	42.02	.06	40.63	.46	39.33		
.87	45.08	.27	43.48	.67	41.99	.07	40.60	.47	39.29		
.88	45.04	.28	43.44	.68	41.95	.08	40.56	.48	39.26		
.89	45.00	.29	43.40	.69	41.92	.09	40.53	.49	39.23		

APPENDIX B

TABLE III. Change in Surface Power, in Dioptres, when Radius (r_1) is Changed to New Radius (r_2), for Plastics (n = 1.49) in Air

Initial radius r_1 mm	New radius (r_2) mm																			
	7.0 (D)	7.1	7.2	7.3	7.4	7.5	7.6	7.7	7.8	7.9	8.0	8.1	8.2	8.3	8.4	8.5	8.6	8.7	8.8	8.9
9.0	15.56	14.57	13.62	12.68	11.78	10.89	10.03	9.20	8.38	7.59	6.81	6.05	5.32	4.60	3.89	3.21	2.54	1.88	1.24	0.62
8.9	14.94	13.95	13.00	12.06	11.16	10.27	9.41	8.58	7.76	6.97	6.19	5.43	4.70	3.98	3.27	2.59	1.92	1.26	0.62	
8.8	14.32	13.33	12.38	11.44	10.54	9.65	8.79	7.96	7.14	6.35	5.57	4.81	4.08	3.36	2.65	1.97	1.30	0.64		
8.7	13.68	12.69	11.74	10.80	9.90	9.01	8.15	7.32	6.50	5.71	4.93	4.17	3.44	2.72	2.01	1.33	0.66			
8.6	13.02	12.03	11.08	10.14	9.24	8.35	7.49	6.66	5.84	5.05	4.27	3.51	2.78	2.06	1.35	0.67				
8.5	12.35	11.36	10.41	9.47	8.57	7.68	6.82	5.99	5.17	4.38	3.60	2.84	2.02	1.39	0.68					
8.4	11.67	10.68	9.73	8.79	7.89	7.00	6.14	5.31	4.49	3.70	2.92	2.16	1.43	0.71						
8.3	10.96	9.97	9.02	8.08	7.18	6.29	5.03	4.60	3.78	2.99	2.21	1.45	0.72							
8.2	10.24	9.25	8.30	7.36	6.46	5.57	4.71	3.88	3.06	2.27	1.49	0.73								
8.1	9.51	8.52	7.57	6.63	5.73	4.84	3.98	3.15	2.33	1.54	0.76									
8.0	8.75	7.76	6.81	5.87	4.97	4.08	3.22	2.39	1.57	0.78										
7.9	7.97	6.98	6.03	5.09	4.19	3.30	2.44	1.61	0.79											
7.8	7.18	6.19	5.24	4.30	3.40	2.51	1.65	0.82												
7.7	6.36	5.37	4.42	3.48	2.58	1.69	0.83													
7.6	5.53	4.54	3.59	2.65	1.75	0.86														
7.5	4.67	3.68	2.73	1.79	0.89															
7.4	3.78	2.79	1.84	0.90																
7.3	2.88	1.89	0.94																	
7.2	1.94	0.95																		
7.1	0.99																			

APPENDIX B

TABLE IV. Change in Reduced Vergence Due to Thickness for a Given Initial Vergence and Refractive Index of 1.49 (Plastics in Air)
(In each cell, the upper figure applies to divergent light, and the lower figure to convergent light)

Initial vergence	Thickness (mm)															
	.01	.02	.03	.04	.05	.06	.07	.08	.09	.10	.11	.12	.13	.14	.15	.16
D 100.0	.07	.13	.20	.27	.34	.40	.47	.54	.60	.67	.74	.80	.86	.93	1.00	1.06
	.07	.14	.20	.27	.34	.41	.48	.54	.61	.68	.75	.82	.88	.95	1.02	1.09
98.0	.06	.13	.19	.26	.32	.38	.45	.51	.58	.64	.70	.77	.83	.89	.96	1.02
	.06	.13	.20	.26	.32	.39	.46	.52	.58	.65	.72	.78	.85	.91	.98	1.05
96.0	.06	.12	.18	.24	.30	.37	.43	.49	.55	.61	.67	.73	.79	.85	.92	.98
	.06	.12	.19	.25	.31	.37	.43	.50	.56	.62	.68	.75	.81	.87	.94	1.00
94.0	.06	.12	.18	.24	.30	.35	.41	.47	.53	.59	.65	.71	.76	.82	.88	.94
	.06	.12	.18	.24	.30	.36	.42	.48	.54	.60	.66	.72	.78	.84	.90	.96
92.0	.06	.11	.17	.22	.28	.34	.39	.45	.50	.56	.62	.67	.73	.78	.84	.90
	.06	.11	.17	.23	.28	.34	.40	.46	.51	.57	.63	.69	.74	.80	.86	.92
90.0	.05	.11	.16	.22	.27	.32	.38	.43	.49	.54	.59	.65	.70	.75	.80	.86
	.06	.11	.16	.22	.28	.33	.38	.44	.50	.55	.60	.66	.72	.77	.82	.88
88.0	.05	.10	.16	.21	.26	.31	.36	.42	.47	.52	.57	.62	.67	.72	.78	.83
	.05	.10	.16	.21	.26	.31	.36	.42	.47	.52	.57	.63	.68	.73	.78	.84
86.0	.05	.10	.15	.20	.24	.29	.34	.39	.44	.49	.54	.59	.64	.69	.74	.78
	.05	.10	.15	.20	.25	.30	.35	.40	.45	.50	.55	.60	.65	.70	.76	.81
84.0	.05	.09	.14	.19	.24	.28	.33	.38	.42	.47	.52	.56	.61	.66	.70	.75
	.05	.10	.14	.19	.24	.29	.34	.38	.43	.48	.53	.58	.62	.67	.72	.77
82.0	.04	.09	.14	.18	.22	.27	.32	.36	.40	.45	.49	.54	.58	.63	.67	.71
	.04	.09	.14	.18	.22	.27	.32	.36	.40	.45	.50	.54	.59	.63	.68	.73
80.0	.04	.09	.13	.17	.22	.26	.30	.34	.39	.43	.47	.51	.56	.60	.64	.68
	.04	.09	.13	.17	.22	.26	.30	.34	.39	.43	.47	.52	.56	.61	.65	.69
78.0	.04	.08	.12	.16	.20	.25	.29	.33	.37	.41	.45	.49	.53	.57	.61	.65
	.04	.08	.12	.16	.20	.25	.29	.33	.37	.41	.45	.49	.54	.58	.62	.66
76.0	.04	.08	.12	.16	.20	.23	.27	.31	.35	.39	.43	.47	.50	.54	.58	.62
	.04	.08	.12	.16	.20	.23	.27	.31	.35	.39	.43	.47	.51	.55	.58	.62
74.0	.04	.07	.11	.15	.18	.22	.26	.30	.33	.37	.41	.44	.48	.51	.55	.59
	.04	.07	.11	.15	.18	.22	.26	.30	.33	.37	.41	.44	.48	.52	.56	.59
72.0	.04	.07	.10	.14	.18	.21	.24	.28	.32	.35	.38	.42	.45	.49	.52	.55
	.04	.07	.10	.14	.18	.21	.24	.28	.32	.35	.38	.42	.46	.49	.52	.56
70.0	.03	.07	.10	.13	.16	.20	.23	.26	.30	.33	.36	.39	.43	.46	.49	.52
	.03	.07	.10	.13	.16	.20	.23	.26	.30	.33	.36	.40	.43	.46	.50	.51
68.0	.03	.06	.09	.12	.16	.19	.22	.25	.28	.31	.34	.37	.40	.43	.46	.50
	.03	.06	.09	.12	.16	.19	.22	.25	.28	.31	.34	.37	.41	.44	.47	.50
66.0	.03	.06	.09	.12	.14	.17	.20	.23	.26	.29	.32	.35	.38	.41	.44	.46
	.03	.06	.09	.12	.15	.17	.20	.23	.26	.29	.32	.35	.38	.41	.44	.47
64.0	.03	.05	.08	.11	.14	.16	.19	.22	.24	.27	.30	.33	.35	.38	.41	.44
	.03	.06	.08	.11	.14	.17	.20	.22	.25	.28	.31	.33	.36	.39	.42	.44
62.0	.03	.05	.08	.10	.13	.16	.18	.21	.23	.26	.28	.31	.34	.36	.38	.41
	.03	.05	.08	.10	.13	.16	.18	.21	.23	.26	.29	.31	.34	.36	.39	.42
60.0	.02	.05	.07	.10	.12	.14	.17	.19	.22	.24	.26	.29	.31	.34	.36	.38
	.02	.05	.07	.10	.12	.14	.17	.19	.22	.24	.26	.29	.32	.34	.36	.39
58.0	.02	.04	.07	.09	.11	.13	.15	.18	.20	.22	.24	.27	.29	.31	.34	.36
	.02	.05	.07	.09	.12	.14	.16	.18	.21	.23	.25	.28	.30	.32	.34	.37
56.0	.02	.04	.06	.08	.10	.13	.15	.17	.19	.21	.23	.25	.27	.29	.32	.34
	.02	.04	.06	.08	.10	.13	.15	.17	.19	.21	.23	.25	.27	.29	.32	.34
54.0	.02	.04	.06	.08	.10	.11	.13	.15	.17	.19	.21	.23	.25	.27	.29	.31
	.02	.04	.06	.08	.10	.12	.14	.16	.18	.20	.22	.24	.26	.28	.30	.31
52.0	.02	.04	.05	.07	.09	.11	.13	.14	.16	.18	.20	.22	.23	.25	.27	.29
	.02	.04	.05	.07	.09	.11	.13	.14	.16	.18	.20	.22	.24	.26	.28	.29
50.0	.02	.03	.05	.07	.08	.10	.12	.14	.15	.17	.19	.20	.22	.23	.25	.27
	.02	.03	.05	.07	.08	.10	.12	.14	.15	.17	.19	.20	.22	.24	.26	.27
48.0	.02	.03	.04	.06	.08	.09	.10	.12	.14	.15	.17	.18	.20	.21	.23	.25
	.02	.03	.05	.06	.08	.10	.11	.13	.14	.16	.18	.19	.20	.22	.24	.25
46.0	.01	.03	.04	.06	.07	.08	.10	.11	.13	.14	.15	.17	.18	.20	.21	.22
	.01	.03	.04	.06	.07	.08	.10	.11	.13	.14	.16	.17	.18	.20	.22	.23
44.0	.01	.03	.04	.05	.06	.08	.09	.10	.12	.13	.14	.16	.17	.18	.20	.21
	.01	.03	.04	.05	.06	.08	.09	.10	.12	.13	.14	.16	.17	.18	.20	.21
42.0	.01	.02	.04	.05	.06	.07	.08	.10	.11	.12	.13	.14	.16	.17	.18	.19
	.01	.02	.04	.05	.06	.07	.08	.10	.11	.12	.13	.14	.16	.17	.18	.19
40.0	.01	.02	.03	.04	.06	.07	.08	.09	.10	.11	.12	.13	.14	.15	.16	.17
	.01	.02	.03	.04	.06	.07	.08	.09	.10	.11	.12	.13	.14	.15	.16	.18

APPENDIX B (continued)

TABLE IV. Change in Reduced Vergence Due to Thickness for a Given Initial Vergence and Refractive Index of 1.49 (Plastics in Air)
(In each cell, the upper figure applies to divergent light, and the lower figure to convergent light)

.17	.18	.19	.20	.21	.22	.23	.24	.25	.26	.27	.28	.29	.30	.31	.32	.33	.34
1.12	1.19	1.26	1.32	1.38	1.45	1.52	1.58	1.64	1.71	1.78	1.84	1.90	1.97	2.03	2.10	2.16	2.23
1.16	1.22	1.29	1.36	1.43	1.50	1.57	1.64	1.70	1.77	1.84	1.91	1.98	2.05	2.12	2.19	2.26	2.33
1.08	1.14	1.21	1.27	1.33	1.40	1.46	1.52	1.58	1.65	.171	1.77	1.84	1.90	1.96	2.02	2.08	2.14
1.11	1.18	1.24	1.31	1.38	1.44	1.51	1.57	1.64	1.71	1.77	1.84	1.90	1.97	2.04	2.11	2.17	2.24
1.04	1.10	1.16	1.22	1.28	1.34	1.40	1.46	1.52	1.58	1.64	1.70	1.76	1.82	1.88	1.94	2.00	2.06
1.06	1.12	1.19	1.25	1.31	1.38	1.44	1.51	1.57	1.63	1.70	1.76	1.83	1.89	1.96	2.02	2.08	2.15
1.00	1.05	1.11	1.17	1.23	1.29	1.34	1.40	1.46	1.52	1.58	1.63	1.69	1.75	1.81	1.86	1.92	1.97
1.02	1.08	1.14	1.20	1.26	1.32	1.38	1.44	1.50	1.57	1.63	1.69	1.75	1.81	1.87	1.93	2.00	2.06
.95	1.01	1.06	1.12	1.18	1.23	1.28	1.34	1.40	1.45	1.50	1.56	1.62	1.67	1.72	1.78	1.84	1.89
.98	1.03	1.09	1.15	1.21	1.27	1.33	1.39	1.44	1.50	1.56	1.62	1.68	1.74	1.80	1.86	1.92	1.98
.91	.96	1.02	1.07	1.12	1.18	1.23	1.28	1.34	1.39	1.44	1.49	1.55	1.60	1.65	1.70	1.76	1.81
.94	.99	1.04	1.10	1.16	1.21	1.27	1.32	1.38	1.44	1.49	1.55	1.60	1.66	1.72	1.77	1.83	1.89
.88	.91	.98	1.03	1.08	1.13	1.18	1.23	1.28	1.33	1.38	1.43	1.48	1.53	1.58	1.63	1.68	1.73
.89	.94	1.00	1.05	1.10	1.16	1.21	1.27	1.32	1.37	1.43	1.48	1.54	1.59	1.64	1.70	1.75	1.81
.83	.88	.93	.98	1.03	1.08	1.12	1.17	1.22	1.27	1.32	1.36	1.41	1.46	1.51	1.56	1.60	1.65
.86	.91	.96	1.01	1.06	1.11	1.16	1.21	1.26	1.32	1.37	1.42	1.47	1.52	1.57	1.62	1.67	1.72
.80	.85	.89	.94	.99	1.03	1.08	1.12	1.17	1.22	1.26	1.31	1.35	1.40	1.44	1.49	1.54	1.58
.82	.86	.91	.96	1.01	1.06	1.11	1.16	1.20	1.25	1.30	1.35	1.40	1.45	1.50	1.55	1.60	1.65
.76	.80	.85	.89	.93	.98	1.02	1.07	1.11	1.15	1.20	1.24	1.29	1.33	1.37	1.42	1.46	1.51
.77	.82	.86	.91	.96	1.00	1.05	1.10	1.14	1.19	1.24	1.29	1.33	1.38	1.43	1.47	1.52	1.57
.72	.77	.81	.85	.89	.93	.98	1.02	1.06	1.10	1.14	1.19	1.23	1.27	1.31	1.35	1.39	1.43
.74	.78	.83	.87	.91	.96	1.00	1.05	1.09	1.13	1.18	1.22	1.27	1.31	1.36	1.40	1.44	1.49
.69	.73	.77	.81	.85	.89	.93	.97	1.01	1.05	1.09	1.13	1.17	1.21	1.25	1.29	1.33	1.37
.70	.75	.79	.83	.87	.91	.95	.99	1.04	1.08	1.12	1.16	1.20	1.24	1.28	1.33	1.37	1.41
.66	.69	.73	.77	.81	.85	.88	.92	.96	1.00	1.04	1.07	1.11	1.15	1.19	1.22	1.26	1.30
.66	.70	.74	.78	.82	.86	.90	.94	.98	1.02	1.06	1.10	1.14	1.18	1.22	1.26	1.30	1.34
.62	.66	.69	.73	.77	.80	.84	.87	.91	.95	.98	1.02	1.05	1.09	1.12	1.16	1.20	1.23
.63	.67	.70	.74	.78	.82	.85	.89	.93	.97	1.01	1.04	1.08	1.12	1.16	1.20	1.23	1.27
.59	.62	.66	.69	.72	.76	.79	.83	.86	.89	.93	.96	1.00	1.03	1.06	1.10	1.13	1.17
.60	.63	.66	.70	.74	.77	.81	.84	.88	.92	.95	.99	1.02	1.06	1.10	1.13	1.17	1.20
.55	.59	.62	.65	.68	.71	.75	.78	.81	.84	.87	.91	.94	.97	1.00	1.03	1.07	1.10
.56	.59	.63	.66	.69	.73	.76	.80	.83	.86	.90	.93	.97	1.00	1.03	1.07	1.10	1.14
.53	.56	.59	.62	.65	.68	.71	.74	.77	.80	.83	.86	.89	.92	.95	.98	1.01	1.04
.53	.57	.60	.63	.66	.69	.72	.75	.78	.82	.85	.88	.91	.94	.97	1.00	1.04	1.07
.49	.52	.55	.58	.61	.64	.67	.70	.72	.75	.78	.81	.84	.87	.90	.93	.95	.98
.50	.53	.56	.59	.62	.65	.68	.71	.74	.77	.80	.83	.86	.89	.92	.95	.98	1.00
.47	.49	.52	.55	.58	.60	.63	.65	.68	.71	.73	.76	.78	.81	.84	.86	.89	.92
.47	.50	.52	.55	.58	.61	.64	.67	.70	.72	.75	.78	.81	.84	.87	.90	.92	.95
.44	.46	.48	.51	.54	.56	.58	.61	.64	.66	.68	.71	.74	.76	.79	.81	.84	.86
.44	.47	.49	.52	.55	.57	.60	.62	.65	.68	.70	.73	.75	.78	.81	.83	.86	.89
.41	.43	.46	.48	.50	.53	.55	.58	.60	.62	.65	.67	.70	.72	.74	.77	.79	.81
.42	.44	.46	.49	.51	.54	.56	.59	.61	.63	.66	.68	.71	.73	.76	.78	.80	.83
.38	.40	.43	.45	.47	.49	.52	.54	.56	.58	.60	.63	.65	.67	.69	.71	.74	.76
.39	.41	.44	.46	.48	.51	.53	.55	.58	.60	.62	.64	.67	.69	.71	.74	.76	.78
.36	.38	.40	.42	.44	.46	.48	.50	.52	.54	.56	.58	.60	.62	.64	.66	.68	.70
.36	.38	.40	.42	.44	.46	.49	.51	.53	.55	.57	.60	.62	.64	.66	.68	.70	.72
.33	.35	.37	.39	.41	.43	.45	.47	.48	.50	.52	.54	.56	.58	.60	.62	.64	.66
.33	.35	.37	.39	.41	.43	.45	.47	.49	.51	.53	.55	.57	.59	.61	.63	.65	.67
.31	.32	.34	.36	.38	.40	.41	.43	.45	.47	.49	.50	.52	.54	.56	.58	.59	.61
.31	.33	.35	.37	.39	.41	.42	.44	.46	.48	.50	.51	.53	.55	.57	.59	.61	.63
.28	.30	.31	.33	.35	.36	.38	.40	.42	.43	.45	.47	.48	.50	.52	.53	.55	.56
.29	.31	.32	.34	.36	.37	.39	.41	.42	.44	.46	.48	.49	.51	.53	.54	.56	.58
.26	.28	.29	.31	.32	.34	.36	.37	.38	.40	.42	.43	.44	.46	.48	.49	.50	.52
.26	.28	.30	.31	.33	.34	.36	.37	.39	.41	.42	.44	.45	.47	.49	.50	.52	.53
.24	.25	.27	.28	.29	.31	.32	.34	.35	.36	.38	.39	.41	.42	.43	.45	.46	.48
.24	.26	.28	.29	.30	.32	.33	.35	.36	.37	.39	.40	.42	.43	.44	.46	.48	.49
.22	.23	.25	.26	.27	.29	.30	.31	.32	.34	.35	.36	.38	.39	.40	.41	.43	.44
.22	.23	.25	.26	.27	.29	.30	.31	.32	.34	.35	.36	.38	.39	.40	.42	.43	.45
.20	.22	.23	.24	.25	.26	.27	.28	.30	.31	.32	.33	.34	.35	.36	.37	.39	.40
.20	.22	.23	.24	.25	.26	.28	.29	.30	.31	.32	.34	.35	.36	.37	.38	.40	.41
.18	.19	.20	.21	.22	.23	.24	.25	.26	.28	.29	.30	.31	.32	.33	.34	.35	.36
.19	.20	.21	.22	.23	.24	.25	.26	.27	.28	.29	.30	.31	.32	.33	.34	.35	.36

APPENDIX B (continued)

TABLE IV. Change in Reduced Vergence Due to Thickness for a Given Initial Vergence and Refractive Index of 1.49 (Plastics in Air)
(In each cell, the upper figure applies to divergent light, and the lower figure to convergent light)

Initial vergence	Thickness (mm)															
D	.35	.36	.37	.38	.39	.40	.41	.42	.43	.44	.45	.46	.47	.48	.49	.50
100.00	2.29	2.35	2.42	2.48	2.55	2.61	2.67	2.74	2.80	2.87	2.93	2.99	3.06	3.12	3.19	3.25
	2.40	2.48	2.55	2.62	2.69	2.76	2.83	2.90	2.97	3.04	3.12	3.19	3.26	3.33	3.40	3.47
98.00	2.20	2.27	2.33	2.39	2.45	2.51	2.57	2.63	2.69	2.75	2.82	2.88	2.94	3.00	3.06	3.12
	2.31	2.38	2.45	2.51	2.58	2.65	2.72	2.79	2.85	2.92	2.99	3.06	3.13	3.19	3.26	3.33
96.00	2.12	2.17	2.23	2.29	2.35	2.41	2.47	2.53	2.59	2.65	2.70	2.76	2.82	2.88	2.94	3.00
	2.22	2.28	2.34	2.41	2.48	2.54	2.61	2.67	2.74	2.80	2.87	2.94	3.00	3.07	3.13	3.20
94.0	2.03	2.09	2.14	2.20	2.25	2.31	2.37	2.42	2.48	2.53	2.59	2.65	2.70	2.76	2.81	2.87
	2.12	2.18	2.24	2.31	2.37	2.43	2.49	2.56	2.62	2.68	2.74	2.81	2.87	2.93	3.00	3.06
92.00	1.94	2.00	2.06	2.11	2.16	2.22	2.27	2.33	2.38	2.44	2.49	2.54	2.60	2.65	2.71	2.76
	2.04	2.09	2.15	2.21	2.27	2.33	2.39	2.45	2.51	2.57	2.63	2.69	2.75	2.81	2.87	2.93
90.00	1.86	1.91	1.96	2.02	2.07	2.12	2.17	2.22	2.28	2.33	2.38	2.43	2.48	2.54	2.59	2.64
	1.94	2.00	2.06	2.12	2.17	2.23	2.29	2.34	2.40	2.46	2.52	2.57	2.63	2.69	2.74	2.80
88.0	1.78	1.83	1.88	1.93	1.98	2.03	2.08	2.13	2.18	2.23	2.28	2.32	2.37	2.42	2.47	2.52
	1.86	1.91	1.97	2.02	2.08	2.13	2.18	2.24	2.30	2.35	2.40	2.46	2.52	2.57	2.62	2.68
86.0	1.70	1.75	1.80	1.84	1.89	1.94	1.99	2.03	2.08	2.13	2.18	2.22	2.27	2.32	2.36	2.41
	1.78	1.83	1.88	1.93	1.98	2.03	2.08	2.14	2.19	2.24	2.30	2.35	2.40	2.45	2.51	2.55
84.00	1.62	1.67	1.72	1.76	1.80	1.85	1.90	1.94	1.98	2.03	2.08	2.12	2.16	2.21	2.26	2.30
	1.70	1.74	1.79	1.84	1.89	1.94	1.99	2.04	2.09	2.14	2.19	2.24	2.29	2.34	2.39	2.44
82.0	1.55	1.59	1.64	1.68	1.73	1.77	1.81	1.86	1.90	1.94	1.98	2.03	2.07	2.11	2.16	2.20
	1.62	1.66	1.71	1.76	1.80	1.85	1.90	1.94	1.99	2.04	2.08	2.13	2.18	2.23	2.27	2.32
80.0	1.48	1.52	1.56	1.60	1.64	1.68	1.72	1.76	1.80	1.84	1.88	1.93	1.97	2.01	2.05	2.09
	1.54	1.58	1.62	1.67	1.72	1.76	1.80	1.85	1.90	1.94	1.98	2.03	2.08	2.12	2.16	2.21
78.0	1.40	1.44	1.48	1.52	1.56	1.60	1.64	1.68	1.72	1.76	1.80	1.83	1.87	1.91	1.95	1.99
	1.46	1.50	1.54	1.58	1.63	1.67	1.71	1.76	1.80	1.84	1.88	1.93	1.97	2.01	2.06	2.10
76.0	1.34	1.37	1.41	1.45	1.48	1.52	1.56	1.59	1.63	1.67	1.70	1.74	1.78	1.82	1.85	1.89
	1.38	1.42	1.46	1.50	1.54	1.58	1.62	1.66	1.70	1.74	1.78	1.83	1.87	1.91	1.95	1.99
74.0	1.26	1.30	1.34	1.37	1.40	1.44	1.48	1.51	1.54	1.58	1.62	1.65	1.68	1.72	1.76	1.79
	1.31	1.35	1.39	1.42	1.46	1.50	1.54	1.58	1.61	1.65	1.69	1.73	1.77	1.80	1.84	1.88
72.0	1.20	1.23	1.27	1.30	1.34	1.37	1.40	1.44	1.47	1.50	1.54	1.57	1.60	1.63	1.67	1.70
	1.24	1.28	1.31	1.35	1.38	1.42	1.46	1.49	1.53	1.56	1.60	1.64	1.67	1.71	1.74	1.78
70.0	1.13	1.16	1.19	1.23	1.26	1.29	1.32	1.35	1.39	1.42	1.45	1.48	1.51	1.55	1.58	1.61
	1.17	1.20	1.24	1.27	1.31	1.34	1.37	1.41	1.44	1.48	1.51	1.54	1.58	1.61	1.65	1.68
68.0	1.07	1.10	1.13	1.16	1.19	1.22	1.25	1.28	1.31	1.34	1.37	1.40	1.43	1.46	1.49	1.52
	1.10	1.13	1.16	1.20	1.23	1.26	1.29	1.33	1.36	1.39	1.42	1.46	1.49	1.52	1.56	1.59
66.0	1.01	1.04	1.07	1.09	1.12	1.15	1.18	1.21	1.23	1.26	1.29	1.32	1.35	1.37	1.40	1.43
	1.04	1.07	1.10	1.13	1.16	1.19	1.22	1.25	1.28	1.31	1.34	1.37	1.40	1.43	1.46	1.49
64.0	.94	.97	1.00	1.03	1.05	1.08	1.11	1.13	1.16	1.19	1.22	1.24	1.27	1.30	1.32	1.35
	.98	1.01	1.04	1.06	1.09	1.12	1.15	1.18	1.20	1.23	1.26	1.29	1.32	1.34	1.37	1.40
62.0	.89	.92	.94	.97	.99	1.02	1.04	1.07	1.09	1.12	1.14	1.16	1.19	1.21	1.24	1.26
	.92	94	.97	1.00	1.02	1.05	1.08	1.10	1.13	1.16	1.18	1.21	1.24	1.27	1.29	1.32
60.0	.84	.86	.88	.90	.93	.95	.97	1.00	1.02	1.04	1.06	1.09	1.11	1.13	1.16	1.18
	.86	.88	.90	.93	.96	.98	1.00	1.03	1.06	1.08	1.10	1.13	1.16	1.18	1.20	1.23
58.0	.78	.80	.82	.85	.87	.89	.91	.93	.96	.98	1.00	1.02	1.04	1.07	1.09	1.11
	.80	.83	.85	.87	.90	.92	.94	.97	.99	1.01	1.04	1.06	1.08	1.10	1.13	1.15
56.0	.72	.75	.77	.79	.81	.83	.85	.87	.89	.91	.93	.95	.97	.99	1.01	1.03
	.74	.77	.79	.81	.83	.85	.87	.89	.92	.94	.96	.98	1.00	1.03	1.05	1.07
54.0	.68	.69	.71	.73	.75	.77	.79	.81	.83	.85	.86	.88	.90	.92	.94	.96
	.69	.71	.73	.75	.77	.79	.81	.83	.85	.87	.90	.92	.94	.96	.98	1.00
52.0	.63	.65	.67	.68	.70	.72	.74	.75	.77	.79	.80	.82	.84	.86	.87	.89
	.64	.66	.68	.70	.72	.74	.76	.78	.79	.81	.83	.85	.87	.88	.90	.92
50.0	.58	.60	.61	.63	.64	.66	.68	.69	.71	.73	.74	.76	.78	.80	.81	.83
	.60	.61	.63	.65	.66	.68	.70	.71	.73	.75	.76	.78	.80	.82	.83	.85
48.0	.54	.55	.56	.58	.60	.61	.62	.64	.66	.67	.68	.70	.72	.73	.74	.76
	.55	.57	.58	.60	.61	.63	.65	.66	.68	.69	.71	.73	.74	.76	.77	.79
46.0	.49	.50	.52	.53	.55	.56	.57	.59	.60	.62	.63	.64	.66	.67	.69	.70
	.50	.52	.54	.55	.56	.58	.59	.61	.62	.64	.65	.66	.68	.69	.71	.72
44.0	.45	.46	.47	.49	.50	.51	.52	.54	.55	.56	.58	.59	.60	.61	.63	.64
	.46	.47	.49	.50	.52	.53	.54	.56	.57	.58	.60	.61	.62	.63	.65	.66
42.0	.41	.42	.43	.45	.46	.47	.48	.49	.50	.51	.52	.54	.55	.56	.57	.58
	.42	.43	.44	.46	.47	.48	.49	.50	.52	.53	.54	.55	.56	.58	.59	.60
40.0	.37	.38	.39	.40	.41	.42	.43	.44	.45	.46	.48	.49	.50	.51	.52	.53
	.38	.39	.40	.41	.42	.43	.44	.45	.46	.47	.48	.50	.51	.52	.53	.54

APPENDIX B (continued)

TABLE IV. Change in Reduced Vergence Due to Thickness for a Given Initial Vergence and Refractive Index of 1.49 (Plastics in Air)
(In each cell, the upper figure applies to divergent light, and the lower figure to convergent light)

.51	.52	.53	.54	.55	.56	.57	.58	.59	.60	.61	.62	.63	.64	.65	.66	.67	.68
3.31	3.37	3.44	3.50	3.56	3.62	3.68	3.75	3.81	3.87	3.93	3.99	4.06	4.12	4.18	4.24	4.30	4.37
3.54	3.62	3.69	3.76	3.84	3.91	3.98	4.05	4.13	4.20	4.27	4.35	4.42	4.49	4.56	4.64	4.71	4.78
3.18	3.24	3.30	3.36	3.42	3.48	3.54	3.60	3.66	3.72	3.78	3.84	3.90	3.96	4.02	4.07	4.13	4.19
3.40	3.47	3.54	3.61	3.68	3.75	3.82	3.89	3.96	4.03	4.10	4.17	4.24	4.31	4.38	4.45	4.52	4.59
3.06	3.11	3.17	3.23	3.28	3.34	3.40	3.46	3.51	3.57	3.63	3.68	3.74	3.80	3.86	3.91	3.97	4.03
3.27	3.33	3.40	3.46	3.53	3.60	3.66	3.73	3.79	3.86	3.93	3.99	4.06	4.13	4.20	4.26	4.33	4.40
2.93	2.98	3.04	3.09	3.15	3.21	3.26	3.32	3.37	3.43	3.48	3.54	3.60	3.65	3.70	3.76	3.82	3.87
3.12	3.19	3.25	3.32	3.38	3.44	3.51	3.57	3.64	3.70	3.76	3.83	3.89	3.96	4.02	4.08	4.15	4.21
2.81	2.87	2.92	2.97	3.02	3.08	3.13	3.18	3.24	3.29	3.34	3.39	3.45	3.50	3.55	3.60	3.65	3.71
2.99	3.05	3.11	3.17	3.24	3.30	3.36	3.42	3.48	3.54	3.60	3.66	3.73	3.79	3.85	3.91	3.97	4.04
2.69	2.74	2.79	2.84	2.90	2.95	3.00	3.05	3.10	3.15	3.20	3.25	3.30	3.35	3.40	3.45	3.50	3.55
2.86	2.92	2.97	3.03	3.09	3.15	3.21	3.26	3.32	3.38	3.44	3.50	3.56	3.62	3.68	3.73	3.79	3.85
2.57	2.62	2.67	2.72	2.76	2.81	2.86	2.91	2.96	3.01	3.06	3.11	3.15	3.20	3.25	3.30	3.35	3.39
2.74	2.79	2.84	2.90	2.96	3.01	3.06	3.12	3.18	3.23	3.29	3.34	3.40	3.45	3.51	3.57	3.62	3.68
2.46	2.50	2.55	2.60	2.64	2.69	2.74	2.79	2.83	2.88	2.93	2.97	3.02	3.06	3.11	3.16	3.20	3.25
2.61	2.67	2.72	2.77	2.82	2.88	2.93	2.98	3.04	3.09	3.14	3.20	3.25	3.30	3.36	3.41	3.46	3.51
2.34	2.39	2.44	2.48	2.52	2.57	2.62	2.66	2.70	2.75	2.79	2.84	2.88	2.93	2.97	3.01	3.06	3.10
2.49	2.54	2.59	2.64	2.69	2.74	2.79	2.84	2.89	2.94	2.99	3.04	3.09	3.14	3.20	3.25	3.30	3.35
2.24	2.28	2.33	2.37	2.41	2.45	2.49	2.54	2.58	2.62	2.66	2.70	2.75	2.79	2.83	2.87	2.91	2.96
2.37	2.42	2.46	2.51	2.56	2.61	2.66	2.70	2.75	2.80	2.85	2.90	2.95	3.00	3.04	3.09	3.14	3.19
2.13	2.17	2.21	2.25	2.30	2.34	2.38	2.42	2.46	2.50	2.54	2.58	2.62	2.66	2.70	2.74	2.78	2.82
2.26	2.30	2.34	2.39	2.44	2.48	2.52	2.57	2.62	2.66	2.71	2.75	2.80	2.84	2.89	2.94	2.98	3.03
2.03	2.07	2.11	2.15	2.18	2.22	2.26	2.30	2.34	2.38	2.42	2.46	2.49	2.53	2.57	2.61	2.65	2.68
2.14	2.19	2.23	2.27	2.32	2.36	2.40	2.44	2.49	2.53	2.57	2.62	2.66	2.71	2.75	2.79	2.84	2.88
1.93	1.96	2.00	2.04	2.08	2.11	2.15	2.19	2.22	2.26	2.30	2.33	2.37	2.40	2.44	2.48	2.51	2.55
2.03	2.07	2.11	2.15	2.20	2.24	2.28	2.32	2.36	2.40	2.44	2.48	2.52	2.56	2.60	2.65	2.69	2.73
1.82	1.86	1.90	1.93	1.96	2.00	2.04	2.07	2.10	2.14	2.18	2.21	2.24	2.28	2.32	2.35	2.38	2.42
1.92	1.96	2.00	2.04	2.08	2.11	2.15	2.19	2.23	2.27	2.31	2.35	2.39	2.43	2.47	2.51	2.55	2.59
1.73	1.77	1.80	1.83	1.86	1.90	1.93	1.96	2.00	2.03	2.06	2.10	2.13	2.16	2.20	2.23	2.26	2.29
1.82	1.85	1.89	1.93	1.96	2.00	2.04	2.08	2.11	2.15	2.19	2.22	2.26	2.30	2.34	2.37	2.41	2.45
1.64	1.67	1.70	1.73	1.76	1.80	1.83	1.86	1.89	1.92	1.95	1.98	2.01	2.04	2.08	2.11	2.14	2.17
1.72	1.75	1.78	1.82	1.86	1.89	1.92	1.96	2.00	2.03	2.06	2.10	2.14	2.17	2.20	2.24	2.28	2.31
1.55	1.58	1.61	1.64	1.66	1.69	1.72	1.75	1.78	1.81	1.84	1.87	1.90	1.93	1.96	1.99	2.02	2.05
1.62	1.65	1.69	1.72	1.75	1.78	1.81	1.85	1.88	1.91	1.94	1.98	2.01	2.04	2.08	2.11	2.14	2.17
1.46	1.49	1.51	1.54	1.57	1.60	1.63	1.65	1.68	1.71	1.74	1.76	1.79	1.82	1.84	1.87	1.90	1.93
1.52	1.55	1.58	1.61	1.64	1.68	1.71	1.74	1.77	1.80	1.83	1.86	1.89	1.92	1.96	1.99	2.02	2.05
1.38	1.40	1.43	1.45	1.48	1.51	1.53	1.56	1.58	1.61	1.64	1.66	1.69	1.71	1.74	1.77	1.79	1.82
1.43	1.46	1.49	1.52	1.54	1.57	1.60	1.63	1.66	1.69	1.72	1.75	1.78	1.81	1.84	1.86	1.89	1.92
1.28	1.31	1.34	1.36	1.38	1.41	1.44	1.46	1.48	1.51	1.53	1.56	1.58	1.61	1.63	1.65	1.68	1.70
1.35	1.37	1.40	1.43	1.46	1.48	1.51	1.54	1.56	1.59	1.62	1.64	1.67	1.70	1.72	1.75	1.78	1.81
1.20	1.23	1.25	1.28	1.30	1.32	1.35	1.37	1.40	1.42	1.44	1.46	1.49	1.51	1.53	1.55	1.57	1.60
1.26	1.28	1.31	1.33	1.36	1.39	1.41	1.44	1.46	1.49	1.52	1.54	1.56	1.59	1.62	1.64	1.66	1.69
1.13	1.15	1.18	1.20	1.22	1.24	1.26	1.29	1.31	1.33	1.35	1.37	1.40	1.42	1.44	1.46	1.48	1.51
1.17	1.20	1.22	1.25	1.27	1.29	1.32	1.34	1.37	1.39	1.41	1.44	1.46	1.48	1.50	1.53	1.55	1.57
1.05	1.07	1.09	1.11	1.13	1.15	1.17	1.19	1.21	1.23	1.25	1.27	1.29	1.31	1.34	1.36	1.38	1.40
1.09	1.11	1.14	1.16	1.18	1.20	1.22	1.24	1.27	1.29	1.31	1.33	1.36	1.38	1.40	1.42	1.44	1.47
.98	1.00	1.02	1.04	1.06	1.07	1.09	1.11	1.13	1.15	1.17	1.19	1.21	1.23	1.24	1.26	1.28	1.30
1.02	1.04	1.06	1.08	1.10	1.12	1.14	1.16	1.18	1.20	1.22	1.24	1.26	1.28	1.30	1.33	1.35	1.37
.91	.93	.94	.96	.98	1.00	1.02	1.03	1.05	1.07	1.09	1.10	1.12	1.14	1.16	1.17	1.19	1.21
.94	.96	.98	1.00	1.02	1.03	1.05	1.07	1.09	1.11	1.13	1.15	1.17	1.19	1.20	1.22	1.24	1.26
.85	.86	.88	.89	.91	.93	.94	.96	.97	.99	1.01	1.02	1.04	1.05	1.07	1.09	1.10	1.12
.87	.89	.90	.92	.94	.96	.98	.99	1.01	1.03	1.05	1.06	1.08	1.10	1.12	1.13	1.15	1.17
.78	.79	.80	.82	.84	.85	.86	.88	.90	.91	.92	.94	.96	.97	.98	1.00	1.02	1.03
.81	.82	.84	.85	.87	.89	.90	.92	.93	.95	.97	.98	1.00	1.01	1.03	1.05	1.06	1.08
.71	.73	.74	.76	.77	.78	.80	.81	.83	.84	.85	.87	.88	.89	.90	.92	.93	.94
.74	.75	.76	.78	.80	.81	.82	.84	.86	.87	.88	.90	.92	.93	.94	.96	.98	.99
.65	.67	.68	.69	.70	.72	.73	.74	.76	.77	.78	.79	.81	.82	.83	.84	.85	.87
.67	.69	.70	.71	.72	.74	.75	.76	.78	.79	.80	.82	.83	.85	.86	.87	.89	.90
.59	.60	.62	.63	.64	.65	.66	.68	.69	.70	.71	.72	.73	.74	.76	.77	.78	.79
.61	.62	.64	.65	.66	.67	.68	.70	.71	.72	.73	.75	.76	.77	.78	.80	.81	.82
.54	.55	.56	.57	.58	.59	.60	.61	.62	.63	.64	.65	.66	.67	.68	.70	.71	.72
.55	.56	.57	.58	.60	.61	.62	.63	.64	.65	.66	.67	.69	.70	.71	.72	.73	.75

APPENDIX B (continued)

TABLE IV. Change in Reduced Vergence Due to Thickness for a Given Initial Vergence and Refractive Index of 1.49 (Plastics in Air)
(In each cell, the upper figure applies to divergent light, and the lower figure to convergent light)

Initial vergence	Thickness (mm)															
D	.69	.70	.71	.72	.73	.74	.75	.76	.77	.78	.79	.80	.81	.82	.83	.84
100.0	4.43 4.86	4.49 4.93	4.55 5.00	4.61 5.08	4.67 5.15	4.73 5.23	4.80 5.30	4.86 5.37	4.92 5.45	4.98 5.52	5.04 5.60	5.10 5.67	5.16 5.75	5.22 5.82	5.28 5.90	5.34 5.97
98.0	4.25 4.66	4.31 4.73	4.37 4.80	4.43 4.87	4.49 4.94	4.55 5.01	4.60 5.08	4.66 5.16	4.72 5.23	4.78 5.30	4.84 5.37	4.90 5.44	4.96 5.51	5.02 5.59	5.07 5.66	5.13 5.73
96.0	4.08 4.46	4.14 4.53	4.20 4.60	4.25 4.67	4.31 4.74	4.37 4.81	4.42 4.88	4.48 4.94	4.54 5.01	4.60 5.08	4.65 5.15	4.71 5.22	4.76 5.29	4.82 5.36	4.88 5.43	4.93 5.50
94.0	3.92 4.28	3.98 4.34	4.03 4.41	4.09 4.47	4.14 4.54	4.20 4.60	4.25 4.67	4.30 4.74	4.36 4.80	4.41 4.87	4.47 4.93	4.52 5.00	4.57 5.07	4.63 5.13	4.68 5.20	4.73 5.26
92.0	3.76 4.10	3.81 4.16	3.86 4.22	3.91 4.28	3.97 4.35	4.02 4.41	4.07 4.47	4.12 4.53	4.17 4.59	4.23 4.66	4.28 4.72	4.33 4.78	4.38 4.84	4.43 4.91	4.48 4.97	4.53 5.03
90.0	3.60 3.91	3.65 3.97	3.70 4.03	3.75 4.09	3.80 4.15	3.85 4.21	3.90 4.27	3.95 4.33	4.00 4.39	4.05 4.45	4.10 4.51	4.15 4.57	4.20 4.63	4.25 4.69	4.30 4.75	4.35 4.81
88.0	3.44 3.73	3.49 3.79	3.54 3.85	3.59 3.90	3.63 3.96	3.68 4.02	3.73 4.08	3.78 4.13	3.83 4.19	3.87 4.25	3.92 4.30	3.97 4.36	4.02 4.42	4.06 4.48	4.11 4.53	4.16 4.59
86.0	3.29 3.57	3.34 3.62	3.39 3.67	3.43 3.73	3.48 3.78	3.52 3.84	3.57 3.89	3.62 3.94	3.66 4.00	3.71 4.05	3.75 4.11	3.80 4.16	3.84 4.22	3.89 4.27	3.94 4.32	3.98 4.38
84.0	3.15 3.40	3.19 3.45	3.23 3.50	3.28 3.55	3.32 3.61	3.36 3.66	3.40 3.71	3.45 3.76	3.49 3.81	3.53 3.87	3.58 3.92	3.62 3.97	3.66 4.02	3.71 4.07	3.75 4.13	3.80 4.18
82.0	3.00 3.24	3.04 3.29	3.08 3.34	3.12 3.39	3.17 3.44	3.21 3.49	3.25 3.54	3.29 3.58	3.33 3.63	3.38 3.68	3.42 3.73	3.46 3.78	3.50 3.83	3.54 3.88	3.58 3.93	3.62 3.98
80.0	2.86 3.07	2.90 3.12	2.94 3.17	2.98 3.21	3.02 3.26	3.06 3.31	3.10 3.36	3.13 3.40	3.17 3.45	3.21 3.50	3.25 3.54	3.29 3.59	3.33 3.64	3.37 3.68	3.41 3.73	3.45 3.78
78.0	2.72 2.93	2.76 2.97	2.80 3.01	2.84 3.06	2.87 3.10	2.91 3.15	2.95 3.19	2.99 3.23	3.03 3.28	3.06 3.32	3.10 3.37	3.14 3.41	3.18 3.46	3.21 3.50	3.25 3.54	3.29 3.59
76.0	2.58 2.77	2.62 2.81	2.66 2.85	2.69 2.89	2.73 2.94	2.76 2.98	2.80 3.02	2.84 3.06	2.87 3.10	2.91 3.15	2.94 3.19	2.98 3.23	3.02 3.27	3.05 3.32	3.09 3.36	3.12 3.40
74.0	2.46 2.63	2.49 2.67	2.52 2.71	2.56 2.75	2.59 2.79	2.63 2.83	2.66 2.86	2.69 2.90	2.73 2.94	2.76 2.98	2.80 3.02	2.83 3.06	2.86 3.10	2.90 3.14	2.93 3.18	2.97 3.22
72.0	2.33 2.48	2.36 2.52	2.39 2.56	2.42 2.60	2.46 2.63	2.49 2.67	2.52 2.71	2.55 2.75	2.58 2.79	2.62 2.82	2.65 2.86	2.68 2.90	2.71 2.94	2.74 2.97	2.78 3.01	2.81 3.05
70.0	2.20 2.34	2.23 2.38	2.26 2.42	2.29 2.45	2.32 2.48	2.35 2.52	2.38 2.56	2.42 2.59	2.45 2.62	2.48 2.66	2.51 2.70	2.54 2.73	2.57 2.77	2.60 2.80	2.63 2.84	2.66 2.87
68.0	2.08 2.21	2.11 2.24	2.14 2.27	2.17 2.31	2.20 2.34	2.23 2.38	2.26 2.41	2.28 2.44	2.31 2.48	2.34 2.51	2.37 2.55	2.40 2.58	2.43 2.61	2.46 2.65	2.48 2.68	2.51 2.71
66.0	1.95 2.08	1.98 2.11	2.01 2.14	2.04 2.17	2.06 2.20	2.09 2.23	2.12 2.26	2.15 2.30	2.18 2.33	2.20 2.36	2.23 2.39	2.26 2.42	2.29 2.45	2.31 2.48	2.34 2.52	2.37 2.55
64.0	1.84 1.95	1.87 1.98	1.90 2.01	1.92 2.04	1.95 2.07	1.97 2.10	2.00 2.13	2.03 2.16	2.05 2.19	2.08 2.22	2.10 2.25	2.13 2.28	2.16 2.31	2.18 2.34	2.20 2.37	2.23 2.40
62.0	1.73 1.83	1.75 1.86	1.78 1.89	1.80 1.92	1.82 1.94	1.85 1.97	1.88 2.00	1.90 2.03	1.92 2.06	1.95 2.08	1.98 2.11	2.00 2.14	2.02 2.17	2.05 2.19	2.07 2.22	2.10 2.25
60.0	1.62 1.72	1.64 1.74	1.66 1.77	1.69 1.79	1.71 1.82	1.73 1.84	1.76 1.87	1.78 1.90	1.80 1.92	1.82 1.95	1.85 1.97	1.87 2.00	1.89 2.03	1.92 2.05	1.94 2.08	1.96 2.10
58.0	1.53 1.60	1.55 1.62	1.57 1.64	1.59 1.67	1.61 1.69	1.63 1.72	1.66 1.74	1.68 1.76	1.70 1.79	1.72 1.81	1.74 1.84	1.76 1.86	1.78 1.88	1.80 1.91	1.82 1.94	1.84 1.96
56.0	1.42 1.49	1.44 1.51	1.46 1.53	1.48 1.56	1.50 1.58	1.52 1.60	1.54 1.62	1.55 1.65	1.57 1.67	1.59 1.69	1.61 1.72	1.63 1.74	1.65 1.76	1.67 1.78	1.69 1.81	1.71 1.83
54.0	1.32 1.39	1.34 1.41	1.36 1.43	1.38 1.45	1.39 1.47	1.41 1.49	1.43 1.51	1.45 1.53	1.47 1.55	1.48 1.57	1.50 1.59	1.52 1.61	1.54 1.63	1.56 1.65	1.58 1.67	1.60 1.69
52.0	1.22 1.28	1.24 1.30	1.26 1.32	1.27 1.34	1.29 1.36	1.31 1.38	1.32 1.40	1.34 1.41	1.36 1.43	1.38 1.45	1.39 1.47	1.41 1.49	1.43 1.51	1.44 1.53	1.46 1.55	1.48 1.57
50.0	1.13 1.18	1.15 1.20	1.17 1.22	1.18 1.24	1.20 1.25	1.21 1.27	1.23 1.29	1.25 1.31	1.26 1.33	1.28 1.34	1.29 1.36	1.31 1.38	1.33 1.40	1.34 1.42	1.36 1.43	1.37 1.45
48.0	1.04 1.09	1.06 1.11	1.08 1.13	1.09 1.14	1.10 1.16	1.12 1.17	1.14 1.19	1.15 1.21	1.16 1.22	1.18 1.24	1.20 1.25	1.21 1.27	1.22 1.29	1.24 1.30	1.25 1.32	1.27 1.33
46.0	.96 1.00	.97 1.02	.98 1.03	1.00 1.05	1.01 1.06	1.03 1.08	1.04 1.09	1.05 1.10	1.07 1.12	1.08 1.13	1.10 1.15	1.11 1.16	1.12 1.18	1.14 1.19	1.15 1.20	1.16 1.22
44.0	.88 .92	.89 .93	.90 .94	.92 .96	.93 .97	.94 .98	.96 1.00	.97 1.01	.98 1.02	.99 1.03	1.01 1.05	1.02 1.06	1.03 1.07	1.04 1.09	1.06 1.10	1.07 1.12
42.0	.80 .84	.81 .85	.82 .86	.83 .87	.85 .89	.86 .90	.87 .91	.88 .92	.89 .93	.91 .95	.92 .96	.93 .97	.94 .98	.95 .99	.96 1.01	.97 1.02
40.0	.73 .76	.74 .77	.75 .78	.76 .79	.77 .80	.78 .81	.79 .82	.80 .84	.81 .85	.82 .86	.83 .87	.84 .88	.85 .89	.86 .90	.87 .91	.88 .92

APPENDIX B (continued)

TABLE IV. *Change in Reduced Vergence Due to Thickness for a Given Initial Vergence and Refractive Index of 1.49 (Plastics in Air)*
(In each cell, the upper figure applies to divergent light, and the lower figure to convergent light)

.85	.86	.87	.88	.89	.90	.91	.92	.93	.94	.95	.96	.97	.98	.99	1.00	1.01	1.02
5.40 / 6.05	5.46 / 6.13	5.52 / 6.20	5.58 / 6.28	5.64 / 6.35	5.70 / 6.43	5.76 / 6.51	5.82 / 6.58	5.88 / 6.66	5.94 / 6.73	6.00 / 6.81	6.05 / 6.89	6.11 / 6.96	6.17 / 7.04	6.23 / 7.11	6.29 / 7.19	6.35 / 7.27	6.41 / 7.35
5.19 / 5.80	5.25 / 5.88	5.31 / 5.95	5.36 / 6.02	5.42 / 6.10	5.48 / 6.17	5.54 / 6.24	5.59 / 6.32	5.65 / 6.39	5.71 / 6.46	5.76 / 6.54	5.82 / 6.61	5.88 / 6.68	5.94 / 6.75	5.99 / 6.83	6.05 / 6.90	6.11 / 6.97	6.16 / 7.05
4.98 / 5.56	5.04 / 5.63	5.10 / 5.70	5.15 / 5.77	5.20 / 5.84	5.26 / 5.91	5.32 / 5.98	5.37 / 6.05	5.42 / 6.12	5.48 / 6.19	5.54 / 6.26	5.59 / 6.33	5.64 / 6.40	5.70 / 6.47	5.76 / 6.54	5.81 / 6.61	5.86 / 6.68	5.92 / 6.75
4.78 / 5.33	4.84 / 5.40	4.89 / 5.46	4.94 / 5.53	5.00 / 5.59	5.05 / 5.66	5.10 / 5.73	5.16 / 5.79	5.21 / 5.86	5.26 / 5.93	5.32 / 6.00	5.37 / 6.06	5.42 / 6.13	5.47 / 6.20	5.53 / 6.26	5.58 / 6.33	5.63 / 6.40	5.68 / 6.47
4.58 / 5.10	4.64 / 5.16	4.69 / 5.22	4.74 / 5.28	4.79 / 5.35	4.84 / 5.41	4.89 / 5.47	4.94 / 5.54	4.99 / 5.60	5.04 / 5.67	5.10 / 5.73	5.15 / 5.79	5.20 / 5.86	5.25 / 5.92	5.30 / 6.00	5.35 / 6.05	5.40 / 6.12	5.45 / 6.18
4.40 / 4.87	4.44 / 4.93	4.49 / 4.99	4.54 / 5.05	4.59 / 5.11	4.64 / 5.17	4.69 / 5.23	4.74 / 5.29	4.79 / 5.36	4.84 / 5.42	4.88 / 5.48	4.93 / 5.54	4.98 / 5.60	5.03 / 5.67	5.08 / 5.73	5.13 / 5.79	5.18 / 5.85	5.23 / 5.91
4.20 / 4.65	4.25 / 4.71	4.30 / 4.77	4.35 / 4.82	4.39 / 4.88	4.44 / 4.94	4.49 / 5.00	4.53 / 5.06	4.58 / 5.11	4.63 / 5.17	4.68 / 5.23	4.72 / 5.29	4.77 / 5.35	4.82 / 5.40	4.86 / 5.46	4.91 / 5.52	4.96 / 5.58	5.00 / 5.64
4.02 / 4.44	4.07 / 4.49	4.12 / 4.54	4.16 / 4.60	4.20 / 4.66	4.25 / 4.71	4.29 / 4.77	4.34 / 4.82	4.38 / 4.88	4.43 / 4.93	4.47 / 4.99	4.51 / 5.05	4.56 / 5.10	4.60 / 5.16	4.65 / 5.21	4.69 / 5.27	4.73 / 5.33	4.78 / 5.38
3.84 / 4.23	3.88 / 4.28	3.93 / 4.33	3.97 / 4.39	4.02 / 4.44	4.06 / 4.49	4.10 / 4.54	4.14 / 4.60	4.19 / 4.65	4.23 / 4.70	4.27 / 4.76	4.31 / 4.81	4.35 / 4.86	4.40 / 4.91	4.44 / 4.97	4.48 / 5.02	4.52 / 5.07	4.56 / 5.13
3.66 / 4.02	3.71 / 4.07	3.75 / 4.12	3.79 / 4.17	3.83 / 4.22	3.87 / 4.27	3.91 / 4.32	3.95 / 4.37	3.99 / 4.42	4.03 / 4.47	4.08 / 4.52	4.12 / 4.58	4.16 / 4.63	4.20 / 4.68	4.24 / 4.73	4.28 / 4.78	4.32 / 4.83	4.36 / 4.88
3.49 / 3.82	3.53 / 3.87	3.57 / 3.92	3.61 / 3.97	3.65 / 4.01	3.69 / 4.06	3.73 / 4.11	3.77 / 4.16	3.81 / 4.20	3.85 / 4.25	3.88 / 4.30	3.92 / 4.35	3.96 / 4.40	4.00 / 4.44	4.04 / 4.49	4.08 / 4.54	4.12 / 4.59	4.16 / 4.64
3.32 / 3.64	3.36 / 3.68	3.40 / 3.72	3.44 / 3.77	3.47 / 3.82	3.51 / 3.86	3.55 / 3.90	3.58 / 3.95	3.62 / 4.00	3.66 / 4.04	3.69 / 4.08	3.73 / 4.13	3.77 / 4.18	3.81 / 4.22	3.84 / 4.26	3.88 / 4.31	3.92 / 4.36	3.95 / 4.40
3.16 / 3.44	3.20 / 3.49	3.23 / 3.53	3.27 / 3.57	3.30 / 3.62	3.34 / 3.66	3.38 / 3.70	3.41 / 3.74	3.44 / 3.79	3.48 / 3.83	3.52 / 3.87	3.55 / 3.91	3.58 / 3.95	3.62 / 4.00	3.66 / 4.04	3.69 / 4.08	3.72 / 4.12	3.76 / 4.17
3.00 / 3.26	3.03 / 3.30	3.07 / 3.34	3.10 / 3.38	3.14 / 3.42	3.17 / 3.46	3.20 / 3.50	3.24 / 3.54	3.27 / 3.58	3.30 / 3.62	3.34 / 3.66	3.37 / 3.71	3.40 / 3.75	3.43 / 3.79	3.47 / 3.83	3.50 / 3.87	3.53 / 3.91	3.57 / 3.95
2.84 / 3.08	2.87 / 3.12	2.90 / 3.16	2.94 / 3.20	2.97 / 3.23	3.00 / 3.27	3.03 / 3.30	3.06 / 3.35	3.10 / 3.39	3.13 / 3.43	3.16 / 3.46	3.19 / 3.50	3.22 / 3.54	3.26 / 3.58	3.29 / 3.62	3.32 / 3.66	3.35 / 3.70	3.38 / 3.74
2.69 / 2.91	2.72 / 2.95	2.75 / 2.98	2.78 / 3.02	2.81 / 3.05	2.84 / 3.09	2.87 / 3.13	2.90 / 3.16	2.93 / 3.20	2.96 / 3.23	2.99 / 3.27	3.02 / 3.31	3.05 / 3.34	3.08 / 3.38	3.11 / 3.41	3.14 / 3.45	3.17 / 3.49	3.20 / 3.52
2.54 / 2.74	2.57 / 2.78	2.60 / 2.81	2.62 / 2.84	2.65 / 2.88	2.68 / 2.91	2.71 / 2.94	2.74 / 2.98	2.77 / 3.01	2.80 / 3.05	2.82 / 3.08	2.85 / 3.11	2.88 / 3.15	2.91 / 3.18	2.94 / 3.22	2.97 / 3.25	3.00 / 3.28	3.03 / 3.32
2.40 / 2.58	2.42 / 2.61	2.45 / 2.64	2.48 / 2.68	2.50 / 2.71	2.53 / 2.74	2.56 / 2.77	2.58 / 2.80	2.61 / 2.84	2.64 / 2.87	2.66 / 2.90	2.69 / 2.93	2.72 / 2.96	2.75 / 3.00	2.77 / 3.03	2.80 / 3.06	2.83 / 3.09	2.85 / 3.12
2.26 / 2.42	2.28 / 2.45	2.30 / 2.48	2.33 / 2.51	2.36 / 2.54	2.38 / 2.57	2.41 / 2.60	2.43 / 2.63	2.46 / 2.66	2.48 / 2.69	2.51 / 2.72	2.54 / 2.75	2.56 / 2.78	2.59 / 2.81	2.61 / 2.84	2.64 / 2.87	2.66 / 2.90	2.69 / 2.93
2.12 / 2.28	2.14 / 2.30	2.17 / 2.33	2.19 / 2.36	2.22 / 2.38	2.24 / 2.41	2.26 / 2.44	2.29 / 2.47	2.31 / 2.49	2.34 / 2.52	2.36 / 2.55	2.38 / 2.58	2.41 / 2.61	2.43 / 2.63	2.46 / 2.66	2.48 / 2.69	2.50 / 2.72	2.53 / 2.75
1.98 / 2.13	2.01 / 2.16	2.03 / 2.18	2.05 / 2.21	2.08 / 2.23	2.10 / 2.26	2.12 / 2.29	2.14 / 2.31	2.17 / 2.34	2.19 / 2.36	2.21 / 2.39	2.23 / 2.42	2.25 / 2.44	2.28 / 2.47	2.30 / 2.49	2.32 / 2.52	2.34 / 2.55	2.36 / 2.57
1.86 / 1.98	1.89 / 2.01	1.91 / 2.04	1.93 / 2.06	1.95 / 2.08	1.97 / 2.11	1.99 / 2.13	2.01 / 2.16	2.03 / 2.18	2.05 / 2.21	2.08 / 2.23	2.10 / 2.25	2.12 / 2.28	2.14 / 2.30	2.16 / 2.33	2.18 / 2.35	2.20 / 2.37	2.22 / 2.40
1.73 / 1.85	1.75 / 1.87	1.77 / 1.89	1.79 / 1.92	1.81 / 1.94	1.83 / 1.96	1.85 / 1.98	1.87 / 2.01	1.89 / 2.03	1.91 / 2.05	1.93 / 2.08	1.95 / 2.10	1.97 / 2.12	1.99 / 2.14	2.01 / 2.17	2.03 / 2.19	2.05 / 2.21	2.07 / 2.24
1.62 / 1.72	1.63 / 1.74	1.65 / 1.76	1.67 / 1.78	1.69 / 1.80	1.71 / 1.82	1.73 / 1.84	1.75 / 1.86	1.76 / 1.88	1.78 / 1.90	1.80 / 1.92	1.82 / 1.95	1.84 / 1.97	1.85 / 1.99	1.87 / 2.01	1.89 / 2.03	1.91 / 2.05	1.93 / 2.07
1.50 / 1.59	1.51 / 1.61	1.53 / 1.63	1.55 / 1.65	1.56 / 1.67	1.58 / 1.69	1.60 / 1.71	1.61 / 1.73	1.63 / 1.75	1.65 / 1.77	1.66 / 1.78	1.68 / 1.80	1.70 / 1.82	1.72 / 1.84	1.73 / 1.86	1.75 / 1.88	1.77 / 1.90	1.78 / 1.92
1.39 / 1.47	1.41 / 1.49	1.42 / 1.51	1.44 / 1.52	1.45 / 1.54	1.47 / 1.56	1.49 / 1.58	1.50 / 1.60	1.51 / 1.61	1.53 / 1.63	1.55 / 1.65	1.56 / 1.67	1.57 / 1.69	1.59 / 1.70	1.61 / 1.72	1.62 / 1.74	1.64 / 1.76	1.65 / 1.78
1.28 / 1.35	1.29 / 1.37	1.31 / 1.38	1.32 / 1.40	1.34 / 1.41	1.35 / 1.43	1.36 / 1.45	1.38 / 1.46	1.40 / 1.48	1.41 / 1.50	1.42 / 1.52	1.44 / 1.53	1.46 / 1.55	1.47 / 1.57	1.48 / 1.58	1.50 / 1.60	1.51 / 1.62	1.53 / 1.63
1.18 / 1.24	1.19 / 1.25	1.20 / 1.26	1.21 / 1.28	1.23 / 1.30	1.24 / 1.31	1.25 / 1.33	1.27 / 1.34	1.28 / 1.36	1.30 / 1.37	1.31 / 1.39	1.32 / 1.41	1.34 / 1.42	1.35 / 1.44	1.37 / 1.45	1.38 / 1.47	1.39 / 1.48	1.41 / 1.50
1.08 / 1.13	1.09 / 1.14	1.10 / 1.16	1.12 / 1.17	1.13 / 1.19	1.14 / 1.20	1.15 / 1.21	1.16 / 1.23	1.18 / 1.24	1.19 / 1.26	1.20 / 1.27	1.21 / 1.28	1.22 / 1.30	1.24 / 1.31	1.25 / 1.33	1.26 / 1.34	1.27 / 1.35	1.28 / 1.37
.98 / 1.03	1.00 / 1.04	1.01 / 1.05	1.02 / 1.07	1.03 / 1.08	1.04 / 1.09	1.05 / 1.10	1.06 / 1.12	1.07 / 1.13	1.08 / 1.14	1.10 / 1.16	1.11 / 1.17	1.12 / 1.18	1.13 / 1.19	1.14 / 1.21	1.15 / 1.22	1.16 / 1.23	1.17 / 1.24
.89 / .94	.90 / .95	.91 / .96	.92 / .97	.93 / .98	.94 / .99	.95 / 1.00	.96 / 1.01	.97 / 1.02	.98 / 1.03	1.00 / 1.04	1.01 / 1.06	1.02 / 1.07	1.03 / 1.08	1.04 / 1.09	1.05 / 1.10	1.06 / 1.11	1.07 / 1.12

TABLE IV. Change in Reduced Vergence Due to Thickness for a Given Initial Vergence and Refractive Index of 1.49 (Plastics in Air)
(In each cell, the upper figure applies to divergent light, and the lower figure to convergent light)

Initial vergence	Thickness (mm)															
	1.03	1.04	1.05	1.06	1.07	1.08	1.09	1.10	1.11	1.12	1.13	1.14	1.15	1.16	1.17	1.18
D 100.0	6.46	6.52	6.58	6.64	6.70	6.75	6.81	6.87	6.93	6.99	7.04	7.10	7.16	7.22	7.28	7.33
	7.42	7.50	7.58	7.66	7.74	7.81	7.89	7.97	8.05	8.13	8.21	8.29	8.36	8.44	8.52	8.60
98.0	6.22	6.27	6.33	6.39	6.44	6.50	6.55	6.61	6.67	6.72	6.78	6.83	6.89	6.95	7.00	7.06
	7.12	7.20	7.27	7.34	7.42	7.49	7.57	7.64	7.72	7.79	7.87	7.94	8.02	8.10	8.17	8.25
96.0	5.97	6.03	6.08	6.13	6.19	6.24	6.30	6.35	6.40	6.46	6.51	6.57	6.62	6.67	6.73	6.78
	6.82	6.89	6.96	7.04	7.11	7.18	7.25	7.32	7.39	7.46	7.54	7.61	7.68	7.75	7.82	7.90
94.0	5.74	5.79	5.84	5.89	5.94	6.00	6.05	6.10	6.15	6.20	6.26	6.31	6.36	6.41	6.46	6.52
	6.53	6.60	6.67	6.74	6.81	6.87	6.94	7.01	7.08	7.15	7.22	7.29	7.36	7.42	7.49	7.56
92.0	5.50	5.55	5.60	5.65	5.70	5.75	5.80	5.85	5.90	5.95	6.00	6.05	6.10	6.15	6.20	6.25
	6.24	6.31	6.38	6.44	6.50	6.57	6.64	6.70	6.77	6.83	6.90	6.96	7.03	7.10	7.16	7.23
90.0	5.27	5.32	5.37	5.42	5.47	5.51	5.56	5.61	5.66	5.70	5.75	5.80	5.84	5.89	5.94	5.99
	5.98	6.04	6.10	6.16	6.22	6.29	6.35	6.41	6.47	6.53	6.60	6.66	6.72	6.78	6.84	6.91
88.0	5.05	5.09	5.14	5.19	5.23	5.28	5.32	5.37	5.42	5.46	5.50	5.55	5.60	5.64	5.68	5.73
	5.70	5.76	5.82	5.87	5.93	5.99	6.05	6.11	6.17	6.23	6.29	6.35	6.41	6.47	6.53	6.59
86.0	4.82	4.87	4.91	4.95	5.00	5.04	5.09	5.13	5.17	5.22	5.26	5.31	5.35	5.39	5.44	5.48
	5.44	5.49	5.55	5.61	5.66	5.72	5.77	5.83	5.89	5.94	6.00	6.06	6.12	6.17	6.23	6.29
84.0	4.61	4.65	4.69	4.73	4.77	4.82	4.86	4.90	4.94	4.98	5.03	5.07	5.11	5.15	5.19	5.24
	5.18	5.23	5.28	5.34	5.39	5.44	5.50	5.55	5.60	5.66	5.72	5.77	5.82	5.88	5.94	5.99
82.0	4.40	4.44	4.48	4.52	4.56	4.60	4.64	4.68	4.72	4.76	4.80	4.84	4.88	4.92	4.96	5.00
	4.93	4.98	5.03	5.08	5.13	5.18	5.23	5.28	5.33	5.38	5.44	5.49	5.54	5.59	5.64	5.70
80.0	4.19	4.23	4.27	4.31	4.35	4.38	4.42	4.46	4.50	4.54	4.57	4.61	4.65	4.69	4.73	4.76
	4.68	4.73	4.78	4.83	4.88	4.92	4.97	5.02	5.07	5.12	5.17	5.22	5.26	5.31	5.36	5.41
78.0	3.99	4.03	4.06	4.10	4.14	4.18	4.21	4.25	4.29	4.32	4.36	4.39	4.43	4.47	4.50	4.54
	4.45	4.49	4.54	4.59	4.63	4.68	4.72	4.77	4.82	4.86	4.91	4.95	5.00	5.05	5.09	5.14
76.0	3.80	3.83	3.86	3.90	3.94	3.97	4.00	4.04	4.07	4.11	4.14	4.18	4.21	4.24	4.28	4.31
	4.21	4.26	4.30	4.34	4.39	4.43	4.48	4.52	4.56	4.61	4.65	4.70	4.74	4.78	4.83	4.87
74.0	3.60	3.63	3.66	3.70	3.73	3.76	3.80	3.83	3.86	3.90	3.93	3.96	4.00	4.03	4.06	4.09
	3.99	4.03	4.08	4.12	4.16	4.20	4.24	4.28	4.32	4.36	4.40	4.44	4.48	4.53	4.57	4.61
72.0	3.41	3.44	3.48	3.51	3.54	3.57	3.60	3.63	3.66	3.69	3.73	3.76	3.79	3.82	3.85	3.89
	3.77	3.81	3.85	3.89	3.93	3.96	4.00	4.04	4.08	4.12	4.16	4.20	4.24	4.27	4.31	4.35
70.0	3.23	3.26	3.29	3.32	3.35	3.38	3.41	3.44	3.47	3.50	3.53	3.56	3.59	3.62	3.65	3.68
	3.56	3.59	3.63	3.67	3.70	3.74	3.77	3.81	3.85	3.88	3.92	3.96	4.00	4.03	4.07	4.11
68.0	3.05	3.08	3.11	3.14	3.17	3.19	3.22	3.25	3.28	3.31	3.33	3.36	3.39	3.42	3.45	3.47
	3.35	3.39	3.42	3.45	3.49	3.52	3.56	3.59	3.62	3.66	3.70	3.73	3.76	3.80	3.84	3.87
66.0	2.88	2.91	2.94	2.96	2.99	3.02	3.04	3.07	3.10	3.12	3.15	3.17	3.20	3.23	3.25	3.28
	3.16	3.19	3.22	3.25	3.28	3.32	3.35	3.38	3.41	3.45	3.48	3.51	3.54	3.58	3.61	3.64
64.0	2.72	2.74	2.76	2.79	2.82	2.84	2.86	2.89	2.92	2.94	2.96	2.99	3.02	3.04	3.06	3.09
	2.96	2.99	3.02	3.05	3.08	3.11	3.14	3.17	3.20	3.23	3.26	3.29	3.32	3.36	3.39	3.42
62.0	2.55	2.57	2.60	2.62	2.64	2.66	2.69	2.71	2.73	2.76	2.78	2.81	2.83	2.85	2.88	2.90
	2.77	2.80	2.83	2.86	2.89	2.91	2.94	2.97	3.00	3.03	3.06	3.09	3.12	3.14	3.17	3.20
60.0	2.39	2.41	2.43	2.45	2.47	2.50	2.52	2.54	2.56	2.59	2.61	2.63	2.66	2.68	2.70	2.72
	2.60	2.62	2.65	2.68	2.70	2.73	2.75	2.78	2.81	2.83	2.86	2.89	2.92	2.94	2.97	3.00
58.0	2.24	2.26	2.28	2.31	2.33	2.35	2.37	2.39	2.41	2.43	2.45	2.47	2.50	2.52	2.54	2.56
	2.42	2.45	2.47	2.49	2.52	2.54	2.57	2.59	2.62	2.64	2.66	2.69	2.72	2.74	2.76	2.79
56.0	2.09	2.11	2.12	2.14	2.16	2.18	2.20	2.22	2.24	2.26	2.28	2.30	2.32	2.34	2.36	2.38
	2.26	2.28	2.30	2.33	2.35	2.37	2.40	2.42	2.44	2.46	2.49	2.51	2.53	2.55	2.57	2.60
54.0	1.94	1.96	1.98	2.00	2.02	2.03	2.05	2.07	2.09	2.11	2.12	2.14	2.16	2.18	2.20	2.21
	2.09	2.11	2.14	2.16	2.18	2.20	2.22	2.24	2.26	2.28	2.31	2.33	2.35	2.37	2.39	2.42
52.0	1.80	1.82	1.84	1.85	1.87	1.89	1.90	1.92	1.94	1.95	1.97	1.99	2.00	2.02	2.04	2.06
	1.94	1.96	1.98	2.00	2.02	2.04	2.06	2.08	2.10	2.12	2.14	2.16	2.18	2.19	2.21	2.23
50.0	1.67	1.68	1.70	1.72	1.73	1.75	1.76	1.78	1.80	1.81	1.83	1.84	1.86	1.88	1.89	1.91
	1.79	1.81	1.83	1.85	1.87	1.88	1.90	1.92	1.94	1.96	1.97	1.99	2.01	2.03	2.05	2.06
48.0	1.54	1.56	1.57	1.58	1.60	1.61	1.63	1.64	1.66	1.67	1.68	1.70	1.72	1.73	1.74	1.76
	1.65	1.66	1.68	1.70	1.71	1.73	1.74	1.76	1.78	1.79	1.81	1.83	1.84	1.86	1.88	1.90
46.0	1.42	1.43	1.44	1.46	1.47	1.48	1.50	1.51	1.52	1.54	1.55	1.56	1.58	1.59	1.60	1.61
	1.52	1.53	1.54	1.56	1.58	1.59	1.60	1.62	1.64	1.65	1.66	1.68	1.70	1.71	1.72	1.74
44.0	1.30	1.31	1.32	1.33	1.34	1.36	1.37	1.38	1.39	1.41	1.42	1.43	1.44	1.46	1.47	1.48
	1.38	1.40	1.41	1.42	1.44	1.45	1.47	1.48	1.49	1.51	1.52	1.54	1.55	1.56	1.58	1.59
42.0	1.18	1.19	1.20	1.22	1.23	1.24	1.25	1.26	1.27	1.28	1.29	1.30	1.32	1.33	1.34	1.35
	1.26	1.27	1.28	1.29	1.30	1.32	1.33	1.34	1.35	1.37	1.38	1.39	1.40	1.42	1.43	1.44
40.0	1.08	1.09	1.10	1.11	1.12	1.13	1.14	1.15	1.16	1.17	1.18	1.19	1.20	1.21	1.22	1.23
	1.14	1.15	1.16	1.17	1.18	1.20	1.21	1.22	1.23	1.24	1.25	1.26	1.28	1.29	1.30	1.31

APPENDIX B (continued)

TABLE IV. Change in Reduced Vergence Due to Thickness for a Given Initial Vergence and Refractive Index of 1.49 (Plastics in Air)
(In each cell, the upper figure applies to divergent light, and the lower figure to convergent light)

1.19	1.20	1.21	1.22	1.23	1.24	1.25	1.26	1.27	1.28	1.29	1.30	1.31	1.32	1.33	1.34	1.35	1.36
7.39 / 8.68	7.45 / 8.76	7.51 / 8.84	7.56 / 8.92	7.62 / 9.00	7.68 / 9.08	7.74 / 9.16	7.79 / 9.24	7.85 / 9.32	7.91 / 9.40	7.96 / 9.48	8.02 / 9.56	8.08 / 9.64	8.13 / 9.72	8.19 / 9.80	8.25 / 9.88	8.30 / 9.96	8.36 / 10.05
7.11 / 8.32	7.17 / 8.40	7.22 / 8.48	7.28 / 8.55	7.34 / 8.63	7.39 / 8.70	7.44 / 8.78	7.50 / 8.86	7.56 / 8.93	7.61 / 9.01	7.66 / 9.08	7.72 / 9.16	7.77 / 9.24	7.83 / 9.32	7.88 / 9.39	7.94 / 9.47	7.99 / 9.55	8.04 / 9.63
6.84 / 7.97	6.89 / 8.04	6.94 / 8.11	7.00 / 8.19	7.05 / 8.26	7.10 / 8.34	7.16 / 8.41	7.21 / 8.48	7.26 / 8.56	7.31 / 8.63	7.37 / 8.71	7.42 / 8.78	7.47 / 8.85	7.52 / 8.93	7.58 / 9.00	7.63 / 9.08	7.68 / 9.15	7.73 / 9.22
6.57 / 7.63	6.62 / 7.70	6.67 / 7.77	6.72 / 7.84	6.77 / 7.91	6.82 / 7.98	6.87 / 8.05	6.92 / 8.12	6.97 / 8.19	7.02 / 8.26	7.07 / 8.33	7.12 / 8.40	7.17 / 8.47	7.22 / 8.54	7.27 / 8.61	7.32 / 8.68	7.38 / 8.76	7.43 / 8.83
6.30 / 7.29	6.35 / 7.36	6.40 / 7.43	6.45 / 7.49	6.50 / 7.56	6.55 / 7.63	6.60 / 7.70	6.64 / 7.76	6.69 / 7.83	6.74 / 7.90	6.79 / 7.96	6.84 / 8.03	6.89 / 8.10	6.94 / 8.17	6.98 / 8.23	7.03 / 8.30	7.08 / 8.37	7.13 / 8.44
6.03 / 6.97	6.08 / 7.03	6.13 / 7.09	6.17 / 7.16	6.22 / 7.22	6.27 / 7.29	6.32 / 7.35	6.36 / 7.41	6.41 / 7.48	6.46 / 7.54	6.50 / 7.61	6.55 / 7.67	6.60 / 7.73	6.64 / 7.80	6.69 / 7.86	6.74 / 7.93	6.78 / 7.99	6.83 / 8.05
5.78 / 6.65	5.82 / 6.71	5.86 / 6.77	5.91 / 6.83	5.96 / 6.89	6.00 / 6.95	6.04 / 7.02	6.09 / 7.08	6.14 / 7.14	6.18 / 7.20	6.22 / 7.26	6.27 / 7.32	6.32 / 7.38	6.36 / 7.44	6.40 / 7.50	6.45 / 7.56	6.50 / 7.62	6.54 / 7.69
5.53 / 6.34	5.57 / 6.40	5.61 / 6.46	5.66 / 6.52	5.70 / 6.57	5.74 / 6.63	5.78 / 6.69	5.83 / 6.75	5.87 / 6.81	5.91 / 6.86	5.96 / 6.92	6.00 / 6.98	6.04 / 7.04	6.09 / 7.10	6.13 / 7.15	6.17 / 7.21	6.22 / 7.27	6.26 / 7.35
5.28 / 6.04	5.32 / 6.10	5.36 / 6.15	5.49 / 6.21	5.45 / 6.26	5.49 / 6.32	5.53 / 6.37	5.57 / 6.42	5.61 / 6.48	5.66 / 6.53	5.70 / 6.59	5.74 / 6.64	5.78 / 6.70	5.82 / 6.75	5.86 / 6.81	5.90 / 6.86	5.94 / 6.92	5.98 / 6.98
5.04 / 5.75	5.08 / 5.80	5.12 / 5.85	5.16 / 5.90	5.20 / 5.96	5.24 / 6.01	5.28 / 6.06	5.31 / 6.11	5.35 / 6.16	5.39 / 6.22	5.43 / 6.27	5.47 / 6.32	5.51 / 6.37	5.55 / 6.43	5.59 / 6.48	5.63 / 6.53	5.67 / 6.58	5.71 / 6.64
4.80 / 5.46	4.84 / 5.51	4.88 / 5.56	4.92 / 5.61	4.95 / 5.66	4.99 / 5.71	5.03 / 5.76	5.07 / 5.80	5.11 / 5.85	5.14 / 5.90	5.18 / 5.95	5.22 / 6.00	5.26 / 6.05	5.29 / 6.10	5.33 / 6.15	5.37 / 6.20	5.40 / 6.25	5.44 / 6.30
4.57 / 5.18	4.61 / 5.23	4.65 / 5.28	4.68 / 5.32	4.72 / 5.37	4.75 / 5.42	4.79 / 5.46	4.83 / 5.51	4.86 / 5.56	4.90 / 5.61	4.93 / 5.65	4.97 / 5.70	5.01 / 5.75	5.04 / 5.79	5.08 / 5.84	5.11 / 5.89	5.15 / 5.94	5.19 / 5.98
4.35 / 4.92	4.38 / 4.96	4.42 / 5.00	4.45 / 5.05	4.48 / 5.09	4.52 / 5.14	4.56 / 5.18	4.59 / 5.22	4.62 / 5.27	4.66 / 5.31	4.70 / 5.36	4.73 / 5.40	4.76 / 5.44	4.80 / 5.49	4.83 / 5.53	4.87 / 5.58	4.90 / 5.62	4.93 / 5.66
4.13 / 4.65	4.16 / 4.69	4.19 / 4.73	4.23 / 4.77	4.26 / 4.82	4.29 / 4.86	4.32 / 4.90	4.36 / 4.94	4.39 / 4.98	4.42 / 5.03	4.46 / 5.07	4.49 / 5.11	4.52 / 5.15	4.55 / 5.19	4.59 / 5.24	4.62 / 5.28	4.65 / 5.32	4.68 / 5.36
3.92 / 4.39	3.95 / 4.43	3.98 / 4.47	4.01 / 4.51	4.04 / 4.55	4.07 / 4.59	4.10 / 4.63	4.14 / 4.67	4.17 / 4.71	4.20 / 4.75	4.23 / 4.79	4.26 / 4.83	4.29 / 4.87	4.32 / 4.91	4.35 / 4.95	4.38 / 4.99	4.41 / 5.02	4.44 / 5.06
3.71 / 4.14	3.74 / 4.18	3.77 / 4.22	3.80 / 4.25	3.83 / 4.29	3.86 / 4.33	3.88 / 4.36	3.91 / 4.40	3.94 / 4.44	3.97 / 4.48	4.00 / 4.51	4.03 / 4.55	4.06 / 4.59	4.09 / 4.63	4.12 / 4.66	4.15 / 4.70	4.18 / 4.74	4.20 / 4.78
3.50 / 3.90	3.53 / 3.94	3.56 / 3.98	3.59 / 4.01	3.61 / 4.04	3.64 / 4.08	3.67 / 4.12	3.70 / 4.15	3.73 / 4.18	3.75 / 4.22	3.78 / 4.26	3.81 / 4.29	3.84 / 4.32	3.86 / 4.36	3.89 / 4.40	3.92 / 4.43	3.94 / 4.46	3.97 / 4.50
3.30 / 3.68	3.33 / 3.71	3.36 / 3.74	3.38 / 3.77	3.41 / 3.81	3.43 / 3.84	3.46 / 3.87	3.49 / 3.90	3.51 / 3.93	3.54 / 3.97	3.56 / 4.00	3.59 / 4.03	3.62 / 4.06	3.64 / 4.10	3.67 / 4.13	3.69 / 4.16	3.72 / 4.20	3.75 / 4.23
3.12 / 3.45	3.14 / 3.48	3.16 / 3.51	3.19 / 3.54	3.21 / 3.57	3.24 / 3.60	3.26 / 3.64	3.28 / 3.67	3.31 / 3.70	3.33 / 3.73	3.36 / 3.76	3.38 / 3.79	3.40 / 3.82	3.43 / 3.85	3.46 / 3.88	3.48 / 3.91	3.50 / 3.94	3.53 / 3.97
2.93 / 3.23	2.95 / 3.26	2.97 / 3.29	3.00 / 3.32	3.02 / 3.35	3.04 / 3.38	3.06 / 3.40	3.09 / 3.43	3.11 / 3.46	3.13 / 3.49	3.16 / 3.52	3.18 / 3.55	3.20 / 3.58	3.23 / 3.61	3.25 / 3.64	3.27 / 3.67	3.30 / 3.70	3.32 / 3.72
2.75 / 3.02	2.77 / 3.05	2.79 / 3.08	2.81 / 3.10	2.83 / 3.13	2.85 / 3.15	2.88 / 3.18	2.90 / 3.21	2.92 / 3.23	2.94 / 3.26	2.96 / 3.28	2.98 / 3.31	3.00 / 3.34	3.02 / 3.36	3.05 / 3.39	3.07 / 3.42	3.09 / 3.44	3.11 / 3.47
2.58 / 2.82	2.60 / 2.84	2.62 / 2.86	2.64 / 2.89	2.66 / 2.92	2.68 / 2.94	2.70 / 2.96	2.72 / 2.99	2.74 / 3.02	2.76 / 3.04	2.78 / 3.06	2.80 / 3.09	2.82 / 3.12	2.84 / 3.14	2.86 / 3.16	2.88 / 3.19	2.90 / 3.22	2.93 / 3.24
2.40 / 2.62	2.42 / 2.64	2.44 / 2.66	2.46 / 2.69	2.48 / 2.71	2.50 / 2.74	2.52 / 2.76	2.53 / 2.78	2.55 / 2.81	2.57 / 2.83	2.59 / 2.86	2.61 / 2.88	2.63 / 2.90	2.65 / 2.93	2.67 / 2.95	2.69 / 2.97	2.70 / 3.00	2.72 / 3.02
2.23 / 2.44	2.25 / 2.46	2.27 / 2.48	2.29 / 2.50	2.30 / 2.52	2.32 / 2.54	2.34 / 2.56	2.36 / 2.59	2.38 / 2.61	2.39 / 2.63	2.41 / 2.65	2.43 / 2.67	2.45 / 2.69	2.47 / 2.71	2.48 / 2.74	2.50 / 2.76	2.52 / 2.78	2.54 / 2.80
2.07 / 2.25	2.09 / 2.27	2.11 / 2.29	2.12 / 2.31	2.14 / 2.33	2.16 / 2.35	2.18 / 2.37	2.19 / 2.39	2.21 / 2.41	2.23 / 2.43	2.24 / 2.45	2.26 / 2.47	2.28 / 2.49	2.29 / 2.51	2.31 / 2.53	2.32 / 2.55	2.34 / 2.57	2.36 / 2.59
1.92 / 2.08	1.94 / 2.10	1.95 / 2.12	1.97 / 2.14	1.99 / 2.15	2.00 / 2.17	2.01 / 2.19	2.03 / 2.21	2.05 / 2.23	2.06 / 2.26	2.07 / 2.28	2.09 / 2.30	2.11 / 2.32	2.12 / 2.34	2.13 / 2.35	2.15 / 2.37	2.17 / 2.39	2.18 / 2.39
1.78 / 1.91	1.79 / 1.93	1.80 / 1.95	1.82 / 1.96	1.83 / 1.98	1.85 / 2.00	1.86 / 2.02	1.87 / 2.03	1.89 / 2.05	1.90 / 2.07	1.92 / 2.08	1.93 / 2.10	1.94 / 2.12	1.96 / 2.13	1.97 / 2.15	1.99 / 2.17	2.00 / 2.18	2.01 / 2.20
1.63 / 1.76	1.64 / 1.77	1.65 / 1.78	1.67 / 1.80	1.68 / 1.82	1.69 / 1.83	1.70 / 1.84	1.72 / 1.86	1.73 / 1.88	1.74 / 1.89	1.76 / 1.90	1.77 / 1.92	1.78 / 1.94	1.80 / 1.95	1.81 / 1.97	1.82 / 1.98	1.84 / 2.00	1.85 / 2.02
1.50 / 1.61	1.51 / 1.62	1.52 / 1.63	1.53 / 1.65	1.55 / 1.66	1.56 / 1.68	1.57 / 1.69	1.58 / 1.70	1.59 / 1.72	1.61 / 1.73	1.62 / 1.75	1.63 / 1.76	1.64 / 1.77	1.65 / 1.79	1.67 / 1.80	1.68 / 1.82	1.69 / 1.83	1.70 / 1.84
1.36 / 1.46	1.37 / 1.47	1.38 / 1.48	1.39 / 1.50	1.40 / 1.51	1.41 / 1.52	1.42 / 1.54	1.44 / 1.55	1.45 / 1.56	1.46 / 1.57	1.47 / 1.59	1.48 / 1.60	1.49 / 1.61	1.50 / 1.63	1.51 / 1.64	1.52 / 1.65	1.54 / 1.66	1.55 / 1.68
1.24 / 1.32	1.25 / 1.33	1.26 / 1.34	1.27 / 1.35	1.28 / 1.37	1.29 / 1.38	1.30 / 1.39	1.31 / 1.40	1.32 / 1.41	1.33 / 1.43	1.34 / 1.44	1.35 / 1.45	1.36 / 1.46	1.37 / 1.47	1.38 / 1.48	1.39 / 1.49	1.40 / 1.50	1.41 / 1.52

APPENDIX B

APPENDIX B (continued)

TABLE IV. Change in Reduced Vergence Due to Thickness for a Given Initial Vergence and Refractive Index of 1.49 (Plastics in Air)
(In each cell, the upper figure applies to divergent light, and the lower figure to convergent light)

Initial vergence	Thickness (mm)													
	1.37	1.38	1.39	1.40	1.41	1.42	1.43	1.44	1.45	1.46	1.47	1.48	1.49	1.50
D 100.0	8.42 / 10.13	8.48 / 10.21	8.53 / 10.29	8.59 / 10.37	8.65 / 10.45	8.70 / 10.53	8.76 / 10.62	8.81 / 10.70	8.87 / 10.78	8.93 / 10.86	8.98 / 10.94	9.04 / 11.03	9.09 / 11.11	9.15 / 11.19
98.0	8.10 / 9.71	8.15 / 9.78	8.21 / 9.86	8.26 / 9.94	8.31 / 10.02	8.37 / 10.10	8.42 / 10.18	8.48 / 10.26	8.53 / 10.34	8.58 / 10.41	8.64 / 10.49	8.69 / 10.57	8.75 / 10.65	8.80 / 10.73
96.0	7.78 / 9.30	7.84 / 9.37	7.89 / 9.45	7.94 / 9.52	7.99 / 9.60	8.04 / 9.67	8.10 / 9.74	8.15 / 9.82	8.20 / 9.90	8.25 / 9.97	8.30 / 10.04	8.36 / 10.12	8.41 / 10.20	8.46 / 10.27
94.0	7.48 / 8.90	7.53 / 8.97	7.58 / 9.04	7.63 / 9.11	7.68 / 9.18	7.73 / 9.25	7.78 / 9.33	7.83 / 9.40	7.88 / 9.47	7.93 / 9.54	7.98 / 9.61	8.03 / 9.69	8.08 / 9.76	8.13 / 9.83
92.0	7.18 / 8.51	7.22 / 8.57	7.27 / 8.64	7.32 / 8.71	7.37 / 8.78	7.42 / 8.85	7.46 / 8.91	7.51 / 8.98	7.56 / 9.05	7.61 / 9.12	7.66 / 9.19	7.70 / 9.25	7.75 / 9.32	7.80 / 9.39
90.0	6.88 / 8.12	6.93 / 8.18	6.97 / 8.25	7.02 / 8.31	7.07 / 8.38	7.11 / 8.44	7.16 / 8.51	7.20 / 8.57	7.25 / 8.64	7.30 / 8.71	7.34 / 8.77	7.39 / 8.84	7.43 / 8.90	7.48 / 8.97
88.0	6.58 / 7.75	6.63 / 7.81	6.68 / 7.87	6.72 / 7.93	6.76 / 7.99	6.81 / 8.05	6.85 / 8.12	6.90 / 8.18	6.94 / 8.24	6.98 / 8.30	7.03 / 8.36	7.07 / 8.43	7.12 / 8.49	7.16 / 8.55
86.0	6.30 / 7.39	6.34 / 7.44	6.39 / 7.50	6.43 / 7.56	6.47 / 7.62	6.51 / 7.68	6.56 / 7.74	6.60 / 7.80	6.64 / 7.86	6.68 / 7.91	6.72 / 7.97	6.77 / 8.03	6.81 / 8.09	6.85 / 8.15
84.0	6.02 / 7.03	6.06 / 7.09	6.10 / 7.14	6.14 / 7.20	6.18 / 7.26	6.22 / 7.31	6.26 / 7.37	6.30 / 7.42	6.34 / 7.48	6.39 / 7.54	6.43 / 7.59	6.47 / 7.65	6.51 / 7.70	6.55 / 7.76
82.0	5.75 / 6.69	5.79 / 6.74	5.83 / 6.80	5.87 / 6.85	5.91 / 6.90	5.95 / 6.96	5.98 / 7.01	6.02 / 7.06	6.06 / 7.12	6.10 / 7.17	6.14 / 7.22	6.17 / 7.27	6.21 / 7.33	6.25 / 7.38
80.0	5.48 / 6.35	5.52 / 6.40	5.55 / 6.45	5.59 / 6.50	5.63 / 6.55	5.66 / 6.60	5.70 / 6.65	5.74 / 6.70	5.78 / 6.76	5.81 / 6.81	5.85 / 6.86	5.89 / 6.91	5.92 / 6.96	5.96 / 7.01
78.0	5.22 / 6.03	5.26 / 6.08	5.29 / 6.12	5.33 / 6.17	5.36 / 6.22	5.40 / 6.27	5.43 / 6.31	5.47 / 6.36	5.50 / 6.41	5.54 / 6.46	5.57 / 6.51	5.61 / 6.55	5.64 / 6.60	5.68 / 6.65
76.0	4.97 / 5.71	5.00 / 5.75	5.04 / 5.80	5.07 / 5.84	5.10 / 5.89	5.14 / 5.93	5.17 / 5.98	5.20 / 6.02	5.24 / 6.07	5.27 / 6.12	5.30 / 6.16	5.33 / 6.21	5.37 / 6.25	5.40 / 6.30
74.0	4.71 / 5.40	4.75 / 5.45	4.78 / 5.49	4.81 / 5.53	4.84 / 5.57	4.87 / 5.62	4.91 / 5.66	4.94 / 5.70	4.97 / 5.74	5.00 / 5.79	5.03 / 5.83	5.07 / 5.87	5.10 / 5.92	5.13 / 5.96
72.0	4.47 / 5.10	4.50 / 5.14	4.53 / 5.18	4.56 / 5.22	4.59 / 5.26	4.62 / 5.30	4.65 / 5.34	4.68 / 5.38	4.72 / 5.42	4.75 / 5.47	4.78 / 5.51	4.81 / 5.55	4.84 / 5.59	4.87 / 5.63
70.0	4.23 / 4.82	4.26 / 4.85	4.29 / 4.89	4.32 / 4.93	4.35 / 4.97	4.38 / 5.01	4.41 / 5.04	4.44 / 5.08	4.46 / 5.12	4.49 / 5.16	4.52 / 5.20	4.55 / 5.23	4.58 / 5.27	4.61 / 5.31
68.0	4.00 / 4.54	4.03 / 4.57	4.05 / 4.60	4.08 / 4.64	4.11 / 4.68	4.14 / 4.71	4.16 / 4.75	4.19 / 4.78	4.22 / 4.82	4.25 / 4.86	4.28 / 4.89	4.30 / 4.93	4.33 / 4.96	4.36 / 5.00
66.0	3.77 / 4.26	3.80 / 4.29	3.82 / 4.33	3.85 / 4.36	3.88 / 4.39	3.90 / 4.43	3.93 / 4.46	3.95 / 4.50	3.98 / 4.53	4.01 / 4.56	4.03 / 4.60	4.06 / 4.63	4.08 / 4.67	4.11 / 4.70
64.0	3.56 / 4.00	3.58 / 4.03	3.60 / 4.06	3.63 / 4.09	3.65 / 4.12	3.68 / 4.15	3.70 / 4.19	3.73 / 4.22	3.75 / 4.25	3.77 / 4.28	3.80 / 4.31	3.82 / 4.35	3.85 / 4.38	3.87 / 4.41
62.0	3.34 / 3.75	3.36 / 3.78	3.39 / 3.81	3.41 / 3.84	3.43 / 3.87	3.46 / 3.90	3.48 / 3.93	3.50 / 3.96	3.52 / 3.98	3.55 / 4.01	3.57 / 4.04	3.59 / 4.07	3.62 / 4.10	3.64 / 4.13
60.0	3.13 / 3.50	3.16 / 3.53	3.18 / 3.55	3.20 / 3.58	3.22 / 3.61	3.24 / 3.64	3.27 / 3.66	3.29 / 3.69	3.31 / 3.72	3.33 / 3.75	3.35 / 3.78	3.38 / 3.80	3.40 / 3.83	3.42 / 3.86
58.0	2.95 / 3.26	2.97 / 3.29	2.99 / 3.32	3.01 / 3.34	3.03 / 3.37	3.05 / 3.39	3.07 / 3.42	3.09 / 3.44	3.11 / 3.47	3.13 / 3.50	3.15 / 3.52	3.17 / 3.55	3.19 / 3.57	3.21 / 3.60
56.0	2.74 / 3.04	2.76 / 3.06	2.78 / 3.09	2.80 / 3.11	2.82 / 3.13	2.84 / 3.16	2.86 / 3.18	2.88 / 3.21	2.90 / 3.23	2.91 / 3.25	2.93 / 3.28	2.95 / 3.30	2.97 / 3.33	2.99 / 3.35
54.0	2.56 / 2.82	2.57 / 2.85	2.59 / 2.87	2.61 / 2.89	2.62 / 2.91	2.64 / 2.93	2.66 / 2.95	2.68 / 2.97	2.70 / 3.00	2.71 / 3.02	2.73 / 3.04	2.75 / 3.06	2.76 / 3.08	2.78 / 3.10
52.0	2.37 / 2.61	2.39 / 2.63	2.40 / 2.65	2.42 / 2.67	2.44 / 2.69	2.45 / 2.71	2.47 / 2.73	2.49 / 2.75	2.50 / 2.77	2.52 / 2.79	2.54 / 2.81	2.56 / 2.83	2.57 / 2.85	2.59 / 2.87
50.0	2.19 / 2.41	2.21 / 2.42	2.23 / 2.44	2.24 / 2.46	2.26 / 2.48	2.27 / 2.50	2.29 / 2.52	2.30 / 2.54	2.32 / 2.56	2.34 / 2.57	2.35 / 2.59	2.37 / 2.61	2.38 / 2.63	2.40 / 2.65
48.0	2.03 / 2.22	2.04 / 2.24	2.06 / 2.25	2.07 / 2.27	2.08 / 2.29	2.10 / 2.30	2.11 / 2.32	2.13 / 2.34	2.14 / 2.36	2.15 / 2.37	2.17 / 2.39	2.18 / 2.41	2.20 / 2.42	2.21 / 2.44
46.0	1.86 / 2.03	1.87 / 2.05	1.89 / 2.06	1.90 / 2.08	1.91 / 2.10	1.93 / 2.11	1.94 / 2.12	1.96 / 2.14	1.97 / 2.16	1.98 / 2.17	2.00 / 2.18	2.01 / 2.20	2.03 / 2.22	2.04 / 2.23
44.0	1.71 / 1.86	1.73 / 1.87	1.74 / 1.89	1.75 / 1.90	1.76 / 1.91	1.77 / 1.93	1.79 / 1.94	1.80 / 1.96	1.81 / 1.97	1.82 / 1.98	1.83 / 2.00	1.85 / 2.01	1.86 / 2.03	1.87 / 2.04
42.0	1.56 / 1.69	1.57 / 1.70	1.58 / 1.72	1.59 / 1.73	1.60 / 1.74	1.61 / 1.75	1.62 / 1.77	1.63 / 1.78	1.64 / 1.79	1.66 / 1.80	1.67 / 1.81	1.68 / 1.83	1.69 / 1.84	1.70 / 1.85
40.0	1.42 / 1.53	1.43 / 1.54	1.44 / 1.55	1.45 / 1.56	1.46 / 1.57	1.47 / 1.58	1.48 / 1.60	1.49 / 1.61	1.50 / 1.62	1.51 / 1.63	1.52 / 1.64	1.53 / 1.66	1.54 / 1.67	1.55 / 1.68

APPENDIX B

TABLE V. Surface Powers in Air for n = 1.336 (Tears), r = radius of curvature, F = surface power

r mm	F Dioptres	r mm	F Dioptres	r mm	F Dioptres	r mm	F Dioptres	r mm	F Dioptres	r mm	F Dioptres	r mm	F Dioptres
4.90	68.57	5.30	63.40	5.70	58.95−	6.10	55.08	6.50	51.69	6.90	48.70	7.30	46.03
.91	68.43	.31	63.28	.71	58.84	.11	54.99	.51	51.61	.91	48.63	.31	45.96
.92	68.29	.32	63.16	.72	58.74	.12	54.90	.52	51.53	.92	48.55+	.32	45.90
.93	68.15	.33	63.04	.73	58.64	.13	54.81	.53	51.45+	.93	48.48	.33	45.84
.94	68.02	.34	62.92	.74	58.54	.14	54.72	.54	51.38	.94	48.41	.34	45.78
.95	67.88	.35	62.80	.75	58.43	.15	54.63	.55	51.30	.95	48.35−	.35	45.71
.96	67.74	.36	62.69	.76	58.33	.16	54.55−	.56	51.22	.96	48.28	.36	45.65+
.97	67.61	.37	62.57	.77	58.23	.17	54.46	.57	51.14	.97	48.21	.37	45.59
.98	67.47	.38	62.45+	.78	58.13	.18	54.37	.58	51.06	.98	48.14	.38	45.53
.99	67.33	.39	62.34	.79	58.03	.19	54.28	.59	50.99	.99	48.07	.39	45.47
5.00	67.20	5.40	62.22	5.80	57.93	6.20	54.19	6.60	50.91	7.00	48.00	7.40	45.41
.01	67.07	.41	62.11	.81	57.83	.21	54.11	.61	50.83	.01	47.93	.41	45.34
.02	66.93	.42	61.99	.82	57.73	.22	54.02	.62	50.76	.02	47.86	.42	45.28
.03	66.80	.43	61.88	.83	57.63	.23	53.93	.63	50.68	.03	47.80	.43	45.22
.04	66.67	.44	61.76	.84	57.53	.24	53.85−	.64	50.60	.04	47.73	.44	45.16
.05	66.53	.45	61.65+	.85	57.44	.25	53.76	.65	50.53	.05	47.66	.45	45.10
.06	66.40	.46	61.54	.86	57.34	.26	53.67	.66	50.45+	.06	47.59	.46	45.04
.07	66.27	.47	61.43	.87	57.24	.27	53.59	.67	50.37	.07	47.52	.47	44.98
.08	66.14	.48	61.31	.88	57.14	.28	53.50	.68	50.30	.08	47.46	.48	44.92
.09	66.01	.49	61.20	.89	57.05−	.29	53.42	.69	50.22	.09	47.39	.49	44.86
5.10	65.88	5.50	61.09	5.90	56.95−	6.30	53.33	6.70	50.15−	7.10	47.32	7.50	44.80
.11	65.75+	.51	60.98	.91	56.85+	.31	53.25−	.71	50.07	.11	47.26	.51	44.74
.12	65.62	.52	60.87	.92	56.76	.32	53.16	.72	50.00	.12	47.19	.52	44.68
.13	65.50	.53	60.76	.93	56.66	.33	53.08	.73	49.93	.13	47.12	.53	44.62
.14	65.37	.54	60.65−	.94	56.57	.34	53.00	.74	49.85+	.14	47.06	.54	44.56
.15	65.24	.55	60.54	.95	56.47	.35	52.91	.75	49.78	.15	46.99	.55	44.50
.16	65.12	.56	60.43	.96	56.38	.36	52.83	.76	49.70	.16	46.93	.56	44.44
.17	64.99	.57	60.32	.97	56.28	.37	52.75−	.77	49.63	.17	46.86	.57	44.39
.18	64.86	.58	60.22	.98	56.19	.38	52.66	.78	49.56	.18	46.80	.58	44.33
.19	64.74	.59	60.11	.99	56.09	.39	52.58	.79	49.48	.19	46.73	.59	44.27
5.20	64.62	5.60	60.00	6.00	56.00	6.40	52.50	6.80	49.41	7.20	46.67	7.60	44.21
.21	64.49	.61	59.89	.01	55.91	.41	52.42	.81	49.34	.21	46.60	.61	44.15+
.22	64.37	.62	59.79	.02	55.81	.42	52.34	.82	49.27	.22	46.54	.62	44.09
.23	64.24	.63	59.68	.03	55.72	.43	52.26	.83	49.19	.23	46.47	.63	44.04
.24	64.12	.64	59.57	.04	55.63	.44	52.17	.84	49.12	.24	46.41	.64	43.98
.25	64.00	.65	59.47	.05	55.54	.45	52.09	.85	49.05	.25	46.34	.65	43.92
.26	63.88	.66	59.36	.06	55.45−	.46	52.01	.86	48.98	.26	46.28	.66	43.86
.27	63.76	.67	59.26	.07	55.35+	.47	51.93	.87	48.91	.27	46.22	.67	43.81
.28	63.64	.68	59.15+	.08	55.26	.48	51.85+	.88	48.84	.28	46.15+	.68	43.75−
.29	63.52	.69	59.05+	.09	55.17	.49	51.77	.89	48.77	.29	46.09	.69	43.69

r mm	F Dioptres	r mm	F Dioptres	r mm	F Dioptres	r mm	F Dioptres	r mm	F Dioptres	r mm	F Dioptres	r mm	F Dioptres
7.70	43.64	8.10	41.48	8.50	39.53	8.90	37.75+	9.30	36.13	9.70	34.64	10.50	32.00
.71	43.58	.11	41.43	.51	39.48	.91	37.71	.31	36.09	.71	34.60	10.55	31.85−
.72	43.52	.12	41.38	.52	39.44	.92	37.67	.32	36.05+	.72	34.57	10.60	31.70
.73	43.47	.13	41.33	.53	39.39	.93	37.63	.33	36.01	.73	34.53	10.65	31.55−
.74	43.41	.14	41.28	.54	39.34	.94	37.58	.34	35.97	.74	34.50	10.70	31.40
.75	43.35+	.15	41.23	.55	39.30	.95	37.54	.35	35.94	.75	34.46	10.75	31.26
.76	43.30	.16	41.18	.56	39.25+	.96	37.50	.36	35.90	.76	34.43	10.80	31.11
.77	43.24	.17	41.13	.57	39.21	.97	37.46	.37	35.86	.77	34.39	10.85	30.97
.78	43.19	.18	41.08	.58	39.16	.98	37.42	.38	35.82	.78	34.36	10.90	30.83
.79	43.13	.19	41.03	.59	39.12	.99	37.37	.39	35.78	.79	34.32	10.95	30.68
7.80	43.08	8.20	40.98	8.60	39.07	9.00	37.33	9.40	35.74	9.80	34.29	11.00	30.55−
.81	43.02	.21	40.93	.61	39.02	.01	37.29	.41	35.71	.81	34.25	11.05	30.41
.82	42.97	.22	40.88	.62	38.98	.02	37.25+	.42	35.67	.82	34.22	11.10	30.27
.83	42.91	.23	40.83	.63	38.93	.03	37.21	.43	35.63	.83	34.18	11.15	30.13
.84	42.86	.24	40.78	.64	38.89	.04	37.17	.44	35.59	.84	34.15−	11.20	30.00
.85	42.80	.25	40.73	.65	38.84	.05	37.13	.45	35.56	.85	34.11	11.25	29.87
.86	42.75−	.26	40.68	.66	38.80	.06	37.09	.46	35.52	.86	34.08	11.30	29.73
.87	42.69	.27	40.63	.67	38.75+	.07	37.05−	.47	35.48	.87	34.04	11.35	29.60
.88	42.64	.28	40.58	.68	38.71	.08	37.00	.48	35.44	.88	34.01	11.40	29.47
.89	42.59	.29	40.53	.69	38.67	.09	36.96	.49	35.41	.89	33.97	11.45	29.34
7.90	42.53	8.30	40.48	8.70	38.62	9.10	36.92	9.50	35.37	9.90	33.94	11.50	29.22
.91	42.48	.31	40.43	.71	38.58	.11	36.88	.51	35.33	.91	33.91	11.55	29.09
.92	42.42	.32	40.38	.72	38.53	.12	36.84	.52	35.29	.92	33.87	11.60	28.97
.93	42.37	.33	40.34	.73	38.49	.13	36.80	.53	35.26	.93	33.84	11.65	28.84
.94	42.32	.34	40.29	.74	38.44	.14	36.76	.54	35.22	.94	33.80	11.70	28.72
.95	42.26	.35	40.24	.75	38.40	.15	36.72	.55	35.18	.95	33.77	11.75	28.60
.96	42.21	.36	40.19	.76	38.36	.16	36.68	.56	35.15−	.96	33.73	11.80	28.47
.97	42.16	.37	40.14	.77	38.31	.17	36.64	.57	35.11	.97	33.70	11.85	28.35+
.98	42.11	.38	40.10	.78	38.27	.18	36.60	.58	35.07	.98	33.67	11.90	28.24
.99	42.05+	.39	40.05−	.79	38.23	.19	36.56	.59	35.04	.99	33.63	11.95	28.12
8.00	42.00	8.40	40.00	8.80	38.18	9.20	36.52	9.60	35.00	10.00	33.60	12.00	28.00
.01	41.95−	.41	39.95+	.81	38.14	.21	36.48	.61	34.96	10.05	33.43	12.05	27.88
.02	41.90	.42	39.91	.82	38.10	.22	36.44	.62	34.93	10.10	33.27	12.10	27.77
.03	41.84	.43	39.86	.83	38.05+	.23	36.40	.63	34.89	10.15	33.10	12.15	27.65+
.04	41.79	.44	39.81	.84	38.01	.24	36.36	.64	34.85+	10.20	32.94	12.20	27.54
.05	41.74	.45	39.76	.85	37.97	.25	36.32	.65	34.82	10.25	32.78	12.25	27.43
.06	41.69	.46	39.72	.86	37.92	.26	36.28	.66	34.78	10.30	32.62	12.30	27.32
.07	41.64	.47	39.67	.87	37.88	.27	36.25−	.67	34.75−	10.35	32.46	12.35	27.21
.08	41.58	.48	39.62	.88	37.84	.28	36.21	.68	34.71	10.40	32.31	12.40	27.10
.09	41.53	.49	39.58	.89	37.80	.29	36.17	.69	34.67	10.45	32.15	12.45	26.99
												12.50	26.88

APPENDIX B

TABLE VI. Change in Surface Power, in Dioptres, When Radius (r_1) is Changed to New Radius (r_2), for Liquid Lens ($n = 1.336$) in Air

Initial radius r_1 mm	New radius (r_2) mm																			
	7.0	7.1	7.2	7.3	7.4	7.5	7.6	7.7	7.8	7.9	8.0	8.1	8.2	8.3	8.4	8.5	8.6	8.7	8.8	8.9
9.0	10.67	9.99	9.34	8.70	8.08	7.47	6.88	6.31	5.75	5.20	4.67	4.15	3.65	3.15	2.67	2.20	1.74	1.29	0.85	0.42
8.9	10.25	9.57	8.92	8.28	7.66	7.05	6.46	5.89	5.33	4.78	4.25	3.73	3.23	2.73	2.25	1.78	1.32	0.87	0.43	
8.8	9.82	9.14	8.49	7.85	7.23	6.62	6.03	5.46	4.90	4.35	3.82	3.30	2.80	2.30	1.82	1.35	0.89	0.44		
8.7	9.38	8.70	8.05	7.41	6.76	6.18	5.59	5.02	4.46	3.91	3.38	2.86	2.36	1.86	1.38	0.91	0.45			
8.6	8.93	8.25	7.60	6.96	6.34	5.73	5.14	4.57	4.01	3.46	2.93	2.41	1.91	1.41	0.93	0.46				
8.5	8.47	7.79	7.14	6.50	5.88	5.27	4.68	4.11	3.55	3.00	2.47	1.95	1.45	0.95	0.47					
8.4	8.00	7.32	6.67	6.03	5.41	4.80	4.21	3.64	3.08	2.53	2.00	1.48	0.98	0.48						
8.3	7.52	6.84	6.19	5.55	4.93	4.32	3.73	3.16	2.60	2.05	1.52	1.00	0.50							
8.2	7.02	6.34	5.69	5.05	4.43	3.82	3.23	2.66	2.10	1.55	1.02	0.50								
8.1	6.52	5.84	5.19	4.55	3.93	3.32	2.73	2.16	1.60	1.05	0.52									
8.0	6.00	5.32	4.67	4.03	3.41	2.80	2.21	1.64	1.08	0.53										
7.9	5.47	4.79	4.14	3.50	2.88	2.27	1.68	1.11	0.55											
7.8	4.92	4.24	3.59	2.95	2.33	1.72	1.13	0.56												
7.7	4.36	3.68	3.03	2.39	1.77	1.16	0.57													
7.6	3.79	3.11	2.46	1.82	1.20	0.59														
7.5	3.20	2.52	1.87	1.23	0.61															
7.4	2.59	1.91	1.26	0.62																
7.3	1.97	1.29	0.64																	
7.2	1.33	0.65																		
7.1	0.68																			

APPENDIX B

TABLE VII. Change in Reduced Vergence due to Thickness for a Given Initial Vergence and Refractive Index of 1.336 (Liquid Lens in Air) (Where there are two figures in one cell, the upper figure applies to divergent light and the lower figure to convergent light)

Initial vergence	Thickness (mm)				Initial vergence	Thickness (mm)			
	0.05	0.10	0.15	0.20		0.05	0.10	0.15	0.20
D 20.00	.01	.03	.05	.06	42.00	.06	.13	.20	.27
21.00	.02	.03	.05	.07	43.00	.07	.14	.21	.28
22.00	.02	.04	.05	.07	44.00	.07	.15	.22	.29
23.00	.02	.04	.06	.08	45.00	.07	.15	.23	.31
24.00	.02	.04	.06	.09	46.00	.08	.16	.24	.32
25.00	.02	.05	.07	.09	47.00	.08	.17	.25	.33
26.00	.03	.05	.08	.10	48.00	.08	.17	.26	.35
27.00	.03	.05	.08	.11	49.00	.09	.18	.27	.36
28.00	.03	.06	.09	.12	50.00	.09	.19	.28	.38
29.00	.03	.06	.09	.13	51.00	.10	.20	.29	.39
30.00	.03	.07	.10	.14	52.00	.10	.20	.30	.41
31.00	.04	.07	.11	.14	53.00	.10	.21	.31	.42
32.00	.04	.08	.12	.15	54.00	.11	.22	.33	.44
33.00	.04	.08	.12	.16	55.00	.11	.23	.34	.46
34.00	.04	.09	.13	.17	56.00	.12	.24	.35	.47 / .48
35.00	.05	.09	.14	.18	57.00	.12	.24	.37	.49 / .50
36.00	.05	.10	.15	.20	58.00	.13	.25	.38	.51 / .52
37.00	.05	.10	.15	.21	59.00	.13	.26	.39	.53 / .53
38.00	.05	.11	.16	.22	60.00	.14	.27	.41	.54 / .55
39.00	.05	.11	.17	.23	61.00	.14	.28	.42	.56 / .57
40.00	.06	.12	.18	.24	62.00	.14	.29	.43	.58
41.00	.06	.13	.19	.25					

APPENDIX B

TABLE VIII. Change in Surface Power (in dioptres) when Radius (r_1) is Changed to New Radius (r_2), for Liquid Lens ($n = 1.336$), in Contact with Plastics ($n = 1.49$). (Thus $n_R = 0.154$)

Initial radius (r_1) mm	New radius (r_2) mm																			
	7.0	7.1	7.2	7.3	7.4	7.5	7.6	7.7	7.8	7.9	8.0	8.1	8.2	8.3	8.4	8.5	8.6	8.7	8.8	8.9
9.0	4.89	4.58	4.28	3.99	3.70	3.42	3.15	2.89	2.63	2.38	2.14	1.90	1.67	1.44	1.22	1.01	0.80	0.59	0.39	0.19
8.9	4.70	4.39	4.09	3.80	3.51	3.23	2.96	2.70	2.44	2.19	1.95	1.71	1.48	1.25	1.03	0.82	0.61	0.40	0.20	
8.8	4.50	4.19	3.89	3.60	3.31	3.03	2.76	2.50	2.24	1.99	1.75	1.51	1.28	1.05	0.83	0.62	0.41	0.20		
8.7	4.30	3.99	3.69	3.40	3.11	2.83	2.56	2.30	2.04	1.79	1.55	1.31	1.08	0.85	0.63	0.42	0.21			
8.6	4.09	3.78	3.48	3.19	2.90	2.62	2.35	2.09	1.83	1.58	1.34	1.10	0.87	0.64	0.42	0.21				
8.5	3.88	3.57	3.27	2.98	2.69	2.41	2.14	1.88	1.62	1.37	1.13	0.89	0.66	0.43	0.21					
8.4	3.67	3.36	3.06	2.77	2.48	2.20	1.93	1.67	1.41	1.16	0.92	0.68	0.45	0.22						
8.3	3.45	3.14	2.84	2.55	2.26	1.98	1.71	1.45	1.19	0.94	0.70	0.46	0.23							
8.2	3.22	2.91	2.61	2.32	2.03	1.75	1.48	1.22	0.96	0.71	0.47	0.23								
8.1	2.99	2.68	2.38	2.09	1.80	1.52	1.25	0.99	0.73	0.48	0.24									
8.0	2.75	2.44	2.14	1.85	1.56	1.28	1.01	0.75	0.49	0.24										
7.9	2.51	2.20	1.90	1.61	1.32	1.04	0.77	0.51	0.25											
7.8	2.26	1.95	1.65	1.36	1.07	0.79	0.52	0.26												
7.7	2.00	1.69	1.39	1.10	0.81	0.53	0.26													
7.6	1.74	1.43	1.13	0.84	0.55	0.27														
7.5	1.47	1.16	0.86	0.57	0.28															
7.4	1.19	0.88	0.58	0.29																
7.3	0.90	0.59	0.29																	
7.2	0.61	0.30																		
7.1	0.31																			

APPENDIX B

TABLE IX. Surface Powers in Air for Plastics Material of n = 1.560 (as used for fused bifocal contact lens segments)

r mm	F Dioptres	Difference in F for 0.01 change in r	r mm	F Dioptres	Difference in F for 0.01 change in r
5.00	112.0000		7.00	80.0000	
		0.2196			0.1127
.10	109.8039		.10	78.8732	
		0.2112			0.1095
.20	107.6923		.20	77.7778	
		0.2032			0.1066
.30	105.6604		.30	76.7123	
		0.1957			0.1037
.40	103.7037		.40	75.6757	
		0.1886			0.1009
.50	101.8182		.50	74.6667	
		0.1818			0.0982
.60	100.0000		.60	73.6842	
		0.1754			0.0957
.70	98.2456		.70	72.7273	
		0.1694			0.0932
.80	96.5517		.80	71.7949	
		0.1636			0.0909
.90	94.9153		.90	70.8861	
		0.1582			0.0886
6.00	93.3333		8.00	70.0000	
		0.1530			0.0864
.10	91.8033		.10	69.1358	
		0.1481			0.0843
.20	90.3226		.20	68.2927	
		0.1434			0.0823
.30	88.8889		.30	67.4699	
		0.1389			0.0803
.40	87.5000		.40	66.6667	
		0.1346			0.0784
.50	86.1538		.50	65.8824	
		0.1305			0.0766
.60	84.8484		.60	65.1163	
		0.1266			0.0748
.70	83.5821		.70	64.3678	
		0.2290			0.0731
.80	82.3529		.80	63.6364	
		0.1194			0.0715
.90	81.1594		.90	62.9213	
		0.1159			0.0699
7.00	80.0000		9.00	62.2223	

APPENDIX B

*TABLE X. Surface Powers in Tears (n = 1.336) for Plastics Material of n = 1.560
(as used for fused bifocal contact lens segments)*

r mm	F Dioptres	Difference in F for 0.01 change in r	r mm	F Dioptres	Difference in F for 0.01 change in r
5.00	44.8000		7.00	32.0000	
		0.0878			0.0451
.10	43.9216		.10	31.5493	
		0.0845—			0.0438
.20	43.0769		.20	31.1111	
		0.0813			0.0426
.30	42.2642		.30	30.6849	
		0.0783			0.0415
.40	41.4815—		.40	30.2703	
		0.0754			0.0404
.50	40.7273		.50	29.8667	
		0.0727			0.0393
.60	40.0000		.60	29.4737	
		0.0702			0.0383
.70	39.2982		.70	29.0909	
		0.0678			0.0373
.80	38.6207		.80	28.7180	
		0.0655—			0.0364
.90	37.9661		.90	28.3544	
		0.0633			0.0354
6.00	37.3333		8.00	28.0000	
		0.0612			0.0346
.10	36.7213		.10	27.6543	
		0.0592			0.0337
.20	36.1290		.20	27.3171	
		0.0573			0.0329
.30	35.5556		.30	26.9880	
		0.0556			0.0321
.40	35.0000		.40	26.6667	
		0.0539			0.0314
.50	34.4615+		.50	26.3530	
		0.0522			0.0306
.60	33.9394		.60	26.0465+	
		0.0507			0.0299
.70	33.4328		.70	25.7471	
		0.0492			0.0292
.80	32.9412		.80	25.4546	
		0.0477			0.0286
.90	32.4638		.90	25.1685+	
		0.0464			0.0280
7.00	32.0000		9.00	24.8889	

APPENDIX B

TABLE XI. Fused Bifocal Lens Contact Surface Powers for a Refractor Index Difference of 1.560–1.490; and Change in Surface Power for radius, r mm, when Refractive Index Changes from 1.490 to 1.560 (as on the back surface of a fused bifocal, back surface segment contact lens)

r mm	F Dioptres	Difference in F for 0.01 change in r	r mm	F Dioptres	Difference in F for 0.01 change in r
5.00	14.0000		7.00	10.0000	
		0.0275			0.0141
.10	13.7255−		.10	9.8592	
		0.0264			0.0137
.20	13.4615+		.20	9.7222	
		0.0254			0.0133
.30	13.2075+		.30	9.5890	
		0.0244			0.0130
.40	12.9630		.40	9.4595−	
		0.0236			0.0126
.50	12.7273		.50	9.3333	
		0.0227			0.0123
.60	12.5000		.60	9.2105	
		0.0219			0.0120
.70	12.2807		.70	9.0909	
		0.0212			0.0116
.80	12.0690		.80	8.9744	
		0.0205			0.0114
.90	11.8644		.90	8.8608	
		0.0198			0.0111
6.00	11.6667		8.00	8.7500	
		0.0191			0.0108
.10	11.4754		.10	8.6420	
		0.0185			0.0105
.20	11.2903		.20	8.5366	
		0.0179			0.0103
.30	11.1111		.30	8.4337	
		0.0174			0.0100
.40	10.9375		.40	8.3333	
		0.0168			0.0098
.50	10.7692		.50	8.2353	
		0.0163			0.0096
.60	10.6061		.60	8.1395+	
		0.0158			0.0094
.70	10.4478		.70	8.0460	
		0.0154			0.0092
.80	10.2941		.80	7.9545+	
		0.0149			0.0089
.90	10.1449		.90	7.8652	
		0.0145			0.0087
7.00	10.0000		9.00	7.7778	

APPENDIX B

TABLE XII. Contact Surface Radii (in mm) for Fused Bifocal Corneal Lenses for Refractive Indices of 1.490 (Main Lens) and 1.560 (Fused Segment), for Various Back Central Optic Radii and Near Additions

Bifocal contact lenses (n_1 = 1.490; n_2 = 1.560) (See Figure 4.26)

	Radius (r_1) of contact surface required to give the following additions Near addition in Dioptres						
r_2 = BCOR mm	+1.00	+1.50	+2.00	+2.50	+3.00	+3.50	+4.00
6.00	5.5263	5.3164	5.1219	4.9412	4.7727	4.6154	4.4681
.10	5.6110	5.3948	5.1947	5.0088	4.8358	4.6743	4.5233
.20	5.6955+	5.4729	5.2670	5.0760	4.8984	4.7328	4.5781
.30	5.7798	5.5507	5.3390	5.1429	4.9606	4.7909	4.6324
.40	5.8639	5.6281	5.4106	5.2093	5.0224	4.8485−	4.6862
.50	5.9477	5.7053	5.4819	5.2754	5.0838	4.9057	4.7396
.60	6.0313	5.7822	5.5529	5.3410	5.1448	4.9624	4.7925
.70	6.1147	5.8588	5.6235−	5.4063	5.2053	5.0187	4.8450
.80	6.1979	5.9352	5.6938	5.4713	5.2655−	5.0746	4.8971
.90	6.2809	6.0112	5.7637	5.5358	5.3253	5.1301	4.9488
7.00	6.3636	6.0870	5.8333	5.6000	5.3846	5.1852	5.0000
.10	6.4461	6.1624	5.9026	5.6638	5.4436	5.2398	5.0508
.20	6.5285+	6.2376	5.9716	5.7273	5.5022	5.2941	5.1012
.30	6.6106	6.3126	6.0402	5.7904	5.5604	5.3480	5.1512
.40	6.6925−	6.3872	6.1085−	5.8531	5.6182	5.4014	5.2008
.50	6.7742	6.4616	6.1765−	5.9155	5.6757	5.4546	5.2500
.60	6.8557	6.5356	6.2441	5.9775+	5.7328	5.5073	5.2988
.70	6.9369	6.6094	6.3115−	6.0392	5.7895−	5.5596	5.3472
.80	7.0180	6.6830	6.3785−	6.1005+	5.8458	5.6115−	5.3952
.90	7.0988	6.7562	6.4452	6.1615+	5.9018	5.6631	5.4429
8.00	7.1795−	6.8293	6.5116	6.2222	5.9574	5.7143	5.4902
.10	7.2599	6.9020	6.5777	6.2825	6.0127	5.7651	5.5371
.20	7.3401	6.9745−	6.6435+	6.3425	6.0676	5.8156	5.5837
.30	7.4202	7.0467	6.7090	6.4022	6.1223	5.8657	5.6299
.40	7.5000	7.1187	6.7742	6.4616	6.1765−	5.9155+	5.6757
.50	7.5796	7.1903	6.8391	6.5205+	6.2304	5.9649	5.7212
.60	7.5111	7.1287	6.7833	6.4698	6.1840	5.9224	5.7663
.70	7.7382	7.3329	6.9679	6.6376	6.3371	6.0627	5.8111
.80	7.8173	7.4039	7.0320	6.6957	6.3901	6.1111	5.8555+
.90	7.8960	7.4745−	7.0956	6.7534	6.4426	6.1592	5.8996
9.00	7.9747	7.5449	7.1591	6.8108	6.4948	6.2069	5.9434

APPENDIX C
SAGITTA
in mm

Radii in mm	Optic diameters (chords) in mm																				
	3.0	3.2	3.4	3.6	3.8	4.0	4.2	4.4	4.6	4.8	5.0	5.2	5.4	5.6	5.8	6.0	6.2	6.4	6.6	6.8	7.0
5.00	0.230	0.263	0.298	0.335	0.375	0.417	0.462	0.510	0.560	0.614	0.670	0.729	0.792	0.858	0.927	1.000	1.077	1.158	1.244	1.334	1.429
5.25	0.219	0.250	0.283	0.318	0.356	0.396	0.438	0.483	0.531	0.581	0.633	0.689	0.748	0.809	0.874	0.942	1.013	1.088	1.167	1.250	1.337
5.50	0.209	0.238	0.269	0.303	0.339	0.377	0.417	0.459	0.504	0.551	0.601	0.653	0.708	0.766	0.827	0.890	0.957	1.027	1.100	1.177	1.257
5.75	0.199	0.227	0.257	0.289	0.323	0.359	0.397	0.438	0.480	0.525	0.572	0.621	0.673	0.728	0.785	0.845	0.907	0.973	1.041	1.113	1.188
6.00	0.191	0.217	0.246	0.276	0.309	0.343	0.380	0.418	0.458	0.501	0.546	0.593	0.642	0.693	0.747	0.804	0.863	0.925	0.989	1.056	1.127
6.25	0.183	0.209	0.236	0.265	0.296	0.329	0.364	0.400	0.439	0.479	0.522	0.566	0.613	0.662	0.714	0.767	0.823	0.881	0.942	1.006	1.072
6.50	0.175	0.200	0.226	0.254	0.284	0.315	0.349	0.384	0.421	0.459	0.500	0.543	0.587	0.634	0.683	0.734	0.787	0.842	0.900	0.960	1.023
6.75	0.169	0.193	0.218	0.245	0.273	0.303	0.335	0.369	0.404	0.441	0.480	0.521	0.564	0.608	0.655	0.703	0.754	0.807	0.862	0.919	0.978
7.00	0.163	0.185	0.210	0.235	0.263	0.292	0.322	0.355	0.389	0.424	0.462	0.501	0.542	0.584	0.629	0.675	0.724	0.774	0.827	0.881	0.938
7.10	0.160	0.183	0.207	0.232	0.259	0.289	0.318	0.349	0.383	0.418	0.455	0.493	0.533	0.575	0.619	0.665	0.713	0.762	0.814	0.867	0.923
7.20	0.158	0.180	0.204	0.229	0.255	0.283	0.313	0.344	0.377	0.412	0.448	0.486	0.525	0.567	0.610	0.655	0.702	0.750	0.801	0.853	0.908
7.30	0.156	0.178	0.201	0.225	0.252	0.279	0.309	0.339	0.372	0.406	0.441	0.479	0.518	0.558	0.601	0.645	0.691	0.739	0.788	0.840	0.894
7.40	0.154	0.175	0.198	0.222	0.248	0.275	0.304	0.335	0.367	0.400	0.435	0.472	0.510	0.550	0.592	0.635	0.681	0.728	0.777	0.827	0.880
7.50	0.152	0.173	0.195	0.219	0.245	0.272	0.300	0.330	0.361	0.394	0.429	0.465	0.503	0.542	0.583	0.626	0.671	0.717	0.765	0.815	0.867
7.60	0.150	0.170	0.193	0.216	0.241	0.268	0.296	0.325	0.356	0.389	0.423	0.459	0.496	0.535	0.575	0.617	0.661	0.707	0.754	0.803	0.854
7.70	0.148	0.168	0.190	0.213	0.238	0.264	0.292	0.321	0.352	0.384	0.417	0.452	0.489	0.527	0.567	0.608	0.652	0.696	0.743	0.791	0.841
7.80	0.146	0.166	0.188	0.211	0.235	0.261	0.288	0.317	0.347	0.378	0.411	0.446	0.482	0.520	0.559	0.600	0.642	0.687	0.732	0.780	0.829
7.90	0.144	0.164	0.185	0.208	0.232	0.257	0.284	0.313	0.342	0.373	0.406	0.440	0.476	0.513	0.552	0.592	0.634	0.677	0.722	0.769	0.818

Radii in mm	Optic diameters (chords) in mm																				
	7.2	7.4	7.6	7.8	8.0	8.2	8.4	8.6	8.8	9.0	9.2	9.4	9.6	9.8	10.0	10.2	10.4	10.6	10.8	11.0	11.2
5.00	1.530	1.637	1.750	1.871	2.000	2.138	2.287	2.449	2.625	2.821	3.040	3.294	3.600	4.005	5.000						
5.25	1.429	1.525	1.628	1.735	1.850	1.971	2.100	2.238	2.386	2.546	2.720	2.911	3.123	3.365	3.649	4.004	4.527				
5.50	1.342	1.431	1.524	1.622	1.725	1.834	1.949	2.071	2.200	2.338	2.485	2.643	2.815	3.002	3.209	3.441	3.708	4.030	4.456	5.500	
5.75	1.266	1.349	1.435	1.525	1.619	1.719	1.823	1.933	2.048	2.171	2.300	2.438	2.584	2.741	2.911	3.094	3.296	3.520	3.775	4.073	4.445
6.00	1.200	1.277	1.357	1.440	1.528	1.619	1.715	1.816	1.921	2.031	2.148	2.270	2.400	2.537	2.683	2.839	3.007	3.188	3.385	3.602	3.846
6.25	1.141	1.213	1.288	1.366	1.448	1.533	1.622	1.714	1.811	1.913	2.019	2.130	2.247	2.370	2.500	2.637	2.783	2.938	3.103	3.281	3.475
6.50	1.088	1.156	1.226	1.300	1.377	1.456	1.539	1.626	1.716	1.810	1.908	2.010	2.117	2.229	2.347	2.470	2.600	2.737	2.882	3.036	3.200
6.75	1.040	1.104	1.171	1.241	1.313	1.388	1.466	1.547	1.631	1.718	1.810	1.905	2.004	2.108	2.215	2.328	2.446	2.570	2.700	2.837	2.981
7.00	0.997	1.058	1.121	1.187	1.255	1.326	1.400	1.476	1.556	1.638	1.724	1.813	1.905	2.001	2.101	2.205	2.314	2.427	2.546	2.670	2.800
7.10	0.980	1.040	1.103	1.167	1.234	1.303	1.375	1.450	1.528	1.608	1.692	1.778	1.868	1.962	2.059	2.160	2.266	2.376	2.490	2.610	2.735
7.20	0.965	1.023	1.084	1.148	1.213	1.281	1.352	1.425	1.501	1.580	1.661	1.746	1.833	1.925	2.019	2.118	2.220	2.327	2.438	2.553	2.675
7.30	0.949	1.007	1.067	1.129	1.193	1.260	1.329	1.401	1.475	1.552	1.632	1.714	1.800	1.889	1.981	2.077	2.177	2.280	2.388	2.500	2.617
7.40	0.935	0.991	1.050	1.111	1.174	1.240	1.307	1.378	1.450	1.525	1.603	1.684	1.768	1.855	1.945	2.038	2.135	2.236	2.340	2.449	2.563
7.50	0.920	0.976	1.034	1.094	1.156	1.220	1.286	1.355	1.426	1.500	1.576	1.655	1.737	1.822	1.910	2.001	2.095	2.193	2.295	2.401	2.511
7.60	0.907	0.961	1.018	1.077	1.138	1.201	1.266	1.333	1.403	1.475	1.550	1.628	1.708	1.791	1.876	1.965	2.057	2.153	2.252	2.355	2.462
7.70	0.893	0.947	1.003	1.061	1.120	1.182	1.246	1.313	1.381	1.452	1.525	1.601	1.679	1.760	1.844	1.931	2.021	2.114	2.211	2.311	2.415
7.80	0.880	0.933	0.988	1.045	1.104	1.164	1.227	1.292	1.360	1.429	1.501	1.575	1.652	1.731	1.813	1.898	1.986	2.077	2.172	2.269	2.370
7.90	0.868	0.920	0.974	1.030	1.088	1.147	1.209	1.273	1.339	1.407	1.477	1.550	1.625	1.703	1.784	1.867	1.953	2.042	2.134	2.229	2.328

Radii in mm	Optic diameters (chords) in mm																	
	11.4	11.6	11.8	12.00	12.25	12.50	12.75	13.00	13.25	13.50	13.75	14.00	14.25	14.50	14.75	15.00	15.25	15.50	15.75	16.00
5.00																				
5.25																				
5.50																				
5.75	4.993																			
6.00	4.127	4.464	4.909	6.000																
6.25	3.686	3.921	4.188	4.500	5.006	6.250														
6.50	3.376	3.566	3.772	4.000	4.324	4.715	5.231	6.500												
6.75	3.134	3.297	3.471	3.658	3.913	4.200	4.531	4.930	5.457	6.750										
7.00	2.937	3.081	3.233	3.394	3.612	3.848	4.109	4.402	4.740	5.146	5.683	7.000								
7.10	2.867	3.005	3.150	3.304	3.509	3.731	3.974	4.243	4.547	4.898	5.327	5.913								
7.20	2.801	2.934	3.073	3.220	3.415	3.625	3.853	4.103	4.381	4.695	5.061	5.515	6.163							
7.30	2.739	2.867	3.001	3.142	3.328	3.528	3.743	3.977	4.234	4.520	4.846	5.229	5.711	6.447						
7.40	2.681	2.804	2.933	3.069	3.247	3.438	3.642	3.863	4.103	4.367	4.662	5.000	5.401	5.918	6.792					
7.50	2.626	2.745	2.870	3.000	3.172	3.354	3.549	3.759	3.984	4.231	4.503	4.807	5.158	5.580	6.136	7.500				
7.60	2.573	2.689	2.809	2.935	3.101	3.276	3.462	3.662	3.876	4.108	4.360	4.640	4.955	5.320	5.764	6.371				
7.70	2.523	2.635	2.752	2.874	3.034	3.001	3.382	3.572	3.776	3.995	4.232	4.492	4.780	5.106	5.487	5.956	6.628			
7.80	2.476	2.585	2.698	2.816	2.970	3.133	3.306	3.488	3.683	3.891	4.116	4.359	4.626	4.923	5.260	5.658	6.157	6.918		
7.90	2.430	2.536	2.646	2.761	2.911	3.068	3.234	3.410	3.598	3.795	4.008	4.238	4.498	4.762	5.068	5.418	5.834	6.397	7.272	

Radii in mm	Optic diameters (chords) in mm																					
	3.0	3.2	3.4	3.6	3.8	4.0	4.2	4.4	4.6	4.8	5.0	5.2	5.4	5.6	5.8	6.0	6.2	6.4	6.6	6.8	7.0	7.2
8.00	0.142	0.162	0.183	0.205	0.229	0.254	0.281	0.308	0.338	0.369	0.401	0.434	0.469	0.506	0.544	0.584	0.625	0.668	0.712	0.758	0.806	0.856
8.10	0.140	0.160	0.180	0.203	0.226	0.251	0.277	0.305	0.333	0.364	0.395	0.429	0.463	0.499	0.537	0.576	0.617	0.659	0.703	0.748	0.795	0.844
8.20	0.138	0.158	0.178	0.200	0.223	0.248	0.274	0.301	0.329	0.359	0.390	0.423	0.457	0.493	0.530	0.568	0.609	0.650	0.693	0.738	0.784	0.833
8.30	0.137	0.156	0.176	0.198	0.220	0.245	0.270	0.297	0.325	0.355	0.385	0.418	0.451	0.487	0.523	0.561	0.601	0.642	0.684	0.728	0.774	0.821
8.40	0.135	0.154	0.174	0.195	0.218	0.242	0.267	0.292	0.321	0.350	0.381	0.413	0.446	0.480	0.516	0.554	0.593	0.633	0.675	0.719	0.764	0.811
8.50	0.133	0.152	0.172	0.193	0.215	0.239	0.264	0.290	0.317	0.346	0.376	0.407	0.440	0.474	0.510	0.547	0.585	0.625	0.667	0.710	0.754	0.800
8.60	0.132	0.150	0.170	0.191	0.213	0.236	0.260	0.286	0.313	0.342	0.371	0.402	0.435	0.469	0.504	0.540	0.578	0.618	0.658	0.701	0.744	0.790
8.70	0.130	0.148	0.168	0.188	0.210	0.233	0.257	0.283	0.310	0.338	0.367	0.398	0.430	0.463	0.498	0.534	0.571	0.610	0.650	0.692	0.735	0.780
8.80	0.129	0.147	0.166	0.186	0.208	0.230	0.254	0.279	0.306	0.334	0.363	0.393	0.424	0.457	0.492	0.527	0.564	0.602	0.642	0.683	0.726	0.770
8.90	0.127	0.145	0.164	0.184	0.205	0.228	0.251	0.276	0.302	0.330	0.358	0.388	0.419	0.452	0.486	0.521	0.557	0.595	0.634	0.675	0.717	0.761
9.00	0.126	0.143	0.162	0.182	0.203	0.225	0.248	0.273	0.299	0.326	0.354	0.384	0.415	0.447	0.480	0.515	0.551	0.588	0.627	0.667	0.708	0.751
9.10	0.125	0.142	0.160	0.180	0.201	0.223	0.246	0.270	0.296	0.322	0.350	0.379	0.410	0.441	0.474	0.509	0.544	0.581	0.619	0.659	0.700	0.742
9.20	0.123	0.140	0.158	0.178	0.198	0.220	0.243	0.267	0.292	0.319	0.346	0.375	0.405	0.436	0.469	0.503	0.538	0.574	0.612	0.651	0.692	0.734
9.30	0.122	0.139	0.157	0.176	0.196	0.218	0.240	0.264	0.289	0.315	0.342	0.371	0.401	0.432	0.464	0.497	0.532	0.568	0.605	0.644	0.684	0.725
9.40	0.121	0.137	0.155	0.174	0.194	0.215	0.238	0.261	0.286	0.312	0.339	0.367	0.396	0.427	0.459	0.492	0.526	0.561	0.598	0.636	0.676	0.717
9.50	0.119	0.136	0.153	0.172	0.192	0.213	0.235	0.258	0.283	0.308	0.335	0.363	0.392	0.422	0.453	0.486	0.520	0.555	0.592	0.629	0.668	0.709
9.60	0.118	0.134	0.152	0.170	0.190	0.211	0.233	0.256	0.280	0.305	0.331	0.359	0.388	0.417	0.448	0.481	0.514	0.549	0.585	0.622	0.661	0.701
9.70	0.117	0.133	0.150	0.169	0.188	0.208	0.230	0.253	0.277	0.302	0.328	0.355	0.383	0.413	0.444	0.476	0.509	0.543	0.579	0.615	0.653	0.693
9.80	0.116	0.132	0.149	0.167	0.186	0.206	0.228	0.250	0.274	0.298	0.324	0.351	0.379	0.409	0.439	0.470	0.503	0.537	0.572	0.609	0.646	0.685
9.90	0.114	0.130	0.147	0.165	0.184	0.204	0.225	0.248	0.271	0.295	0.321	0.348	0.375	0.404	0.434	0.465	0.498	0.531	0.566	0.602	0.639	0.678

Radii in mm	Optic diameters (chords) in mm																					
	7.4	7.6	7.8	8.0	8.2	8.4	8.6	8.8	9.0	9.2	9.4	9.6	9.8	10.0	10.2	10.4	10.6	10.8	11.0	11.2	11.4	11.6
8.00	0.907	0.960	1.015	1.072	1.131	1.191	1.254	1.319	1.386	1.455	1.526	1.600	1.676	1.755	1.836	1.921	2.008	2.097	2.191	2.287	2.387	2.490
8.10	0.894	0.947	1.001	1.057	1.114	1.174	1.236	1.299	1.365	1.433	1.503	1.575	1.650	1.727	1.807	1.890	1.975	2.063	2.154	2.248	2.345	2.446
8.20	0.882	0.934	0.987	1.042	1.099	1.157	1.218	1.280	1.345	1.412	1.481	1.552	1.625	1.701	1.779	1.860	1.943	2.029	2.118	2.210	2.305	2.403
8.30	0.870	0.921	0.973	1.027	1.083	1.141	1.201	1.262	1.326	1.391	1.459	1.529	1.601	1.675	1.752	1.831	1.913	1.997	2.084	2.174	2.267	2.363
8.40	0.859	0.909	0.960	1.014	1.069	1.125	1.184	1.245	1.307	1.371	1.438	1.507	1.577	1.650	1.725	1.803	1.883	1.966	2.051	2.139	2.230	2.324
8.50	0.848	0.897	0.948	1.000	1.054	1.110	1.168	1.227	1.289	1.352	1.418	1.485	1.554	1.626	1.700	1.776	1.855	1.936	2.019	2.105	2.194	2.286
8.60	0.837	0.885	0.935	0.987	1.040	1.095	1.152	1.211	1.271	1.334	1.398	1.464	1.532	1.603	1.675	1.750	1.827	1.907	1.989	2.073	2.160	2.250
8.70	0.826	0.874	0.923	0.974	1.027	1.081	1.137	1.195	1.254	1.316	1.379	1.444	1.511	1.580	1.652	1.725	1.801	1.879	1.959	2.042	2.127	2.215
8.80	0.816	0.863	0.911	0.962	1.013	1.067	1.122	1.179	1.238	1.298	1.360	1.424	1.490	1.558	1.629	1.701	1.775	1.852	1.931	2.012	2.096	2.182
8.90	0.806	0.852	0.900	0.950	1.001	1.053	1.108	1.164	1.221	1.281	1.342	1.405	1.470	1.537	1.606	1.677	1.750	1.825	1.903	1.983	2.065	2.149
9.00	0.796	0.842	0.889	0.938	0.988	1.040	1.094	1.149	1.206	1.264	1.325	1.387	1.451	1.517	1.584	1.654	1.726	1.800	1.876	1.954	2.035	2.118
9.10	0.786	0.831	0.878	0.926	0.976	1.027	1.080	1.134	1.191	1.248	1.308	1.369	1.432	1.497	1.563	1.632	1.703	1.775	1.850	1.927	2.006	2.088
9.20	0.777	0.821	0.868	0.915	0.964	1.015	1.067	1.120	1.176	1.233	1.291	1.351	1.413	1.477	1.543	1.611	1.680	1.752	1.825	1.901	1.979	2.059
9.30	0.768	0.812	0.857	0.904	0.953	1.002	1.054	1.107	1.161	1.217	1.275	1.334	1.396	1.458	1.523	1.590	1.658	1.728	1.801	1.875	1.952	2.030
9.40	0.759	0.802	0.847	0.894	0.941	0.990	1.041	1.093	1.147	1.202	1.259	1.318	1.378	1.440	1.504	1.569	1.637	1.706	1.777	1.850	1.925	2.003
9.50	0.750	0.793	0.837	0.883	0.930	0.979	1.029	1.080	1.133	1.188	1.244	1.302	1.361	1.422	1.485	1.550	1.616	1.684	1.754	1.826	1.900	1.976
9.60	0.742	0.784	0.828	0.873	0.920	0.968	1.017	1.068	1.120	1.174	1.229	1.286	1.345	1.405	1.467	1.530	1.596	1.663	1.732	1.803	1.875	1.950
9.70	0.733	0.775	0.819	0.863	0.909	0.956	1.005	1.055	1.107	1.160	1.215	1.271	1.329	1.388	1.449	1.512	1.576	1.642	1.710	1.780	1.851	1.925
9.80	0.725	0.767	0.809	0.853	0.899	0.946	0.994	1.043	1.094	1.147	1.201	1.256	1.313	1.371	1.432	1.493	1.557	1.622	1.689	1.758	1.828	1.901
9.90	0.717	0.758	0.801	0.844	0.889	0.935	0.983	1.032	1.082	1.134	1.187	1.241	1.298	1.355	1.415	1.476	1.538	1.602	1.668	1.736	1.806	1.877

Radii in mm	Optic diameters (chords) in mm																					
	11.8	12.00	12.25	12.50	12.75	13.00	13.25	13.50	13.75	14.00	14.25	14.50	14.75	15.00	15.25	15.50	15.75	16.00	17.00	18.00	19.00	20.00
8.00	2.597	2.708	2.854	3.006	3.167	3.336	3.516	3.706	3.909	4.127	4.362	4.618	4.900	5.216	5.579	6.016	6.591	8.000				
8.10	2.550	2.658	2.800	2.948	3.103	3.267	3.440	3.623	3.817	4.024	4.247	4.488	4.750	5.041	5.367	5.745	6.204	6.831				
8.20	2.505	2.611	2.748	2.892	3.043	3.201	3.368	3.544	3.731	3.929	4.141	4.369	4.615	4.885	5.183	5.521	5.914	6.400				
8.30	2.462	2.565	2.699	2.839	2.985	3.139	3.300	3.470	3.650	3.840	4.043	4.259	4.492	4.745	5.021	5.329	5.678	6.089				
8.40	2.421	2.521	2.652	2.788	2.930	3.079	3.236	3.500	3.574	3.757	3.951	4.158	4.379	4.617	4.876	5.160	5.477	5.839				
8.50	2.381	2.479	2.606	2.739	2.878	3.023	3.175	3.334	3.502	3.678	3.865	4.063	4.274	4.500	4.744	5.018	5.301	5.628	8.500			
8.60	2.343	2.439	2.563	2.693	2.828	2.969	3.116	3.271	3.433	3.604	3.784	3.974	4.176	4.392	4.623	4.872	5.144	5.444	7.292			
8.70	2.306	2.400	2.522	2.648	2.780	2.917	3.061	3.211	3.369	3.534	3.708	3.891	4.085	4.291	4.511	4.747	5.002	5.281	6.845			
8.80	2.271	2.363	2.481	2.605	2.734	2.868	3.008	3.154	3.307	3.467	3.635	3.812	3.999	4.197	4.407	4.631	4.873	5.134	6.522			
8.90	2.237	2.327	2.443	2.564	2.690	2.821	2.957	3.099	3.248	3.404	3.567	3.738	3.918	4.108	4.310	4.524	4.753	5.000	6.262			
9.00	2.204	2.292	2.406	2.524	2.647	2.775	2.908	3.047	3.192	3.343	3.501	3.667	3.842	4.025	4.219	4.424	4.643	4.877	6.042	9.000		
9.10	2.172	2.258	2.370	2.486	2.605	2.731	2.816	2.997	3.139	3.285	3.439	3.600	3.769	3.946	4.133	4.331	4.540	4.763	5.850	7.755		
9.20	2.141	2.226	2.335	2.449	2.567	2.689	2.817	2.949	3.087	3.230	3.380	3.536	3.700	3.872	4.052	4.242	4.443	4.657	5.680	7.292		
9.30	2.111	2.194	2.302	2.413	2.529	2.649	2.773	2.903	3.037	3.177	3.323	3.475	3.634	3.801	3.976	4.159	4.353	4.558	5.526	6.957		
9.40	2.082	2.164	2.270	2.379	2.492	2.610	2.732	2.858	2.990	3.126	3.269	3.417	3.572	3.733	3.903	4.080	4.267	4.464	5.386	6.687		
9.50	2.054	2.135	2.238	2.345	2.457	2.572	2.691	2.815	2.944	3.077	3.216	3.361	3.512	3.669	3.833	4.006	4.186	4.377	5.257	6.459	9.500	
9.60	2.027	2.106	2.208	2.313	2.422	2.535	2.652	2.774	2.900	3.030	3.166	3.307	3.454	3.608	3.767	3.935	4.110	4.293	5.138	6.259	8.218	
9.70	2.001	2.078	2.178	2.282	2.389	2.500	2.615	2.734	2.857	2.985	3.118	3.256	3.399	3.549	3.704	3.867	4.037	4.215	5.027	6.082	7.740	
9.80	1.975	2.051	2.150	2.252	2.357	2.466	2.579	2.695	2.816	2.941	3.071	3.206	3.346	3.492	3.644	3.802	3.967	4.140	4.923	5.922	7.394	
9.90	1.950	2.025	2.122	2.222	2.326	2.433	2.543	2.658	2.776	2.899	3.027	3.159	3.296	3.438	3.586	3.740	3.900	4.068	4.825	5.776	7.114	

APPENDIX C (continued)
SAGITTA
in mm

Radii in mm	Optic diameters (chords) in mm																
	5.0	5.2	5.4	5.6	5.8	6.0	6.2	6.4	6.6	6.8	7.0	7.2	7.4	7.6	7.8	8.0	8.2
10.00	0.318	0.344	0.371	0.400	0.430	0.461	0.493	0.526	0.560	0.596	0.633	0.670	0.710	0.750	0.792	0.835	0.879
10.25	0.310	0.335	0.362	0.390	0.419	0.449	0.480	0.512	0.546	0.580	0.616	0.653	0.691	0.730	0.771	0.813	0.856
10.50	0.302	0.327	0.353	0.380	0.408	0.438	0.468	0.500	0.532	0.566	0.601	0.636	0.674	0.712	0.751	0.792	0.834
10.75	0.295	0.319	0.345	0.371	0.399	0.427	0.457	0.487	0.519	0.552	0.586	0.621	0.657	0.694	0.732	0.772	0.813
11.00	0.288	0.312	0.337	0.362	0.389	0.417	0.446	0.476	0.507	0.539	0.572	0.606	0.641	0.677	0.715	0.753	0.793
11.25	0.282	0.305	0.329	0.354	0.380	0.408	0.436	0.465	0.495	0.527	0.559	0.592	0.626	0.661	0.698	0.736	0.774
11.50	0.275	0.298	0.321	0.346	0.372	0.398	0.426	0.454	0.484	0.514	0.546	0.578	0.611	0.646	0.681	0.718	0.756
11.75	0.269	0.292	0.315	0.339	0.364	0.390	0.416	0.444	0.473	0.503	0.534	0.566	0.598	0.632	0.666	0.702	0.739
12.00	0.263	0.285	0.308	0.331	0.356	0.381	0.407	0.435	0.463	0.492	0.522	0.553	0.585	0.618	0.651	0.686	0.722
12.25	0.258	0.279	0.302	0.325	0.349	0.373	0.399	0.426	0.453	0.481	0.511	0.541	0.573	0.605	0.638	0.672	0.707
12.50	0.253	0.273	0.295	0.318	0.341	0.365	0.390	0.417	0.443	0.471	0.500	0.530	0.560	0.592	0.624	0.657	0.692
12.75	0.248	0.268	0.289	0.312	0.335	0.358	0.383	0.408	0.435	0.462	0.490	0.519	0.549	0.580	0.612	0.644	0.677
13.00	0.243	0.263	0.283	0.305	0.328	0.351	0.375	0.400	0.426	0.452	0.480	0.508	0.538	0.568	0.599	0.631	0.663
13.25	0.238	0.258	0.278	0.299	0.322	0.344	0.368	0.393	0.418	0.444	0.471	0.498	0.527	0.557	0.587	0.619	0.651
13.50	0.234	0.253	0.273	0.294	0.315	0.338	0.361	0.385	0.410	0.435	0.462	0.489	0.517	0.546	0.576	0.606	0.638
13.75	0.229	0.248	0.268	0.288	0.309	0.332	0.354	0.378	0.402	0.427	0.453	0.480	0.507	0.536	0.565	0.595	0.626
14.00	0.225	0.244	0.263	0.283	0.304	0.325	0.348	0.371	0.394	0.419	0.445	0.471	0.498	0.526	0.554	0.584	0.614
14.25	0.221	0.239	0.258	0.278	0.298	0.320	0.342	0.364	0.388	0.412	0.437	0.463	0.489	0.516	0.544	0.573	0.603
14.50	0.217	0.235	0.254	0.273	0.293	0.314	0.335	0.358	0.381	0.404	0.429	0.454	0.480	0.507	0.534	0.563	0.592
14.75	0.214	0.231	0.249	0.268	0.288	0.308	0.330	0.352	0.374	0.398	0.422	0.447	0.472	0.498	0.525	0.553	0.581
15.00	0.210	0.227	0.245	0.264	0.283	0.303	0.324	0.345	0.368	0.390	0.414	0.438	0.463	0.489	0.516	0.543	0.571
15.25	0.207	0.224	0.241	0.259	0.278	0.298	0.318	0.340	0.362	0.384	0.407	0.431	0.456	0.481	0.507	0.534	0.562
15.50	0.203	0.220	0.237	0.255	0.274	0.293	0.313	0.334	0.355	0.378	0.400	0.424	0.448	0.473	0.499	0.525	0.552
15.75	0.200	0.216	0.233	0.251	0.269	0.288	0.308	0.329	0.350	0.372	0.394	0.417	0.441	0.466	0.491	0.517	0.543
16.00	0.197	0.213	0.229	0.247	0.265	0.284	0.303	0.323	0.344	0.365	0.388	0.410	0.434	0.458	0.483	0.508	0.534
17.00	0.185	0.200	0.216	0.232	0.249	0.267	0.285	0.304	0.323	0.343	0.364	0.386	0.408	0.430	0.453	0.477	0.502

Radii in mm	Optic diameters (chords) in mm																
	8.4	8.6	8.8	9.0	9.2	9.4	9.6	9.8	10.0	10.2	10.4	10.6	10.8	11.0	11.2	11.4	11.6
10.00	0.925	0.972	1.020	1.070	1.121	1.173	1.227	1.283	1.340	1.398	1.458	1.520	1.583	1.648	1.715	1.784	1.854
10.25	0.900	0.946	0.992	1.041	1.090	1.141	1.193	1.247	1.302	1.359	1.417	1.477	1.538	1.601	1.665	1.731	1.799
10.50	0.877	0.921	0.966	1.013	1.061	1.111	1.161	1.213	1.267	1.322	1.378	1.436	1.495	1.556	1.618	1.682	1.747
10.75	0.854	0.897	0.942	0.987	1.034	1.082	1.131	1.182	1.234	1.287	1.341	1.397	1.455	1.514	1.574	1.636	1.699
11.00	0.833	0.875	0.918	0.963	1.008	1.055	1.103	1.152	1.202	1.254	1.307	1.361	1.417	1.474	1.532	1.592	1.653
11.25	0.814	0.854	0.896	0.940	0.984	1.029	1.076	1.124	1.172	1.223	1.274	1.327	1.381	1.436	1.493	1.551	1.611
11.50	0.794	0.834	0.875	0.917	0.960	1.004	1.050	1.096	1.144	1.193	1.243	1.294	1.347	1.400	1.456	1.512	1.570
11.75	0.777	0.815	0.855	0.896	0.938	0.981	1.025	1.071	1.117	1.165	1.214	1.263	1.315	1.367	1.420	1.475	1.532
12.00	0.759	0.797	0.836	0.876	0.917	0.959	1.002	1.046	1.091	1.138	1.185	1.234	1.284	1.335	1.387	1.440	1.495
12.25	0.743	0.780	0.818	0.857	0.897	0.938	0.980	1.023	1.067	1.112	1.159	1.206	1.255	1.304	1.355	1.407	1.460
12.50	0.727	0.763	0.800	0.838	0.877	0.917	0.958	1.000	1.044	1.088	1.133	1.179	1.227	1.275	1.325	1.375	1.427
12.75	0.712	0.747	0.784	0.821	0.859	0.897	0.938	0.979	1.022	1.065	1.109	1.154	1.200	1.248	1.296	1.345	1.396
13.00	0.697	0.732	0.767	0.804	0.841	0.879	0.919	0.959	1.000	1.042	1.085	1.129	1.175	1.221	1.268	1.316	1.366
13.25	0.684	0.717	0.752	0.788	0.824	0.862	0.900	0.940	0.980	1.021	1.063	1.107	1.151	1.195	1.242	1.289	1.337
13.50	0.670	0.703	0.737	0.772	0.808	0.845	0.882	0.921	0.960	1.000	1.042	1.084	1.127	1.171	1.216	1.262	1.309
13.75	0.658	0.690	0.723	0.757	0.792	0.828	0.865	0.903	0.942	0.981	1.021	1.063	1.105	1.148	1.192	1.237	1.283
14.00	0.645	0.677	0.709	0.743	0.777	0.813	0.849	0.886	0.923	0.962	1.002	1.042	1.083	1.126	1.169	1.213	1.258
14.25	0.633	0.665	0.697	0.729	0.763	0.797	0.833	0.869	0.906	0.944	0.983	1.022	1.063	1.104	1.147	1.190	1.234
14.50	0.622	0.652	0.684	0.716	0.749	0.783	0.818	0.853	0.889	0.926	0.964	1.003	1.043	1.084	1.125	1.167	1.211
14.75	0.611	0.641	0.672	0.704	0.736	0.769	0.803	0.838	0.873	0.910	0.947	0.986	1.024	1.064	1.104	1.146	1.189
15.00	0.600	0.630	0.660	0.691	0.723	0.755	0.789	0.823	0.858	0.894	0.930	0.968	1.006	1.045	1.085	1.125	1.167
15.25	0.590	0.619	0.649	0.679	0.711	0.743	0.775	0.809	0.843	0.878	0.914	0.951	0.989	1.027	1.066	1.105	1.146
15.50	0.580	0.608	0.638	0.668	0.698	0.730	0.762	0.795	0.829	0.863	0.898	0.934	0.971	1.009	1.047	1.086	1.126
15.75	0.570	0.598	0.627	0.657	0.687	0.718	0.750	0.782	0.815	0.849	0.883	0.919	0.955	0.992	1.030	1.068	1.107
16.00	0.561	0.589	0.617	0.646	0.676	0.706	0.737	0.769	0.801	0.835	0.869	0.903	0.939	0.975	1.012	1.050	1.088
17.00	0.527	0.553	0.579	0.606	0.634	0.663	0.692	0.721	0.752	0.783	0.815	0.847	0.880	0.914	0.949	0.984	1.020

APPENDIX C (continued)

SAGITTA

in mm

Radii in mm	Optic diameters (chords) in mm																
	11.8	12.00	12.25	12.50	12.75	13.00	13.25	13.50	13.75	14.00	14.25	14.50	14.75	15.00	15.25	15.50	15.75
10.00	1.926	2.000	2.095	2.194	2.295	2.401	2.509	2.622	2.738	2.859	2.983	3.113	3.247	3.386	3.530	3.680	3.837
10.25	1.868	1.940	2.031	2.126	2.224	2.325	2.429	2.536	2.648	2.763	2.881	3.004	3.132	3.263	3.400	3.542	3.689
10.50	1.814	1.883	1.972	2.063	2.157	2.254	2.354	2.457	2.564	2.674	2.787	2.905	3.026	3.152	3.281	3.416	3.555
10.75	1.764	1.830	1.916	2.004	2.094	2.188	2.284	2.383	2.486	2.591	2.700	2.813	2.929	3.049	3.172	3.300	3.432
11.00	1.716	1.780	1.863	1.948	2.036	2.126	2.219	2.315	2.413	2.515	2.619	2.727	2.839	2.953	3.072	3.194	3.320
11.25	1.672	1.734	1.814	1.896	1.981	2.068	2.158	2.250	2.345	2.443	2.544	2.648	2.755	2.865	2.978	3.095	3.216
11.50	1.629	1.689	1.767	1.847	1.929	2.013	2.100	2.189	2.281	2.376	2.473	2.573	2.676	2.782	2.891	3.004	3.119
11.75	1.589	1.648	1.723	1.800	1.880	1.962	2.046	2.132	2.221	2.313	2.407	2.503	2.603	2.705	2.810	2.918	3.030
12.00	1.551	1.608	1.681	1.756	1.833	1.913	1.995	2.078	2.165	2.253	2.344	2.438	2.534	2.633	2.734	2.838	2.945
12.25	1.515	1.570	1.641	1.715	1.790	1.867	1.946	2.028	2.111	2.197	2.285	2.376	2.469	2.564	2.662	2.763	2.867
12.50	1.480	1.534	1.603	1.675	1.748	1.823	1.900	1.979	2.060	2.144	2.229	2.317	2.407	2.500	2.595	2.693	2.793
12.75	1.448	1.500	1.568	1.637	1.708	1.781	1.856	1.933	2.012	2.093	2.177	2.262	2.349	2.439	2.531	2.626	2.723
13.00	1.416	1.467	1.533	1.601	1.670	1.742	1.815	1.890	1.967	2.046	2.126	2.209	2.294	2.382	2.471	2.563	2.657
13.25	1.386	1.436	1.501	1.567	1.634	1.704	1.775	1.848	1.923	2.000	2.079	2.159	2.242	2.327	2.414	2.503	2.599
13.50	1.358	1.407	1.469	1.534	1.600	1.668	1.737	1.809	1.882	1.957	2.033	2.112	2.193	2.275	2.360	2.446	2.535
13.75	1.331	1.379	1.440	1.503	1.567	1.633	1.701	1.771	1.842	1.915	1.990	2.067	2.145	2.226	2.308	2.392	2.478
14.00	1.304	1.351	1.411	1.473	1.536	1.600	1.667	1.735	1.804	1.876	1.949	2.023	2.100	2.178	2.259	2.341	2.425
14.25	1.279	1.325	1.383	1.444	1.506	1.569	1.634	1.700	1.768	1.838	1.909	1.982	2.057	2.133	2.212	2.292	2.374
14.50	1.255	1.300	1.357	1.416	1.478	1.539	1.602	1.667	1.733	1.802	1.871	1.943	2.016	2.090	2.167	2.245	2.325
14.75	1.232	1.276	1.332	1.390	1.449	1.509	1.572	1.635	1.700	1.767	1.835	1.905	1.976	2.049	2.124	2.200	2.278
15.00	1.209	1.252	1.308	1.364	1.422	1.482	1.542	1.605	1.668	1.734	1.800	1.868	1.938	2.010	2.083	2.157	2.233
15.25	1.188	1.230	1.284	1.340	1.396	1.455	1.514	1.575	1.638	1.701	1.767	1.834	1.902	1.972	2.043	2.116	2.191
15.50	1.167	1.208	1.262	1.316	1.372	1.429	1.487	1.547	1.608	1.671	1.735	1.800	1.867	1.935	2.005	2.077	2.150
15.75	1.147	1.188	1.240	1.294	1.348	1.404	1.461	1.520	1.580	1.641	1.704	1.768	1.833	1.900	1.969	2.039	2.110
16.00	1.128	1.168	1.219	1.271	1.325	1.380	1.436	1.494	1.552	1.613	1.674	1.737	1.801	1.867	1.934	2.002	2.072
17.00	1.057	1.094	1.142	1.191	1.241	1.292	1.344	1.398	1.452	1.508	1.565	1.623	1.683	1.744	1.806	1.869	1.934

Radii in mm	Optic diameters (chords) in mm														
	16.0	17.0	18.0	19.0	20.0	21.0	22.0	23.0	24.0	25.0	26.0	27.0	28.0	29.0	30.0
10.00	4.000	4.638	5.641	6.878	10.000										
10.25	3.842	4.522	5.345	6.401	8.000										
10.50	3.699	4.336	5.092	6.028	7.298	10.500									
10.75	3.569	4.169	4.871	5.719	6.805	8.445									
11.00	3.450	4.018	4.675	5.455	6.417	7.721	11.000								
11.25	3.340	3.880	4.500	5.224	6.096	7.211	8.892								
11.50	3.239	3.754	4.341	5.019	5.821	6.810	8.221	11.500							
11.75	3.144	3.638	4.196	4.835	5.581	6.476	7.619	9.339							
12.00	3.056	3.529	4.063	4.669	5.367	6.191	7.204	8.572	12.000						
12.25	2.973	3.429	3.940	4.516	5.175	5.940	6.859	8.030	9.788						
12.50	2.895	3.335	3.825	4.376	5.000	5.718	6.563	7.601	9.000	12.500					
12.75	2.822	3.247	3.719	4.246	4.840	5.517	6.303	7.244	8.442	10.238					
13.00	2.753	3.164	3.619	4.126	4.693	5.335	6.072	6.938	8.000	9.429	13.000				
13.25	2.688	3.086	3.526	4.014	4.557	5.168	5.863	6.669	7.632	8.855	10.688				
13.50	2.626	3.012	3.438	3.908	4.431	5.015	5.674	6.429	7.315	8.401	9.860	13.500			
13.75	2.567	2.942	3.355	3.810	4.313	4.872	5.500	6.213	6.937	8.022	9.271	11.140			
14.00	2.511	2.876	3.276	3.717	4.202	4.740	5.340	6.016	6.789	7.695	8.804	10.292	14.000		
14.25	2.458	2.813	3.202	3.629	4.095	4.616	5.191	5.835	6.565	7.408	8.414	9.688	11.592		
14.50	2.407	2.753	3.131	3.546	4.000	4.500	5.053	5.668	6.361	7.152	8.077	9.208	10.725	14.500	
14.75	2.358	2.695	3.064	3.467	3.907	4.391	4.923	5.514	6.173	6.920	7.781	8.808	10.106	12.046	
15.00	2.311	2.641	3.000	3.392	3.820	4.288	4.802	5.369	6.000	6.708	7.517	8.462	9.615	11.159	15.000
15.25	2.267	2.589	2.939	3.321	3.736	4.191	4.688	5.234	5.839	6.514	7.277	8.157	9.203	10.526	12.500
15.50	2.224	2.539	2.881	3.253	3.657	4.098	4.580	5.108	5.689	6.335	7.059	7.884	8.848	10.023	11.595
15.75	2.183	2.491	2.825	3.189	3.582	4.011	4.478	4.988	5.549	6.168	6.858	7.638	8.535	9.601	10.948
16.00	2.144	2.445	2.771	3.126	3.510	3.927	4.381	4.876	5.417	6.013	6.673	7.412	8.254	9.236	10.432
17.00	2.000	2.278	2.578	2.920	3.252	3.630	4.039	4.480	4.958	5.478	6.046	6.668	7.356	8.126	9.000

APPENDIX D

**Back and Front Vertex Powers for various centre thicknesses and back optic radii,
calculated on the basis of a refractive index of 1.49.**

Centre thickness 0.08 mm

Back Vertex Powers in D	Front Vertex Powers in D for Back Optic Radii in mm of:							
	5.0	6.0	7.0	7.5	8.0	8.5	9.0	10.0
+ 20	19.77	19.81	19.83	19.84	19.85	19.86	19.86	19.87
19	18.78	18.82	18.84	18.85	18.86	18.86	18.87	18.88
18	17.80	17.83	17.85	17.86	17.87	17.87	17.88	17.89
17	16.81	16.84	16.86	16.87	16.87	16.88	16.89	16.90
16	15.82	15.85	15.87	15.88	15.88	15.89	15.89	15.90
15	14.83	14.86	14.88	14.88	14.89	14.90	14.90	14.91
14	13.84	13.87	13.89	13.89	13.90	13.90	13.91	13.92
13	12.86	12.88	12.89	12.90	12.91	12.91	12.92	12.92
12	11.87	11.89	11.90	11.91	11.91	11.92	11.92	11.93
11	10.88	10.90	10.91	10.92	10.92	10.93	10.93	10.94
10	9.89	9.91	9.92	9.93	9.93	9.93	9.94	9.94
9	8.90	8.92	8.93	8.93	8.94	8.94	8.94	8.95
8	7.91	7.93	7.94	7.94	7.94	7.95	7.95	7.96
7	6.92	6.94	6.95	6.95	6.95	6.95	6.96	6.96
6	5.94	5.95	5.95	5.96	5.96	5.96	5.96	5.97
5	4.95	4.96	4.96	4.96	4.97	4.97	4.97	4.97
4	3.96	3.96	3.97	3.97	3.97	3.98	3.98	3.98
3	2.97	2.97	2.98	2.98	2.98	2.98	2.98	2.98
2	1.98	1.98	1.99	1.99	1.99	1.99	1.99	1.99
1	0.99	0.99	0.99	0.99	0.99	0.99	0.99	1.00
0	0.00	0.00	0.00	0.00	0.00	0.00	0.00	0.00
− 1	0.99	0.99	0.99	0.99	0.99	0.99	0.99	1.00
2	1.98	1.98	1.99	1.99	1.99	1.99	1.99	1.99
3	2.97	2.97	2.98	2.98	2.98	2.98	2.98	2.99
4	3.96	3.97	3.97	3.97	3.98	3.98	3.98	3.98
5	4.95	4.96	4.96	4.97	4.97	4.97	4.97	4.98
6	5.94	5.95	5.96	5.96	5.96	5.97	5.97	5.97
7	6.93	6.94	6.95	6.95	6.96	6.96	6.96	6.97
8	7.92	7.93	7.94	7.95	7.95	7.95	7.96	7.96
9	8.91	8.93	8.94	8.94	8.95	8.95	8.95	8.96
10	9.90	9.92	9.93	9.94	9.94	9.94	9.95	9.95
11	10.89	10.91	10.92	10.93	10.93	10.94	10.94	10.95
12	11.88	11.90	11.92	11.92	11.93	11.93	11.94	11.95
13	12.87	12.90	12.91	12.92	12.92	12.93	12.93	12.94
14	13.86	13.89	13.91	13.91	13.92	13.92	13.93	13.94
15	14.86	14.88	14.90	14.91	14.91	14.92	14.93	14.93
16	15.85	15.87	15.89	15.90	15.91	15.92	15.92	15.93
17	16.84	16.87	16.88	16.90	16.90	16.91	16.92	16.93
18	17.83	17.86	17.88	17.89	17.90	17.91	17.91	17.92
19	18.82	18.85	18.88	18.89	18.90	18.90	18.91	18.92
20	19.81	19.85	19.87	19.88	19.89	19.90	19.91	19.92
21	20.80	20.84	20.87	20.88	20.89	20.89	20.90	20.91
22	21.80	21.83	21.86	21.87	21.88	21.89	21.90	21.91
23	22.79	22.83	22.86	22.87	22.88	22.89	22.89	22.91
24	23.78	23.82	23.85	23.86	23.87	23.88	23.89	23.91
25	24.77	24.82	24.85	24.86	24.87	24.88	24.89	24.90
26	25.76	25.81	25.84	25.86	25.87	25.88	25.89	25.90
27	26.76	26.80	26.84	26.85	26.86	26.86	26.88	26.90
28	27.75	27.80	27.83	27.85	27.86	27.87	27.88	27.90
29	28.74	28.79	28.83	28.84	28.86	28.87	28.88	28.89
30	29.73	29.79	29.82	29.84	29.85	29.86	29.87	29.89

APPENDIX D (continued)

Centre thickness 0.10 mm

Back Vertex Powers in D	Front Vertex Powers in D for Back Optic Radii in mm of:							
	5.0	6.0	7.0	7.5	8.0	8.5	9.0	10.00
+ 20	19.71	19.76	19.79	19.80	19.81	19.82	19.83	19.84
19	18.73	18.77	18.80	18.81	18.82	18.83	18.84	18.85
18	17.74	17.78	17.81	17.82	17.83	17.84	17.85	17.86
17	16.76	16.80	16.82	16.83	16.84	16.85	16.86	16.87
16	15.78	15.81	15.83	15.84	15.85	15.86	15.87	15.88
15	14.79	14.82	14.85	14.85	14.86	14.87	14.88	14.89
14	13.81	13.84	13.86	13.87	13.87	13.88	13.89	13.90
13	12.82	12.85	12.87	12.88	12.88	12.89	12.89	12.90
12	11.83	11.86	11.88	11.89	11.89	11.90	11.90	11.91
11	10.85	10.87	10.89	10.90	10.90	10.91	10.91	10.92
10	9.86	9.89	9.90	9.91	9.91	9.92	9.92	9.93
9	8.88	8.90	8.91	8.92	8.92	8.93	8.93	8.94
8	7.89	7.91	7.92	7.93	7.93	7.93	7.94	7.94
7	6.91	6.92	6.93	6.94	6.94	6.94	6.95	6.95
6	5.92	5.93	5.94	5.95	5.95	5.95	5.95	5.96
5	4.93	4.94	4.95	4.96	4.96	4.96	4.96	4.97
4	3.95	3.96	3.96	3.96	3.97	3.97	3.97	3.97
3	2.96	2.97	2.97	2.97	2.98	2.98	2.98	2.98
2	1.97	1.98	1.98	1.98	1.98	1.98	1.99	1.99
1	0.99	0.99	0.99	0.99	0.99	0.99	0.99	0.99
0	0.00	0.00	0.00	0.00	0.00	0.00	0.00	0.00
− 1	0.99	0.99	0.99	0.99	0.99	0.99	0.99	0.99
2	1.97	1.98	1.98	1.98	1.98	1.99	1.99	1.99
3	2.96	2.97	2.97	2.97	2.98	2.98	2.98	2.98
4	3.95	3.96	3.96	3.97	3.97	3.97	3.97	3.98
5	4.94	4.95	4.96	4.96	4.96	4.96	4.97	4.97
6	5.92	5.94	5.95	5.95	5.95	5.96	5.96	5.96
7	6.91	6.93	6.94	6.94	6.95	6.95	6.95	6.96
8	7.90	7.92	7.93	7.94	7.94	7.94	7.95	7.95
9	8.89	8.91	8.92	8.93	8.93	8.94	8.94	8.95
10	9.88	9.90	9.91	9.92	9.93	9.93	9.93	9.94
11	10.87	10.89	10.91	10.91	10.92	10.92	10.93	10.94
12	11.85	11.88	11.90	11.91	11.91	11.92	11.92	11.93
13	12.84	12.87	12.89	12.90	12.91	12.91	12.92	12.93
14	13.83	13.86	13.88	13.89	13.90	13.91	13.91	13.92
15	14.82	14.85	14.88	14.89	14.89	14.90	14.91	14.92
16	15.81	15.84	15.87	15.88	15.89	15.89	15.90	15.91
17	16.80	16.83	16.86	16.87	16.88	16.89	16.90	16.91
18	17.79	17.83	17.85	17.87	17.87	17.88	17.89	17.90
19	18.78	18.82	18.85	18.86	18.87	18.88	18.89	18.90
20	19.77	19.81	19.84	19.85	19.86	19.87	19.88	19.90
21	20.76	20.80	20.83	20.85	20.86	20.87	20.88	20.89
22	21.75	21.79	21.83	21.84	21.85	21.86	21.87	21.89
23	22.74	22.79	22.82	22.84	22.85	22.86	22.87	22.89
24	23.73	23.78	23.81	23.83	23.84	23.85	23.86	23.88
25	24.72	24.77	24.81	24.82	24.84	24.85	24.86	24.88
26	25.71	25.76	25.80	25.82	25.83	25.85	25.86	25.88
27	26.70	26.76	26.80	26.81	26.83	26.84	26.85	26.87
28	27.69	27.75	27.79	27.81	27.82	27.84	27.85	27.87
29	28.68	28.74	28.79	28.80	28.82	28.83	28.85	28.87
30	29.67	29.73	29.78	29.80	29.82	29.83	29.84	29.86

APPENDIX D (continued)

Centre thickness 0.12 mm

Back Vertex Powers in D	Front Vertex Powers in D for Back Optic Radii in mm of:							
	5.0	6.0	7.0	7.5	8.0	8.5	9.0	10.0
+ 20	19.66	19.71	19.75	19.76	19.77	19.78	19.79	19.81
19	18.68	18.72	18.76	18.77	18.79	18.80	18.81	18.82
18	17.69	17.74	17.77	17.79	17.80	17.81	17.82	17.83
17	16.71	16.76	16.79	16.80	16.81	16.82	16.83	16.84
16	15.73	15.77	15.80	15.81	15.82	15.83	15.84	15.85
15	14.75	14.79	14.81	14.83	14.84	14.84	14.85	14.86
14	13.77	13.80	13.83	13.84	13.85	13.86	13.86	13.88
13	12.78	12.82	12.84	12.85	12.86	12.87	12.87	12.89
12	11.80	11.83	11.85	11.86	11.87	11.88	11.88	11.89
11	10.82	10.85	10.87	10.88	10.88	10.89	10.90	10.90
10	9.84	9.86	9.88	9.89	9.89	9.90	9.91	9.91
9	8.85	8.88	8.89	8.90	8.91	8.91	8.92	8.92
8	7.87	7.89	7.91	7.91	7.92	7.92	7.93	7.93
7	6.89	6.91	6.92	6.92	6.93	6.93	6.94	6.94
6	5.90	5.92	5.93	5.94	5.94	5.94	5.95	5.95
5	4.92	4.93	4.94	4.95	4.95	4.95	4.95	4.96
4	3.94	3.95	3.95	3.96	3.96	3.96	3.96	3.97
3	2.95	2.96	2.97	2.97	2.97	2.97	2.97	2.98
2	1.97	1.97	1.98	1.98	1.98	1.98	1.98	1.98
1	0.98	0.99	0.99	0.99	0.99	0.99	0.99	0.99
0	0.00	0.00	0.00	0.00	0.00	0.00	0.00	0.00
− 1	0.98	0.99	0.99	0.99	0.99	0.99	0.99	0.99
2	1.97	1.97	1.98	1.98	1.98	1.98	1.98	1.99
3	2.95	2.96	2.97	2.97	2.97	2.97	2.98	2.98
4	3.94	3.95	3.96	3.96	3.96	3.96	3.97	3.97
5	4.92	4.94	4.95	4.95	4.95	4.96	4.96	4.96
6	5.91	5.93	5.94	5.94	5.94	5.95	5.95	5.96
7	6.90	6.91	6.93	6.93	6.94	6.94	6.94	6.95
8	7.88	7.90	7.92	7.92	7.93	7.93	7.94	7.94
9	8.87	8.89	8.91	8.91	8.92	8.92	8.93	8.94
10	9.85	9.88	9.90	9.90	9.91	9.92	9.92	9.93
11	10.84	10.87	10.89	10.90	10.90	10.91	10.91	10.92
12	11.82	11.86	11.88	11.89	11.89	11.90	11.91	11.92
13	12.81	12.84	12.87	12.88	12.89	12.89	12.90	12.91
14	13.80	13.83	13.86	13.87	13.88	13.89	13.89	13.91
15	14.78	14.82	14.85	14.86	14.87	14.88	14.89	14.90
16	15.77	15.81	15.84	15.85	15.86	15.87	15.88	15.90
17	16.76	16.80	16.83	16.85	16.86	16.87	16.88	16.89
18	17.75	17.79	17.82	17.84	17.85	17.86	17.87	17.89
19	18.73	18.78	18.82	18.83	18.84	18.85	18.86	18.88
20	19.72	19.77	19.81	19.82	19.84	19.85	19.86	19.88
21	20.71	20.76	20.80	20.82	20.83	20.84	20.85	20.87
22	21.70	21.75	21.79	21.81	21.82	21.84	21.85	21.87
23	22.68	22.74	22.79	22.80	22.82	22.83	22.84	22.86
24	23.67	23.73	23.78	23.80	23.81	23.83	23.84	23.86
25	24.66	24.72	24.77	24.79	24.81	24.82	24.83	24.85
26	25.65	25.72	25.76	25.78	25.80	25.81	25.83	25.85
27	26.64	26.71	26.76	26.78	26.79	26.81	26.82	26.85
28	27.63	27.70	27.75	27.77	27.79	27.80	27.82	27.84
29	28.61	28.69	28.74	28.76	28.78	28.80	28.81	28.84
30	29.60	29.68	29.74	29.76	29.78	29.80	29.81	29.84

APPENDIX D (continued)

Centre thickness 0.14 mm

Back Vertex Powers in D	Front Vertex Powers in D for Back Optic Radii in mm of:							
	5.0	6.0	7.0	7.5	8.0	8.5	9.0	10.00
+ 20	19.60	19.66	19.70	19.72	19.74	19.75	19.76	19.78
19	18.62	18.68	18.72	18.74	18.75	18.76	18.77	18.79
18	17.64	17.70	17.74	17.75	17.77	17.78	17.79	17.81
17	16.67	16.72	16.75	16.77	16.78	16.79	16.80	16.82
16	15.69	15.73	15.77	15.78	15.79	15.80	15.81	15.83
15	14.71	14.75	14.78	14.80	14.81	14.82	14.83	14.84
14	13.73	13.77	13.80	13.81	13.82	13.83	13.84	13.85
13	12.75	12.79	12.82	12.83	12.84	12.85	12.85	12.87
12	11.77	11.81	11.83	11.84	11.85	11.86	11.87	11.88
11	10.79	10.82	10.85	10.86	10.86	10.87	10.88	10.89
10	9.81	9.84	9.86	9.87	9.88	9.88	9.89	9.90
9	8.83	8.86	8.88	8.88	8.89	8.90	8.90	8.91
8	7.85	7.87	7.89	7.90	7.90	7.91	7.91	7.92
7	6.87	6.89	6.90	6.91	6.92	6.92	6.92	6.93
6	5.89	5.91	5.92	5.92	5.93	5.93	5.94	5.94
5	4.91	4.92	4.93	4.94	4.94	4.94	4.95	4.95
4	3.93	3.94	3.95	3.95	3.95	3.96	3.96	3.96
3	2.95	2.95	2.96	2.96	2.97	2.97	2.97	2.97
2	1.96	1.97	1.97	1.98	1.98	1.98	1.98	1.98
1	0.98	0.99	0.99	0.99	0.99	0.99	0.99	0.99
0	0.00	0.00	0.00	0.00	0.00	0.00	0.00	0.00
− 1	0.98	0.99	0.99	0.99	0.99	0.99	0.99	0.99
2	1.96	1.97	1.97	1.98	1.98	1.98	1.98	1.98
3	2.95	2.96	2.96	2.96	2.97	2.97	2.97	2.97
4	3.93	3.94	3.95	3.95	3.96	3.96	3.96	3.97
5	4.91	4.93	4.94	4.94	4.95	4.95	4.95	4.96
6	5.89	5.91	5.93	5.93	5.94	5.94	5.94	5.95
7	6.88	6.90	6.91	6.92	6.93	6.93	6.93	6.94
8	7.86	7.89	7.90	7.91	7.92	7.92	7.93	7.93
9	8.84	8.87	8.89	8.90	8.91	8.91	8.92	8.93
10	9.83	9.86	9.88	9.89	9.90	9.90	9.91	9.92
11	10.81	10.84	10.87	10.88	10.89	10.89	10.90	10.91
12	11.80	11.83	11.86	11.87	11.88	11.88	11.89	11.90
13	12.78	12.82	12.85	12.86	12.87	12.88	12.88	12.90
14	13.76	13.81	13.84	13.85	13.86	13.87	13.88	13.89
15	14.75	14.79	14.83	14.84	14.85	14.86	14.87	14.88
16	15.73	15.78	15.82	15.83	15.84	15.85	15.86	15.88
17	16.72	16.77	16.81	16.82	16.83	16.84	16.85	16.87
18	17.70	17.76	17.80	17.81	17.83	17.84	17.85	17.87
19	18.69	18.75	18.79	18.80	18.82	18.83	18.84	18.86
20	19.67	19.73	19.78	19.79	19.81	19.82	19.83	19.85
21	20.66	20.72	20.77	20.79	20.80	20.82	20.83	20.85
22	21.65	21.71	21.76	21.78	21.79	21.81	21.82	21.84
23	22.63	22.70	22.75	22.77	22.79	22.80	22.82	22.84
24	23.62	23.69	23.74	23.76	23.78	23.80	23.81	23.83
25	24.60	24.68	24.73	24.75	24.77	24.79	24.80	24.83
26	25.59	25.67	25.72	25.75	25.77	25.78	25.80	25.83
27	26.58	26.66	26.72	26.74	26.76	26.78	26.79	26.82
28	27.56	27.65	27.71	27.73	27.75	27.77	27.79	27.82
29	28.55	28.64	28.70	28.73	28.75	28.77	28.78	28.81
30	29.54	29.63	29.69	29.72	29.74	29.76	29.78	29.81

APPENDIX D

APPENDIX D (continued)

Centre thickness 0.16 mm

Back Vertex Powers in D	Front Vertex Powers in D for Back Optic Radii in mm of:							
	5.0	6.0	7.0	7.5	8.0	8.5	9.0	10.00
+ 20	19.54	19.61	19.66	19.68	19.70	19.71	19.73	19.75
19	18.57	18.63	18.68	18.70	18.72	18.73	18.74	18.76
18	17.59	17.66	17.70	17.72	17.73	17.75	17.76	17.78
17	16.62	16.68	16.72	16.73	16.75	16.76	16.77	16.79
16	15.64	15.70	15.74	15.75	15.77	15.78	15.79	15.81
15	14.67	14.72	14.75	14.77	14.78	14.79	14.80	14.82
14	13.69	13.74	13.77	13.79	13.80	13.81	13.82	13.83
13	12.71	12.76	12.79	12.80	12.81	12.82	12.83	12.85
12	11.74	11.78	11.81	11.82	11.83	11.84	11.85	11.86
11	10.76	10.80	10.82	10.84	10.84	10.85	10.86	10.87
10	9.78	9.82	9.84	9.85	9.86	9.87	9.87	9.89
9	8.81	8.84	8.86	8.87	8.87	8.88	8.89	8.90
8	7.83	7.86	7.87	7.88	7.89	7.90	7.90	7.91
7	6.85	6.87	6.89	6.90	6.90	6.91	6.91	6.92
6	5.87	5.89	5.91	5.91	5.92	5.92	5.93	5.93
5	4.89	4.91	4.92	4.93	4.93	4.94	4.94	4.95
4	3.92	3.93	3.94	3.94	3.95	3.95	3.95	3.96
3	2.94	2.95	2.95	2.96	2.96	2.96	2.96	2.97
2	1.96	1.97	1.97	1.97	1.97	1.98	1.98	1.98
1	0.98	0.98	0.99	0.99	0.99	0.99	0.99	0.99
0	0.00	0.00	0.00	0.00	0.00	0.00	0.00	0.00
− 1	0.98	0.98	0.99	0.99	0.99	0.99	0.99	0.99
2	1.96	1.97	1.97	1.97	1.97	1.98	1.98	1.98
3	2.94	2.95	2.96	2.96	2.96	2.96	2.97	2.97
4	3.92	3.93	3.94	3.95	3.95	3.95	3.96	3.96
5	4.90	4.92	4.93	4.93	4.94	4.94	4.95	4.95
6	5.88	5.90	5.92	5.92	5.93	5.93	5.93	5.94
7	6.86	6.88	6.90	6.91	6.91	6.92	6.92	6.93
8	7.84	7.87	7.89	7.90	7.90	7.91	7.91	7.92
9	8.82	8.85	8.88	8.88	8.89	8.90	8.90	8.92
10	9.80	9.84	9.86	9.87	9.88	9.89	9.90	9.91
11	10.79	10.82	10.85	10.86	10.87	10.88	10.89	10.90
12	11.77	11.81	11.84	11.85	11.86	11.87	11.88	11.89
13	12.75	12.79	12.83	12.84	12.85	12.86	12.87	12.88
14	13.73	13.78	13.81	13.83	13.84	13.85	13.86	13.88
15	14.71	14.76	14.80	14.82	14.83	14.84	14.85	14.87
16	15.70	15.75	15.79	15.81	15.82	15.83	15.84	15.86
17	16.68	16.74	16.78	16.79	16.81	16.82	16.83	16.85
18	17.66	17.72	17.77	17.78	17.80	17.81	17.83	17.85
19	18.64	18.71	18.76	18.77	18.79	18.81	18.82	18.84
20	19.63	19.70	19.75	19.76	19.78	19.80	19.81	19.83
21	20.61	20.68	20.73	20.76	20.77	20.79	20.80	20.83
22	21.60	21.67	21.72	21.75	21.77	21.78	21.80	21.82
23	22.58	22.66	22.71	22.74	22.76	22.77	22.79	22.82
24	23.56	23.65	23.70	23.73	23.75	23.77	23.78	23.81
25	24.55	24.63	24.69	24.72	24.74	24.76	24.78	24.81
26	25.53	25.62	25.69	25.71	25.73	25.75	25.77	25.80
27	26.52	26.61	26.68	26.70	26.73	26.75	26.76	26.80
28	27.50	27.60	27.67	27.69	27.72	27.74	27.76	27.79
29	28.49	28.59	28.66	28.69	28.71	28.73	28.75	28.79
30	29.47	29.58	29.65	29.68	29.70	29.73	29.75	29.78

APPENDIX D (continued)

Centre thickness 0.18 mm

Back Vertex Powers in D	Front Vertex Powers in D for Back Optic Radii in mm of:							
	5.0	6.0	7.0	7.5	8.0	8.5	9.0	10.0
+ 20	19.49	19.56	19.62	19.64	19.66	19.68	19.69	19.72
19	18.52	18.59	18.64	18.66	18.68	18.70	18.71	18.73
18	17.54	17.61	17.66	17.68	17.70	17.71	17.73	17.75
17	16.57	16.64	16.68	16.70	16.72	16.73	16.74	16.77
16	15.60	15.66	15.70	15.72	15.74	15.75	15.76	15.78
15	14.63	14.68	14.72	14.74	14.75	14.77	14.78	14.80
14	13.65	13.71	13.74	13.76	13.77	13.78	13.79	13.81
13	12.68	12.73	12.76	12.78	12.79	12.80	12.81	12.83
12	11.70	11.75	11.78	11.80	11.81	11.82	11.83	11.84
11	10.73	10.77	10.80	10.81	10.83	10.83	10.84	10.86
10	9.76	9.79	9.82	9.83	9.84	9.85	9.86	9.87
9	8.78	8.82	8.84	8.85	8.86	8.87	8.87	8.89
8	7.81	7.84	7.86	7.87	7.88	7.88	7.89	7.90
7	6.83	6.86	6.88	6.89	6.89	6.90	6.90	6.91
6	5.86	5.88	5.90	5.90	5.91	5.91	5.92	5.93
5	4.88	4.90	4.91	4.92	4.92	4.93	4.93	4.94
4	3.91	3.92	3.93	3.94	3.94	3.94	3.95	3.95
3	2.93	2.94	2.95	2.95	2.96	2.96	2.96	2.96
2	1.95	1.96	1.97	1.97	1.97	1.97	1.97	1.98
1	0.98	0.98	0.98	0.98	0.99	0.99	0.99	0.99
0	0.00	0.00	0.00	0.00	0.00	0.00	0.00	0.00
− 1	0.98	0.98	0.98	0.99	0.99	0.99	0.99	0.99
2	1.95	1.96	1.97	1.97	1.97	1.97	1.97	1.98
3	2.93	2.94	2.95	2.95	2.96	2.96	2.96	2.97
4	3.91	3.92	3.94	3.94	3.94	3.95	3.95	3.96
5	4.89	4.91	4.92	4.93	4.93	4.93	4.94	4.94
6	5.87	5.89	5.90	5.91	5.92	5.92	5.93	5.93
7	6.84	6.87	6.89	6.90	6.90	6.91	6.92	6.92
8	7.82	7.85	7.87	7.88	7.89	7.90	7.90	7.91
9	8.80	8.84	8.86	8.87	8.88	8.89	8.89	8.90
10	9.78	9.82	9.85	9.86	9.87	9.87	9.88	9.90
11	10.76	10.80	10.83	10.84	10.85	10.86	10.87	10.89
12	11.74	11.78	11.82	11.83	11.84	11.85	11.86	11.88
13	12.72	12.77	12.80	12.82	12.83	12.84	12.85	12.87
14	13.70	13.75	13.79	13.81	13.82	13.83	13.84	13.86
15	14.68	14.74	14.78	14.79	14.81	14.82	14.83	14.85
16	15.66	15.72	15.76	15.78	15.80	15.81	15.82	15.84
17	16.64	16.70	16.75	16.77	16.79	16.80	16.81	16.84
18	17.62	17.69	17.74	17.76	17.78	17.79	17.80	17.83
19	18.60	18.67	18.73	18.75	18.77	18.78	18.80	18.82
20	19.58	19.66	19.71	19.74	19.76	19.77	19.79	19.81
21	20.56	20.64	20.70	20.73	20.75	20.76	20.78	20.81
22	21.55	21.63	21.69	21.71	21.74	21.75	21.77	21.80
23	22.53	22.62	22.68	22.70	22.73	22.75	22.76	22.79
24	23.51	23.60	23.67	23.69	23.72	23.74	23.76	23.79
25	24.49	24.59	24.66	24.68	24.71	24.73	24.75	24.78
26	25.47	25.57	25.65	25.67	25.70	25.72	25.74	25.78
27	26.46	26.56	26.64	26.67	26.69	26.71	26.74	26.77
28	27.44	27.55	27.63	27.66	27.68	27.71	27.73	27.77
29	28.42	28.54	28.62	28.65	28.68	28.70	28.72	28.76
30	29.41	29.52	29.61	29.64	29.67	29.69	29.72	29.76

APPENDIX D (continued)

Centre thickness 0.20 mm

Back Vertex Powers in D	Front Vertex Powers in D for Back Optic Radii in mm of:							
	5.0	6.0	7.0	7.5	8.0	8.5	9.0	10.0
+ 20	19.43	19.52	19.58	19.60	19.62	19.64	19.66	19.69
19	18.46	18.54	18.60	18.62	18.64	18.66	18.68	18.71
18	17.49	17.57	17.62	17.65	17.67	17.68	17.70	17.72
17	16.52	16.60	16.65	16.67	16.69	16.70	16.72	16.74
16	15.55	15.62	15.67	15.69	15.71	15.72	15.74	15.76
15	14.58	14.65	14.69	14.71	14.73	14.74	14.75	14.78
14	13.61	13.67	13.72	13.73	13.75	13.76	13.77	13.79
13	12.64	12.70	12.74	12.75	12.77	12.78	12.79	12.81
12	11.67	11.71	11.76	11.77	11.79	11.80	11.81	11.83
11	10.70	10.75	10.78	10.79	10.81	10.82	10.83	10.84
10	9.73	9.77	9.80	9.81	9.82	9.83	9.84	9.86
9	8.76	8.80	8.82	8.83	8.84	8.85	8.86	8.87
8	7.79	7.82	7.84	7.85	7.86	7.87	7.88	7.89
7	6.81	6.84	6.86	6.87	6.88	6.89	6.89	6.90
6	5.84	5.87	5.88	5.89	5.90	5.90	5.91	5.92
5	4.89	4.89	4.90	4.91	4.92	4.92	4.92	4.93
4	3.90	3.91	3.92	3.93	3.93	3.94	3.94	3.95
3	2.92	2.93	2.94	2.95	2.95	2.95	2.96	2.96
2	1.95	1.96	1.96	1.97	1.97	1.97	1.97	1.97
1	0.97	0.98	0.98	0.98	0.98	0.99	0.99	0.99
0	0.00	0.00	0.00	0.00	0.00	0.00	0.00	0.00
− 1	0.97	0.98	0.98	0.98	0.98	0.99	0.99	0.99
2	1.95	1.96	1.96	1.97	1.97	1.97	1.97	1.97
3	2.92	2.94	2.95	2.95	2.95	2.96	2.96	2.96
4	3.90	3.92	3.93	3.93	3.94	3.94	3.94	3.95
5	4.87	4.90	4.91	4.92	4.92	4.93	4.93	4.94
6	5.85	5.88	5.89	5.90	5.91	5.91	5.92	5.93
7	6.83	6.86	6.88	6.89	6.89	6.90	6.91	6.92
8	7.80	7.84	7.86	7.87	7.88	7.89	7.89	7.90
9	8.78	8.82	8.84	8.86	8.86	8.87	8.88	8.89
10	9.76	9.80	9.83	9.84	9.85	9.86	9.87	9.88
11	10.73	10.78	10.81	10.83	10.84	10.85	10.86	10.89
12	11.71	11.76	11.80	11.81	11.82	11.84	11.85	11.86
13	12.69	12.74	12.78	12.80	12.81	12.82	12.83	12.85
14	13.66	13.72	13.77	13.78	13.80	13.81	13.82	13.84
15	14.64	14.71	14.75	14.77	14.79	14.80	14.81	14.83
16	15.62	15.69	15.74	15.76	15.77	15.79	15.80	15.83
17	16.60	16.67	16.72	16.74	16.76	16.78	16.79	16.82
18	17.58	17.65	17.71	17.73	17.75	17.77	17.78	17.81
19	18.56	18.64	18.70	18.72	18.74	18.76	18.77	18.80
20	19.54	19.62	19.68	19.71	19.73	19.75	19.76	19.79
21	20.52	20.61	20.67	20.69	20.72	20.74	20.75	20.79
22	21.50	21.59	21.66	21.68	21.71	21.73	21.75	21.78
23	22.48	22.57	22.64	22.67	22.70	22.72	22.74	22.77
24	23.46	23.56	23.63	23.66	23.69	23.71	23.73	23.76
25	24.44	24.54	24.62	24.65	24.68	24.70	24.72	24.76
26	25.42	25.53	25.61	25.64	25.67	25.69	25.71	25.75
27	26.40	26.51	26.60	26.63	26.66	26.68	26.71	26.75
28	27.38	27.50	27.58	27.62	27.65	27.68	27.70	27.74
29	28.36	28.48	28.57	28.61	28.64	28.67	28.69	28.73
30	29.34	29.47	29.56	29.60	29.63	29.66	29.69	29.73

APPENDIX D (continued)

Centre thickness 0.22 mm

Back Vertex Powers in D	Front Vertex Powers in D for Back Optic Radii in mm of:							
	5.0	6.0	7.0	7.5	8.0	8.5	9.0	10.0
+ 20	19.38	19.47	19.54	19.56	19.59	19.61	19.63	19.66
19	18.41	18.50	18.56	18.59	18.61	18.63	18.65	18.68
18	17.44	17.53	17.59	17.61	17.63	17.65	17.67	17.70
17	16.48	16.56	16.61	16.64	16.66	16.67	16.69	16.72
16	15.51	15.59	15.64	15.66	15.68	15.69	15.71	15.73
15	14.54	14.61	14.66	14.68	14.70	14.72	14.73	14.75
14	13.58	13.64	13.69	13.71	13.72	13.74	13.75	13.77
13	12.61	12.67	12.71	12.73	12.74	12.76	12.77	12.79
12	11.64	11.70	11.74	11.75	11.77	11.78	11.79	11.81
11	10.67	10.72	10.76	10.77	10.79	10.80	10.81	10.83
10	9.70	9.75	9.78	9.80	9.81	9.82	9.83	9.84
9	8.73	8.78	8.81	8.82	8.83	8.84	8.85	8.86
8	7.76	7.80	7.83	7.84	7.85	7.86	7.86	7.88
7	6.80	6.83	6.85	6.86	6.87	6.88	6.88	6.89
6	5.83	5.85	5.87	5.88	5.89	5.89	5.90	5.91
5	4.86	4.88	4.90	4.90	4.91	4.91	4.92	4.93
4	3.88	3.90	3.92	3.92	3.93	3.93	3.93	3.94
3	2.91	2.93	2.94	2.94	2.95	2.95	2.95	2.96
2	1.94	1.95	1.96	1.96	1.96	1.97	1.97	1.97
1	0.97	0.98	0.98	0.98	0.98	0.98	0.98	0.99
0	0.00	0.00	0.00	0.00	0.00	0.00	0.00	0.00
− 1	0.97	0.98	0.98	0.98	0.98	0.98	0.98	0.99
2	1.94	1.95	1.96	1.96	1.97	1.97	1.97	1.97
3	2.92	2.93	2.94	2.94	2.95	2.95	2.95	2.96
4	3.89	3.91	3.92	3.93	3.93	3.94	3.94	3.95
5	4.86	4.89	4.90	4.91	4.91	4.92	4.92	4.93
6	5.84	5.86	5.88	5.89	5.90	5.90	5.91	5.92
7	6.81	6.84	6.87	6.87	6.88	6.89	6.90	6.91
8	7.78	7.82	7.85	7.86	7.87	7.88	7.88	7.90
9	8.76	8.80	8.83	8.84	8.85	8.86	8.87	8.88
10	9.73	9.78	9.81	9.82	9.84	9.85	9.86	9.87
11	10.71	10.76	10.79	10.81	10.82	10.83	10.84	10.86
12	11.68	11.74	11.78	11.79	11.81	11.82	11.83	11.85
13	12.66	12.72	12.76	12.78	12.79	12.81	12.82	12.84
14	13.63	13.70	13.74	13.76	13.78	13.79	13.81	13.83
15	14.61	14.68	14.73	14.75	14.77	14.78	14.79	14.82
16	15.58	15.66	15.71	15.73	15.75	15.77	15.78	15.81
17	16.56	16.64	16.70	16.72	16.74	16.76	16.77	16.80
18	17.54	17.62	17.68	17.70	17.73	17.74	17.76	17.79
19	18.51	18.60	18.67	18.69	18.71	18.73	18.75	18.78
20	19.49	19.58	19.65	19.68	19.70	19.72	19.74	19.77
21	20.47	20.57	20.64	20.66	20.69	20.71	20.73	20.76
22	21.45	21.55	21.62	21.65	21.68	21.70	21.72	21.76
23	22.42	22.53	22.61	22.64	22.67	22.69	22.71	22.75
24	23.40	23.51	23.59	23.63	23.66	23.68	23.70	23.74
25	24.38	24.50	24.58	24.62	24.64	24.67	24.69	24.73
26	25.36	25.48	25.57	25.60	25.63	25.66	25.69	25.73
27	26.34	26.47	26.56	26.59	26.62	26.65	26.68	26.72
28	27.32	27.45	27.54	27.58	27.61	27.64	27.67	27.71
29	28.30	28.43	28.53	28.57	28.60	28.63	28.66	28.71
30	29.28	29.42	29.52	29.56	29.60	29.63	29.65	29.70

APPENDIX D (continued)

Centre thickness 0.24 mm

Back Vertex Powers in D	Front Vertex Powers in D for Back Optic Radii in mm of:							
	5.0	6.0	7.0	7.5	8.0	8.5	9.0	10.0
+ 20	19.32	19.42	19.49	19.52	19.55	19.57	19.59	19.63
19	18.36	18.45	18.52	18.55	18.57	18.60	18.62	18.65
18	17.40	17.49	17.55	17.58	17.60	17.62	17.64	17.67
17	16.43	16.52	16.58	16.60	16.62	16.64	16.66	16.69
16	15.47	15.55	15.61	15.63	15.65	15.67	15.68	15.71
15	14.50	14.58	14.63	14.65	14.67	14.69	14.71	14.73
14	13.54	13.61	13.66	13.68	13.70	13.71	13.73	13.75
13	12.57	12.64	12.69	12.70	12.72	12.74	12.75	12.77
12	11.61	11.67	11.71	11.73	11.74	11.76	11.77	11.79
11	10.64	10.70	10.74	10.75	10.77	10.78	10.79	10.81
10	9.68	9.73	9.76	9.78	9.79	9.80	9.81	9.83
9	8.71	8.76	8.79	8.80	8.81	8.82	8.83	8.85
8	7.74	7.78	7.81	7.82	7.83	7.84	7.85	7.87
7	6.78	6.81	6.84	6.85	6.86	6.86	6.87	6.88
6	5.81	5.84	5.86	5.87	5.88	5.88	5.89	5.90
5	4.84	4.87	4.89	4.89	4.90	4.91	4.91	4.92
4	3.87	3.89	3.91	3.92	3.92	3.92	3.93	3.94
3	2.91	2.92	2.93	2.94	2.94	2.94	2.95	2.95
2	1.94	1.95	1.96	1.96	1.96	1.96	1.97	1.97
1	0.97	0.97	0.98	0.98	0.98	0.98	0.98	0.98
0	0.00	0.00	0.00	0.00	0.00	0.00	0.00	0.00
− 1	0.97	0.97	0.98	0.98	0.98	0.98	0.98	0.99
2	1.94	1.95	1.96	1.96	1.96	1.96	1.97	1.97
3	2.91	2.92	2.94	2.94	2.94	2.95	2.95	2.96
4	3.88	3.90	3.91	3.92	3.93	3.93	3.93	3.94
5	4.85	4.88	4.89	4.90	4.91	4.91	4.92	4.93
6	5.82	5.85	5.87	5.88	5.89	5.90	5.90	5.91
7	6.79	6.83	6.85	6.86	6.87	6.88	6.89	6.90
8	7.76	7.80	7.83	7.84	7.85	7.86	7.87	7.89
9	8.74	8.78	8.81	8.83	8.84	8.85	8.86	8.87
10	9.71	9.76	9.79	9.81	9.82	9.83	9.84	9.86
11	10.68	10.74	10.78	10.79	10.81	10.82	10.83	10.85
12	11.65	11.71	11.76	11.77	11.79	11.80	11.82	11.84
13	12.63	12.69	12.74	12.76	12.77	12.79	12.80	12.82
14	13.60	13.67	13.72	13.74	13.76	13.77	13.79	13.81
15	14.57	14.65	14.70	14.72	14.74	14.76	14.78	14.80
16	15.55	15.63	15.69	15.71	15.73	15.75	15.76	15.79
17	16.52	16.61	16.67	16.69	16.72	16.73	16.75	16.78
18	17.50	17.59	17.65	17.68	17.70	17.72	17.74	17.77
19	18.47	18.57	18.64	18.66	18.69	18.71	18.73	18.76
20	19.45	19.55	19.62	19.65	19.67	19.70	19.72	19.75
21	20.42	20.53	20.60	20.63	20.66	20.69	20.71	20.74
22	21.40	21.51	21.59	21.62	21.65	21.67	21.70	21.73
23	22.37	22.49	22.57	22.61	22.64	22.66	22.69	22.73
24	23.35	23.47	23.56	23.59	23.62	23.65	23.68	23.72
25	24.33	24.45	24.54	24.58	24.61	24.64	24.67	24.71
26	25.30	25.43	25.53	25.57	25.60	25.63	25.66	25.70
27	26.28	26.42	26.52	26.56	26.59	26.62	26.65	26.69
28	27.26	27.40	27.50	27.54	27.58	27.61	27.64	27.69
29	28.24	28.38	28.49	28.53	28.57	28.60	28.63	28.68
30	29.21	29.37	29.48	29.52	29.56	29.59	29.62	29.67

APPENDIX D (continued)

Centre thickness 0.26 mm

Back Vertex Powers in D	Front Vertex Powers in D for Back Optic Radii in mm of:									
	5.0	5.5	6.0	6.5	7.0	7.5	8.0	8.5	9.0	10.0
+ 20	19.27	19.33	19.38	19.42	19.45	19.48	19.51	19.54	19.56	19.60
19	18.31	18.36	18.41	18.45	18.48	18.51	18.54	18.56	18.58	18.62
18	17.35	17.40	17.44	17.48	17.51	17.54	17.57	17.59	17.61	17.64
17	16.39	16.44	16.48	16.51	16.54	16.57	16.59	16.61	16.63	16.66
16	15.42	15.47	15.51	15.54	15.57	15.60	15.62	15.64	15.66	15.69
15	14.46	14.51	14.54	14.58	14.60	14.63	14.65	14.67	14.68	14.71
14	13.50	13.54	13.58	13.61	13.63	13.65	13.67	13.69	13.71	13.73
13	12.54	12.58	12.61	12.64	12.66	12.68	12.70	12.71	12.73	12.75
12	11.58	11.61	11.64	11.67	11.69	11.71	11.72	11.74	11.75	11.77
11	10.61	10.65	10.67	10.70	10.72	10.73	10.75	10.76	10.77	10.79
10	9.65	9.68	9.70	9.73	9.74	9.76	9.77	9.79	9.80	9.81
9	8.69	8.71	8.74	8.75	8.77	8.79	8.80	8.81	8.82	8.83
8	7.72	7.75	7.77	7.78	7.80	7.81	7.82	7.83	7.84	7.85
7	6.76	6.78	6.80	6.81	6.82	6.84	6.84	6.85	6.86	6.87
6	5.79	5.81	5.83	5.84	5.85	5.86	5.87	5.88	5.88	5.89
5	4.83	4.84	4.86	4.87	4.88	4.88	4.89	4.90	4.90	4.91
4	3.86	3.88	3.89	3.89	3.90	3.91	3.91	3.92	3.92	3.93
3	2.90	2.91	2.92	2.92	2.93	2.93	2.94	2.94	2.94	2.95
2	1.93	1.94	1.94	1.95	1.95	1.95	1.96	1.96	1.96	1.97
1	0.97	0.97	0.97	0.97	0.98	0.98	0.98	0.98	0.98	0.98
0	0.00	0.00	0.00	0.00	0.00	0.00	0.00	0.00	0.00	0.00
− 1	0.97	0.97	0.97	0.97	0.98	0.98	0.98	0.98	0.98	0.98
2	1.93	1.94	1.95	1.95	1.95	1.96	1.96	1.96	1.96	1.97
3	2.90	2.91	2.92	2.92	2.93	2.93	2.94	2.94	2.95	2.95
4	3.87	3.88	3.89	3.90	3.91	3.91	3.92	3.92	3.93	3.94
5	4.84	4.85	4.87	4.88	4.88	4.89	4.90	4.91	4.91	4.92
6	5.81	5.82	5.84	5.85	5.86	5.87	5.88	5.89	5.89	5.91
7	6.76	6.80	6.81	6.83	6.84	6.85	6.86	6.87	6.88	6.89
8	7.74	7.77	7.79	7.80	7.82	7.83	7.84	7.85	7.86	7.88
9	8.71	8.74	8.76	8.78	8.80	8.81	8.82	8.84	8.85	8.86
10	9.68	9.71	9.74	9.76	9.78	9.79	9.81	9.82	9.83	9.85
11	10.65	10.69	10.71	10.74	10.76	10.77	10.79	10.80	10.81	10.84
12	11.62	11.66	11.69	11.71	11.74	11.76	11.77	11.79	11.80	11.82
13	12.60	12.63	12.67	12.69	12.72	12.74	12.76	12.77	12.79	12.81
14	13.57	13.61	13.64	13.67	13.70	13.72	13.74	13.76	13.77	13.80
15	14.54	14.58	14.62	14.66	14.68	14.70	14.72	14.74	14.76	14.79
16	15.51	15.56	15.60	15.63	15.66	15.69	15.71	15.73	15.74	15.77
17	16.48	16.53	16.57	16.61	16.64	16.67	16.69	16.71	16.73	16.76
18	17.45	17.51	17.55	17.59	17.62	17.65	17.68	17.70	17.72	17.75
19	18.43	18.48	18.53	18.57	18.61	18.64	18.66	18.69	18.71	18.74
20	19.40	19.46	19.51	19.55	19.59	19.62	19.65	19.67	19.69	19.73
21	20.37	20.44	20.49	20.53	20.57	20.60	20.63	20.66	20.68	20.72
22	21.35	21.41	21.47	21.51	21.55	21.59	21.62	21.65	21.67	21.71
23	22.32	22.39	22.45	22.50	22.54	22.57	22.61	22.63	22.66	22.70
24	23.30	23.37	23.43	23.48	23.52	23.56	23.59	23.62	23.65	23.69
25	24.27	24.34	24.41	24.46	24.51	24.55	24.58	24.61	24.64	24.69
26	25.25	25.32	25.39	25.44	25.49	25.53	25.57	25.60	25.63	25.68
27	26.22	26.30	26.37	26.43	26.48	26.52	26.56	26.59	26.62	26.67
28	27.20	27.28	27.35	27.41	27.46	27.51	27.54	27.58	27.61	27.66
29	28.17	28.26	28.33	28.39	28.45	28.49	28.53	28.57	28.60	28.65
30	29.15	29.24	29.31	29.38	29.43	29.48	29.52	29.56	29.59	29.65

APPENDIX D (continued)

Centre thickness 0.28 mm

Back Vertex Powers in D	Front Vertex Powers in D for Back Optic Radii in mm of:									
	5.0	5.5	6.0	6.5	7.0	7.5	8.0	8.5	9.0	10.0
+ 20	19.21	19.28	19.33	19.37	19.41	19.45	19.48	19.50	19.52	19.56
19	18.26	18.32	18.37	18.41	18.45	18.48	18.51	18.53	18.55	18.59
18	17.30	17.35	17.40	17.42	17.48	17.51	17.53	17.56	17.58	17.61
17	16.34	16.39	16.44	16.48	16.51	16.54	16.56	16.59	16.61	16.64
16	15.38	15.43	15.47	15.51	15.54	15.57	15.59	15.61	15.63	15.66
15	14.42	14.47	14.51	14.54	14.57	14.60	14.62	14.64	14.66	14.69
14	13.46	13.51	13.55	13.58	13.60	13.63	13.65	13.67	13.68	13.71
13	12.50	12.55	12.58	12.61	12.63	12.66	12.68	12.69	12.71	12.73
12	11.54	11.58	11.61	11.64	11.66	11.69	11.70	11.72	11.73	11.76
11	10.58	10.62	10.65	10.67	10.69	10.71	10.73	10.74	10.76	10.78
10	9.62	9.96	9.68	9.70	9.72	9.74	9.76	9.77	9.78	9.80
9	8.66	8.69	8.72	8.74	8.75	8.77	8.78	8.79	8.80	8.82
8	7.70	7.73	7.75	7.77	7.78	7.80	7.81	7.82	7.83	7.84
7	6.74	6.76	6.78	6.80	6.81	6.82	6.83	6.84	6.85	6.86
6	5.78	5.80	5.81	5.83	5.84	5.85	5.86	5.87	5.87	5.88
5	4.82	4.89	4.85	4.86	4.87	4.88	4.88	4.89	4.90	4.91
4	3.85	3.87	3.88	3.89	3.89	3.90	3.91	3.91	3.92	3.92
3	2.89	2.90	2.91	2.92	2.92	2.93	2.93	2.93	2.94	2.94
2	1.93	1.93	1.94	1.94	1.95	1.95	1.95	1.96	1.96	1.96
1	0.96	0.97	0.97	0.97	0.97	0.98	0.98	0.98	0.98	0.98
0	0.00	0.00	0.00	0.00	0.00	0.00	0.00	0.00	0.00	0.00
− 1	0.96	0.97	0.97	0.97	0.97	0.98	0.98	0.98	0.98	0.98
2	1.93	1.94	1.94	1.95	1.95	1.95	1.96	1.96	1.96	1.96
3	2.89	2.90	2.91	2.92	2.92	2.93	2.93	2.94	2.94	2.95
4	3.86	3.87	3.88	3.89	3.90	3.91	3.91	3.92	3.92	3.93
5	4.83	4.84	4.85	4.87	4.88	4.88	4.89	4.90	4.90	4.91
6	5.79	5.81	5.83	5.84	5.85	5.86	5.87	5.88	5.89	5.90
7	6.76	6.78	6.80	6.82	6.83	6.84	6.85	6.86	6.87	6.88
8	7.73	7.75	7.77	7.79	7.81	7.82	7.83	7.84	7.85	7.87
9	8.69	8.72	8.75	8.77	8.78	8.80	8.81	8.82	8.83	8.85
10	9.66	9.69	9.72	9.74	9.76	9.78	9.79	9.81	9.82	9.84
11	10.63	10.66	10.69	10.72	10.74	10.76	10.77	10.79	10.80	10.82
12	11.60	11.63	11.67	11.69	11.72	11.74	11.76	11.77	11.78	11.81
13	12.56	12.61	12.64	12.67	12.70	12.72	12.74	12.75	12.77	12.80
14	13.53	13.58	13.62	13.65	13.67	13.70	13.72	13.74	13.75	13.78
15	14.50	14.55	14.59	14.62	14.65	14.70	14.70	14.72	14.74	14.77
16	15.47	15.52	15.57	15.60	15.63	15.66	15.69	15.71	15.72	15.76
17	16.44	16.50	16.54	16.58	16.61	16.64	16.67	16.69	16.71	16.74
18	17.41	17.47	17.52	17.56	17.59	17.63	17.65	17.68	17.70	17.73
19	18.38	18.44	18.50	18.54	18.58	18.61	18.64	18.66	18.68	18.72
20	19.36	19.42	19.47	19.52	19.56	19.59	19.62	19.65	19.67	19.71
21	20.33	20.39	20.45	20.50	20.54	20.57	20.61	20.63	20.66	20.70
22	21.30	21.37	21.43	21.48	21.52	21.56	21.59	21.62	21.65	21.69
23	22.27	22.34	22.41	22.46	22.50	22.54	22.58	22.61	22.63	22.68
24	23.24	23.32	23.38	23.44	23.49	23.53	23.56	23.59	23.62	23.67
25	24.22	24.30	24.36	24.42	24.47	24.51	24.55	24.58	24.61	24.66
26	25.19	25.27	25.34	25.40	25.45	25.50	25.54	25.57	25.60	25.65
27	26.16	26.25	26.32	26.38	26.44	26.48	26.52	26.56	26.59	26.64
28	27.14	27.23	27.30	27.37	27.42	27.47	27.51	27.55	27.58	27.64
29	28.11	28.20	28.28	28.35	28.41	28.45	28.50	28.54	28.57	28.63
30	29.09	29.18	29.26	29.33	29.39	29.44	29.49	29.53	29.56	29.62

APPENDIX D (continued)

Centre thickness 0.30 mm

Back Vertex Powers in D	Front Vertex Powers in D for Back Optic Radii in mm of:									
	5.0	5.5	6.0	6.5	7.0	7.5	8.0	8.5	9.0	10.0
+ 20	19.16	19.23	19.28	19.33	19.37	19.41	19.44	19.47	19.49	19.53
19	18.20	18.27	18.32	18.37	18.41	18.44	18.47	18.50	18.52	18.56
18	17.25	17.31	17.36	17.40	17.44	17.47	17.50	17.53	17.55	17.59
17	16.29	16.35	16.40	16.44	16.48	16.51	16.53	16.56	16.58	16.61
16	15.34	15.39	15.44	15.48	15.51	15.54	15.56	15.59	15.61	15.64
15	14.38	14.43	14.48	14.51	14.54	14.57	14.59	14.61	14.63	14.66
14	13.43	13.47	13.51	13.55	13.58	13.60	13.62	13.64	13.66	13.69
13	12.47	12.51	12.55	12.58	12.61	12.63	12.65	12.67	12.69	12.71
12	11.51	11.55	11.59	11.62	11.64	11.66	11.68	11.70	11.71	11.74
11	10.56	10.59	10.62	10.65	10.67	10.69	10.71	10.73	10.74	10.76
10	9.60	9.63	9.66	9.68	9.71	9.72	9.74	9.75	9.77	9.79
9	8.64	8.67	8.70	8.72	8.74	8.75	8.77	8.78	8.79	8.81
8	7.68	7.71	7.73	7.75	7.77	7.78	7.79	7.81	7.82	7.83
7	6.72	6.75	6.77	6.78	6.80	6.81	6.82	6.83	6.84	6.85
6	5.76	5.78	5.80	5.82	5.83	5.84	5.85	5.86	5.86	5.88
5	4.80	4.82	4.84	4.85	4.86	4.87	4.87	4.88	4.89	4.90
4	3.84	3.86	3.87	3.88	3.89	3.89	3.90	3.91	3.91	3.92
3	2.88	2.89	2.90	2.91	2.92	2.92	2.93	2.93	2.93	2.94
2	1.92	1.93	1.94	1.94	1.94	1.95	1.95	1.95	1.96	1.96
1	0.96	0.96	0.97	0.97	0.97	0.97	0.98	0.98	0.98	0.98
0	0.00	0.00	0.00	0.00	0.00	0.00	0.00	0.00	0.00	0.00
− 1	0.96	0.97	0.97	0.97	0.97	0.97	0.98	0.98	0.98	0.98
2	1.92	1.93	1.94	1.94	1.95	1.95	1.95	1.96	1.96	1.96
3	2.89	2.90	2.91	2.91	2.92	2.92	2.93	2.93	2.94	2.94
4	3.85	3.86	3.88	3.88	3.89	3.90	3.91	3.91	3.92	3.93
5	4.81	4.83	4.84	4.86	4.87	4.88	4.88	4.89	4.90	4.91
6	5.78	5.80	5.81	5.83	5.84	5.85	5.86	5.87	5.88	5.89
7	6.74	6.76	6.79	6.80	6.82	6.83	6.84	6.85	6.86	6.87
8	7.71	7.73	7.76	7.77	7.79	7.81	7.82	7.83	7.84	7.86
9	8.67	8.70	8.73	8.75	8.77	8.78	8.80	8.81	8.82	8.84
10	9.64	9.67	9.70	9.72	9.74	9.76	9.78	9.79	9.80	9.83
11	10.60	10.64	10.67	10.70	10.72	10.74	10.76	10.77	10.79	10.81
12	11.57	11.61	11.64	11.67	11.70	11.72	11.74	11.75	11.77	11.80
13	12.53	12.58	12.62	12.65	12.67	12.70	12.72	12.74	12.75	12.78
14	13.50	13.55	13.59	13.62	13.65	13.68	13.70	13.72	13.74	13.77
15	14.47	14.52	14.56	14.60	14.63	14.66	14.68	14.70	14.72	14.75
16	15.44	15.49	15.54	15.57	15.61	15.64	15.66	15.69	15.71	15.74
17	16.40	16.46	16.51	16.55	16.59	16.62	16.65	16.67	16.69	16.73
18	17.37	17.43	17.49	17.53	17.57	17.60	17.63	17.65	17.68	17.71
19	18.34	18.41	18.46	18.51	18.55	18.58	18.61	18.64	18.66	18.70
20	19.31	19.38	19.44	19.48	19.53	19.56	19.59	19.62	19.65	19.69
21	20.28	20.35	20.41	20.46	20.51	20.54	20.58	20.61	20.63	20.68
22	21.25	21.32	21.39	21.44	21.49	21.53	21.56	21.59	21.62	21.67
23	22.22	22.30	22.36	22.42	22.47	22.51	22.55	22.58	22.61	22.66
24	23.19	23.27	23.34	23.40	23.45	23.49	23.53	23.57	23.60	23.65
25	24.16	24.25	24.32	24.38	24.43	24.48	24.52	24.55	24.58	24.64
26	25.13	25.22	25.30	25.36	25.41	25.46	25.50	25.54	25.57	25.63
27	26.10	26.20	26.27	26.34	26.40	26.45	26.49	26.53	26.56	26.62
28	27.08	27.17	27.25	27.32	27.38	27.43	27.48	27.51	27.55	27.61
29	28.05	28.15	28.23	28.30	28.36	28.42	28.46	28.50	28.54	28.60
30	29.02	29.12	29.21	29.28	29.35	29.40	29.45	29.49	29.53	29.59

APPENDIX D

APPENDIX D (continued)

Centre thickness 0.32 mm

Back Vertex Powers in D	Front Vertex Powers in D for Back Optic Radii in mm of:									
	5.0	5.5	6.0	6.5	7.0	7.5	8.0	8.5	9.0	10.0
+ 20	19.10	19.18	19.24	19.29	19.33	19.37	19.40	19.43	19.46	19.50
19	18.15	18.22	18.28	18.33	18.37	18.40	18.44	18.46	18.49	18.53
18	17.20	17.27	17.32	17.36	17.40	17.44	17.47	17.50	17.52	17.56
17	16.25	16.31	16.36	16.40	16.44	16.47	16.50	16.53	16.55	16.59
16	15.30	15.35	15.40	15.44	15.48	15.51	15.54	15.56	15.58	15.62
15	14.34	14.40	14.44	14.48	14.51	14.54	14.57	14.59	14.61	14.64
14	13.39	13.44	13.48	13.52	13.55	13.58	13.60	13.62	13.64	13.67
13	12.44	12.48	12.52	12.55	12.58	12.61	12.63	12.65	12.67	12.70
12	11.48	11.52	11.56	11.59	11.62	11.64	11.66	11.68	11.69	11.72
11	10.53	10.57	10.60	10.63	10.65	10.67	10.69	10.71	10.72	10.75
10	9.57	9.61	9.64	9.66	9.69	9.71	9.72	9.74	9.75	9.77
9	8.62	8.65	8.68	8.70	8.72	8.74	8.75	8.76	8.78	8.80
8	7.66	7.69	7.71	7.73	7.75	7.77	7.78	7.79	7.80	7.82
7	6.71	6.73	6.75	6.77	6.78	6.80	6.81	6.82	6.83	6.85
6	5.75	5.77	5.79	5.80	5.82	5.83	5.84	5.85	5.86	5.87
5	4.79	4.81	4.82	4.84	4.85	4.86	4.87	4.87	4.88	4.89
4	3.83	3.85	3.86	3.87	3.88	3.89	3.89	3.90	3.91	3.91
3	2.88	2.89	2.90	2.90	2.91	2.92	2.92	2.93	2.93	2.94
2	1.92	1.92	1.93	1.94	1.94	1.94	1.95	1.95	1.95	1.96
1	0.96	0.96	0.97	0.97	0.97	0.97	0.97	0.98	0.98	0.98
0	0.00	0.00	0.00	0.00	0.00	0.00	0.00	0.00	0.00	0.00
− 1	0.96	0.96	0.97	0.97	0.97	0.97	0.97	0.98	0.98	0.98
2	1.92	1.93	1.93	1.94	1.94	1.95	1.95	1.95	1.96	1.96
3	2.88	2.89	2.90	2.91	2.91	2.92	2.92	2.93	2.93	2.94
4	3.84	3.85	3.87	3.88	3.89	3.89	3.90	3.91	3.91	3.92
5	4.80	4.82	4.83	4.85	4.86	4.87	4.88	4.88	4.89	4.90
6	5.76	5.78	5.80	5.82	5.83	5.84	5.85	5.86	5.87	5.88
7	6.72	6.75	6.77	6.79	6.80	6.82	6.83	6.84	6.85	6.87
8	7.69	7.72	7.74	7.76	7.78	7.79	7.81	7.82	7.83	7.85
9	8.65	8.68	8.71	8.73	8.75	8.77	8.79	8.80	8.81	8.83
10	9.61	9.65	9.68	9.70	9.73	9.75	9.76	9.78	9.79	9.81
11	10.58	10.62	10.65	10.68	10.70	10.72	10.74	10.76	10.77	10.80
12	11.54	11.58	11.62	11.65	11.68	11.70	11.72	11.74	11.75	11.78
13	12.50	12.55	12.59	12.62	12.65	12.68	12.70	12.72	12.74	12.77
14	13.47	13.52	13.56	13.60	13.63	13.66	13.68	13.70	13.72	13.75
15	14.43	14.49	14.53	14.57	14.61	14.63	14.66	14.68	14.70	14.74
16	15.40	15.46	15.51	15.55	15.58	15.61	15.64	15.66	15.69	15.72
17	16.37	16.43	16.48	16.52	16.56	16.59	16.62	16.65	16.67	16.71
18	17.33	17.40	17.45	17.50	17.54	17.57	17.60	17.63	17.65	17.70
19	18.30	18.37	18.43	18.47	18.52	18.55	18.59	18.61	18.64	18.68
20	19.27	19.34	19.40	19.45	19.49	19.53	19.57	19.60	19.62	19.67
21	20.23	20.31	20.37	20.43	20.47	20.51	20.55	20.58	20.61	20.66
22	21.20	21.28	21.35	21.40	21.45	21.50	21.53	21.57	21.60	21.65
23	22.17	22.25	22.32	22.38	22.43	22.48	22.52	22.55	22.58	22.63
24	23.14	23.22	23.30	23.36	23.41	23.46	23.50	23.54	23.57	23.62
25	24.11	24.20	24.27	24.34	24.39	24.44	24.49	24.52	24.56	24.61
26	25.08	25.17	25.25	25.32	25.38	25.43	25.47	25.51	25.54	25.60
27	26.05	26.14	26.23	26.30	26.36	26.41	26.46	26.50	26.53	26.59
28	27.02	27.12	27.20	27.28	27.34	27.39	27.44	27.48	27.52	27.58
29	27.99	28.09	28.18	28.26	28.32	28.38	28.43	28.47	28.51	28.58
30	28.96	29.07	29.16	29.24	29.30	29.36	29.41	29.46	29.50	29.57

APPENDIX D (continued)

Centre thickness 0.34 mm

Back Vertex Powers in D	Front Vertex Powers in D for Back Optic Radii in mm of:									
	5.0	5.5	6.0	6.5	7.0	7.5	8.0	8.5	9.0	10.0
+ 20	19.05	19.13	19.19	19.24	19.29	19.33	19.37	19.40	19.43	19.47
19	18.10	18.17	18.23	18.28	18.33	18.37	18.40	18.43	18.46	18.50
18	17.15	17.22	17.28	17.33	17.37	17.41	17.44	17.47	17.49	17.53
17	16.20	16.27	16.32	16.37	16.41	16.44	16.47	16.50	16.52	16.56
16	15.25	15.31	15.37	15.41	15.45	15.48	15.51	15.53	15.55	15.59
15	14.30	14.36	14.41	14.45	14.48	14.51	14.54	14.56	14.59	14.62
14	13.35	13.41	13.45	13.49	13.52	13.55	13.57	13.60	13.62	13.65
13	12.40	12.45	12.49	12.53	12.56	12.58	12.61	12.63	12.65	12.68
12	11.45	11.50	11.53	11.57	11.59	11.62	11.64	11.66	11.68	11.70
11	10.50	10.54	10.58	10.60	10.63	10.65	10.67	10.69	10.71	10.73
10	9.55	9.58	9.62	9.64	9.67	9.69	9.70	9.72	9.73	9.76
9	8.59	8.63	8.66	8.68	8.70	8.72	8.74	8.75	8.76	8.78
8	7.64	7.67	7.70	7.72	7.74	7.75	7.77	7.78	7.79	7.81
7	6.69	6.71	6.74	6.75	6.77	6.79	6.80	6.81	6.82	6.84
6	5.73	5.76	5.78	5.79	5.81	5.82	5.83	5.84	5.85	5.86
5	4.78	4.80	4.81	4.83	4.84	4.85	4.86	4.87	4.87	4.89
4	3.82	3.84	3.85	3.86	3.87	3.88	3.89	3.89	3.90	3.91
3	2.87	2.88	2.89	2.90	2.90	2.91	2.92	2.92	2.93	2.93
2	1.91	1.92	1.93	1.93	1.94	1.94	1.94	1.95	1.95	1.96
1	0.96	0.96	0.96	0.97	0.97	0.97	0.97	0.97	0.98	0.98
0	0.00	0.00	0.00	0.00	0.00	0.00	0.00	0.00	0.00	0.00
− 1	0.96	0.96	0.96	0.97	0.97	0.97	0.97	0.97	0.98	0.98
2	1.91	1.92	1.93	1.93	1.94	1.94	1.95	1.95	1.95	1.96
3	2.87	2.88	2.89	2.90	2.91	2.91	2.92	2.93	2.93	2.94
4	3.83	3.85	3.86	3.87	3.88	3.89	3.89	3.90	3.91	3.92
5	4.79	4.81	4.82	4.84	4.85	4.86	4.87	4.88	4.88	4.90
6	5.75	5.77	5.79	5.81	5.82	5.83	5.84	5.85	5.86	5.88
7	6.71	6.73	6.76	6.78	6.79	6.81	6.82	6.83	6.84	6.86
8	7.67	7.70	7.72	7.75	7.76	7.78	7.80	7.81	7.82	7.84
9	8.63	8.66	8.69	8.72	8.74	8.76	8.77	8.79	8.80	8.82
10	9.59	9.63	9.66	9.69	9.71	9.73	9.75	9.76	9.78	9.80
11	10.55	10.59	10.63	10.66	10.68	10.71	10.73	10.74	10.76	10.79
12	11.51	11.56	11.60	11.63	11.66	11.68	11.70	11.72	11.74	11.77
13	12.47	12.52	12.57	12.60	12.63	12.66	12.68	12.70	12.72	12.75
14	13.44	13.49	13.54	13.57	13.61	13.64	13.66	13.68	13.70	13.74
15	14.40	14.46	14.51	14.55	14.58	14.61	14.64	14.66	14.68	14.72
16	15.36	15.42	15.48	15.52	15.56	15.59	15.62	15.64	15.67	15.71
17	16.33	16.39	16.45	16.49	16.53	16.57	16.60	16.63	16.65	16.69
18	17.29	17.36	17.42	17.47	17.51	17.55	17.58	17.61	17.63	17.68
19	18.26	18.33	18.39	18.44	18.49	18.53	18.56	18.59	18.62	18.66
20	19.22	19.30	19.36	19.42	19.46	19.50	19.54	19.57	19.60	19.65
21	20.19	20.27	20.33	20.39	20.44	20.48	20.52	20.56	20.59	20.64
22	21.15	21.24	21.31	21.37	21.42	21.47	21.50	21.54	21.57	21.62
23	22.12	22.21	22.28	22.34	22.40	22.45	22.49	22.52	22.56	22.61
24	23.09	23.18	23.26	23.32	23.38	23.43	23.47	23.51	23.54	23.60
25	24.05	24.15	24.23	24.30	24.36	24.41	24.45	24.49	24.53	24.59
26	25.02	25.12	25.20	25.28	25.34	25.39	25.44	25.48	25.52	25.58
27	25.99	26.09	26.18	26.25	26.32	26.37	26.42	26.46	26.50	26.57
28	26.96	27.06	27.16	27.23	27.30	27.36	27.41	27.45	27.49	27.56
29	27.93	28.04	28.13	28.21	28.28	28.34	28.39	28.44	28.48	28.55
30	28.90	29.01	29.11	29.19	29.26	29.32	29.38	29.43	29.47	29.54

APPENDIX D (continued)

Centre thickness 0.36 mm

Back Vertex Powers in D	Front Vertex Powers in D for Back Optic Radii in mm of:									
	5.0	5.5	6.0	6.5	7.0	7.5	8.0	8.5	9.0	10.0
+ 20	19.00	19.08	19.14	19.20	19.25	19.29	19.33	19.36	19.39	19.44
19	18.05	18.13	18.19	18.24	18.29	18.33	18.37	18.40	18.43	18.47
18	17.10	17.18	17.24	17.29	17.33	17.37	17.40	17.43	17.46	17.51
17	16.16	16.23	16.28	16.33	16.37	16.41	16.44	16.47	16.50	16.54
16	15.21	15.27	15.33	15.37	15.41	15.45	15.48	15.50	15.53	15.57
15	14.26	14.32	14.37	14.42	14.45	14.49	14.51	14.54	14.56	14.60
14	13.32	13.37	13.42	13.46	13.49	13.52	13.55	13.57	13.59	13.63
13	12.37	12.42	12.46	12.50	12.53	12.56	12.59	12.61	12.63	12.66
12	11.42	11.47	11.51	11.54	11.57	11.60	11.62	11.64	11.66	11.69
11	10.47	10.51	10.55	10.58	10.61	10.63	10.65	10.67	10.69	10.72
10	9.52	9.56	9.59	9.62	9.65	9.67	9.69	9.70	9.72	9.74
9	8.57	8.61	8.64	8.66	8.69	8.70	8.72	8.74	8.75	8.77
8	7.62	7.65	7.68	7.70	7.72	7.74	7.75	7.77	7.78	7.80
7	6.67	6.70	6.72	6.74	6.76	6.77	6.79	6.80	6.81	6.83
6	5.72	5.74	5.76	5.78	5.79	5.81	5.82	5.83	5.84	5.85
5	4.77	4.79	4.80	4.82	4.83	4.84	4.85	4.86	4.87	4.88
4	3.81	3.83	3.84	3.85	3.86	3.87	3.88	3.89	3.89	3.90
3	2.86	2.87	2.88	2.89	2.90	2.91	2.91	2.92	2.92	2.93
2	1.91	1.92	1.92	1.93	1.93	1.94	1.94	1.95	1.95	1.95
1	0.95	0.96	0.96	0.96	0.97	0.97	0.97	0.97	0.97	0.98
0	0.00	0.00	0.00	0.00	0.00	0.00	0.00	0.00	0.00	0.00
− 1	0.95	0.96	0.96	0.96	0.97	0.97	0.97	0.97	0.97	0.98
2	1.91	1.92	1.92	1.93	1.94	1.94	1.94	1.95	1.95	1.95
3	2.87	2.88	2.89	2.90	2.90	2.91	2.92	2.92	2.93	2.93
4	3.82	3.84	3.85	3.86	3.87	3.88	3.89	3.90	3.90	3.91
5	4.78	4.80	4.81	4.83	4.84	4.85	4.86	4.87	4.88	4.89
6	5.73	5.76	5.78	5.80	5.81	5.82	5.84	5.85	5.85	5.87
7	6.69	6.72	6.74	6.76	6.78	6.80	6.81	6.82	6.83	6.85
8	7.65	7.68	7.71	7.73	7.75	7.77	7.78	7.80	7.81	7.83
9	8.61	8.64	8.67	8.70	8.72	8.74	8.76	8.77	8.79	8.81
10	9.57	9.61	9.64	9.67	9.69	9.72	9.73	9.75	9.77	9.79
11	10.52	10.57	10.61	10.64	10.67	10.69	10.71	10.73	10.74	10.77
12	11.48	11.53	11.57	11.61	11.64	11.66	11.69	11.71	11.72	11.76
13	12.44	12.50	12.54	12.58	12.61	12.64	12.66	12.69	12.70	12.74
14	13.40	13.46	13.51	13.55	13.58	13.61	13.64	13.66	13.69	13.72
15	14.37	14.43	14.48	14.52	14.56	14.59	14.62	14.64	14.67	14.70
16	15.33	15.39	15.45	15.49	15.53	15.57	15.60	15.62	15.65	15.69
17	16.29	16.36	16.42	16.46	16.51	16.54	16.58	16.60	16.63	16.67
18	17.25	17.32	17.38	17.44	17.48	17.52	17.55	17.58	17.61	17.66
19	18.21	18.29	18.35	18.41	18.46	18.50	18.53	18.57	18.59	18.64
20	19.18	19.26	19.33	19.38	19.43	19.48	19.51	19.55	19.58	19.63
21	20.14	20.22	20.30	20.36	20.41	20.46	20.49	20.53	20.56	20.62
22	21.10	21.19	21.27	21.33	21.39	21.43	21.48	21.51	21.55	21.60
23	22.07	22.16	22.24	22.31	22.36	22.41	22.46	22.50	22.53	22.59
24	23.03	23.13	23.21	23.28	23.34	23.39	23.44	23.48	23.52	23.58
25	24.00	24.10	24.19	24.26	24.32	24.37	24.42	24.46	24.50	24.57
26	24.96	25.07	25.16	25.23	25.30	25.36	25.40	25.45	25.49	25.55
27	25.93	26.04	26.13	26.21	26.28	26.34	26.39	26.43	26.47	26.54
28	26.90	27.01	27.11	27.19	27.26	27.32	27.37	27.42	27.46	27.53
29	27.87	27.98	28.08	28.17	28.24	28.30	28.36	28.41	28.45	28.52
30	28.83	28.95	29.06	29.14	29.22	29.28	29.34	29.39	29.44	29.51

APPENDIX D (continued)

Centre thickness 0.38 mm

Back Vertex Powers in D	Front Vertex Powers in D for Back Optic Radii in mm of:									
	5.0	5.5	6.0	6.5	7.0	7.5	8.0	8.5	9.0	10.0
+ 20	18.94	19.03	19.10	19.16	19.21	19.25	19.29	19.33	19.36	19.41
19	18.00	18.08	18.15	18.20	18.25	18.30	18.33	18.37	18.40	18.45
18	17.06	17.13	17.20	17.25	17.30	17.34	17.37	17.40	17.43	17.48
17	16.11	16.18	16.24	16.30	16.34	16.38	16.41	16.44	16.47	16.51
16	15.17	15.24	15.29	15.34	15.38	15.42	15.45	15.48	15.50	15.55
15	14.22	14.29	14.34	14.39	14.42	14.46	14.49	14.51	14.54	14.58
14	13.28	13.34	13.39	13.43	13.47	13.50	13.53	13.55	13.57	13.61
13	12.33	12.39	12.44	12.47	12.51	12.54	12.56	12.59	12.61	12.64
12	11.39	11.44	11.48	11.52	11.55	11.58	11.60	11.62	11.64	11.67
11	10.44	10.49	10.53	10.56	10.59	10.61	10.64	10.65	10.67	10.70
10	9.50	9.54	9.57	9.60	9.63	9.65	9.67	9.69	9.70	9.73
9	8.55	8.59	8.62	8.64	8.67	8.69	8.71	8.72	8.74	8.76
8	7.60	7.63	7.66	7.69	7.71	7.72	7.74	7.75	7.77	7.79
7	6.65	6.68	6.71	6.73	6.75	6.76	6.77	6.79	6.80	6.82
6	5.70	5.73	5.75	5.77	5.78	5.80	5.81	5.82	5.83	5.84
5	4.75	4.77	4.79	4.81	4.82	4.83	4.84	4.85	4.86	4.87
4	3.80	3.82	3.84	3.85	3.86	3.87	3.87	3.88	3.89	3.90
3	2.85	2.87	2.88	2.89	2.89	2.90	2.91	2.91	2.92	2.92
2	1.90	1.91	1.92	1.92	1.93	1.93	1.94	1.94	1.95	1.95
1	0.95	0.96	0.96	0.96	0.97	0.97	0.97	0.97	0.97	0.98
0	0.00	0.00	0.00	0.00	0.00	0.00	0.00	0.00	0.00	0.00
− 1	0.95	0.96	0.96	0.96	0.97	0.97	0.97	0.97	0.97	0.98
2	1.91	1.91	1.92	1.93	1.93	1.94	1.94	1.94	1.95	1.95
3	2.86	2.87	2.88	2.89	2.90	2.91	2.91	2.92	2.92	2.93
4	3.81	3.83	3.84	3.85	3.87	3.87	3.88	3.89	3.90	3.91
5	4.77	4.79	4.80	4.82	4.83	4.84	4.85	4.86	4.87	4.88
6	5.72	5.75	5.77	5.78	5.80	5.81	5.83	5.84	5.85	5.86
7	6.67	6.70	6.73	6.75	6.77	6.78	6.80	6.81	6.82	6.84
8	7.63	7.66	7.69	7.72	7.74	7.76	7.77	7.79	7.80	7.82
9	8.59	8.62	8.66	8.68	8.71	8.73	8.75	8.76	8.78	8.80
10	9.54	9.58	9.62	9.65	9.68	9.70	9.72	9.74	9.75	9.78
11	10.50	10.55	10.59	10.62	10.65	10.67	10.69	10.71	10.73	10.76
12	11.46	11.51	11.55	11.59	11.62	11.65	11.67	11.69	11.71	11.74
13	12.41	12.47	12.52	12.56	12.59	12.62	12.64	12.67	12.69	12.72
14	13.37	13.43	13.48	13.52	13.56	13.59	13.62	13.65	13.67	13.71
15	14.33	14.39	14.45	14.49	14.53	14.57	14.60	14.62	14.65	14.69
16	15.29	15.36	15.42	15.46	15.51	15.54	15.57	15.60	15.63	15.67
17	16.25	16.32	16.38	16.43	16.48	16.52	16.55	16.58	16.61	16.65
18	17.21	17.29	17.35	17.41	17.45	17.49	17.53	17.56	17.59	17.64
19	18.17	18.25	18.32	18.38	18.43	18.47	18.51	18.54	18.57	18.62
20	19.13	19.22	19.29	19.35	19.40	19.45	19.49	19.52	19.55	19.61
21	20.09	20.18	20.26	20.32	20.38	20.43	20.47	20.50	20.54	20.59
22	21.06	21.15	21.23	21.30	21.35	21.40	21.45	21.49	21.52	21.58
23	22.02	22.12	22.20	22.27	22.33	22.38	22.43	22.47	22.51	22.57
24	22.98	23.08	23.17	23.25	23.31	23.36	23.41	23.45	23.49	23.55
25	23.95	24.05	24.14	24.22	24.28	24.34	24.39	24.43	24.47	24.54
26	24.91	25.02	25.11	25.19	25.26	25.32	25.37	25.42	25.46	25.53
27	25.87	25.94	26.09	26.17	26.24	26.30	26.36	26.40	26.45	26.52
28	26.84	26.96	27.06	27.14	27.22	27.28	27.34	27.39	27.43	27.51
29	27.80	27.93	28.03	28.12	28.20	28.26	28.32	28.37	28.42	28.50
30	28.77	28.90	29.01	29.10	29.18	29.25	29.31	29.36	29.41	29.49

APPENDIX D

APPENDIX D (continued)

Centre thickness 0.40 mm

Back Vertex Powers in D	Front Vertex Powers in D for Back Optic Radii in mm of:									
	5.0	5.5	6.0	6.5	7.0	7.5	8.0	8.5	9.0	10.0
+ 20	18.89	18.98	19.05	19.11	19.17	19.22	19.26	19.29	19.33	19.38
19	17.95	18.03	18.10	18.16	18.21	18.26	18.30	18.33	18.36	18.42
18	17.01	17.09	17.16	17.21	17.26	17.30	17.34	17.37	17.40	17.45
17	16.07	16.14	16.21	16.26	16.31	16.35	16.38	16.41	16.44	16.49
16	15.13	15.20	15.26	15.31	15.35	15.39	15.42	15.45	15.48	15.52
15	14.19	14.25	14.31	14.35	14.40	14.43	14.46	14.49	14.51	14.56
14	13.24	13.30	13.36	13.40	13.44	13.47	13.50	13.53	13.55	13.59
13	12.30	12.36	12.41	12.45	12.48	12.51	12.54	12.56	12.59	12.62
12	11.36	11.41	11.46	11.49	11.53	11.55	11.58	11.60	11.62	11.65
11	10.41	10.46	10.50	10.54	10.57	10.59	10.62	10.64	10.65	10.69
10	9.47	9.51	9.55	9.58	9.61	9.63	9.65	9.67	9.69	9.72
9	8.52	8.56	8.60	8.63	8.65	8.67	8.69	8.71	8.72	8.75
8	7.58	7.61	7.64	7.67	7.69	7.71	7.73	7.74	7.76	7.78
7	6.63	6.64	6.69	6.71	6.73	6.75	6.76	6.78	6.79	6.81
6	5.69	5.71	5.74	5.76	5.77	5.79	5.80	5.81	5.82	5.84
5	4.74	4.76	4.78	4.80	4.81	4.82	4.83	4.84	4.85	4.87
4	3.79	3.81	3.83	3.84	3.85	3.86	3.87	3.88	3.88	3.89
3	2.85	2.86	2.87	2.88	2.89	2.90	2.90	2.91	2.91	2.92
2	1.90	1.91	1.91	1.92	1.93	1.93	1.94	1.94	1.94	1.95
1	0.95	0.95	0.96	0.96	0.96	0.97	0.97	0.97	0.97	0.97
0	0.00	0.00	0.00	0.00	0.00	0.00	0.00	0.00	0.00	0.00
− 1	0.95	0.95	0.96	0.96	0.96	0.97	0.97	0.97	0.97	0.97
2	1.90	1.91	1.92	1.92	1.93	1.93	1.94	1.94	1.94	1.95
3	2.85	2.86	2.88	2.88	2.89	2.90	2.91	2.91	2.92	2.93
4	3.80	3.82	3.83	3.85	3.86	3.87	3.88	3.88	3.89	3.90
5	4.75	4.78	4.79	4.81	4.82	4.84	4.85	4.86	4.86	4.88
6	5.71	5.73	5.75	5.77	5.79	5.80	5.82	5.83	5.84	5.86
7	6.66	6.69	6.72	6.74	6.76	6.77	6.79	6.80	6.81	6.83
8	7.61	7.65	7.68	7.70	7.72	7.74	7.76	7.77	7.79	7.81
9	8.57	8.60	8.64	8.67	8.69	8.71	8.73	8.75	8.76	8.79
10	9.52	9.56	9.60	9.63	9.66	9.68	9.71	9.72	9.74	9.77
11	10.47	10.52	10.56	10.60	10.63	10.66	10.68	10.70	10.72	10.75
12	11.43	11.48	11.53	11.57	11.60	11.63	11.65	11.67	11.69	11.73
13	12.38	12.44	12.49	12.53	12.57	12.60	12.63	12.65	12.67	12.71
14	13.34	13.40	13.46	13.50	13.54	13.57	13.60	13.63	13.65	13.69
15	14.30	14.36	14.42	14.47	14.51	14.55	14.58	14.60	14.63	14.67
16	15.25	15.33	15.39	15.44	15.48	15.52	15.55	15.58	15.61	15.65
17	16.21	16.29	16.35	16.41	16.45	16.49	16.53	16.56	16.59	16.64
18	17.17	17.25	17.32	17.38	17.43	17.47	17.51	17.54	17.57	17.62
19	18.13	18.21	18.29	18.35	18.40	18.44	18.48	18.52	18.55	18.60
20	19.09	19.18	19.25	19.32	19.37	19.42	19.46	19.50	19.53	19.59
21	20.05	20.14	20.22	20.29	20.35	20.40	20.44	20.48	20.51	20.57
22	21.01	21.11	21.19	21.26	21.32	21.37	21.42	21.46	21.49	21.56
23	21.97	22.07	22.16	22.23	22.29	22.35	22.40	22.44	22.48	22.54
24	22.93	23.04	23.13	23.20	23.27	23.33	23.38	23.42	23.46	23.53
25	23.89	24.00	24.10	24.18	24.25	24.31	24.36	24.41	24.45	24.52
26	24.85	24.97	25.07	25.15	25.22	25.29	25.34	25.39	25.43	25.51
27	25.82	25.94	26.04	26.13	26.20	26.26	26.32	26.37	26.42	26.49
28	26.78	26.90	27.01	27.10	27.18	27.24	27.30	27.36	27.40	27.48
29	27.74	27.87	27.98	28.08	28.16	28.23	28.29	28.34	28.39	28.47
30	28.71	28.84	28.96	29.05	29.13	29.21	29.27	29.33	29.38	29.46

APPENDIX D (continued)

Centre thickness 0.50 mm

Back Vertex Powers in D	Front Vertex Powers in D for Back Optic Radii in mm of:										
	5.0	5.5	6.0	6.5	7.0	7.5	8.0	8.5	9.0	9.5	10.0
+ 20	18.63	18.73	18.82	18.90	18.97	19.03	19.08	19.12	19.16	19.20	19.23
19	17.70	17.80	17.89	17.96	18.03	18.08	18.13	18.17	18.21	18.24	18.28
18	16.77	16.87	16.95	17.02	17.08	17.14	17.18	17.22	17.26	17.29	17.32
17	15.85	15.94	16.02	16.08	16.14	16.19	16.23	16.27	16.30	16.34	16.36
16	14.92	15.01	15.08	15.14	15.19	15.24	15.28	15.32	15.35	15.38	15.41
15	13.99	14.07	14.14	14.20	14.25	14.29	14.33	14.37	14.40	14.43	14.45
14	13.06	13.14	13.20	13.26	13.30	13.34	13.38	13.41	13.44	13.47	13.49
13	12.13	12.20	12.26	12.31	12.36	12.40	12.43	12.46	12.48	12.51	12.53
12	11.20	11.27	11.32	11.37	11.41	11.45	11.48	11.50	11.53	11.55	11.57
11	10.27	10.33	10.38	10.43	10.46	10.50	10.52	10.55	10.57	10.59	10.61
10	9.34	9.40	9.44	9.48	9.52	9.54	9.57	9.59	9.61	9.63	9.65
9	8.41	8.46	8.50	8.54	8.57	8.59	8.62	8.64	8.65	8.67	8.69
8	7.48	7.52	7.56	7.59	7.62	7.64	7.66	7.68	7.70	7.71	7.72
7	6.55	6.58	6.62	6.64	6.67	6.69	6.71	6.72	6.74	6.75	6.76
6	5.61	5.65	5.67	5.70	5.72	5.73	5.75	5.76	5.78	5.79	5.80
5	4.68	4.71	4.73	4.75	4.77	4.78	4.79	4.80	4.81	4.82	4.83
4	3.74	3.77	3.79	3.80	3.81	3.83	3.84	3.85	3.85	3.86	3.87
3	2.81	2.83	2.84	2.85	2.86	2.87	2.88	2.88	2.89	2.90	2.90
2	1.87	1.88	1.89	1.90	1.91	1.91	1.92	1.92	1.93	1.93	1.94
1	0.94	0.94	0.95	0.95	0.95	0.96	0.96	0.96	0.96	0.97	0.97
0	0.00	0.00	0.00	0.00	0.00	0.00	0.00	0.00	0.00	0.00	0.00
− 1	0.94	0.94	0.95	0.95	0.96	0.96	0.96	0.96	0.97	0.97	0.97
2	1.88	1.89	1.90	1.90	1.91	1.92	1.92	1.93	1.93	1.93	1.94
3	2.82	2.83	2.85	2.86	2.87	2.88	2.88	2.89	2.90	2.90	2.91
4	3.75	3.78	3.79	3.81	3.82	3.84	3.85	3.86	3.86	3.87	3.88
5	4.69	4.72	4.75	4.76	4.78	4.80	4.81	4.82	4.83	4.84	4.85
6	5.64	5.67	5.70	5.72	5.74	5.76	5.77	5.79	5.80	5.81	5.82
7	6.58	6.61	6.65	6.67	6.70	6.72	6.74	6.75	6.77	6.78	6.79
8	7.52	7.56	7.60	7.63	7.66	7.68	7.70	7.72	7.74	7.75	7.76
9	8.46	8.51	8.55	8.59	8.62	8.64	8.67	8.69	8.71	8.72	8.74
10	9.40	9.46	9.51	9.54	9.58	9.61	9.63	9.66	9.68	9.69	9.71
11	10.35	10.41	10.46	10.50	10.54	10.57	10.60	10.63	10.65	10.67	10.69
12	11.29	11.36	11.41	11.46	11.50	11.54	11.57	11.60	11.62	11.64	11.66
13	12.24	12.31	12.37	12.42	12.46	12.50	12.54	12.57	12.59	12.62	12.64
14	13.18	13.26	13.32	13.38	13.43	13.47	13.50	13.54	13.57	13.59	13.62
15	14.13	14.21	14.28	14.34	14.39	14.43	14.47	14.51	14.54	14.57	14.59
16	15.08	15.16	15.24	15.30	15.36	15.40	15.44	15.48	15.51	15.54	15.57
17	16.02	16.12	16.20	16.26	16.32	16.37	16.41	16.45	16.49	16.52	16.55
18	16.97	17.07	17.15	17.22	17.29	17.34	17.39	17.43	17.46	17.50	17.53
19	17.92	18.02	18.11	18.19	18.25	18.31	18.36	18.40	18.44	18.47	18.51
20	18.87	18.98	19.07	19.15	19.22	19.28	19.33	19.38	19.42	19.45	19.49
21	19.82	19.93	20.03	20.12	20.19	20.25	20.30	20.35	20.39	20.43	20.47
22	20.77	20.89	20.99	21.08	21.15	21.22	21.28	21.33	21.37	21.41	21.45
23	21.72	21.85	21.95	22.05	22.12	22.19	22.25	22.30	22.35	22.39	22.43
24	22.67	22.81	22.92	23.01	23.09	23.16	23.23	23.28	23.33	23.38	23.42
25	23.63	23.76	23.88	23.98	24.06	24.14	24.20	24.26	24.31	24.36	24.40
26	24.58	24.72	24.84	24.95	25.03	25.11	25.18	25.24	25.29	25.34	25.38
27	25.53	25.68	25.81	25.91	26.01	26.09	26.16	26.22	26.27	26.32	26.37
28	26.49	26.64	26.77	26.88	26.98	27.06	27.13	27.20	27.26	27.31	27.35
29	27.44	27.60	27.74	27.85	27.95	28.04	28.11	28.18	28.24	28.29	28.34
30	28.40	28.56	28.70	28.82	28.92	29.01	29.09	29.16	29.22	29.28	29.33

APPENDIX D (continued)

Centre thickness 0.60 mm

Back Vertex Powers in D	Front Vertex Powers in D for Back Optic Radii in mm of:										
	5.0	5.5	6.0	6.5	7.0	7.5	8.0	8.5	9.0	9.5	10.0
+ 20	18.27	18.49	18.60	18.69	18.77	18.84	18.90	18.95	19.00	19.04	19.08
19	17.46	17.57	17.68	17.77	17.84	17.91	17.96	18.01	18.06	18.10	18.14
18	16.54	16.66	16.75	16.84	16.91	16.97	17.02	17.07	17.12	17.15	17.19
17	15.63	15.74	15.83	15.91	15.97	16.03	16.08	16.13	16.17	16.21	16.24
16	14.72	14.82	14.90	14.98	15.04	15.10	15.14	15.19	15.23	15.26	15.29
15	13.80	13.90	13.98	14.05	14.11	14.16	14.20	14.24	14.28	14.31	14.34
14	12.89	12.98	13.05	13.12	13.17	13.22	13.26	13.30	13.33	13.36	13.39
13	11.97	12.05	12.12	12.18	12.24	12.28	12.32	12.35	12.39	12.41	12.44
12	11.06	11.13	11.20	11.25	11.30	11.34	11.38	11.41	11.44	11.46	11.49
11	10.14	10.21	10.27	10.32	10.36	10.40	10.43	10.46	10.49	10.51	10.53
10	9.22	9.28	9.34	9.38	9.42	9.46	9.49	9.51	9.54	9.56	9.58
9	8.30	8.36	8.41	8.45	8.48	8.51	8.54	8.57	8.59	8.61	8.62
8	7.38	7.43	7.48	7.51	7.54	7.57	7.60	7.62	7.64	7.65	7.67
7	6.46	6.51	6.54	6.58	6.60	6.63	6.65	6.67	6.68	6.70	6.71
6	5.54	5.58	5.61	5.64	5.66	5.68	5.70	5.72	5.73	5.74	5.76
5	4.62	4.65	4.68	4.70	4.72	4.74	4.75	4.77	4.78	4.79	4.80
4	3.70	3.72	3.75	3.76	3.78	3.79	3.80	3.82	3.82	3.83	3.84
3	2.77	2.79	2.81	2.82	2.83	2.85	2.85	2.86	2.87	2.88	2.88
2	1.85	1.86	1.87	1.88	1.89	1.90	1.90	1.91	1.91	1.92	1.92
1	0.93	0.93	0.94	0.94	0.95	0.95	0.95	0.96	0.96	0.96	0.96
0	0.00	0.00	0.00	0.00	0.00	0.00	0.00	0.00	0.00	0.00	0.00
− 1	0.93	0.93	0.94	0.94	0.95	0.95	0.95	0.96	0.96	0.96	0.96
2	1.85	1.87	1.88	1.89	1.89	1.90	1.91	1.91	1.92	1.92	1.93
3	2.78	2.80	2.82	2.83	2.84	2.85	2.86	2.87	2.88	2.88	2.89
4	3.71	3.73	3.76	3.77	3.79	3.80	3.82	3.83	3.84	3.85	3.85
5	4.64	4.67	4.70	4.72	4.74	4.76	4.77	4.79	4.80	4.81	4.82
6	5.57	5.60	5.64	5.67	5.69	5.71	5.73	5.74	5.76	5.77	5.78
7	6.50	6.54	6.58	6.61	6.64	6.66	6.69	6.70	6.72	6.74	6.75
8	7.43	7.48	7.52	7.56	7.59	7.62	7.64	7.67	7.69	7.70	7.72
9	8.36	8.42	8.47	8.51	8.54	8.58	8.60	8.63	8.65	8.67	8.69
10	9.29	9.36	9.41	9.46	9.50	9.53	9.56	9.59	9.61	9.64	9.66
11	10.22	10.30	10.36	10.41	10.45	10.49	10.52	10.55	10.58	10.60	10.63
12	11.16	11.24	11.30	11.36	11.41	11.45	11.48	11.52	11.55	11.57	11.60
13	12.09	12.18	12.25	12.31	12.36	12.41	12.45	12.48	12.51	12.54	12.57
14	13.03	13.12	13.20	13.26	13.32	13.37	13.41	13.45	13.48	13.51	13.54
15	13.96	14.06	14.14	14.21	14.27	14.33	14.37	14.41	14.45	14.48	14.51
16	14.90	15.00	15.09	15.17	15.23	15.29	15.34	15.38	15.42	15.45	15.49
17	15.84	15.95	16.04	16.12	16.19	16.25	16.30	16.35	16.39	16.43	16.46
18	16.78	16.89	16.99	17.07	17.15	17.21	17.27	17.32	17.36	17.40	17.43
19	17.72	17.84	17.94	18.03	18.11	18.17	18.23	18.28	18.33	18.37	18.41
20	18.66	18.78	18.89	18.99	19.07	19.14	19.20	19.25	19.30	19.35	19.39
21	19.60	19.73	19.85	19.94	20.03	20.10	20.17	20.23	20.28	20.32	20.36
22	20.54	20.68	20.80	20.90	20.99	21.07	21.14	21.20	21.25	21.30	21.34
23	21.48	21.63	21.75	21.86	21.95	22.04	22.11	22.17	22.23	22.28	22.32
24	22.42	22.58	22.71	22.82	22.92	23.00	23.08	23.14	23.20	23.25	23.30
25	23.36	23.53	23.66	23.78	23.88	23.97	24.05	24.12	24.18	24.23	24.28
26	24.31	24.48	24.62	24.74	24.85	24.94	25.02	25.09	25.15	25.21	25.26
27	25.25	25.43	25.58	25.70	25.81	25.91	25.99	26.07	26.13	26.19	26.25
28	26.20	26.38	26.54	26.67	26 78	26.88	26.97	27.04	27.11	27.17	27.23
29	27.15	27.33	27.49	27.63	27.75	27.85	27.94	28.02	28.09	28.15	28.21
30	28.09	28.29	28.45	28.59	28.72	28.82	28.91	28.90	29.07	29.14	29.20

APPENDIX D (continued)

Centre thickness 0.70 mm

Back Vertex Powers in D	Front Vertex Powers in D for Back Optic Radii in mm of:										
	5.0	5.5	6.0	6.5	7.0	7.5	8.0	8.5	9.0	9.5	10.0
+ 20	18.12	18.26	18.38	18.49	18.58	18.66	18.73	18.79	18.84	18.89	18.94
19	17.22	17.36	17.47	17.57	17.66	17.73	17.80	17.86	17.91	17.96	18.00
18	16.32	16.45	16.56	16.65	16.74	16.81	16.87	16.92	16.97	17.02	17.06
17	15.42	15.54	15.65	15.74	15.81	15.88	15.94	15.99	16.04	16.08	16.12
16	14.52	14.63	14.73	14.82	14.89	14.95	15.01	15.06	15.10	15.14	15.18
15	13.62	13.73	13.82	13.90	13.97	14.02	14.08	14.12	14.16	14.20	14.23
14	12.72	12.82	12.90	12.98	13.04	13.10	13.14	13.19	13.23	13.26	13.29
13	11.81	11.91	11.99	12.05	12.11	12.17	12.21	12.25	12.29	12.33	12.35
12	10.91	11.00	11.07	11.13	11.19	11.23	11.28	11.31	11.35	11.38	11.40
11	10.00	10.08	10.15	10.21	10.26	10.30	10.34	10.38	10.41	10.43	10.46
10	9.10	9.17	9.23	9.29	9.33	9.37	9.41	9.44	9.46	9.49	9.51
9	8.19	8.25	8.31	8.36	8.40	8.44	8.47	8.50	8.52	8.54	8.56
8	7.29	7.34	7.39	7.44	7.47	7.50	7.53	7.56	7.58	7.60	7.62
7	6.38	6.43	6.47	6.51	6.54	6.57	6.59	6.62	6.63	6.65	6.67
6	5.47	5.51	5.55	5.58	5.61	5.63	5.65	5.67	5.69	5.70	5.72
5	4.56	4.60	4.63	4.65	4.68	4.70	4.71	4.73	4.74	4.76	4.77
4	3.65	3.68	3.70	3.72	3.74	3.76	3.77	3.79	3.80	3.81	3.82
3	2.74	2.76	2.78	2.79	2.81	2.82	2.83	2.84	2.85	2.86	2.86
2	1.83	1.84	1.85	1.86	1.87	1.88	1.89	1.89	1.90	1.91	1.91
1	0.91	0.92	0.93	0.93	0.94	0.94	0.94	0.95	0.95	0.95	0.96
0	0.00	0.00	0.00	0.00	0.00	0.00	0.00	0.00	0.00	0.00	0.00
− 1	0.91	0.92	0.93	0.93	0.94	0.94	0.95	0.95	0.95	0.95	0.96
2	1.83	1.84	1.86	1.87	1.88	1.88	1.89	1.90	1.90	1.91	1.91
3	2.75	2.77	2.79	2.80	2.82	2.83	2.84	2.85	2.86	2.86	2.87
4	3.66	3.69	3.72	3.74	3.76	3.77	3.79	3.80	3.81	3.82	3.83
5	4.58	4.62	4.65	4.67	4.70	4.72	4.74	4.75	4.77	4.78	4.79
6	5.50	5.54	5.58	5.61	5.64	5.66	5.70	5.72	5.74	5.75
7	6.42	6.47	6.51	6.55	6.58	6.61	6.64	6.66	6.68	6.69	6.71
8	7.34	7.40	7.45	7.49	7.53	7.56	7.59	7.61	7.63	7.65	7.67
9	8.26	8.33	8.38	8.43	8.47	8.51	8.54	8.57	8.59	8.61	8.64
10	9.18	9.25	9.32	9.37	9.42	9.46	9.49	9.52	9.55	9.58	9.60
11	10.10	10.18	10.25	10.31	10.36	10.41	10.45	10.48	10.51	10.54	10.56
12	11.03	11.12	11.19	11.25	11.31	11.36	11.40	11.44	11.47	11.50	11.53
13	11.95	12.05	12.13	12.20	12.26	12.31	12.36	12.40	12.43	12.47	12.50
14	12.88	12.98	13.07	13.14	13.21	13.26	13.31	13.36	13.40	13.43	13.46
15	13.80	13.91	14.01	14.09	14.16	14.22	14.27	14.32	14.36	14.40	14.43
16	14.73	14.85	14.95	15.03	15.11	15.17	15.23	15.28	15.32	15.36	15.40
17	15.66	15.78	15.89	15.98	16.06	16.13	16.19	16.24	16.29	16.33	16.37
18	16.58	16.72	16.83	16.93	17.01	17.08	17.15	17.21	17.26	17.30	17.34
19	17.51	17.66	17.78	17.88	17.97	18.04	18.11	18.17	18.22	18.27	18.31
20	18.44	18.59	18.72	18.83	18.92	19.00	19.07	19.13	19.19	19.24	19.29
21	19.38	19.53	19.66	19.78	19.87	19.96	20.03	20.10	20.16	20.21	20.26
22	20.31	20.47	20.61	20.73	20.83	20.92	21.00	21.07	21.13	21.19	21.24
23	21.24	21.41	21.56	21.68	21.79	21.88	21.96	22.04	22.10	22.16	22.21
24	22.17	22.35	22.50	22.63	22.74	22.84	22.93	23.00	23.07	23.13	23.19
25	23.11	23.29	23.45	23.59	23.70	23.80	23.89	23.97	24.04	24.11	24.17
26	24.04	24.24	24.40	24.54	24.66	24.77	24.86	24.94	25.02	25.08	25.14
27	24.98	25.18	25.35	25.50	25.62	25.73	25.83	25.92	25.99	26.06	26.12
28	25.92	26.12	26.30	26.45	26.58	26.70	26.80	26.89	26.97	27.04	27.10
29	26.85	27.07	27.25	27.41	27.55	27.66	27.77	27.86	27.94	28.02	28.08
30	27.79	28.02	28.21	28.37	28.51	28.63	28.74	28.83	28.92	29.00	29.07

APPENDIX D (continued)

Centre thickness 0.80 mm

Back Vertex Powers in D	Front Vertex Powers in D for Back Optic Radii in mm of:										
	5.0	5.5	6.0	6.5	7.0	7.5	8.0	8.5	9.0	9.5	10.0
+ 20	17.87	18.03	18.17	18.29	18.39	18.48	18.55	18.62	18.69	18.74	18.79
19	16.98	17.14	17.27	17.38	17.48	17.56	17.64	17.70	17.76	17.81	17.86
18	16.10	16.24	16.37	16.47	16.57	16.65	16.72	16.78	16.83	16.88	16.93
17	15.21	15.35	15.47	15.57	15.65	15.73	15.80	15.85	15.91	15.95	16.00
16	14.32	14.46	14.56	14.66	14.74	14.81	14.87	14.93	14.98	15.02	15.06
15	13.44	13.56	13.66	13.75	13.83	13.89	13.95	14.00	14.05	14.09	14.13
14	12.55	12.66	12.76	12.84	12.91	12.97	13.03	13.08	13.12	13.16	13.20
13	11.66	11.76	11.85	11.93	12.00	12.05	12.10	12.15	12.19	12.23	12.26
12	10.76	10.86	10.95	11.02	11.08	11.13	11.18	11.22	11.26	11.29	11.32
11	9.87	9.96	10.04	10.10	10.16	10.21	10.25	10.29	10.33	10.36	10.38
10	8.98	9.06	9.13	9.19	9.24	9.29	9.33	9.36	9.39	9.42	9.44
9	8.09	8.16	8.22	8.28	8.32	8.36	8.40	8.43	8.46	8.48	8.50
8	7.19	7.26	7.31	7.36	7.40	7.44	7.47	7.50	7.52	7.54	7.56
7	6.30	6.35	6.40	6.44	6.48	6.51	6.54	6.56	6.58	6.60	6.62
6	5.40	5.45	5.49	5.53	5.56	5.58	5.61	5.63	5.65	5.66	5.68
5	4.50	4.54	4.58	4.61	4.63	4.66	4.68	4.69	4.71	4.72	4.74
4	3.60	3.64	3.66	3.69	3.71	3.73	3.74	3.76	3.77	3.78	3.79
3	2.70	2.73	2.75	2.77	2.78	2.80	2.81	2.82	2.83	2.84	2.84
2	1.80	1.82	1.83	1.85	1.86	1.87	1.87	1.88	1.89	1.89	1.90
1	0.90	0.91	0.92	0.92	0.93	0.93	0.94	0.94	0.94	0.95	0.95
0	0.00	0.00	0.00	0.00	0.00	0.00	0.00	0.00	0.00	0.00	0.00
− 1	0.90	0.91	0.92	0.92	0.93	0.93	0.94	0.94	0.94	0.95	0.95
2	1.81	1.82	1.84	1.85	1.86	1.87	1.88	1.88	1.89	1.90	1.90
3	2.71	2.74	2.76	2.78	2.79	2.80	2.82	2.83	2.84	2.85	2.85
4	3.62	3.65	3.68	3.70	3.72	3.74	3.76	3.77	3.78	3.80	3.81
5	4.52	4.57	4.60	4.63	4.66	4.68	4.70	4.72	4.73	4.75	4.76
6	5.43	5.48	5.52	5.56	5.59	5.62	5.64	5.66	5.68	5.70	5.71
7	6.34	6.40	6.45	6.49	6.53	6.56	6.59	6.61	6.63	6.65	6.67
8	7.25	7.32	7.37	7.42	7.46	7.50	7.53	7.56	7.58	7.61	7.63
9	8.16	8.23	8.30	8.35	8.40	8.44	8.48	8.51	8.54	8.56	8.59
10	9.07	9.15	9.23	9.29	9.34	9.38	9.42	9.46	9.49	9.52	9.54
11	9.98	10.08	10.15	10.22	10.28	10.33	10.37	10.41	10.44	10.48	10.50
12	10.90	11.00	11.08	11.15	11.22	11.27	11.32	11.36	11.40	11.43	11.47
13	11.81	11.92	12.01	12.09	12.16	12.22	12.27	12.32	12.36	12.39	12.43
14	12.73	12.84	12.94	13.03	13.10	13.16	13.22	13.27	13.31	13.35	13.39
15	13.64	13.77	13.87	13.96	14.04	14.11	14.17	14.22	14.27	14.31	14.35
16	14.56	14.69	14.81	14.90	14.99	15.06	15.12	15.18	15.23	15.28	15.32
17	15.48	15.62	15.74	15.84	15.93	16.01	16.08	16.14	16.19	16.24	16.28
18	16.40	16.55	16.67	16.78	16.88	16.96	17.03	17.10	17.15	17.20	17.25
19	17.32	17.47	17.61	17.72	17.82	17.91	17.99	18.06	18.12	18.17	18.22
20	18.24	18.40	18.55	18.67	18.77	18.86	18.94	19.02	19.08	19.14	19.19
21	19.20	19.33	19.48	19.61	19.72	19.82	19.90	19.98	20.04	20.10	20.16
22	20.08	20.27	20.42	20.55	20.67	20.77	20.86	20.94	21.01	21.07	21.13
23	21.00	21.20	21.36	21.50	21.62	21.73	21.82	21.90	21.98	22.04	22.10
24	21.93	22.13	22.30	22.45	22.57	22.68	22.78	22.87	22.94	23.01	23.08
25	22.86	23.06	23.24	23.39	23.53	23.64	23.74	23.83	23.91	23.98	24.05
26	23.78	24.00	24.19	24.34	24.48	24.60	24.71	24.80	24.88	24.96	25.02
27	24.71	24.94	25.13	25.29	25.44	25.56	25.67	25.77	25.85	25.93	26.00
28	25.64	25.87	26.07	26.24	26.39	26.52	26.63	26.73	26.82	26.90	26.98
29	26.57	26.81	27.02	27.19	27.35	27.48	27.60	27.70	27.80	27.88	27.96
30	27.50	27.75	27.96	28.15	28.31	28.44	28.57	28.67	28.77	28.86	28.94

APPENDIX D (continued)

Centre thickness 0.90 mm

Back Vertex Powers in D	Front Vertex Powers in D for Back Optic Radii in mm of:										
	5.0	5.5	6.0	6.5	7.0	7.5	8.0	8.5	9.0	9.5	10.0
+ 20	17.63	17.81	17.96	18.09	18.20	18.30	18.38	18.46	18.53	18.59	18.65
19	16.75	16.92	17.07	17.19	17.30	17.39	17.48	17.55	17.61	17.67	17.73
18	15.88	16.04	16.18	16.30	16.40	16.49	16.57	16.63	16.70	16.75	16.80
17	15.01	15.16	15.29	15.40	15.50	15.58	15.65	15.72	15.78	15.83	15.88
16	14.13	14.28	14.40	14.50	14.59	14.67	14.74	14.80	14.86	14.91	14.95
15	13.26	13.39	13.51	13.60	13.69	13.76	13.83	13.89	13.94	13.98	14.03
14	12.38	12.51	12.61	12.70	12.78	12.85	12.91	12.97	13.02	13.06	13.10
13	11.50	11.62	11.72	11.80	11.88	11.94	12.00	12.05	12.09	12.13	12.17
12	10.62	10.73	10.82	10.90	10.97	11.03	11.08	11.13	11.17	11.21	11.24
11	9.74	9.84	9.93	10.00	10.06	10.12	10.16	10.21	10.25	10.28	10.31
10	8.86	8.95	9.03	9.10	9.15	9.20	9.25	9.28	9.32	9.35	9.38
9	7.98	8.06	8.13	8.19	8.24	8.29	8.33	8.36	8.39	8.42	8.45
8	7.10	7.17	7.23	7.28	7.33	7.37	7.41	7.44	7.46	7.49	7.51
7	6.22	6.28	6.33	6.38	6.42	6.45	6.48	6.51	6.54	6.56	6.58
6	5.33	5.38	5.43	5.47	5.50	5.53	5.56	5.58	5.60	5.62	5.64
5	4.44	4.49	4.53	4.56	4.59	4.61	4.64	4.66	4.67	4.69	4.70
4	3.56	3.59	3.62	3.65	3.67	3.69	3.71	3.73	3.74	3.75	3.76
3	2.67	2.70	2.72	2.74	2.76	2.77	2.79	2.80	2.81	2.82	2.83
2	1.78	1.80	1.81	1.83	1.84	1.85	1.86	1.87	1.87	1.88	1.88
1	0.89	0.90	0.91	0.91	0.92	0.93	0.93	0.93	0.94	0.94	0.94
0	0.00	0.00	0.00	0.00	0.00	0.00	0.00	0.00	0.00	0.00	0.00
− 1	0.89	0.90	0.91	0.92	0.92	0.93	0.93	0.93	0.94	0.94	0.94
2	1.79	1.80	1.82	1.83	1.84	1.85	1.86	1.87	1.88	1.88	1.89
3	2.68	2.71	2.73	2.75	2.77	2.78	2.80	2.81	2.82	2.83	2.84
4	3.57	3.61	3.64	3.67	3.69	3.71	3.73	3.74	3.76	3.77	3.78
5	4.47	4.52	4.55	4.59	4.62	4.64	4.66	4.68	4.70	4.72	4.73
6	5.37	5.42	5.47	5.51	5.54	5.57	5.60	5.62	5.64	5.66	5.68
7	6.26	6.33	6.38	6.43	6.47	6.51	6.54	6.56	6.59	6.61	6.63
8	7.16	7.24	7.30	7.35	7.40	7.44	7.47	7.51	7.53	7.56	7.58
9	8.06	8.15	8.22	8.28	8.33	8.37	8.41	8.45	8.48	8.51	8.54
10	8.97	9.06	9.13	9.20	9.26	9.31	9.35	9.39	9.43	9.46	9.49
11	9.87	9.97	10.05	10.13	10.19	10.25	10.30	10.34	10.38	10.41	10.44
12	10.77	10.88	10.97	11.05	11.12	11.18	11.24	11.29	11.33	11.37	11.40
13	11.67	11.79	11.90	11.98	12.06	12.12	12.18	12.23	12.28	12.32	12.36
14	12.58	12.71	12.82	12.91	12.99	13.06	13.13	13.18	13.23	13.28	13.32
15	13.49	13.62	13.74	13.84	13.93	14.01	14.07	14.13	14.18	14.23	14.28
16	14.39	14.54	14.67	14.77	14.87	14.95	15.02	15.08	15.14	15.19	15.24
17	15.30	15.46	15.59	15.71	15.80	15.89	15.97	16.03	16.10	16.15	16.20
18	16.21	16.38	16.52	16.64	16.74	16.84	16.92	16.99	17.05	17.11	17.16
19	17.12	17.30	17.45	17.57	17.68	17.78	17.87	17.94	18.01	18.07	18.13
20	18.03	18.22	18.38	18.51	18.63	18.73	18.82	18.90	18.97	19.03	19.09
21	18.95	19.14	19.31	19.45	19.57	19.68	19.77	19.85	19.93	20.00	20.06
22	19.86	20.06	20.24	20.38	20.51	20.63	20.72	20.81	20.89	20.96	21.03
23	20.77	20.99	21.17	21.32	21.46	21.58	21.68	21.77	21.85	21.93	21.99
24	21.69	21.91	22.10	22.26	22.40	22.53	22.63	22.73	22.82	22.89	22.96
25	22.61	22.84	23.04	23.20	23.35	23.48	23.59	23.69	23.78	23.86	23.93
26	23.52	23.77	23.97	24.15	24.30	24.43	24.55	24.65	24.75	24.83	24.91
27	24.44	24.69	24.91	25.09	25.25	25.39	25.51	25.62	25.71	25.80	25.88
28	25.36	25.62	25.85	26.04	26.20	26.34	26.47	26.58	26.68	26.77	26.85
29	26.28	26.55	26.79	26.98	27.15	27.30	27.43	27.55	27.65	27.75	27.83
30	27.21	27.49	27.72	27.93	28.10	28.26	28.39	28.51	28.62	28.72	28.81

APPENDIX D (continued)

Centre thickness 1.00 mm

Back Vertex Powers in D	Front Vertex Powers in D for Back Optic Radii in mm of:										
	5.0	5.5	6.0	6.5	7.0	7.5	8.0	8.5	9.0	9.5	10.0
+ 20	17.39	17.58	17.75	17.89	18.01	18.12	18.22	18.30	18.38	18.45	18.51
19	16.53	16.72	16.87	17.01	17.13	17.23	17.32	17.40	17.47	17.53	17.59
18	15.67	15.85	16.00	16.12	16.23	16.33	16.42	16.49	16.56	16.62	16.68
17	14.81	14.97	15.12	15.24	15.34	15.43	15.51	15.59	15.65	15.71	15.76
16	13.95	14.10	14.24	14.35	14.45	14.54	14.61	14.68	14.74	14.79	14.84
15	13.08	13.23	13.35	13.46	13.55	13.64	13.71	13.77	13.83	13.88	13.92
14	12.22	12.36	12.47	12.57	12.66	12.73	12.80	12.86	12.91	12.96	13.00
13	11.35	11.48	11.59	11.68	11.76	11.83	11.89	11.95	12.00	12.04	12.08
12	10.49	10.60	10.70	10.79	10.86	10.93	10.99	11.04	11.08	11.12	11.16
11	9.62	9.73	9.82	9.90	9.97	10.02	10.08	10.12	10.17	10.20	10.24
10	8.75	8.85	8.93	9.00	9.07	9.12	9.17	9.21	9.25	9.28	9.31
9	7.88	7.97	8.04	8.11	8.16	8.21	8.26	8.29	8.33	8.36	8.39
8	7.01	7.09	7.15	7.21	7.26	7.30	7.34	7.38	7.41	7.44	7.46
7	6.14	6.20	6.26	6.31	6.36	6.40	6.43	6.46	6.49	6.51	6.53
6	5.26	5.32	5.37	5.42	5.45	5.49	5.51	5.54	5.56	5.58	5.60
5	4.39	4.44	4.48	4.52	4.55	4.57	4.60	4.62	4.64	4.66	4.67
4	3.51	3.55	3.59	3.61	3.64	3.66	3.68	3.70	3.71	3.73	3.74
3	2.64	2.67	2.69	2.71	2.73	2.75	2.76	2.78	2.79	2.80	2.81
2	1.76	1.78	1.80	1.81	1.82	1.83	1.84	1.85	1.86	1.87	1.87
1	0.88	0.89	0.90	0.91	0.91	0.92	0.92	0.93	0.93	0.93	0.94
0	0.00	0.00	0.00	0.00	0.00	0.00	0.00	0.00	0.00	0.00	0.00
− 1	0.88	0.89	0.90	0.91	0.91	0.92	0.92	0.93	0.93	0.93	0.94
2	1.76	1.78	1.80	1.81	1.83	1.84	1.85	1.86	1.86	1.87	1.88
3	2.65	2.68	2.70	2.72	2.74	2.76	2.77	2.79	2.80	2.81	2.82
4	3.53	3.57	3.60	3.63	3.66	3.68	3.70	3.72	3.73	3.75	3.76
5	4.42	4.47	4.51	4.54	4.58	4.60	4.63	4.65	4.67	4.69	4.70
6	5.30	5.36	5.41	5.46	5.50	5.53	5.56	5.58	5.61	5.63	5.65
7	6.19	6.26	6.32	6.37	6.42	6.45	6.49	6.52	6.55	6.57	6.59
8	7.08	7.16	7.23	7.29	7.34	7.38	7.42	7.45	7.49	7.51	7.54
9	7.97	8.06	8.14	8.20	8.26	8.31	8.35	8.39	8.43	8.46	8.49
10	8.86	8.96	9.05	9.12	9.18	9.24	9.29	9.33	9.37	9.40	9.44
11	9.75	9.86	9.96	10.04	10.11	10.17	10.22	10.27	10.31	10.35	10.39
12	10.65	10.77	10.87	10.96	11.03	11.10	11.16	11.21	11.26	11.30	11.34
13	11.54	11.67	11.78	11.88	11.96	12.03	12.10	12.15	12.20	12.25	12.29
14	12.44	12.58	12.70	12.80	12.89	12.97	13.03	13.10	13.15	13.20	13.24
15	13.33	13.48	13.61	13.72	13.82	13.90	13.97	14.04	14.10	14.15	14.20
16	14.23	14.39	14.53	14.65	14.75	14.84	14.92	14.99	15.05	15.10	15.16
17	15.13	15.30	15.45	15.57	15.68	15.77	15.86	15.93	16.00	16.06	16.11
18	16.03	16.21	16.37	16.50	16.61	16.71	16.80	16.88	16.95	17.01	17.07
19	16.93	17.12	17.29	17.43	17.55	17.65	17.75	17.83	17.90	17.97	18.03
20	17.83	18.03	18.21	18.35	18.48	18.59	18.69	18.78	18.86	18.93	18.99
21	18.74	18.95	19.13	19.28	19.42	19.54	19.64	19.73	19.82	19.89	19.96
22	19.64	19.86	20.05	20.22	20.36	20.48	20.59	20.69	20.77	20.85	20.92
23	20.55	20.78	20.98	21.15	21.30	21.43	21.54	21.64	21.73	21.81	21.89
24	21.45	21.70	21.91	22.08	22.24	22.37	22.49	22.60	22.69	22.78	22.85
25	22.36	22.61	22.83	23.02	23.18	23.32	23.44	23.55	23.65	23.74	23.82
26	23.27	23.54	23.76	23.96	24.12	24.27	24.40	24.51	24.61	24.71	24.79
27	24.18	24.46	24.69	24.89	25.07	25.22	25.35	25.47	25.58	25.67	25.76
28	25.09	25.38	25.62	25.83	26.01	26.17	26.31	26.43	26.54	26.64	26.73
29	26.01	26.30	26.55	26.77	26.96	27.12	27.27	27.39	27.51	27.61	27.71
30	26.92	27.23	27.49	27.71	27.91	28.07	28.22	28.36	28.48	28.58	28.68

APPENDIX D (continued)

Centre thickness 1.10 mm

Back Vertex Powers in D	Front Vertex Powers in D for Back Optic Radii in mm of:										
	5.0	5.5	6.0	6.5	7.0	7.5	8.0	8.5	9.0	9.5	10.0
+ 20	17.16	17.37	17.55	17.70	17.83	17.95	18.05	18.14	18.23	18.30	18.37
19	16.31	16.51	16.68	16.83	16.95	17.06	17.16	17.25	17.33	17.40	17.46
18	15.46	15.65	15.81	15.95	16.07	16.18	16.27	16.35	16.43	16.49	16.55
17	14.61	14.79	14.95	15.08	15.19	15.29	15.38	15.45	15.52	15.59	15.64
16	13.76	13.93	14.08	14.20	14.31	14.40	14.48	14.56	14.62	14.68	14.73
15	12.91	13.07	13.21	13.32	13.42	13.51	13.59	13.66	13.72	13.77	13.82
14	12.06	12.21	12.33	12.44	12.54	12.62	12.69	12.75	12.81	12.86	12.91
13	11.21	11.34	11.46	11.56	11.65	11.72	11.79	11.85	11.91	11.95	12.00
12	10.35	10.48	10.59	10.68	10.76	10.83	10.89	10.95	11.00	11.04	11.08
11	9.49	9.61	9.71	9.80	9.87	9.93	9.99	10.04	10.09	10.13	10.17
10	8.64	8.74	8.83	8.91	8.98	9.04	9.09	9.14	9.18	9.21	9.25
9	7.78	7.87	7.96	8.03	8.09	8.14	8.19	8.23	8.27	8.30	8.33
8	6.92	7.00	7.08	7.14	7.19	7.24	7.28	7.32	7.35	7.38	7.41
7	6.06	6.13	6.20	6.25	6.30	6.34	6.38	6.41	6.44	6.46	6.49
6	5.20	5.26	5.32	5.36	5.40	5.44	5.47	5.50	5.52	5.54	5.57
5	4.33	4.39	4.43	4.47	4.51	4.53	4.56	4.58	4.61	4.62	4.64
4	3.47	3.51	3.55	3.58	3.61	3.63	3.65	3.67	3.69	3.70	3.72
3	2.60	2.64	2.66	2.69	2.71	2.73	2.74	2.75	2.77	2.78	2.79
2	1.74	1.76	1.78	1.79	1.81	1.82	1.83	1.84	1.85	1.85	1.86
1	0.87	0.88	0.89	0.90	0.90	0.91	0.92	0.92	0.92	0.93	0.93
0	0.00	0.00	0.00	0.00	0.00	0.00	0.00	0.00	0.00	0.00	0.00
− 1	0.87	0.88	0.89	0.90	0.91	0.91	0.92	0.92	0.93	0.93	0.93
2	1.74	1.76	1.78	1.80	1.81	1.82	1.83	1.84	1.85	1.86	1.87
3	2.61	2.65	2.67	2.70	2.72	2.74	2.75	2.77	2.78	2.79	2.80
4	3.49	3.53	3.57	3.60	3.63	3.65	3.67	3.69	3.71	3.72	3.74
5	4.36	4.42	4.46	4.50	4.54	4.57	4.59	4.62	4.64	4.66	4.67
6	5.24	5.30	5.36	5.41	5.45	5.48	5.52	5.54	5.57	5.59	5.61
7	6.12	6.19	6.26	6.31	6.36	6.40	6.44	6.47	6.50	6.53	6.55
8	7.00	7.08	7.16	7.22	7.27	7.32	7.36	7.40	7.44	7.47	7.49
9	7.88	7.97	8.06	8.13	8.19	8.24	8.29	8.33	8.37	8.41	8.44
10	8.76	8.87	8.96	9.04	9.11	9.17	9.22	9.27	9.31	9.35	9.38
11	9.64	9.76	9.86	9.95	10.02	10.09	10.15	10.20	10.25	10.29	10.33
12	10.52	10.65	10.76	10.86	10.94	11.01	11.08	11.14	11.19	11.23	11.27
13	11.41	11.55	11.67	11.77	11.86	11.94	12.01	12.07	12.13	12.18	12.22
14	12.29	12.45	12.58	12.69	12.78	12.87	12.94	13.01	13.07	13.12	13.17
15	13.18	13.34	13.48	13.60	13.71	13.80	13.88	13.95	14.01	14.07	14.12
16	14.07	14.24	14.39	14.52	14.63	14.73	14.81	14.89	14.96	15.02	15.07
17	14.96	15.14	15.30	15.44	15.56	15.66	15.75	15.83	15.90	15.97	16.03
18	15.85	16.05	16.21	16.36	16.48	16.59	16.69	16.77	16.85	16.92	16.98
19	16.74	16.95	17.13	17.28	17.41	17.53	17.63	17.72	17.80	17.87	17.94
20	17.64	17.85	18.04	18.20	18.34	18.46	18.57	18.67	18.75	18.83	18.90
21	18.53	18.76	18.96	19.12	19.27	19.40	19.51	19.61	19.70	19.78	19.86
22	19.43	19.67	19.87	20.05	20.20	20.34	20.46	20.56	20.66	20.74	20.82
23	20.32	20.58	20.79	20.98	21.14	21.28	21.40	21.51	21.61	21.70	21.78
24	21.22	21.49	21.71	21.90	22.07	22.22	22.35	22.46	22.57	22.66	22.74
25	22.12	22.40	22.63	22.83	23.01	23.16	23.30	23.42	23.52	23.62	23.71
26	23.02	23.31	23.55	23.76	23.95	24.10	24.24	24.37	24.48	24.58	24.67
27	23.92	24.22	24.48	24.69	24.88	25.05	25.20	25.33	25.44	25.55	25.64
28	24.83	25.14	25.40	25.63	25.82	26.00	26.15	26.28	26.40	26.51	26.61
29	25.73	26.05	26.33	26.56	26.77	26.94	27.10	27.24	27.37	27.48	27.58
30	26.64	26.97	27.26	27.50	27.71	27.89	28.06	28.20	28.33	28.45	28.55

APPENDIX D (continued)

Centre thickness 1.20 mm

Back Vertex Powers in D	Front Vertex Powers in D for Back Optic Radii in mm of:										
	5.0	5.5	6.0	6.5	7.0	7.5	8.0	8.5	9.0	9.5	10.0
+ 20	16.93	17.15	17.35	17.51	17.65	17.78	17.89	17.99	18.08	18.16	18.23
19	16.09	16.31	16.49	16.65	16.78	16.90	17.01	17.10	17.19	17.26	17.33
18	15.26	16.46	15.63	15.78	15.91	16.03	16.13	16.21	16.29	16.37	16.43
17	14.42	14.61	14.78	14.92	15.04	15.15	15.24	15.32	15.40	15.47	15.53
16	13.58	13.76	13.92	14.05	14.17	14.27	14.36	14.43	14.51	14.57	14.63
15	12.74	12.91	13.06	13.18	13.29	13.38	13.47	13.54	13.61	13.67	13.72
14	11.90	12.06	12.20	12.31	12.41	12.50	12.58	12.65	12.71	12.77	12.82
13	11.06	11.21	11.33	11.44	11.54	11.62	11.69	11.75	11.81	11.86	11.91
12	10.22	10.35	10.47	10.57	10.66	10.73	10.80	10.86	10.91	10.96	11.00
11	9.37	9.50	9.60	9.70	9.78	9.85	9.91	9.96	10.01	10.05	10.10
10	8.53	8.64	8.74	8.82	8.89	8.96	9.01	9.06	9.11	9.15	9.18
9	7.68	7.78	7.87	7.95	8.01	8.07	8.12	8.16	8.20	8.24	8.27
8	6.83	6.92	7.00	7.07	7.13	7.18	7.22	7.26	7.30	7.33	7.36
7	5.98	6.06	6.13	6.19	6.24	6.28	6.32	6.36	6.39	6.42	6.44
6	5.13	5.20	5.26	5.31	5.35	5.39	5.42	5.45	5.48	5.51	5.53
5	4.28	4.34	4.39	4.43	4.46	4.50	4.52	4.55	4.57	4.59	4.61
4	3.43	3.47	3.51	3.54	3.57	3.60	3.62	3.64	3.66	3.68	3.69
3	2.57	2.61	2.64	2.66	2.68	2.70	2.72	2.73	2.75	2.76	2.77
2	1.72	1.74	1.76	1.78	1.79	1.80	1.81	1.82	1.83	1.84	1.85
1	0.86	0.87	0.88	0.89	0.90	0.90	0.91	0.91	0.92	0.92	0.93
0	0.00	0.00	0.00	0.00	0.00	0.00	0.00	0.00	0.00	0.00	0.00
− 1	0.86	0.87	0.88	0.89	0.90	0.90	0.91	0.91	0.92	0.92	0.93
2	1.72	1.74	1.76	1.78	1.80	1.81	1.82	1.83	1.84	1.85	1.85
3	2.58	2.62	2.65	2.67	2.70	2.71	2.73	2.75	2.76	2.77	2.78
4	3.45	3.49	3.53	3.57	3.60	3.62	3.64	3.66	3.68	3.70	3.71
5	4.31	4.37	4.42	4.46	4.50	4.53	4.56	4.58	4.61	4.63	4.65
6	5.18	5.25	5.31	5.36	5.40	5.44	5.47	5.51	5.53	5.56	5.58
7	6.05	6.13	6.20	6.26	6.31	6.35	6.39	6.43	6.46	6.49	6.51
8	6.91	7.01	7.09	7.15	7.21	7.27	7.31	7.35	7.39	7.42	7.45
9	7.78	7.89	7.98	8.05	8.12	8.18	8.23	8.28	8.32	8.35	8.39
10	8.66	8.77	8.87	8.96	9.03	9.10	9.15	9.20	9.25	9.29	9.33
11	9.53	9.66	9.76	9.86	9.94	10.01	10.08	10.13	10.18	10.23	10.27
12	10.40	10.54	10.66	10.76	10.85	10.93	11.00	11.06	11.12	11.17	11.21
13	11.28	11.43	11.56	11.67	11.77	11.85	11.93	11.99	12.05	12.11	12.15
14	12.15	12.32	12.46	12.58	12.68	12.77	12.85	12.93	12.99	13.05	13.10
15	13.03	13.21	13.36	13.49	13.60	13.70	13.78	13.86	13.93	13.99	14.05
16	13.91	14.10	14.26	14.40	14.52	14.62	14.71	14.79	14.87	14.93	14.99
17	14.79	14.99	15.16	15.31	15.43	15.55	15.64	15.73	15.81	15.88	15.94
18	15.67	15.89	16.07	16.22	16.35	16.47	16.58	16.67	16.75	16.83	16.90
19	16.56	16.78	16.97	17.13	17.28	17.40	17.51	17.61	17.70	17.78	17.85
20	17.44	17.68	17.88	18.05	18.20	18.33	18.45	18.55	18.64	18.73	18.80
21	18.33	18.57	18.79	18.97	19.13	19.26	19.38	19.49	19.59	19.68	19.76
22	19.22	19.47	19.70	19.89	20.05	20.20	20.32	20.44	20.54	20.63	20.71
23	20.10	20.38	20.61	20.81	20.98	21.13	21.26	21.38	21.49	21.59	21.67
24	20.99	21.28	21.52	21.73	21.91	22.07	22.21	22.33	22.44	22.54	22.63
25	21.89	22.18	22.43	22.65	22.84	23.00	23.15	23.28	23.40	23.50	23.60
26	22.78	23.09	23.35	23.57	23.77	23.94	24.09	24.23	24.35	24.46	24.56
27	23.67	23.99	24.27	24.50	24.70	24.88	25.04	25.18	25.31	25.42	25.52
28	24.57	24.90	25.18	25.43	25.64	25.82	25.99	26.13	26.26	26.38	26.49
29	25.46	25.81	26.10	26.36	26.58	26.77	26.94	27.09	27.22	27.35	27.46
30	26.36	26.72	27.02	27.28	27.51	27.71	27.89	28.05	28.19	28.31	28.43

APPENDIX D (continued)

Centre thickness 1.30 mm

Back Vertex Powers in D	Front Vertex Powers in D for Back Optic Radii in mm of:										
	5.0	5.5	6.0	6.5	7.0	7.5	8.0	8.5	9.0	9.5	10.0
+ 20	16.71	16.94	17.15	17.32	17.48	17.61	17.73	17.83	17.93	18.01	18.09
19	15.88	16.11	16.30	16.47	16.62	16.74	16.86	16.96	17.05	17.13	17.20
18	15.06	15.27	15.46	15.62	15.75	15.88	15.98	16.08	16.16	16.24	16.31
17	14.23	14.44	14.61	14.76	14.89	15.01	15.11	15.20	15.28	15.35	15.42
16	13.41	13.60	13.76	13.90	14.03	14.13	14.23	14.31	14.39	14.46	14.52
15	12.58	12.76	12.91	13.05	13.16	13.26	13.35	13.43	13.50	13.57	13.62
14	11.75	11.92	12.06	12.19	12.29	12.39	12.47	12.55	12.61	12.67	12.73
13	10.92	11.08	11.21	11.32	11.42	11.51	11.59	11.66	11.72	11.78	11.83
12	10.09	10.23	10.36	10.46	10.55	10.64	10.71	10.77	10.83	10.88	10.93
11	9.25	9.39	9.50	9.60	9.68	9.76	9.82	9.88	9.93	9.98	10.02
10	8.42	8.54	8.64	8.73	8.81	8.88	8.94	8.99	9.04	9.08	9.12
9	7.58	7.69	7.79	7.87	7.94	8.00	8.05	8.10	8.14	8.18	8.22
8	6.75	6.84	6.93	7.00	7.06	7.11	7.16	7.20	7.24	7.28	7.31
7	5.91	5.99	6.07	6.13	6.18	6.23	6.27	6.31	6.34	6.37	6.40
6	5.07	5.14	5.20	5.26	5.30	5.34	5.38	5.41	5.44	5.47	5.49
5	4.23	4.29	4.34	4.38	4.42	4.46	4.49	4.51	4.54	4.56	4.58
4	3.38	3.43	3.47	3.51	3.54	3.57	3.59	3.61	3.63	3.65	3.67
3	2.54	2.58	2.61	2.64	2.66	2.68	2.70	2.71	2.73	2.74	2.75
2	1.70	1.72	1.74	1.76	1.77	1.79	1.80	1.81	1.82	1.83	1.84
1	0.85	0.86	0.87	0.88	0.89	0.89	0.90	0.91	0.91	0.92	0.92
0	0.00	0.00	0.00	0.00	0.00	0.00	0.00	0.00	0.00	0.00	0.00
− 1	0.85	0.86	0.87	0.88	0.89	0.90	0.90	0.91	0.91	0.92	0.92
2	1.70	1.72	1.75	1.76	1.78	1.79	1.81	1.82	1.83	1.83	1.84
3	2.55	2.59	2.62	2.65	2.67	2.69	2.71	2.73	2.74	2.75	2.77
4	3.41	3.46	3.50	3.53	3.57	3.59	3.62	3.64	3.66	3.68	3.69
5	4.26	4.32	4.38	4.42	4.46	4.49	4.52	4.55	4.58	4.60	4.62
6	5.12	5.19	5.25	5.31	5.36	5.40	5.43	5.47	5.50	5.52	5.55
7	5.97	6.06	6.14	6.20	6.25	6.30	6.35	6.38	6.42	6.45	6.49
8	6.83	6.93	7.02	7.09	7.15	7.21	7.26	7.30	7.34	7.38	7.41
9	7.69	7.81	7.90	7.98	8.05	8.12	8.17	8.22	8.26	8.30	8.34
10	8.56	8.68	8.79	8.88	8.96	9.03	9.09	9.14	9.19	9.23	9.27
11	9.42	9.56	9.67	9.77	9.86	9.94	10.00	10.06	10.12	10.17	10.21
12	10.28	10.43	10.56	10.67	10.77	10.85	10.92	10.99	11.05	11.10	11.15
13	11.15	11.31	11.45	11.57	11.67	11.76	11.84	11.91	11.98	12.04	12.09
14	12.02	12.19	12.34	12.47	12.58	12.68	12.76	12.84	12.91	12.97	13.03
15	12.89	13.07	13.23	13.37	13.49	13.59	13.69	13.77	13.84	13.91	13.97
16	13.76	13.96	14.13	14.27	14.40	14.51	14.61	14.70	14.78	14.85	14.92
17	14.63	14.84	15.02	15.18	15.31	15.43	15.54	15.63	15.72	15.79	15.86
18	15.50	15.73	15.92	16.08	16.23	16.35	16.47	16.57	16.65	16.73	16.81
19	16.38	16.61	16.82	16.99	17.14	17.28	17.40	17.50	17.59	17.68	17.76
20	17.25	17.50	17.72	17.90	18.06	18.20	18.33	18.44	18.54	18.63	18.71
21	18.13	18.39	18.62	18.81	18.98	19.13	19.26	19.38	19.48	19.57	19.66
22	19.01	19.28	19.52	19.72	19.90	20.06	20.19	20.32	20.42	20.52	20.61
23	19.89	20.18	20.43	20.64	20.82	20.99	21.13	21.26	21.37	21.47	21.57
24	20.77	21.07	21.33	21.55	21.75	21.92	22.07	22.20	22.32	22.43	22.53
25	21.65	21.97	22.24	22.47	22.67	22.85	23.00	23.14	23.27	23.38	23.48
26	22.54	22.87	23.15	23.39	23.60	23.78	23.95	24.09	24.22	24.34	24.44
27	23.42	23.76	24.06	24.31	24.53	24.72	24.89	25.04	25.17	25.29	25.41
28	24.31	24.66	24.97	25.23	25.46	25.65	25.83	25.99	26.13	26.25	26.37
29	25.20	25.57	25.88	26.15	26.39	26.59	26.78	26.94	27.08	27.22	27.33
30	26.09	26.47	26.80	27.08	27.32	27.53	27.72	27.89	28.04	28.18	28.30

APPENDIX D (continued)

Centre thickness 1.40 mm

Back Vertex Powers in D	Front Vertex Powers in D for Back Optic Radii in mm of:										
	5.0	5.5	6.0	6.5	7.0	7.5	8.0	8.5	9.0	9.5	10.0
+ 20	16.49	16.74	16.96	17.14	17.30	17.45	17.57	17.68	17.78	17.87	17.96
19	15.68	15.92	16.12	16.30	16.45	16.59	16.71	16.81	16.91	16.99	17.07
18	14.86	15.09	15.29	15.45	15.60	15.73	15.84	15.94	16.03	16.11	16.19
17	14.05	14.26	14.45	14.61	14.75	14.87	14.97	15.07	15.16	15.23	15.30
16	13.23	13.44	13.61	13.76	13.89	14.00	14.11	14.20	14.28	14.35	14.42
15	12.42	12.61	12.77	12.91	13.03	13.14	13.24	13.32	13.40	13.46	13.53
14	11.60	11.78	11.93	12.06	12.18	12.28	12.36	12.44	12.51	12.58	12.64
13	10.78	10.95	11.09	11.21	11.32	11.41	11.49	11.56	11.63	11.69	11.74
12	9.96	10.11	10.24	10.36	10.45	10.54	10.62	10.68	10.75	10.80	10.85
11	9.14	9.28	9.40	9.50	9.59	9.67	9.74	9.80	9.86	9.91	9.96
10	8.31	8.44	8.55	8.64	8.73	8.80	8.86	8.92	8.97	9.02	9.06
9	7.49	7.60	7.70	7.79	7.86	7.93	7.98	8.03	8.08	8.12	8.16
8	6.66	6.77	6.85	6.93	6.99	7.05	7.10	7.15	7.19	7.23	7.26
7	5.83	5.92	6.00	6.07	6.13	6.18	6.22	6.26	6.30	6.33	6.36
6	5.01	5.08	5.15	5.21	5.26	5.30	5.34	5.37	5.40	5.43	5.45
5	4.17	4.24	4.29	4.34	4.38	4.42	4.45	4.48	4.51	4.53	4.55
4	3.34	3.39	3.44	3.48	3.51	3.54	3.56	3.59	3.61	3.63	3.64
3	2.51	2.55	2.58	2.61	2.63	2.66	2.68	2.69	2.71	2.72	2.73
2	1.67	1.70	1.72	1.74	1.76	1.77	1.79	1.80	1.81	1.82	1.83
1	0.84	0.85	0.86	0.87	0.88	0.89	0.89	0.90	0.90	0.91	0.91
0	0.00	0.00	0.00	0.00	0.00	0.00	0.00	0.00	0.00	0.00	0.00
− 1	0.84	0.85	0.86	0.87	0.88	0.89	0.90	0.90	0.91	0.91	0.92
2	1.68	1.71	1.73	1.75	1.76	1.78	1.79	1.80	1.81	1.82	1.83
3	2.52	2.56	2.59	2.62	2.65	2.67	2.69	2.71	2.72	2.74	2.75
4	3.37	3.42	3.46	3.50	3.53	3.56	3.59	3.61	3.63	3.65	3.67
5	4.21	4.28	4.33	4.38	4.42	4.46	4.49	4.52	4.55	4.57	4.59
6	5.06	5.14	5.20	5.26	5.31	5.35	5.39	5.43	5.46	5.49	5.51
7	5.91	6.00	6.08	6.14	6.20	6.25	6.30	6.34	6.38	6.41	6.44
8	6.75	6.86	6.95	7.03	7.09	7.15	7.20	7.25	7.29	7.33	7.36
9	7.61	7.72	7.82	7.91	7.99	8.05	8.11	8.16	8.21	8.25	8.29
10	8.46	8.59	8.70	8.80	8.88	8.96	9.02	9.08	9.13	9.18	9.22
11	9.31	9.46	9.58	9.69	9.78	9.86	9.93	10.00	10.05	10.11	10.15
12	10.17	10.33	10.46	10.58	10.68	10.77	10.85	10.92	10.98	11.04	11.09
13	11.02	11.20	11.34	11.47	11.58	11.67	11.76	11.84	11.90	11.97	12.02
14	11.88	12.07	12.23	12.36	12.48	12.58	12.68	12.76	12.83	12.90	12.96
15	12.74	12.94	13.11	13.26	13.38	13.49	13.59	13.68	13.76	13.83	13.90
16	13.60	13.82	14.00	14.15	14.29	14.41	14.51	14.61	14.69	14.77	14.84
17	14.47	14.69	14.88	15.05	15.19	15.32	15.43	15.53	15.62	15.70	15.78
18	15.33	15.57	15.77	15.95	16.10	16.24	16.36	16.46	16.56	16.64	16.72
19	16.20	16.45	16.67	16.85	17.01	17.15	17.28	17.39	17.49	17.58	17.67
20	17.06	17.33	17.56	17.75	17.92	18.07	18.21	18.32	18.43	18.53	18.61
21	17.93	18.21	18.45	18.66	18.84	18.99	19.13	19.26	19.37	19.47	19.56
22	18.80	19.10	19.35	19.56	19.75	19.92	20.06	20.19	20.31	20.42	20.51
23	19.67	19.98	20.25	20.47	20.67	20.84	20.99	21.13	21.25	21.36	21.46
24	20.55	20.87	21.14	21.38	21.59	21.77	21.93	22.07	22.20	22.31	22.42
25	21.42	21.76	22.05	22.29	22.51	22.69	22.86	23.01	23.14	23.26	23.37
26	22.30	22.65	22.95	23.20	23.43	23.62	23.80	23.95	24.09	24.22	24.33
27	23.18	23.54	23.85	24.12	24.35	24.55	24.74	24.90	25.04	25.17	25.29
28	24.06	24.43	24.76	25.03	25.28	25.49	25.67	25.84	25.99	26.13	26.25
29	24.94	25.33	25.66	25.95	26.20	26.42	26.62	26.79	26.95	27.08	27.21
30	25.82	26.23	26.57	26.87	27.13	27.36	27.56	27.74	27.90	28.04	28.18

APPENDIX D (continued)

Centre thickness 1.50 mm

Back Vertex Powers in D	Front Vertex Powers in D for Back Optic Radii in mm of:										
	5.0	5.5	6.0	6.5	7.0	7.5	8.0	8.5	9.0	9.5	10.0
+ 20	16.27	16.54	16.77	16.96	17.13	17.28	17.41	17.53	17.64	17.73	17.82
19	15.47	15.72	15.94	16.03	16.29	16.43	16.56	16.67	16.77	16.86	16.95
18	14.67	14.91	15.12	15.29	15.45	15.58	15.70	15.81	15.91	15.99	16.07
17	13.87	14.10	14.29	14.46	14.60	14.73	14.84	14.94	15.04	15.12	15.19
16	13.06	13.28	13.46	13.62	13.76	13.88	13.98	14.08	14.16	14.24	14.31
15	12.26	12.46	12.63	12.78	12.91	13.02	13.12	13.21	13.29	13.36	13.43
14	11.45	11.64	11.80	11.94	12.06	12.16	12.26	12.34	12.42	12.48	12.55
13	10.64	10.82	10.97	11.10	11.21	11.31	11.39	11.47	11.54	11.60	11.66
12	9.83	9.99	10.13	10.25	10.36	10.45	10.53	10.60	10.66	10.72	10.77
11	9.02	9.17	9.30	9.41	9.50	9.59	9.66	9.73	9.78	9.84	9.89
10	8.21	8.34	8.46	8.56	8.65	8.72	8.79	8.85	8.90	8.95	9.00
9	7.40	7.52	7.62	7.71	7.79	7.86	7.92	7.97	8.02	8.06	8.10
8	6.58	6.69	6.78	6.86	6.93	6.99	7.04	7.09	7.14	7.17	7.21
7	5.76	5.81	5.94	6.01	6.07	6.12	6.17	6.21	6.25	6.28	6.32
6	4.94	5.03	5.10	5.15	5.21	5.25	5.29	5.33	5.36	5.39	5.42
5	4.12	4.19	4.25	4.30	4.34	4.38	4.42	4.45	4.47	4.50	4.52
4	3.30	3.36	3.40	3.44	3.48	3.51	3.54	3.56	3.58	3.60	3.62
3	2.48	2.52	2.55	2.58	2.61	2.63	2.65	2.67	2.69	2.70	2.72
2	1.65	1.68	1.70	1.72	1.74	1.76	1.77	1.78	1.79	1.80	1.81
1	0.83	0.84	0.85	0.86	0.87	0.88	0.89	0.89	0.90	0.90	0.91
0	0.00	0.00	0.00	0.00	0.00	0.00	0.00	0.00	0.00	0.00	0.00
− 1	0.83	0.84	0.86	0.87	0.87	0.88	0.89	0.89	0.90	0.91	0.91
2	1.66	1.69	1.71	1.73	1.75	1.76	1.78	1.79	1.80	1.81	1.82
3	2.49	2.53	2.57	2.60	2.63	2.65	2.67	2.69	2.70	2.72	2.73
4	3.33	3.38	3.43	3.47	3.50	3.54	3.56	3.59	3.61	3.63	3.65
5	4.16	4.23	4.29	4.34	4.38	4.42	4.46	4.49	4.52	4.54	4.56
6	5.00	5.08	5.15	5.21	5.27	5.31	5.35	5.39	5.42	5.45	5.48
7	5.84	5.93	6.02	6.09	6.15	6.20	6.25	6.30	6.33	6.37	6.40
8	6.68	6.79	6.88	6.96	7.03	7.10	7.15	7.20	7.25	7.29	7.32
9	7.52	7.64	7.75	7.84	7.92	7.99	8.05	8.11	8.16	8.20	8.25
10	8.36	8.50	8.62	8.72	8.81	8.89	8.96	9.02	9.07	9.12	9.17
11	9.21	9.36	9.49	9.60	9.70	9.79	9.86	9.93	9.99	10.05	10.10
12	10.05	10.22	10.36	10.48	10.59	10.69	10.77	10.84	10.91	10.97	11.03
13	10.90	11.08	11.24	11.37	11.49	11.59	11.68	11.76	11.83	11.90	11.96
14	11.75	11.94	12.11	12.26	12.38	12.49	12.59	12.68	12.75	12.82	12.89
15	12.60	12.81	12.99	13.14	13.28	13.40	13.50	13.59	13.68	13.75	13.82
16	13.45	13.68	13.87	14.03	14.18	14.30	14.41	14.51	14.60	14.68	14.76
17	14.31	14.54	14.75	14.92	15.08	15.21	15.33	15.44	15.53	15.62	15.70
18	15.16	15.41	15.63	15.82	15.98	16.12	16.25	16.36	16.46	16.55	16.64
19	16.02	16.29	16.52	16.71	16.88	17.03	17.17	17.29	17.39	17.49	17.58
20	16.88	17.16	17.40	17.61	17.79	17.95	18.09	18.21	18.33	18.43	18.52
21	17.74	18.03	18.29	18.51	18.70	18.86	19.01	19.14	19.26	19.37	19.46
22	18.60	18.91	19.18	19.40	19.60	19.78	19.94	20.07	20.20	20.31	20.41
23	19.47	19.79	20.07	20.31	20.52	20.70	20.86	21.01	21.14	21.25	21.36
24	20.33	20.67	20.96	21.21	21.43	21.62	21.79	21.94	22.08	22.20	22.31
25	21.20	21.50	21.85	22.11	22.34	22.54	22.72	22.88	23.02	23.15	23.26
26	22.07	22.43	22.75	23.02	23.26	23.47	23.65	23.82	23.96	24.10	24.22
27	22.94	23.32	23.65	23.93	24.18	24.39	24.58	24.76	24.91	25.05	25.17
28	23.81	24.21	24.55	24.84	25.10	25.32	25.52	25.70	25.86	26.00	26.13
29	24.68	25.09	25.45	25.76	26.02	26.25	26.46	26.64	26.81	26.96	27.09
30	25.56	25.98	26.35	26.66	26.94	27.18	27.40	27.59	27.76	27.91	28.05

APPENDIX D (continued)

Centre thickness 1.60 mm

Back Vertex Powers in D	Front Vertex Powers in D for Back Optic Radii in mm of:										
	5.0	5.5	6.0	6.5	7.0	7.5	8.0	8.5	9.0	9.5	10.0
+ 20	16.06	16.34	16.58	16.78	16.96	17.12	17.26	17.39	17.50	17.60	17.69
19	15.27	15.54	15.76	15.96	16.13	16.28	16.41	16.53	16.64	16.73	16.82
18	14.48	14.73	14.95	15.13	15.30	15.44	15.57	15.68	15.78	15.87	15.95
17	13.69	13.93	14.13	14.31	14.46	14.60	14.71	14.82	14.92	15.00	15.08
16	12.90	13.12	13.31	13.48	13.62	13.75	13.86	13.96	14.05	14.13	14.21
15	12.10	12.31	12.49	12.65	12.78	12.90	13.01	13.10	13.19	13.26	13.33
14	11.31	11.50	11.67	11.82	11.94	12.06	12.15	12.24	12.32	12.39	12.46
13	10.51	10.69	10.85	10.98	11.10	11.21	11.30	11.38	11.45	11.52	11.58
12	9.71	9.88	10.02	10.15	10.26	10.35	10.44	10.51	10.58	10.64	10.70
11	8.91	9.06	9.20	9.31	9.41	9.50	9.58	9.65	9.71	9.77	9.82
10	8.11	8.25	8.37	8.47	8.57	8.65	8.72	8.78	8.84	8.89	8.93
9	7.30	7.43	7.54	7.63	7.72	7.79	7.85	7.91	7.96	8.01	8.05
8	6.50	6.61	6.71	6.79	6.87	6.93	6.99	7.04	7.08	7.12	7.16
7	5.69	5.79	5.88	5.95	6.01	6.07	6.12	6.16	6.20	6.24	6.27
6	4.88	4.97	5.04	5.10	5.16	5.21	5.25	5.29	5.32	5.35	5.38
5	4.07	4.14	4.21	4.26	4.30	4.34	4.38	4.41	4.44	4.47	4.49
4	3.26	3.32	3.37	3.41	3.45	3.48	3.51	3.53	3.56	3.58	3.60
3	2.45	2.49	2.53	2.56	2.59	2.61	2.63	2.65	2.67	2.69	2.70
2	1.63	1.66	1.69	1.71	1.73	1.74	1.76	1.77	1.78	1.79	1.80
1	0.82	0.83	0.84	0.86	0.86	0.87	0.88	0.89	0.89	0.90	0.90
0	0.00	0.00	0.00	0.00	0.00	0.00	0.00	0.00	0.00	0.00	0.00
− 1	0.82	0.83	0.85	0.86	0.87	0.87	0.88	0.89	0.89	0.90	0.90
2	1.64	1.67	1.69	1.72	1.73	1.75	1.76	1.78	1.79	1.80	1.81
3	2.46	2.51	2.54	2.58	2.60	2.63	2.65	2.67	2.69	2.70	2.72
4	3.29	3.35	3.39	3.44	3.47	3.51	3.54	3.56	3.59	3.61	3.63
5	4.11	4.19	4.25	4.30	4.35	4.39	4.42	4.46	4.49	4.51	4.54
6	4.94	5.03	5.10	5.17	5.22	5.27	5.31	5.35	5.39	5.42	5.45
7	5.77	5.87	5.96	6.03	6.10	6.16	6.21	6.25	6.29	6.33	6.36
8	6.60	6.72	6.82	6.90	6.98	7.04	7.10	7.15	7.20	7.24	7.28
9	7.43	7.56	7.68	7.77	7.86	7.93	8.00	8.06	8.11	8.16	8.20
10	8.27	8.41	8.54	8.64	8.74	8.82	8.89	8.96	9.02	9.07	9.12
11	9.10	9.26	9.40	9.52	9.62	9.71	9.79	9.87	9.93	9.99	10.04
12	9.94	10.11	10.27	10.39	10.51	10.61	10.69	10.77	10.84	10.91	10.97
13	10.78	10.97	11.13	11.27	11.39	11.50	11.60	11.68	11.76	11.83	11.89
14	11.62	11.82	12.00	12.15	12.28	12.40	12.50	12.59	12.68	12.75	12.82
15	12.46	12.68	12.87	13.03	13.17	13.30	13.41	13.51	13.60	13.68	13.75
16	13.31	13.54	13.74	13.91	14.07	14.20	14.32	14.42	14.52	14.60	14.68
17	14.15	14.40	14.62	14.80	14.96	15.10	15.23	15.34	15.44	15.53	15.61
18	15.00	15.26	15.49	15.68	15.86	16.01	16.14	16.26	16.37	16.46	16.55
19	15.85	16.13	16.37	16.57	16.75	16.91	17.05	17.18	17.29	17.39	17.49
20	16.70	16.99	17.25	17.46	17.65	17.82	17.97	18.10	18.22	18.33	18.43
21	17.55	17.86	18.13	18.36	18.56	18.73	18.89	19.03	19.15	19.27	19.37
22	18.40	18.73	19.01	19.25	19.46	19.64	19.81	19.95	20.09	20.20	20.31
23	19.26	19.60	19.89	20.14	20.36	20.56	20.73	20.88	21.02	21.14	21.26
24	20.12	20.47	20.78	21.04	21.27	21.47	21.65	21.81	21.96	22.09	22.20
25	20.98	21.35	21.67	21.94	22.18	22.39	22.58	22.75	22.90	23.03	23.15
26	21.84	22.22	22.56	22.84	23.09	23.31	23.51	23.68	23.84	23.98	24.11
27	22.70	23.10	23.45	23.74	24.00	24.23	24.44	24.62	24.78	24.93	25.06
28	23.56	23.98	24.34	24.65	24.92	25.16	25.37	25.55	25.72	25.88	26.01
29	24.43	24.86	25.24	25.55	25.84	26.08	26.30	26.49	26.67	26.83	26.97
30	25.30	25.75	26.13	26.46	26.75	27.01	27.24	27.44	27.62	27.78	27.93

Table I—Solutions and Drops for Use with Hard Lenses

(Most soft lens solutions may also be used for hard lenses (*see Table II*). However, for lens materials other than poly-methyl methacrylate the manufacturer's instructions regarding solutions should be followed, as lenses containing silicone and cellulose acetate butyrate, for example, may not be compatible with all preservatives.)

Name of solution and sizes available	Manufacturer	Preservatives with percentage concentration	Remarks
Soaking solutions (which may also be used for cleaning)			
Contique Cleaning and Soaking, 120 ml	Alcon (Contique)	B Cl 0.02; EDTA 0.1	
Clean-N-Soak, 120 ml	Allergan	PMN 0.004	
Soakare, 120 ml	Allergan	B Cl 0.01; EDTA 0.25	
Soquette, 10 ml, 120 ml	Barnes-Hind	B Cl 0.01; EDTA 0.2	
Contacare Cleaning and Soaking, 120 ml	Barnes-Hind	B Cl 0.01; EDTA 0.2	
Contactasoak, 7 ml, 120 ml	Contactasol	B Cl 0.004; EDTA 0.1; CHX 0.006	
Duo-Flow Cleaning and Soaking, 120 ml	Cooper	B Cl 0.013; EDTA 0.25	
Hoya Hard Daily Soaking/Cleaning, 120 ml	Hoya	B Cl ?; EDTA ?	
Kelsoak, 10 ml, 120 ml	Kelvin	B Cl 0.01; EDTA 0.1	
C-Thru Hard Soaking/Cleaning, 110 ml	Optimedic	B Cl 0.02; EDTA 0.1	
Optrex Soaking, 120 ml	Optrex	B Cl 0.02; THI 0.004	
Steri-Soak, 110 ml	Sauflon Pharmaceuticals	B Cl 0.002; EDTA 0.1; CHLB 0.4	
Transoak, 10 ml, 120 ml	Smith and Nephew Pharmaceuticals	B Cl 0.01; EDTA 0.2	
Wetting solutions (which may also be used for re-wetting on the eye)			
Adapt, 2 ml, 15 ml	Alcon (Burton, Parsons)	EDTA 0.05; THI 0.002	
Dualwet, 60 ml	Alcon (Contique)	B Cl 0.01; EDTA 0.05	
Liquifilm Wetting, 60 ml	Allergan	B Cl 0.004; EDTA ?	
Presert, 15 ml	Allergan	B Cl 0.004; EDTA 0.02	
Barnes-Hind Wetting, 35 ml, 60 ml	Barnes-Hind	B Cl 0.004; EDTA 0.02	

Key — B Cl Benzalkonium Chloride; CHLB Chlorbutol; CHX Chlorhexidine Gluconate; EDTA Ethylenediamine Tetraacetic Acid; PHE Phenylephrine Hydrochloride; PMN Phenylmercuric Nitrate; THI Thiomersalate; Z S Zinc Sulphate; ? Concentration not available

Table I (continued)

Name of solution and sizes available	Manufacturer	Preservatives with percentage concentration	Remarks
Contactasol, 7 ml, 60 ml	Contactasol	B Cl 0.004; EDTA 0.1; CHX 0.006	
Hy-Flow, 60 ml	Cooper	B Cl 0.01; EDTA 0.025	
Kelvinol, 10 ml, 58 ml	Kelvin	B Cl 0.005; EDTA 0.1	
C-Thru Hard Lens Wetting, 70 ml	Optimedic	EDTA 0.1; THI 0.004	
Optrex Wetting, 55 ml	Optrex	B Cl 0.01; THI 0.004	
Steri-Clens, 65 ml	Sauflon Pharmaceuticals	EDTA 0.1; THI 0.004	Suitable for cleaning
Transol, 10 ml, 50 ml	Smith and Nephew Pharmaceuticals	B Cl 0.004; EDTA 0.02	

Combined soaking and wetting solutions (which may also be used for cleaning)

Soaclens, 10 ml, 120 ml	Alcon (Burton, Parsons)	EDTA 0.1; THI 0.004	
Total, 60 ml, 120 ml	Allergan	B Cl ?; EDTA ?	
One Solution, 90 ml	Barnes-Hind	B Cl 0.01; EDTA 0.02	
Barnes-Hind Wetting and Soaking, 120 ml	Barnes-Hind	B Cl 0.005; EDTA 0.1	
K-Lens, 230 ml	Maws	CHX 0.005	

Cleaning solutions (see also **Soft lens cleaning solutions**, Table II)

Clens, 10 ml, 60 ml	Alcon (Burton, Parsons)	B Cl 0.02; EDTA 0.1	
Contique Hard Cleaning, 30 ml	Alcon (Contique)	B Cl 0.02	
Titan, 30 ml	Barnes-Hind	B Cl ?; EDTA ?	
Gel Clean, 30g tube	Barnes-Hind	THI 0.004	
Contactaclean, 20 ml	Contactasol	B Cl 0.004; EDTA 0.1; CHX 0.006	
D-Film, 25 ml	Cooper	B Cl 0.013; EDTA 0.1	
Hoya Hard Cleaner, 60 ml	Hoya	EDTA ?	

Key — B Cl Benzalkonium Chloride; CHLB Chlorbutol; CHX Chlorhexidine Gluconate; EDTA Ethylenediamine Tetraacetic Acid; PHE Phenylephrine Hydrochloride; PMN Phenylmercuric Nitrate; THI Thiomersalate; Z S Zinc Sulphate; ? Concentration not available

Table I (continued)

Name of solution and sizes available	Manufacturer	Preservatives with percentage concentration	Remarks
Re-wetting solutions (*see also* **Soft lens re-wetting solutions,** *Table II*)			
Blink-N-Clean, 7.5 ml, 15 ml	Allergan	CHLB 0.5	
Comfort Drops, 15 ml	Barnes Hind	B Cl 0.005; EDTA 0.02	
Solpro, 15 ml	Contactasol	B Cl 0.004; CHX 0.006; EDTA 0.1	Intended for artificial eyes
Aqua-Flow, 25 ml	Cooper	B Cl 0.005; EDTA 0.025	
Transdrop, 10 ml	Smith and Nephew Pharmaceuticals	B Cl 0.004	
Artificial tears drops (which may also be used for re-wetting hard lenses)			
Adsorbotear, 15 ml	Alcon (Burton, Parsons)	EDTA 0.05; THI 0.002	Pharmacy Medicine
Tears Naturale, 15 ml	Alcon (Contique)	B Cl 0.01; EDTA 0.05	Pharmacy Medicine
Isoptoplain, 15 ml	Alcon	B Cl 0.01	Pharmacy Medicine
Isoptoalkaline, 15 ml	Alcon	B Cl 0.01	Pharmacy Medicine
Liquifilm Tears, 15 ml	Allergan	CHLB 0.5	Pharmacy Medicine
Neoteers, 15 ml	Barnes-Hind	EDTA 0.02; THI 0.004	Pharmacy Medicine. Awaiting a product licence
Conjunctival decongestants (*see also Table III*) (These are all Pharmacy Medicines)			
Isoptofrin, 15 ml	Alcon	B Cl 0.01	Contains PHE 0.12 per cent
Zincfrin, 15 ml	Alcon	B Cl 0.01	PHE 0.12 per cent; Z S 0.25 per cent
Prefrin, 15 ml	Allergan	B Cl 0.004	PHE 0.12 per cent
Eyeclear, 20 ml	Contactasol	B Cl 0.004	PHE 0.12 per cent
Miscellaneous solutions			
O_2 Care, 100 ml	Contactasol	EDTA 0.02; THI 0.002	For Menicon O_2 hard lenses
Eyesoothe, 120 ml with eyebath	Contactasol	B Cl 0.004	Eye lotion contains PHE 0.01 per cent

Key — B Cl Benzalkonium Chloride; CHLB Chlorbutol; CHX Chlorhexidine Gluconate; EDTA Ethylenediamine Tetraacetic Acid; PHE Phenylephrine Hydrochloride; PMN Phenylmercuric Nitrate; THI Thiomersalate; Z S Zinc Sulphate; ? Concentration not available

Table II—Solutions and Drops for Use with Soft Lenses

(Most soft lens solutions may also be used for hard lenses (*see Table I*). However, for lens materials other than polymethyl methacrylate the manufacturer's instructions regarding solutions should be followed, as lenses containing silicone and cellulose acetate butyrate, for example, may not be compatible with all preservatives. The same caution should be observed with any soft lens made of a new material, as preservatives may bind to the material, and cleaning solutions and systems might alter the lens parameters.)

Name of solution and sizes available	Manufacturer	Preservatives with percentage concentration	Remarks

Disinfecting and storage (soaking) solutions (these are basically saline, except where indicated)

Hydrophilic lenses

Name of solution and sizes available	Manufacturer	Preservatives with percentage concentration	Remarks
Ami-10, 40 ml, 200 ml	Abatron	CHX 0.005; EDTA 0.01; THI 0.001	
Flexsol, 10 ml, 45 ml, 120 ml, 175 ml	Alcon (Burton, Parsons)	CHX 0.005; EDTA 0.1; THI 0.001	
Flexcare, 250 ml	Alcon (Burton, Parsons)	CHX 0.005; EDTA 0.1; THI 0.001	
Contigel, 120 ml	Alcon (Contique)	CHX 0.005; EDTA 0.02; THI 0.0005	
Pliacide, 7.5 ml* used with	Alcon (Contique)	IOD 0.1	Not for use with lenses of greater than 53 per cent water content
Nutraflow, 110 ml	Alcon (Contique)	EDTA 0.1; S A 0.1	
Hydrocare Soaking and Cleaning, 120 ml, 240 ml	Allergan	ATAC 0.03; THI 0.002	
Hexidin, 120 ml, 240 ml	Barnes-Hind	EDTA 0.02; CHX 0.005; THI 0.001	
Bausch and Lomb Disinfecting, 120 ml, 250 ml	Bausch and Lomb	CHX 0.005; EDTA 0.1; THI 0.001	
Soflens Soaking, 120 ml, 240 ml	Bausch and Lomb	ATAC 0.03; THI 0.002	
Lensept, 240 ml (Septicon system)* used with	British American Optical		Hydrogen peroxide, 3 per cent solution used for 20 minutes followed by soaking in Lensrins with platinum disc to neutralize residual hydrogen peroxide
Lensrins, 240 ml	British American Optical	EDTA 0.1; THI 0.001	

Key — ATAC Alkyl Triethanol Ammonium Chloride; B A Benzoic Acid; CHX Chlorhexidine Gluconate; EDTA Ethylenediamine Tetraacetic Acid; IOD Iodine; NIPA Nipastat; PMN Phenylmercuric Nitrate; POV Povidone; S A Sorbic Acid; S P Sodium Perborate; THI Thiomersalate; * not saline

Table II (continued)

Name of solution and sizes available	Manufacturer	Preservatives with percentage concentration	Remarks
Hydrosoak, 20 ml, 120 ml	Contactasol	CHX 0.0025; EDTA 0.1; THI 0.0025	
Mirasoak, 120 ml	Cooper	CHX 0.008; EDTA 0.1	
Hydron Soft Lens Soaking, 120 ml	Hydron Europe	CHX 0.0025; EDTA 0.1; THI 0.0025	
ICN Unicare, 25 ml, 240 ml	ICN Pharmaceuticals	EDTA ?; THI ?	
Medisoak, 35 ml, 120 ml	Kelvin	CHX 0.0025; EDTA 0.1; THI 0.0025	
C-Thru Storage, 110 ml	Optimedic	CHX 0.005; EDTA 0.1; THI 0.001	
Optrex Soft Lens Soak, 120 ml	Optrex	CHX 0.005; EDTA 0.001; THI 0.002	
Steri-Sal, 110 ml	Sauflon Pharmaceuticals	CHX 0.001; EDTA 0.1; THI 0.002	
Steri-Soft, 110 ml	Sauflon Pharmaceuticals	EDTA 0.1; NIPA 0.01	
Transoft tablets*	Smith and Nephew Pharmaceuticals	POV; IOD	Not for use with lenses of greater than 53 per cent water content
used with			
Transoft, 120 ml	Smith and Nephew Pharmaceuticals	B A 0.079	
Silicone lenses			
Silicolens, 120 ml	Alcon (Burton, Parsons)	EDTA 0.1; THI 0.004	
Consil Wetting and Storage, 90 ml	Barnes-Hind	CHX 0.005; EDTA 0.1; THI 0.001	

Key — ATAC Alkyl Triethanol Ammonium Chloride; B A Benzoic Acid; CHX Chlorhexidine Gluconate; EDTA Ethylenediamine Tetraacetic Acid; IOD Iodine; NIPA Nipastat; PMN Phenylmercuric Nitrate; POV Povidone; S A Sorbic Acid; S P Sodium Perborate; THI Thiomersalate; *not saline

Table II (continued)

Name of solution and sizes available	Manufacturer	Preservatives with percentage concentration	Suitable for boiling
Preserved saline solution (which is used for rinsing) (Most of the disinfecting and storage solutions are basically preserved normal saline solutions, also suitable for rinsing)			
Boil-N-Soak, 240 ml	Alcon (Burton, Parsons)	EDTA 0.1; THI 0.001	Yes
Normol, 10 ml, 45 ml, 175 ml, 250 ml	Alcon (Burton, Parsons)	CHX 0.005; EDTA 0.1; THI 0.001	No
Thermosal, 250 ml	Alcon (Burton, Parsons)	EDTA 0.1; THI 0.001	Yes
Nutraflow, 110 ml	Alcon (Contique)	EDTA 0.1; S A 0.1	Yes
Hydrocare Boiling and Rinsing, 240 ml*	Allergan	EDTA ?; THI 0.001	Yes
Preserved Saline, 240 ml*	Allergan	EDTA ?; THI 0.001	Yes
Soft-Therm, 240 ml	Barnes-Hind	EDTA 0.1; THI 0.001	Yes
Soflens Saline, 120 ml, 250 ml	Bausch and Lomb	EDTA 0.1; THI 0.001	Yes
Lensrins, 240 ml	British American Optical	EDTA 0.1; THI 0.01	No
Solar, 120 ml	Contactasol	EDTA 0.1; THI 0.001	Yes
Mirasol, 120 ml	Cooper	EDTA 0.1; S A 0.1; THI 0.001	No
ICN Eyefresh, 240 ml	ICN Pharmaceuticals	EDTA ?; THI 0.001	No
C-Thru Rinsing, 110 ml	Optimedic	EDTA 0.1; THI 0.001	Yes
Optrex Soft Lens Rinse, 120 ml	Optrex	CHX 0.0025; EDTA 0.001; THI 0.001	No

*These are identical solutions

(Also available are Soft Salt Granules in packets, made by Hoya. They are preserved with EDTA and used with distilled water to make up normal saline solution for heat disinfection)

Key — ATAC Alkyl Triethanol Ammonium Chloride; B A Benzoic Acid; CHX Chlorhexidine Gluconate; EDTA Ethylenediamine Tetraacetic Acid; IOD Iodine; NIPA Nipastat; PMN Phenylmercuric Nitrate; POV Povidone; S A Sorbic Acid; S P Sodium Perborate; THI Thiomersalate

Table II (continued)

Name of solution and sizes available	Manufacturer	Preservatives with percentage concentration	Remarks
Sterile unpreserved saline solution (for rinsing and heat disinfection)			
Amidose, 30 ml	Abatron	—	In screw-capped tubes
Hydron Non-preserved Sterile Saline, 250 ml	Hydron Europe	—	Aerosol can
Normasol, 25 ml	Prebbles Medical	—	Sachets
Salettes, 10 ml	Sauflon Pharmaceuticals	—	Sachets
Daily cleaning solutions (for use on removal of the lenses from the eyes) (These solutions may also be used with hard lenses, subject to the provisions stated in *Table I*)			
Hydrophilic lenses			
Amiclean gel, 15 ml	Abatron	PMN 0.002	Screw-capped tube
Amiclean solution, 10 ml, 60 ml	Abatron	CHX 0.005; EDTA 0.01; THI 0.01	
Preflex, 10 ml, 45 ml	Alcon (Burton, Parsons)	EDTA 0.2; THI 0.004	
Pliagel, 25 ml	Alcon (Contique)	EDTA 0.5; S A 0.1	
LC 65, 15 ml, 60 ml	Allergan	EDTA ?; THI 0.001	
Cleaner No. 4 (Softmate), 35 ml	Barnes-Hind	EDTA 0.2; THI 0.004	
Daily Cleaner, 45 ml	Bausch and Lomb	EDTA 0.2; THI 0.004	
Hydroclean, 20 ml	Contactasol	CHX 0.0025; EDTA 0.1; THI 0.0025	
Solar Cleaning, 20 ml	Contactasol	EDTA 0.1; THI 0.001	For use prior to heat disinfection
Miraflow, 25 ml	Cooper	?	
Hoya Soft Cleaner, 60 ml	Hoya	CHX ?; EDTA ?	
Hydron Soft Lens Cleaning, 20 ml	Hydron Europe	CHX 0.0025; EDTA 0.1; THI 0.0025	
Mediclean, 20 ml, 35 ml	Kelvin	CHX 0.0025; EDTA 0.1; THI 0.0025	
C-Thru Cleaning, 70 ml	Optimedic	EDTA 0.2; THI 0.004	

Key — ATAC Alkyl Triethanol Ammonium Chloride; B A Benzoic Acid; CHX Chlorhexidine Gluconate; EDTA Ethylenediamine Tetraacetic Acid; IOD Iodine; NIPA Nipastat; PMN Phenylmercuric Nitrate; POV Povidone; S A Sorbic Acid; S P Sodium Perborate; THI Thiomersalate

Table II (continued)

Name of solution and sizes available	Manufacturer	Preservatives with percentage concentration	Remarks
Optrex Soft Lens Clean, 120 ml	Optrex	CHX 0.005; EDTA 0.001; THI 0.002	
Steri-Solv, 65 ml	Sauflon Pharmaceuticals	EDTA 0.1; THI 0.004	
Transoft, 10 ml	Smith and Nephew Pharmaceuticals	B A 0.1	
Transgele	Smith and Nephew Pharmaceuticals	—	In sachets
Silicone lenses			
Silclens, 45 ml	Alcon (Burton, Parsons)	EDTA 0.2; THI 0.004	
Consil Clean, 35 ml	Barnes-Hind	THI 0.001	

Occasional cleaners (those which do not involve heating are also suitable for hard lenses)

Amiclair tablets used with Amiclair-O, 200 ml, sterile purified water	Abatron	EDTA ?	Contains the chelating agent EDTA, and 3 enzymes; a lipase, and 2 proteases, one being pronase for removal of lipids, mucin and protein
Clean-O-Gel, powder in pouches	Alcon (Burton, Parsons)		Contains a lipase and surfactant
Liprofin, powder in sachets	Alcon (Burton, Parsons)		Oxidizing agent used hot or cold. Unsuitable for Menicon soft lenses. For practitioner use only
Ren-O-Gel, powder; No. 1, 50 g (alkaline); No. 2, 75 g (acid)	Alcon (Contique)		Oxidizing agent using heat. For practitioner use only. No longer available in U.K.
Hydrocare Protein (Enzyme) Remover Tablets	Allergan		Contains papain, a proteolytic enzyme
Hexaclean, 90 ml, 120 ml	Barnes-Hind	EDTA 0.1; THI 0.001	
Soflens Protein Remover Tablets	Bausch and Lomb		Contains papain for protein removal
Duragel Reconditioning Tablets	Cooper		Contains dichloro-isocyanurate

Key — ATAC Alkyl Triethanol Ammonium Chloride; B A Benzoic Acid; CHX Chlorhexidine Gluconate; EDTA Ethylenediamine Tetraacetic Acid; IOD Iodine; NIPA Nipastat; PMN Phenylmercuric Nitrate; POV Povidone; S A Sorbic Acid; S P Sodium Perborate; THI Thiomersalate

Table II (continued)

Name of solution and sizes available	Manufacturer	Preservatives with percentage concentration	Remarks
Optrex Soft Lens Protein Remover Tablets	Optrex		For protein removal
used with			
Optrex Soft Lens Clean, 120 ml	Optrex	CHX 0.005; EDTA 0.001; THI 0.002	
Monoclens powder in sachets	Sauflon Pharmaceuticals	EDTA ?; S P	Oxidizing system using heat. For practitioner use only
Monoclens C 40, 60 ml tube	Sauflon Pharmaceuticals	EDTA ?	Removes calcium deposits

Re-wetting solutions (these may also be used for hard lenses)

Name of solution and sizes available	Manufacturer	Preservatives with percentage concentration	Remarks
Amilis Wetting, 20 ml	Abatron	PMN 0.003	
Adapettes, 2 ml, 15 ml	Alcon (Burton, Parsons)	EDTA 0.1; THI 0.004	
Soft Lens Comfort Drops, 15 ml	Barnes-Hind	EDTA 0.1; THI 0.004	
Bausch and Lomb Lubricant, 15 ml	Bausch and Lomb	EDTA 0.1; THI 0.004	
Hydrosol, 20 ml	Contactasol	CHX 0.0025; EDTA 0.1; THI 0.0025	Intended to be rubbed into lens surfaces prior to wear
Clerz, 25 ml	Cooper	EDTA 0.1; S A 0.1	
Hydron Soft Lens Comfort, 20 ml	Hydron Europe	CHX 0.0025; EDTA 0.1; THI 0.0025	
C-Thru Rewetting, 15 ml	Optimedic	EDTA 0.1; THI 0.002	
Steri-Lette, 4 ml, 15 ml	Sauflon Pharmaceuticals	EDTA 0.1; THI 0.002	

Key — ATAC Alkyl Triethanol Ammonium Chloride; B A Benzoic Acid; CHX Chlorhexidine Gluconate; EDTA Ethylenediamine Tetraacetic Acid; IOD Iodine; NIPA Nipastat; PMN Phenylmercuric Nitrate; POV Povidone; S A Sorbic Acid; S P Sodium Perborate; THI Thiomersalate

Table III—Drugs used in contact lens practice (*see* footnote on page 81 for reference to proprietary names etc.)

Drug	Concentrations used (percentage)	Legal category	Use by ophthalmic opticians	Available in single dose units
Topical anaesthetics				
Amethocaine Hydrochloride	0.5, 1.0	POM	U	Yes
Proxymetacaine Hydrochloride	0.5	POM	U	No
Oxybuprocaine Hydrochloride	0.4	POM	U	Yes
Lignocaine Hydrochloride	4.0	POM	U	Only combined with fluorescein 0.25 per cent
Conjunctival decongestants (vaso-constrictors) (*see also Table I*)				
Adrenaline Acid Tartrate	0.1	P	U/S	No
Naphazoline Hydrochloride	0.1	POM	U/S	No
Xylometazoline Hydrochloride with Antazoline Sulphate	0.05 / 0.5	P	U/S	No
Diagnostic staining agents				
Fluorescein Sodium	1.0, 2.0	P	U/S	Yes, and as paper strips
Rose Bengal	1.0	P	U/S	Yes
Chemotherapeutic (antimicrobial) agents				
Drops				
Framycetin Sulphate	0.5	POM	U	No
Mafenide Propionate	5.0	POM	U/S	No
Sulphacetamide Sodium	10.0, 15.0, 20.0, 30.0	POM	U/S	Only in 10 per cent strength

Key — P Pharmacy Medicine; POM Prescription Only Medicine; U Use Only; U/S Use and Supply for Prophylaxis Only

Table III (continued)

Drug	Concentrations used (percentage)	Legal category	Use by ophthalmic opticians	Available in single dose units
Sulphacetamide Sodium with Zinc Sulphate and Cetrimide	5.0 0.1 0.01	POM	U/S	No
Propamidine Isethionate	0.1	P	U/S	No
Ointments				
Framycetin Sulphate	0 5	POM	U	No
Sulphacetamide Sodium	2.5, 6.0, 10.0	POM	U/S	No
Dibromopropamidine Isethionate	0.15	P	U/S	No
Miscellaneous agents				
Hypertonic saline solution				
Sodium Chloride	2.0, 5.0	POM*	U*	No

*This preparation is awaiting a product licence and these are the expected categories

Key — P Pharmacy Medicine; POM Prescription Only Medicine; U Use Only; U/S Use and Supply for Prophylaxis Only

Chapter 13

Contact Lens Materials

B. J. Tighe

INTRODUCTION

It is perhaps not immediately obvious that the use of polymers for contact lenses in recent years represents an example of the biomedical application of synthetic materials. It is, nonetheless, quite true for just as the use of quite similar materials in joint replacement, heart valves, membrane oxygenators and haemodialysis membranes presents specific problems associated with, for example, their biocompatibility, strength and permeability so, in contact lens usage, the question of the material design to give a balance of properties appropriate to the environment in which the material will ultimately be used is of prime importance. The situation is obviously less critical in the case of lenses intended for daily wear only, than it is in the case of extended or 'continuous' wear lenses. In both cases, however, very similar properties to those mentioned above in connection with other biomedical applications are involved.

The contact lens, of course, does have certain unique features which tend to set it apart from other areas of biomedicine. The design and fitting of the lens can play an overriding part in governing the patients' response to a given material, although this is to a large extent offset by the relative ease of insertion and removal of the device. Thus, it is much easier in this than most other fields to compare the response of reasonably large numbers of patients to different materials under conditions in which variables related to design and fitting have been isolated. For this reason, the research carried out in recent years into the use of hydrogel polymers in contact lenses has provided information on a wide range of materials of this type which will greatly assist future work on their use in other biomedical applications.

The historical aspect of the development of contact lens materials is quite interesting. Glass was used exclusively for some years and it was conventional for lenses to be individually ground. When polymethyl methacrylate began to replace glass in the 1940's it was because of its toughness, optical properties and physiological inactivity coupled with ease of processing by existing turning techniques. It was not, therefore, in any sense a purpose-designed polymer and yet, as will be seen it possesses a combination of properties that are difficult to surpass in a thermoplastic or conventional elastomeric polymer. There have been many attempts to find alternative materials but it was not until the class of polymers known as hydrogels appeared on the scene that any serious competitor emerged. In order to appreciate the reasons for this, it is necessary to review briefly some of the general characteristics of 'polymers', which is a general term for a group of materials that includes plastics (both thermoplastics and thermosetting), fibres, rubbers (or more correctly elastomers) and hydrogels.

CLASSIFICATION OF CONTACT LENS MATERIALS

We can all readily appreciate the differences in behaviour between gases, liquids and solids. It is helpful to consider the difference in molecular make-up of these three groups before dealing with polymers as a particular class of solid materials.

In gases, we are dealing with a collection of individual small molecules well separated from each other and moving rapidly and randomly in the space that encloses them. The resistance that a gas offers to anything moving through it is, therefore, negligible. When we move to liquids we are talking about a 'condensed' phase and although the molecules are still small individual entities, the resistance to motion within them is greater. (Think, for example, of the difference in ease of movement in the air and in a swimming pool.) Motion in a liquid can be likened to placing a hand into a large bag of ball-bearings or marbles. There is some resistance, but the hand can move by displacing the ball-bearings if the force that it exerts is greater than the force of attraction between the individual ball-bearings.

In the case of solid materials the individual molecules are packed more efficiently. Alternatively, it could be said that the forces of attraction between them have increased. In the absence of reasonably strong deforming forces, the material retains its shape whereas a liquid, of course, will take the shape of the vessel into which it is poured – being deformed simply by the force of gravity. There are within this group of solid materials all sorts of different behaviours ranging from that of toffee or thick treacle to that of metals. Toffee and treacle are in some aspects liquid-like in their behaviour and in some respects resemble solids.

If solids, then, are materials in which the constituent molecules are well packed together we have to consider in more detail the way in which the molecules are packed or associated or bonded together since this will play a large part in determining the strength of the material in question. Metals, ceramics or glasses, and polymers represent three different types of solid material in which the constituent atoms or molecules are in some way linked together. The ways in which they are linked together are quite different and so we get different types of behaviour in passing from one class to another.

The unique properties that polymers have arise from the ability of certain atoms to bond together to form stable covalent bonds. Foremost amongst the atoms that can do this is carbon (C) which can link together with four other atoms either of its own kind or alternatively atoms of, for example, hydrogen (H), oxygen (O), nitrogen (N), sulphur (S) or chlorine (Cl). It is because of this unique property of carbon that most of the polymers that we are concerned with fall within the realm of what is called organic chemistry or the chemistry of carbon compounds. These polymers may be purely natural (such as cellulose), modified natural polymers (such as cellulose acetate) or completely synthetic (such as polymethyl methacrylate).

The single characteristic that unites these and other polymers is the fact that, as the name (polymer) suggests, they are composed of many units linked together in long chains. Thus, if we can imagine a molecule of oxygen and a molecule of water enlarged to the size of a tennis ball (the molecular size of water and oxygen is very similar) a molecule of polymethyl methacrylate on the same scale would be of similar cross-sectional diameter but anything up to 200 feet in length. It is the gigantic length of polymers (sometimes called macromolecules) in relation to their cross-sectional diameter that gives them their unique properties.

Most of the polymers that we shall be concerned with are synthetic and prepared from monomers by the process of polymerization. In this way, the simplest polymer, polyethylene, is obtained by polymerization of ethylene monomer.

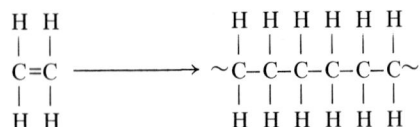

$$\begin{array}{c} H\ \ H \\ |\ \ | \\ C=C \\ |\ \ | \\ H\ \ H \end{array} \longrightarrow \begin{array}{c} H\ H\ H\ H\ H\ H \\ |\ |\ |\ |\ |\ | \\ \sim C\!-\!C\!-\!C\!-\!C\!-\!C\!-\!C\!\sim \\ |\ |\ |\ |\ |\ | \\ H\ H\ H\ H\ H\ H \end{array}$$

This is more usually represented by a general equation showing the conversion of n ethylene units to a polyethylene chain that is n units long, that is:

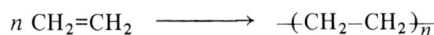

$$n\ CH_2{=}CH_2 \longrightarrow \ (\!-CH_2{-}CH_2\!-)_{\overline{n}}$$

In a commercial polymer n might have a value of several thousand.

The polymerization of methyl methacrylate can be shown in a similar manner.

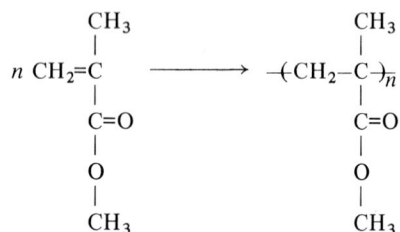

$$n\ CH_2{=}\!\!\begin{array}{c} CH_3 \\ | \\ C \\ | \\ C{=}O \\ | \\ O \\ | \\ CH_3 \end{array} \longrightarrow \ (\!-CH_2{-}\!\!\begin{array}{c} CH_3 \\ | \\ C \\ | \\ C{=}O \\ | \\ O \\ | \\ CH_3 \end{array}\!\!-)_{\overline{n}}$$

The structure enclosed within the bracket is known as the 'repeating unit' and it is conventional when writing the name of the polymer to indicate precisely what this is. Thus, we should write poly(ethylene) or poly(methyl methacrylate) but since these are well known commercial polymers the brackets are often omitted. The same is true of polystyrene

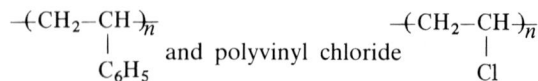

$$(\!-CH_2{-}\!\!\begin{array}{c} CH \\ | \\ C_6H_5 \end{array}\!\!-)_{\overline{n}} \quad \text{and polyvinyl chloride} \quad (\!-CH_2{-}\!\!\begin{array}{c} CH \\ | \\ Cl \end{array}\!\!-)_{\overline{n}}$$

To indicate that a polymer contains more than one type of repeating unit obtained by polymerizing together two different monomers the term 'copolymer' is used. Thus, by copolymerizing styrene and methyl methacrylate a styrene-methyl methacrylate copolymer is obtained. This would more correctly be described as poly(methyl methacrylate-costyrene). Although the term copolymer is a general one and can be used to describe polymers obtained from mixtures of more than two monomers the term 'terpolymer' is frequently used for the specific case of a polymer produced by the polymerization of three monomers. The more common usage, however, is that involving copolymer to describe a polymer obtained from at least (but not necessarily exactly) two different monomers.

Perhaps the best way of visualizing the way in which polymer molecules arrange themselves is by taking several pieces of string to represent individual molecules. The most usual arrangement will be a random one in which the pieces of string are loosely entangled (in a heap or ball rather than being extended). It is the interaction and entanglement of the individual molecules in this way that gives polymers their characteristic physical properties. By changing the chemical nature of the polymer chain and their arrangement together we can change the physical properties and thus obtain either flexible, elastomeric behaviour or, at the other extreme, hard glassy behaviour.

These variations arise from differences in mobility of the constituent polymer chains. Thus, at very low temperatures all polymers are hard and glassy. As the temperature is raised, however, the thermal energy of the system increases and eventually the individual polymer chains will possess enough energy to begin to undergo rotation. If we think of the tangled string as a plate of spaghetti at this point, the rotational energy that it achieves would be enough to give it the mobility of a plate of worms. In terms of physical properties this corresponds to a change from glassy behaviour to rubbery or leathery behaviour. For this reason the temperature at which this occurs is known as the 'glass-rubber transition temperature' (T_g). The actual temperature at which the transition occurs will depend on the chemical nature of the polymer. Thus, for natural rubber it is below 0°C and for polymethyl methacrylate it is above 100°C. For this reason at room temperature natural rubber is readily deformed whereas polymethyl methacrylate is glassy.

There are several additional subtleties involved in the design of polymers that have the ability to undergo the large deformation with instantaneous recovery which is characteristic of ideal elastomeric behaviour. Despite this, the principle of intramolecular mobility and the glass transition temperature is the fundamental factor and provides an adequate basis for understanding the difference between 'hard' and 'soft' lens materials.

There is another important way in which a hard glassy thermoplastic material such as polymethyl methacrylate or polyvinyl chloride can be converted into a flexible material and that is by the incorporation of a 'plasticizer'. This is a mobile component, often an organic liquid having a high boiling point, that will act as an 'internal lubricant'. Its presence separates the polymer chains, and allows them to move more freely. Its function is to lower the temperature at which the transition from glassy to flexible behaviour takes place.

Thus, polyvinyl chloride in its unmodified state is a rigid glassy material and will be familiar as the clear corrugated roofing material used on car ports and similar domestic extensions. When a plasticizer is incorporated the material is converted into the flexible material used for example as 'vinyl' seat coverings in cars and general domestic applications. In these cases, pigments and various processing aids will also have been added in order to enable the polymer to be produced in a variety of colours and textures.

An almost identical principle is involved in the formation of so-called 'hydrogel' polymers. The structure of polymethyl methacrylate can be made more hydrophilic by the incorporation of hydroxyl groups. The simplest structure that can be made in this way is poly(2-hydroxyethyl methacrylate) which is obtained by polymerizing 2-hydroxyethyl methacrylate monomer:

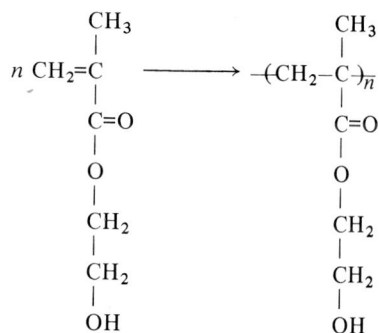

$$n \ \underset{\substack{\displaystyle | \\ \displaystyle C=O \\ \displaystyle | \\ \displaystyle O \\ \displaystyle | \\ \displaystyle CH_2 \\ \displaystyle | \\ \displaystyle CH_2 \\ \displaystyle | \\ \displaystyle OH}}{CH_2=C-CH_3} \longrightarrow \underset{\substack{\displaystyle | \\ \displaystyle C=O \\ \displaystyle | \\ \displaystyle O \\ \displaystyle | \\ \displaystyle CH_2 \\ \displaystyle | \\ \displaystyle CH_2 \\ \displaystyle | \\ \displaystyle OH}}{(CH_2-C-CH_3)_n}$$

The monomer and polymer are often referred to as HEMA and polyHEMA* respectively.

In the dry state polymethyl methacrylate and poly(2-hydroxyethyl methacrylate) have very similar characteristics – both are hard glassy polymers as their structures would indicate. Whereas polymethyl methacrylate is relatively unaffected by water, however, (it absorbs approximately 0.5 per cent of its own weight) the more hydrophilic poly(2-

*In clinical practice the term 'HEMA' is used for simplicity but actually refers to 'polyHEMA'.

hydroxyethyl methacrylate) swells to form an elastic hydrogel. The water acts as a plasticizer in the manner previously described. It behaves as an 'internal lubricant' and allows the chains to move more freely with respect to each other, and as a result the glass transition temperature of the hydrogel is well below room temperature whereas that of the dehydrated polymer is about 100°C.

It is necessary to describe one more molecular feature that is required in elastic polymers (both hydrogels and synthetic elastomers), that is the 'cross-link'. So far polymer chains have been considered to be individual molecular species unattached to each other. In some cases, however, it is necessary to link individual chains to their neighbours at intervals along each polymer backbone. In this way, a polymer 'network' is formed and the frequency at which these linkages occur is called the 'cross-link density'. The necessity for doing this can

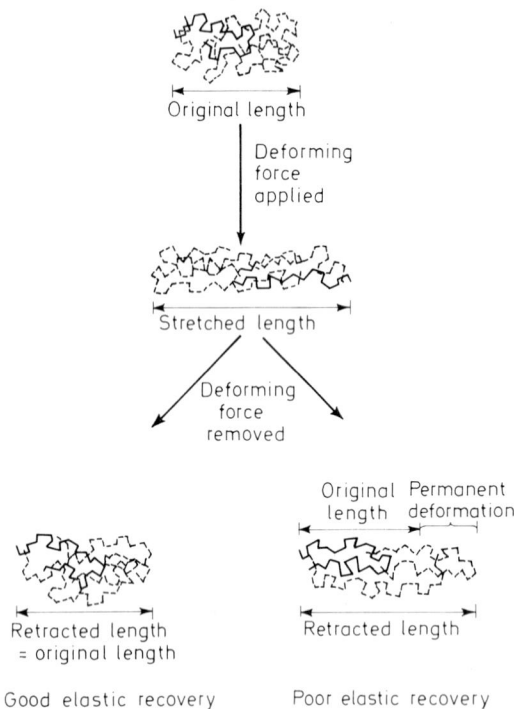

Figure 13.1—Diagrammatic representation of the deformation of entangled polymer chains illustrating both good and poor elastic recovery

be best understood by considering *Figure 13.1* which illustrates good and bad elastic behaviour. To obtain good elastic behaviour the chains must be mobile enough to change their positions when a deforming force is applied but they also need some restraining

links to ensure that they are able to return to their original positions. The incorporation of an excessively large number of cross-links will of course restrict deformability and destroy elastic behaviour. For good elastic behaviour, the upper limit of cross-link density is in the region of one cross-link per hundred backbone atoms. The theoretical basis of elastic behaviour in polymers is of course much more complex than this but the simplified picture given above enables the behaviour exhibited by the types of polymer that are important in contact lens usage to be understood.

THE NATURE OF POLYMERIC MATERIALS

It is convenient to consider the polymers that have been used or suggested for use as contact lens materials under three headings: (1) thermoplastics; (2) synthetic elastomers; and (3) hydrogels. Each group has its own characteristic advantages and disadvantages which may be best illustrated by taking a typical member of each group and making a comparative list of appropriate properties.

(1) The thermoplastics are the group of polymers that are capable of being shaped or moulded under the application of heat and pressure but which at room temperature are fairly rigid, possibly showing some flexibility, but certainly not elastic. Foremost amongst this group is polymethyl methacrylate which, since its introduction in the 1940s, has been the most widely used contact lens material. It is apparent that several of its advantageous properties are shared by other thermoplastics. Amongst these properties are optical clarity, processability, toughness and ease of sterilization. On the other hand, the rigidity and virtual impermeability to oxygen must certainly count as disadvantages, and prevent the material from being considered for anything other than daily wear. The rigidity and impermeability to oxygen are obviously interrelated since although rigidity is a prime factor in producing discomfort it does permit the lens to be fitted in such a manner as to promote the flow of tears fluid behind the lens thus compensating for the absence of oxygen transmission through the lens itself. This does mean, however, that attempts to reduce the rigidity of the lens material to any marked extent have the consequence of requiring a greater permeability of the lens to oxygen. It is largely to improve on the behaviour of polymethyl methacrylate in these two areas that other polymers have been suggested as replacements.

At first sight the task of finding an improved material would not seem too difficult since almost all thermoplastics are less rigid and more oxygen permeable than polymethyl methacrylate. Materials patented for contact lens use range from simple structures such as polyethylene (Studies Inc., 1969) and polyvinyl chloride (Rosen, 1969) to complex copolymers of tetrafluoroethylene with perfluoro-2-methylene-4-methyl-1,3-dioxolane or with hexafluoroacetone and ethylene (Dupont, 1971). None of these materials has, however, achieved any success largely because of inadequate surface properties, a point which will be elaborated in due course. More promising results have been obtained with both poly(4-methyl pent-1-ene), a form of which is known commercially as TPX (Kamath, 1970),

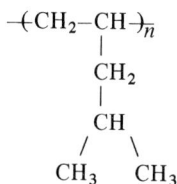

$$\text{---}(\text{CH}_2\text{---}\text{CH})_n\text{---}$$
$$|$$
$$\text{CH}_2$$
$$|$$
$$\text{CH}$$
$$/ \quad \backslash$$
$$\text{CH}_3 \quad \text{CH}_3$$

and with cellulose esters such as cellulose acetate butyrate.

The structures of cellulose such as cellulose acetate, cellulose acetate butyrate or cellulose acetate propionate are quite different from those of the carbon-backbone polymers previously considered. Cellulose itself consists of a series of rings or cyclic structures linked together by oxygen atoms.

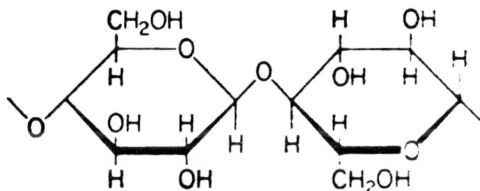

The hydroxyl groups in the polymer can be partially or completely reacted. If all three hydroxyl groups in each ring are acetylated the resultant polymer is the well known cellulose triacetate, which will be familiar as the textile fibre 'Tricel'.

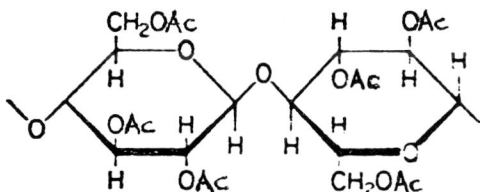

Two variations now become apparent. In the first place, some of the hydroxyl groups may be left unreacted (the average number of hydroxyl groups per ring that have been reacted is referred to as the 'degree of substitution'). Secondly, propionyl (CH_3CH_2CO-) or butyryl ($CH_3CH_2CH_2CO$-) groups may be used wholly or partially in place of acetyl groups. Cellulose acetate butyrate therefore describes the case in which we have some acetyl, some butyryl and usually some free hydroxyl groups. This highlights one of the problems with this material in that, unlike polymethyl methacrylate and other polymers previously discussed, it does not have a fixed composition. For this reason, supplies from different sources can have somewhat different properties. In general, higher concentrations of free hydroxyl groups will result in a greater tendency to take up water and will produce rather more hydrophilic surfaces. On the other hand, increasing the relative concentrations of butyryl groups produces rather greater flexibility and a slight increase in oxygen permeability.

Poly(4-methyl pent-1-ene) and cellulose acetate butyrate resemble each other in many ways. Both polymers are less rigid and less brittle than polymethyl methacrylate – they can conveniently be described as tougher. It is debatable, however, as to whether the greater flexibility is of any substantial advantage in relation to comfort. Poly(4-methyl pent-1-ene) is unique in having a glass transition temperature between room temperature and the temperature of the eye ($Tg \simeq 29°C$). In principle this should mean that the polymer is more resistant to deformation and damage during handling at room temperature but when placed in the eye its flexibility and therefore comfort should increase. In practice, however, the increase in flexibility makes virtually no difference to comfort. This will be clarified when the effect of rigidity modulus on lens comfort and visual performance is discussed (page 384). The most relevant point is that the flexibility associated with these two polymers is very much less than that associated with elastomers and hydrogels.

The oxygen permeability of both cellulose acetate butyrate and poly(4-methyl pent-1-ene) is appreciably (of the order of one hundred times) greater than that of polymethyl methacrylate. This is not as advantageous as it may seem at first sight, however, since even in the case of poly(4-methyl pent-1-ene) which is by far the more permeable of the two, a lens of minimal centre thickness prevents normal functioning of the cornea during the closed eye condition. This point will be discussed in more detail in the general context of oxygen permeability requirements (page 389).

In certain other respects, cellulose acetate butyrate has some advantages over poly(4-methyl pent-1-ene). Although it has a variable composition this does mean that it is possible to produce a grade of polymer that will be adequately wettable and able to sustain a film of tears fluid. On the other hand, poly(4-methyl pent-1-ene) lenses have to undergo surface treatment to enable them to do this. In addition, cellulose acetate butyrate is somewhat easier to process.

On balance there is no dramatic advantage over polymethyl methacrylate in the case of either poly(4-methyl pent-1-ene) or cellulose acetate butyrate. Neither polymer is sufficiently flexible to produce substantially greater comfort and neither polymer has a sufficiently high oxygen permeability to permit its overnight use in the closed eye condition. Both polymers can be used as alternatives to polymethyl methacrylate, however, and individual practitioners may have personal preferences in this respect. Some of the problems associated with surface treatment of flexible thermoplastics and results of a clinical trial with poly(4-methyl pent-1-ene) have been presented in more detail elsewhere (Larke, Pedley and Tighe, 1973; Larke *et al.*, 1973; Ng, Pedley and Tighe, 1976).

(2) The synthetic elastomers are the group of polymers which are not only flexible but show rubber-like behaviour. That is, they are capable of being compressed or stretched and when the deforming force is removed they instantaneously return to their original shape. They consist of polymer chains that possess high mobility and which are cross-linked at intervals along the polymer backbones. Their properties are in many ways intermediate between those of thermoplastics and hydrogels. Thus, they possess to a degree the toughness associated with the former group of materials and the softness of the latter. In this sense they are ideal candidates for contact lens usage. Unfortunately, however, they possess one inherent disadvantage. The molecular features required for true elastic behaviour invariably produce polymers with hydrophobic surfaces. All polymers in this group require some form of surface treatment, therefore, to render them sufficiently hydrophilic for use as contact lenses. In general, it has been the absence of a suitably permanent treatment that has prevented their use on a wide scale.

In addition to natural rubber itself many synthetic elastomers have been patented in connection with contact lens manufacture (Dow Corning, 1971). These include ethylene propylene terpolymer (EPT) which may be simply represented as

$$(CH_2-CH_2-CH_2-\overset{\overset{\displaystyle CH_3}{|}}{CH})_n$$

cis-polybutadiene

$$\overset{}{-}(CH_2 \quad\quad CH_2)_{\overline{n}}$$
$$\quad \backslash \quad\quad /$$
$$\quad CH=CH$$

and cis-polyisoprene

$$\overset{}{-}(CH_2 \quad\quad CH_2)_{\overline{n}}$$
$$\quad \backslash \quad\quad /$$
$$\quad CH=C$$
$$\quad\quad\quad |$$
$$\quad\quad\quad CH_3$$

which is synthetic natural rubber.

Although these polymers have oxygen permeabilities which are more than one hundred times greater than that of polymethyl methacrylate the most significant member of this group has an oxygen permeability which is over one thousand times greater than that of polymethyl methacrylate. For this reason this polymer, silicone rubber or poly-(dimethyl siloxane), has received considerable attention as a potential contact lens material.

$$\overset{\quad\quad CH_3}{\underset{\quad\quad CH_3}{-(O-\overset{|}{\underset{|}{Si}})_{\overline{n}}}}$$

The high oxygen permeability arises from the backbone of alternate silicone and oxygen atoms which has not only great freedom of rotation but a much higher solubility for oxygen than polymers with all-carbon backbones.

Surface-treated silicone rubber lenses were developed in the mid-1960's (Becker, 1966; Dow Corning, 1967) and found clinically to have little effect on corneal respiration (Hill and Schloessler, 1967; Burns, Roberts and Rich, 1971). Despite the apparent attraction of a soft yet tough, highly oxygen permeable material, problems have been encountered in its clinical use (Bitonte and Keates, 1972). Not the least of these is the fact that surface treatments tend to be non-permanent and to cause some reduction in the optical qualities of the lens surface. Despite this it is to be anticipated that an adequate surface-treatment technique will be developed in the course of time. Lenses made of current materials (page 462, Chapter 14) have yet to be proven. In conclusion it is appropriate to note that because of the nature of the materials, elastomer lenses are normally produced by some form of compression moulding technique.

(3) The third and final group, hydrogels, is also potentially the largest. These are hydrophilic polymers which are plasticized by the water that they absorb and can be conveniently described as soft, elastic, water-containing gels. The first of these to achieve commercial significance, polyHEMA, was developed by Wichterle and his co-workers in

Czechoslovakia as a general purpose surgical material, (Wichterle and Lim, 1960, 1961, 1965). PolyHEMA is in many ways typical of other hydrogels and unfortunately the terms have been used synonymously on many occasions. The range of properties obtainable with hydrogels is, however, extremely wide and with this class of material, more than any other, it is possible to 'purpose-design' or 'tailor-make' polymers for contact lens use. Before discussing the extent to which it is possible to design a hydrogel specifically for this purpose, it is important to make some quantitative assessment of property requirements.

PROPERTIES OF CONTACT LENS MATERIALS

The following properties are amongst the most important in affecting the performance of materials as contact lenses.

Density
Refractive index
Optical transmittance
Dimensional stability with respect to: time, temperature, pH and tonicity
Surface hydrophilicity or wettability
Water content
Mechanical properties, including tensile strength, tear strength and rigidity modulus
Permeability to oxygen, carbon dioxide, etc.
Biocompatibility
Toxicity and chemical stability
Method and ease of sterilization

The relative importance of the various properties will depend on whether the lens is intended for daily wear or continuous wear. In addition, some properties such as refractive index and density vary by relatively small amounts within the range of polymers that are otherwise suitable for contact lens use. Consequently, the potential value of a material as a lens material is not greatly affected by its density or refractive index.

Similarly, the dimensional stability of a material with respect to changes in temperature is less important than the reversibility of any changes that occur. This aspect of lens behaviour will usually be most important during heat sterilization procedures, if these are employed. To a lesser extent, some dimensional changes with changing pH and tonicity can be tolerated provided that such changes are reversible and small over the range of pH and tonicity encountered in the eye. Dimensional stability with respect to time is extremely important since instability will result in irreversible flattening or distortion of the lens. Dimensional instability in

so-called 'hard' lens materials is invariably the result of strain induced during lens manufacture.

One of the problems associated with the measurement of mechanical properties of lens materials is that no single property measurement reflects accurately the 'in use' situation. Thus, 'tensile strength' indicates the resistance of the material to deformation under tension, 'tear strength' the resistance of the material to tear propagation from a notch or imperfection and 'rigidity modulus' the resistance to deformation under compression. The first two give some indication of the behaviour of a material during handling whilst the third indicates the extent to which the eyelid will deform it. Thus, a 'hard' or rigid material would have a high rigidity modulus whereas a 'soft' material would have a much lower value. Whilst a low rigidity modulus is associated with greater comfort, in extreme cases poor visual stability is encountered, thus setting a lower limit to this property.

Attempts have been made to define the properties of the 'ideal contact lens' (Kamath, 1969) but in view of the divergence of clinical preference in relation to the wide range of lenses presently available such an approach is unlikely to succeed. It is possible, however, to define acceptable ranges of certain situations (that is, daily wear, continuous wear, hard lenses, soft lenses). It is useful in doing this to compare the properties of a representative member of each of the three classes of material previously discussed, bearing in mind the difference between the typical member chosen and other members of that group previously referred to (for example, cellulose acetate butyrate, poly(4-methyl pent-1-ene), ethylene propylene terpolymer). It is also useful to include for comparison the properties of the cornea although collection of the relevant information in this case is not easy (Kamath, 1969; Anderton, 1973; Tighe, 1976).

A comparison of various properties of polymethyl methacrylate, poly(dimethyl siloxane) or silicone rubber, polyHEMA hydrogel and the cornea is presented in *Table 13.1*. In the light of these figures and the preceding discussion it will be apparent that relatively few properties are absolutely critical in determining whether or not a material is suitable for contact lens use. From the point of view of lens description, rigidity modulus and surface wettability will be sufficient to define the material (in the commonly used terms) as hard hydrophobic, soft hydrophobic or soft hydrophilic (corresponding to each of the three classes). In addition, the oxygen permeability will indicate whether the material is suitable for daily wear only or may be investigated as an extended wear candidate. Most of the other properties are either relatively unimportant or affect only convenience of use and ease of handling

TABLE 13.1 Properties of Representative Contact Lens Materials
(all reported at 25°C unless otherwise stated)

	Polymethyl methacrylate (thermoplastics)	Silicone rubber (elastomers)	PolyHEMA (hydrogels)	Cornea
Density (g cm^{-3})	1.18	1.10	1.16	1.03
Refractive index	1.49	1.43	1.43	1.37
Dimensional stability with respect to: Time Temperature pH Toxicity	Generally good unless strain induced during processing	Generally good	Generally good	
Surface wettability Critical surface tension (dyne cm^{-1})	39	25	$\simeq 50$	$\simeq 30$
Equilibrium water contact angle (°)	65–70	$\simeq 96$	$\simeq 20$	$\simeq 47$
Water content (%)	$\simeq 0.5$	$\simeq 0$	$\simeq 39$	$\simeq 8$
Tensile strength (dyne cm^{-2})	$\simeq 50 \times 10^7$	$\simeq 10 \times 10^7$	$\simeq 0.5 \times 10^7$	$\simeq 5 \times 10^7$
Rigidity modulus (dyne cm^{-2})	$\simeq 1 \times 10^{10}$	$\simeq 8 \times 10^7$	$\simeq 5 \times 10^7$	$\simeq 10 \times 10^7$
Tear strength (g mm^{-1})	Strong but brittle	$\simeq 2000$	$\simeq 10$	$\simeq 1500$
Oxygen permeability (0.1 mm thick sample) Pg (cc(STP)mm cm^{-2} sec^{-1} cm Hg^{-1})	$\simeq 1 \times 10^{10}$	$\simeq 5000 \times 10^{-10}$	—	—
Pd (cc(STP)mm cm^{-2} sec^{-1} cm Hg^{-1})	$\simeq 1 \times 10^{-10}$	$\simeq 1500 \times 10^{-10}$	75×10^{-10}	$\simeq 300 \times 10^{-10}$

(tensile and tear strengths for example). In either case, absolute limits cannot be put on their magnitude although in the case of both tear and tensile strengths it should be as high as possible.

If an alternative approach is taken, that of considering the contact lens as an extension of the cornea, a similar conclusion is reached. Thus, the lens must allow the cornea to respire normally, it must resist the deforming force of the eyelid and it must permit a continuous tear film to be maintained on the lens. These factors can be discussed in terms of oxygen permeability, rigidity modulus and surface wettability (or critical surface tension). Some attempt must therefore be made to put quantitative limits on these very important properties.

RIGIDITY MODULUS

The value of the rigidity modulus indicates the force (stress) necessary to compress (strain) the material by a given amount. It is therefore a bulk property

and has units of 'force per unit area' such as lbs in^{-2} or dynes cm^{-2}. Although this gives a good indication of the flexibility of the material, it bears no relationship to properties that are measured in tension, such as tensile strength and tear strength. Some indication of the way in which the rigidity modulus is related to comfort and visual performance is given in *Figure 13.2*. The two latter parameters are expressed in arbitrary units since a general rather than precise relationship is intended.

It is apparent from the figure that there are two regions (A and C) in which the visual performance has markedly deteriorated. Region C corresponds to the very low rigidity modulus associated with some hydrogels, often of high water content. In this case, the poor visual performance is due to the inability of the material to adequately resist the deforming force of the eyelid. Region A corresponds to flexible thermoplastics that have poor elastic recovery. Plasticized polyvinyl chloride of the type encountered in vinyl seat coverings is an example of polymers showing this behaviour. Here the material is insufficiently rigid for the lens to be fitted as a

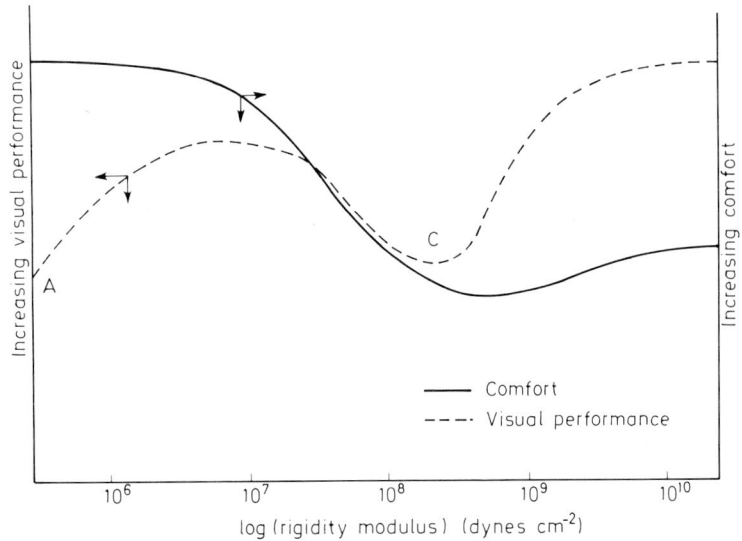

Figure 13.2—The general relationship between the rigidity modulus of a contact lens material and the comfort and visual performance of the lens

conventional hard lens but insufficiently flexible and elastic to be accommodated to the corneal profile in the way that conventional 'soft' lenses are.

This illustrates the difficulty in achieving a balance between comfort, visual performance and flexibility and in particular the problems associated with a 'semi-rigid' lens which would of course otherwise have many attractive features. In practical terms, materials in regions C and A are unsuitable for contact lens usage. Although the exact limits are difficult to define, it is apparent from clinical studies that poly(4-methyl pent-1-ene) or TPX is approaching the point where reduced rigidity (in comparison with polymethyl methacrylate) results in some loss in visual performance when conventional fitting techniques are used (Larke, Pedley and Tighe, 1973; Larke *et al.*, 1973; Ng, Pedley and Tighe, 1976).

Rigidity modulus and related measurements have been made on a wide range of contact lens materials using a micro-indentation apparatus (Ng, 1974; Tighe, 1976). This technique enables samples of similar thickness to that of contact lenses (0.1–0.4 mm) to be studied. Rigidity modulus measurements are made by measuring the deformation produced in the sample by a spherical indenter to which a series of loads are applied. *Figure 13.3* illustrates the relationship between log load and log indentation for a spherical indenter of 0.16 mm radius. Materials of decreasing rigidity are found on moving from left to right and it is relevant to note that the cornea corresponds to line G in this figure. From this figure it is also easy to appreciate that under a load (say, 1 g) that causes moderate deformation of elastomers, hydrogels and the cornea (F–H), the effect on the

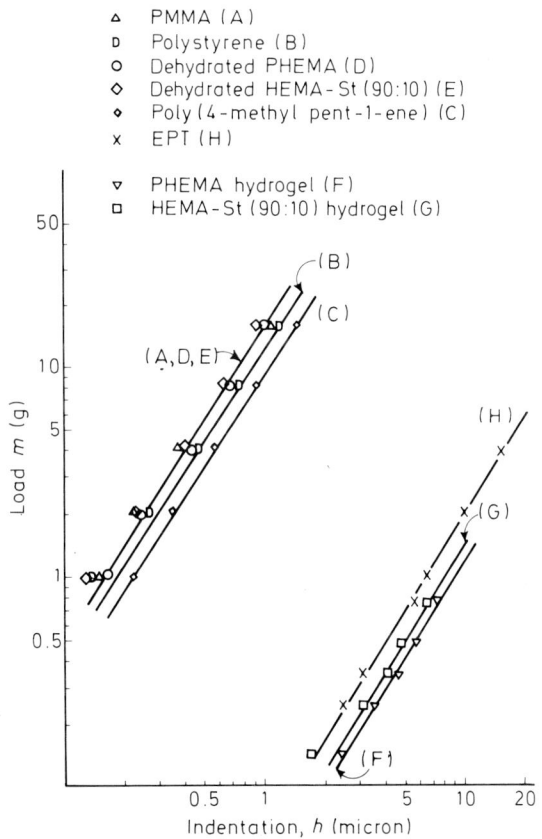

Figure 13.3—Micro-indentation studies. The correlation of a log(load) with log(indentation) for various materials

group of thermoplastics (A–E) is negligible. Thus, although we can detect manually the difference in flexibility or rigidity between, say, polymethyl methacrylate and a 'semi-rigid' plastic such as poly(4-methyl pent-1-ene), the cornea is unable to detect any difference.

This point is illustrated more clearly when the micro-indentation technique is used with a flat-ended indenter and load calibrated to produce a pressure similar to that exerted by the eyelid ($\simeq 2.6 \times 10^4$ dynes cm^{-2}). Using this procedure the deformation and recovery of polymer samples of contact lens thickness under eyelid load can be studied. No detectable deformation is produced in any of the thermoplastic polymers previously discussed. It must be remembered, however, that this is compression of a supported material and not 'flattening' of an unsupported lens which does begin to occur with less rigid polymers.

Indentation studies of this type under eyelid load correlate well with clinical studies. Although the ideal elastic behaviour exhibited (*Figure 13.4*) by synthetic elastomers under these low loads is preferable, appreciable deviations from this situation still produce acceptable clinical behaviour. Thus, materials whose behaviour is more time-dependent (that is, less than instantaneous deformation and recovery) produce acceptable visual stability levels in

Although water content plays a large part in controlling the mechanical properties of hydrogels it is only one of several factors. It is possible to produce very stable high (> 70 per cent) water content gels. The elastic behaviour and rigidity of hydrogels is closely governed by monomer structure and effective cross-link density, which includes not only covalent cross-links but also ionic, polar and steric interchain forces. In general, making hydrogels with good elastic response and reasonable rigidity is very much less of a problem than overcoming the poor tear strength of such materials.

SURFACE WETTABILITY AND CRITICAL SURFACE TENSION

This subject has been discussed in some detail both in relation to contact lens materials in general and the problems associated with the surface treatment of polymers in particular (Larke, Pedley and Tighe (1973); Ng, Pedley and Tighe, 1976). The wetting of contact lenses is important because the maintenance of a pre-corneal tears film in the form of a thin

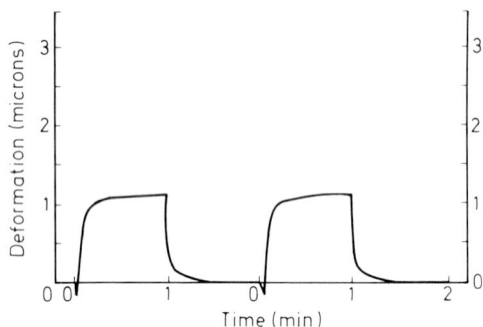

Figure 13.4—Deformation properties of ethylene-propylene terpolymer under eyelid pressure

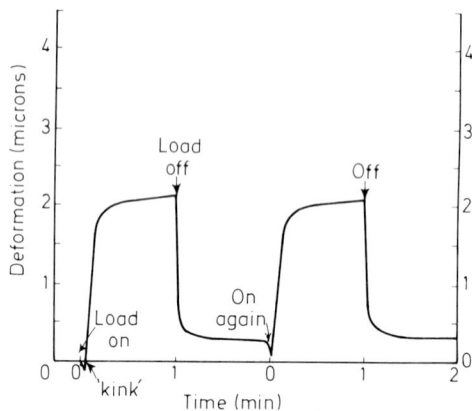

Figure 13.5—Deformation properties of poly(HEMA) under eyelid pressure

lenses provided that the overall deformation is not more than about 2 per cent. PolyHEMA itself shows reasonably good elastic behaviour under eyelid load as illustrated in *Figure 13.5*.

Hydrogels whose deformational behaviour is characterized by large ($\simeq 5$ per cent) and rapid initial deformation that does not reach equilibrium within one minute and shows poor recovery, invariably give rise to lenses whose visual stability is unacceptable. Some early, fragile, high water content hydrogel lenses tended to behave in this way.

capillary layer has long been recognized as a primary requirement for the physiological compatibility of lens and patient. Defining in quantitative terms the surface characteristics that are necessary to produce this behaviour has, however, only relatively recently been attempted.

The terms hydrophilic and hydrophobic have been widely and often misleadingly used in this connection. When used to refer to bulk properties they mean simply water-loving and water-hating respectively. In this sense a dehydrated hydrogel can be said to be hydrophilic since it imbibes water to form a gel. When the terms are used in connection with surfaces they have a more specific meaning. The term hydrophilic used in this sense means that water will spread spontaneously on the surface, whereas hydrophobic implies that water will not spontaneously spread on the surface. Many contact lens materials are referred to as hydrophilic when by this definition they are not so. The position is complicated by the fact that when contact lens materials are referred to, the implication is that they are wetted by tears fluid rather than by water itself.

and the contact angle (θ) is the angle enclosed by the surface and the tangent to the droplet-surface interface (*Figure 13.6*). Thus, a liquid which spontaneously wets or spreads on a surface has a contact angle of zero. A hydrophilic surface then is one on which water exhibits a zero contact angle.

The wetting of the cornea by tears fluid can be treated in a similar way although it is a much more complex process. The epithelial surface is, itself, too hydrophobic to be spontaneously wetted by tears (Mishima, 1965) and is thought to be covered by a lipid layer (Ehlers, 1965). The resultant surface would itself be relatively hydrophobic and the most satisfactory hypothesis to explain the fact that tears wet the cornea is that the conjunctival glycoproteins also adsorb on the corneal surface thus rendering it wettable. Although the structure and function of tears is complex (for example, Mishima and Maurice, 1961; Wolff, 1976), for the purpose of studying interactions with polymers we can consider the fluid to be an aqueous liquid whose surface tension has been reduced to approximately 46 dynes cm^{-1} by the presence of surfactants or wetting agents. It should be noted, however, that this value

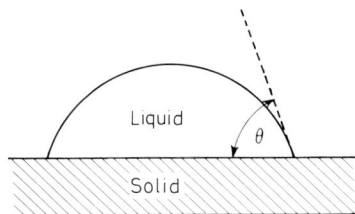

Figure 13.6–Droplet of liquid resting at equilibrium on a solid surface showing the contact angle (θ)

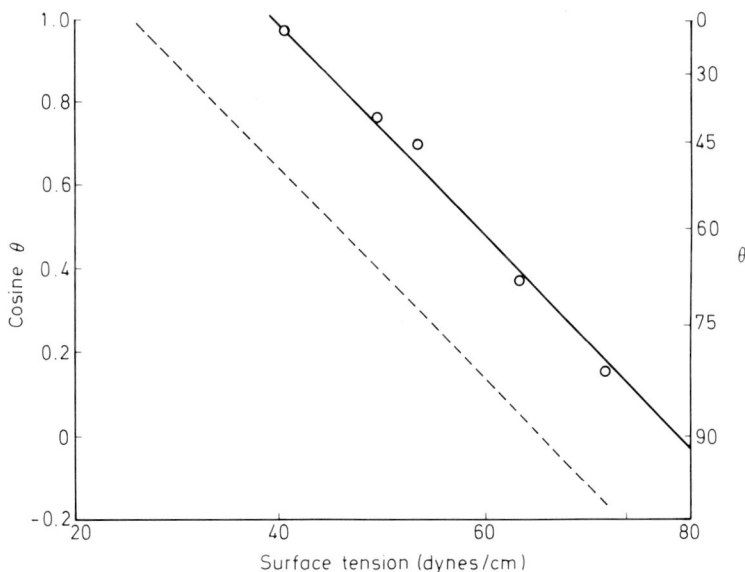

Figure 13.7—Determination of the critical surface tension of polymers by the method of Fox and Zisman illustrating the difference in wettability and critical surface tension of polymethyl methacrylate (———) and silicone rubber (- - - - - -)

These then are some of the aspects of the subject that must be taken into account.

The most convenient way of assessing wettability is by the contact angle. The simplest method for measuring this is by observing the formation of a sessile drop of liquid (delivered, for example, by a hypodermic syringe) on the solid surface. The image of the droplet may be projected or photographed

for the surface tension of tears fluid (Miller, 1969) has been thought by some workers to be too high (Lemp *et al.*, 1970). The surface tension of pure water by comparison is 72.8 dynes cm^{-1}.

The contact angles produced by a series of liquids of differing surface tensions on a solid surface can be used to obtain a parameter that is characteristic of the wettability of that surface. This parameter, the critical surface tension of the solid surface, was first defined by Fox and Zisman (1950) and has been used as a convenient way of predicting tears film stability (Larke et al., 1973; Ng, Pedley and Tighe, 1976).

An example is shown in *Figure 13.7*. Here the cosine of the contact angle (cos θ) is plotted against the surface tension for a series of liquids. The experimental results are obtained by observation of sessile droplet behaviour as shown in *Figure 13.6*. It will be observed that the line can be extrapolated to θ=0 (the point at which spontaneous spreading of the liquid or wetting of the surface would occur). The corresponding value on the surface tension axis is referred to as the critical surface tension of the solid (γ_c). All liquids of surface tension equal to or less than γ_c will spontaneously wet the surface. The figure illustrates the fact that tears fluid having a surface tension of 46 dynes cm^{-1} or slightly lower is only just able to wet the polymethyl methacrylate sample used in this experiment. The practice of using viscous wetting solution with methyl methacrylate lenses helps to establish the necessary continuous tears film on insertion. By contrast the silicone rubber sample shown on the same graph would require a liquid having a much lower surface tension ($\simeq$ 25 dynes cm^{-1}) in order for it to be spontaneously wetted. The function of surface treatment of this type of polymer is to increase the critical surface tension of the material.

Variations in the slope and indeed the shape of plots of the type shown in *Figure 13.7* do occur especially when liquids capable of hydrogen bonding with the surface are used, as they must be in contact lens work. Failure to take this into account has resulted in calculated values for the critical surface tension of the cornea that are excessively low. Even when this fact is taken into account it will be seen that the critical surface tension of the cornea ($\gamma_c \simeq$ 35 dynes cm^{-1}) is similar to, but somewhat lower than that of polymethyl methacrylate ($\gamma_c \simeq 39$ dynes cm^{-1}). There are three important observations that must be made on these figures.

The first point that requires clarification is the fact that these surfaces are unexpectedly wetted by a liquid of higher surface tension (46 dynes cm^{-1}). We can obviously take into account the fact that 46 dynes cm^{-1} is thought to be a conservatively high estimate of the surface tension of tears fluid and the unique nature of the corneal surface. The most important reason, however, since it applies to all surfaces, is the occurrence of a phenomenon known as contact angle hysteresis. This is the difference between the advancing contact angle observed when a liquid boundary advances over a clean dry solid surface and the receding contact angle observed when a liquid boundary recedes from a previously

wetted surface. The former (advancing) value is used in *in vitro* experimental work because it is far more reproducible. The latter value, which is significantly lower is, however, important in the *in vivo* contact lens situation. This is because the establishment of the tears film, corresponding to the advancing contact angle, is assisted mechanically by the eyelid and sometimes by the use of wetting solutions. The receding angle, however, dictates whether the formed film will be stable or will break up on the lens surface.

It is important to note that this difference, although significant, is relatively small and is not sufficient to sustain tears films on polymers having critical surface tensions significantly lower than polymethyl methacrylate. This raises the second point. Although there are many alternative thermoplastic polymers that might compete with polymethyl methacrylate in contact lens use, there are very few (suitable in other respects) that share its similarity in critical surface tension to the cornea. This is probably the major single reason that polymethyl methacrylate occupies the unique position that it does. Of the alternative hard lens materials currently available, only cellulose acetate butyrate possesses similar surface properties without surface treatment. The problems associated with surface treatment of various alternative thermoplastics to make their surfaces sufficiently wettable for contact lens use have been recently discussed (Ng, Pedley and Tighe, 1976). Clinical studies in conjunction with surface treatment of polymers (Larke et al., 1973; Pedley, 1976) indicate that for a material to be useful for contact lens fabrication it should have an equilibrium advancing contact angle (θ) with water of not greater than 65–70 degrees. This is, in fact, a better single criterion than the critical surface tension because of the aforementioned effects of polarity and hydrogen bonding on the determination of the latter.

Although it might be anticipated that hydrogel polymers would present no problems in relation to wettability, this is not the case and relates to third point arising from critical surface tension data. Although hydrogels are readily wetted by tears fluid and are capable of sustaining a tears fluid layer, they present a considerable problems in their tendency to accumulate proteinaceous and other material (for example, Cureton, 1973) on the lens surface during use. In addition to any specific interaction of such debris with functional groups on the surface of the polymer there is a general principle involved. This is the observation (for example, Schonhorn, 1972) that the adhesion of a mobile phase to a solid substrate increases as the surface becomes more wettable (that is, as its critical surface tension increases). There is then a desirable limit to the wettability of polymers for contact lens use. Hydrogels are not truly hydrophilic (in terms of the precise definition stated earlier) since they exhibit an equilibrium advancing contact angle of around 20 degrees. If this value could be raised, however, it would be possible to retain wettability by tears fluid whilst decreasing the problems of lens cleaning. Perhaps the best analogy here is that of non-stick domestic pan linings. Scrambled egg, which in some respects resembles the proteinaceous debris in question, adheres strongly to high energy metal surfaces but relatively weakly to the low energy poly(tetrafluoroethylene) surfaces used as pan coatings. It has been recently shown (Barnes et al., 1974; Pedley and Tighe, 1974) that by structural modification it is possible to produce hydrogels whose critical surface tensions are substantially lower (that is, less wettable by tears fluid) that would be predicted from their water contents and bulk structural considerations.

OXYGEN PERMEABILITY

The importance of oxygen to corneal metabolism is well known and the physiological consequences of oxygen deprivation in this respect are discussed in Chapter 2. Notable contributions to our knowledge of the effect of contact lenses of different types have been made over a considerable period by R. M. Hill (Hill and Fatt, 1964; Hill, 1966; Hill and Schloessler, 1967; Hill and Augsburger, 1971). A great deal of confused information has been published, however, on the actual values of oxygen permeability for different contact lens materials, particularly hydrogels.

The first point to note is that conventional 'gaseous' oxygen permeability coefficients (P_g) obtained for the transport of oxygen from the gas phase through the polymer film to another gas phase are not applicable to contact lens work. Values determined in this way are of great value in the food packaging industry, for example, and commercial apparatus for this type of measurement is readily obtainable. Measurements made in this way are inapplicable in the present context because (a) materials such as hydrogels are progressively dehydrated under these conditions and will give completely erroneous results, and more important, (b) these methods do not simulate the actual situation of the contact lens on the eye. In order to do this it is necessary to measure the transport of oxygen dissolved in one aqueous phase through the polymer and into another aqueous phase. This value is referred to as the 'dissolved' oxygen permeability coefficient (P_d).

The experimental difficulties associated with these measurements on samples that are often fragile are quite severe. Although measurements on thermoplastics and elastomers are easier to make than on hydrogels, there is with all hydrophobic polymers a barrier effect resulting from the interfacial tension between the polymer and aqueous phase. In order to obtain (P_d) values on such polymers, therefore, measurements on samples of various thicknesses must be made. Because of this barrier effect, hydrophobic polymers transport oxygen much less efficiently from water phase to water phase (as in the eye) than from gas phase to gas phase. This has meant that over-optimistic predictions have been made for polymers such as ethyl cellulose, polystyrene and poly(4-methyl pent-1-ene) on the basis of their quoted gas–gas (P_g) permeabilities. When measurements of the 'dissolved' oxygen permeabilities have been made, however, the disappointing clinical performance of such materials is understood.

A description of suitable apparatus for 'dissolved' oxygen permeability measurements has been given (Ng, 1974; Ng and Tighe, 1976a) and its application to both hydrogels (Ng and Tighe, 1976b) and non-hydrogels (Ng, Pedley and Tighe, 1976) discussed. Measurements were made at both 25°C and 34°C, that is, at room temperature and the temperature of the cornea respectively.

The relationship of corneal oxygen requirement to the thickness and dissolved oxygen permeability coefficient (P_d) of a material can be approached in various ways. The minimum partial pressure of oxygen (sometimes called oxygen tension) required at the anterior surface of the epithelium is generally taken to be somewhere in the range 11–19 mm quoted by Polse and Mandell (1970). Taking an average value (15 mm) it can be assumed that this is the minimum oxygen tension required behind a contact lens during both open and closed eye conditions. This value can then be inserted (as p_2) in a relationship (Fatt and St Helen, 1971) which enables the oxygen flux (F) across the epithelial surface under a tight fitting contact lens to be determined, that is:

$$F = \alpha p_2{}^\beta$$

In this equation α and β are two empirical constants having the values $\alpha = 0.24 \times 10^{-6}$ cc (STP) cm^{-2} sec^{-1} (mm Hg)$^{-0.5}$ and $\beta = 0.5$. This calculation indicates that the critical (or minimum) oxygen flux through a contact lens should be 0.93×10^{-6} cc (STP) cm^{-2} sec^{-1}. In alternative units this is approximately 3.5×10^{-6} 1 cm^{-2} hr^{-1}. This value compares well with independently determined values which range from $2.8 \rightarrow 7.8 \times 10^{-6}$ 1 cm^{-2} hr^{-1} and can, therefore, be taken as a minimum but sufficient oxygen flux (F) to maintain corneal transparency. (For explanation of units see Addendum, page 397.)

One way in which this information can be used is by comparing it with values obtained from the equation relating oxygen flux, thickness, and dissolved oxygen permeability coefficient for contact lenses.

$$F = \frac{Pd}{L} \times \Delta p$$

L is contact lens thickness and Δp is the pressure difference across the lens. Since the minimum partial pressure of oxygen behind the lens has been taken as 15 mm and since the generally accepted values for open and closed eye in the absence of a lens (Fatt and Bieber, 1968) are 155 mm and 55 mm respectively,

Δp (open eye)   = 140 mm Hg

Δp (closed eye) = 40 mm Hg

Pedley (1976) has pointed out, on good evidence, that these values could, in fact, be as low as 107 mm Hg and 28 mm Hg respectively but for the present calculation the earlier values will be used.

Figure 13.8 shows the result of this calculation for various contact lens materials and must be used in conjunction with the 'critical' F value of 0.93×10^{-6} cc (STP) cm^{-2} sec^{-1}. The first point of interest is the boundary effect seen clearly here with the hydrophobic materials. It is because of this that the gaseous oxygen permeability coefficients give a misleadingly optimistic picture of the suitability of a polymer for contact lens use. In the case of a poly(4-methyl pent-1-ene) lens of 0.1 mm centre thickness the 'dissolved' permeability coefficient is about half the 'gaseous' figure. Using the latter figures one would predict that such a lens might just allow the cornea to respire normally even in the closed eye condition. Not only is this situation impossible with a lens of this thickness but as the figure shows, reducing lens thickness is of virtually no value since the boundary effect is the controlling factor at this point. Although silicone rubber shows a boundary effect its oxygen permeability is so high that this does not interfere with the oxygen flux requirements of the cornea.

PolyHEMA hydrogel having an equilibrium water content of 39 per cent and a 'dissolved' oxygen permeability coefficient of 145×10^{-10} cc (STP) mm cm^{-2} sec^{-1} cm Hg^{-1} at 34°C and in the form of a contact lens 0.2 mm thick would give an oxygen flux just sufficient for the corneal requirement in the open eye condition but quite insufficient in the closed eye situation. Bearing in mind that polyHEMA lenses are frequently thicker than this

and Pedley's suggestion that the figure for the pressure difference across the lens should be reduced somewhat, the prediction is seen to be consistent with the fact that it is clinically desirable to avoid tight fitting for daily wear with these lenses. The material is of course unsuitable for continuous wear with lenses of realistic centre thickness.

An alternative approach is to take the experimentally determined figures for the oxygen consumption of the cornea under normal conditions and calculate the relationship between oxygen permeability coefficient (P_g) and lens thickness. This has been done by Ng (1974) for both open eye and closed eye conditions and used as a basis for predicting continuous wear requirements (Ng and

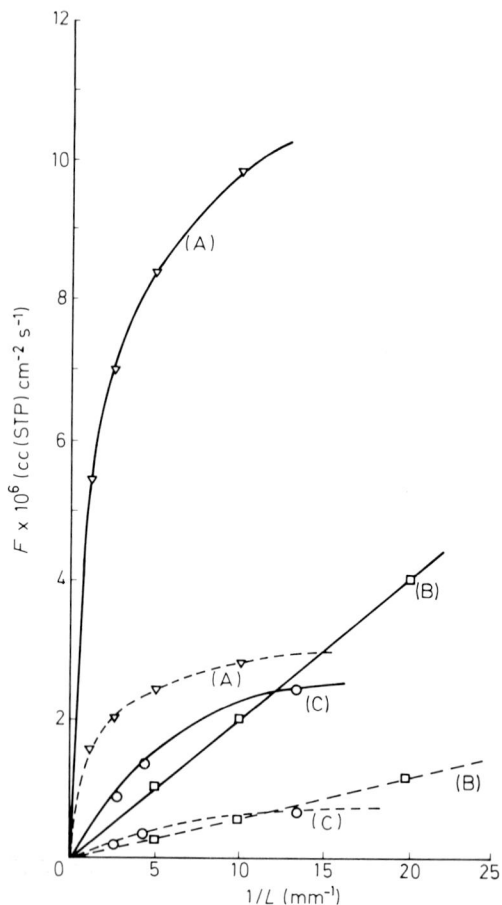

Figure 13.8—The correlation of oxygen flux (F) through the contact lens with inverse of lens thickness (L) at 34°C for various materials under open (———) and closed (- - - - -) eye conditions. (A) Silicone rubber. (B) PolyHEMA. (C) Poly (4-methyl pent-1-ene)

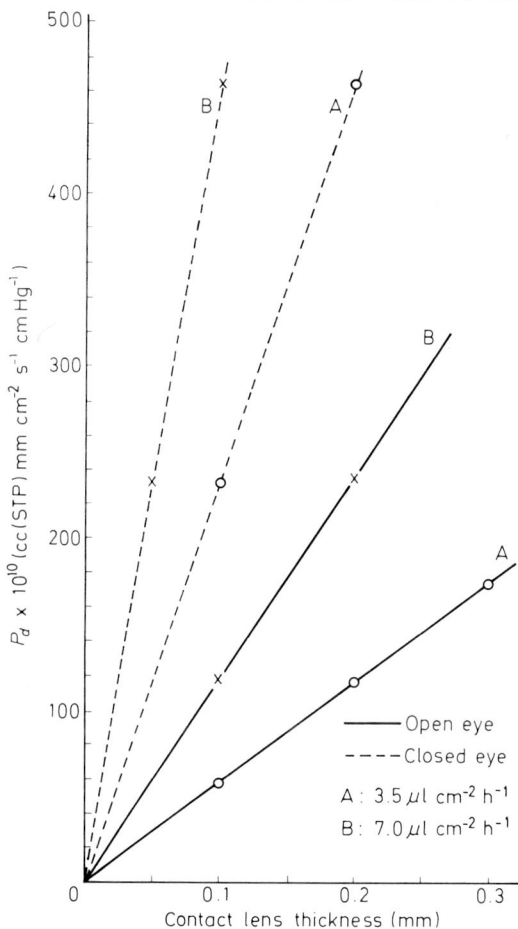

Figure 13.9—Theoretical prediction of required contact lens thickness from the 'dissolved' oxygen permeability coefficient for an oxygen flux of 3.5 or 7.0 μl cm^{-2} hr^{-1} under both open (————) and closed (- - - - - -) eye conditions, at 34°C

Tighe, 1976b). The relationship is shown in *Figure 13.9* for the range of corneal oxygen consumption figures suggested by various workers. This figure indicates that for lenses having a centre thickness of the order of 0.15 mm the minimum dissolved oxygen permeability coefficient (P_d) requirements for open and closed eye conditions are 80 and 320×10^{-10} cc (STP) mm cm^{-2} sec^{-1} cm Hg^{-1} respectively. It is interesting to note that the latter figure is of the same order as values quoted for the oxygen permeability of corneal tissue.

In predictive work of this kind many assumptions must be made. These are more fully discussed with references given but it is important to note that factors such as eyeball movement during sleep, the variations in the solubility of oxygen in tears fluid and person-to-person variation as well as diurnal variation in oxygen consumption rate have been neglected.

HYDROGELS AND THE CONCEPT OF CONTINUOUS WEAR LENSES

It has already been observed that hydrogels form the largest group of polymers in contact lens applications. This is because combinations of monomers capable of producing hydrogel polymers are virtually limitless. Hydrophilic monomers which have been used or patented for use include the following.

2-hydroxyethyl acrylate and methacrylate
2- and 3-hydroxypropyl acrylate and methacrylate
acrylic acid and methacrylic acid
acrylamide and N-substituted acrylamides
methacrylamide and N-substituted methacrylamides
N-vinyl pyrrolidone and other N-vinyl lactams
glycidyl acrylate and methacrylate
2-aminoethyl acrylate and methacrylate.

These can be copolymerized in various combinations with each other and with hydrophobic monomers such as:

methyl, ethyl or propyl acrylate or methacrylate
methoxyethyl or ethoxyethyl acrylate or methacrylate
styrene or substituted styrenes.

Some of these monomers have been mentioned previously. Of the others, the following are particularly important.

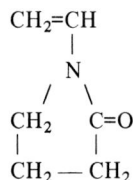

$$CH_2=CH$$
$$|$$
$$N$$
$$/ \quad \backslash$$
$$CH_2 \quad C=O$$
$$| \qquad |$$
$$CH_2 — CH_2$$

N-vinyl pyrrolidone

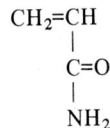

$$CH_2=CH$$
$$|$$
$$C=O$$
$$|$$
$$NH_2$$

Acrylamide

$$CH_3$$
$$|$$
$$CH_2{=}C$$
$$|$$
$$C{=}O$$
$$|$$
$$O$$
$$|$$
$$CH_2$$
$$|$$
$$CH_2$$
$$|$$
$$OCH_3$$

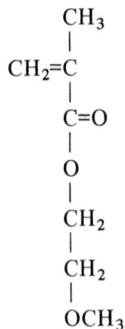

Methoxyethyl methacrylate

The incorporation of cross-links is usually achieved by copolymerizing small (of the order of 1 per cent quantities of divinyl compounds such as:

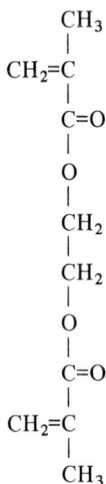

$$CH_3$$
$$|$$
$$CH_2{=}C$$
$$|$$
$$C{=}O$$
$$|$$
$$O$$
$$|$$
$$CH_2$$
$$|$$
$$CH_2$$
$$|$$
$$O$$
$$|$$
$$C{=}O$$
$$|$$
$$CH_2{=}C$$
$$|$$
$$CH_3$$

ethylene glycol dimethacrylate with the monomer mixture. Hydrogels formed in this way (that is, in which the network is linked together by primary chemical bonds) are the only satisfactory type for contact lens usage. There are, however, other classes of hydrogel (for example polyelectrolyte complexes and microcrystalline gels such as those of cellulose or collagen) which either because of fabrication difficulties or instability under conditions of changing pH and tonicity are unsuitable for this application. A survey of the earlier literature on various types of hydrogels and its relevance to contact lens work can be found elsewhere (Larke, Ng and Tighe, 1971).

From the previous discussion on the desirable ranges of various properties under both open eye and closed eye conditions, available on the cornea and its possible use as a model structure, and a knowledge of the way in which the various available monomers govern the properties of the hydrogels that they produce, it should be possible to assess the feasibility of designing a hydrogel for use as a continuous wear lens.

WATER CONTENT

This is the most important single property of a hydrogel and is more correctly called the equilibrium water content (EWC). Some confusion has arisen between this term and 'water uptake'. If a dry polymer takes up its own weight of water its equilibrium water content which is defined as:

$$\frac{\text{weight of water}}{\text{weight of hydrated gel}} \times 100 \text{ per cent}$$

will be 50 per cent. It is important to define the temperature at which the measurement was made and whether this was made in pure water or saline solution. It will become apparent that the water content of a gel measured in water at 20°C can be quite different from its value at eye temperature and in isotonic saline solution.

PolyHEMA hydrogel has an equilibrium water content of approximately 39 per cent (depending on conditions of measurement). This can be progressively reduced by copolymerizing with increasing amounts of a hydrophobic monomer such as methyl methacrylate or styrene. It can, on the other hand, be progressively increased by copolymerizing with increasing amounts of a more hydrophilic monomer such as vinyl pyrrolidone or acrylamide. Vinyl pyrrolidone and acrylamide can alternatively be copolymerized with, for example, methyl methacrylate. The water contents of the resultant polymers are dependent on the relative proportions of hydrophilic and hydrophobic monomers. Leaving aside the sophistications of graft versus random copolymerization and spin cast versus bulk polymerized materials we can use this as a basis for categorizing available lens materials.

The largest single group consists of lenses which are essentially polyHEMA. This includes Snoflex 38, Hydron, Hydroflex, Aoflex, Soflens and Weicon. The second category contains materials in which the water contents are lower than that of polyHEMA. This would typically be achieved by incorporation of a small amount of hydrophobic monomer with a resulting increase in toughness and some relatively slight loss in flexibility and oxygen permeability. An example of a material in this category is Consoft (29 per cent water content). The final group, which is expanding rapidly, consists of polymers in which a more hydrophilic monomer, usually N-vinyl pyrrolidone but occasionally acrylamide, is combined with one or more of the other hydrophilic or hydrophobic monomers to produce a polymer having a higher water content than that of polyHEMA. Examples of materials in this group are Bionite, Permalens, Snoflex 50 and the various grades of Sauflon. Some of the factors affecting and consequences of water content can now be examined using the properties listed in *Table 13.1* as a basis.

DENSITY

The density of hydrogel polymers depends on both the water content and the monomer composition. Very low water content (and fairly rigid) gels containing styrene as the hydrophobic monomer have the greatest densities of the common hydrogels. These are around 1.22 g cc^{-1} at 10 per cent water content and 20°C. Typical copolymers containing HEMA and the more hydrophilic monomers decrease progressively from around 1.16 at 38 per cent water content to around 1.05 at 75 per cent water content (all at 20°C).

REFRACTIVE INDEX

Refractive index again decreases progressively with increasing water content. The variation is almost linear with water content, and the results for hydrogels of the various types indicated above lie within a fairly narrow, almost rectilinear band, decreasing from 1.46 to 1.48 at 20 per cent water content to 1.37–1.38 at 75 per cent water content. This point is illustrated in *Figure 13.10*.

OPTICAL TRANSMITTANCE

Transparency is obviously the main requisite of a hydrogel for contact lens use but not all hydrogels are optically transparent. Translucence and opacity in hydrogels is associated with microphase separation of water thereby producing regions of differing refractive index within the gel. Although it is possible to synthesize hydrogels that show this type of behaviour (for example, by making copolymers with large blocks or segments of hydrophobic and hydrophilic monomers rather than randomly dispersing them) in contact lens usage the accidental and unwanted onset of translucency is of greater importance. This is usually associated with sudden or large changes in temperature which induce the gel to absorb excessive quantities of water. This point, which will be illustrated with respect to the thermal stability of hydrogels is, fortunately, normally reversible.

DIMENSIONAL STABILITY

Since the linear swell and volume swell shown by hydrogels on hydration is a direct consequence of the volume of water absorbed, any phenomena that cause a change in water content will cause a change in lens dimensions. PolyHEMA is an extremely stable hydrogel and variations in temperature, pH and tonicity have relatively little effect on its water content. The use of monomers that are more hydrophilic invariably incurs some penalty in this respect whether the monomer is more hydrophilic because of a basic nitrogen atom (as in N-vinyl pyrrolidone and acrylamide) or an acidic hydrogen atom (as in methacrylic and acrylic acid). The precise combination of monomers used can have a marked effect on the stability of the material. This is illustrated with respect to temperature changes in *Figure 13.11*. Note here (a) the uniquely regular behaviour of polyHEMA, (b) the decrease in water content in other cases between 20 and 40°C (a phenomenon shown by many hydrogels and which is

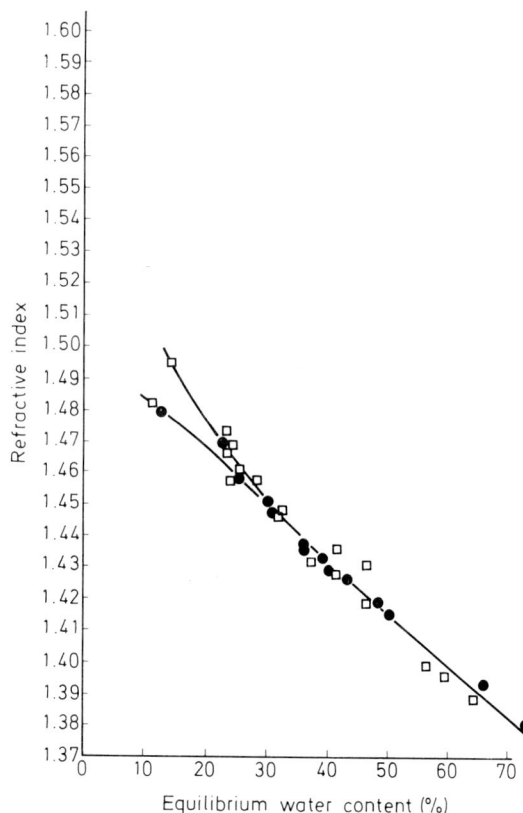

Figure 13.10—Refractive indices of various hydrogels as a function of their equilibrium water contents at 20°C (●) 34°C (□)

attributable to an increase in hydrophobic interaction or bonding in the gel), and (c) the dramatic increase in water content with concurrent onset of translucency shown by some compositions. This type of instability would obviously be most undesirable in a lens that was to be heat sterilized since, although the behaviour is reversible it leads to progressive deterioration of the polymer network.

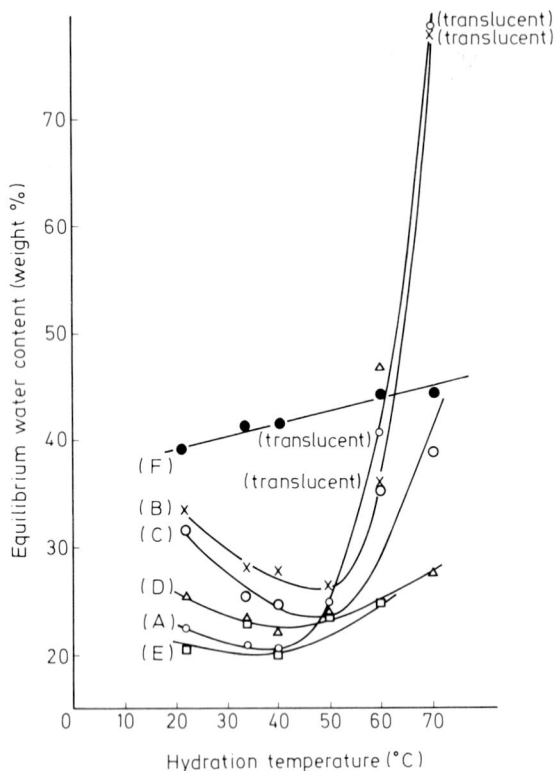

Figure 13.11–Effect of temperature on the equilibrium water contents of various hydrogels based on hydroxy propyl methacrylate and vinyl pyrrolidone. (A) HPMA. (B) HPMA – VP (80:20). (C) HPMA – VP (80:20) + (1%) EGDMA. (D) HPMA – VP (80:20) + (5%) EGDMA. (E) HPMA – VP (80:20) + (10%) EGDMA. The gels are cross-linked with ethylene glycol dimethacrylate. PolyHEMA (F) is shown for comparison

The figure illustrates in addition the effect of cross-link density on water content. Increasing the cross-link density reduces the rotational freedom of the chains, thereby restricting the ability of the polymer network to expand in response to temperature changes.

The sensitivity of water content to tonicity is similarly affected by monomer structure. This is illustrated in *Figure 13.12* which shows the effect of

vinyl pyrrolidone incorporation. In general, hydrogels show some small decrease in water content when the equilibration solution is changed from pure water to isotonic saline solution. It should be emphasized, however, that this does not in any way argue against the use of vinyl pyrrolidone. These changes, and others induced by changing the nature of the storage solution, are much greater than changes brought about by tonicity variations in the eye.

Variations with respect to pH are much more marked and monomer dependent, minima in water content often being observed with varying pH. The pH changes involved, however, ($\simeq$ 2–10) are much greater than those occurring diurnally or on a patient-to-patient basis on the eye. It is relevant to point out that reputable material manufacturers are well aware of the types of dimensional instability discussed above and will avoid monomer compositions showing unacceptable behaviour.

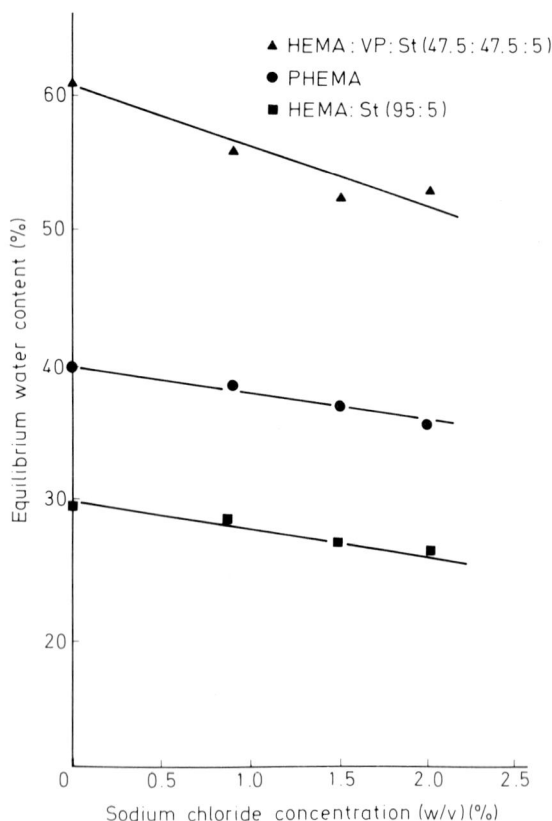

Figure 13.12—The equilibrium water contents of some hydrogels in hydrating solutions of various sodium chloride concentrations at 20°C

SURFACE WETTABILITY

This topic has been previously discussed in some detail. It is apparent that hydrogels do not suffer any deficiencies in terms of inadequate wettability and that it may be desirable to reduce their ability in this respect. One related factor that contributes to the comfort of hydrogels is the low coefficient of friction between the lens and the eyelid. This frictional interaction is much greater with elastomers of similar bulk rigidity (such as ethylene propylene terpolymer and silicone rubber) even after surface treatment.

MECHANICAL PROPERTIES

In its dehydrated state, polyHEMA (and, indeed, most other hydrogel forming polymers) is hard and brittle, resembling polymethyl methacrylate. When swollen in water, however, it becomes soft and rubber-like with a very low tear and tensile strength. This lack of mechanical strength has, of course, a profound effect on the lifetime of the lens. Although the water content has a marked effect on mechanical strength, the chemical structure of the polymer can also play a large part in determining its value. This can be best illustrated by comparing the tensile strength of polyHEMA with that of cellophane. Bixler and Michaels (1968) have reported that cellophane with a water content of 55 per cent has a tensile modulus of nearly five times and an ultimate tensile strength of over fifty times that of polyHEMA.

Unfortunately, one of the easiest ways of preparing hydrogels having improved mechanical properties involves the use of structures that are extremely sensitive to temperature, pH and tonicity. Nonetheless, by use of modified monomer combinations and cross-linking agents high water content (> 70 per cent) polymers having reasonable stability and elasticity can be prepared. It will be apparent that there are now commercially available high water content lenses which are vastly superior in strength to the earlier generation of fragile gels of similar water content based on HEMA-vinyl pyrrolidone. Unfortunately, however, the problem of poor tear strength is fundamental to these materials and although improvements can be expected miracles can not.

OXYGEN PERMEABILITY

This topic has also been discussed at some length and it is only necessary at this point to indicate that oxygen permeability of hydrogels is governed by the

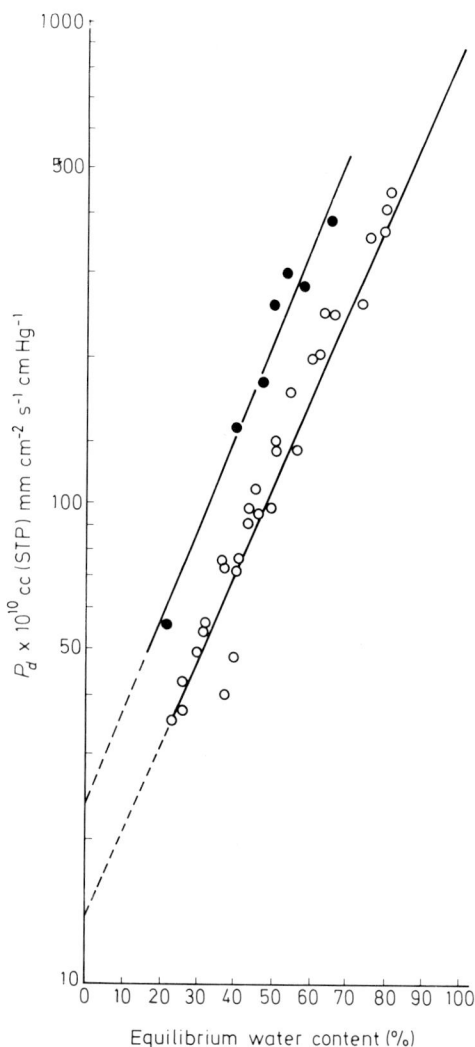

Figure 13.13—The variation of log dissolved oxygen permeability coefficient (P_d) as a function of water content for various hydrogels at 25° ($\bigcirc$) and 34° ($\bullet$)

water content (Ng and Tighe, 1976b). This is illustrated by Figure 13.13 which shows the variation in P_d with water content for hydrogels of various compositions, at 25 and 34°C. Although the increase in oxygen permeability coefficient with this change in temperature is quite marked (a factor of approximately two), this may not be representative of the change in P_d for a given hydrogel. The reason for this is the previously discussed observation that many hydrogels decrease in water content with increasing temperature in this region. To determine the oxygen permeability of a hydrogel at 34°C from this graph, then, it is necessary to use the value of the water content determined at that temperature. Thus, a value for P_d of 350×10^{-10} cc (STP) mm cm^{-2} sec^{-1} cm Hg^{-1} at 34°C would be given by a gel having a water content of something over 60 per cent at that temperature. The water content of that same gel at 25°C might, however, be nearer 70 per cent. According to the corneal requirement predictions discussed earlier, this would represent the minimum water content required for an extended wear lens having a centre thickness of around 0.15 mm.

WATER PERMEABILITY AND PORE RADIUS

Hydrogels are porous materials and the average pore radius can be measured and calculated in various ways. Homogeneous (transparent) hydrogels of the type discussed here show a distribution of pore sizes about the mean or average value and the magnitude of the average pore radius increases with increasing water content. The increase becomes much more marked at higher water contents as illustrated by the following values corresponding to the water contents following them in brackets: 4.0Å (40 per cent), 6.0Å (60 per cent), 20Å (80 per cent), 30Å (85 per cent). The fact that this is only an average value and that larger than average pores occur explains the fact that fluorescein (molecular radius 5.5Å) is known to be absorbed into polyHEMA hydrogel.

This indication of the order of magnitude of pore sizes occurring in hydrogels is of value in predicting the types of species that are likely to diffuse in and possibly become trapped or concentrated (by interaction) within the porous structure. It is particularly important in this respect that lenses should only be exposed to solutions specifically recommended for that material. There is still (Paul, 1973) dispute as to whether the diffusion of water through hydrogels is due entirely to self-diffusion or partially (at high water contents) to viscous flow. Whichever mechanism is responsible it seems inescapable that tears fluid exchange with the lens occurs and contributes to the compatibility of the lens with the eye. It is relevant to note that water and oxygen are of similar molecular size and that the permeability coefficients for water and oxygen are of the same order when expressed in the same units. Further the water permeability coefficient increases by a factor of approximately 4 in moving from polyHEMA to a 60 per cent water content gel and by a factor of

approximately 60 in moving to an 80 per cent water content gel.

CONCLUSIONS

It is apparent from this review of materials that the problem of describing an ideal material is an impossible one. A lens for daily wear, to withstand repeated handling and sterilization routines will be much more durable if chosen from the thermoplastic or synthetic elastomer category. The problems associated with materials in these groups that differ significantly from the representative member listed in *Table 13.1* have been discussed and it is apparent that until surface treatment techniques are considerably improved the choice lies between polymethyl methacrylate and cellulose acetate butyrate. Much more clinical experience is available with the former material and the only marked advantage that cellulose acetate butyrate has on the basis of physical properties is an improved oxygen permeability. Since its (P_d) is only approximately one-quarter of that of poly(4-methyl pent-1-ene) it will be apparent from *Figure 13.8* that it cannot transmit sufficient oxygen to supply the cornea during daily wear without the assistance of tears flow behind the lens. Nonetheless, in the final analysis it is the preference of patient and practitioner that governs the success or otherwise of a given material. Such factors as lens design, as well as curvature and power changes with dehydration on the eye are outside the scope of this chapter, but are dealt with fully in Chapter 4, Volume 1, and Chapters 14 and 16 as appropriate. However, these factors too, influence the success of any given material.

In predicting the properties required for an extended or continuous wear lens it will be apparent that the superior biocompatibility of hydrogels makes them the obvious choice. The corneal oxygen requirement is the major initial stumbling block and the predictive work described here, with all its attendant approximations, indicates that a material must have an equilibrium water content measured in isotonic saline solution at 34°C of not less than 60 per cent in order to be considered. With the temperature and tonicity effects observed with the more hydrophilic monomers that are needed to obtain this figure, the corresponding water content at 25°C in water will probably be in the region of 70 per cent. Such a material may be expected to give reasonable visual stability and resistance to handling under normal conditions but to have relatively poor tear strength. The major problem still to be overcome is modification of the hydrogel surface to reduce the adhesion of mucus and related debris.

ADDENDUM

UNITS AND TERMS IN PERMEABILITY AND MECHANICAL PROPERTY MEASUREMENTS

Manufacturers' literature and, indeed, work by independent authors express properties in a variety of terms and units. This addendum provides some explanatory notes and conversion factors.

MECHANICAL PROPERTIES

The strength of a material is usually defined in terms of the force per unit area required to cause failure under the particular test procedure (that is, tensile, tear, impact, shear). The modulus, on the other hand, is defined as the stress (that is, force per unit area) required to produce a unit strain (deformation) in the direction of the force (for example, tensile modulus, rigidity modulus). Several different units of stress are used (tsi – tons weight per square inch; psi – pounds weight per square inch; kg or kgf mm^{-2} – kilograms weight per square millimetre; and dyne cm^{-2} – dynes per square centimetre). In Great Britain and Europe, SI (Systeme Internationale) units have recently been adopted. The SI unit of stress is Nm^{-2} (newtons per square metre), but this is an extremely small quantity and MNm^{-2} (mega newtons per square metre, equal to 10^6Nm^{-2}) is a more useful unit.

The various units are related as follows: 1 dyne $cm^{-2} = 0.1Nm^{-2} = 10^{-7}MNm^{-2} = 1.45 \times 10^{-5}$ psi $= 6.46 \times 10^{-9}$ tsi $= 1.02 \times 10^{-8}$ kgmm^{-2}. Thus, in order to convert a strength or modulus expressed in dyne cm^{-2} to other units it should be multiplied by the appropriate factor, and to convert values in other units to dynes cm^{-2} the values should be divided by the appropriate factor.

In contact lens work tear strength (which is rather unusual in being expressed in terms of the force required to propagate a tear of unit length) is usually presented in units of grams per millimetre (g mm^{-1}).

OXYGEN PERMEABILITY

The most important term in this work is the oxygen permeability coefficient, P, which is the amount of gas passing in unit time through a unit area of membrane subjected to a unit gas pressure gradient (that is, pressure difference per unit thickness) across the membrane. The difference between 'dissolved' and 'gaseous' coefficients (P_d and P_g) is discussed in the text (see page 389). The units in both cases are cc(STP) mm cm^{-2} sec^{-1} cm Hg^{-1} or one of the equivalents listed below. The oxygen permeability coefficient is equal to the product of the oxygen diffusion coefficient (D) and its solubility (S), that is, $P = D \times S$. The units of D are simply cm^2 sec^{-1} and those of S, cc cm^{-3} cm Hg^{-1}, for example, cc(O_2) per $cm^3(H_2O)$ per cm Hg.

Two additional terms that are sometimes used are oxygen flux (F), which is the volume of gass passing per unit time through unit area of a membrane under given experimental conditions (for example, pressure difference, temperature) and oxygen transmission rate (TR) which is the amount of gas passing in unit time through a unit area of a membrane of given thickness under unit gas pressure gradient. The units of F are typically cc cm^{-2} sec^{-1} and those of TR, cc(STP) cm^{-2} sec^{-1} cm Hg^{-1}. In order to convert transmission rates (sometimes referred to as transmissibility, see Chapter 14, page 445) to permeability coefficients the value is simply multiplied by sample thickness; for example, $TR \times$ sample thickness $= P$.

To convert oxygen flux values to permeability coefficients it is first necessary to change the volume of gas to its value under conditions of standard temperature and pressure (STP) and then to multiply by sample thickness and divide by the oxygen pressure gradient across the sample; for example, F (converted to STP) $\times$ sample thickness $\times$ 1/oxygen pressure gradient $= P$.

The units of P are preferably cc(STP) mm cm^{-2} sec^{-1} cm Hg^{-1} but may contain alternative terms for thickness (cm, mm), time (min^{-1}, hr^{-1}, day^{-1}), volume (ml, cm^3), area (m^2, 100 in^2) or pressure gradient (atm^{-1}, mm Hg^{-1}). In addition, units are sometimes 'simplified' by dividing or multiplying top and bottom by a common facture such as cm or mm. One of the most common examples is the conversion:

$$\frac{cc(STP)\ cm}{sec\ cm^2\ mm\ Hg} \times \frac{cm}{cm} = \frac{cc(STP)\ cm^2}{sec\ cm^3\ mm\ Hg}$$

The two sets are identical but the right-hand units may now be expressed as:

$$\frac{ml\ O_2\ cm^2}{sec\ ml\ mm\ Hg}$$

or   (cm^2/sec)(ml O_2/ml $\times$ mm Hg)
as used by Fatt (see Chapter 14)

When dealing with strange or unrecognizable units it is advisable to (a) change ml to cm^3 and (b) try multiplying both top and bottom of the equation by the same factor

$$(\text{for example,} \quad \frac{cm}{cm} \quad)$$

until one of the recognizable forms of units listed below is reached. Remember also that the value quoted may be an oxygen flux or transmission rate, especially if the determination was carried out on a lens. In such cases the quoted figure must be multiplied by sample thickness, or thickness and pressure gradient, as indicated above.

The more commonly encountered units of oxygen permeability are related as shown below.

1 cc(STP) mm cm^{-2} sec^{-1} cm Hg^{-1}
or cm^3(STP) mm cm^{-2} sec^{-1} cm Hg^{-1}
or cm mm sec^{-1} cm Hg^{-1}

  is equivalent to

0.1 cc(STP) cm cm^{-2} sec^{-1} cm Hg^{-1}
or cm^3(STP) cm cm^{-2} sec^{-1} cm Hg^{-1}
or cm^2 sec^{-1} cm Hg^{-1}
or cm^3(STP) cm^{-1} sec^{-1} cm Hg^{-1}

  is equivalent to

0.1 cc(STP) mm cm^{-2} sec^{-1} mm Hg^{-1}
or cm^3(STP) mm cm^{-2} sec^{-1} mm Hg^{-1}
or cm mm sec^{-1} mm Hg^{-1}
or (cm^2/sec)(ml O/ml mm Hg) as illustrated in the example above

is equivalent to

0.01 cc(STP) cm cm^{-2} sec^{-1} mm Hg^{-1}
or cm^3(STP) cm cm^{-2} sec^{-1} mm Hg^{-1}
or cm^2 sec^{-1} mm Hg^{-1}
or cm^3(STP) cm^{-1} sec^{-1} mm Hg^{-1}

  is equivalent to

7.6 cc (STP) cm cm^{-2} sec^{-1} atm^{-1}
or cm^3(STP) cm cm^{-2} sec^{-1} atm^{-1}
or cm^2 sec^{-1} atm^{-1}
or cm^3(STP) cm^{-1} sec^{-1} atm^{-1}

  is equivalent to

2.59 $\times$ 10^{12} cc(STP) ml day^{-1} m^{-2} atm^{-1}
or cm^3(STP) ml day^{-1} m^{-2} atm^{-1}

  is equivalent to

16.5 $\times$ 10^{10} cc(STP) ml day^{-1} (100 in)$^{-2}$ atm^{-1}

  is equivalent to

1.02 $\times$ 10^{10} in^3 ml day^{-1} (100 in)$^{-2}$ atm^{-1}

  is equivalent to

7.69 $\times$ 10^{-6} cm^4 sec^{-1} dyne^{-1}

ACKNOWLEDGEMENTS

I am grateful for valuable discussions and for the excellent research work carried out on these and other aspects of the biomedical applications of polymers by Derek Pedley, Chiong Ng, Peter Skelly and Andrew Barnes and to Mrs M. Husbands for typing the manuscript.

REFERENCES

Anderton, J. (1973). *Consideration of the cornea as a model for the design and synthesis of polymers for continuous-wear contact lenses.* M.Sc. Thesis, Department of Chemistry, University of Aston, Birmingham

Barnes, A., Ensor, R., Ng, C.O., Pedley, D. G. and Tighe, B. J. (1974). 'Wettability phenomena in synthetic hydrogels for contact lens applications.' Paper presented at 5th European Symposium on Fluorine Chemistry, Aviemore, Scotland

Becker, W. E. (1966). 'Corneal contact lens fabricated from silicone rubber.' *U.S. Patent* 3,228,741

Bitonte, J. L. and Keates, R. H. (1972). *A Symposium on the Future of Flexible Lenses vs. Rigid Lenses.* St. Louis: Mosby

Bixler, H. J. and Michaels, A. S. (1968). 'Polyelectrolyte complexes.' In *Kirk-Othmer Encyclopaedia of Chemical Technology,* 2nd ed., Vol. 16. New York: Interscience

Burns, R. P., Roberts, H. and Rich, L. F. (1971). 'Effect of silicone contact lenses on corneal epithelial metabolism.' *Am. J. Ophthal.* **71**, 486–489

Cureton, G. L. (1973). 'New perspectives on solutions for hard and soft contact lenses. *Mfg Optics Int.* **26**, 503–511

Dow Corning Corporation (1967). 'Hydrophilic silicone rubber.' *British Patent* 1,229,608

E. I. Dupont de Nemours and Company (1971). 'Contact lenses.' *British Patent* 1,254,567

Ehlers, N. (1965). 'The precorneal film. Biomicroscopical histological and chemical investigations.' *Acta Ophthal. (Kbh)* Suppl. 81

Fatt, I. and Bieber, M. T. (1968). 'The steady state distribution of oxygen and carbon dioxide in the *in vivo* cornea. 1: The open eye in air and the closed eye.' *Exp. Eye Res.* **7**, 103–112

Fatt, I. and St. Helen, R. (1971). 'Oxygen tension under and oxygen-permeable contact lens.' *Am. J. Optom.* **48**, 545–555

Fox, H. W. and Zisman, W. A. (1950). 'The spreading of liquids on low energy surfaces.' *J. Colloid Sci.* **5**, 514–531

Hill, R. M. (1966). 'Effects of a silicone rubber lens on corneal respiration.' *J. Am. optom. Ass.* **37**, 1119–1121

Hill, R. M. and Augsburger, A. (1971). 'Oxygen tensions at the epithelial surface with a contact lens *in situ*.' *Am. J. Optom.* **48**, 416–418

Hill, R. M. and Fatt, I. (1964). 'Oxygen measurements under a contact lens.' *Am. J. Optom.* **41**, 382–387

Hill, R. M. and Schoessler, J. (1967). 'Optical membranes of silicone rubber.' *J. Am. optom. Ass.* **38**, 480–483

Kamath, P. M. (1969). 'Physical and chemical attributes of an ideal contact lens.' *Contacto* **13**(4), 29–34

Kamath, P. M. (1970). 'Rigid gas permeable plastic contact lens.' *U.S. Patent* 3,551,035

Larke, J. R., Ng. C. O. and Tighe, B. J. (1971). 'Hydrogel polymers in contact lens applications: Parts I and II. A survey of existing literature.' *Optician* **162**(4206), 12–16 and (4207), 12–16

Larke, J. R., Pedley, D. G. and Tighe, B. J. (1973). 'Polymers in contact lens applications: Parts III and IV, Wettability phenomena.' *Optician***166**(4300), 32–39 and (4301), 21–30

Larke, J. R., Pedley, D. G., Smith., P. and Tighe, B. J. (1973). 'A semi-rigid contact lens.' *Ophthal. Optician* **13**, 1065–1067

Lempe, M. A., Holly, F. J., Iwata, S. and Dohlman, C. H. (1970). 'The precorneal tear film: I. Factors in spreading and maintaining a continuous tear film over the corneal surface.' *Archs Ophthal.* **83**, 89–94

Miller, D. (1969). 'Measurement of the surface tension of tears.' *Archs Ophthal.* **82**, 386–371

Mishima, S. (1965). 'Some physiological aspects of the precorneal tear film.' **73**, 233–241

Mishima, S. and Maurice, B. M. (1961). 'The effect of normal evaporation on the eye.' *Exp. Eye. Res.* **1**, 46–52

Ng, C. O. (1974). *Hydrogel polymers in contact lens applications.* Ph.D. Thesis, Department of Chemistry, University of Aston, Birmingham

Ng, C. O. and Tighe, B. J. (1976a). 'Polymers in contact lens applications: V. Design and calibration of a technique for dissolved oxygen permeability measurements.' *Br. Polym. J.* **8**, 78–82

Ng, C. O. and Tighe, B. J. (1976b). 'Polymers in contact lens applications: VI. The dissolved oxygen permeability of hydrogels and the design of materials for use in continuous-wear lenses.' *Br. Polym. J.* **8**, 118–123

Ng, C. O., Pedley, D. G. and Tighe, B. J. (1976). 'Polymers in contact lens applications: VII. Oxygen permeability and surface hydrophilicity of poly(4-methylpent-1-ene) and related polymers.' *Br. Polym. J.* **8**, 124–130

Paul, D. R. (1973). 'Relation between hydraulic permeability and diffusion in homogeneous swollen membranes.' *J. Polym. Sci. Polym. Phys. Edn.* **11**, 289–296

Pedley, D. G. (1976). *Hydrophilic Polymers.* Ph.D. Thesis, Department of Chemistry, University of Aston, Birmingham

Pedley, D. G. and Tighe, B. J. (1974). 'Hydrogel-forming polymers.' *British Patent. Prov. Spec.,* 40464/74

Polse, K. A. and Mandell, R. B. (1970). 'Critical oxygen tension at the corneal surface.' *Archs Ophthal.* **84**, 505–508

Rosen, H. (1969). 'Contact lens with flexible central portion.' *U.S. Patent* 3,468,602

Schonhorn, H. (1972). 'Wetting phenomena pertaining to adhesion.' In *Progress in Membrane and Surface Science,* pp. 121–137. New York and London: Academic Press

Studies Inc. (1969). 'Flexible polyethylene contact lens.' *U.S. Patent* 3,431,046

Tighe, B. J. (1976). 'The design of polymers for contact lens applications.' Based on paper at symposium entitled: 'Polymers in biomedical applications.' Presented at Brunel University, May, 1974. *Br. Polym. J.* **8**, 71–77

Wichterle, O. and Lim, D. (1960). 'Hydrophilic gels for biological use.' *Nature* **185**, 117–118

Wichterle, O. and Lim, D. (1961). 'Process for producing three-dimensional hydrophilic highpolymers.' *U.S. Patent* 2,976,576

Wichterle, O. and Lim, D. (1965). 'Cross-linked hydrophilic articles and polymers made therefrom.' *U.S. Patent* 3,220,960

Wolff, E. (1976). *Anatomy of the Eye and Orbit,* 7th ed. London: H. K. Lewis

Chapter 14

Soft Lens Fitting

A. P. Gasson

INTRODUCTION

During the last ten years hydrophilic lenses have been the fastest developing aspect of a constantly changing contact lens world. This has been due to improvements and changes in polymers and materials, techniques of manufacture, cleaning and disinfection procedures and methods of fitting. Within this time span the status of soft lenses has changed from occasional experimental use in difficult cases to a routine and indispensable part of contact lens practice.

Since their introduction, in addition to brand names, the new lenses have become known by a variety of descriptions such as 'soft', 'hydrophilic', 'hydrogel', 'gel', 'flexible', 'pliable', and 'supple' in order to distinguish them from corneal lenses which have now been described as 'hard', 'stable' 'rigid' or 'firm'. 'Soft' (defined as 'yielding to pressure') and 'hard', with the advantage of simplicity, have both become the most acceptable and widely used terms. 'Hydrophilic' (water loving), although applicable to most lenses mentioned in this chapter, is not a strictly accurate description, since it is more properly used to define the surface characteristics of a material in relation to the angle of contact, or wetting angle. It is a term which can also be applied to corneal lenses, so that a hydrophobic hard lens may be coated to become hydrophilic. Conversely, a flexible silicone lens is extremely hydrophobic unless the surface is treated to become hydrophilic. The term 'hydrogel' signifies a material made from a hydrogel polymer, which absorbs and binds water into its molecular structure. It usefully describes those lenses mentioned as having a percentage water content, although not all hydrogels need necessarily be soft. Within the category of hydrogels there are a great many individual polymers, some of which,

such as HEMA, have themselves become generic. *Figure 14.1* shows how a soft lens with a thin edge may be virtually invisible on an eye, and *Figure 14.2* shows that a soft lens with good tensile strength can withstand considerable abuse.

HISTORICAL BACKGROUND

The first soft lenses were produced in Czechoslovakia by Wichterle and Lim, two polymer chemists from the Prague Institute of Macro-Molecular Physics. Having worked in association with Dreifus, they reported that certain hydrogels developed for biological application could successfully be used for the manufacture of contact lenses (Wichterle and Lim, 1960). The early lenses, known as Geltact or Spofa, were made by spin-casting from hydroxyethyl methacrylate (HEMA). They were successful in a country which had no hard lens industry, but when compared by foreign researchers with their own corneal lenses, they were found to be difficult to fit and to give unsatisfactory vision. The material was of variable quality and the life span short. They nevertheless represent an important milestone in the history of contact lenses, for they provided the impetus to the rest of the world for the vast programmes of research and development undertaken since that time into new materials and lens forms. This has resulted in soft lenses now being routinely fitted in practice as an acceptable form of visual correction.

The rights to the Czechoslovakian lens were acquired in 1965 by the American company, National Patents Development Corporation, who in turn, during 1966, licensed Bausch and Lomb in the United States to its continued manufacture by the spin-casting process. At the same time production of lenses was started in various other countries around the world by the more usual method of lathe-cutting under the name of Hydron, as well as using the same HEMA material for many other applications such as biological implants. Bausch and Lomb spent five years in improving and developing all aspects of the

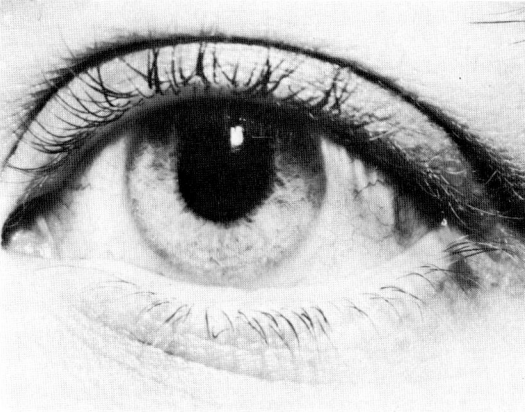

Figure 14.1—An eye wearing a small semi-scleral (or large corneal size) soft lens with an ultra-thin edge

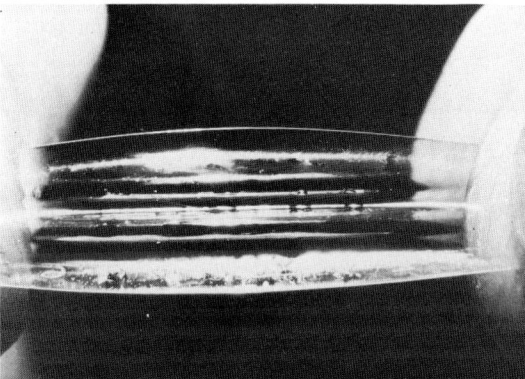

Figure 14.2–The elastic property of a low water content hydrophilic lens being stretched

spin-cast lens, and eventually gained approval from the U.S. Food and Drugs Administration (FDA) in March, 1971.

In the mid-1960's a great many non-HEMA materials were investigated and the Bionite lens appeared in 1969, together with the then new method of semi-scleral fitting.

In the United Kingdom Sauflon material was investigated as long ago as 1968, and fitted to patients in 1970, at about the same time as early Permalenses were first fitted by de Carle (de Carle, 1972). Bionite was first prescribed in 1971, Hydron

early in 1972, and the Bausch and Lomb Soflens in July, 1972. Since then there has been a proliferation of new materials, mostly HEMA-based. These have been accompanied by the development of such allied technologies as lens disinfection, storage and cleaning, whilst many of the earlier lens forms have already disappeared because of their unsatisfactory clinical performance.

THE ADVANTAGES OF SOFT CONTACT LENSES

There are numerous advantages which soft lenses of all types possess in common; they are as follows.

Greater Comfort

Hydrophilic lenses are in nearly all cases significantly more comfortable than hard lenses, patients frequently stating that they can scarcely feel the lens' presence even from the first moment of insertion. With all types of contact lens there are two different adaptation processes involved. The first is that of the lids to the sensation caused by the presence of a foreign body in the eye; the second is that of the cornea to changes in its normal metabolism. It is the reduction or even complete absence of lid sensation which allows a hydrophilic lens to be immediately comfortable. The softness of the lens material is certainly concerned with this initial comfort, but just as important is the hydrophilic nature of the lens surface, so that the lid is in contact with a smooth, moist surface which gives a very similar sensation to that of the cornea itself. Soft lenses of smaller than corneal size tend to be unstable in fitting and, because of their excessive movement, can be as irritating as hard lenses. They have therefore evolved in their design to be the same size as the cornea or greater. Stability, currently achieved through a relatively large overall size, is a very important requirement for comfort, for exactly the same reason that a scleral lens is usually quite comfortable on initial insertion, because there is no differential sensation of the lid making and breaking contact with the edge of the lens. Manufacturing considerations are also important, and the lens edge must be thin and well formed.

Ease of Adaptation

Soft lens wearers are normally able to adapt to their lenses within a very few days. This is due to the physical and chemical properties of the hydrogel material, and to the absence of lid sensation as mentioned above. There is no disincentive to proper blinking, and tears exchange readily occurs by the pumping action of the lids on a well-fitting lens. The cornea therefore receives an adequate supply of oxygen with minimum disturbance to its normal metabolism.

Normal Head Posture and Facial Expression

Abnormal head posture and unnatural facial expressions are commonly seen with hard lens wearers in the early stages of adaptation. Because of the initial comfort, soft lens wearers generally look perfectly natural from the beginning of their wearing schedule.

Longer Wearing Time

Hydrophilic lenses can frequently be worn for longer periods of time than corneal lenses. This is especially true of those patients who have achieved only limited success with hard lenses.

Lower Incidence of Corneal Oedema

Corneal oedema is seen less frequently with soft lens wearers, and even if present it is usually only of a mild degree and difficult to detect.

Rare Occurrence of the 'Over-Wear Syndrome'

Because oedema is so much less of a problem with a well-fitting lens, patients who wear soft lenses for excessively long periods are unlikely to suffer severe epithelial damage and the 'over-wear syndrome'. Moderate stinging and burning with conjunctival injection is sometimes encountered, but this usually disappears rapidly when the lenses are removed. Over-wear is normally self-limiting with soft lenses, because discomfort usually occurs before they have caused any severe epithelial damage.

Absence of Spectacle Blur

It is uncommon for spectacle blur to occur with hydrophilic lenses because under normal circumstances they do not produce significant changes in keratometer readings. Even if oedema is present with an increase in corneal thickness, it is uniform and extends from limbus to limbus with little or no localized change in radius or physical distortion of

corneal curvature as occurs with hard corneal lenses. Even when small changes of corneal curvature do occur, these are not permanent (Hill, 1975, 1976a).

The absence of noticeable spectacle blur means that patients can change from soft lenses to spectacles whenever they wish, and that the long-term clinical management of their spectacle refraction is straightforward. This can be undertaken at any convenient time, without requiring lenses to be removed for a specified number of hours or days.

Maintenance of Corneal Sensitivity

The wearing of hard lenses can cause a temporary but significant loss of corneal sensitivity. This potentially dangerous situation does not occur with soft lenses to anything like the same extent; the sensitivity loss is only half that of hard lenses (Millodot, 1971, 1974, 1976).

Lower Incidence of Corneal Staining

Because hydrophilic lenses are soft, large and stable, corneal insult of the sort inherent in the use of a hard lens, such as apical, arcuate and 3 and 9 o'clock staining, is not commonly encountered.

Occasional Wear

The ease of adaptation and the absence of spectacle blur mean that soft lenses are ideal for patients who wish to wear contact lenses irregularly for sporting or social occasions.

Absence of Photophobia and Lacrimation

The typically adaptive photophobia and lacrimation found with corneal lenses is almost invariably absent with hydrophilic lenses.

Lower Incidence of Flare

Because of their large optic diameter, patients rarely complain of flare or peripheral reflections when wearing soft lenses.

Less Difficulty with Dust and Foreign Bodies

Because the lenses are of corneal diameter, or greater, they effectively protect the eye against dust and wind. Except on insertion – for it is quite easy to inadvertently place a lens on the eye with a speck of dust – patients wearing soft lenses are rarely troubled by foreign bodies.

Lower Risk of Loss

Losses of hydrophilic lenses normally occur during handling and not from the eye. They do not fall out except in cases of extreme dehydration, and they are not easily ejected by eye rubbing or lid tension; nor are they generally dislodged onto the sclera.

Therapeutic Uses

Hydrophilic lenses are proving effective in treating several pathological conditions. These include bullous keratopathy, the dry eye syndromes, corneal burns and sterile indolent ulcers. Apart from their use as a corneal bandage, they have also been employed as a drug release mechanism (Hillman, 1976).

The Successful Refitting of Hard Lens Failures

Perhaps the major advantage of soft lenses is that it is now possible to successfully refit many patients who have previously failed with hard lenses. The instant comfort of soft lenses when compared with the earlier irritation occasioned by their hard lenses proves a reassuring factor in deciding many patients to recommence contact lens wear.

DISADVANTAGES OF SOFT CONTACT LENSES

Despite their many advantages, soft lenses have several drawbacks which must be carefully evaluated for each patient.

Distance Vision

Visual acuity is often not as good as that obtained with hard lenses. Poor vision generally relates to uncorrected astigmatism, but may also result from limitations imposed by lens geometry.

Near Vision

It is quite common for patients to complain of poor near vision, whilst distance acuity is perfectly satisfactory (see page 410).

Variable Vision

Visual acuity can vary with hydrophilic lenses as a result of fluctuations from blinking, or because of environmental factors affecting their fitting characteristics (see page 410).

Breakage and Tearing

Soft lenses can suffer from breakage, tears, and edge nicks. The frequency and need for lens replacements depends on the tensile strength and water content of the lens, as well as the handling ability of the patient.

Lens Ageing and Surface Degradation

Hydrophilic lenses suffer from discoloration and the deposition of mucoprotein and calcium on their surfaces. Lenses eventually become uncomfortable,

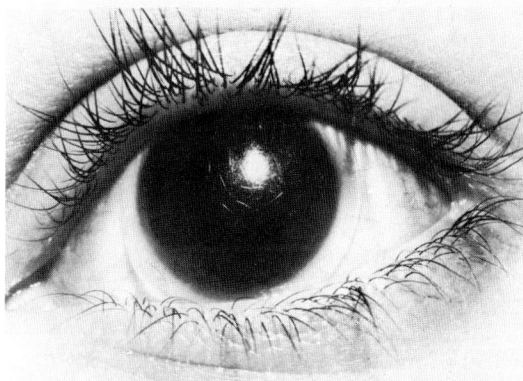

(a)

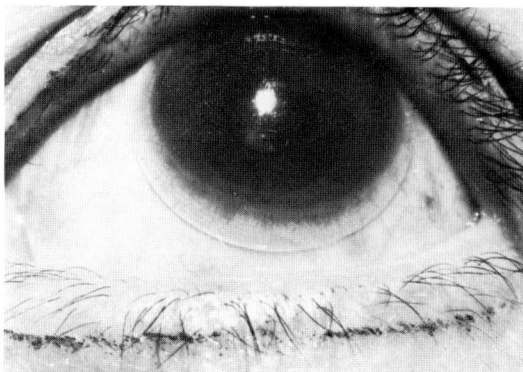

(b)

Figure 14.3–(a) Surface scratching of an old loosely fitting low water content soft lens. (b) A two-year-old low water content soft lens with pitted surface

their fitting characteristics alter, and they can give reduced visual acuity. Lenses showing surface scratching and pitting are shown in *Figure 14.3a* and *b*.

Difficulty of Cleaning

The various cleaning processes which have been introduced must be applied with painstaking regularity if they are to be effective. They are frequently expensive and time-consuming.

The Need for Lens Disinfection

Hydrophilic lenses must be disinfected daily to avoid the risk of contamination by microorganisms. Many patients find boiling an unacceptable procedure, whilst others develop an adverse reaction to solutions. The efficacy of both methods has been criticized (Bernstein and Maddox, 1973; Bernstein, Stow and Maddox, 1973; Norton *et al.*, 1974).

Unknown but Limited Life Span

It is not possible to predict with certainty the life span of any given soft lens, but it is almost invariably less than that for a hard lens.

The Inability to Modify Soft Lenses

It has not proved practicable to modify either the power or fitting parameters of soft lenses. If the patient's refractive error should alter, a new lens becomes necessary.

Difficulty of Lens Checking and Verification

Methods for checking and verification of soft lenses have not yet proved straightforward for speedy use in the consulting room. Practitioners have been obliged to rely on the manufacturer's quality and control and skill in checking.

Vascularization and Other Pathological Complications

Long-term wear of hydrophilic lenses has produced limbal vascularization and nodules in a small number of patients. Secondary vernal conjunctivitis causing papillae of the upper palpebral conjunctiva and general conjunctival injection is another sequel to soft lens wear, as are stromal and endothelial disturbances of the cornea with rare cases of apparent endothelial detachment and of nummular keratitis (Allansmith *et al.*, 1977; Mackie, 1977). *Colour Plates XIX–XXII* show these conditions.

Chemical Contamination

It is possible for a hydrophilic lens to absorb chemicals into its naturally porous structure if worn in a polluted environment. These chemicals may be retained and become a future source of ocular irritation. It is not generally safe to use eyedrops while wearing soft lenses, since the preservatives may be similarly absorbed.

Increased Cost

Greater costs are incurred by both practitioner and patient when soft lenses are fitted.

PATIENT AND LENS SELECTION

With so many advantages and disadvantages, careful discussion is required with patients at the first consultation to determine their full history and discover their reasons for wanting to wear contact lenses. These aspects are fully covered in Chapters 7 and 8, Volume 1.

Generally, if a patient has not already tried a hard lens and is willing to persevere with the normal range of adaptive symptoms, a corneal lens should be the first choice. If patients have already failed with hard lenses, or their tolerance looks unpromising at the initial consultation, then soft lenses can be tried straight away. There are, in fact, many instances where a soft lens is the obvious choice with which to commence fitting. The various factors in evaluating this decision of hard or soft may be considered briefly under the headings of Ocular Factors and Non-ocular Factors.

Ocular Factors

Considerations here are the type and degree of astigmatism, the standard of vision likely to be obtained with a soft lens and, just as important, the standard of vision actually required by the patient. There is little point in insisting that a patient should obtain 6/5 acuity with a hard lens, when 6/9 is perhaps perfectly adequate for his or her needs. Corneal and lid sensitivity, accounting for the majority of hard lens failures, are equally important factors. A soft lens may well prove the answer in the type of case where a small corneal lens gives flare, but where a corneal lens of larger overall size causes oedema which cannot be resolved by improvements to the fit, or by fenestrations, or in which the fenestrations themselves are the cause of visual disturbance. Hydrophilic lenses should be considered for hyperopes and low myopes who may be unhappy with a corneal lens because of the relative thickness and weight, which in turn give rise to excessive lens mobility on blinking. Pupil size is important because flare with hard lenses is nearly always avoided with the larger optic diameter of a soft lens. Patients with awkward anatomical features for corneal lenses, such as proptosed eyes, a low lower lid position, or a decentred corneal apex may prove much more successful with a hydrophilic lens.

The presence of any abnormal ocular condition and other factors such as tears flow, should also be considered.

Non-ocular Factors

It is essential to determine from patients the reason for wanting contact lenses, and the regularity of wearing schedule which they intend to adopt. The irregular or intermittent wearer is ideally suited to soft lenses, particularly if sporting requirements demand a stable fitting. Economic factors must be taken into account, not only the higher fees for initial fitting, but also the long-term costs of future lens replacements, accessory solutions and cleaning agents. Geographic locations and working environment are important; whether they are hot or cold, humid or dry, dusty or clean, and whether they are likely to contain noxious fumes or chemicals. Airline crews have noted difficulty in the low humidity of aircraft cabins; Arias (1968, 1973) mentioned problems encountered in the high altitude of Mexico. This is not surprising, for Hill (1976b) has shown that in Mexico City the percentage of oxygen in the atmosphere is only 16 per cent compared with 21 per cent at sea level. On the summit of Mount Everest it is only 7 per cent, but Clarke (1976) has reported the successful use of Permalenses at up to 24,000 feet, some 5000 feet below the summit. In Australia something over 75 per cent of contact lenses fitted are hydrophilic because of their greater comfort in the dust and heat (Gilford, 1975).

The availability of lens disinfecting solutions, saline and distilled water must also be ascertained. Psychological factors should be considered for those patients who need the sense of security of a stable fitting lens which it is almost impossible to dislodge from the eye by accident, or for those who are temperamentally unsuitable to undergo the slow adaptation process required by hard lenses. Many patients find the insertion and removal of soft lenses rather easier than hard lenses.

CLASSIFICATION OF SOFT LENSES

Soft lenses can be classified in a number of different ways, as follows.

According to Method of Manufacture

Hydrophilic lenses were originally divided into spun-cast and lathe-cut. In practice, only the Bausch and Lomb Soflens and the original Czechoslovakian lenses are spun-cast, whereas almost all of the many other varieties are lathe-cut. The original 14.5 mm series of Bausch and Lomb Soflenses were hybrid in character, being lathe-cut after initial spin-casting. Silicone lenses are compression moulded in the same way as some hard lenses.

According to Water Content and Polymer

In this context the following definitions are used.

$$\% \text{ water content} = \frac{\text{wt of fully hydrated lens} - \text{wt of fully dehydrated lens}}{\text{wt of fully hydrated lens}} \times 100\%$$

British Standards recommend that this should apply to lenses under equilibrium conditions with normal physiological saline solution at a temperature of $20° \pm 0.5°C$.

$$\% \text{ water uptake} = \frac{\text{wt of fully hydrated lens} - \text{wt of fully dehydrated lens}}{\text{wt of fully dehydrated lens}} \times 100\%$$

Thus, a lens with a water content of 38 per cent has a water uptake of approximately 61 per cent. Care must be exercised when interpreting brand names which include a numerical suffix, since these do not always accurately reflect the water content. For example, Snoflex 50 and Mollitor 35 have true water contents of respectively 52 and 30 per cent.

Water contents vary from 3 to 85 per cent with an equally varied range of polymers, although nearly all of the successful lenses currently being fitted are HEMA-based. These include Menicon (Toyo material, 30 per cent) at the low end of the scale; Burton Parsons (35 per cent); the pure HEMA's, Hydron and Soflens (38 per cent); the cross-linked HEMA's, Aoflex, Aosoft, Hydroflex, and Weicon, (38–42 per cent). Low water content lenses are predominantly fitted at the moment because of their greater tensile strength and longer life span. They have the further advantage that they can be made thinner, because of their smaller swell factor during hydration. In addition, the various cleaning and rejuvenating agents have in the main been developed for HEMA-based materials.

The higher water content lenses are represented by Duragel, Permalens, Sauflon, Softcon and Snoflex. The 55 per cent Softcon (originally known as Bionite) is a graft polymer of polyHEMA and polyvinyl pyrrolidone. It has gained FDA approval as a corneal bandage lens. Sauflon, on the other hand, is a copolymer of polymethyl methacrylate and N-vinyl pyrrolidone, and is available in standard water contents of 55, 68 and 80 per cent. The first two are used mainly for daily wear, and the latter for 'continuous' wear. Duragel is available with water contents of 60 and 75 per cent for daily wear and extended wear respectively. Cross-linked terpolymers include Snoflex (52 per cent) for daily wear, and Permalens (74 per cent), containing N-vinyl pyrrolidone, for extended wear.

According to Size

On a purely clinical level lenses may be better classified according to overall size, depending on whether they are of semi-scleral or corneal diameter. The semi-scleral group includes Aoflex, Flexicon, Hydroflex, Hydron, Sauflon 70, Softcon, Snoflex and Weicon. They are normally fitted with overall sizes of between 13.00 mm and 16.00 mm,

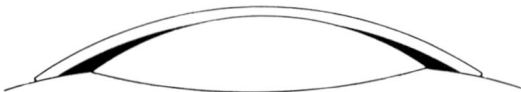

Figure 14.4—A semi-scleral soft lens giving apical and scleral touch but bridging the limbus region

and with back central optic radii from 0.6 mm to 1.50 mm flatter than flattest 'K'.* Their fitting philosophy is to give deliberate apical touch with further support beyond the limbus where they overlap on to the sclera (*see Figure 14.4*). The corneal group includes Aoflex/mini, Aosoft, Duragel, Hydran, Hydroflex/m, Permalens, Sauflex, Sauflon PW, Snoflex 50, Soflens, Mericon Soft

* 'K' is used to refer to the keratometer radius reading.

and Weicon/mini. These lenses have overall sizes between 11.5 and 13.5 mm to give complete corneal coverage but with minimum overlap. Back central optic radii are generally about 0.3 mm flatter than flattest 'K', but may be anything from 0.6 mm steeper to 0.6 mm flatter than 'K'.

According to Fitting Philosophy

Daily wear hydrophilic lenses may currently be grouped according to the way they are fitted into three distinct fitting philosophies, as follows.

CORNEAL DIAMETER LENSES

These are of low to medium water content, and are manufactured from materials of consistent quality to give reproducible lenses with good durability. They are small and thin to give a minimum of interference with the normal corneal metabolism, and excellent cosmetic appearance. They can be recommended for the majority of straightforward cases; patients with poor handling ability, particularly those with small palpebral apertures; and most of those cases prone to oedema with hard lenses. They may be contra-indicated for some patients with tight lids and shallow corneo-scleral junctions if these cause lens decentration and consequent visual problems, or peripheral arcuate staining. Patients with sensitive lids may find adaptation difficult because of the sensation experienced each time the lid margin crosses the edge of the lens on blinking.

SEMI-SCLERAL LENSES – LOW WATER CONTENT

These often give greater stability of vision and fit than corneal diameter lenses, and may be successful for patients with sensitive lids or limbus. They are also manufactured from consistent materials so that reproducibility and durability are good. They can be recommended for most straightforward myopic eyes, and are more likely to give satisfactory visual acuity than the corneal-sized lenses in cases of moderate astigmatism. Semi-scleral lenses necessarily have a greater thickness than corneal lenses, and may therefore be contra-indicated for patients with corneas susceptible to oedema. Many hard lens failures come within this category, so that a low water content semi-scleral lens is not necessarily the ideal choice for these patients, particularly if they are hyperopes or low to medium myopes, where the lens geometry is thickest and least flexible. Cosmetically, semi-scleral lenses are rather more noticeable in wear.

SEMI-SCLERAL LENSES – HIGH WATER CONTENT

Since not all patients can be satisfactorily fitted by the first two groups – perhaps failing with the one for visual reasons, and with the other because of oedema – a third type of lens is required. High water content semi-scleral lenses give not only stable fitting and vision, but also a much greater oxygen permeability, and in theory are potentially capable of successfully fitting the widest range of patients. They can be recommended for the majority of cases, including moderate degrees of astigmatism, and eyes prone to corneal oedema. In practice they must be contra-indicated for those with poor lens handling ability, for whom the breakage rate can be very high. Such lenses deteriorate with age more rapidly than those with low water content, and they are more susceptible to dimensional changes as a result of alterations in environmental conditions such as temperature and humidity. Reproducibility has also been found to be a problem because they are more difficult to manufacture and the material is more susceptible to variation between one batch and another.

It is significant that a fourth group of lenses is now beginning to emerge. These are of corneal diameter and high water content and represent the results of materials research and improved manufacturing methods.

VISUAL CONSIDERATIONS

The refractive result obtained with soft lenses, as opposed to hard lenses or spectacles, is neither fixed nor absolute. It may be of extreme variability, changing from moment to moment, or from day to day, depending on external environment and lens fitting and performance. The visual standard is very much a subjective interpretation by the patient, and does not necessarily correlate with the Snellen acuity on the letter chart. Applegate and Massof (1975), for example, found marked changes in contrast sensitivity although the visual acuity remained the same, stressing that acuity is only one aspect of visual performance. Similar conclusions were reached by Rosenblum and Leach (1975) with Bausch and Lomb Soflens patients. The defining of visual acuity therefore represents something of a problem, since the quality of vision is just as important as the precise number of lines read on the test chart. In some circumstances a good 6/9 may be more acceptable than a poor 6/6, so that Snellen acuity is not always a reliable guide to a patient's potential visual success with soft lenses. Practitioners are obliged to place more than usual reliance on the patient's subjective impression as to whether vision is good enough for his needs. This is especially true of near vision, and this factor must always be considered in relation to the patient's work and visual requirements. Variations of vision with hydrophilic lenses can be due to several different causes, as follows.

ENVIRONMENTAL FACTORS

The basic lens dimensions of back central optic radius, overall size and thickness can all vary with environmental factors. These include such ocular effects as temperature, pH and tonicity of the tears as well as the volume of tears produced. Some of these are in turn influenced by external factors such as ambient temperature, humidity, atmospheric pressure or the state of the lens when placed on the eye.

Generally, lenses manufactured from HEMA-based polymers undergo smaller variations than those made from high water content materials, as, for example, with the effect of temperature. Tonicity has been investigated by Poster and Skolnik (1974), who demonstrated a 1.6 per cent decrease in size when a Bausch and Lomb Soflens was taken from distilled water and placed in isotonic saline solution. A further decrease of 2.8 per cent occurred when the lens was transferred to hypertonic, 1.8 per cent, saline solution. Eriksen, Randeri and Ster (1972) also showed changes of size with polyHEMA lenses, but significantly greater changes with Bionite lenses. They also found that pH had little effect on the dimensions of polyHEMA lenses, but gave a measurable decrease in size for Bionite in acidic solution. Harris and Mock (1974) were able to demonstrate changes in both power and light transmission according to the tonicity of lens storage solutions. Ford (1974) has shown how the degree of lens hydration, and all of these other influences, can summate to give a significant error of power when a lens has fully settled on the cornea.

LENS FLEXURE AND OPTICAL CONSIDERATIONS (see also Chapter 4 in Volume 1, and Chapter 16)

A second possible cause of power change is the effect of lens flexure. This has been argued for all types of lenses, whether corneal or semi-scleral, and occurs when a flexible lens fitted either flatter or steeper than 'K' bends to conform to the corneal curvature. Wichterle (1967) gave a mathematical analysis of this effect, and in 1967 Vincent (Blackstone, 1968) reported that in practice the original Czechoslovakian lenses increased their effective negative power when allowed to steepen, and vice versa. Sarver, Ashley and Van Every (1974) described how a thin corneal-sized soft lens with back and front surface radii of 8.00 mm and 8.50 mm respectively increased its power from –3.25 D to –4.00 D when allowed to steepen by 1.00 mm, and he has proposed the term 'supplemental power effect'. This represents the total change in power, due first to lens flexure, and secondly to a liquid lens if the posterior surface of the contact lens fails to conform to the front surface of the cornea. In practice any supplemental power effect is likely to be created by a combination of these two causes, with the greater proportion resulting from flexure. On the assumption of a plano liquid lens, a constant centre thickness, and a change in front and back surface curvatures of exactly the same proportion, Strachan (1973) calculated the theoretical power changes caused by flexure for semi-scleral lenses; so that if a series of –2.00 D lenses of radii 7.5 mm, 7.8 mm, 8.1 mm and 8.4 mm were placed on the same 7.5 mm cornea, the resultant powers would be –2.00 D, –2.09 D, –2.13 D and –2.21 D. He concluded that both positive and negative lenses increase their power on steepening, in direct proportion to the degree of flexure, and to the power of the original lens. A more recent analysis by Bennett (1976), assuming only that the volume of the lens remains constant, has shown that refractive changes due to flexure are independent of power, and invariably add negative power. This closely agrees with the earlier analysis of Wichterle, as well as with Sarver's clinical findings.

Another variable factor which can affect the power of a hydrophilic lens is refractive index – see Table 4.10, page 111 in Chapter 4, Volume 1. Strachan (1973) evaluated a hypothetical case of a 60 per cent water content lens, with a refractive index of 1.52 in the dry state. When fully hydrated, this lens becomes a mixture of 40 per cent polymer (n = 1.52) and 60 per cent water (n = 1.333), with a resultant refractive index of 1.40. If the lens is in a state of partial dehydration on the eye the refractive index increases, with a consequent change of power. In Strachan's example, a –3.00 D lens becomes –3.12 D and –3.37 D, when the refractive index changes from 1.40 to 1.42 and 1.46 respectively; and conversely a +3.00 D lens alters its power to +3.18 D and +3.55 D respectively. Ford (1976) has demonstrated a typical water loss of 8.79 per cent when a 70 per cent water content soft lens reaches a state of equilibration on the eye, with the refractive index changing from 1.43 to 1.4397.

When a soft lens is placed on an astigmatic cornea, the final refractive result depends on the way in which the lens moulds itself to the corneal topography. If a lens partially dehydrates within the palpebral aperture, there can be an astigmatic power change due to alteration in the refractive index, and to the lens becoming less flexible meridionally, with differential power changes because of the resulting flexure. These effects tend to become very complicated, but they can sometimes partially neutralize corneal astigmatism, reducing it to a level suitable for soft lens fitting.

AGEING EFFECTS

Changes in visual acuity also occur with time and use. Discoloured lenses (*Colour Plate XXIII*), and

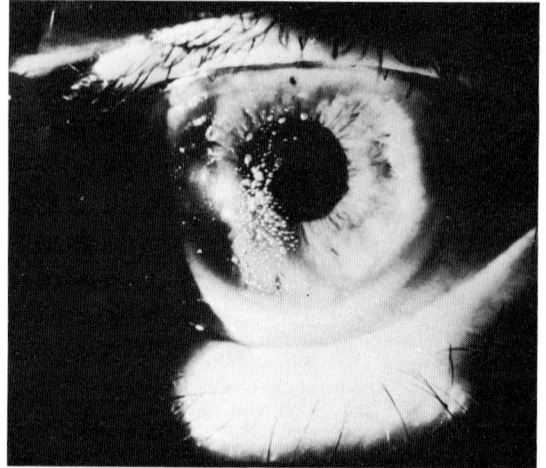

Figure 14.5—White spots (calcium) on a high water content soft lens (reproduced by kind permission of Contact Lenses (Manufacturing) Ltd.)

those affected by mucoprotein or calcium deposits from the tears, are commonly seen (*see Figure 14.5*). Such deposits and discoloration may sometimes cause a serious reduction in visual acuity. The fitting characteristics of these lenses may alter along with their state of hydration on the eye, presumably because of clogged surface pores. Refractive changes have been found, and marked differences shown in the light transmission curves between new and old lenses (Gasson, 1975).

OVER-REFRACTIONS*

The various factors already mentioned – environment, flexure, degree of hydration, ageing and dimensional changes – all combine to give a refractive result at a particular time for a particular set of conditions. It cannot be assumed that this refraction

*A refraction carried out when a contact lens is being worn is termed an 'over-refraction'.

will remain constant and it does frequently change by small amounts. If, for example, a patient should move from indoors to outdoors, temperature and humidity will alter, and the lenses must reach a new state of equilibration on the eye. Usually, no very great concern is caused, although there may be complaints of visual fluctuation, especially in the early days of wear when the tears flow has still not returned to normal.

If the over-refractions are carefully monitored, these changes can be easily demonstrated. Also, cylinder power and axis can both vary widely and apparently at random. There does not seem to be any correlation with 'K' readings (Larke and Sabell, 1971), and Gasson (1975) has shown the same type of variation with a series of different lens types on the same eye, and also with the same lens on the same eye examined on different occasions. It was originally held that thicker lenses would more effectively mask corneal astigmatism, transferring less cylinder through to the anterior surface of the soft lens but this has since been disproved (Morrison, 1973). It is now considered that thinner lenses are likely to give a better visual result, and that thicker lenses should be avoided for physiological, visual, and cosmetic reasons. Gasson (1976) found the acuities with ultra-thin Bausch and Lomb Soflenses of centre thickness only 0.04 mm, to be superior to those achieved with the equivalent lenses of standard thickness 0.14 mm. Morrison (1973) in a study of three HEMA based materials, found that neither thickness, diameter, power, water content nor method of manufacture, seemed to have an appreciable effect on the amount of astigmatism transferred to the front surface of the lens. When a soft lens is placed on the eye, the spherical anterior surface may become an aspheric or irregular curve with different optical qualities. Such effects are not predictable, so that the prescription and quality of vision must be determined empirically by placing lenses on the cornea. Even if the same over-refraction can be demonstrated with quite different designs of lens, it may be only one type of fitting which gives an acceptable visual result to the patient. Stability of vision is important, and semi-scleral lenses are often preferred by patients with higher degrees of astigmatism. It can be demonstrated that the addition of a quite small cylinder, perhaps only –0.50 D, can give a very significant improvement in acuity, eliminating ghosting and distortion. The typically small degree of residual astigmatism which can be easily ignored by both patient and practitioner when prescribing hard lenses, cannot always be so readily discounted with soft lenses. It is also found that the binocular visual acuity is frequently better out of all proportion to the monocular results, so that R. and L. 6/9–, may

well give 6/6+ binocularly. For this reason monocular patients are likely to be rather less happy with their soft lens visual acuity, particularly if they are wearing a toric soft lens where variations in vision are more common.

CORNEAL AND RESIDUAL ASTIGMATISM

Two basic assumptions should be made when assessing the potential success of astigmatic patients being fitted with spherical soft lenses.

(1) Total ocular astigmatism = corneal astigmatism + lenticular astigmatism.

(2) All corneal astigmatism is transferred through the lens to its anterior surface.

Patients may therefore be divided into the following four groups at their initial examination by reference to spectacle correction and 'K' readings.

Spherical Cornea with Spherical Refraction

Rx: –3.00 DS
'K': 7.85 mm along 180, (43.00 D); 7.85 mm along 90, (43.00 D).

This is the ideal situation for contact lens fitting. Vision should be equally good with either hard or soft lenses.

Spherical Cornea with Astigmatic Refraction

Rx: –2.00/–1.75 × 90
'K': 7.85 mm along 180, (43.00 D); 7.90 mm along 90, (42.75 D).

The astigmatism is almost entirely lenticular, so that the visual result is the same with either hard or soft lenses. A front surface toric lens, hard or soft, should be used to correct the 1.50 D of residual astigmatism.

Astigmatic Cornea with Astigmatic Refraction

Rx: –2.00/–1.75 × 180
'K': 7.80 mm along 180, (43.25 D); 7.50 mm along 90, (45.00 D).

All of the astigmatism is corneal, so that a spherical hard lens, or a toroidal soft lens should be fitted.

Astigmatic Cornea with Spherical Refraction

Rx: –3.00 DS
'K': 7.80 mm along 180, (43.25 D); 7.50 mm along 90, (45.00 D).

In this example there is 1.75 D of with-the-rule

corneal astigmatism together with an equivalent degree of against-the-rule lenticular astigmatism, to give a resultant spherical refraction. A hard lens would leave a residual cylinder of -1.75×90. A soft lens, *because* it transfers all of the corneal astigmatism through to its front surface without optically neutralizing it, is the lens of choice.

These theoretical considerations should be confirmed by clinical observation with a soft lens placed on the eye. The arbitrary figure of 1.50 D ocular astigmatism is frequently given as the upper limit for which good visual acuity can be obtained with a spherical hydrophilic lens. In practice this limit can be as low as 0.50 D or 0.75 D for patients who are critical observers, accustomed to good vision and required by their occupation to undertake exacting visual tasks. Conversely, satisfactory acuity has occasionally been obtained with cylinders as high as 4.00 D for less critical and strongly motivated patients. In these cases the distance visual acuity is usually more acceptable than that for near. However, with such high astigmatism success is unlikely, and patients should not be unduly encouraged. Nevertheless, it is worthwhile trying a spherical lens, especially with those for whom all other considerations, including perhaps hard lens failure, indicate a soft lens, and where time and expense rule out a toric soft lens fitting. In order to make a proper assessment, trial lenses should be as close as possible to the expected prescription. Because lenses are fitted flatter than flattest 'K', the most satisfactory vision is usually obtained for myopic patients with the least negative focal line on the retina, rather than with the predicted best vision sphere. For example, spectacle Rx $-3.50/-1.00 \times 180$; likely BVP of soft lens: -3.50 DS. In borderline cases, plano-cylindrical spectacles can be worn for critical vision and driving, and cylinders may be incorporated into a normal presbyopic correction.

NEAR VISION PROBLEMS

When prescribing soft lenses, near vision should be carefully assessed as a separate function from distance acuity. Frequently, patients who can wear soft lenses comfortably and see well for distance, find their near vision completely unsatisfactory. Clinical results show that the deciding factor for soft lens success or failure can often be the quality of near vision, especially if it interferes with work or study. There are many causes of near vision difficulty. Stone (1967), in an assessment of this problem with hard lenses, suggested four main reasons, as follows.

(1) Alteration in the accommodation-convergence relationship.
(2) Reduced size of palpebral aperture.
(3) Reduced evaporation of tears.
(4) Alteration in corneal curvature during convergence.

From their very nature, the last three of these effects are likely to be of greater significance with hydrophilic lenses, but there are several other more important possible causes, any or all of which could produce problems.

(1) Questionable acuity for distance.
(2) Lid pressure, causing irregular buckling or flexure of the lens with the eyes in the near vision position.
(3) Irregular astigmatism at near.
(4) Reduced blink rate, causing drying of the lens surface.
(5) Changes in scleral topography during convergence.
(6) A decentred lens.
(7) A poor fitting.

VISUAL ADVANTAGES OF SOFT LENSES

Despite all the visual problems which can arise, the majority of patients do achieve a good and worthwhile standard of vision. Indeed, many claim that their quality of vision and field of view are better with soft lenses than with either hard lenses or spectacles. Their size and stability of fitting ensure that hydrophilic lenses have certain natural advantages over corneal lenses. There is a significant reduction in the incidence of flare and peripheral reflections, especially at night or in dim illumination when the pupils are enlarged. Patients adapting to soft lenses, which have relatively large optic diameters, rarely complain of the flare so commonly observed with hard lenses. For those with naturally large pupils and where corneal lenses cannot be made to give satisfactory centration a hydrophilic lens may be the only means of eliminating intolerable visual disturbance. Many patients wearing conventionally fitted hard lenses of positive or low negative power find the constantly altering vision, which is unstable after blinking, quite unacceptable. The soft lens with its very limited vertical movement nearly always provides a satisfactory solution.

SPECIAL METHODS APPLICABLE TO SOFT LENS FITTING

Soft lens fitting employs certain techniques additional to those routinely used with hard lenses.

SLIT LAMP TECHNIQUES

Pachymetry (*see* Chapter 5, Volume 1)

If increased corneal thickness is to be used as a potential indicator of oedema, a pachymeter attachment to the slit lamp is required (Stone, 1974).

Photography (*see* Chapter 6, Volume 1)

The use of clinical photography permits a permanent record to be maintained of the eye and its vascular state prior to fitting.

Graticules

A calibrated graticule in the slit lamp eyepiece can be used to assess both the corneal diameter, and the overall size of a soft lens in wear.

PLACIDO DISC, AND KLEIN KERATOSCOPE

These simple devices permit a qualitative assessment to be made of the regularity of the anterior surface of a soft lens whilst it is being worn. Any

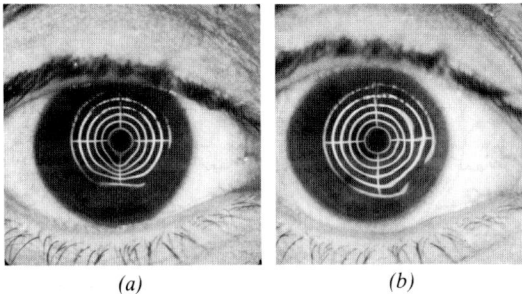

(a)   *(b)*

Figure 14.6—Photokeratoscopy showing distortion from the front surfaces of steeply fitted soft lenses during wear. (a) A high water content 'extended' wear lens of corneal size. (b) A low water content semi-scleral lens

noticeable distortion of image quality suggests a poor fitting, and is likely to be accompanied by poor subjective acuity (*see Figure 14.6a* and *b*).

LENS VERIFICATION

The instruments for this purpose are fully described in Chapter 15, but those commonly used for reasonably fast verification in the consulting room are: test spheres for radius and overall size; a soft lens radiuscope, either dry or wet cell; a vertex distance compensator for use with a focimeter; and a projection magnifier for diameter measurements and for assessing lens condition. The last-named is particularly useful in the consulting room, for demonstrating to patients any flaws which may have developed in the surfaces or edge of a lens.

CONSULTING ROOM PROCEDURES AND EQUIPMENT

Practitioners must ensure a readily available supply of normal saline solution. This may be obtained in made-up form in either bottles or sacs as used in hospitals for drip-feeding (*see* page 73, Chapter 3, Volume 1). Such saline solution may or may not be preserved. Alternatively, a less expensive method is to prepare it fresh each day with salt tablets and distilled water. The solution must then be boiled to make sure that it is sterile. This is the same procedure as that normally recommended to patients, except that a larger calibrated bottle is more usefully employed.

Lenses are most easily extracted from their vials by means of soft-ended plastics tweezers or a glass rod. For the more fragile high water content lenses, the complete contents of the vial should be tipped into a small dish. This has the additional advantage of making sure that the storage solution is changed on each occasion that the lens is used, and is therefore a good procedure to adopt with any type of lens. Additional screw-cap 10 cc bottles are useful for storing patients' lenses when they are removed during an after-care examination, or if lenses are retained for cleaning and rejuvenation. For the latter purpose a small hot-plate or magnetic stirrer may be required, together with a large heat sterilizer or autoclave for disinfecting several trial lenses at the same time. The smaller pharmaceutical vials require a crimping device for re-sealing their metal caps. Since many soft lenses are not marked and are therefore unidentifiable without time-consuming measurement, self-adhesive labels are extremely useful for the identification of lenses temporarily stored in otherwise plain bottles. A selection of lens vials is shown in *Figure 14.7*.

ASSESSMENT OF TEARS FLOW

It is important to be able to recognize dry-eyed patients with inadequate tears flow, as they are very likely to develop into problem cases. Schirmer's Test (*Figure 14.8*) is the most commonly used method of measuring tears output and is described in Chapter 2, Volume 1, page 53. However, it is not

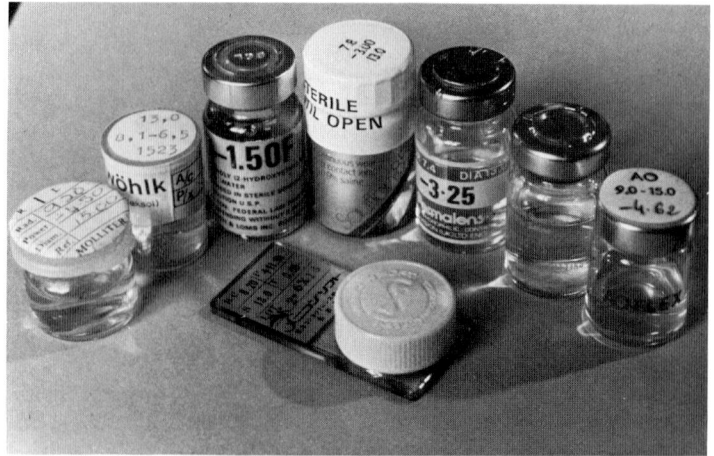

Figure 14.7—A selection of vials for soft lenses as supplied by various manufacturers

always a reliable method, unless very carefully carried out, and other tests are probably preferable. Ordinary fluorescein canbe used as a simple diagnostic test by observing the break-up time of the pre-corneal film which is normally about 8 μm (microns) thick (Rengstorff, 1974). A small drop of fluorescein is instilled into the lower fornix, and the patient instructed to blink several times, and then stare straight ahead. Observation is made with the slit lamp at about x15 magnification, using the blue filter. Break-up of the pre-corneal film is easily seen by the presence of dark areas against the otherwise bright green background as shown in *Colour Plate XXVb*. A break-up time of 10–60 seconds is fairly common. If it is more rapid than 10 seconds, a deficiency of either the volume or wetting properties of the tears is indicated (*see* Chapter 7, Volume 1).

Norn (1974) has described a more elaborate, quantitative, procedure, whereby fluorescein is mixed with 1 per cent rose bengal. The colour of the composite stain is evaluated according to a time scale related to the dilution effect of tears flow on a single 10 μl drop instilled into the conjunctival sac (*Table 14.1*). Observation with the slit lamp is made on the lacrimal rivus in the central portion of the lower lid after exactly 5 minutes. Ford (1974) has further extended this technique to give the predicted water loss from a hydrophilic lens during wear,

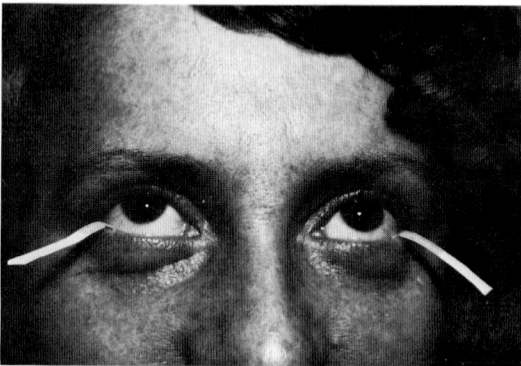

(a)

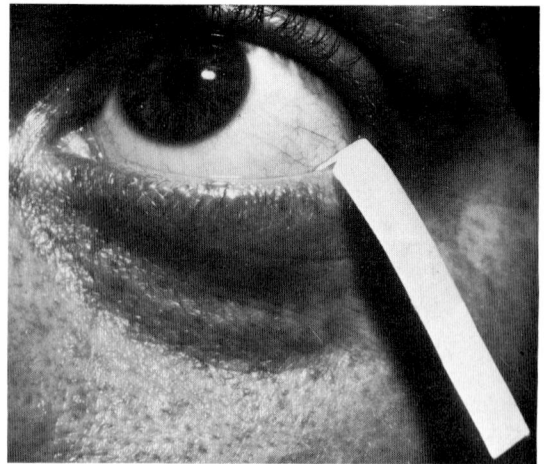

(b)

Figure 14.8—Schirmer's test showing how the tears fluid wets the paper strips. (a) Being carried out on both eyes at once. (b) Close-up of one eye. This is best carried out on one eye at a time with the patient looking up and in, as shown in (b). The normal output for a young adult is 15 mm of the paper strip wetted in 5 minutes or 10 mm wetted in 3 minutes. Measurement is made from the notch at the lid margin

Table 14.1–Tears Dilution Test (After Norn and Ford)

Group	Colour	Dilution	Indicated tears flow per hour	Water loss (from 70 per cent water contact lens)
1	Intense red	Insignificant	<0.18 ml (3 drops)	
2	Pale red	4–1	0.36 ml (6 drops)	13–23 per cent
3	Intense orange	16–1	1.8 ml (30.6 drops)	5–12 per cent
4	Weak orange	64–1	7.6 ml (128 drops)	<5 per cent
5	Yellow	256–1	30.6 ml (520 drops)	

thereby enabling him to calculate the probable change of power caused by lens dehydration.

Norn (1974) has also discussed the use of bromothymol blue as a pH indicator for the tears in the range 6.8–7.6, as shown in *Table 14.2*. The colour is assessed after exactly 5 seconds, before carbon dioxide from the tears renders the lacrimal rivus more alkaline.

ASSESSMENT OF LIMBAL TOPOGRAPHY

Chapters 9, 10 and 11 (Volume 1) on scleral and corneal lens fitting commenced by stressing the respective importance of scleral and corneal topography. In the fitting of soft lenses these factors are no less important, but practitioners are also concerned with those aspects of global topography which it is least easy to quantify and measure. These are the diameter of the cornea, the rate of flattening of the corneal periphery and the configuration of the corneo-scleral junction, all of which can only be assessed by observation rather than by direct measurement. They can often account for the unusual behaviour of a soft lens, and explain why two eyes with the same refractive error and keratometric readings may require soft lenses with completely different specifications in order to establish a satisfactory fit.

Corneal diameter is usually measured as the visible iris diameter, and varies from 10 to 14 mm, with an average of 12 mm. Direct measurement with, for example, a graticule in the slit lamp eyepiece, only gives an assessment of the dimensions concerned, since it is not truly possible to ascertain exactly where the cornea finishes and the sclera begins. The horizontal axis is normally longer than the vertical by about 0.5–1.0 mm. The effective corneal diameter is perhaps best evaluated by placing a corneal soft lens of known overall size on the eye and examining it *in situ*.

Peripheral flattening of the cornea can be studied with the topographic keratometer (Sampson and Soper, 1970), but this can be time-consuming to undertake routinely. Alternatively, the Photo-Electric Keratoscope (PEK) may be used (Bibby, 1976). Limbal topography can also be assessed by observing the continuity of a slit beam as it crosses the corneo-scleral junction, and is most easily seen with a vertical slit at the lower limbus with the patient looking upwards. The reflection of a Placido disc at the limbus is also helpful in assessing its contour (*Figure 14.9*) in which the patient's gaze is directed slightly upwards. A corneal diameter lens

Table 14.2–Bromothymol Blue as a pH Indicator for Tears

pH	Colour of tears
≤6.8	Yellow
7.0	Yellowish-green
7.2	Green
7.4	Greenish-blue
≥7.6	Blue

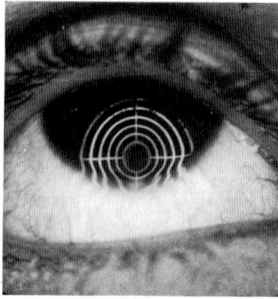

Figure 14.9—Limbal topography as shown by reflection from an A.I.M. photokeratoscope. The patient is looking up at the fourth ring from the centre

on an eye with a shallow corneo-scleral junction typically decentres and lags more easily than when the junction is well defined.

THE USE OF FLUORESCEIN IN FITTING

Ordinary fluorescein with a molecular weight of 376.27 cannot be used with hydrophilic lenses because it will be absorbed into the porous structure of the material. Except for high water content polymers, from which the colour may gradually fade, the lenses can be permanently stained. Since the fluorescein in any case rapidly spreads behind, in front and within the lens, it would be of little use. There have now appeared various forms of high molecular weight fluorescein, such as Fluoflex and Fluorexon, whose molecular size is sufficiently great to prevent immediate penetration into the soft lens material. Fluorexon was introduced in 1972 by Refojo and others (Refojo, Korb and Silverman, 1972; Refojo, Miller and Fiore, 1972). It has a molecular weight of 710.47 and the full chemical name is bis-(N,N-bis (carboxymethyl)-aminoethyl) – fluorescein tetrasodium (Refojo, Miller and Fiore, 1972; Mossé and Scott, 1976). The degree of fluorescence, however, is much less than with standard fluorescein, and the fitting pattern difficult to observe and of doubtful value with a standard ultra-violet light. Poster (1977) found much better clinical results using Kodak Wratten filter No. 47. Nevertheless, such dyes have been recommended for use in practice to demonstrate tears flow (Rocher, 1977). One or two drops are instilled into the lower fornix, and the eye observed after a few blinks. If fluorescein can then be seen beneath the lens, it confirms that an interchange of tears occurs on blinking. If no fluorescein is observed, it suggests that the fitting is too tight, and the lens periphery is creating a seal where the edge of the lens rests against the bulbar conjunctiva.

CLINICAL ROUTINE

The complete clinical routine in the consulting room consists of the following steps, elaborated further in Chapters 7 and 8, Volume 1, and on subsequent pages here, and in Chapter 16.

(1) The taking of general and optical history.

(2) A complete routine refraction examination, including all the usual procedures such as ophthalmoscopy and tests of binocular function.

(3) Keratometry.

(4) Preliminary external eye examination, including slit lamp examination and other techniques as outlined on page 410 onwards.

(5) Discussion with the patient of lens types, and the decision to fit soft rather than other types of contact lens.

(6) The decision as to which variety of soft lens should be fitted or tried initially.

(7) Insertion of lenses.

(8) Initial assessment of fitting and vision.

(9) Tolerance trial.

(10) Re-assessment of vision, fitting and lens type.

(11) Re-examination with slit lamp.

(12) Ordering of lenses.

(13) Dispensing of lenses and patient instruction.

(14) After-care examinations.

PRELIMINARY EXAMINATION

The first important steps are refraction, recording of monocular and binocular acuities and keratometry. These are all especially important with soft lens fitting, because an early assessment of visual suitability has to be made with respect to corneal and refractive astigmatism. A detailed slit lamp examination should then be made, paying particular attention to the limbus and perilimbal blood vessels. If it is intended to insert soft lenses shortly afterwards, fluorescein and rose bengal should not be used at this stage. However, they should be employed where the possibility of some prevailing corneal or conjunctival condition is indicated, warranting a more definite diagnosis before fitting can be safely commenced. Thus, in cases where these dyes are used, to prevent their absorption into the lens, the conjunctival sac should be irrigated with saline solution afterwards and fitting delayed for at least two hours. External eye examination should include eversion of the upper lid to confirm the normality of the palpebral conjunctiva (Allansmith *et al.*, 1977), and an assessment of the patient's tears flow, either by Schirmer's test or, better, by direct observation of the pre-corneal film (McDonald, 1969). An estimate of the horizontal corneal diameter is made and, if part of the normal routine, clinical photography and pachymetry are carried out prior to fitting.

INSERTION OF LENSES

Lenses may be inserted by the practitioner in a variety of ways. Those of corneal size may be handled in much the same way as a hard lens, and placed directly onto the cornea. Lenses are, however, temporarily unstable at the moment of insertion if an air bubble should be trapped behind, and they may be expelled by an involuntary blink. The risk of this occurring is reduced if patients are requested to look down with gentle eye closure after insertion. A second method is for the patient to look upwards at some suitable fixation target, and then to place the lens onto the inferior sclera, from which it will position itself correctly on the cornea when the eye turns to the primary position. A further method, and probably the most suitable for the larger, semi-scleral lenses, is to have the patient look down and nasally, whilst the lens is placed on the upper temporal sclera. It may then easily be slid across into the correct position. In some cases, where the palpebral aperture is small, it may be necessary to partially fold the lens between finger and thumb so as to effectively reduce its overall size during insertion. Alternatively, it is sometimes helpful to balance the lens between the first and second fingers during insertion, particularly if it is a high positive lens, and unstable on only one finger because of its weight and the steep curvature of the lenticular portion of the front surface. In all cases, there is less likelihood of the lens falling off the practitioner's finger or fingers if the patient's head is tilted slightly forward.

Certain of the proprietary solutions for storing hydrophilic lenses may cause some degree of stinging, so that lenses should be cleaned and rinsed with normal saline solution prior to insertion. This also removes any particles which may be present on the lens surfaces. Care should be taken to avoid touching the back surface of the lens after it has been rinsed. Once the lens has assumed its correctly centred position on the cornea the patient should be no more than slightly aware of its presence. Any significant level of discomfort is likely to be due to a foreign body trapped behind the lens. This may have been a speck of dust or make-up carried in, for example, from the eyelashes, or it may have been already present in the tears film and subsequently trapped by the lens. If discomfort is only mild, and patients sometimes describe this foreign body sensation as stinging, the lens should be slid onto the temporal sclera with a circular motion, and allowed to recentre. This wiping action is usually sufficient to eliminate the cause of the discomfort, but if it persists the lens should be removed from the eye, cleaned and re-inserted. Removal can sometimes be effected by the hard lens method of applying lid tension, but a much simpler technique is to slide the lens onto either the temporal or inferior sclera from where it is pinched directly out of the eye. Although not ideal, suction holders can be used, if necessary, as described in Chapter 8, Volume 1.

INITIAL ASSESSMENT OF FITTING AND VISION

When a hydrophilic lens is removed from its vial it is fully hydrated with the maximum water uptake permitted by its particular storage medium. The lens, in settling on the eye, loses water by evaporation from its anterior surface, and by the squeezing action of the eyelids. Some part, but not all, of this water loss is replenished by normal tears flow, until a state of equilibrium has been achieved for the

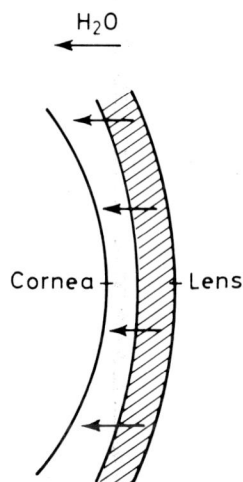

Figure 14.10—A soft lens stored in hypotonic saline solution adhering to the cornea due to the osmotic pressure difference which encourages water to enter the cornea from the lens. The application of normal saline solution eventually restores the osmotic balance permitting the lens to be removed

environmental conditions prevailing in the consulting room. At the same time, the lens is adjusting to the temperature of the cornea, and to the pH and tonicity of the tears. The movement of the lens, and therefore its fitting characteristics, unless grossly loose or tight cannot be reliably judged for at least 20 minutes, until this state of equilibrium on the cornea has been reached. The vision, on the other hand, if it is going to prove satisfactory usually settles within the first 5 minutes, although the refractive result is not necessarily accurate after so short a time. If the visual acuity is initially poor it is unlikely to improve and the lens should be changed.

In some instances, particularly with the smaller and less rigid corneal diameter lenses, false fitting results can occur. A lens sometimes settles within its storage vial so as to adhere to the base, neck or lid. It therefore has a temporarily distorted shape, unrelated to its true fitting parameters, and its behaviour on the eye may be very different from that of the same lens in an unstressed state. Similarly, if a lens has been disinfected by heating and not allowed sufficient time to cool and revert to its proper shape, it may well appear to fit too tightly. The same effect can be produced by a lens stored in hypotonic saline solution, which may sometimes even give a temporary osmotic adhesion to the cornea, requiring the liberal application of normal saline solution for release. This situation is illustrated in *Figure 14.10*.

CHARACTERISTICS OF A GOOD FITTING

A lens which is fitting well is comfortable in all directions of gaze, gives complete corneal coverage, and appears properly centred. Normal blinking results in about 1 mm of vertical movement when the eye is in the primary position. The lens lags by up to 1.5 mm on lateral movements of the eye, and also when looking upwards. Vision is good, remaining stable on blinking. Refraction gives a precise

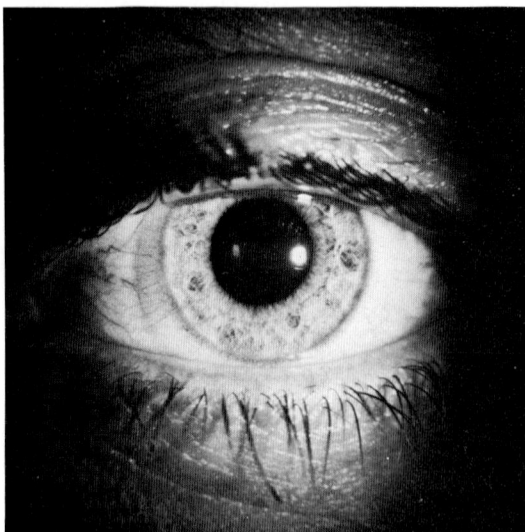

Figure 14.11—Nasal scleral indentation following the wearing of a tight semi-scleral lens

end-point, correlating with the BVP of the spectacles. The retinoscopy reflex is crisp and sharp both before and after a blink. Keratometry of the front surface of the lens on the eye shows the mires to be stable and undistorted. The slit lamp shows no irritation of the limbal vessels or compression of the conjunctiva.

CHARACTERISTICS OF A STEEP (TIGHT) FITTING

A lens fitting too steeply gives little or no movement either on blinking, or as the eye changes fixation. Initially, a tight fitting is quite comfortable, sometimes more so than a correct fit, because a completely immobile lens produces the minimum of lid sensation. Centration is usually good, although a corneal-sized lens may sometimes assume a decentred position. This is easily differentiated from a decentred flat fitting because of the lack of movement. The slit lamp may show irritation of the conjunctival or limbal vessels and, with very tight semi-scleral lenses, an annular ring of conjunctival compression may be seen, which is often visible even after the lens has been removed (*Figure 14.11*).

A steep fitting soft lens vaults the corneal apex, but is momentarily pressed onto the eye on blinking. Vision is therefore unstable and of poor quality, although showing some transient improvement after a blink. Subjective refraction is difficult, with no clearly defined end-point, and more negative power than predicted may be required because of a positive liquid lens. Retinoscopy reflex and keratometer mires both show irregular distortions such as those indicated by photokeratoscopy in *Figure 14.6a* and *b*. They may also improve momentarily on blinking.

CHARACTERISTICS OF A FLAT FITTING

A flat fitting is more easily diagnosed because of the absence of proper centration, greater lens mobility on blinking, and excessive lag on lateral eye movements as shown in *Figure 14.12*. Such a fit is often very uncomfortable, especially on looking upwards, when the lens may slide down 3 mm or more, and catch against the upper lid on blinking. In the primary position, lower lid sensation is experienced if the lens sags, and discomfort is accentuated if the lens is so flat that the periphery buckles to give edge stand-off. Vision and over-refraction are variable, but nevertheless may still give a satisfactory result. The retinoscopy reflex may be clear centrally but with peripheral distortion. Keratometry mires change according to lens movement, showing an

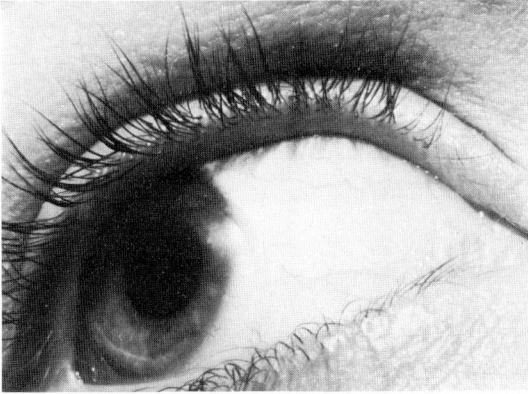

Figure 14.12—A flat-fitting spun-cast lens of corneal size showing excessive lag on temporal excursion of the eye. The edge of the lens is clearly visible

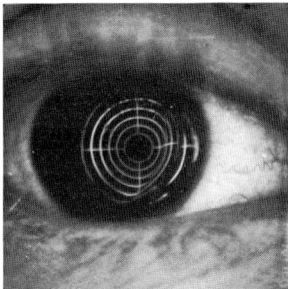

Figure 14.13—An eye wearing a flat-fitting low water content lens of corneal size. The photokeratoscope shows up the peripheral distortion

eccentric shape on blinking. *Figure 14.13* shows the photokeratoscope image from a flat lens, the peripheral distortion being most marked.

The above information is summarized in *Table 14.3*.

METHODS OF OBSERVING THE FIT

Lens movement and position are most easily observed with white light by using the slit lamp and low magnification. The action of the lens edge on blinking can be judged in relation to the position of the limbal vessels. In some eyes with rather loose conjunctival tissue, however, the appearance can be misleading. Movement of possibly even a tightly fitted lens maybe attributed to the lens when it is, in fact, motion of the bulbar conjunctiva. A further indication of fit may be obtained by using ×35 or ×40 magnification and observing the passage of

blood through the limbal vessels beneath the lens edge, to ensure that there is no obstruction to its normal steady flow. Without a slit lamp, lens movement is best seen by directing the beam from a hand-held pen torch, not necessarily from in front, but from the side or below so that the junction of the lenticular portion of the lens casts an easily observed annular light pattern and shadow onto the iris background (*see Colour Plate XXIV*). The movement of this is more easily discernible than that of the lens itself. A further simple test for semi-scleral lenses is to slide the lens gently onto the temporal sclera, two-thirds of the way off the cornea, and to observe the way in which it recentres. A correctly fitting lens has a quick recovery movement, whereas that of a flat fitting is considerably more sluggish. A steep lens, although recentring sharply, may be difficult to slide off the cornea.

Since most fitting criteria relate to lens movement and quality of vision, the two most important fitting instruments become the slit lamp and the retinoscope.

TOLERANCE TRIAL

Once the initial fitting characteristics have been confirmed as satisfactory, ideally the next stage of the clinical routine is a long tolerance trial of about 4 hours, using lenses of power as nearly correct as possible. A stock system of lenses with a wide range of variables is most suitable for this purpose. Patients can then be sent away to do a whole morning's or afternoon's work in their usual daily environment, carrying out their normal visual tasks. In this way a fairly reliable assessment is possible of their potential success, and latent problems such as dry eyes or near vision difficulty may be discovered. A long tolerance trial is especially important for previous hard lens failures so that on the one hand the practitioner can be sure of a satisfactory result, and on the other, the patient may be reassured with regard to contact lenses in the light of earlier failure. After the trial, fitting and refraction are carefully re-assessed. Any marked deterioration in visual acuity suggests the fitting was too steep. This can occur when the initial increased tears output permits exaggerated lens movement to be observed at first and then, when the tears flow returns to normal, the fit is seen to be tight. Examination of the eye itself should confirm the absence of corneal oedema and striae, punctate epithelial staining with fluorescein, limbal and conjunctival irritation and scleral indentation. If any elevations of the upper palpebral conjunctiva had been previously noted, the lids should be everted to make sure that there is no staining of these areas with fluorescein.

Table 14.3–Fitting Characteristics of Soft Lenses

	Good fit	*Steep fit*	*Flat fit*
Comfort	Good	Good, initially	Poor
Centration	Good, with complete corneal coverage	Usually good, may be decentred, but no recovery on blinking	Poor
Movement on blinking	Up to 1.0 mm	Less than 0.5 mm	Excessive, over 2.0 mm
Movement on upwards gaze	Up to 1.5 mm	Little or none	Excessive, over 3.0 mm
Movement on lateral gaze	Up to 1.5 mm	Little or none	Excessive, over 3.0 mm
Vision	Good	Poor and variable, momentary improvement on blinking	Variable, may improve on staring after blinking
Over-refraction	Precise end-point, power correlates with BVP of spectacle *Rx*	Poorly defined end-point, positive liquid lens	Variable, negative liquid lens
Retinoscopy reflex	Clear reflex, before and after blinking	Poor and distorted, central shadow, momentarily improved on blinking	Variable, may be clear centrally with peripheral distortion
Slit lamp after settling	No limbal injection or scleral indentation	Conjunctival or limbal injection, scleral indentation	Localized limbal injection, possible edge stand-off
Keratometer mires	Sharp, stable before and after blinking	Irregular, momentary improvement on blinking	Variable and eccentric, changing on blinking
Placido disc	Regular image	Irregular image anywhere but at the edge of the lens	Irregular image, more often peripheral only but occasionally central as well

At this stage the clinical decision can usually be made as to whether the patient is suitable for hydrophilic lenses. In cases of doubt, either visual or physiological, the tolerance trial should be repeated on another occasion. If possible, patients are loaned lenses of optimum fitting and power for several days, in order to extend the trial period. This procedure is straightforward if lenses are fitted from stock, or if the manufacturer concerned operates a lens exchange system.

In ordering the final lenses, it is advantageous, whenever feasible, to prescribe the same for right and left eyes. There is then no problem of identification if lenses are inadvertently switched by the patient.

LENS TYPES AND METHODS OF FITTING

It is not possible in this chapter to include a detailed description of the fitting procedures for each and every soft lens currently available. Earlier lens designs have been improved on or discontinued whilst new varieties are constantly being introduced.

The lenses described here, although mostly relating to an individual laboratory, have been chosen as typical examples of the many lenses of the same general type. Thus, Snoflex 38 is typical of low water content semi-scleral lenses; Sauflon of high water content semi-scleral lenses; and Hydroflex/m of low water content corneal fittings. It should therefore be possible to deduce the fitting method for any soft lens not specifically named here, by relating it to the general fitting principles described. Certain types, such as Bausch and Lomb Soflenses, are unique in their approach and must be considered separately.

A list of commonly available lenses is shown in *Table 14.4* together with some of their salient features, and *Figure 14.14a* shows the relationship between the equivalent oxygen performance and lens thickness for some of the available hydrophilic and hard lens materials (cf. Chapter 13, pages 389 and 395, and page 444 of this chapter). *Figure 14.14b* gives an idea of the relationship between equivalent oxygen performance and oxygen permeability over a similar range of lens thickness, the figures being based on a pilot study by Loshaek and Hill (1977). They point out that the information given in this figure is based on a limited amount of data, and may need slight amendment as more data become available.

SEMI-SCLERAL LENSES*

SNOFLEX 38

Snoflex 38 lenses were introduced to the United Kingdom early in 1972 under the original name of Hydron. They are now manufactured by Smith and Nephew, and are typical of other low water content semi-scleral lenses. Hydron is the registered trademark of the National Patents Development Corporation, the American company which acquired the manufacturing and distribution rights for those

---

*British Standard 3521:1979 refers to the lenses to be described under this heading (which is commonly used in the United Kingdom) as soft hydrophilic scleral lenses.

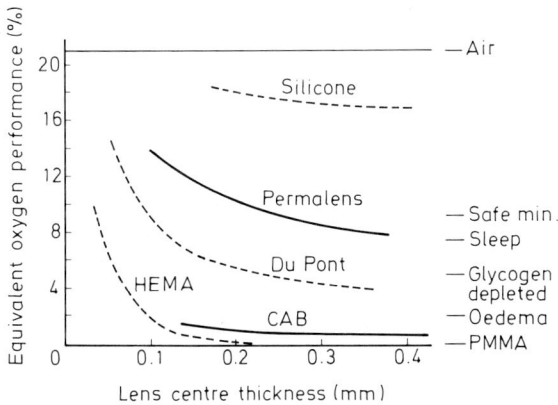

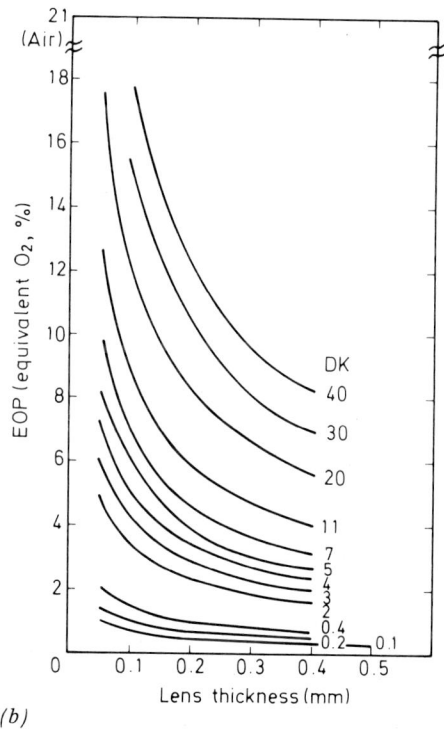

(a)   *(b)*

Figure 14.14–(a) A comparison of the equivalent oxygen performances of several general classes of hard and soft contact lens materials. Performances vary within a given class depending on differences in the particular material and lens fabrication techniques used by each manufacturing laboratory. No account has been taken of any mechanical 'pump' effect under the lens. (By 'equivalent oxygen performance' is meant that the cornea responds as if it were in an atmosphere containing that particular percentage of oxygen) (after Hill, R. M. 1977.) (b) The calculated curves of equivalent oxygen performance (EOP) responses anticipated for materials with various permeability constants (DK) measured at 23°C in units $\times 10^{-11}$ (cm^2/sec) (ml O$_2$/ml mm Hg), over the range of lens thicknesses shown (after Loshaek and Hill, 1977)

Table 14.4—Salient Features of Some Commonly Available Soft Lenses

Name of lens	Manufacturer (of polymer)	Nature of polymer	Water content (percentage)	Oxygen permeability $\times 10^{-11}$ (cm²/sec) (ml O_2/ml mm Hg) at 20°C unless otherwise stated	Fitting method	Remarks
Aoflex	American Optical	HEMA	40.0	7.3	Large Semi-scleral	
Aoflex/mini	American Optical	HEMA	40.0	7.3	Corneal	
Aosoft	American Optical	Terpolymer of HEMA NVP MMA	42.5	Not available	Corneal	Also supplied under the name Aquaflex
Aquaflex	UCO Optics	Terpolymer of HEMA NVP MMA	42.5	Not available	Corneal	Also supplied under the name Aosoft
Consoft	Toyo	HEMA	29.6 34.6	5.85	Corneal Corneal	
Duragel	Global Vision Ltd.	Amido-amino copolymer with tertiary amines	60.0 75.0	13.9 34.9*	Corneal Corneal	Suitable for extended wear
Durasoft	Wesley-Jessen	HEMA copolymer	30.0	3.0 at 25°C	Corneal	
Flexsol 35	Burton Parsons	HEMA	35.0	Not available	Large Semi-scleral	
Hoya	Hoya Lens Corporation	HEMA copolymer	35.0	Not available	Corneal	
Hydrocurve	Soft Lenses Inc.	HEMA + NVP	45.0	Not available	Semi-scleral	
Hydrocurve 11	Soft Lenses Inc.	HEMA + acrylamide	45.0	Not available	Semi-scleral	
Hydroflex	Wöhlk-Contact-Linsen	HEMA	38.6	7.3*	Large Semi-scleral	
Hydroflex/m	Wöhlk-Contact-Linsen	HEMA	38.6	7.3*	Corneal	
Hydroflex 72	Wöhlk-Contact-Linsen	HEMA	72.0	26.9*	Semi-scleral	Bandage lens
Hydron	Hydron Europe	HEMA	38.6	8.0*	Semi-scleral	

Name	Manufacturer	Material			Design	Notes
Hydron mini	Hydron Europe	HEMA	38.6	8.0*	Corneal	
Menicon–Soft	Toyo	HEMA	29.6	5.85	Corneal	
Permalens	Cooper Vision	Terpolymer of HEMA+NVP+MA	74.0	34.3*	Corneal (steeper than 'K')	Designed for continuous wear
Scanlens	Scanlens	PMMA + PVP	72.0	31.0*	Corneal	
Sauflex	Contact Lenses (Manufacturing)	Terpolymer with VP + PMMA	55.0	13.0	Corneal	
Sauflon 70	Contact Lenses (Manufacturing)	Copolymer with VP + PMMA	68.0	30.5*	Semi-scleral or corneal	
Sauflon PW	Contact Lenses (Manufacturing)	Copolymer of VP + PMMA	80.0	48.6*	Corneal	Designed for continuous wear. Originally known as Sauflon 85
Snoflex 38	Smith & Nephew	HEMA	38.6	8.0*	Semi-scleral	Originally called Hydron
Snowflex 38/SD	Smith & Nephew	HEMA	38.6	8.0*	Corneal	
Snoflex 50	Smith & Nephew	Terpolymer of VP + MMA + 3-methoxy-2-hydroxy-propyl methacrylate	52.0	10.5	Large Semi-scleral	
Soflens	Bausch & Lomb	HEMA	38.6	8.0*	Corneal Semi-scleral	Spun-cast Lathe-cut
Softcon	American Optical	PVP + HEMA	55.0		Semi-scleral	Originally known as Bionite
Weicon	Titmus Eurocon	HEMA	38.6	7.3*	Large Semi-scleral	
Weicon/mini	Titmus Eurocon	HEMA	38.6	7.3*	Corneal	
Weicon 60	Titmus Eurocon	Copolymer of HEMA + PVP	59.0	16.5	Corneal	Single fitting parameter
Weicon 72	Titmus Eurocon	+ others	72.0	27.5	Semi-scleral	
Silflex	Wöhlk-Contact-Linsen	Silicone	xxxxx	79.8	Corneal	
Tessicon	Titmus Eurocon	Silicone	xxxxx	69.0	Corneal	

Figures marked * by courtesy of Morris and Fatt (1977)

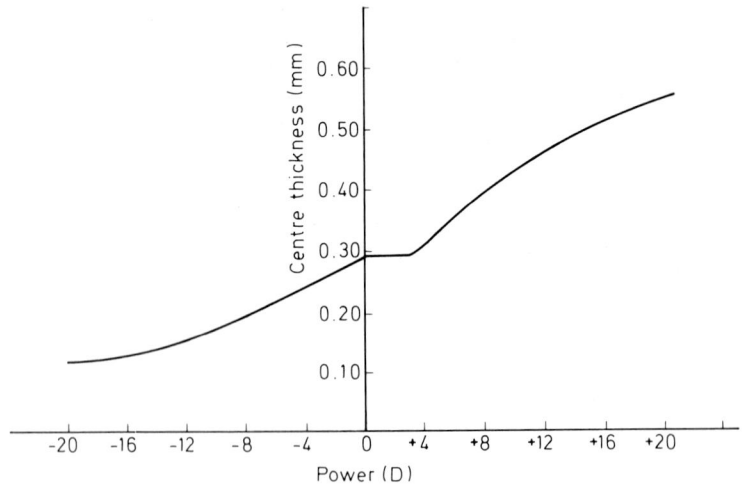

Figure 14.15–Variation of centre thickness with power for Hydron Europe in the hydrated state

lenses originally developed in Czechoslovakia. The various companies around the world which manufacture lenses from Hydron material have each developed their own version of lens geometry, so that a lens produced in the United Kingdom is not necessarily the same as one of similar specification from, for example, Europe or Australia.

All Snoflex 38 and Hydron lenses, however, are made from 2-hydroxyethyl methacrylate (HEMA). In addition, a plastics monomer, ethylene glycol di-methacrylate (EDMA or EGDMA) is employed as the cross-linking agent, and it is this which determines such factors as water content and swell factor. Physical and mechanical properties are as follows.

Density	1.17 g/cc
Tensile modulus	0.2 dynes/cm^2 $\times$ 10^7
Tensile strength	0.3 dynes/cm^2 $\times$ 10^7
Tear resistance	50 g/mm
Optical transmission	95 per cent
Refractive index	1.51 (dry)
	1.43 (wet)
Oxygen permeability	8.0×10^{-11}(cm^2/sec) (ml O^2/ml $\times$ mm Hg)
Water permeability	approximately 10 cm^4/dynes $\times$ 10^{15}
Chemical nature	HEMA cross-linked polymer
Water content	38 per cent
Linear swell factor	19 per cent

Lenses are manufactured according to the tolerances shown in *Table 14.5*.

Lens Geometry

All lenses are of lenticular construction to provide adequate control of centre thickness and front optic diameter. The graph in *Figure 14.15* relates specifically to Hydron Europe lenses, and shows how the centre thickness varies with respect to power, from 0.12 mm at –20.00 D to 0.55 mm at +20.00 D. *Figure 14.16*, also for Hydron Europe lenses, shows how the front optic diameter of both positive and negative lenses varies inversely with power from a

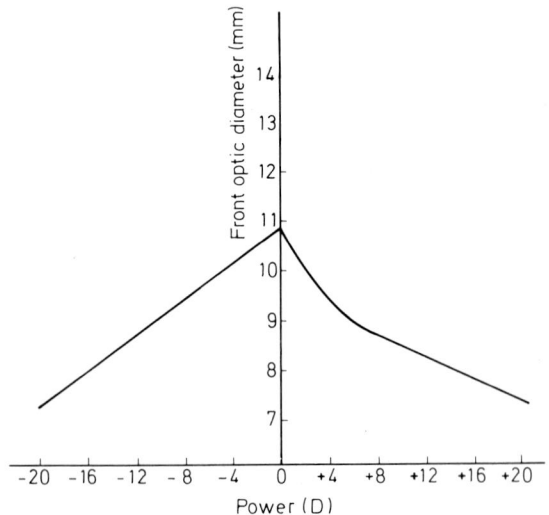

Figure 14.16–Variation of front optic diameter with power for Hydron Europe lenses in the hydrated state

maximum value of 10.8 mm for a plano lens. *Table 14.6* gives similar values for Snoflex 38 lenses. The geometry and thickness of the edge remain constant throughout the power range.

The peripheral curve on the posterior surface for all lenses is 0.6 mm wide, with a radius of 12.25 mm. A typical Snoflex 38 lens could be described according to British Standards recommended method of specification as C2/8.70:13.30/12.25:14.50 −3.50 D, but this is almost invariably written as 8.70:14.50 −3.50 D. *Figure 14.17a–d* shows examples of geometric construction.

Table 14.5–Tolerances of Hydron Lenses

	Dry	*Hydrated*
Radius	±0.04 mm	±0.05 mm
Thickness	±0.02 mm	±0.024 mm
Overall size	±0.05 mm	±0.06 mm
Power	±0.12 D	±0.14 D

Table 14.6–Thickness and Front Central Optic Diameter Relative to Power for Snoflex 38 Lenses Manufactured by Smith & Nephew Optical Ltd.

		Thickness (mm)	
BVP (D)	*FCOD (mm)*	*Centre*	*Edge and junction*
Plano	10.30	0.27	0.18
−3.00	10.90	0.27	0.18
−6.00	10.20	0.18	0.18
−10.00	9.40	0.18	0.18
−20.00	9.40	0.18	0.18
+3.00	10.10	0.31	0.18
+6.00	10.10	0.43	0.18
+12.00	9.50	0.61	0.18
+20.00	9.50	0.85	0.18

Fitting Set and Range of Lens Parameters

Table 14.7 shows the parameters and coding of the basic fitting set. These lenses are supplied in powers of −3.00 D and +4.00 D.

Table 14.7–Basic Parameters of Snoflex 38 Fitting Lenses

BCOR *(mm)*	OS *(mm)*	Lens code
8.10	13.5	0
8.40	13.5	3
8.40	14.0	4
8.40	14.5	5
8.70	14.0	6
8.70	14.5	7
9.00	14.0	8
9.00	14.5	9
9.50	14.5	10
9.50	15.0	11

In addition, there are 10 supplementary standard fittings available.

BCOR *(mm)*	OS *(mm)*			
8.10	–	14.0	14.5	15.0
8.40	–	–	–	15.0
8.70	13.5	–	–	15.0
9.00	13.5	–	–	15.0
9.50	13.5	14.0	–	–

The composition of the basic fitting set is somewhat different from that originally introduced in 1972. Since that time fitting has become appreciably flatter, and has resulted in the elimination of two seldom used lenses of BCOR 8.10 mm, and the introduction of the significantly flatter lens of 9.50 mm BCOR. The large interval between 9.0 mm and 9.50 mm is now filled by a further, non-standard, lens of BCOR 9.25 mm. Snoflex 38 lenses are engraved with a figure and letter for identification purposes. The number represents the fitting code shown in *Table 14.7*. Letters relate to power, based on A = −1.00 D, B = −1.25 D, and so on, throughout the power range to Z. For example, 9.00:14.5 −2.00 is designated 9E. Non-standard specifications are engraved in full on the lens periphery.

Fitting Technique

Most of the early forms of hydrophilic lens made the same size as, or smaller than, the cornea proved to be very unstable because of their relative thickness; they gave poor vision, and were very uncomfortable because of lid sensation. It is for this reason that the 'semi-scleral' method of fitting evolved, in order to give stability of fitting and vision. The technique is totally unlike any of the fitting procedures used with corneal lenses. The intention of the fitting philosophy is to give definite apical touch, with further

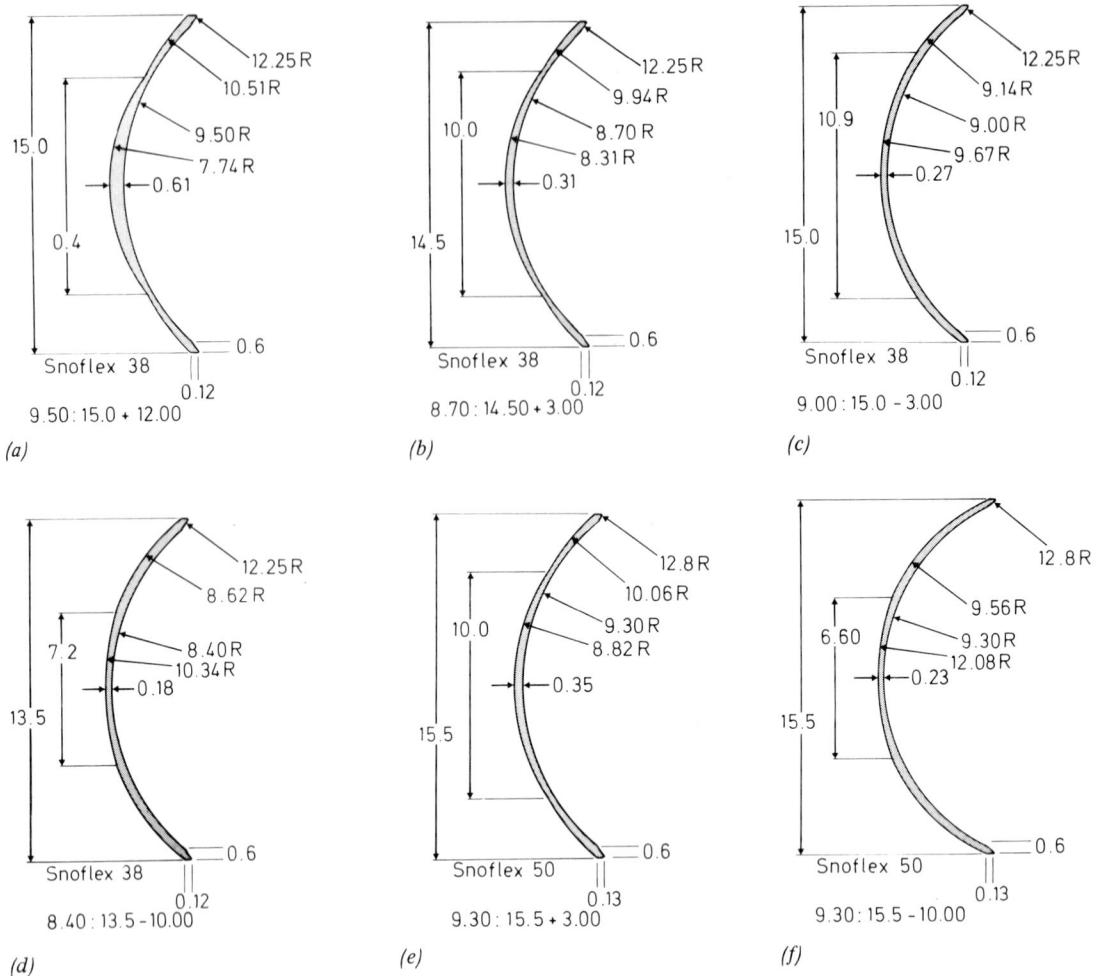

(a)

(b)

(c)

(d)

(e)

(f)

Figure 14.17–Parameters of Snoflex 38 lenses – (a), (b), (c) and (d); and Snoflex 50 lenses – (e) and (f). All dimensions are in mm and where followed by R denote a radius value

support for the lens edge being provided beyond the limbus by the much flatter peripheral curve resting on the sclera. *Figure 14.8* shows how the tears layer is greatest in the area of the corneo-scleral junction, and it is essential that the overall size of the lens is large enough not to interfere with the blood vessels in this limbal region.

Initial lens selection is determined by two factors: the keratometer readings, and the horizontal corneal diameter. In common with most other soft lenses, the fitting of Snoflex 38 lenses has, since their introduction, become both flatter and larger. Originally they were fitted only some 0.6 mm flatter than flattest 'K'. They are now more correctly fitted in the majority of cases 1.0–1.2 mm flatter than

flattest 'K'. The overall size is chosen to be 2 mm or more larger than the visible iris diameter. Thus, if 'K' readings measure 7.60 mm and 7.50 mm, and the iris diameter is 11.8 mm, the initial trial lens selected should be 8.70:14.0. With all hydrophilic lens fitting, and every type of lens, if there is a possible choice between two radii, it is better to commence with the flatter, for three reasons. First, it is much easier to see the movement of a lens which is too flat and therefore excessively mobile, rather than the lack of movement of a steep fitting; secondly, a sharper end-point can be obtained with over-refraction; and thirdly, soft lenses in most cases become tighter in their fitting as they settle.

The fitting characteristics of correct, steep and flat

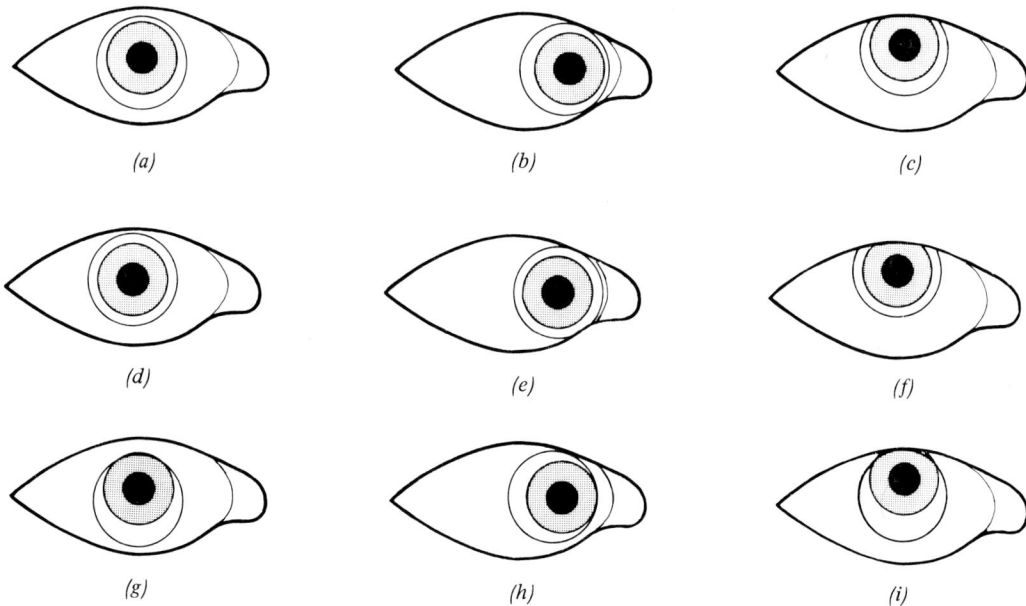

Figure 14.18—Semi-scleral lenses shown with the eye in the primary position, on the left-hand side; looking laterally, in the centre column; and looking upwards, on the right-hand side. The upper three diagrams, (a), (b) and (c), show a correctly fitting lens; the centre three diagrams, (d), (e) and (f), show a tightly fitting lens; and the lower three diagrams, (g), (h) and (i), show a loose fitting lens.

fitting lenses are as described on pages 416–417, and summarized in *Table 14.3. Figure 14.18a–c* shows diagrammatically the limits of acceptable lens movement and position for semi-scleral lenses with the eye in the primary position and in lateral and upward gaze respectively. *Figure 14.18d–f* shows the lack of movement with a tight lens. *Figure 14.18g–i* shows the excessive mobility of a loose fitting lens. In addition, a liquid lens of about –0.50 D is anticipated for a correct lens-cornea relationship.

A steep fitting may be corrected in two ways; either by selecting a lens with a flatter radius, or by employing a smaller overall size. If the initial lens has proved very tight, it may be necessary to combine both of these fitting changes. For example, if a lens of specification 8.7:14.5 is too steep, it may be progressively loosened by the following lenses: 8.7:14.0, 9.0:14.5, and 9.0:14.0. Generally, altering the radius has a greater effect on the fitting than changing the overall size.

Conversely, a flat fitting may be corrected by choosing a steeper radius, or a larger overall size, or possibly both. Thus, 8.70:14.0 may be progressively steepened by the lenses: 8.70:14.5, 8.40:14.0, and 8.40:14.5. A slightly flat fitting Snoflex 38 lens is shown in *Figure 14.19*.

Primary Sagitta

The choice of action required to correct an unsatisfactory semi-scleral fitting has been related by Brailsford (1972), Rocher (1974) and Hodd (1976a)

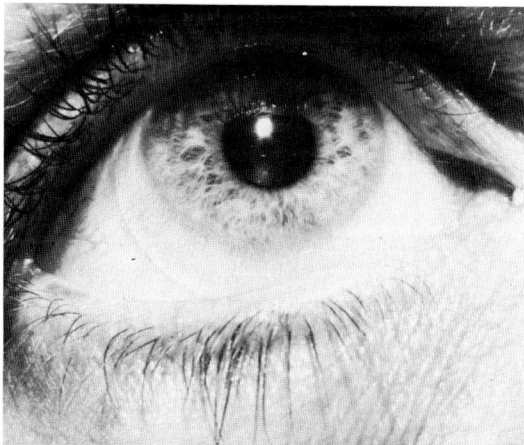

Figure 14.19—A slightly loose semi-scleral Snoflex 38 lens

to the primary sag or sagittal height of the lens in the same way as described for FLOM lenses on page 246, Chapter 10, Volume 1. In this way, a steep lens is corrected by decreasing the sag (flatter radius or smaller overall size), and a flat lens by increasing the sag (steeper radius or larger overall size).

The principle of clinical equivalents therefore also applies as it does to FLOM lenses, so that two lenses of different but related specification may behave in the same way on the same eye. Approximately, a change of radius of 0.3 mm is equivalent to altering the overall size by 0.5 mm. For example, 8.40:13.5 ≃ 8.70:14.0, and 9.0:15.0 ≃ 8.70:14.5. *Table 14.8* shows the primary sagitta for the standard Snoflex 38 parameters. When considering these in relation to fitting characteristics, the absolute value for any given lens is less important than its difference from the lens with which it is being compared.

Table 14.8–Primary Sagitta and Ratio of Sag/Overall Size for Standard Snoflex 38 Fitting Lenses

BCOR (mm)	OS (d) (mm)	Primary sagitta (s) (mm)	s/d
8.10	13.50	3.211	0.238
8.10	14.00	3.540	0.253
8.10	14.50	3.904	0.269
8.10	15.00	4.312	0.287
8.40	13.50	3.055	0.226
8.40	14.00	3.357	0.240
8.40	14.50	3.688	0.254
8.40	15.00	4.053	0.270
8.70	13.50	2.914	0.215
8.70	14.00	3.194	0.228
8.70	14.50	3.499	0.241
8.70	15.00	3.831	0.255
9.00	13.50	2.779	0.206
9.00	14.00	3.040	0.217
9.00	14.50	3.321	0.229
9.00	15.00	3.625	0.242
9.50	13.50	2.631	0.195
9.50	14.00	2.872	0.205
9.50	14.50	3.129	0.216
9.50	15.00	3.406	0.227

Clinical equivalents do not, in fact, have the same primary sag because of their different diameters. Cooke (1976) has suggested that the ratio between primary sag and overall size, as given in column 4 of *Table 14.8*, is more meaningful. Thus, 8.40:14.0, 8.70:14.5, and 9.00:15.0, which may be considered clinically equivalent in terms of their fitting characteristics, have almost the same sag to overall size ratios, of 0.240, 0.241, and 0.242, respectively.

When two lenses of different specification do behave on the eye in the same way, it is more often correct to use the larger and flatter, because this more readily facilitates tears flow beneath the lens with its flexure on blinking. This decision, however, must always be related to the dimensions and anatomical features of the eye being fitted. In some cases, for example, the option to use a smaller lens may not be feasible in practice, if such a lens would cause limbal irritation.

SAUFLON

Sauflon material has been developed by Contact Lenses (Manufacturing) Ltd., since 1968. It differs from most of the other soft lenses in three important respects. First, it is not a HEMA-based material, being a cross-linked copolymer of PMMA and N-vinyl-2-pyrrolidone. This is intended to combine the physical structure of the former, with the abundant hydrophilic sites of the latter, to which water molecules are attached during hydration. Secondly, lenses are available in a variety of water contents. Of these, the most common is Sauflon 70 (water content 68 per cent) for daily wear, Sauflon PW for 'continuous' wear (*see* page 446), and Sauflon 55 where greater tensile strength is required. Thirdly, the material has been made widely available for a variety of laboratories to produce finished lenses of their own individual design. Although great versatility of design is therefore possible, the quality of manufacture and lens geometry depend very much on the particular laboratory concerned. Control of such factors as lens thickness is very important, for two lenses of the same specification but different substance can behave very differently on the eye. It is therefore unwise to order Sauflon lenses from one laboratory while using the fitting set of another. Most of this section relates specifically to Sauflon 70 as manufactured by C.L.M. and reintroduced in 1977 in a modified and somewhat strengthened form.

Chemical and Physical Properties

Chemical composition	Cross-linked copolymer of N-vinyl-2-pyrrolidone and methyl methacrylate.
Water content	68 per cent.
Refractive index	1.54 (dry). 1.39 (wet).
Light transmission	> 95 per cent.
Oxygen permeability	30.5×10^{-11} (cm^2/sec) (ml O_2/ml × mm Hg).
Tensile strength	40 g/mm^2.
Elongation to break	65 per cent.

Fitting Procedures

The majority of Sauflon 70 lenses are used as small semi-sclerals, and the basic fitting principles are very similar to those outlined for Snoflex 38 except that the higher water content and greater lens flexibility permit smaller and tighter fittings without the risk of corneal oedema. There is therefore some overlap of fitting technique with lenses of corneal size. Originally there was no standardization of lens design, and various fitting methods have evolved. Some practitioners preferred to fit 0.4 mm flatter than 'K' and about 1 mm larger than the cornea, whilst others used lenses 1 mm flatter than 'K' and up to 3 mm larger than the cornea. Litvin (1973), with the original Sauflon 70 material, developed the technique of fitting a constant overall size of 13.5 mm and of varying the radius to achieve optimum centration and movement. The composition of the trial set must therefore depend on the method of fitting to which it relates. A common technique with the new Sauflon 70 material is to fit 0.70–0.80 mm flatter than flattest 'K' with overall sizes of 1–2 mm larger than the horizontal corneal diameter, in which case the range of parameters outlined in *Table 14.9* represent a reasonable minimum.

The fitting characteristics of correct, steep and flat lenses are as described on pages 416–417 including *Table 14.3*, and in *Figure 14.18*. Because of their high water content, Sauflon lenses must be allowed longer to settle during fitting evaluation than HEMA lenses. They are more likely to alter their fitting characteristics while reaching a state of equilibration on the cornea, particularly in relation to temperature, which can cause a significant change in lens dimensions. There can be a noticeable tightening of fit as water is lost from the lens by evaporation, especially with dry-eyed patients, for whom the material is in other respects very suitable.

Standard Sauflon 70 lenses are available from C.L.M. in powers from +8.00 D to –8.00 D in 0.25 D steps, with BCOR from 7.80 mm to 9.00 mm in 0.2 mm steps, and three overall sizes of 12.3 mm, 13.0 mm and 13.7 mm. High positive lenses from +8.00 D to +20.00 D in 0.50 D steps may also be

Table 14.9–Parameters of a Minimum Trial Set of Twelve Sauflon 70 Lenses of Low Negative Power

BCOR (mm)	OS (mm)		
8.20	12.30	13.00	
8.40	12.30	13.00	13.70
8.60	12.30	13.00	13.70
8.80		13.00	13.70
9.00		13.00	13.70

obtained in the same BCOR values but only in overall sizes of 13.0 mm and 13.7 mm. Non-standard lenses may be obtained at extra cost.

The main clinical advantage of Sauflon is its high oxygen permeability, which makes it very suitable for fragile corneas, prone to oedema. Indeed, even a tightly fitting lens does not necessarily produce observable corneal oedema, although such a lens may well cause marked scleral indentation and peri-limbal injection. A main disadvantage of the material has been its short life span, because of fragility and ease of contamination, but as the material has now been altered to strengthen it, this should be less of a problem.

Similar to Sauflon 70 are Focus 66 lenses made of Duragel material which closely resembles Sauflon in its fitting characteristics. Negative lenses are made with an overall size of 13.00 mm and centre thickness of 0.10 mm; low positive lenses with an OS of 13.50 mm and t_c of 0.30 mm; and high positive lenticular lenses with an OS of 14.00 mm and t_c of 0.40 mm maximum. Depending on overall size the first lens selected for fitting should be 0.60 mm, 0.80 mm or 1.00 mm flatter than flattest 'K', and should be allowed to settle for 30 minutes before assessing the fit. The lenses are monocurve and are available in the BOR range 7.80–9.20 mm in 0.10 mm steps, with an extension to this range available as special lenses made to prescription. *Table 14.10* shows the recommended fitting set for low negative powered lenses.

Table 14.10–Parameters of a Minimum Trial Set of Ten Focus 66 Lenses of BVP –3.00 D

BCOR (mm)	OS (mm)	
8.00	13.00	
8.20	13.00	13.50
8.40	13.00	13.50
8.60	13.00	13.50
8.80		13.50
9.00		13.50
9.20		13.50

LARGE SEMI-SCLERAL LENSES AND SIMPLIFIED FITTING PROCEDURES

The number of parameters which may be varied in soft lens fitting is significantly less than with hard lenses. Factors such as width and radius of peripheral curve, lenticulation, centre thickness and edge shape are predetermined by most laboratories, allowing only the two main variables of radius (BCOR) and overall size (OS) to be specified. For example, implicit in the prescription 9.00:15.0 –3.00 D, may be a back peripheral curve of radius 10.00

Table 14.11–Typical Parameters of a Large Semi-scleral
Lens Fitting Set

BCOR (mm)	OS (mm)
8.40	15.0
8.60	15.0
8.80	15.0
9.00	15.0
9.20	15.0
9.40	15.0
9.60	15.0

mm, a centre thickness of 0.18 mm, and a front optic
diameter of 12.0 mm. However, many types of
semi-scleral lens are now fitted according to an even
more simplified procedure, by standardizing one of
these main parameters (usually the OS at a fixed
15.0 mm) and altering the only other remaining
variable (usually the BCOR).

The large lenses which can be fitted in this
simplified fashion include Aoflex, the '4' Series
Bausch and Lomb Soflens, Flexol 35, the large
Hydroflex, Mollitor 35, Snoflex and Weicon. Apart
from Snoflex which is fitted differently (*see* page
429) and has a higher water content, these are all
HEMA lenses with low water contents in the 30–40
per cent range. Fitting intervals are usually 0.2 mm,
and a typical fitting set is given in *Table 14.11*. An
example of lens geometry is shown in *Figure 14.20*
which illustrates a large Hydroflex lens.

The initial radius selected in fitting is 1.2 mm to
1.3 mm flatter than flattest 'K'. The overall size is

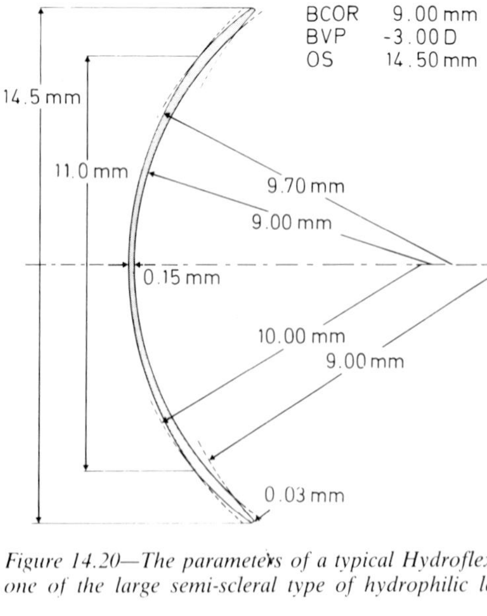

```
BCOR    9.00 mm
BVP    -3.00 D
OS     14.50 mm
```

14.5 mm

11.0 mm

9.70 mm

9.00 mm

0.15 mm

10.00 mm

9.00 mm

0.03 mm

*Figure 14.20—The parameters of a typical Hydroflex lens,
one of the large semi-scleral type of hydrophilic lens.*

3.0–3.5 mm larger than the horizontal corneal
diameter, so that 15.0 mm lenses are fitted in the
majority of cases. The criteria for a correct fitting in
terms of movement, comfort and vision are the same
as those described for other semi-scleral lenses.
These simplified fittings generally have a peripheral
curve 1 mm wide, and 1 mm flatter than the BCOR,

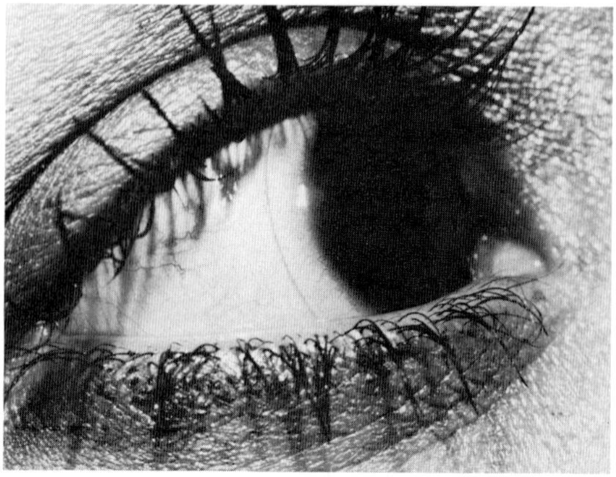

*Figure 14.21—A correctly fitted large semi-scleral lens seen
on lateral gaze*

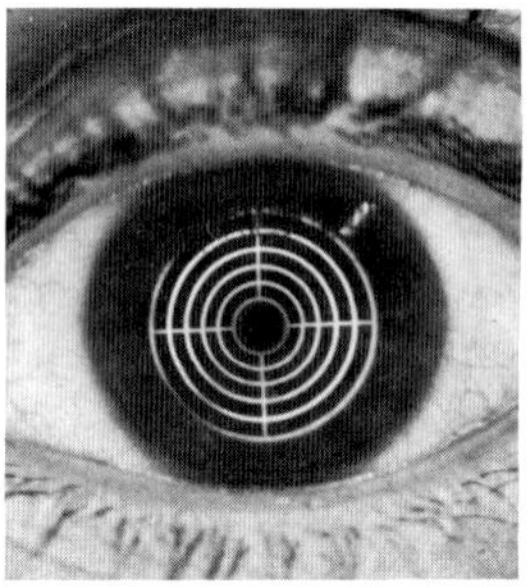

*Figure 14.22—A large semi-scleral lens fitted slightly too
steep (by approximately 0.2 mm). The regularity of the
photokeratoscope image may be deceptively good and mask
the poor fit*

and as long as the lenses are thin, this simplified
approach does provide good initial subjective comfort, and a fairly rapid technique of establishing the
optimum fitting. It is, of course, essential that larger
and smaller overall sizes should be available for the
minority of cases in which 15.0 mm proves unsatisfactory. *Figure 14.21* shows the cosmetic appearance
of a correctly fitting large semi-scleral lens with the
eye looking laterally.

If such large lenses are fitted too steep, they tend
to produce corneal oedema, although other signs of
a steep fit may be absent. (*Figure 14.22* shows a
good photokeratoscopic image achieved with lens
0.2 mm too steep.) If fitted too flat, they can buckle

at the periphery, causing uncomfortable edge stand-off. Excessive lens movement can give unacceptable lower lid sensation.

The main advantages of these lenses are the simplicity of fitting, and their good subjective comfort. They can sometimes produce a satisfactory result where smaller lenses have failed because of discomfort, decentration on the cornea, or poor vision.

Disadvantages are greater difficulty in handling, particularly for those patients with tight lids and small palpebral apertures, cosmetic appearance (*Figure 14.21*), irritation of the lower lid margin if this is positioned abnormally low and a slightly greater tendency for white spot formation on the lens surfaces.

The converse approach to simplified fitting is offered by Snoflex 50 in which only one radius is available, but the overall size is varied to obtain the correct fitting. The lens is not made from HEMA, but from a cross-linked terpolymer of methyl methacrylate, vinyl pyrrolidone, and 3-methoxy-2-hydroxypropyl methacrylate.

Water content	52 per cent.
Linear swell factor at 20°	1.33
Refractive index	1.51 (dry).
	1.41 (wet).
Oxygen permeability at 20°C	10.5×10^{-11} (cm^2/sec) (ml O$_2$·ml / mm Hg).

The fitting philosophy is based on the theory of primary sagitta and clinical equivalents (Cooke, 1976), so that, for example, lenses of specification 9.00:14.5 and 9.30:15.0 should behave in the same way on the eye. Lenses are, in fact, only made with the one BCOR of 9.3 mm, but with five overall sizes of 14.0 mm, 14.5 mm, 15.0 mm, 15.5 mm, and 16.0 mm. These lenses in powers of −3.00 D represent the basic fitting set. Examples of lens geometry are shown in *Figure 14.17e,f.*

Snoflex 50 lenses have the same advantages as the more usual large semi-scleral lenses, together with a slightly improved oxygen permeability as a result of the higher water content. Severe limitations are placed on fittings by the minimum choice of parameters available. Steeper eyes, which are normally smaller in size, require a larger than average lens in order to obtain the required primary sag; conversely, flat eyes, although usually large in size, predictably require smaller lenses.

An example of an even more simplified fitting is the Weicon 60. This high water content lens has not only a single overall size of 13.00 mm but also a constant aspheric back surface approximately equivalent to a spherical radius of 8.20 mm

CORNEAL-SIZED LENSES*

BAUSCH AND LOMB SOFLENS

The Bausch and Lomb Soflens is the only hydrophilic lens manufactured by the spin-casting process, which is exactly the same in principle as the centrifugal technique employed for the original gel lenses from Czechoslovakia, and which is still being used in that particular country. Bausch and Lomb commenced their programme of research and development as early as 1966, in order to make extensive refinements to the basic spinning process. Elaborate techniques to ensure quality control and reproducibility were introduced, and the geometry of the lens redesigned to a sophisticated level.

Bausch and Lomb was the first, and for a long time, the only contact lens manufacturer to have received FDA† approval. This was granted on March 18th, 1971, not specifically for the lens, but for the entire system appertaining to the lens. It therefore included such items as the carrying case, heat disinfection unit and storage vials.

Physical and Chemical Properties

Refractive index	1.43 (wet).
Softening point	120°C.
Visible light transmission	> 97 per cent.
Water content by weight	
Equilibrated in water	41.7 per cent.
Equilibrated in 0.9 per cent saline solution	38.6 per cent.
Linear swell factor	18 per cent.
Oxygen permeability	8.0×10^{-11} (cm^2/sec) (ml O$_2$/ml × mm Hg).
Chemical nature	HEMA cross-linked polymer.

Manufacturing Process

The manufacturing process has been described by Watts (1971) and Wycoff (1972). The monomer mixture and the solvent, glycerol, are introduced into ground and highly polished female moulds,

*British Standard 3521:1979 refers to Soft, Hydrophilic, Corneal Lenses where such lenses are designed to be worn in front of the cornea only.

†FDA is the abbreviation for the United States Department of Health, Education and Welfare, Public Health Service, Food and Drug Administration, 5600 Fishers Lane, Rockville, Maryland 20852, U.S.A.

which are mounted on a central spindle to permit rotation at speed. Polymerization takes place whilst the mould is spinning about its central axis. Water is then pumped in to replace the glycerol and to hydrate the lens, which is afterwards removed manually from the mould for edging. The lenses are extracted for 22 hours in circulating distilled water at 87°C to remove any remaining unreacted monomers, catalyst or water-soluble polymer. After checking, the lenses are finally sealed in 5 cc pharmaceutical vials for autoclaving. The process is different from the moulding or pressing techniques employed by some hard lens manufacturers for two reasons. First, the mould is open, and secondly it is spinning during polymerization.

The spherical curvature of the mould itself determines the anterior surface of the lens which is designated the 'base curve' or 'Series'. The posterior lens surface, which governs the power, is aspheric, due to centrifugal force distributing liquid polymer away from the apex of the mould according to its speed of rotation. A faster speed gives a higher minus lens, and vice versa. The exact shape of the back surface depends on a number of other factors, including the volume of polymer used, surface tension, rate of polymerization and the duration of the polymerization process. The following formula, associated with *Figure 14.23*, has been used:

$$Z = \frac{W^2 \, X^2}{2_g} + K$$

where Z = Distance on vertical axis
X = Distance on horizontal axis
W = Speed of rotation
g = gravity constant
K = a function of surface tension.

The aspheric posterior surface of the lens has been related by Poster (1975) to the mathematical form of an ellipse. Within a particular Series, the surface shape gradually changes from oblate to prolate as the power is increased as indicated in *Figure 14.24*. The change-over, or sphere point occurs with a different power for each Series as shown in *Table 14.12*.

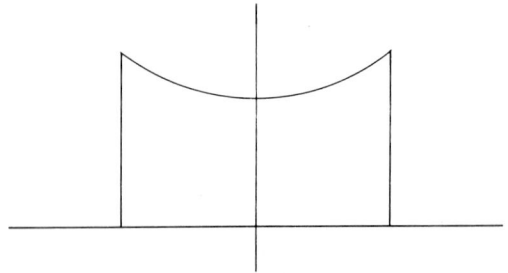

Figure 14.23–Female mould used for spin-casting Bausch and Lomb Soflenses

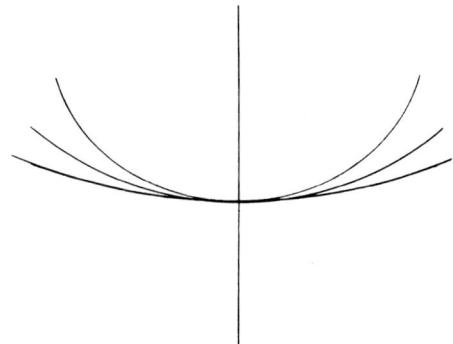

Figure 14.24–Aspheric back surfaces of Bausch and Lomb Soflenses: the steepest curve, associated with the highest negative power, is in the form of the prolate portion of an ellipse, whilst the flattest curve is that of the oblate portion of an ellipse, the intermediate curve being spherical

Table 14.12–Sphere Points* for Different Series of Bausch and Lomb Soflenses

	Series letter						
	B	*F*	*J*	*N*	*B3*	*F3*	*J3*
BVP (D)	−5.50	−3.75	−2.00	−1.25	−3.50	−2.00	−0.50
PAR (mm)	8.10	8.10	8.10	7.90	8.95	8.90	8.90

*Values obtained by calculation.

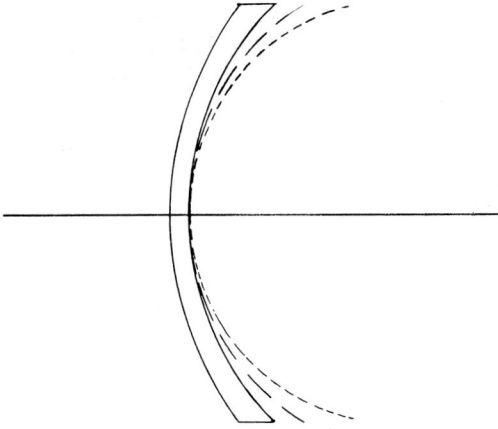

Figure 14.25–Bausch and Lomb Series Soflenses. The front surface radius is constant. Variation in power is achieved by altering the posterior apical radius; the steeper it is, the higher the negative power

The back surface cannot truly be defined as having a BCOR, since only the central 2–3 mm is in fact spherical, and so the term posterior apical radius (PAR) is used. Quoted PAR's are always obtained by calculation, and not by measurement.

Figure 14.25 shows, for the F Series, how progressively higher powers are obtained by using steeper posterior apical radii in conjunction with the constant radius of the front surface. It illustrates the way in which Bausch and Lomb Soflens design, and consequently its method of fitting, has fundamental differences when compared with any other type of lens, either hard or soft. First, the 'base curve' or series is always the anterior surface of the lens; this is the opposite of lathe-cut lenses where the BCOR, sometimes referred to as the 'base curve', is always the posterior surface. Secondly, the power for any given Series is determined by the back surface, also the opposite of all other lenses. In clinical terms it means that the fitting characteristics of the lens are

Table 14.13–Details of Bausch and Lomb Soflenses of 12.5 mm Overall Size

Series	F	+N	U
Overall size (mm)	12.5	12.5	12.5
Power range (D)	–0.25 to –9.50	+0.25 to +17.50	plano to –9.00
Average centre thickness (mm)	0.12	0.19–0.47 (+0.25 to +6.00 D)	0.07
Anterior surface radius (mm)	8.74		8.60
Anterior bevel width (mm)	0.71		0.80
Primary sagitta (mm)	2.837		2.885

Table 14.14–Details of Bausch and Lomb Soflenses of 13.5 mm Overall Size

Series	B3	+B3	U3	O3
Overall size (mm)	13.5	13.5	13.5	13.5
Power range (D)	–0.25 to –20.00	+0.25 to +6.00 (+H3 over this)	plano to –9.00	–1.00 to –9.00
Average centre thickness (mm)	0.12	0.127 to 0.299	0.07	0.035
Anterior surface radius (mm)	9.67	8.74 (FCOD 9.00)	9.15	10.08 (–1.00 and –1.25 D)* 9.55 (–1.50 to –9.00 D)
Anterior bevel width (mm)	1.20	0.83	0.90	1.20
Primary sagitta (mm)	3.10	3.41 to 3.24	3.09	3.12 (–1.00 and –1.25 D)* 3.18 (–1.50 to –9.00 D)

*In the O Series a different mould is used in the lower powers to facilitate handling.

Table 14.15–Details of Bausch and Lomb Soflens of 14.5 mm Overall Size

Series	B4	+B4	U4	O4
Overall size (mm)	14.5	14.5	14.5	14.5
Power range (D)	–0.25 to –9.00	+0.25 to +6.00 (+H4 over this)	–0.25 to –9.00	–1.00 to –9.00
Average centre thickness (mm)	0.12	0.128 to 0.300	0.07	0.035
Anterior surface radius (mm)	10.08	9.47 (FCOD 10.00 mm)	9.07	9.92 (–1.00 to –1.75 D) 8.90 (–2.00 to –9.00 D)
Anterior bevel width (mm)	1.20	0.86	1.05	1.10
Primary sagitta (mm)	4.59	4.65 to 3.48	4.05	3.71–4.10

changed if the power is altered, since a steeper or flatter PAR has been used.

The spin-casting process has certain advantages. It is possible to design and manufacture lenses with a better surface quality and edge shape. Reproducibility and consistency of manufacture are also more easily maintained. On the other hand, the method does impose limitations on the variety of back surface forms which may be conveniently obtained. The entire range of powers for every anterior surface radius is not produced, so that, for example, a correctly fitting high minus lens may not be obtainable in practice if the cornea is very flat.

The earliest lens form produced was the C Series, with a front surface curvature of 8.14 mm, an overall size of 13.5 mm, and a centre thickness which varied according to power. Its thin tapering edges made it a very comfortable lens to wear, but its poor clinical performance meant that it was soon superseded by the N and F Series, which established the pattern for subsequent developments. These lenses, together with the B and J Series which were fitted from 1974, had a constant centre thickness and an overall size of 12.5 mm. *Table 14.13* gives some parameters of the current Series of 12.5 mm OS. In 1976, the B3, F3, and J3 Series were introduced, the numerical suffix '3' designating a larger overall size of 13.6 mm. *Table 14.14* gives details of the current Series. *Table 14.15* shows the parameters of the 14.5 mm overall size lenses which became available in the United Kingdom from 1977. These lenses were significantly different from the earlier Series because the back surface was produced by moulding and the front surface was lathe-cut in the conventional way to provide spherical curvatures. Lenses effectively had fitting intervals of 0.3 mm. All of the Series, except those lenses of 14.5 mm overall size, have this fitting 'base curve' on the front surface rather than the back. *Figure 14.26* shows cross-sectional diagrams of some of the Bausch and Lomb Soflenses Series.

Until 1975 lenses were labelled in silver-coloured vials with what is now termed the 'functional power'. This was always less negative than the true power, and could differ from it by as much as 0.75 D. Lenses are now always specified in BVP. A blue label indicates a 12.5 mm overall size lens; a gold label a 13.6 mm lens; and white a 14.5 mm lens.

The fitting of Bausch and Lomb lenses then evolved from a simple but irrational system with limited lens parameters into a more soundly based fitting philosophy requiring a much greater number of lenses. When only 'N' and 'F' Series were available, with power as the only other variable, the selection of the first lens was based simply on 'K' readings and spectacle refraction (Gasson, 1973). There was no reference to PAR's since the data was at that time unpublished, and it was therefore recommended that corneas of radius 7.50 mm or steeper should be filled with 'N' Series lenses, and corneas flatter than this with 'F' Series lenses: 7.50 mm was considered a 'normal' or average curvature, and to this figure were related the selection procedure, the lens labelling system and power compensations for lens flexure.

The significant changes to make Bausch and Lomb Soflens fitting more scientific took place from the middle of 1974. Practitioners were provided with detailed information about lens geometry, true BVP's, and the calculated PAR's, so that it became possible to relate the curvature of the lens being fitted to that of the cornea. At the same time the B and J Series were introduced to provide four fitting curves for each power which might be required. The fitting intervals of approximately 0.3 mm between the radii of the various Series compared favourably with those of lathe-cut soft lenses, and made possible what has been termed the 'best fit formula'.

The clinical investigations of Touch and Clark (1974) and Touch, Mertz and Seger (1976) assessed the fitting characteristics of a large number of lenses

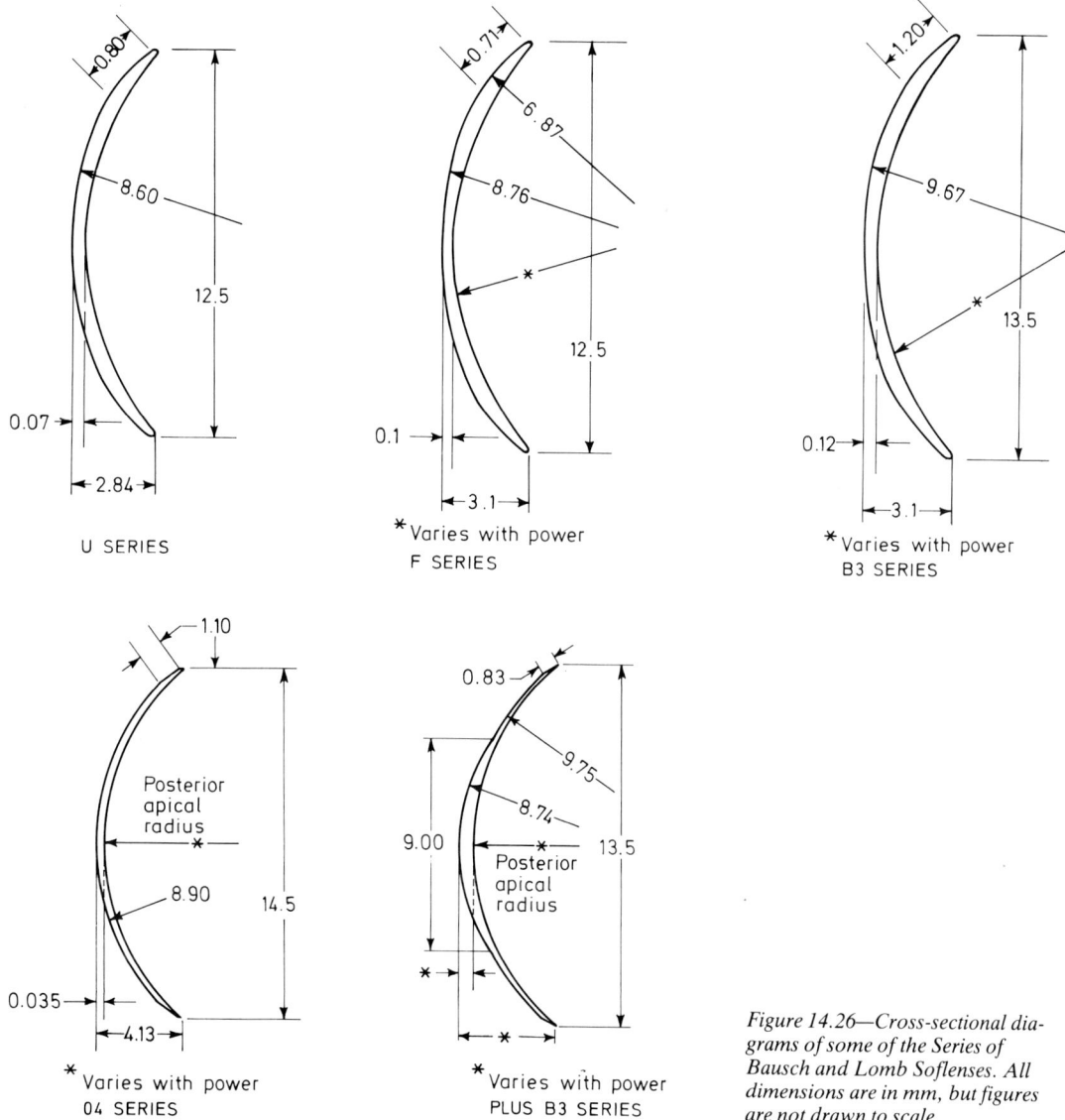

*Varies with power
F SERIES

*Varies with power
B3 SERIES

U SERIES

Posterior apical radius

*Varies with power
04 SERIES

Posterior apical radius

*Varies with power
PLUS B3 SERIES

Figure 14.26—Cross-sectional diagrams of some of the Series of Bausch and Lomb Soflenses. All dimensions are in mm, but figures are not drawn to scale

on a particular group of eyes. The results for all the 12.5 mm overall size Series showed that an optimum fitting was given with, on average, a PAR 0.5 mm flatter than flattest 'K'. With many eyes, because of lens flexure and corneal topography, a range of PAR's could give the same fitting characteristics. The normal range within which there was little change in apparent fitting was about ±0.25 mm, slightly less for N Series and slightly greater for J Series lenses. This was referred to as the 'range of best fits' or 'band width'. The greatest probability of an optimum fitting occurred if the PAR at the centre of this range was 0.5 mm flatter than flattest 'K'.

This is represented for the B Series power range by the dotted line in *Figure 14.27*. The shaded area gives the total band width, and points taken towards the edge of this are less likely to produce a satisfactory fitting.

For example, a –4.50 B lens has a PAR of 8.30 mm, and was expected to be successful for corneal radii between 7.55 mm and 8.05 mm. If it was applied to a spherical cornea of radius 7.80 mm the probability of an optimum fitting was greatest, since the lens was precisely 0.5 mm flatter. If it was then placed on a cornea of central radius 7.60 mm, a successful result was still probable, but less so than

Table 14.16–Back Vertex Powers with Posterior Apical Radii (PAR) and Shape Factors (SF) of Bausch and Lomb 12.5 mm OS and 13.5 mm OS Series Lenses
(All information available at time of going to press)

	12.5 mm OS								13.5 mm OS						
Power (D)	−F PAR (mm)	−F SF	+N PAR (mm)	+N SF	−U PAR (mm)	−U SF	−B3 PAR (mm)	−B3 SF	+B3 PAR (mm)	+B3 SF	−U3 PAR (mm)	−U3 SF	−O3 PAR (mm)	−O3 SF	Power (D)
plano	8.65	1.301	8.15		8.55	1.475	9.60	1.391	8.74	1.236	9.15	1.280			plano
0.25	8.65	1.272	8.15		8.50	1.446	9.55	1.357	8.79	1.255	9.10	1.249			0.25
0.50	8.60	1.242	8.20		8.50	1.418	9.45	1.324	8.83	1.274	9.05	1.219			0.50
0.75	8.55	1.213	8.25		8.45	1.389	9.40	1.291	8.87	1.293	9.00	1.189			0.75
1.00	8.50	1.183	8.25		8.40	1.361	9.35	1.259	8.92	1.313	8.95	1.159	9.85		1.00
1.25	8.45	1.155	8.30		8.35	1.334	9.30	1.227	8.96	1.333	8.90	1.130	9.80		1.25
1.50	8.40	1.126	8.35		8.30	1.306	9.25	1.195	9.00	1.353	8.85	1.101	9.25		1.50
1.75	8.40	1.098	8.35		8.30	1.279	9.20	1.164	9.05	1.373	8.80	1.072	9.20		1.75
2.00	8.35	1.070	8.40		8.25	1.252	9.15	1.133	9.09	1.394	8.75	1.044	9.15		2.00
2.25	8.30	1.042	8.45		8.20	1.225	9.15	1.102	9.14	1.415	8.70	1.016	9.10		2.25
2.50	8.25	1.015	8.50		8.15	1.199	9.10	1.071	9.18	1.436	8.65	0.988	9.05		2.50
2.75	8.20	0.988	8.55		8.10	1.173	9.05	1.041	9.23	1.458	8.60	0.960	9.00		2.75
3.00	8.20	0.961	8.55		8.10	1.147	9.00	1.012	9.27	1.480	8.55	0.933	8.95		3.00
3.25	8.15	0.934	8.60		8.05	1.121	8.95	0.982	9.32	1.502	8.50	0.906	8.90		3.25
3.50	8.10	0.908	8.65		8.00	1.096	8.90	0.953	9.37	1.525	8.45	0.879	8.85		3.50
3.75	8.05	0.882	8.70		7.95	1.071	8.85	0.924	9.42	1.548	8.40	0.852	8.80		3.75
4.00	8.05	0.856	8.75		7.90	1.046	8.80	0.895	9.47	1.572	8.35	0.826	8.75		4.00
4.25	8.00	0.830	8.75		7.90	1.021	8.75	0.867	9.51	1.595	8.30	0.800	8.70		4.25
4.50	7.95	0.804	8.80		7.85	0.996	8.70	0.839	9.56	1.620	8.25	0.774	8.65		4.50
4.75	7.90	0.779	8.85		7.80	0.972	8.65	0.811	9.61	1.644	8.20	0.749	8.60		4.75
5.00	7.85	0.730	8.95		7.75	0.948	8.60	0.757	9.72	1.694	8.10	0.724	8.50		5.00
5.50	7.80	0.681	9.05		7.65	0.900	8.50	0.703	9.82	1.746		0.674	8.40		5.50
6.00	7.70	0.633	7.00			0.854	8.40	0.651				0.625	8.35		6.00
6.50	7.60	0.585	7.05			0.808	8.35	0.599				0.577	8.25		6.50
7.00	7.50	0.539	7.10			0.763	8.25	0.548				0.530	8.20		7.00
7.50	7.45	0.494	7.15			0.718	8.20	0.499				0.483	8.10		7.50
8.00	7.40	0.449	7.20			0.675	8.10	0.450				0.438	8.05		8.00
8.50	7.30	0.405	7.25			0.632	8.05	0.402				0.393	7.95		8.50
9.00		0.362	7.30			0.590	7.95	0.355				0.349			9.00
9.50			7.35				7.90	0.309							9.50
10.00			7.40				7.80	0.264							10.00
10.50			7.45				7.75	0.220							10.50
11.00			7.50				7.65	0.176							11.00
11.50			7.55				7.60	0.133							11.50
12.00			7.60												12.00
12.50			7.65												12.50
13.00			7.70												13.00
13.50			7.75												13.50
14.00			7.80												14.00
14.50			7.90												14.50
15.00			7.95												15.00
15.50			8.00												15.50
16.00			8.05												16.00
16.50			8.10												16.50
17.00			8.15												17.00
17.50															17.50
18.00															18.00
18.50															18.50
19.00															19.00
19.50															19.50
20.00															20.00

Table 14.16 (cont)–Back Vertex Powers with Posterior Apical Radii (PAR) and Shape Factors (SF) of Bausch and Lomb 14.5 mm OS Series Lenses (All information available at time of going to press)

14.5 mm OS

Power (D)	−B4 PAR (mm)	−B4 SF	+B4 PAR (mm)	+B4 SF	U4 PAR (mm)	U4 SF	O4 PAR (mm)	O4 SF	Power (D)
plano									plano
0.25	9.98	1.507	9.48	1.269	8.99	1.248			0.25
0.50	9.92	1.476	9.53	1.291	8.95	1.225			0.50
0.75	9.87	1.446	9.58	1.313	8.90	1.203			0.75
1.00	9.81	1.415	9.63	1.335	8.86	1.181	9.70		1.00
1.25	9.76	1.385	9.68	1.358	8.81	1.159	9.65		1.25
1.50	9.70	1.355	9.73	1.381	8.77	1.137	9.60		1.50
1.75	9.65	1.326	9.79	1.405	8.72	1.116	9.50		1.75
2.00	9.60	1.297	9.84	1.428	8.68	1.095	8.55		2.00
2.25	9.54	1.268	9.89	1.453	8.64	1.074	8.50		2.25
2.50	9.49	1.240	9.95	1.477	8.60	1.053	8.45		2.50
2.75	9.44	1.212	10.00	1.502	8.55	1.032	8.45		2.75
3.00	9.39	1.184	10.06	1.527	8.51	1.012	8.40		3.00
3.25	9.34	1.156	10.11	1.553	8.47	0.992	8.35		3.25
3.50	9.29	1.129	10.17	1.579	8.43	0.972	8.30		3.50
3.75	9.24	1.102	10.22	1.606	8.39	0.952	8.25		3.75
4.00	9.19	1.076	10.28	1.633	8.35	0.932	8.25		4.00
4.25	9.14	1.049	10.34	1.660	8.31	0.913	8.20		4.25
4.50	9.09	1.023	10.40	1.689	8.27	0.894	8.15		4.50
4.75	9.05	0.998	10.46	1.717	8.23	0.874	8.10		4.75
5.00	9.00	0.972	10.52	1.746	8.19	0.856	8.10		5.00
5.50	8.91	0.922	10.64	1.805	8.11	0.818	8.00		5.50
6.00	8.82	0.873	10.77	1.867	8.04	0.782	7.95		6.00
6.50	8.73	0.825			7.97	0.746	7.85		6.50
7.00	8.64	0.778			7.89	0.711	7.80		7.00
7.50	8.56	0.732			7.82	0.676	7.70		7.50
8.00	8.47	0.687			7.75	0.643	7.65		8.00
8.50	8.39	0.642			7.69	0.609	7.60		8.50
9.00	8.31	0.599			7.62	0.577	7.50		9.00

Corneal radius in dioptres

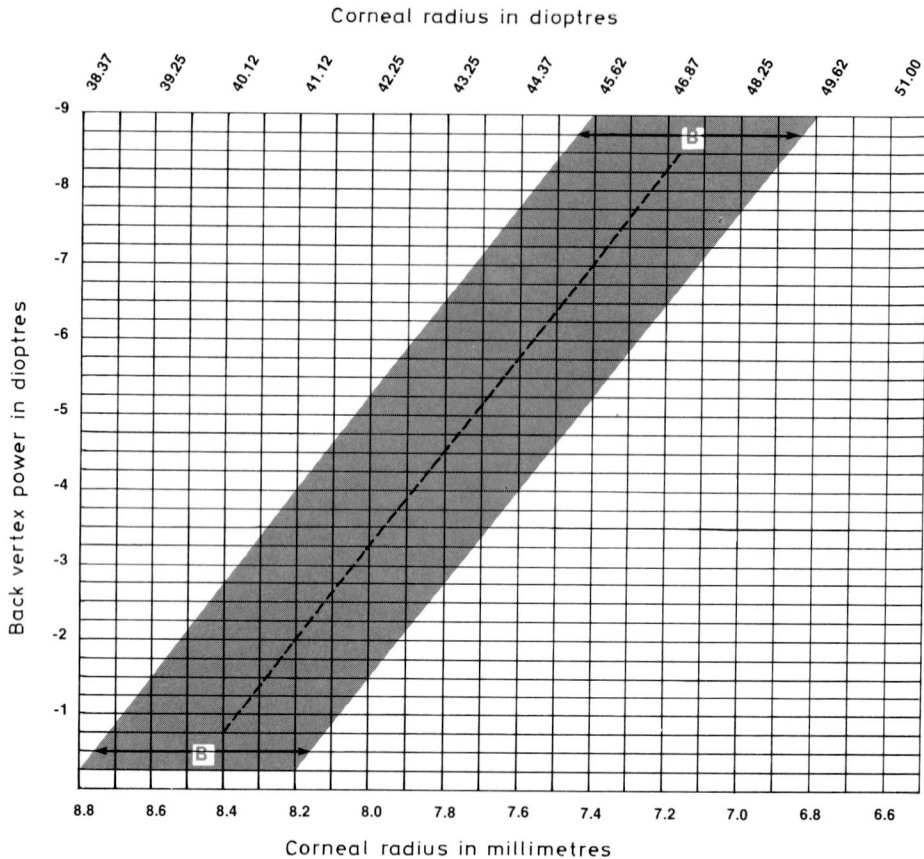

Figure 14.27–Best fit band chart for B Series Bausch and Lomb Soflenses

before, since its 0.2 mm difference from the centre of the band width was towards the expected limit of ±0.25 mm for a good fitting. If the same lens was applied to a cornea of central radius 8.20 mm, a successful result was unlikely because the difference was now 0.4 mm and well outside the normal range of best fits.

A similar analysis for the 13.6 mm (now 13.5 mm) overall size Series showed that the optimum fitting would be given by a PAR some 0.85 mm flatter than flattest 'K', and that the range of best fits was ±0.4 mm.

The lathe-cut 14.5 mm overall size lenses were usually fitted at least 1.2 mm flatter than flattest 'K'.

Initial lens selection now takes into account horizontal corneal diameter (Touch, 1977a), in addition to 'K' readings and the spectacle Rx. In a study of 200 eyes, to find the optimum overall size of Bausch and Lomb Soflenses, Touch (1977b) found that the 13.6 mm lens was fitted in 61 per cent of eyes. Corneas between 11.5 mm and 12.5 mm in

diameter generally required a 13.6 mm lens, whereas those smaller than 11.5 mm were first tried with the 12.5 mm Series. Lens selection was then most easily made from *Table 14.16*, which gave not only the power range for the 12.5 mm and 13.6 mm Series, but also the calculated PAR for each available lens. Lens selector guides were also available to simplify the choice of the initial trial lens.

Example 1
Rx: –2.25 DS
'K': 7.85 mm (spherical)
Corneal diameter: 11.25 mm
OS of required lens = 12.5 mm
Thus, PAR of required lens = 7.85 + 0.50 = 8.35 mm

The value 8.35 is found in the F Series column for a BVP of precisely –2.25 D. The initial lens was therefore –2.25 F.

Example 2
Rx: –3.50/–0.50 × 180
'K': 8.15 mm along 180, 8.10 mm along 90
Corneal diameter: 12.6 mm
OS of required lens = 13.6 mm
Thus, PAR of required lens = 8.15 + 0.85 = 9.00 mm

Moving to the right, along the –3.50 D line, the nearest value to this figure is 8.95 mm in the B3 column. This is well within the 'range of best fits' or 'band width', so that the lens selected was –3.50 B3. If the higher powers of –3.75 D or –4.00 D were found to be necessary to give best possible visual acuity then their PAR values of 8.90 mm and 8.85 mm respectively still fell within the acceptable range for fitting.

Fitting characteristics for Bausch and Lomb lenses are mostly as described in *Table 14.3* (page 418), except that movement on blinking, is up to 0.5 mm, and a little less than with other types of soft lens. It is particularly important to achieve proper centration with complete corneal coverage. A decentred Bausch and Lomb Soflens, because of its aspheric optic, can give very poor visual acuity. It can also result in arcuate staining at the limbus where the lens edge produces a combination of corneal drying and abrasion, as shown in *Colour Plate XXV*. This could easily occur on the nasal side of the cornea of the eye as in *Figure 14.28* which shows a –7.50 F lens

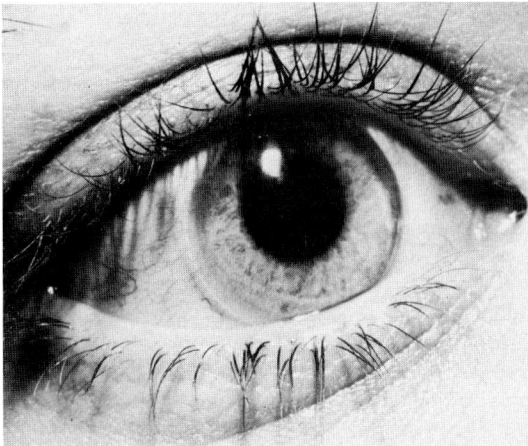

Figure 14.28–A soft lens of corneal size decentred slightly temporally. This can give rise to nasal corneal/limbal drying and abrasion

decentred slightly temporally. Lens decentration might occur with either a loose or a tight fitting, but in the latter case there is no recovery movement on blinking.

In the same way that the fitting concept differs from other types of soft lens, so also do some of the fitting characteristics of an incorrectly fitting lens. For example, a flat fitting lens would normally be expected to ride low on the cornea. With Bausch and Lomb lenses the aspheric back surface produces a high riding lens. Conversely, a steep fitting lens will tend to centre down and out. Some fitting guides, such as the improvement in V.A. in a steep fitting lens when the lids are screwed up, are the same as for the other lens types.

If the first lens proved too flat, it was advised that the fitting could be improved by either changing the Series to the next steeper, which effectively tightened the radius by 0.3 mm, or, uniquely with the Bausch and Lomb Soflens, by increasing the negative power if permitted by the refractive result. In the latter case a lens with a slightly steeper PAR has been used, so that an additional control over the lens movement could be exercised. Approximately, a change in power of 0.25 D was equivalent to a change of radius of 0.05 mm.

If the first lens was too steep – and this could always be suspected if the visual acuity was much worse than anticipated – the next flatter Series was tried, flattening the radius by 0.3 mm. The alternative method was to use a lens of lower negative power which has a flatter PAR.

If adequate centration could not be obtained with the initial overall size, lenses were tried from the next larger Series.

The lathe-cut 14.5 mm overall size lenses were not fitted like the 12.5 mm and 13.6 mm overall size Series, but in the same way as other semi-scleral lenses. They were used as a first choice if the horizontal corneal diameter was greater than 12.5 mm, and were selected to be at least 1.2 mm flatter than flattest 'K'.

There was similarly no 'best fit formula' for low positive and aphakic lenses, where the number of Series was still limited.

An extension to the negative range, in BVPs up to –9.00 D, was then provided by the ultra-thin U, U3 and U4 Series of 12.5 mm, 13.5 mm and 14.5 mm overall size respectively. The front optic radius is 8.60 mm for the U Series, 9.15 mm for the U3 Series, and 9.07 mm for the U4 Series. The PAR in each case depends on the power. The centre thickness of these lenses is 0.07 mm, and despite difficulty with handling they can prove useful in many problem cases.

Because the centre thickness of these lenses is only 0.07 mm they make a very useful alternative in cases of persistent oedema, highly sensitive patients or where tight lids cause centration problems with the normal thickness lenses. This Series is fitted by BVP only, since the lens is sufficiently flexible to conform to almost all corneal curvatures, and the OS is selected as for the other Series. Lens insertion can present more of a problem initially but is most easily achieved by keeping the inserting finger dry.

More recent additions have been the hyper-thin Series, 03 and 04, with a constant centre thickness of 0.035 mm. Additionally, the centration of the negative powered lenses has led to the introduction of thinner, lenticulated positive powered lenses with a negative carrier portion. These are designated +B3, +B4, and +H3 and H4 in the higher power range (+6.50 D and over).

Also available is the 'Plano T' lens which is specifically made for therapeutic purposes (*see* Chapter 24, page 675).

Long-term clinical research has led full circle to a more simplified approach to fitting. Of the presently marketed standard thickness lenses, the B, F and B3 Series have been shown to provide a significantly higher success rate than other standard Series lenses. The F Series lens is preferred over the B Series lens due to a thinner edge design resulting in greater comfort. This improved success rate with these lenses is primarily due to better optical quality. By this is meant that if a lens decentres on an eye, degradation of visual acuity will not be as pronounced as with lenses of the other Series. This optical improvement has been designed into ultra-thin Series lenses as well, and will be designed into all future lenses. The current fitting philosophy has therefore evolved into the more simplified routine shown in *Table 14.17*.

The 14.5 mm Series lenses (B4, U4) are now produced by the spin-casting method as with the other Series. The choice of which centre thickness lens to use depends on practitioner preference and on each individual patient. If the minimum of physiological disruption is necessary (as for oedema-prone patients) then the ultra-thin Series will be the lenses of choice. If, however, the patient's dexterity is poor or the environment is very dry, then the Standard Series lenses should be fitted first. At the present time Bausch and Lomb has been able to identify only two lens parameter variables – overall size and centre thickness – which have a predictable effect on the clinical performance of spun-cast lenses.

HYDROFLEX/m

The Hydroflex 'mini' is manufactured by Wöhlk-Contact-Linsen in Germany from the same HEMA-based material as their large, semi-scleral, Hydroflex lens. It was originally introduced in 1974 as a supplementary lens to the latter, but now represents the great majority of their soft lens production, and has established the strong general trend towards corneal-sized soft lens fitting in preference to semi-scleral lenses. It has been available in the United Kingdom since 1975. The material has the following physical properties.

Refractive index (at 23°C) 1.448
Water content: 38.6 per cent at 23°C.

Swell factor: $\left(\dfrac{1 \text{ wet}}{1 \text{ dry}}\right)^3$ 1.69

Softening temperature 109°C
Elasticity 11.3 mm elastic deformation
Penetration strength 4.81 Newton
Hardness (at 20°C) 85.6 Shore-D-units
Ash content (3 g ashed at 550°C) < 0.1 per cent
Oxygen permeability 7.3×10^{-11} (cm²/sec) (ml O₂/ml × mm Hg)

All lenses are manufactured by lathe-cutting, and are hydrated in normal saline solution of pH 7.0–7.2

Table 14.17–Current Bausch and Lomb Fitting Philosophy

Horizontal visible corneal diameter (mm)	Standard centre thickness Negative powers (t_c 0.12 mm)	Positive powers	Series Ultra-thin centre thicknesses (t_c 0.07 mm)	(t_c 0.035 mm)
< 11.5	F	+N	U	
				O3
11.5–12.0	B3	+B3 (H3 higher powers)	U3	
> 12.0	B4	+B4 (H4 higher powers)	U4	O4

Table 14.18–Parameters of Hydroflex/mini Lenses

Power (D)	Average centre thickness (mm)	Front optic diameter for overall sizes of			
		12.0 mm	*12.5 mm*	*13.0 mm*	*13.5 mm*
Plano to −2.00	0.17	9.5–11.5	10.0–12.0	10.5–12.5	11.0–13.0
−2.25 to −8.00	0.10	8.0– 9.5	8.0–10.0	8.5–10.5	9.0–11.0
−8.25 to −14.00	0.10	8.0	8.0	8.0– 8.5	8.0– 9.0
−14.25 to −30.00	0.09	7.7	7.7	8.0	8.0
+0.25 to +1.75	0.20	11.0	11.5	12.0	12.5
+2.00 to +8.00	0.14	7.7	7.7	7.7	7.7
+8.25 to +14.00	0.20–0.24	7.7	7.7	7.7	7.7
+14.25 to +20.00	0.26	7.7	7.7	7.7	7.7
+20.25 to +30.00	0.34	7.7	7.7	7.7	7.7

Hydroflex/m lenses have no peripheral curve on the posterior surface.
Edge thickness for all lenses is 0.08 mm.
Positive lenses over +2.00 D are lenticular.

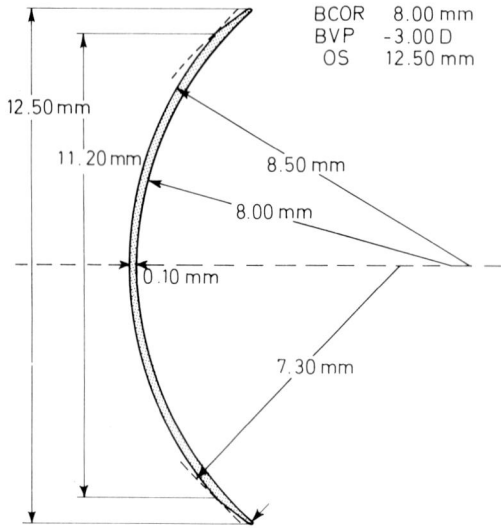

(a)

BCOR   8.00 mm
BVP   -3.00 D
OS   12.50 mm

12.50 mm
11.20 mm
8.50 mm
8.00 mm
0.10 mm
7.30 mm

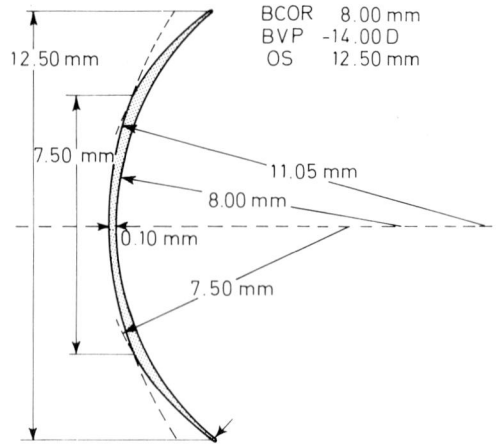

(b)

BCOR   8.00 mm
BVP   -14.00 D
OS   12.50 mm

12.50 mm
7.50 mm
11.05 mm
8.00 mm
0.10 mm
7.50 mm

Figure 14.29–Parameters of typical Hydroflex/m lenses: Cross-sections of (a) An 8.00:12.5 –3.00 lens. (b) An 8.00:12.5 –14.00 lens. (c) An 8.00:12.5 +14.00 lens

over a period of 12 hours. Before hydration, lenses are engraved with a serial number which, although having no clinical significance, serves as a simple means of identification for patient and practitioner.

Lens Geometry

Figure 14.29a,b and *c* shows typical examples of Hydroflex/m geometry for powers of –3.00 D, –14.00 D and +14.00 D. The posterior surface of all lenses is of monocurve construction, there being no peripheral curve. The front surface is lenticulated to allow the production of a very thin lens, so that for

Table 14.19–Basic Fitting Set of 21 Hydroflex/m Lenses

BCOR (mm)		BVP (D)	
	–3.00	–3.00	+3.00
7.5	12.5	–	–
7.7	12.5	13.0	13.0
7.9	12.5	13.0	13.0
8.1	12.5	13.0	13.0
8.3	12.5	13.0	13.0
8.5	12.5	13.0	13.0
8.7	12.5	13.0	13.0
8.9	–	13.0	–

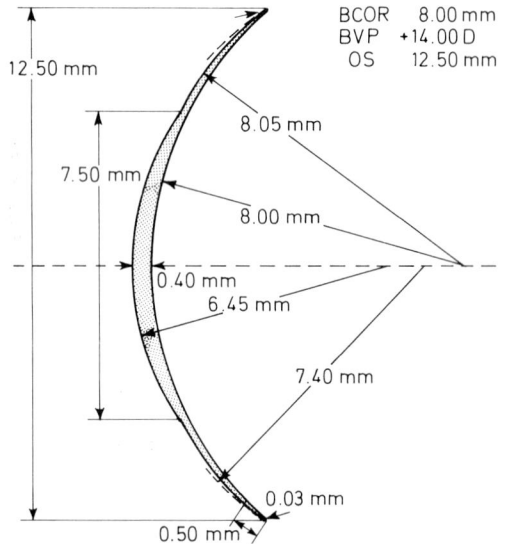

(c)

BCOR   8.00 mm
BVP   +14.00 D
OS   12.50 mm

12.50 mm
8.05 mm
7.50 mm
8.00 mm
0.40 mm
6.45 mm
7.40 mm
0.03 mm
0.50 mm

powers higher than –3.00 D, the centre thickness is 0.10 mm; the edge thickness is 0.08 mm for all powers. *Table 14.18* gives figures for thickness and lenticulation throughout the standard power range of +20.00 D to –20.00 D. The most frequently used overall sizes are 12.5 mm and 13.0 mm, but also available are lenses of 11.5 mm, 12.0 mm and 13.5 mm. The standard interval for fitting steps is 0.2 mm, although it is possible to obtain intermediate radii.

Fitting Sets

The recommended fitting set consists of the lenses shown in *Table 14.19*.

Supplementary sets are available for powers of ±6.00 D and ±14.00 D. With lenses of corneal size it is particularly important to note that hypermetropic eyes cannot be reliably fitted with negative trial lenses because of their very different geometric form.

Fitting Technique

The intention of the fitting philosophy is to provide a properly centred lens which is the same size as, or up to 1 mm larger than, the horizontal corneal diameter, and which gives complete corneal coverage: 12.5 mm overall size lenses usually give a

Table 14.20–Determination of BCOR of First Trial Lens for Hydroflex/m Lenses of Overall Size 12.5 mm

Mean corneal radius (mm)	Value to be added (mm)
7.10–7.49	0.40
7.50–7.89	0.30
7.90–8.29	0.20
8.30–8.60	0.10

satisfactory fitting for corneas up to 12.0 mm, whilst those larger than this may require a 13.0 mm lens. Wöhlk recommend that radius selection should be made according to *Table 14.20*, for 12.5 mm lenses.

Example 1
'K': 7.80 mm (spherical)
Corneal diameter: 11.8 mm
Initial trial lens should be 8.10:12.5 –3.00

Example 2
'K': 7.50 mm along 180, 7.30 mm along 90
Corneal diameter: 11.5 mm
Mean 'K' = 7.40 mm
From *Table 14.20* the theoretical BCOR of the first lens should be 7.8 mm, but as this is not included in the standard fitting set, the next lens flatter is selected. The initial trial lens is therefore 7.90:12.5 –3.00.

Voerste (1976) in a retrospective analysis of 300 eyes substantiated the accuracy of this fitting guide for the majority of cases, but at the same time found that quite wide variations in lens fitting could sometimes be required for corneas of apparently the same central radius. He also found that the majority of lenses with an overall size of 12.5 mm were of

BCOR from 7.70 mm to 8.30 mm, whereas most of the 13.0 mm overall size lenses used were flatter than 8.00 mm BCOR. In addition, he confirmed the validity of the important clinical rule that: a change in radius of 0.2 mm ≡ 0.5 mm change in overall size.

Thus, 7.9:12.5 is clinically equivalent to 8.1:13.0, and 8.5:13.0 is clinically equivalent to 8.3:12.5. This rule must be taken into account when using *Table 14.20* for 13.0 mm lenses.

Example 3
'K': 8.20 mm along 90, 8.00 mm along 180
Corneal diameter: 12.5 mm
Mean 'K' = 8.10 mm. Add 0.2 mm from *Table 14.20* and another 0.2 mm as a 13.0 mm overall size lens is used for the larger corneal diameter. The initial trial lens is therefore 8.5:13.0 –3.00 D.

An alternative, but more approximate method, which usually gives a similar result, is to select the first trial lens with BCOR 0.3 mm flatter than flattest 'K'. The overall size is chosen independently, on the basis of corneal diameter, as before.

Fitting Characteristics of Corneal Soft Lenses

Fitting characteristics are mainly as outlined in *Table 14.3*, page 418. Corneal diameter lenses require careful observation of centration and movement, since they are more significantly influenced by such factors as corneal and limbal topography, lid pressure and the size and position of the palpebral aperture. *Figure 14.30a–d* indicates the four common ways a lens may position on the cornea with the eye in the primary position.

In (*a*) an optimum fitting is shown, with the lens perfectly centred. There should be 0.5–1.0 mm vertical movement on blinking.

In (*b*) the lens is riding slightly high, influenced perhaps by a tight upper lid. This is acceptable as long as the decentration is no more than 0.5 mm, but the fitting may well be improved by choosing a larger lens which is clinically equivalent. It is often possible to achieve a satisfactory fitting with a rather flatter lens than average in this situation, because of the gripping action of the upper lid.

In (*c*) the lens is shown riding in a low position, and generally represents an unsatisfactory fitting. It can occur with a lens which is too small or too flat, in which case there maybe unacceptable lid sensation. It can also result from the downward pressure of a relatively heavy upper lid, creating a fitting which is tight, but initially quite comfortable. After several hours of wear, there is a risk of arcuate staining at the superior limbus, and anoxia because of insufficient tears being pumped beneath the lens from below.

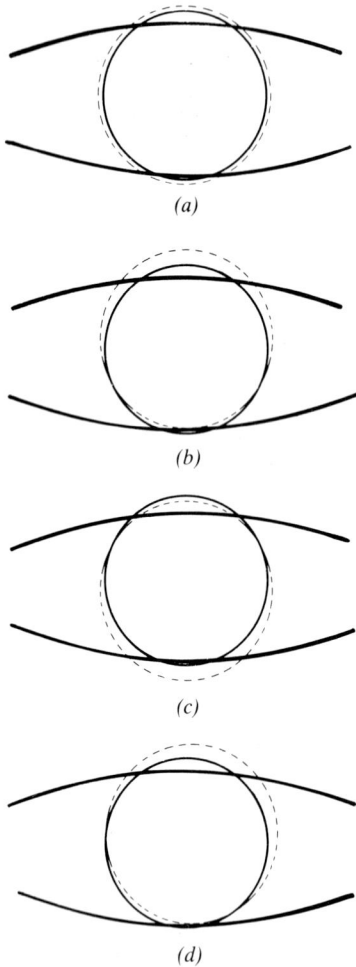

Figure 14.30—The four common positions taken up by soft lenses of corneal size, on an eye in the primary position. (a) Correctly centred. (b) Slightly high. (c) Slightly low. (d) Laterally decentred

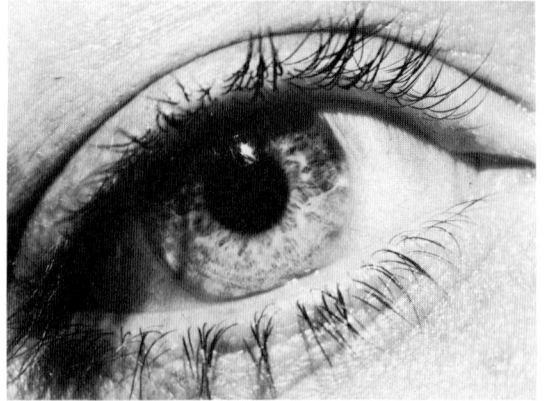

Figure 14.31—Slight nasal displacement of a Hydroflex/m lens estimated to be 0.2 mm too flat

refractive result. Voerste (1976) found that powers should be almost the same as the ocular refraction; 70 per cent were within ±0.25 D, and 90 per cent within ±0.50 D. If the first trial lens proves too mobile, it is usually better to achieve stability by increasing the overall size rather than by steepening the radius. For example, if 'K' is 7.60, and 7.90:12.5 appears too loose, 7.90:13.0 should be tried before 7.70:12.5.

In some instances, an apparently correct fitting may still give persistent subjective awareness, which may only be eliminated by selecting a larger overall size. Positive and high-powered negative lenses are often fitted one step tighter than usual. This compensates, in the former case, for the weight factor and prevents downwards decentration, and,

In (d) the lens is eccentrically located, either because it is too small or too flat, or because of lid pressure combined with a shallow corneo-scleral junction. This is not a very satisfactory fitting, but may sometimes prove acceptable if the decentration is limited to 0.5 mm. A lens with a larger overall size should be tried. Figure 14.31 shows a slightly flat lens locating somewhat nasally, and Figure 14.32 shows its excessive movement on rotation of the eye nasally.

It is particularly important to avoid fitting too steeply, since although comfort and vision may at first be satisfactory, ultimately the visual acuity will deteriorate when the initial excess tears flow returns to normal. A further clue is provided by the

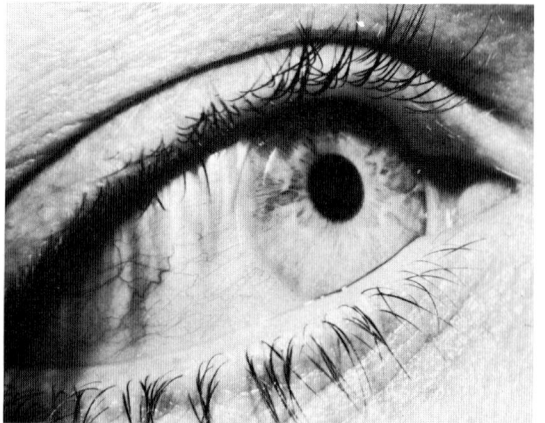

Figure 14.32—The same lens as in Figure 14.31 showing excessive lag on nasal rotation of the eye, confirming the flatness of the fit

in the latter, for any excessive mobility from lid action on the much thicker mid-peripheral portion of the lens.

Hydroflex/m – sd

The super-thin version of the standard Hydroflex/m was introduced in mid-1978, for the solution of some problem cases. Lenses are available in overall sizes of 13.0, 13.5 and 14.5 mm, the former in powers from +10.00 D to –10.00 D, and the latter in the aphakic range from +10.00 D to +20.00 D. The centre thickness of a –3.00 D lens of 13.0 mm overall size is 0.08 mm.

In addition, a high water content material, Hydroflex 65, provides the basis for a range of lenses including the lower power range, aphakic prescriptions, and front surface toric lenses.

Hydroflex/m lenses are available in a range of eight tints. These can also be produced with clear or black pupils from 3 to 6 mm in diameter.

Two versions of back surface toric lens are available, either with prism ballast or truncated (see pages 449 and 452).

MENICON*

Menicon lenses, previously fitted in Japan for several years, have been available in the United Kingdom since 1976. The lens material is a HEMA-based polymer containing vinyl acetate. The relatively low water content of only 29.6 per cent gives a rather tougher material to handle, slightly more stable visual acuity, but less good initial comfort and lower oxygen permeability than many other corneal sized soft lenses. Physical properties are given below.

Water content	29.6 per cent
Water uptake	43 per cent
Linear swelling coefficient	13.7
Oxygen permeability	5.85×10^{-11} (cm²/sec) (ml O₂/ml × mm Hg)
Rubber hardness	28
Refractive index	1.458
Visible light transmission	> 90 per cent
Specific gravity	1.16
Tensile strength	14.5 kg/cm²
Penetration strength	913 g/mm
Thermal conductivity	6.43×10^{-4}

*This section refers to the Menicon '1500' material. The M79 material has a water content of 39% and the separate fitting manual supplied by Menicon should be used.

Fitting Sets

The standard range of lenses consists of BCOR from 7.8 mm to 9.2 mm in steps of 0.2 mm; overall sizes of 12.5 mm and 13.0 mm; and powers of +20.00 D to –20.00 D in steps of 0.25 D. The recommended fitting set is shown in Table 14.21.

Table 14.21–Number of Lenses in the Recommended Menicon Fitting Set, Shown in Terms of BCOR, OS and BVP

BCOR (mm)	OS (mm) and BVP (D)		
	12.5	13.0	13.0
	–3.00	–3.00	+5.00
8.0	1	–	1
8.2	2	1	1
8.4	2	2	1
8.6	2	2	1
8.8	2	2	1
9.0	1	2	–
9.2	–	1	–

Fitting Technique

The fitting technique aims to provide an overall size slightly larger than the horizontal corneal diameter, with the same type of characteristics for centration and movement as other corneal sized soft lenses (see Table 14.3 on page 418, and pages 416–417). The first trial lens may be selected according to Table 14.22.

Phillips (1977) found this guide to be very reliable, but stressed the importance of selecting the flattest fit and smaller overall size where possible, for physiological reasons. The lower water content is more likely to produce a greater incidence of corneal oedema, particularly with the relatively thick positive lenses.

The Toyo material, from which Menicon lenses are made, is also used by various other laboratories

Table 14.22–Selection of First Menicon Trial Lens

Mean 'K' (mm)	BCOR of first trial lens (mm) for OS (mm) of	
	12.5	13.0
6.90 to 7.50	8.20	8.40
7.55 to 7.80	8.40	8.60
7.85 to 8.40	8.60	8.80

to manufacture lenses of different geometries. Such lenses include the N and N (Grosvenor and Callender, 1973), Consoft 2000, and Molliter.

Other corneal diameter soft lenses include Snoflex SD38 (Smith and Nephew); the Hydron Europe 'mini'; the Weicon 'mini' (Titmus-Eurocon); Hoya lenses Durasoft (Wesley-Jessen); Aosoft, previously called Aquaflex (American Optical); and Aoflex mini (American Optical). This last lens is unusual in that it is of tricurve construction.

CONTINUOUS AND EXTENDED WEAR

The development of soft lenses which are suitable for continuous wear represents a significant advance in contact lens practice, since they have important advantages for a great many patients, such as medical cases, aphakics and other poor lens handlers. Many patients are known to have worn hard lenses without removal for long periods of time, but they have frequently caused at least some degree of damage, if not irreversible changes to the cornea. The effects of daily wear soft lenses on the cornea during both sleep and limited continuous wear have shown them to be feasible, but unwise for this purpose for most normal eyes. Studies with such lenses, usually with a water content of about 40 per cent, have demonstrated a morning phase of corneal oedema after overnight wear (Mandell, 1976). Harris, Sanders and Zisman (1975) found a 5 per cent increase in corneal thickness after only 30 minutes of eye closure, and Liebowitz, Laing and Sandstrom (1973) measured a 30 per cent increase after 10 days. Ruben (1974) considered that the possible adverse consequences of continuous wear could include vascularization, infection, epithelial necrosis, endothelial dysfunction and mucus formation. Permanent wear lenses therefore demand considerable caution and very careful patient management if all of the possible difficulties are to be avoided.

The essential requirement for continuous wear is the maintenance of normal corneal physiology, even during closed eye conditions. Holly and Refojo (1972) found the normal consumption of oxygen by the cornea to be 7.0 μl/cm^2/h, and the figure below which its metabolism begins to be adversely affected to be 3.5 μl/cm^2/h. Additionally, Fatt and Bieber (1968) found that the normal value for oxygen tension at the corneal surface is 55 mm Hg under closed eye conditions, although Polse and Mandell (1970) concluded that normal corneal metabolism could be maintained if the oxygen tension did not fall below 11–19 mm Hg (varying between one individual and another). Any lens to be considered for continuous wear must therefore satisfy these requirements, by providing an adequate supply of oxygen to the cornea. This may be achieved in two ways: by means of high water content, since there is a direct relationship between gas permeability and water content for any given material; or by making lenses as thin as possible, because of the further relationship between oxygen flow and lens thickness (Larke and Sabell, 1971; Fatt, 1977). Fatt (1977) has likened the flow of oxygen through a gas permeable soft lens to the flow of electricity through a conductor by the application of an Ohm's law type of analysis. The oxygen tension at the lens-cornea interface is less than that at the front surface of the lens, the drop in oxygen tension being a function of the oxygen permeability (Dk) of the material. D represents the diffusion coefficient, and k the solubility of oxygen for the material. For any given lens the thickness (L) must be taken into account to give the value Dk/L, the 'transmissibility'. (In Chapter 13, page 397, the oxygen permeability is given as P, the oxygen diffusion coefficient as D and its solubility as S, that is $P = D \times S$ instead of Fatt's $Dk = D \times k$, as here. Also the oxygen transmission rate is referred to, in Chapter 13, as TR which corresponds to the 'transmissibility' given here.)

In practical terms, these figures mean that for a 40 per cent water content HEMA lens the cornea's oxygen requirement is met for open and closed eye conditions if the minimum lens thicknesses are 0.14 mm and 0.04 mm respectively. With 70 per cent water content lenses the equivalent values for lens thickness must be 0.47 mm and 0.13 mm respectively (Rocher, 1977). Gasson (1976) found that ultrathin Bausch and Lomb lenses of centre thickness 0.04 mm could be worn continuously, but that they were not ideally suitable for this purpose, discomfort supervening after about 7 days. Danker (1976), in the United States reported that silicone rubber lenses which have virtually zero water content, but extremely high oxygen permeability, have proved suitable for constant wear, and this has been confirmed more recently by patients in the United Kingdom. However, the affinity of mucus deposits for silicone material means that lenses may require removal for cleaning every 6 or 7 days. A distinction may be made between this sort of extended wear, in which lenses are worn overnight for one or several days, and true continuous wear in which lenses are not removed from the eye for several months. The first two soft lenses specifically developed for continuous wear were Permalens and Sauflon PW. Both are high water content and relatively thin, and have been successfully used for this purpose over the last few years. In addition a lens of more recent origin is Duragel 75.

PERMALENS

Permalens was developed by de Carle in 1970, and is manufactured in the United Kingdom by Global Vision. The lens is made from a HEMA-based terpolymer, sometimes referred to as Perfilcon-A containing N-vinyl pyrrolidone. It has a water content of 74 per cent and a swell factor of 1.43. It is important to note that it is only this particular lens which is correctly described by the name Permalens, which has erroneously been used as a generic term.

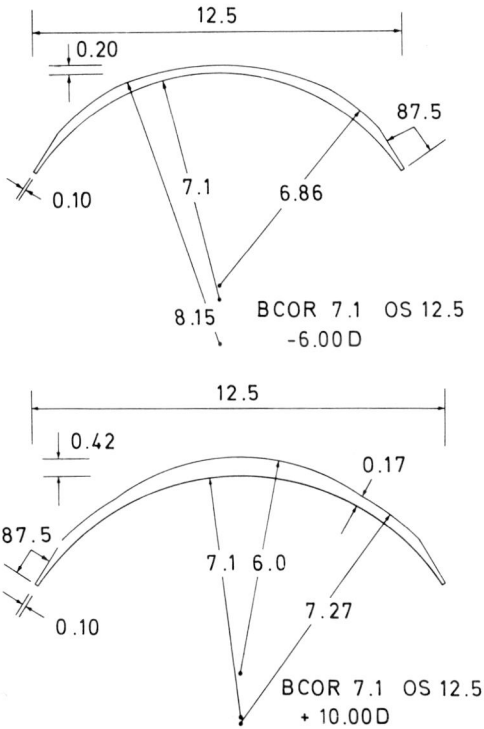

Figure 14.34–A typical Permalens on the eye

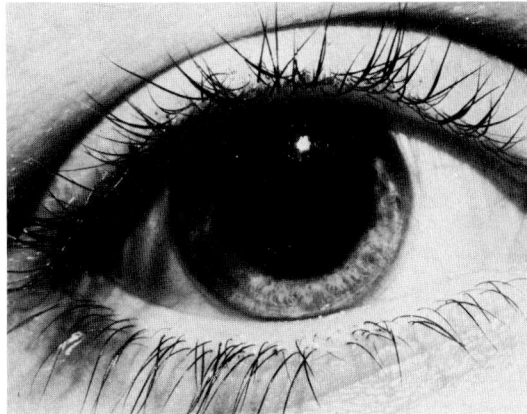

Figure 14.33–The geometry of typical Permalenses. All dimensions are in mm

Lens Geometry and Fitting Set

The posterior surface of the lens is of monocurve construction, whilst the front surface is lenticulated to give as thin a lens as possible. At –3.00 D the centre thickness is 0.15 mm. The geometry of two typical Permalenses is shown in *Figure 14.33* and a typical lens on the eye in *Figure 14.34*.

The basic minus trial set consists of the 7 lenses shown in *Table 14.23*, but fittings are most satisfactorily carried out with the aid of a large stock of lenses, so that lenses of the correct power may be used wherever possible.

Fitting Technique

Permalens is exceptional among soft lenses because it is fitted using back surface radii which may be steeper than the cornea. The lens material is extremely soft so that a properly fitting lens flattens to become effectively an alignment fit. The radius of the initial low negative trial lens is selected to be the first available BCOR steeper than flattest 'K'. Due to their greater centre thickness and, therefore, rigidity, positive lenses are fitted on flattest 'K' or the first available BCOR that is flatter than the flattest 'K', and with a slightly larger OS than negative powered lenses.

Table 14.23–Permalens Range of Parameters for Negative Lenses

BCOR (mm)	OS (mm)			
6.50	12.00			
6.80	12.00	12.50		
7.10		12.50	13.00	
7.40			13.00	
7.70				13.50
8.00				13.50

For negative powered lenses the OS should be 1.0 to 2.0 mm larger than the horizontal VID. For high positive powered lenses the OS should be increased to 2.0 to 3.00 mm larger than VID.

Fittings which are slightly too steep or flat show distortion of keratometer mires from the front surface of the lens. Excessive steepness is indicated where the mires look pear-shaped just before a blink and where vision is improved by the application of lid pressure in screwing up the eyes.

A well fitting Permalens is very comfortable, often more so than a daily wear lens. (Some hypersensitive patients who have been unable to wear any kind of daily wear lens beyond 4 or 5 hours have rapidly achieved all day tolerance, and sometimes continuous wear, with Permalens.) The lens should remain stable on the cornea in all directions of gaze with a minimum of movement, 0.5 mm being

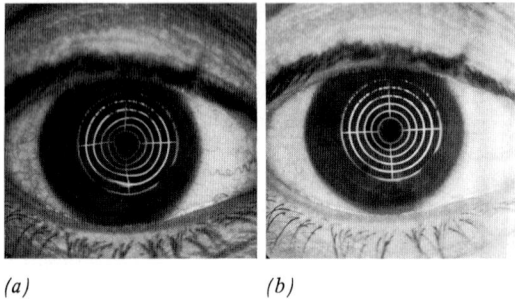

(a)   *(b)*

Figure 14.35—A correctly fitting Permalens showing the photokeratoscope image. (a) Before settling. (b) After settling

the usual limit. Some patients initially experience mild subjective awareness, but this should have disappeared after the first two days. By this time the visual acuity should also have fully settled to give a good refractive result, and the retinoscopy reflex should be sharp. A dark spot in the centre of this reflex indicates a fitting which is too steep. A flat fitting Permalens can be quite uncomfortable; de-centres on the cornea or is too mobile. *Figure 14.35a* and *b* shows the improvement in the photokeratoscope image between a newly inserted and a fully settled Permalens.

SAUFLON PW

Sauflon PW was introduced by Contact Lenses (Manufacturing) Ltd., in 1972. The material, being from the same polymeric family, is chemically similar to Sauflon 70; the higher water content

makes it very suitable for continuous wear, but at the same time lenses are rather too fragile for frequent handling.

Fitting Set

The standard range of available lenses is shown in *Table 14.24*, from which it will be seen that the overall size is constant for any given power.

Table 14.24–Standard Range of Sauflon PW Lenses

BCOR (mm)	OS (mm) for BVP of	
	−10.00 D to +10.75 D	+11.00 D to +20.00 D
7.50	13.00	13.50
7.80	13.00	13.50
8.10	13.00	13.50
8.40	13.00	13.50

A basic fitting set therefore consists of just the four radii in whatever powers are considered appropriate. As with Permalens, however, Sauflon PW is best fitted with the aid of a large stock of lenses. Negative lenses have a centre thickness of 0.2 mm or less. Aphakic lenses have a reduced optic and a +18.00 D lens, for example, has a front optic diameter of 8.00 mm, a centre thickness of 0.35 mm and a carrier portion 0.15 mm thick.

Fitting Technique

The overall size of the lens is predetermined by the manufacturers according to its power, so that fitting consists merely of choosing the correct radius. On average for negative lenses this is approximately 0.2 mm flatter than flattest 'K'. Hodd (1976c) has related the selection of the initial radius to the corneal diameter by means of *Table 14.25*.

Table 14.25–Selection of Initial Radius

Corneal diameter (mm)	Value to be added to mean 'K' (mm) for lenses of	
	13.00 mm	13.50 mm
10.00	0.35	0.40
10.50	0.30	0.35
11.00	0.25	0.30
11.50	0.20	0.25
12.00	0.15	0.20
12.50	0.10	0.15
13.00	0.05	0.10
13.50	Unsuitable	0.05

A correct fitting gives good vision and comfort. A steep fit may also be initially comfortable, but can produce oedematous blurring after overnight wear, together with conjunctival injection and scleral indentation. A flat fitting is easily recognized because of its excessive mobility, and the lens may slip completely off the cornea on blinking.

Sauflon PW has gained wide acceptance in the fitting of aphakics, and continuous wear may be the only method of providing such patients with an acceptable form of visual correction. In some cases both Sauflon PW and Permalens have been fitted at operation (Pierse and Kersley, 1977; de Carle, 1977). Morris (1976) found that with the use of a spectacle correction in astigmatic cases Sauflon PW can give visual acuity as good as with spectacles alone.

DURAGEL 75

Duragel 75 is one of a range of Duragel materials having water contents of 60, 71 and 75 per cent respectively. The 75 per cent water content material is that designed for extended wear but the 71 per cent material may also be used in the thinner, negative powered range.

The material is an amido-amino copolymer with tertiary amines as the hydrophilic sites, and is unrelated to HEMA. The monomers are placed in a vacuum system and exposed to the effects of a low pressure gas discharge. This 'glow discharge' produces low energy electrons which interact with the monomer mixture to produce active chemical sites suitable for the formation of the cross-linked polymer. The process does not therefore depend on the intervention of potentially hazardous and reactive chemical reagents and, additionally, it allows the

polymerization process to be closely controlled. The material is claimed to be much stronger than other hydrogels of equivalent high water content and formulated to minimize chemical interaction of contaminated molecules by the use of stoicheimetric interference. Thus, if the hydrophilic sites are arranged to be well shielded by other parts of the polymer structure, large molecules, such as protein, cannot approach the hydrophilic sites closely enough to interact with them although the sites are readily accessible to small molecules such as water.

The lenses are lathe-cut and, although they may be made to any specification, are available in the 75 per cent water content material in a stock range shown in *Table 14.21*.

Table 14.26–Standard Parameters for Duragel 75

BCOR (mm)	OS (mm)	BVP (D)
8.10	13.50	Afocal to −8.00 D in 0.25 D steps
8.30	13.50	+0.25 D to +8.00 D in 0.25 D steps
8.50	13.50	+8.50 D to +20.00 D in 0.50 D steps

Lenses are fitted 0.5 mm flatter than the flattest 'K'. The flattest lens commensurate with comfort and visual stability is the most suitable fitting and gives rise to the fewest complications. The manufacturers claim a material strength such that even the 75 per cent water content lenses may be used on either a daily or extended wear basis.

Wearing Schedule

Whenever possible, patients for Permalens, Sauflon PW or Duragel 75 are fitted in the morning so that they can be carefully examined after wearing the lenses all day. If everything is satisfactory at this stage they are permitted to wear the lenses overnight, and checked again the following morning. Patients are advised that vision may be hazy for a few minutes on waking. This may be due either to adaptive oedema or to mucus deposits on the lens surface which may be removed by the application of one of the proprietary soft lens solutions. Further examinations take place after 1 week and 1 month, and subsequently at 3 monthly intervals, for lens cleaning and after-care.

Although most patients can sustain continuous wear from the beginning, some practitioners prefer an adaptation period of daily wear for about the first week. This is not feasible, however, for those patients such as aphakics who have been specifically fitted with 'continuous' wear lenses because of handling difficulty. In all cases patients must be shown how to remove lenses, and never to ignore redness, soreness or discomfort, which might presage some more severe ocular response.

Problems with Continuous Wear Lenses

The high water content which makes certain soft lenses suitable for continuous wear is also the main cause of clinical problems. The large swell factor makes the lenses more difficult to manufacture, reproducibility can therefore be unreliable, and fitting unnecessarily time-consuming. The pore size is also larger and so the material is more easily contaminated by proteins and other substances. Handling is difficult because of the softness of the material, lenses are very fragile, and breakages can occur spontaneously while on the eye. Vision can be unsatisfactory with the steeper fittings, and lenses are sometimes rubbed out of the eye during sleep.

Other problems relate to lens ageing. Severe red eyes are usually attributable to dirty lenses which have been worn for too long a period without cleaning, although a similar reaction is sometimes caused by removal of the lens disturbing the corneal epithelium. A very common problem is the large white spot (*Figure 14.5*), from which both Permalens and Sauflon PW suffer. They are calcium in origin, and the phenomenon is worse with patients who have relatively dry eyes and who are partial blinkers. These large discrete deposits usually occur within the area of the exposed palpebral aperture. Their formation appears to be accelerated with Sauflon PW if there is a temperature gradient across a thick lens which is fitting too tightly (Kersley, Kerr and Pierse, 1977), whereas with Permalens, de Carle (1978) has found a more rapid deposition with a loose fitting.

Most of the problems currently encountered would be obviated if continuous wear lenses could be regarded as disposable and replaced at regular intervals of about 6 months. This is borne out by Ruben (1977) who feels that constant wear of soft lenses is more likely to lead to irreversible ocular changes than daily wear, as the latter allows several hours each day in which healing can take place. He gives a considerable list of pathological complications of soft lens wear and, as far as constant wear lenses are concerned, the main causes are infection from the lens itself, from solutions or from some other source. This emphasizes the imperative need

for hygiene in all aspects of lens handling by both patient and practitioner and the desirability of replacing dirty lenses with new ones to minimize the risks of infection.

Indications for Continuous Wear

Despite all the possible difficulties and the great care which must be taken, there are many patients for whom a continuous wear lens is the most suitable, if not the only form of visual correction; they are as follows.

(1) Aphakics. This is perhaps the most important group, because of the large number of potential patients and their great difficulty with lens handling.

(2) Other poor lens handlers.

(3) Medical cases, where the lens is used as a corneal bandage, such as bullous keratopathy, or corneal dystrophy (*see* Chapter 21).

(4) Young children, where it is not feasible to handle lenses on a daily basis, and where a hard lens would be rejected.

(5) In certain occupations or vocational uses where an ametropic patient requires good visual acuity immediately on waking.

(6) Patients who have no facility for soft lens disinfection.

(7) As one component of a low vision aid, where poor visual acuity makes regular handling impossible.

In addition to continuous wear, there are obvious advantages in patients using on a daily basis, lenses which are suitable for extended wear. There is then no risk of problems if a patient inadvertently falls asleep while wearing the lenses, or if travelling prevents their removal for one or two days.

TORIC SOFT LENSES

Several different methods have evolved to deal with the problem of fitting astigmatic patients with soft contact lenses. Such lenses may be of corneal or semi-scleral diameter, and with the toric curve on either the back or front surface. In cases of with-the-rule astigmatism the thickest portions of the correcting toric lens lie at the top and bottom. The normal action of the lids is to rotate the lens 90 degrees off axis to bring the thickest parts of the lens into the horizontal meridian. To prevent this rotation, and to maintain correct orientation of the lens with respect to the cylinder axis, soft lenses must be stabilized on the eye. Three methods have been used for this purpose, either on their own, or in combination: (1) prism ballast; (2) truncation; and (3) 'dynamic stabilization'.

BACK SURFACE TORIC SOFT LENSES

Back surface toric lenses have evolved logically from the fact that most of the astigmatism encountered in contact lens practice is predominantly corneal. It is measurable with the keratometer, and a comparison with the spectacle refraction gives an immediate prediction of the likelihood of visual success. Lenticular astigmatism, however, is not correctable with these lenses, since the back surface toric essentially attempts to neutralize the astigmatic cornea and replace it with the front spherical refracting surface. The lenses are not used merely to provide a better physical fit as is the case with hard lenses. Despite the complexity of the actual lens design, fitting procedures are straightforward, and the toric calculations quite simple.

Two lens designs are possible, having different geometries and fitting techniques. They are prism ballast as with the Hydroflex/m-T, and the Hydrocurve; and the truncation as with the Hydroflex-TS.

With both types of lenses careful consideration must be given to patient selection, since they are not designed to correct lenticular astigmatism. Both the axis and power of the corneal astigmatism should correlate with the spectacle Rx.

The Hydroflex/m-T avoids the use of a fitting set. It is cosmetically superior, being the natural development of the spherical Hydroflex/m, and it is more suitable for very small corneas. Handling is easier, and there is less risk of lid sensation from the lower edge of the lens.

The Hydroflex-TS is less affected by lid pressure and corneal topography, and the use of a fitting set allows the prediction of the way in which the final lens will settle on the eye. It is more suitable for larger corneas and wider palpebral apertures.

PRISM BALLAST

The Hydroflex/m-T is a lens of corneal diameter whose fitting principles are based on those of the Hydroflex/m (Jurgensen, 1977). Stabilization of the astigmatic axis is achieved by means of $1\frac{1}{2}\triangle$ base-down, but this is assisted by the natural stabilization effect of a toric lens surface in apposition to an equivalently toroidal cornea. The front surface at the lower edge is chamfered to maintain good physical comfort. The standard range of lens parameters is shown in *Table 14.27*.

It should be noted that it is not the entire back surface which is toroidal, but only the central optic portion. This is ellipsoidal in shape, the precise dimensions depending on the lens powers and radii; it is larger with a lower cylinder, and vice versa.

Table 14.27–Range of Available Hydroflex/m-T Lenses

BCOR (mm)	7.10 to 9.00 (in steps of 0.10)
Spherical power (D)	+20.00 to −20.00 (in steps of 0.25)
Cylindrical power (D)	−0.50 to −6.00 (in steps of approximately 0.50 determined by astigmatic differences of 0.10 mm)
Overall size (mm)	12.00 to 13.50 (in steps of 0.50)

Figures 14.36 and *14.37* show the construction of a lens of specification: 8.50/7.50 12.50 −3.00 T180.

BCOR	8.50/7.50 mm
Power	−3.00 D
Overall size	12.50 mm
Astigmatic axis	180 degrees
Prism	$1\frac{1}{2}\triangle$ Base-down at 270 degrees

All lenses are engraved at the periphery with two short reference markings, at exactly 90 degrees to the base apex line of the prism. These are unrelated to the actual astigmatic axis of the correction, but serve toidentify and describe the orientation of the lens when worn on the eye. Ideally they should settle at 180 degrees for the first lens.

Fitting Method

Toric trial lenses are not used with the Hydroflex/m-T for two reasons. First, because all of the required fitting parameters can be predicted from a spherical fitting set; and secondly, because the number of variables in terms of radius, power, astigmatic difference and overall size would be so great as to make such a trial set unrealistically large in practice.

Fitting, therefore, proceeds in much the same manner as for a spherical Hydroflex/m. The spectacle correction should be expressed in negative cylinder form, and the fitting carried out with trial lenses of power as near as possible to the BVP of the spherical component. The toric lens ordered to prescription will fit somewhat tighter than the equivalent spherical lens, so that the desired fitting is the flattest and largest which is clinically possible, to ensure proper lens mobility and complete corneal coverage. Approximately, a change of radius of 0.2 mm is clinically equivalent to a change in overall size

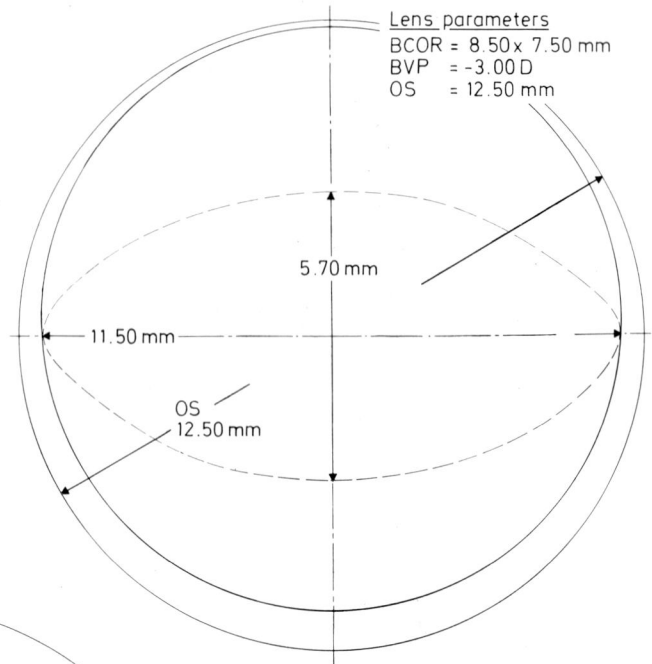

Figure 14.36—Back surface of Hydroflex/m-T lens. The maximum and minimum diameters of the oval toroidal back central optic portion are shown

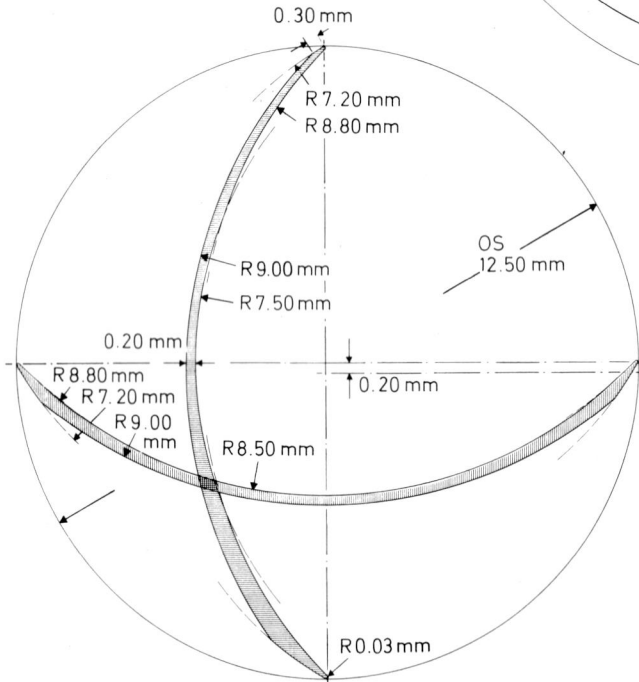

Figure 14.37—Cross-section of a Hydroflex/m-T lens in its principal meridians. Radii are shown prefixed by R

of 0.50 mm. Thus, if the lens 7.90:12.50 gives a satisfactory result, 8.10:13.00 should also be considered. It may well give an equally satisfactory fitting, in which case it would be the preferred specification on which to base the final toric lens.

The sphere, together with the cylinder power and axis, can be taken directly from the spectacle Rx, but are better confirmed by over-refraction with a fully settled trial lens. The astigmatic difference to correct the cylinder is then determined by a simple calculation using *Table 14.28*.

For example, if the best fitting lens 8.10:13.00 has been tried on an eye with a refraction –2.00/–2.00 × 10, the flatter meridian of the lens to be ordered will also be 8.10 mm. This converts to a surface power of –54.91 D from column 2. Adding the cylinder power of –2.00 D gives –56.91 D. The nearest value to this in the table is –57.03 D, which converts back to a radius of 7.80 mm. The complete specification of the toric lens is therefore

$$8.10/7.80 \quad 13.00 \quad -2.00 \quad T10$$

Table 14.28–Radii and Surface Powers for a Refractive Index of 1.4448

BCOR (mm)	Surface power (D)		
		7.80	57.03
		7.90	56.30
		8.00	55.60
		8.10	54.91
6.00	74.13	8.20	54.24
6.10	72.92	8.30	53.59
6.20	71.74	8.40	52.95
6.30	70.60	8.50	52.33
6.40	69.50	8.60	51.72
6.50	68.43	8.70	51.13
6.60	67.39	8.80	50.55
6.70	66.39	8.90	49.98
6.80	65.41	9.00	49.42
6.90	64.46	9.10	48.88
7.00	63.54	9.20	48.35
7.10	62.65	9.30	47.83
7.20	61.78	9.40	47.32
7.30	60.93	9.50	46.82
7.40	60.11	9.60	46.33
7.50	59.31	9.70	45.86
7.60	58.53	9.80	45.39
7.70	57.77	9.90	44.93

In this example the vertex distance has been ignored. With higher powers, this must be taken into account, in which case the two meridional powers must be calculated separately.

This type of calculation gives a satisfactory first lens in a large percentage of cases. However, with a certain number of patients, the influence of lid pressure and corneal topography cause rotation off axis, so that a second lens is required to include an inbuilt compensation for this degree of rotation. This is determined by direct measurement of the reference markings engraved on the lens, whose orientation is most easily observed with the aid of the slit lamp. If the lens in the previous example settles with its toric markings at 165 degrees instead of 180 degrees, the lens should be re-ordered with a T setting of 25 degrees. The assumption is that the second lens will also rotate off axis to the same extent, that is, by 15 degrees, so that the cylinder axis is altered by the same amount, but in the opposite direction to compensate for the rotation which is now expected to occur. The important point is that the engraved markings on the second lens should also settle at 165 degrees and *not* at 180 degrees. It is always the T setting of the cylinder axis which is altered to make the desired compensation.

The refractive effect of a toric lens which has rotated to an incorrect axis can be deduced from *Table 14.29*. For example, a lens incorporating a –2.00 D cylinder which rotates 5 degrees from the correct axis gives a resultant cylinder of –0.50 D at

Table 14.29–Effective Powers and Axes of Mis-aligned Cylinders

Cyl. (D)	Resultant cylinder power for rotation off axis of			
	5 degrees	11 degrees	22 degrees	45 degrees
1.00	0.25	0.37	0.75	1.50
2.00	0.50	0.75	1.50	3.00
3.00	0.75	1.12	2.25	4.50
4.00	1.00	1.62	3.00	6.00
5.00	1.25	2.00	3.75	7.50
6.00	1.50	2.37	4.50	9.00
	43 degrees	38 degrees	33.50 degrees	22.50 degrees

Difference of axis of resultant cylinder from the axis of the correcting cylinder

an axis 43 degrees from that of the axis of the correcting cylinder. Thus, an over-refraction should confirm the degree of mis-alignment seen by observation of the reference markings on the lens. These reference markings are most easily observed with the slit lamp, and an eyepiece containing a protractor-type graticule with degree markings at 5 degree intervals assists in accurately determining their exact location.

A more simplified approach to fitting back surface toric lenses is given by the Hydrocurve lens which has a single overall size of 13.50 mm. The flatter meridian is always of radius 8.60 mm with an astigmatic difference in the back surface to correct either a 1.25 D cylinder or a 2.00 D cylinder. Spherical powers can be obtained from −6.00 D to +3.00 D. Stabilization is by means of 1△ base-down and the base of the prism is identified by a small dot.

When only one toric lens is required, in theory, the spherical lens for the other eye should also include base-down prism to prevent binocular imbalance. In practice, this has seldom been found necessary, and the spherical lens is often initially ordered in the normal way, without prism.

TRUNCATION

The Hydroflex-TS is a truncated semi-scleral lens whose fitting method is based on the large Hydroflex lens. Stabilization of the astigmatic axis is achieved in three ways: by a single 1.5 mm truncation; by 1△ base-down; and by the influence of the toroidal back surface of the lens when applied to an equivalently toroidal cornea. The standard overall size is 14.00 mm in the horizontal meridian (12.50 mm vertically), although 15.00 mm lenses are also available. The range of parameters is shown in *Table 14.30*, although the laboratory will make any specification which is technically possible.

As with the Hydroflex/m-T, the back central optic portion is ellipsoidal in shape, and varies according to the specification of the lens. *Figures 14.38* and *14.39* show the construction of a lens of specification: 9.10/8.10 14.00 −3.00 T180.

BCOR	9.10/8.10 mm
Power	−3.00 DS/−6.00 DC
Overall size	14.00 mm × 12.50 mm
Astigmatic axis	180 degrees
Prism	1△ Base-down at 90 degrees

All lenses are engraved at the periphery with reference markings at 90 degrees to the base apex line of the prism.

Fitting Method

The main difference between fitting the Hydroflex-TS and the m-T is that the TS is fitted with the aid of the trial set shown in *Table 14.31*.

These lenses do not have a toroidal back surface, but are truncated, and engraved with reference markings to determine the orientation of the lens accurately. It means that the effects of corneal topography, lid pressure and the angle of the lower lid margin can be predicted at the fitting stage. This

Table 14.30–Range of Available Hydroflex-TS Lenses

BCOR (mm)	8.10 to 10.00 (in steps of 0.10)
Spherical power (D)	+20.00 to −20.00 (in steps of 0.25)
Cylindrical power (D)	−0.50 to −6.00 (in steps of approximately 0.50, determined by astigmatic differences of 0.10 mm)
Overall size (mm)	14.00 and 15.00

Table 14.31–BCOR and OS of Lenses in the Hydroflex-TS Fitting Set

BCOR (mm)	OS (mm)
8.50	14.00
8.70	14.00
8.90	14.00
9.10	14.00
9.30	14.00
9.50	14.00

Table 14.32–Determining the BCOR of the Initial Hydroflex-TS Trial Lens

Mean corneal radius (mm)	Value to be added (mm)
7.10 to 7.45	1.2
7.50 to 7.85	1.1
7.90 to 8.25	1.0
8.30 to 8.60	0.9

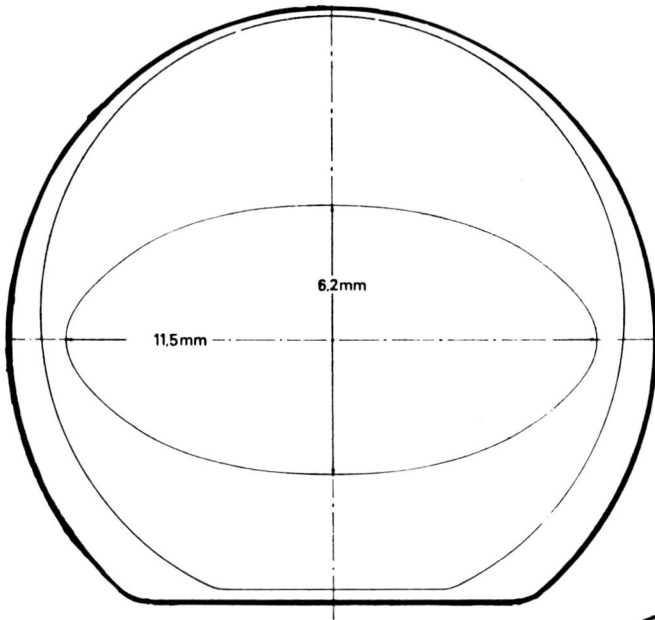

Figure 14.38–Back surface of a Hydroflex-TS lens. The maximum and minimum diameters of the oval toroidal back central optic portion are shown

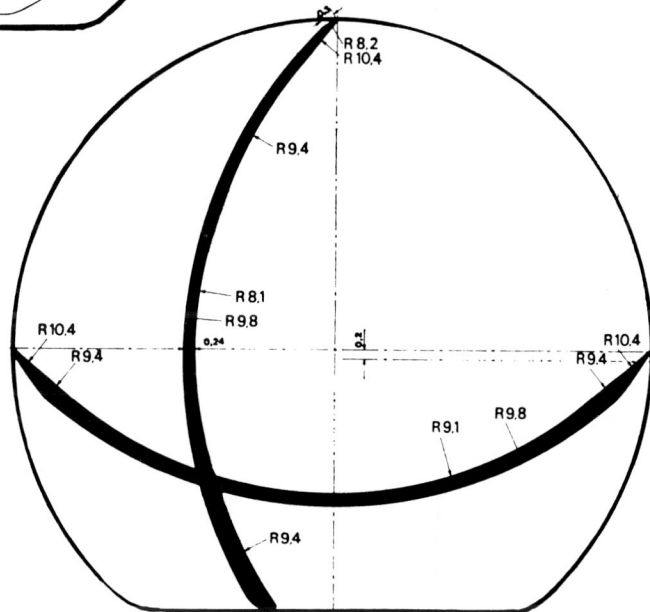

Figure 14.39–Cross-section of a Hydroflex-TS lens in its principal meridians. Overall size is 14.0 mm horizontally and 12.5 mm vertically

therefore reduces the number of lenses which may have to be re-ordered because of rotation off axis.

Selection of the initial trial lens may be made according to *Table 14.32*, but on average the correct fitting is about 0.7 mm flatter than flattest 'K'.

The eventual prescription lens with a toroidal back surface is ordered to be about 0.2 mm steeper than the equivalent spherical trial lens.

A lens which is too flat may rotate on the eye, or ride high, leaving the lower portion of the cornea exposed. A correctly fitting lens should settle with the truncation just resting on the lower lid. Slit lamp examination will then indicate whether or not the line of the truncation and the axis identification markings settle at 180 degrees. With a slightly mobile trial lens, the angle of the lower lid is one of the main influences on the orientation of the lens. For example, if the spectacle Rx is −0.50/−3.50 × 15, and the truncation settles at 10 degrees, the T setting should be ordered as T5, the expectation being that

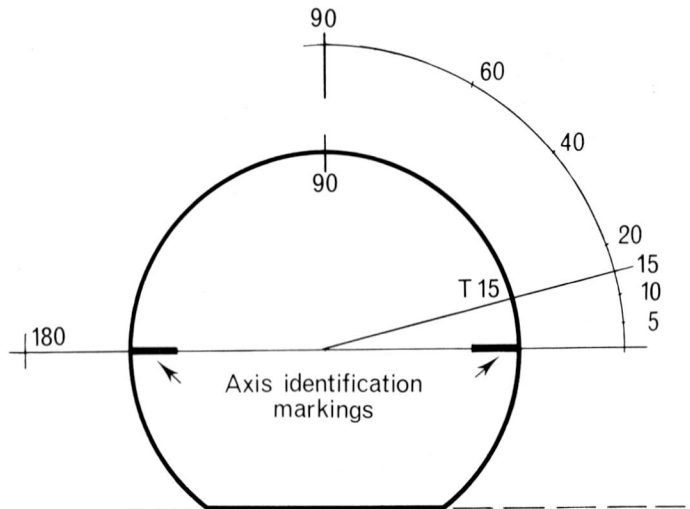

Figure 14.40–Hydroflex-TS Fitting: T 15 lens with axis at 15 degrees before rotation

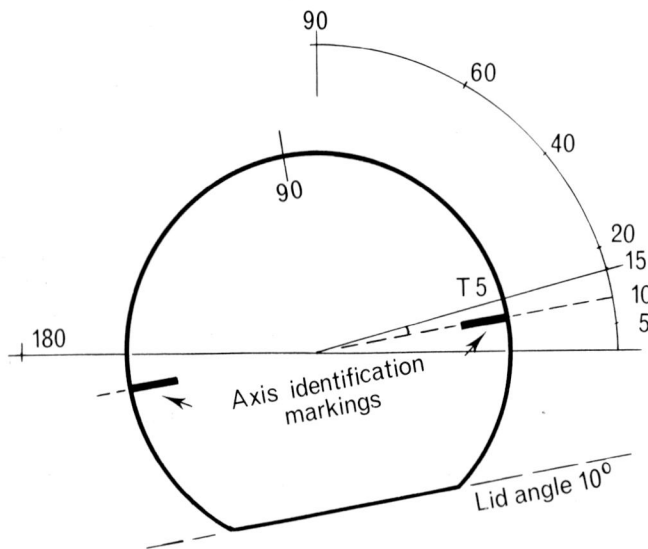

Figure 14.41—Due to rotation of the T 15 lens of Figure 14.40 by 10 degrees, a T 5 lens, after rotation on the eye, is shown correctly orientated with the 180 degrees axis markings located at 10 degrees and the negative cylinder axis (T 5) at 15 degrees

the prescription lens will also settle with its truncation resting on the lower lid at an angle of 10 degrees (*Figures 14.40* and *14.41*).

The astigmatic difference is calculated in the same way as for a Hydroflex/m-T lens, with the aid of *Table 14.28*. Suppose the best fitting trial lens is 9.30:14.00; a radius of 9.30 mm has a surface power of −47.83 D, to which the addition of −3.50 D gives −51.33 D for the steeper meridian. The nearest value to this is −51.13 D, which converts back to a radius of 8.70 mm. The complete specification of the lens is therefore 9.30/8.70   14.00   −0.50   T5.

FRONT SURFACE TORIC LENSES

Front surface torics are capable of correcting both corneal and lenticular astigmatism. Several designs of lens are possible, the methods of stabilization being truncation or 'dynamic stabilization'.

Truncation

The principle of truncation is exactly the same as that employed with hard lenses (page 551), and the truncation may be either single or double (Hodd, 1976d; Van Wauwe, 1977). Sometimes truncation alone is sufficient to achieve stabilization, but single truncated lenses are usually more effective when combined with 1△ base-down. Soft lenses of this type were manufactured in Australia and New Zealand as long ago as 1969. Both high and low water content materials have been used, and the back surface may be either spherical or conocoidal.

The Hydron T lens, manufactured by Hydron Europe, is based on the original aspheric design of Hirst (Pennington, 1977), and can be fitted from the trial set shown in *Table 14.33*. These lenses, although aspheric, are neither astigmatic nor truncated.

Table 14.33–Conocoidal Fitting Set

BCOR (mm)	OS (mm)
7.70	13.50
7.90	13.50
7.90	14.00
8.10	13.50
8.10	14.00
8.30	13.50
8.30	14.00
8.50	14.00
8.50	14.50
8.70	14.50
8.90	14.50

Hodd (1977a) found that conocoidal lenses do not have to be fitted as flat as the equivalent spherical Hydron lens, so that the radius of the initial trial lens is selected to be about 0.7 mm flatter than mean 'K', and with an overall size 2.00–2.50 mm larger than the visible iris diameter. The 1.5 mm truncation prevents small rotations of the final lens, but it also effectively loosens the fitting. The prescription lens is therefore ordered 0.5 mm larger in overall size to compensate for this. As with back surface torics, the truncation should align with the angle of the lower lid. If this is other than horizontal, the axis of the minus cylinder must be compensated in the same way as indicated in *Figures 14.40* and *14.41*.

Dynamic Stabilization

The term 'dynamic stabilization' was first used by Fanti (1975) with the introduction by Titmus-Eurocon of the Weicon-T lens. The fitting technique is based on that of the standard 15.00 mm Weicon lens. The lens design has since been emulated by other laboratories, and consists of chamfering the top and bottom portions of the lens in order to

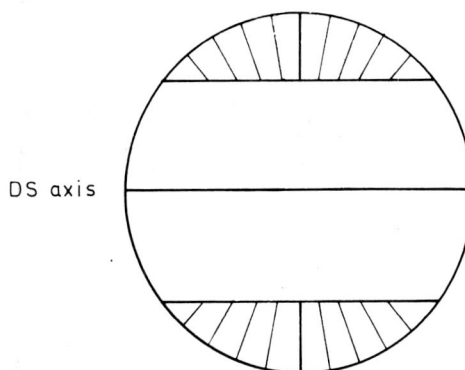

Figure 14.42–The Weicon-T lens showing the DS or 'dynamic stabilization' axis and upper and lower stabilization zones

reduce the thickness where the stabilization zones fit beneath the eyelids. The optic portion is a central 8 mm band which lies within the palpebral aperture. *Figure 14.42* shows the dynamic stabilization or DS axis running across the centre of the lens.

Weicon-T lenses are fitted from the trial set shown in *Table 14.34*. These diagnostic DS-lenses do not have a toroidal front surface, and are of spherical power. The DS axis, however, is clearly engraved between the stabilization zones, so that

Table 14.34–Weicon-T Trial Set

BCOR (mm)	OS (mm)
8.40	15.00
8.60	15.00
8.80	15.00
9.00	15.00
9.20	15.00
9.40	15.00

the orientation of the final prescription lens may be accurately predicted. If the trial lens rotates off axis, the cylinder axis is compensated for according to the same principles as those used with truncated lenses. The terms 'additive inclination' and 'subtractive inclination' have been used for when the DS axis rotates clockwise and counter-clockwise respectively. Approximately 10 minutes should be allowed for stabilization to occur, and the mean of three assessments should be taken. A typical prescription would read: 9.00:15.00 –5.00/–3.00 × 10.

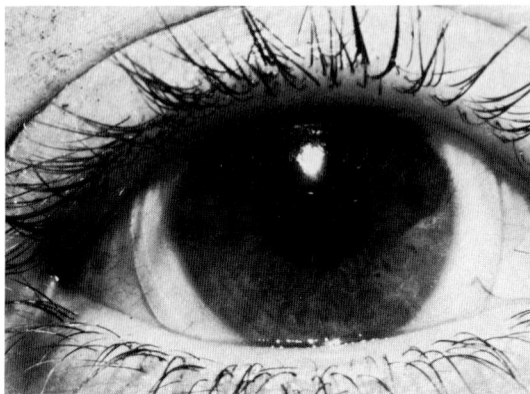

(a)

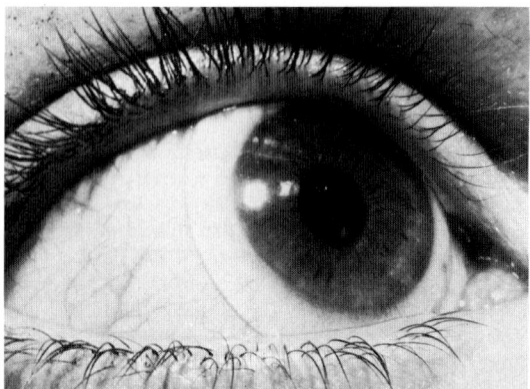

(b)

Figure 14.43–A Weicon-T lens with the eye. (a) In the primary position. (b) Looking nasally

The large overall size of 15.00 mm puts geometric constraints on the range of powers which it is possible to manufacture. Initially these have been restricted to –3.00 D to –20.00 D for spherical powers, and –1.00 D to –4.00 D for cylinders. Hodd (1977b), however, found satisfactory results with lenses of 14.00 mm overall size which permit a considerably extended power range. *Figure 14.43a* and *b* shows the size of a Weicon-T lens. Further details of toric soft lenses are given in Chapter 18.

SPECIAL FEATURES

TINTED AND COSMETIC SOFT LENSES

The need for tinted soft lenses is much less than with hard lenses because of the low incidence of adaptive photophobia. Nevertheless, some laboratories offer a range of tinted lenses, and these can produce an attractive cosmetic effect with some combinations of iris and lens colour. They are also very useful for hypermetropic and aphakic patients who would otherwise find difficulty in locating the position of a misplaced lens.

Table 14.35–Aoflex Tints

	Light transmission (%)		
	Light	*Medium*	*Dark*
Turquoise	80	65	45
Brown	75	50	25
Grey	75	60	20

Aoflex, for example, have produced the tints indicated in *Table 14.35* (Hodd, 1976a), and Hydroflex lenses are available in eight colours. In both cases clear and black occluding pupils may be obtained. Titmus-Eurocon, in addition to tinted lenses, make true cosmetic lenses with an artificial iris pattern, and Menicon have also produced similar lenses. Further details are given in Chapter 24, page 688.

All of these tints may be regarded as permanent, but a temporary method of tinting is the application of non-toxic vegetable dye to a soft lens, which then absorbs the colour into its porous structure. Daily or twice daily applications of the dye are necessary to maintain the colour.

LENS IDENTIFICATION

Several varieties of low water content soft lens have engravings at the periphery. These may be purely for identification, or possibly indicate the complete specification of the lens, and as such are extremely useful. These markings do sometimes attract deposits to the lens surface, and very occasionally fractures may occur at the position of the engraving.

In the main, however, these minor problems are far outweighed by the considerable advantage of having an easy method of identification for both patient and practitioner.

Menicon lenses have the BCOR and OS 'printed' at the lens periphery. This is not visible to the observer when on the eye but can be seen by the practitioner with the slit lamp, and when off the eye. The printing also aids patients detection of inverted lenses.

ULTRA-THIN LENSES

Ultra-thin lenses, with a centre thickness of approximately 0.07 mm in the hydrated state, are produced in overall sizes of 12.5 mm, 13.6 mm and 14.5 mm by Bausch and Lomb, and additionally a range of 'hyper-thin' lenses (t_c 0.035 mm). Wohlk also have a range of 'super-thin' Hydroflex lenses with overall sizes of 13.0 mm and 13.5 mm. Centre thickness is 0.08 mm for minus lenses, and plus powers are also available. A similar lens of centre thickness 0.06 mm has been introduced by Hydron Europe. In general, the advantages of such lenses are as follows.

(1) Better comfort because of the thin edge.

(2) Less oedema because of the reduced centre thickness.

(3) Better centration because of the reduced effect of lid pressure.

(4) Less limbal pressure.

(5) An improvement for many patients with a tendency to conjunctival injection.

Their main disadvantages are occasional difficulty in handling by the patient, and possible reduced lens life.

HARD-SOFT COMBINATION LENSES

Little first described the use of a hard-soft combination lens for keratoconus patients in 1971. The soft lens achieves comfort with an otherwise sensitive cornea, and the hard lens, fitted to match its anterior surface, provides a good visual result. Combination lenses have also been used in fitting pathological cases (Westerhout, 1973 and Chapter 21), and astigmatic patients (Mavani, 1976a,b; Harwood, 1977). Mackay Taylor (1976) has suggested that the hydrophilic-base lens may be fenestrated, channelled or toric edged in order to promote tears flow.

CIRCUMFERENTIAL CHANNELS

Circumferential channels have occasionally been added to low water content lenses during manufacture. The American Hydrocurve lens, made from a copolymer of HEMA and N-vinyl-2-pyrrolidone had a single annular channel 1.0 mm wide and 9.0 mm in diameter, to aid tears flow on blinking (Russell, 1974). The Micro-Molliter, fitted 0.2 mm smaller than the horizontal diameter of the cornea, had two such circumferential grooves. These assisted lens flexure, and gave a close conformation to the corneal curvature. The centre and edge thicknesses of 0.10 mm and 0.06 mm respectively and the enclosed reservoirs of tears permitted extended wear in certain cases whilst causing corneal insult in some others.

INSTRUCTIONS TO PATIENTS

Patients should be given clear instructions, both verbally and in writing. Lens handling is fully described in Chapter 8, Volume 1, but the most important points to be discussed may be listed as follows.

(1) The identification marks on the lenses, if they are engraved.

(2) The wearing schedule. This should be uncomplicated, and a typical example is 4 hours on the first day, increasing by 1 hour extra each day. Positive lenses may well require a slower rate of adaptation.

(3) Lens comfort should be no worse than that already experienced on a tolerance trial, and the eyes should not become unduly red or sore.

(4) The method of lens disinfection.

(5) The solution in the lens case should be changed every day.

(6) The importance of cleaning lenses, and the distinction between cleaning and disinfection.

(7) Spectacle blur should not be experienced.

(8) Hard lens solutions should never be used.

(9) Soft lenses should not be worn if eyedrops or ointment have been prescribed for any reason.

(10) Environments containing fumes, chemicals, or sprays, should be avoided.

(11) The importance of always removing any trace of noxious chemicals from the hands.

(12) Extreme environments in terms of temperature or humidity may temporarily affect both comfort and vision.

(13) If a patient falls asleep or enters certain extreme environments, lenses may give a temporary adhesion to the cornea. This can be released by the application of normal saline solution.

(14) The lens case should be carried at all times, containing the appropriate storage solution.

(15) Lenses are not necessarily spoiled if they dry out, since they recover their normal shape after rehydration, but that they are very fragile when dry.

(16) Patients should bring with them for their first after-care examination both their lens case and their spectacles. They should arrive having worn the lenses for as long as possible on that particular day.

DISINFECTION OF SOFT LENSES

When soft lenses were first fitted, great concern was expressed at the risk of bacterial contamination. Fortunately, amongst all of the other development problems of hydrophilic lenses, the fear of ocular infection has proved largely unfounded. In fact it can be argued that worse problems have been created by the disinfection procedures themselves; by accelerated lens ageing with boiling on the one hand, and hypersensitivity reactions to solutions on the other. Nevertheless, it is essential that every patient is properly advised with respect to the appropriate disinfection and cleaning procedures for his particular type of lens. It is also extremely important that the patient understands the distinction between cleaning and disinfection, since a sterile but 'dirty' lens produces as many problems as a clean contaminated one. Full details of the methods currently employed for lens disinfection are described in Chapter 3, Volume 1, but the two basic approaches are: (1) heat; and (2) chemical.

HEAT

Heat disinfection may be carried out by placing a suitable storage case, containing the lenses in normal saline solution, in boiling water for approximately 15 minutes. Alternatively, a thermostatically controlled heating unit, designed specifically for this purpose, may be used, or the lens case may be placed in a vacuum flask containing water which has just been boiled. These procedures are not truly sterilization, since they fall short of the absolute efficacy of autoclaving, and are better described as pasteurization, asepticizing or, preferably, disinfection.

CHEMICAL

Chemical disinfection is carried out by using a variety of proprietary soft lens solutions. Hard lens solutions, which contain such preservatives as benzalkonium chloride or chlorbutanol, should under no circumstances ever be used with soft lenses because of their propensity to concentrate on and within the hydrophilic material. The active constituents of most soft lens solutions are chlorhexidine and thiomersalate, which are effective against bacteria and fungi respectively. Unfortunately, chlorhexidine also tends to bind to and concentrate within hydrogel materials to a certain extent and particularly to deposits on the lens surface.

Most lenses currently available can be disinfected by either heating or the use of solutions, but the methods should not be mixed. Cases of 'red eye'

reaction have been precipitated by the use of occasional or intermittent boiling in conjunction with a solutions regimen. If changing from solutions to boiling, patients are advised to boil three times on the first occasion in order to extract from the lenses as much of the remaining preservatives as possible. It is also important to note that certain lenses can only be used with a restricted range of solutions. The Weicon 60, for example, can significantly alter its parameters if used with an incompatible solution.

AFTER-CARE

After-care for patients fitted with soft lenses, particularly at their early visits, is very much an extension of the fitting procedure. This is frequently the case with those patients for whom lenses have been fitted and dispensed on the first visit, where a lens may require to be changed for a different fitting or power. The examination is more than usually directed at the lenses while still being worn. A comprehensive treatment of all aspects of after-care is to be found in Chapter 16, but the clinical routine should contain the following steps: (1) discussion with the patient; (2) over-refraction; (3) examination of the lenses *in situ*, with and without magnification; (4) slit lamp examination and staining, with lenses removed; (5) change of lens fitting or lens type, if necessary; and (6) re-appraisal of wearing schedule.

The initial discussion with the patient establishes the wearing time which has been achieved, together with the wearer's subjective appraisal of comfort, distance vision and near vision. The monocular and binocular visual acuities are then recorded, and over-refraction carried out to determine any residual error. The usual importance is given to the quality of the retinoscopy reflex. Lenses are then examined *in situ*, with the keratometer, Placido disc, and slit lamp. The latter is especially important because not only can the fitting best be judged with low to medium magnification, but so also can the general condition of the lens surface. Embedded foreign particles can easily be seen, as can possible deposits from the tears, or contamination from make-up. The integrity of the lens edge is also studied in this manner, as well as its possible effect on the limbal or conjunctival blood vessels. Lenses engraved with identification marks are easily confirmed as being worn both the right way round, and in the correct eye.

Lenses are then removed, cleaned, and placed in the patient's carrying case. It is sometimes necessary at this stage to consider a change of fitting, power, or even lens type. By the time of the first after-care examination, lenses will have been worn for one or two weeks, tears flow will be back to normal, and the fitting may have significantly altered. Usually lenses become tighter rather than looser, so that a reduction in visual acuity, or scleral indentation may have occurred. For physiological reasons it may be necessary to change the type of lens, so that a higher water content material may be indicated; or a semi-scleral used instead of a lens of corneal size. If there is some doubt about the comfort given by a particular lens, it is often instructive to deliberately switch right and left lenses into the opposite eye. If the discomfort follows the lens into the alternate eye, then it must be suspected as being faulty, and replaced. Assuming that no other lenses are to be tried at this consultation, ordinary fluorescein is used and the slit lamp examination continued to confirm the absence of corneal insult.

It is sometimes necessary to change the wearing schedule at this stage. Finally patients are instructed that the lenses may be worn again after a gap of two hours, by which time all traces of fluorescein will have disappeared from the eye.

Severe problems do not arise frequently with hydrophilic lenses, but it should not be assumed that, because they are so soft and flexible, ocular changes do not occur, and practitioners must expect that at least some small percentage of their patients will one day present themselves with, for example, a suddenly contracted red eye. Punctate staining of an adaptive nature is sometimes observed centrally or peripherally. Crescentic areas of stain have been observed in the mid-periphery, and arcuate stains are seen at the limbus with some types of corneal-sized lens; this is due to a combination of corneal drying by the lens edge, and physical abrasion (*see Colour Plate XXVa*). Patients who are hypersensitive to disinfection or cleaning solutions show diffuse punctate erosions in the superficial epithelium; they may or may not exhibit discomfort, photophobia and lacrimation. Striae may be seen as folds in Descemet's membrane (Wechsler, 1974; Katz, 1976). These occur if corneal swelling exceeds 7 per cent (Polse, Mandell and Olsen, 1975). Limbal injection may be observed either in association with these foregoing conditions, or on its own. Long-term soft lens wearers have produced true neo-vascularization spreading from the limbal arcades; arcuate staining near the superior limbus has also occurred accompanied by vascularization caused by the downward pressure of a tight upper lid. Greyish infiltrates have been seen in the corneal stroma considered by some to be localized oedema, and cases of disciform keratitis, nummular keratitis and superficial punctate keratitis have been diagnosed.

Corneal oedema is sometimes present, but compared to that found with hard lenses it is difficult to observe. It is an overall effect, extending from limbus to limbus with no clearly defined edge to be seen against the background of the dark pupil area as found with hard lens wearers. There is usually very little or no change in either the refraction or the 'K' readings, which accounts for the absence of spectacle blur. Carney (1975) found that epithelial anoxia gives both central and peripheral thickness changes, so that there is no actual change in the corneal topography. Mandell (1975) described a linear relationship between corneal thickness increase and corneal oedema. For these reasons pachometry is probably the only sure way of diagnosing the low levels of oedema encountered with soft lenses. Compared with hard lenses, Hamano *et al.* (1975) found less morphological changes in the cornea, and a smaller reduction in glycogen levels.

LENS AGEING

Hydrophilic lenses stored in sealed vials continue to remain in good condition for several years, but once they are worn regularly the constant action of ocular secretions causes lens deterioration in a variety of ways. Unlike hard lenses, ageing effects have now become a more frequent cause of lens replacement than either loss or damage. The degree to which any particular lens is affected depends on several factors, as follows.

(1) The polymer from which the lens is manufactured, so that HEMA lenses age differently from those of higher water content.

(2) The wearing schedule, so that continuous wear lenses are more badly affected than daily wear lenses, and these are, in turn, more badly affected than lenses worn only occasionally.

(3) The nature of the tears chemistry. Some patients' lenses last only a few months, whereas others remain in good condition for several years.

(4) Method of disinfection. Lenses may have a shorter lifespan when sterilized by heating as opposed to solutions.

(5) The regularity and method of cleaning.

(6) The environment in which the lenses are worn.

TYPES OF AGEING EFFECT

Protein Deposition

Most lenses suffer from mucoprotein deposits, although HEMA lenses are more badly affected. Cummings (1973) considered that there is a chemical bonding between the proteins of the tears and the hydroxyl groups of the polymer. Some degree of deposition is therefore inevitable, but heat disinfection compounds the problem by denaturing protein present on the lens surface which has not been removed by proper cleaning. In the early stages a blue-grey film is seen when the lens is observed by oblique illumination against a dark background, or if the patient refrains from blinking and the lens is allowed to partially dry on the eye during slit lamp examination. Eventually large areas of deposit are clearly visible, even without magnification, and the lens becomes discoloured. Loose fittings appear to be more severely affected, as do spun-cast lenses despite their superior degree of surface finish.

Brown Discoloration

High water content lenses very commonly suffer from brown discoloration, even when not disinfected by heat. HEMA lenses can also be affected. Gasson (1975) and Ganju and Cordrey (1976) demonstrated a reduction in light transmission of such discoloured lenses. The brown colour may be due to adrenaline compounds in the tears, or, if the lenses fluoresce under ultra-violet light it may be due to chlorhexidine bound to surface deposits.

White Spots

These are usually considered to be calcium or lipid in origin. They rarely occur with daily wear corneal-sized lenses, and spun-cast lenses are especially good in this respect. Large semi-scleral lenses are more often affected, particularly with patients who are poor blinkers or who have dry eyes. White spots always occur on the front surface of the lens. They may sometimes be observed as a cloud of fine punctate dots, but are more usually seen as quite noticeable discrete white spots scattered irregularly over the lens surface. In severe cases, particularly with continuous wear lenses, they can be extremely large and uncomfortable. These larger deposits are sometimes referred to as 'mulberries'.

Rust Spots

Rust spots affect all types of hydrophilic lens. They are mainly due to atmospheric pollution, but have occasionally been found as a manufacturing fault. Loran (1973) has shown them to be a form of ferrous contamination, and they are more often observed in patients who live or work in industrial areas (see also Chapter 15, Figures 15.22, 15.24 and 15.25).

Surface and Edge Deterioration

Lathe-cut HEMA lenses can develop fissures relating to manufacturing lathe marks (Barradell, 1973), and they gradually suffer from surface scratching. The integrity of the edge, with age, can break down to produce small chips and imperfections, and engraving marks can sometimes become encrusted with deposits (see Figure 15.21, Chapter 15). Lenses affected by protein tend to dry more easily on the eye, and if this occurs unevenly at the periphery, the edge may become crenellated.

Fitting Changes

Lenses with deposits, scratches, or other surface irregularities are more influenced by the mechanical pressure of the upper lid, so that significant changes in fitting characteristics can occur. Usually they become looser, and small lenses may become badly decentred, or high riding because the lens surface tends to adhere to the upper lid. As a consequence apical or peripheral corneal staining is sometimes observed.

Refractive Changes

Old lenses frequently give a reduced standard of vision, not only because of surface deposits, but also as a result of spurious changes in the over-refraction of as much as 1.00 D. If the patient is subsequently checked with a new lens, the refractive change is nearly always found to be unnecessary. This may indicate deposition in the porous structure of the lens possibly giving rise to refractive index and flexure changes.

Patients sometimes produce a severe ocular response to the wearing of contaminated lenses. This may be either corneal, or conjunctival of an allergic follicular nature (Allansmith et al., 1977).

The majority of the foregoing difficulties are resolved by thorough lens cleaning, or replacement. However, it is not possible to predict with any degree of certainty the life-span for a soft lens, although the various cleaning and rejuvenation procedures now available make 2–4 years feasible, compared with only 3–6 months for the earliest forms of hydrophilic lens. Patients should be supplied from the beginning with the appropriate solutions. Ideally, they should use daily a surface acting cleaner effective against mucoprotein, combined with a periodic enzymatic or other cleaning process.

GENERAL COMMENTS ON SOFT LENS PRACTICE

There are now very many types of hydrophilic lens available to the practitioner. They differ in water content, chemical composition, size, geometric construction, method of manufacture and technique of fitting so that they may have little in common, except for the fact that they are described by the adjective 'soft'. They are best regarded as complementary rather than competitive systems, for the question: Which is the best soft lens? does not necessarily have an answer unless it relates to a particular patient, or perhaps even to a particular eye. If it is intended to fit as many patients as possible, it is necessary to have available more than one variety of lens. Lenses of corneal size are certainly preferable in many cases; but semi-scleral lenses are essential in some others, as are lenses with a much higher oxygen permeability for a remaining small percentage. It is not possible to prescribe lenses of one type based on the fitting set of another. A comprehensive range of lenses for one preferred fitting philosophy should therefore be supplemented by at least a minimum set of an alternative method. It is not possible to prescribe only one sort of hard lens, nor is this feasible with soft lenses.

In choosing a soft lens system it is desirable to fit and prescribe those lenses and materials produced by the major soft lens manufacturers, who have carried out the necessary pre-clinical studies to ensure the safety of their lenses, and who continue with research and development into new materials and improved lens designs. It is advantageous to use a lens which is part of a complete system, backed by an easily workable warranty, exchange and replacement scheme. This enables the practitioner to maintain an efficient fitting service, and the patient to have at least some idea of what the future costs might be as a soft lens wearer. Such a system should not be too rigid, for the things which happen to soft lenses can sometimes defy classification.

The material from which lenses are made must be durable and avoid rapid deterioration, and it must withstand patient handling in order that a reasonable life-span may be expected. Good reproducibility is essential and lenses should be capable of being autoclaved, so that any method of disinfection may be used.

The ideal way of prescribing soft lenses, of any variety, is from a substantial lens stock. This largely avoids problems of uncertain manufacturing times, and inconsistent quality. It is re-assuring to have the certain knowledge that any given lens is immediately available within the consulting room, and that a lens which has been successfully worn on a tolerance trial in terms of vision, fitting and comfort can become the patient's own prescription lens. If, however, it is preferred to start with a limited trial set, it should be possible to extend this later by the addition of further fitting modules. Positive as well as negative lenses should be included even in a basic fitting set, as it is not possible to fit one reliably from the other. Lenses with standardized parameters and recommended fitting procedures are preferred in most cases, but any soft lens system should be sufficiently versatile to provide intermediate fitting steps and non-standard lenses where clinically necessary.

SILICONE LENSES

Although they are not hydrophilic, silicone lenses look very much like hydrophilic soft lenses and they are therefore included in this chapter for the sake of completeness. At the time of writing they are newly introduced into the United Kingdom and some of the details which follow may well become rapidly superceded.

Silicone rubber has been investigated as a material for contact lens use since 1962. It is chemically and physiologically inert (Breger, 1971; Elze, 1976), and its very high permeability to oxygen and carbon dioxide, together with its negligible effects on corneal physiology have been demonstrated respectively by Fatt (1969), Fatt and St. Helen (1971), Hill (1966, 1977), Hill and Schoessler (1967) and by Burns, Roberts and Rich (1971). Roth *et al.* (1980), however, have reported on a variety of clinical complications found with these lenses from Germany and Japan.

Silicone lenses differ from PMMA hard lenses in several ways. They can be flexed, stretched and turned inside out; they have excellent elastic properties, partly conform to the shape of the cornea in wear, and have an oxygen permeability several times greater than either HEMA or CAB lenses. They are also unlike hydrophilic lenses because they are extremely tough, and their natural state is dry. Since they do not absorb water to any significant extent, fluorescein can be used in their fitting, and they do not need disinfecting in the same way as soft lenses. Silicone should therefore be regarded as a completely different category of material, which lies somewhere between 'hard' and 'soft', possessing many of the advantages of both. It is best and most simply described by the adjective 'flexible'.

Because of the amorphous nature of the silicone rubber raw materials, lenses are produced by a moulding and vulcanization technique, which also assists in maintaining good reproducibility. The main difficulty with silicone is that its natural surface is extremely hydrophobic, and it has been necessary to devise a method of rendering the surface permanently hydrophilic without interfering with any of its optical or physical properties. The final stage of manufacture is therefore surface treatment by ion bombardment. It is likely that before long there will be a variety of makes of silicone lenses available, and, as with soft lenses, each manufacturer's product will have its own geometry and fitting characteristics.

The first silicone lenses were fitted with an overall size of 10.50 mm, but because of their relatively great centre thickness of 0.30 mm they tended to be low riding (Long, 1972; Black, 1972). More recent lenses such as Silflex (Wöhlk) and Tesicon (*Titmus Eurocon*) are thinner and of approximately corneal size in order to achieve better centration.

Physical Properties of Silicone Material

Hardness	72–77 Shore 'A' units
Penetration strength	47–53 per cent
Refractive index	1.435–1.436
Density at 22°C	1.19–1.2 g/cm^3
Oxygen permeability	79.8 × 10^{-11} (cm^2/sec)
(of Silflex)	(ml O$_2$/ml × mm Hg)

Lens Geometry and Fitting Techniques

The most commonly fitted overall sizes for Silflex are 12.2 mm and 12.7 mm, although 11.7 mm and 13.2 mm lenses are also available. BCOR fitting intervals are 0.1 mm. Tesicon lenses are fitted a little larger and flatter, with overall sizes of 12.7 and 13.5 mm being most commonly used.

Fitting Technique

Lenses, which must be fitted with as much precision and accuracy as a hard lens, should be about the same size as the horizontal corneal diameter, and approximately 0.3 mm smaller than the equivalent HEMA soft lens. BCOR can be selected according to *Table 14.38*.

In practice, most successful fittings are about 0.1 mm flatter than flattest 'K'. A correctly fitting lens gives good centration and about 1 mm of vertical movement on blinking. Fluorescein gives a very distinctive four-part pattern consisting of central touch, surrounded by an annular ring of green,

which is in turn enclosed within a circle of peripheral alignment, adjacent to a narrow band of edge clearance. *Colour Plate XXVI* illustrates this, as does *Figure 14.44*.

With other lenses, the terms 'flat' and 'loose', and 'steep' and 'tight' have been used almost synonymously. With Silflex this is not necessarily accurate, since in some cases flattening the radius can result in a tighter lens, and vice versa. If progressively flatter lenses are applied to the same cornea, four fitting stages can be observed, as follows.

(1) A lens which is too steep is indeed too tight, with little or no movement. It shows marked apical clearance, with fluorescein pooling beneath almost the entire lens. Vision is poor and variable, and the peripheral curve is very narrow or altogether absent.

(2) The next flatter stage is a correct fitting, giving proper centration and movement. The fluorescein pattern is the typical four-part pattern described above and shown in *Colour Plate XXVI* and *Figure 14.44*.

(3) A flatter lens than this may initially be somewhat loose, but on settling can become completely immobile and apparently stuck to the cornea. In the mobile phase the peripheral curve appears excessively wide, and the two rings of fluorescein tend towards each other, and usually coalesce under at least one area of the lens. Subsequently, in the tight phase, all tears flow is excluded from beneath the lens, and there is no discernible fluorescein picture. Patients are perfectly comfortable with such a lens, and still obtain good visual acuity. In some cases this type of fitting produces no corneal insult, even after long periods of wear. In others, lens decentration and corneal abrasion occur, together with the accumulation of debris trapped beneath the lens.

(4) If an even flatter radius is used, the lens definitely does become too loose on the cornea. There is excessive mobility, possibly edge buckling and stand-off, and considerable subjective discomfort. Vision is unstable, and flare may be noticed. Fluorescein shows excessive peripheral clearance and central touch which is harder in appearance than the alignment obtained with an optimum fitting.

It is important to avoid fitting a lens of too large an overall size. Initially comfort is better, with an optimum fluorescein pattern, but eventually the fitting can become too tight as the edge of the lens seals off against the bulbar conjunctiva, preventing tears flow beneath the lens. In general, fitting should proceed in the reverse fashion to that of hydrophilic lenses. Instead of erring on the side of largeness and flatness, the correct fitting should be approached from the direction of smaller and steeper.

The usual fitting routine consists of the following steps.

(1) Normal contact lens preliminaries of refraction, keratometry, and slit lamp examination.

(2) Determination of the effective corneal diameter and the correct overall size of lens.

(3) Selection of the radius for the initial trial lens from 'K' readings.

(4) After 5 minutes, examination of the fitting with white light. Once the overall size has been confirmed as satisfactory, this should normally be kept constant, and only the radius altered in any subsequent changes of fitting.

(5) Examination of fluorescein pattern. In the majority of cases a departure from the optimum picture will ultimately give a lens which becomes too tight (although not necessarily too steep). Lenses must be fitted with precision, and 0.1 mm steps are essential.

(6) After 30 minutes, refraction, and re-examination of fitting.

(7) A longer wearing period or tolerance trial, which may be carried out at the initial fitting, or alternatively, with the patient's actual prescription lenses.

Comfort of Silicone Lenses

Wide differences in comfort are experienced. For most patients the degree of comfort is about two-thirds of the way between hard and soft lenses – much better than hard, but not as immediately comfortable as a well fitting hydrophilic lens. Previous hard lens patients usually find them readily acceptable by comparison, whereas soft lens wearers are nearly all conscious of some degree of lid sensation during the first few days. The patients who find them least acceptable are those who experience discomfort even with a soft lens, sometimes never achieving complete adaptation.

Silicone lenses have proved very suitable in cases of previous failure because of corneal oedema, and the majority of eyes, even when prone to conjunctival injection, remain white throughout the wearing period.

Less variation in comfort is experienced with differing environmental conditions such as temperature and humidity as compared to hydrophilic lenses. Foreign bodies and dust, however, can be a problem, particularly with a loose fitting.

Visual Acuity with Silicone Lenses

Silicone lenses, being truly flexible, mould themselves to conform to the curvature of the central cornea. Any significant degree of toricity is therefore transferred to the anterior surface of the lens, and there is very little masking of astigmatism with a lens of normal thickness. Over-refraction shows the same type of small residual astigmatic error that is found with a hydrophilic lens, but it is far less disturbing to the patient. A better quality and brightness of vision is obtained, and Snellen acuities are often half a line better than that achieved with an equivalent hydrophilic lens. Occasional exceptions occur, but the majority of these relate to an unsatisfactory fitting and are capable of improvement.

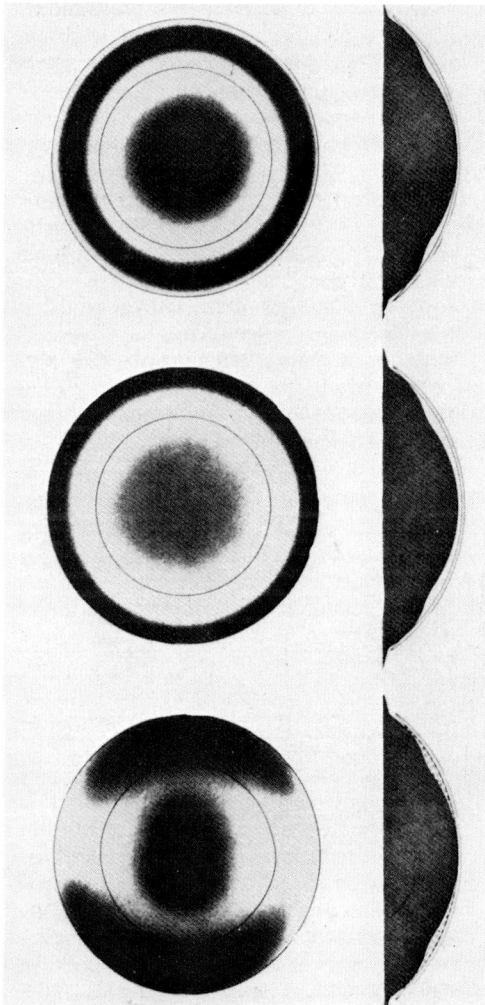

Figure 14.44—Fluorescein patterns (left) and cross-sectional diagrams (right) of Silflex silicone lens fittings. Fluorescein is shown light and touch areas are shown dark. Top — correct fitting. Middle — steep fitting. Bottom — flat fitting (reproduced by kind permission of K. Voerste)

There is very little deterioration of vision towards the end of the day, and spectacle blur is not normally encountered. The greater stability of vision afforded by a more rigid material means that many cases whose visual acuity is unacceptable with a hydrophilic lens can achieve success with silicone. This is especially true for patients with 0.75–1.50 D of astigmatism, whose correction does not warrant a toric hydrophilic lens.

Lens Handling and Storage

Lenses are inserted in the same way as a hard lens, by placing directly onto the cornea. They can also be placed on the temporal sclera and slid across, but unlike a hydrophilic lens this method is much easier if an air bubble is initially allowed to remain beneath the lens. Lenses are not easily removed by pinching from the eye as is done with a hydrophilic soft lens. The most effective technique for the majority of patients is to place the forefinger of each hand on the upper and lower lid margins and to apply simultaneous pressure to the lens edges. This method, together with the application of normal saline solution, very effectively releases the suction of the completely immobile fittings. Silicone lenses tend to be a little less easy to handle than hydrophilic soft lenses, because of the slippery nature of the moist lens surface, but they are most unlikely to be lost directly from the eye, and the strength of the silicone material means that breakage is rarely a problem.

Lenses are stored, and inserted, with a single solution containing 0.004 per cent thiomersalate and 0.1 per cent disodium edetate, which has been specifically developed for its compatibility with silicone. They are not kept in solution in order to maintain hydration, the lenses having a zero water content; nor to sterilize them in the same sense as a hydrophilic lens; but lenses are rather more comfortable if the surfaces are maintained in a hydrophilic state by a suitably viscous fluid. A small minority of patients suffer from a stinging reaction to the

solution, and preserved saline solution is a satisfactory alternative. Lenses are cleaned daily, on removal, by rubbing with a separate cleaning solution which contains 0.004 per cent thiomersalate and 0.2 per cent disodium edetate.

Existing hard lens solutions have not been advocated because the possibility of a reaction would have to be excluded for each and every one. Certainly, solutions containing chlorbutol should not be used, since it has a great affinity to bind to the surface of silicone (Black, 1972).

Indications for Silicone Lenses

Silicone lenses may be recommended for the majority of straightforward patients, but they are particularly indicated where:

(1) Corneal oedema is a problem.
(2) Soft hydrophilic lenses are repeatedly damaged.
(3) Conjunctival injection occurs with hydrophilic lenses.
(4) Visual acuity is unsatisfactory with a soft lens, and with low degrees of astigmatism.
(5) Soft lens solutions cause a hypersensitivity reaction, and boiling is impracticable.
(6) Superior arcuate staining with soft lenses cannot be resolved.
(7) Neo-vascularization has occurred with other forms of contact lens.

Contra-Indications for Silicone Lenses

Despite many clinical advantages, the main problem with many forms of silicone lenses has proven to be the short life span. This has been attributed to the fact that once the surface has been rendered hydrophilic it is also made liable to protein deposition from the tears.

Contra-indications include: (1) patients with sensitive lids who also experience discomfort with soft lenses; and (2) higher degrees of astigmatism, where a toric lens is necessary.

REFERENCES

Allansmith, M. R., Korb, D. R., Greiner, J. V., Henriquez, A. S., Simon, M. A. and Finnemore, V. M. (1977). 'Giant papillary conjunctivitis in contact lens wearers.' *Am. J. Ophthal.* **83**, 697–708
Applegate, R. A. and Massof, R. W. (1975). 'Changes in the contrast sensitivity function induced by contact lens wear.' *Am. J. Optom.* **52**, 840–846

Arias, M. C. (1968). 'Contact lens fitting in high altitudes and/or dry climates.' *Contacto* **12**(3), 10–13
Arias, M. C. (1973). Paper read at Conference of International Society of Contact Lens Specialists, Chateau d'Artigny, Montbazon, France, and reported in *Optician* **166**(4291), 18–19, 23–24
Barradell, M. J. (1973). 'Soft lenses compared.' *Optician* **166**(4304), 39, 43–44

Bennett, A. G. (1976). 'Power changes in soft lenses due to bending.' *Ophthal. Optician* **16**, 939–945

Bernstein, H. N. and Maddox, Y. (1973). 'Evaluation of the "asepticization" procedure for the Soflens hydrophilic contact lens.' *Contact Lens* **4**(3), 3

Bernstein, H. N., Stow, M. N. and Maddox, Y. (1973). 'Evaluation of the asepticization procedure for the Soflens hydrophilic contact lens.' *Canad. J. Ophthal.* **8**, 575–576

Bibby, M. M. (1976). 'Computer-assisted photokeratoscopy and contact lens design.' *Optician* **171**, Part 1, (4423), 37, 39, 41, 43; Part 2, (4424), 11, 14–15, 17; Part 3, (4425), 22–23; Part 4, (4426), 15, 17

Black, C. J. (1972). 'Silicone lens.' Chapter 14 in *Soft Contact Lens*, ed. by Gassett, A. R. and Kaufman, H. E. St. Louis: Mosby, pp. 126–138

Blackstone, M. R. (1968). 'Hydrophilic contact lenses: 1967, 1968 and onwards.' *Optician* **155**, 156–159

Brailsford, M. I. D. (1972). 'The importance of sag heights when fitting Bionite lenses.' *Ophthal. Optician* **12**, 1047–1048

Breger, J. L. (1971). 'The silicone rubber lens.' *Optician* **162**(4189), 12–14

British Standard 5562. (1978). *Specification for Contact Lenses – BS 5562:1978*. London: British Standards Institution

British Standard 3521. (1979). *Glossary of Terms Relating to Ophthalmic Lenses and Spectacle Frames – BS 3521:1979. Part 3. Glossary of Terms Relating to Contact Lenses*. London: British Standards Institution

Burns, R. P., Roberts, H. and Rich, L. F. (1971). 'Effects of silicone contact lenses on corneal epithelial metabolism.' *Am. J. Ophthal.* **71**, 486–489

Carney, L. G. (1975). 'Effect of hypoxia on central and peripheral corneal thickness and corneal topography.' *Austral. J. Optom.* **58**, 61–65

Clarke, C. (1976). 'Contact lenses at high altitude.' *Br. J. Ophthal.* **60**, 479–480

Cooke, G. E. (1975). 'Developing a single base curve soft contact lens.' *Optician* **170**(4407), 13–17

Cooke, G. E. (1976). Personal communication

Cumming, J. S. (1973). 'The future of soft contact lenses.' *Mfg. Optics Internat.* **26**(6), 309–312

Danker, F. (1976). 'The present state of silicone lenses and cellulose acetate butyrate lenses in the United States.' Paper read at meeting of International Society of Contact Lens Specialists, Fuschl, Austria, September, 1976, and reported in *Optician* **172**(4453), 15–16

de Carle, J. (1972). 'Developing hydrophilic lenses for constant wearing.' *Austral. J. Optom.* **55**, 343–346

de Carle, J. (1978). 'Survey of 200 consecutive patients requesting Permalenses in April/May 1976.' *J. Br. contact Lens Ass.* **1**, 3–7

Elze, K. L. (1976). 'Toxicity of soft contact lens material.' *Contact intraocular Lens med. J.* **2**(1), 57–61

Eriksen, S., Randeri, K. and Ster, J. (1972). 'Behaviour of hydrophilic soft contact lenses under stress conditions of pH and tonicities.' In *Symposium on the Flexible Lens*, pp. 213–217, by Bitonte, J. L. and Keates, R. H. St. Louis: Mosby

Fanti, P. (1975). 'The fitting of a soft toroidal contact lens.' *Optician* **169**(4376), 8–9, 13, 15–16

Fatt, I. (1969). 'A pre-clinical study of gas permeable contact lens material.' *Contact Lens* **2**(4), 3–5

Fatt, I. (1977). 'A rational method for the design of gas-permeable soft contact lenses.' *Optician* **173**(4470), 12, 13, 15

Fatt, I. and Bieber, M. T. (1968). 'The steady-state distribution of oxygen and carbon dioxide in the *in vivo* cornea. I: The open eye in air and the closed eye.' *Exper. Eye Res.* **7**, 103–112

Fatt, I. and St. Helen, R. (1971). 'Oxygen tension under an oxygen-permeable contact lens.' *Am. J. Optom.* **48**, 545–555

Ford, M. W. (1974). 'Changes in hydrophilic lenses when placed on an eye.' Paper read at the joint International Congress of The Contact Lens Society and The National Eye Research Foundation, Montreux, Switzerland

Ford, M. W. (1976). 'Computation of the back vertex powers of hydrophilic lenses.' Paper read at the Interdisciplinary Conference on Contact Lenses, Department of Ophthalmic Optics and Visual Science, The City University, London

Ganju, S. N. and Cordrey, P. (1976). 'Removal of adsorbed preservative in soft contact lenses.' *Optician* **171**(4423), 16, 18, 20–21

Gasson, A. P. (1973). 'Clinical experience with the B & L Soflens.' *Ophthal. Optician* **13**, 81–84

Gasson, A. P. (1975). 'Visual considerations with hydrophilic lenses.' *Ophthal. Optician* **15**, 439–448

Gasson, A. P. (1976). 'Fitting evaluation of an ultra-thin Soflens (polymacon) contact lens.' *Optician, Special Supplement, Jan. 1976*, 35–37

Gilford, S. J. W. (1975). 'How atmosphere affects soft lens wearers.' Letter in *Optician* **169**(4375), 30

Grosvenor, T. and Callender, M. (1973). 'The N & N soft contact lens.' *Am. J. Optom.* **50**, 489–498

Hamano, H., Hori, M., Hirayama, K., Kawabe, H. and Mitsunaga, S. (1975). 'Influence of soft and hard contact lenses on the cornea.' *Austral. J. Optom.* **58**, 326–336

Harris, M. G. and Mock, L. G. (1974). 'The effect of saline solutions of various compositions on hydrogel lens dimensions.' *Am. J. Optom.* **51**, 457–464

Harris, M. G., Sanders, T. L. and Zisman, F. (1975). 'Napping while wearing Hydrogel contact lenses.' *Internat. contact Lens Clin.* **2**(1), 84–87

Harwood, L. W. (1977). 'Combination Soflens contact lenses/hard lenses – use on high-toric corneas.' In *Proceedings of the Second National Research Symposium on Soft Contact Lenses*, pp. 131–137. Chicago, Illinois, August 16–17, 1975, Excerpta Medica, Amsterdam, Holland, and Princeton, N.J., U.S.A.

Hill, J. F. (1975). 'A comparison of refractive and keratometric changes during adaptation to flexible and non-flexible contact lenses.' *J. Am. optom. Ass.* **46**, 290–294

Hill, J. F. (1976). 'Changes in corneal curvature and refractive error upon refitting with flatter hydrophilic contact lenses.' *J. Am. optom. Ass.* **47**, 1214–1216

Hill, R. M. (1966). 'Effects of a silicone rubber contact lens on corneal respiration.' *J. Am. optom. Ass.* **37**, 1119–1121

Hill, R. M. (1976). 'Perils of the pump.' *Internat. contact Lens Clin.* **3**(3), 48–49

Hill, R. M. (1977). 'Oxygen permeable contact lenses: how convinced is the cornea?' *Internat. contact Lens Clin.* **4**(2), 34–36

Hill, R. M. and Schoessler, J. (1967). 'Optical membranes of silicone rubber.' *J. Am. optom. Ass.* **38**, 480–483

Hillman, J. S. (1976). 'The use of hydrophilic contact lenses.' *Optician* **172**(4458), 9–11

Hodd, N. F. B. (1976a). 'How to fit soft lenses – No. 6: Vergo group AO: Aoflex.' *Optician* **172**(4449), 15, 17, 20

Hodd, N. F. B. (1976b). 'How to fit soft lenses – No. 8: Global Vision (UK) Ltd: Permalens.' *Optician* **172**(4462), 16, 18

Hodd, N. F. B. (1976c). 'How to fit soft lenses – No. 7: Contact Lenses (Manufacturing) Ltd: Sauflon 85.' *Optician* **172**(4458), 12, 14, 16

Hodd, N. F. B. (1976d). 'Clinical appraisal of toric soft lenses.' *Optician* **172**(4445), 8, 11, 13

Hodd, N. F. B. (1977a). 'How to fit soft lenses – No. 10: toric soft lenses (part 2).' *Optician* **173**(4483), 8, 11–12

Hodd, N. F. B. (1977b). 'A comparison of toric soft lens success.' *Optician* **173**(4487), 29–30, 32

Holly, F. J. and Refojo, M. F. (1972). 'Oxygen permeability of hydrogel contact lenses.' *J. Am. optom. Ass.* **43**, 1173–1180

Jurgensen, G. (1977). 'Fitting the small, soft toric contact lens Hydroflex/m-T.' *Ophthal. Optician* **17**, 539–540, 542

Katz, H. H. (1976). 'A hypothesis for the formation of vertical corneal striae as observed in the wearing of Soflens contact lenses and in keratoconus.' *Am. J. Optom.* **53**, 420–421

Kersley, H. J., Kerr, C. and Pierse, D. (1977). 'Hydrophilic lenses for continuous wear in aphakia: definitive fitting and the problems which can occur.' *Brit. J. Ophthal.* **61**, 38–42

Larke, J. R. and Sabell, A. G. (1971). 'Some basic design concepts of hydrophilic gel contact lenses.' *Br. J. physiol. Optics* **26**, 49–60

Leibowitz, H. M., Laing, R. A. and Sandstrom, M. (1973). 'Continuous wear of hydrophilic contact lenses.' *Archs Ophthal.* **89**, 306–310

Little, I. (1971). 'Soft lenses in keratoconus.' Letter in *Optician,* **162**(4204), 26

Litvin, M. W. (1973). 'Personal experiences in fitting soft contact lenses.' *Optician* **166**(4300), 11–12

Long, W. E. (1972). 'Silicone rubber corneal contact lens.' In *Symposium on the Flexible Lens,* pp. 73–79, ed. by Bitonte, J. L. and keates, R. H. St. Louis: Mosby

Loran, D. F. C. (1973). 'Surface corrosion of hydrogel contact lenses.' *Contact Lens* **4**(4), 3–6, 8, 10

Loshaek, S. and Hill, R. M. (1977). 'Oxygen permeability measurements: correlation between living-eye and electrode-chamber measurements.' *Internat. contact Lens Clin.* **4**(6), 26–29

Mackie, I. A. (1977). 'Complications of soft lenses.' Paper read at Summer Clinical Conference of the British Contact Lens Association, April 1977, Torquay, Devon

Mandell, R. B. (1975). 'Corneal edema and curvature changes from gel changes.' *Internat. contact Lens Clin.* **2**(1), 88–98

Mavani, M. R. (1976a). 'The correction of high astigmatism.' *Optician* **172**(4453), 34

Mavani, M. R. (1976b). 'The concept of the correction of high astigmatism with a combination of hard and soft lenses.' *Contacto* **20**(6), 31–33

McDonald, J. E. (1969). 'Surface phenomena of the tear film.' *Am. J. Ophthal.* **67**, 56–64

McKay Taylor, C. (1976). 'Combining hard and soft lenses with applied fitting techniques.' *Ophthal. Optician* **16**, 356–364

Millodot, M. (1971). 'Corneal sensitivity and contact lenses.' *Optician* **162**(4210), 23–24

Millodot, M. (1974). 'Effect of soft lenses on corneal sensitivity.' *Acta Ophthal.* **52**, 603–608

Millodot, M. (1976). 'Effect of the length of wear of contact lenses on corneal sensitivity.' *Acta Ophthal.* **54**, 721–730

Morris, J. A. (1976). 'Visual results with aphakic 85 per cent Sauflon lenses.' *Optician* **172**(4444), 4, 6

Morris, J. A. and Fatt, I. (1977). 'A survey of gas-permeable contact lenses.' *Optician* **174**(4509), 27–36

Morrison, R. J. (1973). 'Comparative studies: visual acuity with spectacles and flexible lenses, ophthalmometer readings with and without flexible lenses.' *Am. J. Optom.* **50**, 807–809

Mossé, P. and Scott, V. (1976). 'What use is large molecular fluorescein in contact lens fitting?' *Optician Special Supplement, January, 1976,* 15–19

Norn, M. S. (1974). *External Eye, Methods of Examination,* p. 121. Copenhagen: Scriptor

Norton, D. A., Davies, D. J. G., Richardson, N. E. Meakin, B. J. and Keall, A. (1974). 'The antimicrobial efficiencies of contact lens solutions.' *J. Pharm. Pharmacol.* **26**, 841–846. Also reproduced in *Optician* **168**(4360), 14–16

Pennington, N. (1977). 'Toric soft lenses.' *Optician* **174**(4505), 10–12

Phillips, A. J. (1977). 'Menicon – Japan enters the UK contact lens scene.' *Ophthal. Optician* **17**, 200–202

Pierse, D. and Kersley, H. J. (1977). 'Hydrophilic lenses for continuous wear in aphakia: fitting at operation.' *Br. J. Ophthal.* **61**, 34–37

Polse, K. A. and Mandell, R. B. (1970). 'Critical oxygen tension at the corneal surface.' *Archs Ophthal.* **84**, 505–508

Polse, K. A., Mandell, R. B. and Olsen, M. (1975). 'Origin of striate corneal lines.' *Internat. contact Lens Clin.* **3**(3), 85–88

Poster, M. G. (1975). 'A rationale for fitting the Bausch & Lomb Soflens.' *J. Am. optom. Ass.* **46**, 223–227

Poster, M. G. (1977). 'Lens/eye relationships of hydrogel lenses using fluorescein analysis.' Paper read at National Research Symposium on Soft Contact Lenses, August, 1977, Rochester, New York

Poster, M. G. and Skolnik, A. (1974). 'The effects of pH and tonicity change on some parameters of the Soflens.' *J. Am. optom. Ass.* **45**, 311–314

Refojo, M. F., Korb, D. and Silverman, H. (1972). 'Clinical evaluation of new fluorescent dye for hydrogel lenses.' *J. Am. optom. Ass.* **43**, 321–326

Refojo, M. F., Miller, D. and Fiore, A. S. (1972). 'A new fluorescent stain for soft hydrophilic lens fitting.' *Archs Ophthal.* **87**, 275–277

Colour Plate Section

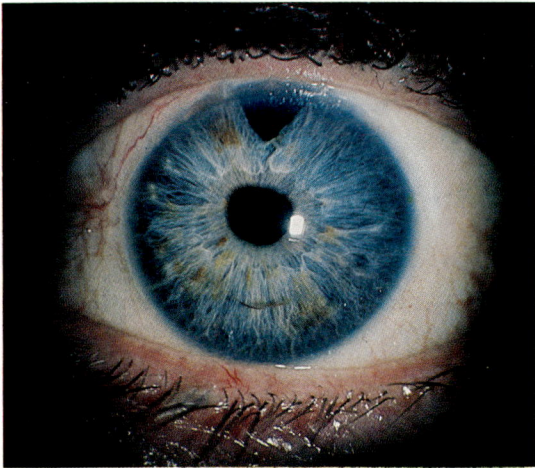

Plate I. General record of external eye prior to fitting. Special features such as the nasal pinguecula, degree of bulbar conjunctival injection, pupil shape and upper peripheral iridectomy can be used for comparison with the appearance of the eye after fitting (reproduced by kind permission of A.P. Gasson)

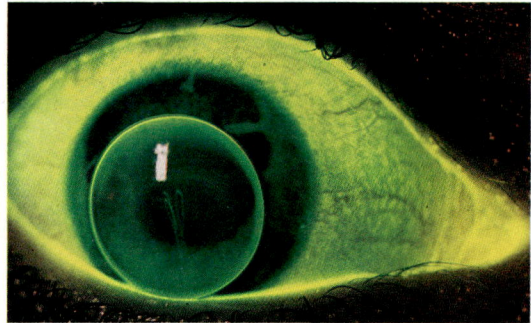

Plate II. A typical 'foreign body' stain. Fluorescein shows up the damaged epithelium along the track taken by the foreign body under the lens. The lens shows a good central alignment fit with a narrow band of peripheral clearance and a fairly sharp transition between the two evidenced by a faint arcuate stain at the centre of the cornea caused by upper lid pressure and downward movement of the lens during blinking

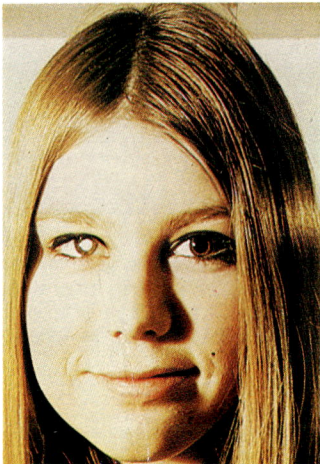

Plate III. A prosthetic corneal lens used to mask an unsightly traumatic cataract. Left: without the lens. Right: with the lens. Similar effects can be achieved with prosthetic soft and scleral lenses (reproduced by kind permission of Mr. R. R. Cockell)

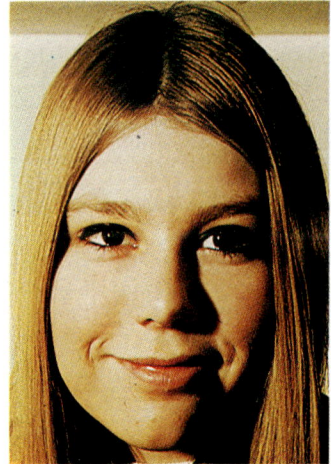

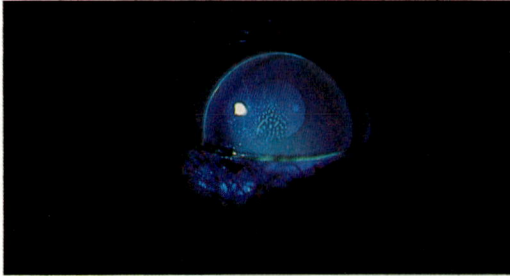

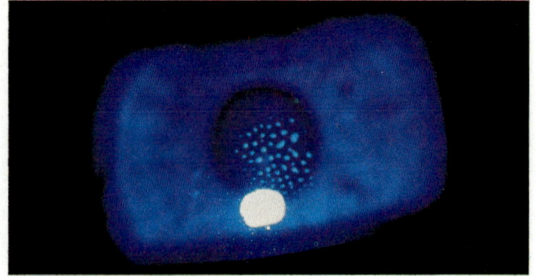

Plate IV. (Left) Small bubbles trapped under a corneal lens have caused furrows and dimples in the epithelium during lens movement. (Right) Fluorescein has collected in these furrows and dimples. The resultant deterioration in vision is known as 'dimple veil'

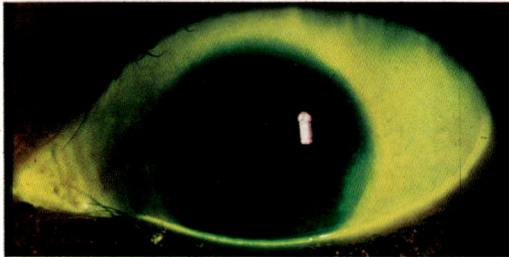

Plate V. 'Three and nine o'clock' corneal staining caused by inadequate wetting of those areas of cornea. Diffuse punctate central staining of the cornea is also present due to apical pressure by a corneal lens

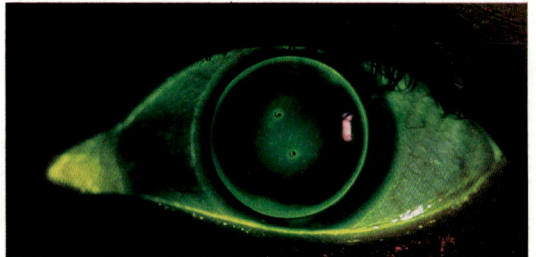

Plate VI. A lens with two 0.3 mm diameter fenestration holes in the central portion, to assist tears interchange and prevent central epithelial oedema in a lens fitted with apical clearance and intermediate bearing in order to give good centration. There is a narrow band of peripheral clearance

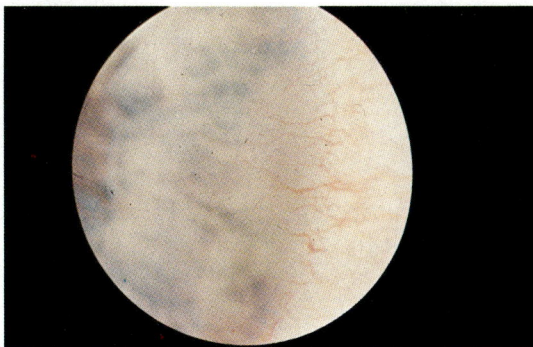

Plate VII. Neovascularization of the cornea following 'three and nine o'clock' corneal drying with corneal lens wear. The same result may occur if a bubble remains stationary under a scleral lens and following the wear of small soft lenses which have caused epithelial drying

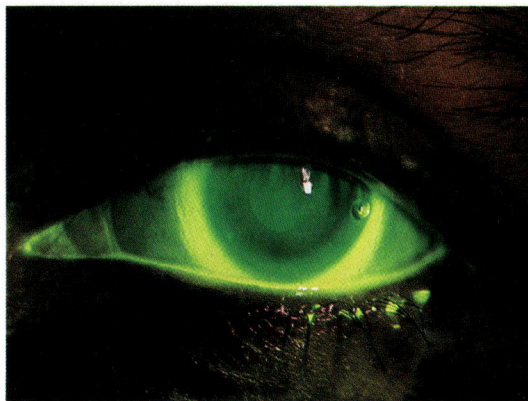

Plate VIII. A fully settled impression scleral lens made by the laminate method. The transition region extends well beyond the limbus giving adequate clearance. The patient is looking down slightly and there is a 'glancing' touch in the mid-periphery of the cornea

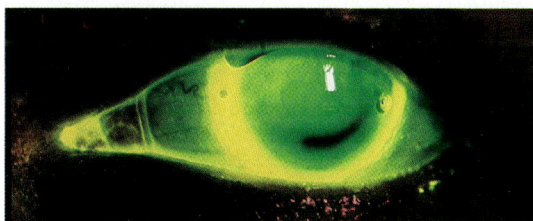

Plate IX. The same lens as Plate VIII showing the introduction of a bubble following an extreme movement of the eye down and to the temporal side. The eye is still looking slightly in that direction and the 'glancing' corneal touch has moved to the lower, mid-temporal cornea

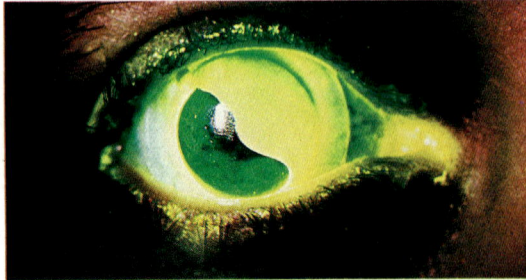

Plate X. The FLOM 8.25/13.00 on an eye with keratometer readings of 7.91 mm along 180, 7.81 mm along 90. The fluorescein picture shows too large and slightly too round a bubble with condensation on the back central optic of the lens. Limbal clearance is insufficient as shown by the touch at the top. The next FLOM to try would be 8.50/13.25 which would give slightly less apical clearance and more limbal clearance. The 0.25 mm increase in diameter would give more apical and limbal clearance, but the extra apical clearance would be more than offset by flattening the radius by 0.25 mm which would also increase the limbal clearance

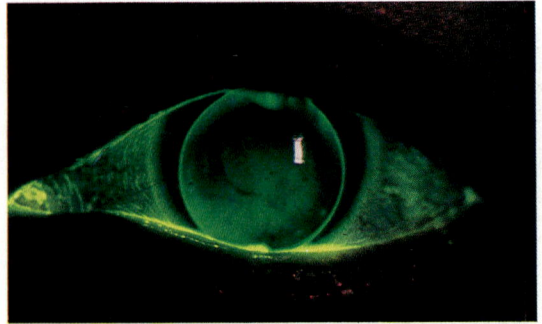

Plate XI. The tricurve lens C3/7.80:7.00/8.30:8.80/12.25: 9.20 on an eye with keratometer readings of 7.91 mm along 180, 7.81 mm along 90. The fluorescein pattern shows slight apical corneal clearance and insufficient peripheral clearance. Such a lens would probably cause central epithelial oedema with steepening of the corneal apex giving rise subsequently to the appearance of apical corneal touch

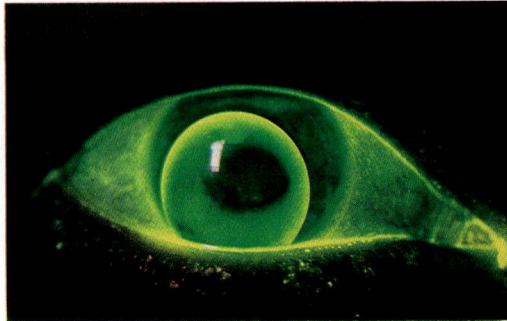

Plate XII. The corneal lens C5/8.10:7.00/8.60:7.60/9.60: 8.20/10.80:8.80/12.25:9.20 on the same eye as in Plate XI. The fluorescein pattern shows the central flat fit with bearing on the apex of the cornea and a slight epithelial abrasion as a result. The lens is riding lower temporally. The lens periphery also appears to have excessive clearance, partially due to the central flat fit

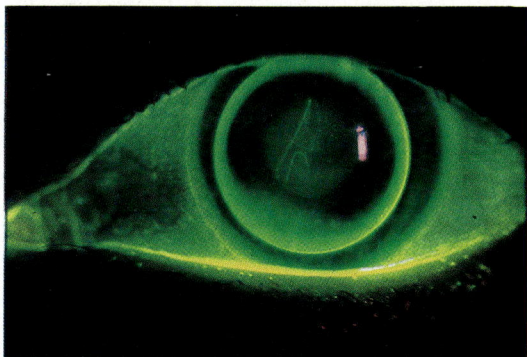

Plate XIII. A pentacurve 'tapered' corneal lens C5/7.85: 7.00/8.35:7.60/9.10:8.20/10.10:8.80/12.25:9.20 on the same eye as in Plate XI. The lens is fitted with the central portion in alignment with the cornea and with gradually increasing peripheral clearance. A foreign body track is also present as shown up by the fluorescein staining

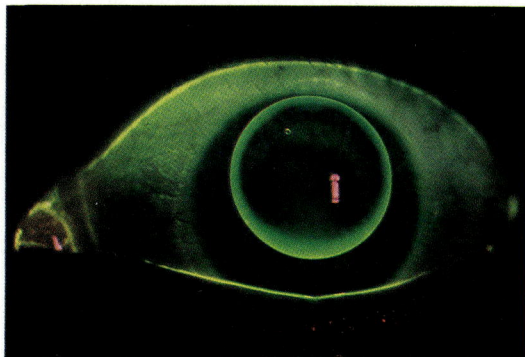

Plate XIV. A 'continuous curve' lens with a single 0.25 mm diameter fenestration hole fitted with very slight central clearance. There is gradually increasing clearance at the periphery, more noticeable at the bottom of the lens which is situated over the central cornea following a blink

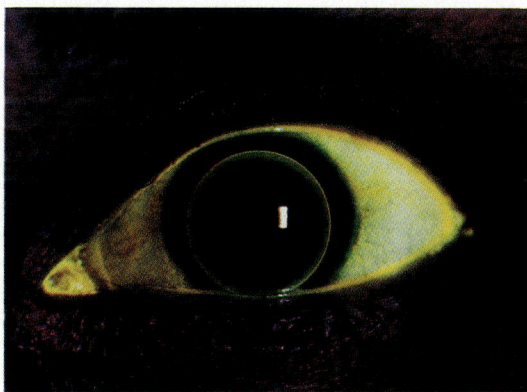

Plate XV. A spherical tetracurve lens on a cornea with spherical keratometer reading. The central and first peripheral curves give an almost matching fit, and the second and third peripheral curves give gradually increasing clearance. To assist tears flow behind the lens the junction between the first and second peripheral curves could be blended to widen slightly the band of peripheral clearance

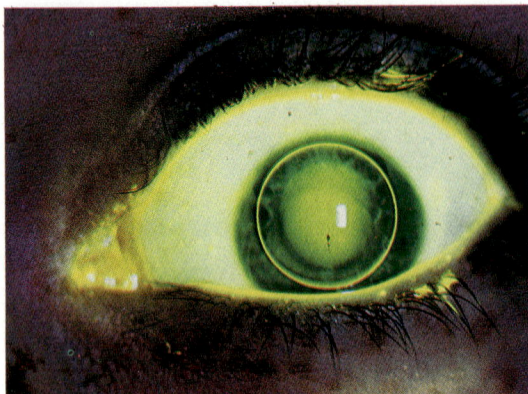

Plate XVI. A 'Bayshore' type interpalpebral corneal lens fitted slightly too steep. It shows excessive central clearance with a small entrapped bubble, alignment of the first peripheral curve and a narrow band of clearance at the lens edge due to the flat second peripheral curve

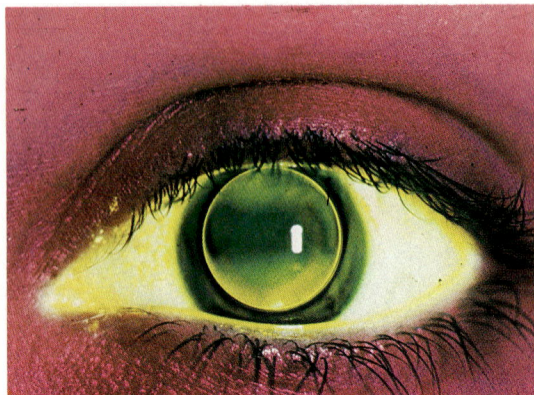

Plate XVII. An interpalpebral spherical corneal lens fitted with the back central portion in alignment with the horizontal meridian of a toroidal cornea having 'with-the-rule' astigmatism

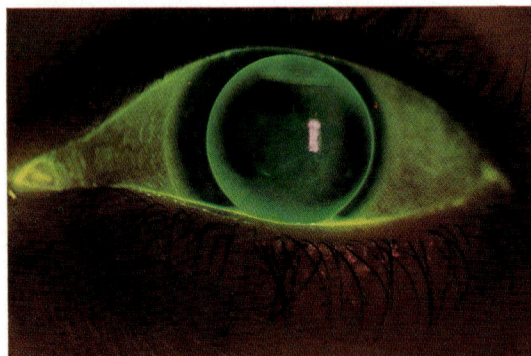

Plate XVIII. A spherical lens fitted with slight apical clearance to a 'with-the-rule' toroidal cornea, the steepest corneal meridian being 70 degrees. The peripheral zone has been fitted slightly steep to prevent too much edge clearance at the top and bottom, in order to minimize discomfort when blinking. There are two crescentic bands of corneal touch on either side of the 160 degrees meridian, and fluorescein shows on the front surface of the top of the lens. Slight central clearance can just be seen along the 70 degrees meridian

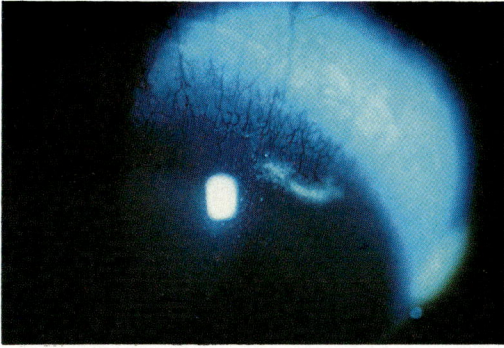

Plate XIX. Limbal vascularization and epithelial hypertrophy due to soft lens wear (reproduced by kind permission of A. P. Gasson)

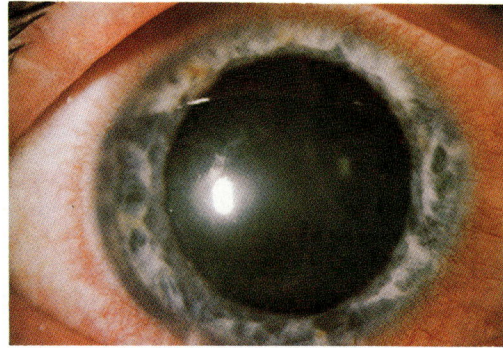

(a)

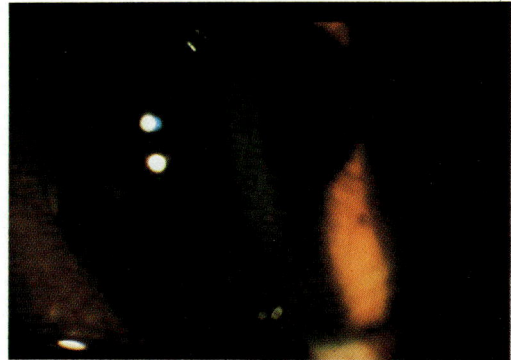

(a)

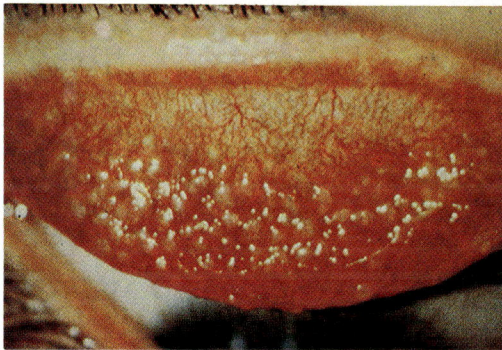

(b)

Plate XXI. (a) Epithelial ring. (b) Endothelial ring. Both conditions are associated with soft lens wear and are associated with pain, discomfort and a red eye. The epithelial condition is protracted but the endothelial ring usually clears quickly (reproduced by kind permission of I. A. Mackie)

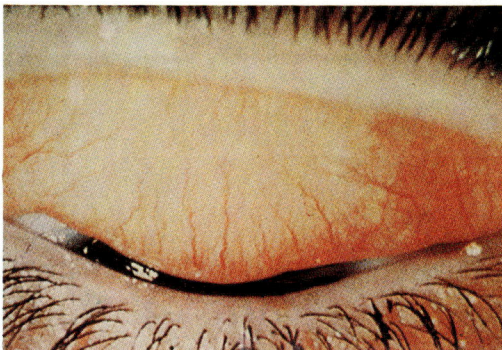

(b)

Plate XX. 'Giant' papillary conjunctivitis of the upper palpebral conjunctiva due to soft contact lens wear (a) compared to the normal (b) (reproduced by kind permission of M. R. Allansmith)

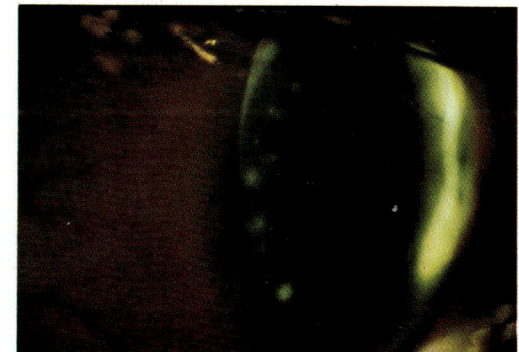

Plate XXII. Nummular keratitis; probably attributable to long-term chronic oedema following soft lens wear (reproduced by kind permission of I. A. Mackie)

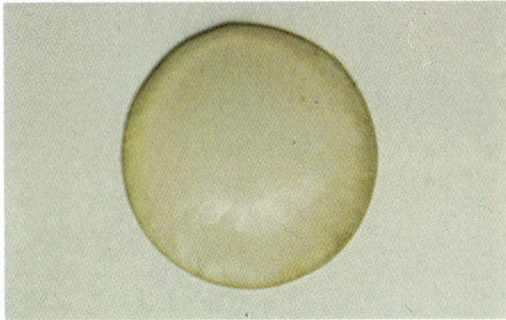

Plate XXIII. Discoloured soft lens (reproduced by kind permission of A. P. Gasson)

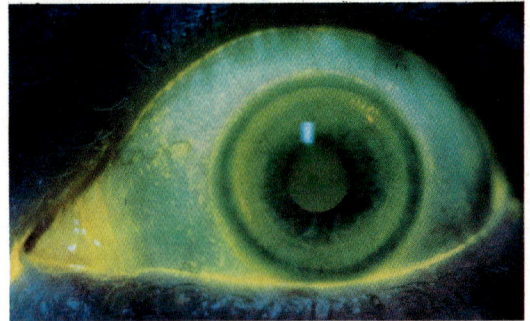

Plate XXVI. Ideal fluorescein pattern of correctly fitting Silflex (silicone) lens (reproduced by kind permission of D. Burns)

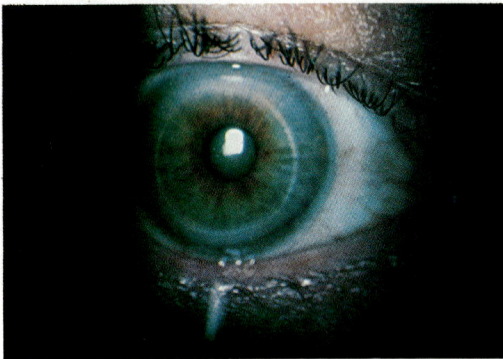

Plate XXIV. Shadows of lenticular junction of a negative powered soft lens visible on the iris. These assist observation of lens movement (reproduced by kind permission of A. P. Gasson)

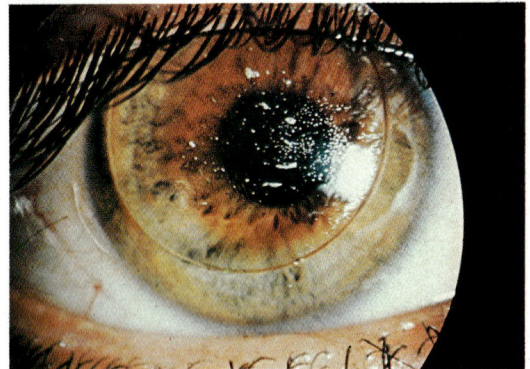

Plate XXVII. Grease and mucus on the scratched front surface of a corneal lens.

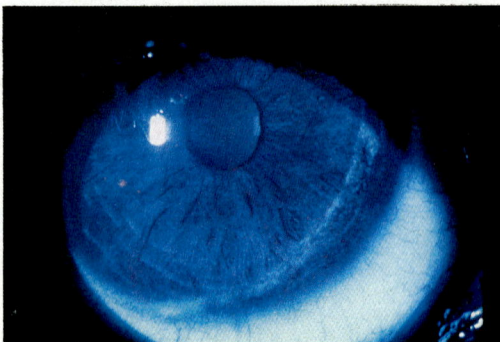

(a)

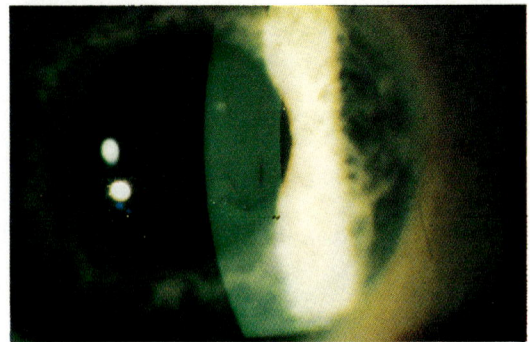

(b)

Plate XXV. (a) Arcuate limbal staining caused by abrasion from a soft lens edge coupled with epithelial dehydration (reproduced by kind permission of Bausch and Lomb Ltd). (b) Initial appearance of a 'dry spot' – in this case a vertical streak – here associated with a recurrent epithelial abrasion just below it (reproduced by kind permission of I. A. Mackie)

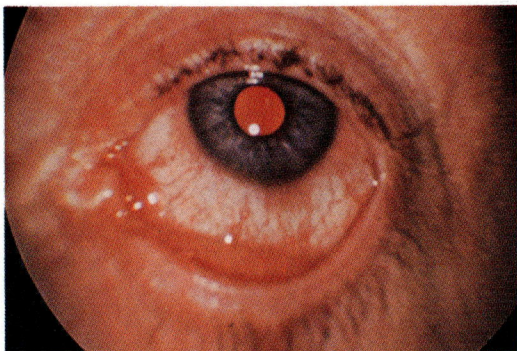

Plate XXVIII. Conjunctival hyperaemia due to the sensitivity response to preservatives in a soft lens storage solution which frequently adhere to mucus deposits on the lens surface (reproduced by kind permission of the London Refraction Hospital)

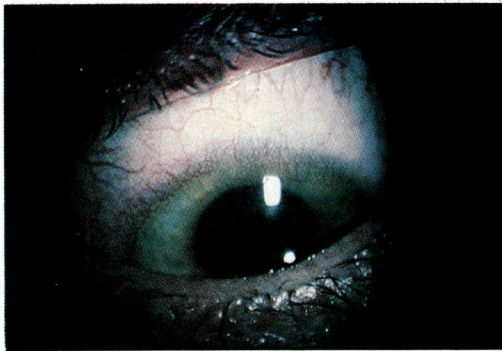

Plate XXXI. Circumferential neovascularization following prolonged oedema associated with soft lens wear (reproduced by kind permission of A. P. Gasson)

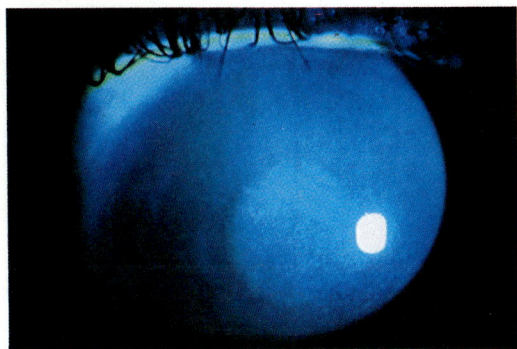

Plate XXIX. Corneal epithelial staining as a result of reaction to preservatives in soft lens cleaning and storage solutions (reproduced by kind permission of Bausch and Lomb Ltd)

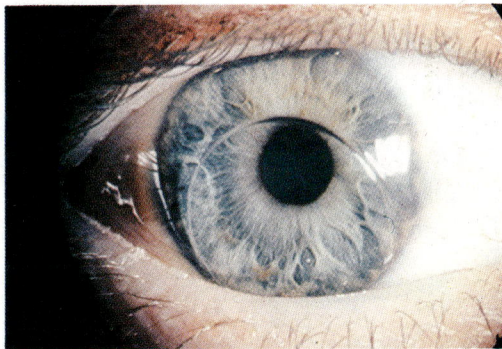

Plate XXXII. Right eye with high corneal astigmatism. Keratometer reading 7.86 mm along 2½, 7.26 mm along 92½. Optimum fit with spherical BCOR showing lens centring very badly

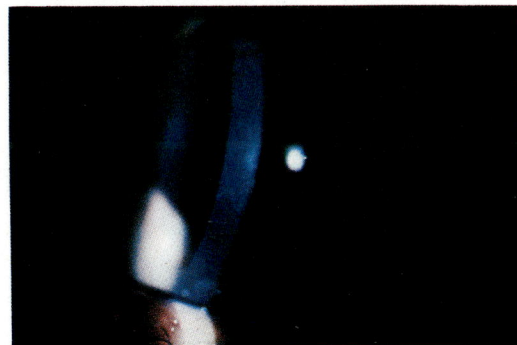

Plate XXX. Vertical striae at the back of the cornea (endothelial folds) shown to the left of an area of stromal and epithelial scarring (reproduced by kind permission of A. P. Gasson)

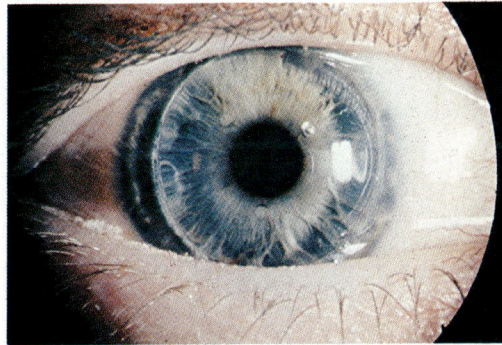

Plate XXXIII. Same right eye as in Plate XXXII wearing an alignment fitted corneal lens utilizing a toroidal back central optic portion of BCOR 7.85 × 7.25 mm. Note: the lens now centres well, but requires fenestration for adequate tears exchange

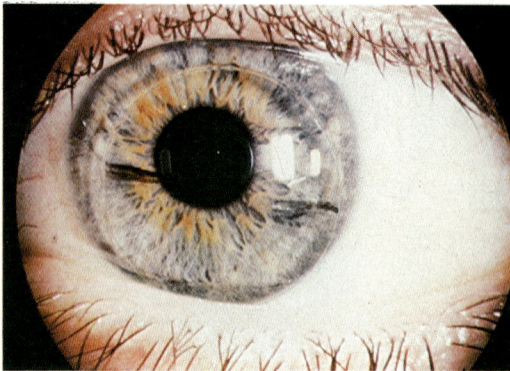

Plate XXXIV. A left lens with a toroidal back central optic portion fitted in alignment. Keratometer reading: 8.16 mm along 175, 7.60 mm along 85. Lens BCOR 8.15 × 7.60 mm. The 8.15 meridian is marked with grease pencil and can be seen aligning well with the 175 meridian. There is no significant rotation, thus permitting accurate correction of residual astigmatism, as well as induced astigmatism, with a front surface cylinder

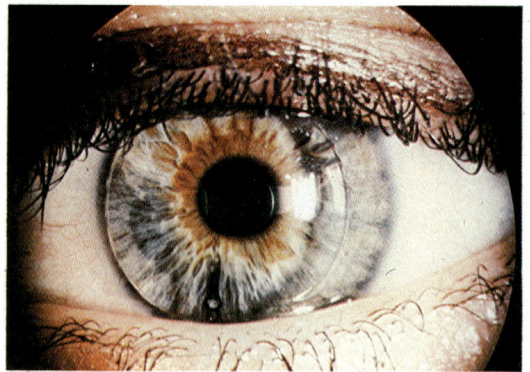

Plate XXXVII. Left eye and prism ballasted corneal lens with base-apex along an average angle of 80°

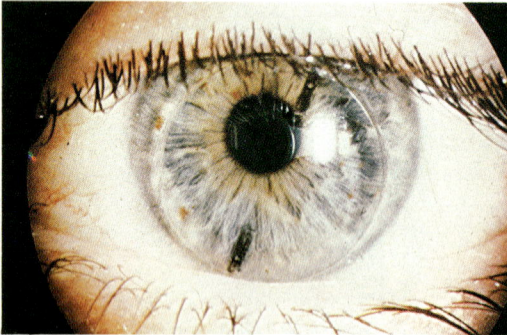

Plate XXXV. Right eye. Keratometer reading: 8.27 mm along 175. 7.70 mm along 85. BCOR 8.25 × 7.70 mm with 8.25 meridian marked with grease pencil. This should be located along the 175 meridian, but, as shown, this lens rotates badly, thus permitting only the accurate correction of induced astigmatism with a front surface cylinder

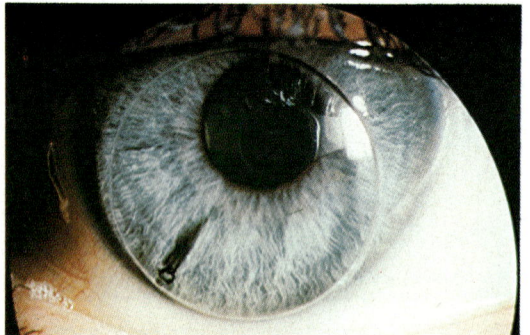

Plate XXXVIII. Right eye and prism ballasted lens with base-apex along 35° (prism base at 215°). This is some 45° off the expected position

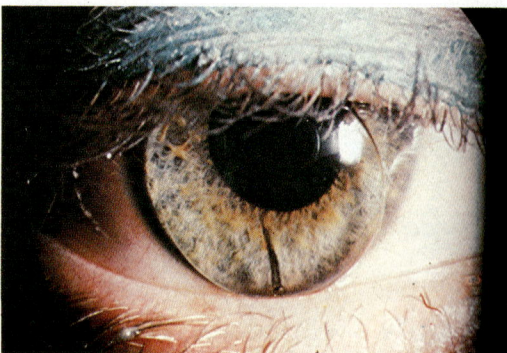

Plate XXXVI. Right eye and prism ballasted corneal lens with base-apex along an average angle of 100°

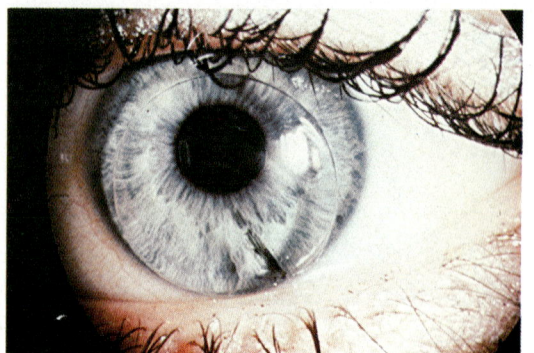

Plate XXXIX. Left eye and prism ballasted lens with base-apex along an angle of 120°. This is some 40° off the expected position

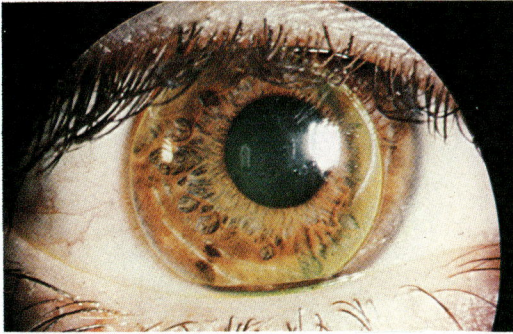

Plate XL. A prism ballasted lens with single truncation. This often proves very successful in preventing unwanted rotation

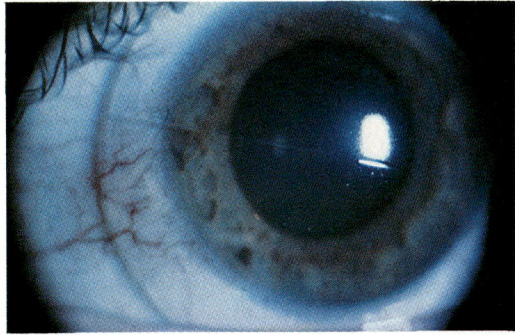

Plate XLIII. A Weicon T trial fitting lens illustrating the engraved line (D.S. axis) with reference to which the cylinder axis is prescribed. The conjunctival injection is normal in this particular patient even in the absence of a contact lens

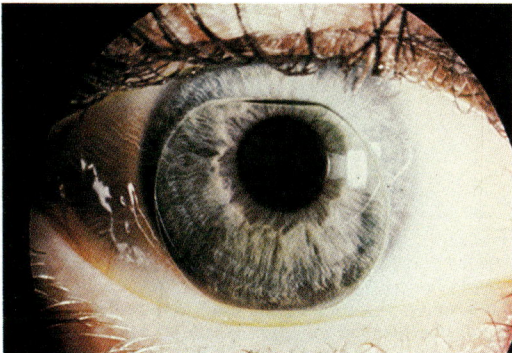

Plate XLI. A double truncated lens without prism. This lens contains a front surface cylinder correction of 1.50 D which remains stable and gives a V.A. of 6/4.5 and complete comfort. The patient had previously had seven other pairs of unsuccessful lenses from various sources

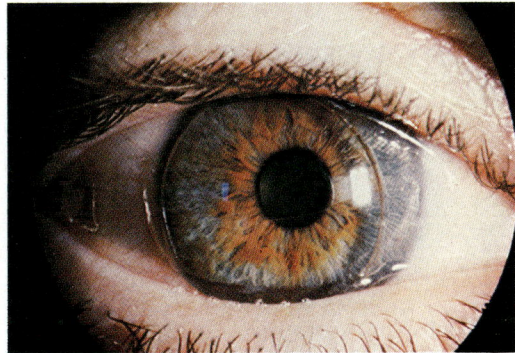

Plate XLIV. A straight top fused bifocal corneal lens correctly positioned for distance vision with the top of the segment slightly overlapping the lower margin of the pupil

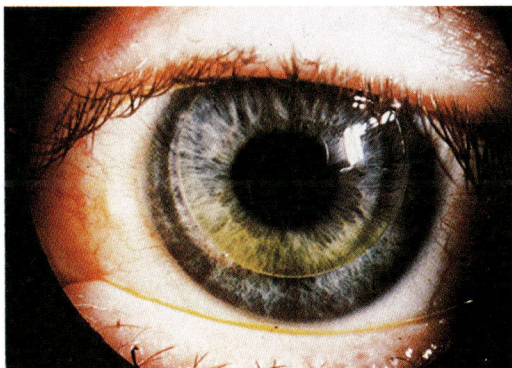

Plate XLII. High corneal astigmatism does not always require correction with a toroidal back central optic portion. This cornea has keratometer readings of 8.23 mm along 180, 7.43 mm along 90. The corneal lens has a BCOR of 8.10 mm and a power of +3.00 D. It centres extremely well and gives a V.A. of 6/4.5

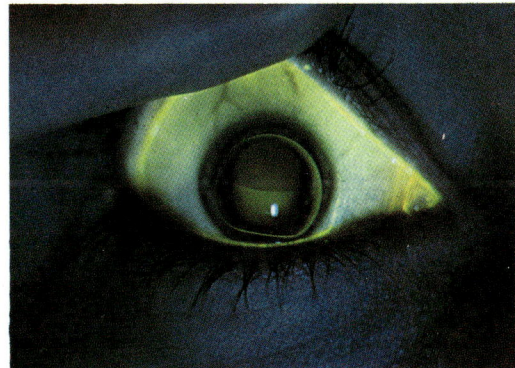

Plate XLV. A crescent fluorescent fused bifocal in a truncated, prism ballasted, corneal lens. The segment half covers the pupil area as the wearer begins to look downwards

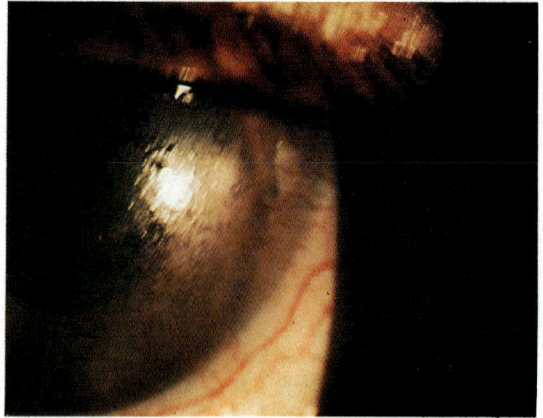

Plate XLVI. Bullous keratopathy. This eye suffered from painful bullae when the condition developed as a sequel to cataract removal. The eye was subsequently treated with HEMA soft lenses which have been worn continuously for four years. The cornea became much clearer despite vascularization, and useful vision is maintained as the lens is made in a full correction for the aphakia. All painful symptoms are relieved although these recur within minutes of the lens being removed

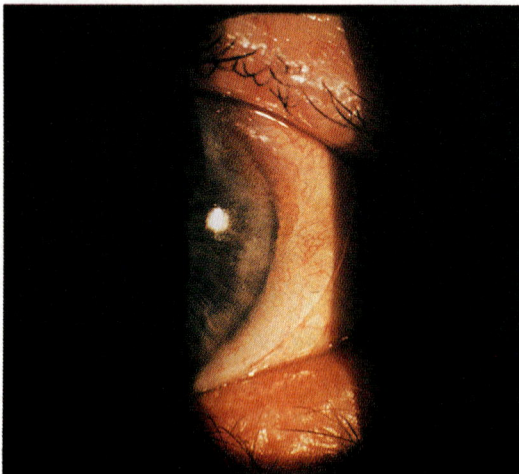

Plate XLVII. Keratopathy of uncertain classification. Both eyes were extremely painful and no therapy other than a soft lens would produce any relief. Vascularization was in evidence before the lenses were fitted but no further deterioration occurred after three years. The corneas remained clear over the pupil and V.A. remained at 6/6

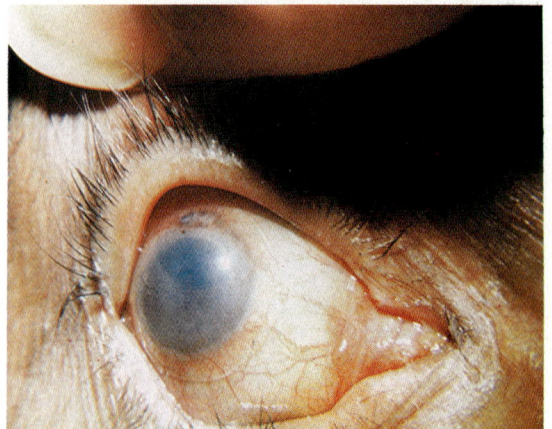

Plate XLVIII. Bullous keratopathy. This patient lived alone many hundreds of miles from ophthalmological or optometric care. Due to his age he was fitted with a large, continuous wear lens of high water content. This relieved all painful symptoms but the vision did not improve. This condition developed as a sequel to cataract surgery

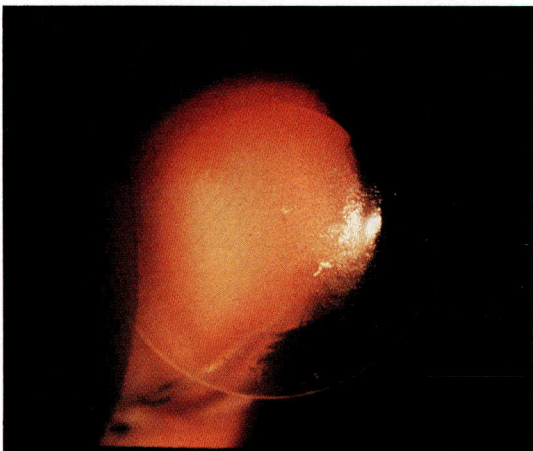

Plate XLIX. Illustrating severe contamination of a HEMA soft lens worn continuously on the eye shown in Colour Plate XLVI. This photograph was taken after the lens had been worn for eight months. If this patient wore a thin lens of the same material then negligible contamination occurred, but all high positive aphakic lenses eventually became contaminated in the manner illustrated

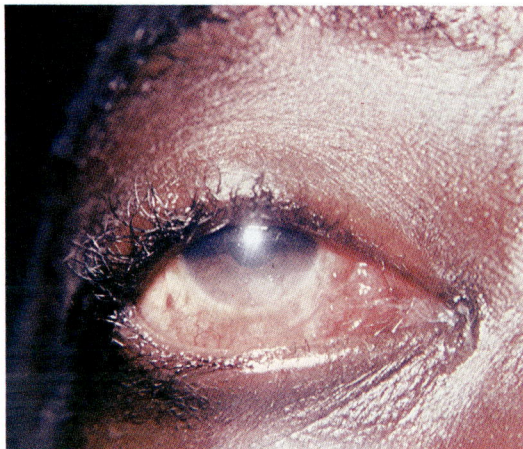

Plate L. Ulceration of the cornea due to inability to close the lids. This patient suffered from proptosis and an inability to move the eyes due to abnormal development of the eye muscles. A soft lens was fitted as a bandage for daily use and the cornea has not ulcerated in the two years that the bandage has been worn. No lens contamination has been seen. The other eye had lid surgery which resulted in the upper lid covering the pupil

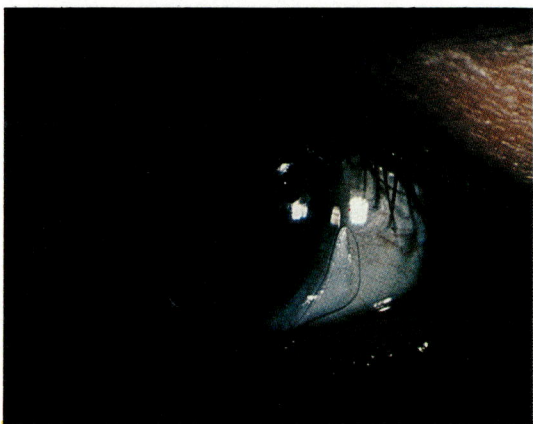

Plate LI. Soft lens worn beneath a scleral lens. In this case a scleral lens could not be produced in a fenestrated form without troublesome bubbles. A high water content soft lens of 12.5 mm overall size was worn under the scleral lens without discomfort and removed all troublesome bubbles

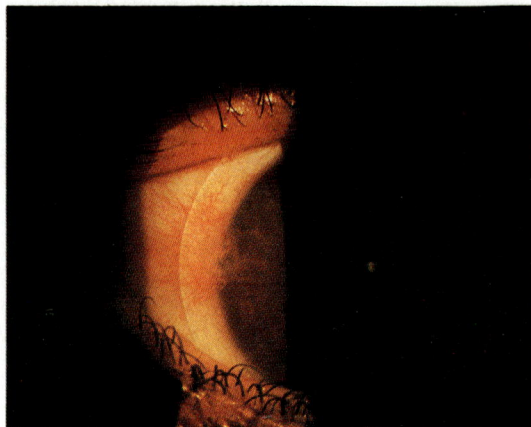

Plate LII. Pterygium. This patient had worn corneal lenses successfully for many years before an enlarging pterygium caused discomfort. The pterygium was excised but a corneal lens was still uncomfortable. Soft lenses, fitted well over the sensitive area were, however, very comfortable although one had to be fitted in toric form

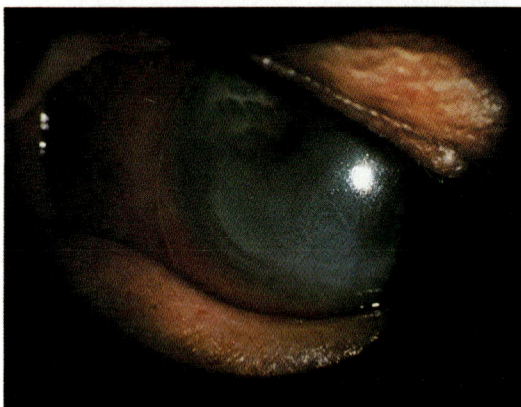

Plate LIII. Herpes ulceration. This patient had unfortunately been treated with cortisone for an ulceration of the cornea. When first seen by the author he was hospitalized, in great pain and using topical anaesthetics hourly to relieve pain. His ophthalmologists were considering enucleating the eye if relief could not be achieved. A soft lens bandage was applied and pain was relieved within four hours. Within 24 hours vision improved considerably and the patient was discharged after three more days in hospital

Plate LIV. Peripheral ulcerative keratitis associated with rheumatoid arthritis. This patient was in severe pain but treatment with a high water content soft lens relieved it entirely. Vision, however, remained unimproved

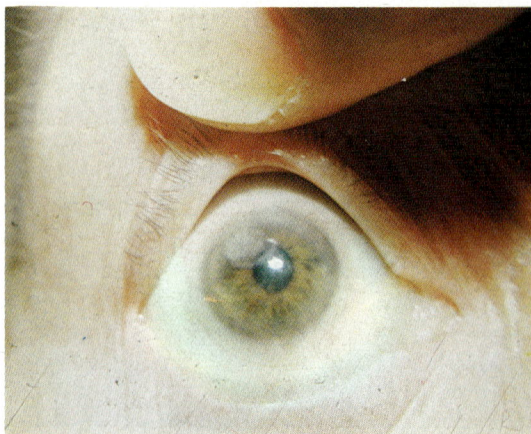

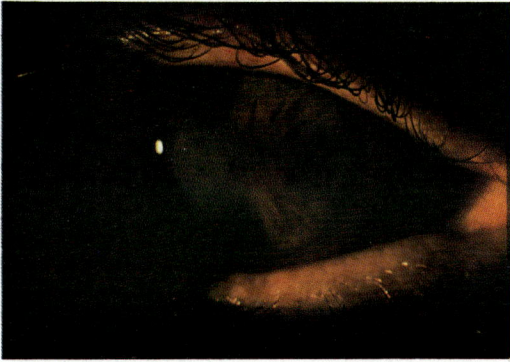

Plate LV. Chronic dendritic corneal ulcer. This patient was treated conventionally for several months without any improvement. A soft lens produced a rapid improvement and after two weeks the cornea had become very regular. Daily wear only was used thereafter and no complications occurred until the lens was lost over a weekend. During the two days of non-use the ulcer recurred and perforated with loss of aqueous. This photograph illustrates the position one week after perforation

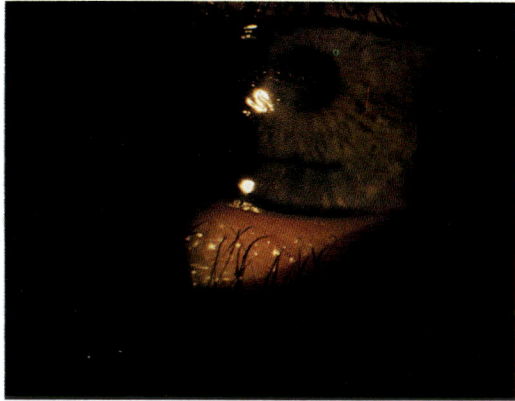

Plate LVI. The same eye as in Colour Plate LV. This illustrates the eye after a further year of continuing daily use of a soft lens after penetration. The considerable increase in transparency of the cornea is evident

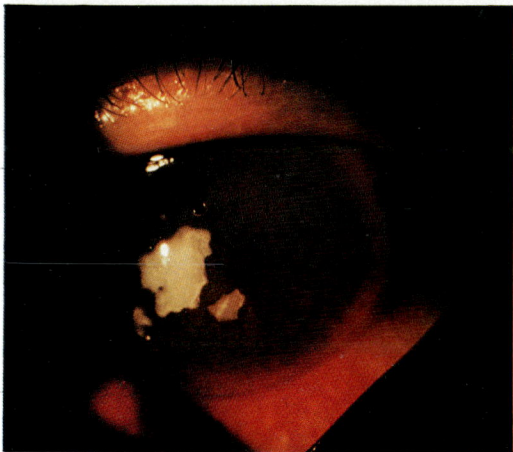

Plate LVII. Recurrent ulceration and cauterization. This patient was first seen with a tarsorrhaphy. A request was made to substitute a soft lens for the tarsorrhaphy. The cornea could be examined through the open lids in the outer canthus region. The lids were opened and a soft lens fitted. Results were good with complete comfort and no recurrence of ulceration. The largest problem proved to be calcium-like deposits which formed on the cornea. Surprisingly the lens did not become contaminated

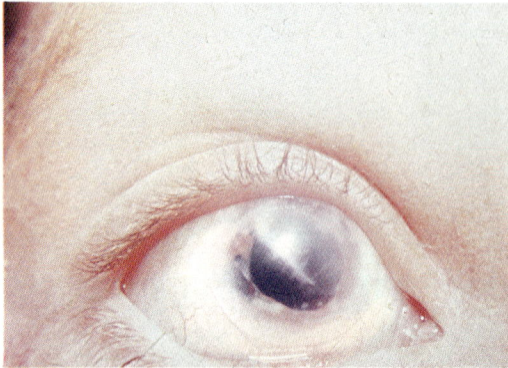

Plate LVIII. Soft lens fitted over scarring caused by a penetrating wound of the eye. Due to the irregularity, a hard corneal lens was not satisfactory and the soft lens acted as a suitable foundation for a 'combination lens'

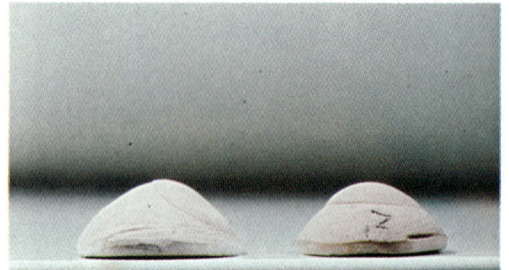

Plate LX. Side view of casts taken from impressions made with a soft lens in situ on the eye. Both successful (right) and unsuccessful (left) impressions are illustrated. The scleral lens is made by pressing the plastic sheet directly onto the cast

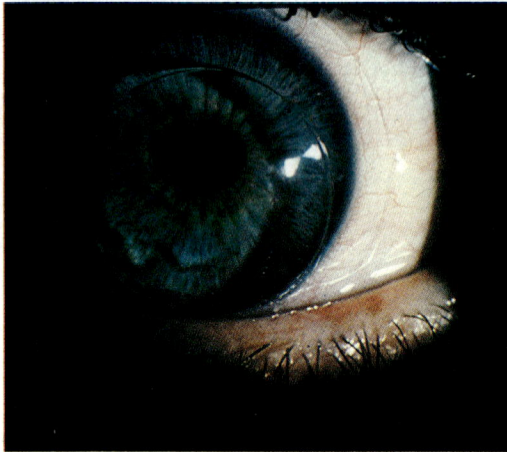

Plate LIX. Illustrating the use of a 'combination lens'. This eye suffers from advanced keratoconus, and orthodox corneal lenses had become useless with the progression of the cone. The corneal lens fitted on top of the soft lens initially produced slight corneal and lid oedema which was relieved by the addition of fenestrations in the corneal lens. Fenestration is seldom necessary in a 'combination lens' system, but if it appears to be indicated the use of a gas permeable corneal lens is usually more effective than fenestration

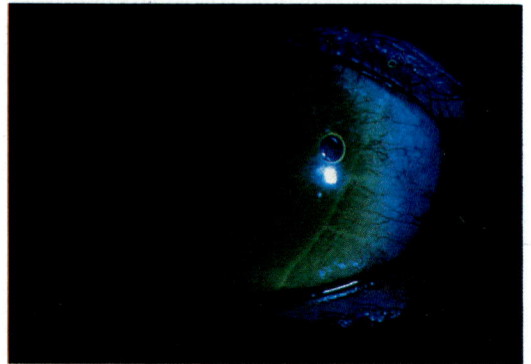

Plate LXI. Fluorescein pattern of scleral lens fitted by taking an impression of an eye wearing a soft lens (as in Colour Plate LX). The lens gives even clearance over the whole cornea.

Rengstorff, R. H. (1974). 'The precorneal tear film; break-up time and location in normal subjects.' *Am. J. Optom.* **51**, 765–769

Rocher, P. (1977). 'Hydrogel lenses and oxygen permeability.' *Optician* **174**(4493), 7–8, 10–11, 13

Rocher, P. and Schwegler, Y. (1974). 'A fitting method for soft hydrophilic lenses based on sagittal height differences.' Paper read at Annual Meeting of American Academy of Optometry, Miami, Florida, December, 1974

Rosenblum, W. M. and leach, N. E. (1975). 'The subjective quality (SQF) of Bausch & Lomb Soflens.' *Am. J. Optom.* **52**, 658–662

Roth, H. W. *et al.* (1980). 'Complication caused by silicon elastomer lenses in West Germany and Japan.' *Contacto* **24**(3), 28–36

Ruben, M. (1974). 'The factors essential for constant wear of a contact lens.' *Optician* **167**(4320), 27–33

Ruben, M. (1977). 'Constant wear v daily wear.' *Optician* **174**(4496), 7, 9, 11

Russell, J. (1974). 'The Hydrocurve contact lens.' *Internat. contact Lens Clin.* **1**(1), 76–88

Sampson, W. G. and Soper, J. W. (1970). 'Keratometry.' Chapter 6 in *Corneal Contact Lenses*, pp. 65–92, 2nd ed. Ed. by Girard, L. J. St. Louis: Mosby

Sarver, M. D., Ashley, D. and Van Every, J. (1974). 'Supplemental power effect of Bausch & Lomb Soflens contact lenses.' *Internat. contact Lens Clin.* **1**(1), 100–109

Stone, Janet (1967). 'Near vision difficulties in non-presbyopic corneal lens wearers.' *Contact Lens J.* **1**(2), 14–16, 24–25

Stone, Janet (1974). 'The measurement of corneal thickness.' *Contact Lens J.* **5**(2), 14–19

Strachan, J. P. F. (1973). 'Some principles of the optics of hydrophilic lenses and geometrical optics applied to flexible lenses.' *Austral. J. Optom.* **56**, 25–33

Touch, A. J. (1977a). 'Selection of lens diameter in fitting soft contact lens patients.' *Optom. Wkly* **68**, 252–255

Touch, A. J. (1977b). 'Study shows 13.6 mm hydrophilic lenses preferred to "best fit".' *Contact Lens J.* **6**(3), 23

Touch, A. J. and Clark, R. (1974). 'The Touch technique for fitting Soflens (polymacon) contact lenses.' Paper read at the Midwest Contact Lens Congress, Chicago, April, 1974, and reviewed in Touch, Mertz and Seger (1976) below

Touch, A. J., Mertz, G. W. and Seger, R. G. (1976). 'The best-fit band theory – two years later.' *Internat. contact Lens Clin.* **3**(4), 32–36

Van Wauwe, L. (1977). 'The aspheric toric Hydron lens – early clinical results.' *Optician* **173**(4470), 8, 10–11

Voerste, K. (1976). 'Analysing the clinical results of fitting a type of soft contact lens.' *Optician* **171**(4414), 15–16, 18, 23

Watts, G. K. (1971). 'Hydrophilic contact lenses – a review.' *Optician* **161**(4174), 10–13

Wechsler, S. (1974). 'Striate corneal lines.' *Am. J. Optom.* **51**, 852–856

Westerhout, D. (1973). ' "The combination lens" and therapeutic uses of soft lenses.' *Contact Lens J.* **4**(5), 3–10, 12, 16–18, 20, 22

Wichterle, O. (1967). 'Changes of refracting power of a soft lens caused by its flattening.' In *Corneal and Scleral Contact Lenses*, The Proceedings of the International Congress, paper 29, pp. 247–256, March 1966, ed. by Girard, L. J. St. Louis: Mosby

Wichterle, O. and Lim, D. (1960). 'Hydrophilic gels for biological use.' *Nature* **185**, 117–118

Wycoff, P. (1972). 'Hydrophilic contact lenses.' *Contact Lens Soc.. Am. J.* **6**(3), 12–21

Chapter 15

The Verification of Soft Contact Lenses

D. F. C. Loran

Hydrogel contact lenses are flexible and if exposed to the atmosphere they dehydrate and alter their contour; thus, conventional methods of measuring hard lens parameters are not applicable to this type of contact lens. As a consequence, practitioners may feel unable to check the specification of these lenses conveniently and this may, in turn, result in frustration and disappointment if a lens received from the laboratory does not provide the expected performance *in situ*. Such a situation is obviously most unsatisfactory and practitioners are urged to verify the parameters of soft contact lenses within the limitations of present instrumentation.

Undoubtedly it is most convenient to check soft lens parameters directly in air using conventional instruments, although such methods may present inaccuracies due to surface deformation, shrinkage of the hydrogel on dehydration and also accumulation of surface moisture. In order to overcome these artifacts liquid cells as shown in *Figures 15.1* and *15.2* have been utilized to measure the parameters of soft lenses.

If hydrogel lenses are mounted in a transparent cell containing a compatible medium such as sterile normal saline solution (without a preservative) then the lens should assume its natural, undistorted form. Masnick and Holden (1972) ascertained that changes in pH and tonicity of the lens environment produced clinically significant alterations in the water content with associated parametric variations. Measurements of the overall size and also primary sag of soft lenses by Poster and Skolnik (1974) indicated that these changes varied with tonicity but not pH, whilst Masnick and Holden (1972) observed

a decrease in overall size in acidic and an increase in overall size in alkaline solutions. Such effects are also likely to vary with the lens material.

In a comprehensive survey Harris, Hall and Dye (1973) checked soft lenses in air and concluded that with the notable exception of radii these parameters could be checked in air with a reasonable degree of accuracy. Mandell (1974a) recommends the following procedure for air measurement of soft lens power.

(1) The lens should be removed from its liquid environment using a sterile spatula or soft plastics-protected forceps.

(2) The lens is then placed on a lint-free tissue and the tissue folded over the uppermost convex surface of the lens.

(3) The lens is transferred onto a dry area of tissue and step (2) repeated to make sure that both surfaces are blotted dry.

(4) The lens is dried in air with forceps.

(5) The lens surfaces are examined macroscopically and if smudges are present the process is repeated.

(6) Although it is probably preferable to check the lens within an overall period of one minute of air exposure (Titmus Eurocon, 1974), the lens essentially maintains its contour within clinical limits for up to four minutes during which time the measurements should be completed.

Before considering the verification of soft contact lenses, however, it is expedient to consider the lens specification which, in turn, is predetermined by the method of manufacture which may be spin-casting, lathe-cutting or moulding.

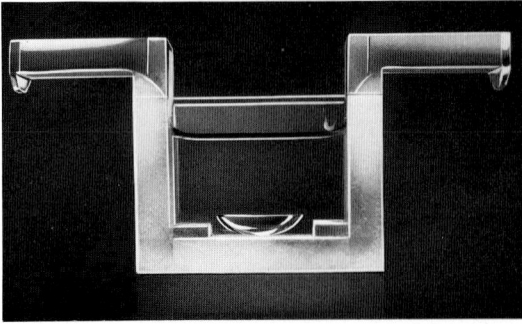

Figure 15.1–Hydrogel lens immersed in normal saline solution in a liquid cell (photograph by courtesy of Söhnges Optik)

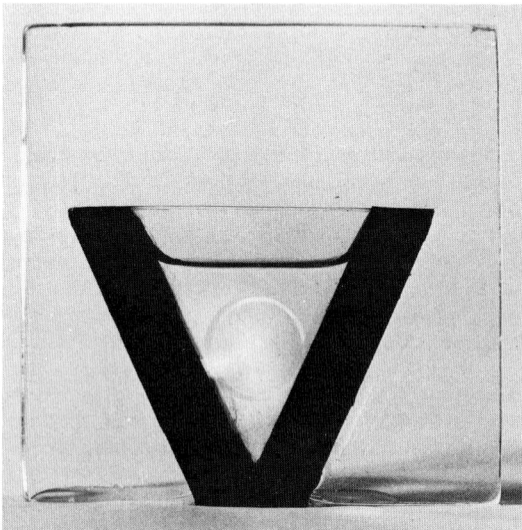

Figure 15.2–Liquid cell, showing transverse section of immersed lens, used to determine power of lens in saline solution, to measure diameters with a band magnifier, or for surface inspection

MANUFACTURE OF HYDROGEL CONTACT LENSES

SPIN-CASTING

The Bausch and Lomb Soflens (Polymacon) is produced by a computer-controlled method of axial spin-casting originally introduced by Wichterle and Lim (1960) for the Czechoslovakian Geltakt lens.

Liquid monomers of 2-hydroxethyl methacrylate and ethylene diglycol methacrylate are stored at a temperature of –5°C and injected through a polythene tube into a rotating female mould where polymerization occurs in a carbon dioxide atmosphere at a temperature of 65°C (Hartstein, 1973).

By controlling three variables; mould diameter, spin-speed and the volume of monomer injected, it is possible to produce a variety of shapes and curves. As illustrated in *Figure 15.3*, the lens is formed front surface downwards through the action of centripetal force and gravity (Bausch and Lomb, 1975). The front curve is therefore determined by the shape of the female mould and at the time of writing the front central optic radii of the Bausch and Lomb Soflens range from 8.60 mm to 10.08 mm and the centre thickness from 0.035 mm to 0.30 mm. These lenses are available in three overall sizes, 12.50 mm, 13.50 mm and 14.50 mm, and are described by a 'Series' code which is currently F, +N, U, B3, +B3, H3, U3, O3, B4, +B4, +H4, U4 and O4. The full specifications of the present Soflenses are given in *Tables 14.13, 14.14* and *14.15*.

As the injection pressure or the speed of rotation is increased more material is projected towards the periphery thereby increasing the edge thickness. Consequently, as negative power is increased for a given Series the back surface steepens and the lens fits more tightly, the reverse occurring as negative power is reduced or positive power is increased.

The spin casting process is fully automatic and produces smooth, reproducible surfaces free from

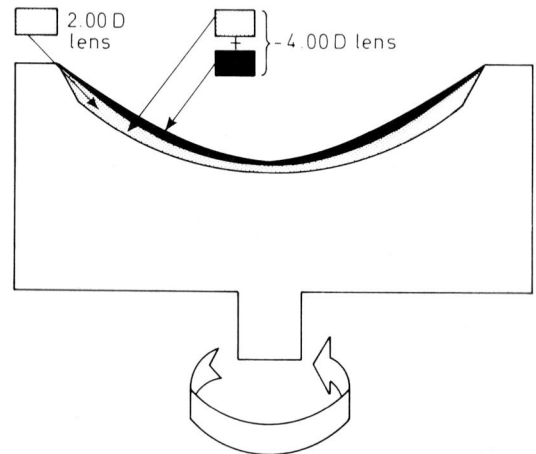

Figure 15.3–Axial spin-casting method of producing the Geltakt and the Bausch and Lomb Soflens by injecting liquid monomers into a rotating mould where polymerization occurs. The lens is indicated by the grey shaded area within the concave mould. The darker area above indicates the lens shape and the additional minus power produced either by a higher speed of mould rotation or a greater injection pressure

tool marks, peripheral grooves and other imperfections which may occur in the polishing and finishing of lathe-cut lenses.

LATHE-CUT LENSES

With the notable exceptions of the Bausch and Lomb Soflens (also the Czechoslovakian Geltakt lens – from which the former is derived) and injection moulded ILC lenses (*see below*) most hydrogel lenses are lathe-cut and polished in a generally similar manner to hard lenses. The front and back optic radii are lathe-cut from stress-free dehydrated buttons, allowance being made for expansion of the polymer on hydration. In the manufacturers' literature lathe-cut lenses are usually specified as follows: *back central optic radius/overall size/back vertex power/thickness.*

MOULDING

A moulded contact lens is produced by pressing, usually between dyes, and is defined as one manufactured basically by a shaping process without the removal of material (British Standards Institution, 1979). Moulded scleral lenses have been produced for many years by heating a Perspex laminate to softening point and it is then pressed onto a hard cast. Kelvin Lenses Ltd., and Wöhlk Contact Linsen currently mould hard corneal lenses both in polymethyl methacrylate and cellulose acetate butyrate.

Providing plastic memory can be controlled then moulding is generally considered to be a satisfactory manufacturing process and may result in relatively thin, smooth and reproducible surfaces. Indeed, most polymers if they are not cross-linked are basically suitable for moulding (Gee, 1980) and consequently this process has also been used to produce soft contact lenses. Silicone lenses such as Tesicon produced by Titmus Eurocon and the Silflex lens produced by Wöhlk Contact Linsen are both moulded and a hydrogel lens manufactured by the International Lens Corporation (ILC) is moulded between dyes from liquid monomers.

Current fitting philosophy appears to be directed towards thin, permeable lenses worn for extended periods and possibly discarded when removed from the eye. If this concept is desired then it is conceivable that moulding could be considered as a suitable manufacturing process to produce relatively inexpensive lenses to fulfil these criteria.

LENS SPECIFICATION

It should be noted, however, that in general both the width of the front and back peripheral curves and also the back peripheral optic radius are fixed parameters. As the overall size is increased the back central optic diameter is also increased by a similar amount and hence it could be argued that in specifying diameters it is unnecessary to specify both the basic optic diameter and the overall size. It might be anticipated, however, that eventually peripheral parameters may be varied and also the radii blended as in hard lenses and therefore a more comprehensive specification might read as follows: *back central optic radius: basic optic diameter/back peripheral optic radius: back hydrogel size/degree of blending/back vertex power/central and/or edge thickness/tint.* Front central optic diameter and front peripheral radius may also be specified where necessary. The British Standards Institution has now published tolerances for soft lens parameters. These and Australian draft standards are shown in *Table 15.1.*

Having considered the parameters it is now in order to consider the quality control of these parameters, namely, radii, diameters and linear parameters, thickness, back vertex power and surfaces.

VERIFICATION PROCEDURES

RADII

The central optic radii are probably the most clinically significant variables in fitting soft contact lenses but paradoxically they are the most difficult to check. An undistorted lens is a necessity for the measurement of soft contact lens radii and because of the inherent flexibility of the material it is preferable, if not essential, to support the lens in a liquid-filled, parallel, flat-surfaced cell in order to determine radii, which may be measured by reflected light, microspherometry or optical gauging.

THE USE OF REFLECTED LIGHT TO DETERMINE SOFT CONTACT LENS RADII

Keratometers

A keratometer is essential in the armamentarium of the contact lens practitioner, and its use has therefore been considered in determining the radii of hydrogel lenses (Chaston, 1973) and an accuracy of ±0.10 mm is claimed (Forst, 1974). It is essential that the lens is mounted in a liquid cell and the mire images are then reflected into the telescope either by a prism as illustrated in *Figure 15.4a* or alternatively by an inclined mirror, as shown in *Figure 15.4b*.

The lens is completely immersed in normal saline solution of refractive index 1.336 but separated from the telescope by air. The contact lens/liquid lens air system thus acts as an equivalent mirror (Chaston, 1973) so that the vertex of the mirror and the centre of curvature of the equivalent mirror are displaced towards each other as illustrated in *Figure 15.5*. Consequently, the measured radius of curvature is

Table 15.1–Standards for the Tolerances of Hydrogel Contact Lenses

Parameter	Draft Australian Standards (1976)	British Standard (1978)
Back central optic radius	±0.05 mm	±0.10 mm (dry) ±0.20 mm (wet)
Back central optic diameter		±0.10 mm (dry)
Peripheral optic radius		±0.10 mm (dry) ±0.20 mm (wet)
Back peripheral optic diameter		±0.20 mm (dry)
Overall size	±0.05 mm (< 50% water) ±0.10 mm (> 50% water)	±0.25 mm (wet)
Front central optic diameter		±0.20 mm (dry) ±0.20 mm (wet)
Central and edge thickness	±0.02 mm (single lens) ±0.03 mm (lens pair)	±0.02 mm (dry) ±0.05 mm (wet)
Back vertex power (in the weaker meridian)	±0.12 D (< 10.00 D) ±0.25 D (> 10.00 D)	±0.25 D (wet, < 10.00 D) ±0.50 D (wet, > 10.00 D)

Table 15.2–Steepest Soft Lens Radii Capable of Checking by Keratometry due to the Limitations Set by the Steep End of the Scale of Various Instruments (*Note:* Keratometer Scales can be Extended (*see* page 474)

Instrument	Steepest scale reading in air = soft lens radius measured in saline solution (mm)	Corresponding soft lens radius in air = radius in saline solution × 1.336 (mm)
Guilbert Routit (topographical)	4.60	6.15
Zeiss (Jena) (East German)	5.00	6.70
Carl Zeiss (West German) (Oberkochen)	5.50	7.35
Gambs	5.50	7.35
Sbisa (Javal Schiotz)	5.60	7.50
American Optical	5.60	7.50
Guilbert Routit (Javal Schiotz)	6.00	8.05
Bausch and Lomb	6.40	8.55

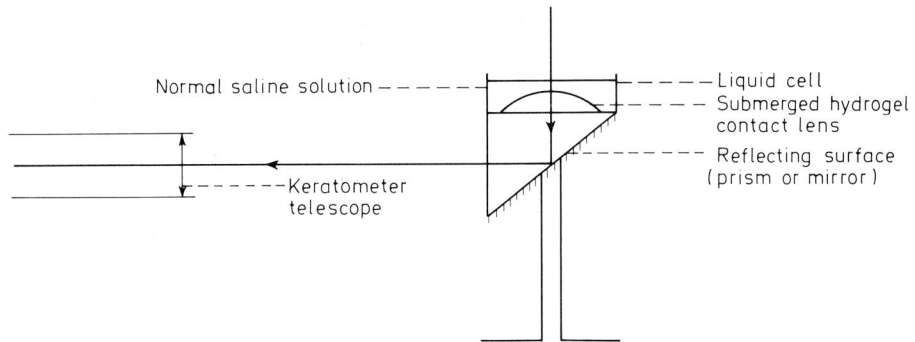

(a)

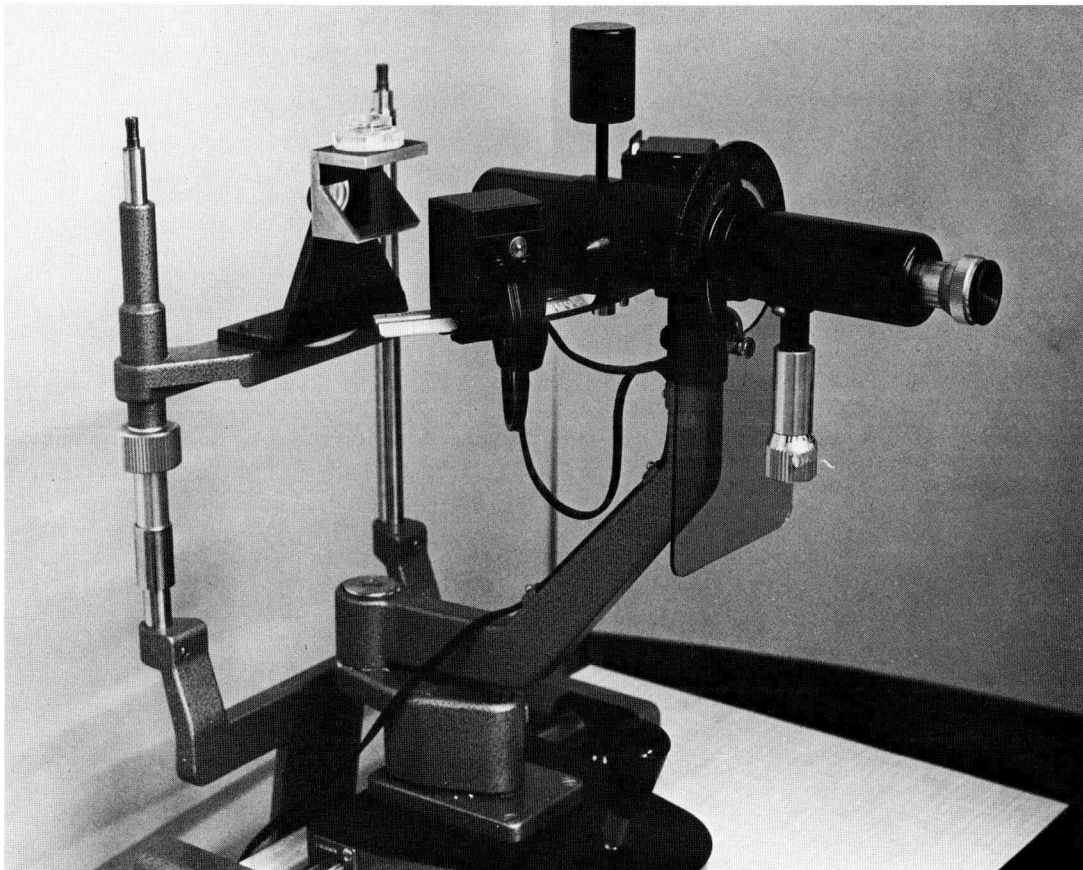

(b)

Figure 15.4–(a) Measurement of the back central optic radius of a soft contact lens by keratometry. (b) Soft contact lens immersed in saline solution and mounted on a Javal-Schiotz keratometer (photograph by courtesy of Smith and Nephew Research Ltd.)

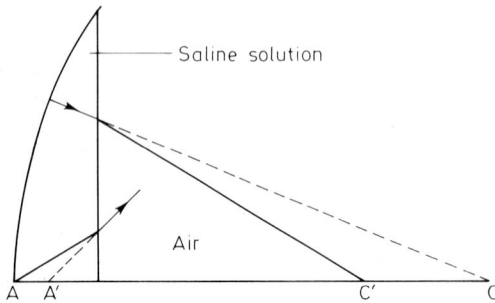

Figure 15.5–The equivalent mirror effect which results in a reduced back central optic radius reading when a liquid-immersed lens is measured by keratometry (Chaston, 1973)

shorter than the true radius of curvature by an amount dependent on the refractive index of the saline solution. Furthermore, a keratometer calibrated for convex surfaces will slightly underestimate the radii of concave surfaces by approximately 0.03 mm (Emsley, 1963; Bennett, 1966).

Therefore: $r = nr' + Y$

where r is the radius of curvature in air
        r' is the radius of curvature in liquid
        n is the refractive index of saline
        solution = 1.336

and Y is the concave compensation factor so that
        $r = \dfrac{4 \times r'}{3} + (\simeq) \; 0.03$

Thus:

$4/3 \times r'$	Corrected values (Bausch and Lomb) for concave surfaces
7.00 mm	7.02 mm
7.50 mm	7.525 mm
8.00 mm	8.030 mm
8.50 mm	8.535 mm

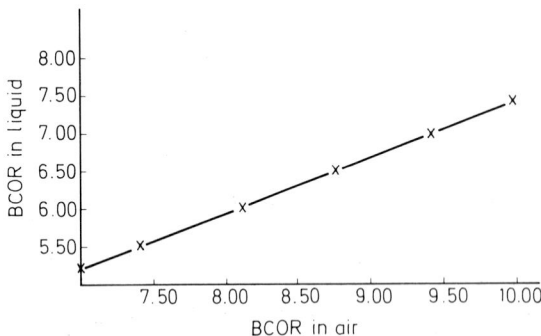

Figure 15.6–Conversion from the back central optic radius measured in saline solution by the keratometer to the back central optic radius in air

The radius of curvature of the lens in air, however, may be more easily determined from a graph as shown in *Figure 15.6*.

It is suggested that an instrument for checking soft lens radii should have a range from 7.40 to 9.50 mm which by liquid immersion is transferred to the range 5.40–7.10 mm. *Table 15.2* illustrates the range of radii of keratometers chosen at random and from this it is noted that the radii are too flat to measure soft lenses in 50 per cent of the instruments. However, as pointed out by Hartstein (1973), it is possible by placing a +1.25 D spherical auxiliary lens over the telescope objective, to extend the range of steeper radii measured by approximately 1.30 mm. This topic is also covered in Chapters 5 and 12, Volume 1.

Further complications, as listed below, arise in the use of keratometers with liquid immersion.

(1) In a liquid environment less light is reflected from each lens surface than when the lens is in air. Fresnel's law for light of normal incidence is:

$$R = \left[\frac{n' - n}{n' + n}\right]^2 \times 100 \text{ per cent}$$

where R is the percentage of reflected light, n is the refractive index of the surrounding medium (= 1.336 for saline solution and 1.00 for air) n' is the refractive index of the second medium (= 1.430 for hydrogel material). In air, therefore, $R = 3.13$ per cent, and in saline solution $R = 0.115$ per cent.

The luminosity of the mires has therefore to be significantly increased to compensate for the reduction in intensity of the reflected light when a lens is measured in a saline solution cell.

(2) In order to increase the luminosity it is feasible that excessive heat could be generated, and Loran (1974) has shown that the manifestation of an increased ambient temperature of the liquid is to steepen the radii. Ideally, soft lens parameters should be checked at the environmental temperature of the conjunctival sac. The temperature of the cornea exceeds that of the atmosphere, but is slightly below body temperature (Mandell, 1974b) although when a soft lens is inserted into the eye a temperature gradient is manifested which may vary from 37°C on the back surface to 20–50°C on the front (Ruben, 1973, 1974). Furthermore, the temperature of the conjunctival sac may vary with factors such as lid closure, blepharospasm and palpebral aperture size (Hill and Leighton, 1964).

(3) If an attempt is made to utilize reflected light to measure the radii of a submerged lens then a double image is formed by reflections at the front and back surfaces of the lens respectively, so that the operator must first identify, and secondly ignore

the unwanted image. The image formed by the surface proximal to the mires will be brighter, and if the back vertex power of the lens is negative the back surface will produce the smaller image; the reverse occurring with positive lenses (Forst, 1974).

Although the above-mentioned limitations are not confined to keratometry it is obvious that this technique is not entirely straight-forward and practice is necessary to achieve the claimed reliability.

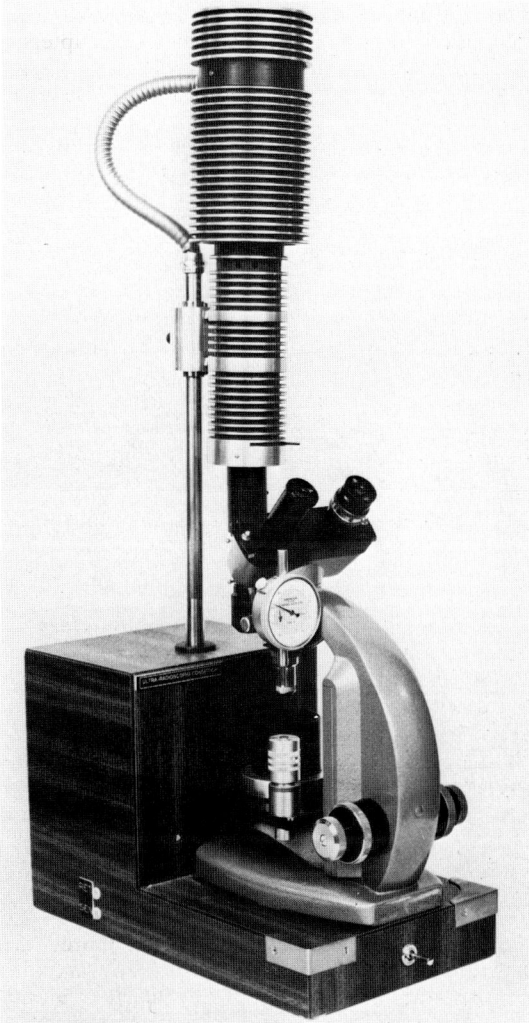

Figure 15.7–The Ultra Radiuscope produced by Conoptica Laboratory, Madrid. The lens is mounted in a liquid cell and the objective is immersed into the saline solution. The back central radius is read directly from the instrument (photograph by courtesy of G. Nissel & Co.)

Radiuscopes

In employing a radiuscope to determine the back central optic radii of a hard lens one immerses the front of the lens in a liquid-filled concave holder which avoids distortion of the lens and also eliminates unwanted reflections from the front surface. A similar technique for hydrogel soft lenses has been suggested by Stone (1975) who recommends blotting the back surface dry and carefully floating the convex surface in a concave holder filled with saline solution. Capillary attraction, however, between the lens and the holder tends to tilt and distort the lens and accumulation of surface moisture often precludes a clear image. Tajiri (1974) has designed a conical corral-type holder which permits a clear radiuscope reading. Its lattice structure is apparently not unlike the basket holder of many hard lens soaking cases, and maintains the lens contour parallel to the saline surface and also acts as a pump to suspend the lens at the liquid-air surface. If a clear image of the radiuscope lamp filament is obtainable the examiner is able to obtain a clear image of the radiuscope target and the radius is determined in the normal way.

A specially designed soft lens radiuscope has been produced by Chamarro Torino (1974) which claims to overcome the previously mentioned difficulties. The Ultra Radiuscope is illustrated in *Figure 15.7* which shows the lens centred in a liquid cell into

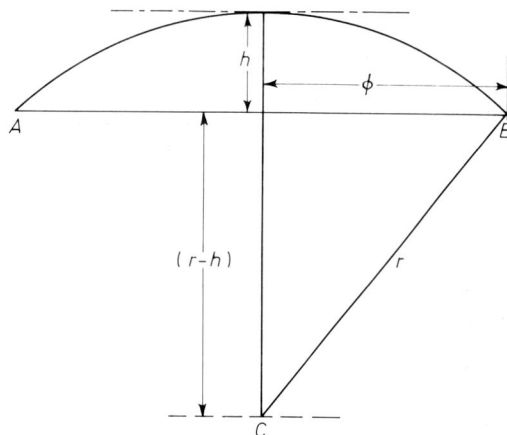

Figure 15.8–Principle of microspherometry

which the waterproof objective lens of a travelling microscope is immersed. Although a high luminosity is required in this instrument the reflected light only travels through a single refracting medium and a direct reading through saline solution is taken in a similar manner to a conventional radiuscope, resulting in a reliability of ± 0.02 mm (Nissel, 1975). In order to attain the required brightness it is necessary to incorporate a 200 watt halogen bulb into the instrument which normally only has a working life of 25 hours, although this can be doubled by using sub-maximum voltage supplied to the instrument in gradual stages (Nissel, 1975).

MICROSPHEROMETRY

Contact lens radii are steep and the curvatures represent a small part of a complete sphere, and in such circumstances one can indirectly determine the radii by microsph_erometry.

In *Figure 15.8*, *AB* represents a small portion of a spherical curve, *C* is the centre of curvature, *r* is the radius of curvature, and *h* is the primary sag for a given chord $2\emptyset$ *so that:*

$$r^2 = \emptyset^2 + (r - h)^2 \text{ and } r = \emptyset^2/2h + h/2$$

Thus, if the chord diameter and the primary sag can be measured for a given segment it is possible to deduce the radius of curvature. This principle is used in the Abbé spherometer and is also utilized in the following instruments.

The Wet Cell Radius Gauge (Contact Lenses (Manufacturing) Ltd.)

This instrument, illustrated in *Figure 15.9* is a magnified vertex depth gauge which permits approximate determination of the back central optic

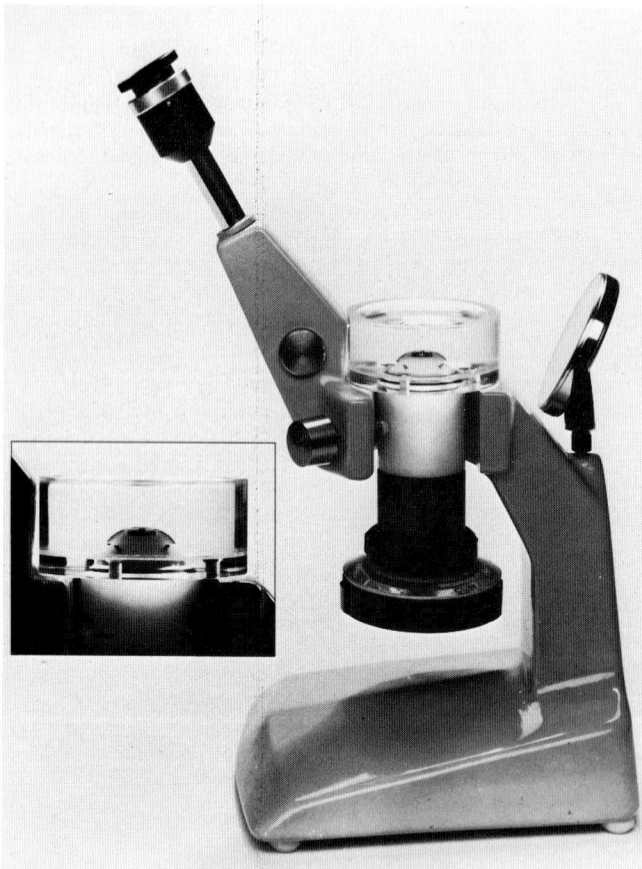

Figure 15.9–The Wet Cell Gauge produced by Contact Lenses (Manufacturing) Ltd., which utilizes microsph_erometry to determine the approximate radius of curvature of a liquid-immersed contact lens. Inset: Soft lens in place in saline cell. The support ring, oblique centring posts and central probe can be seen (photograph by courtesy of Contact Lenses (Manufacturing) Ltd.)

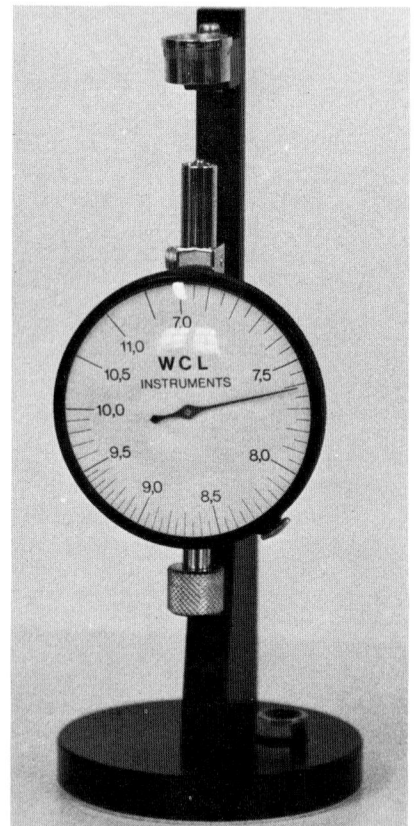

Figure 15.10–The Wöhlk Microsph2erometer determines the primary sag for a predetermined chord diameter of a soft contact lens in air. The back central optic radius which corresponds to a specific sag height is directly read off a clock dial (photograph by courtesy of Wöhlk-Contact-Lenses, Crowborough, Sussex)

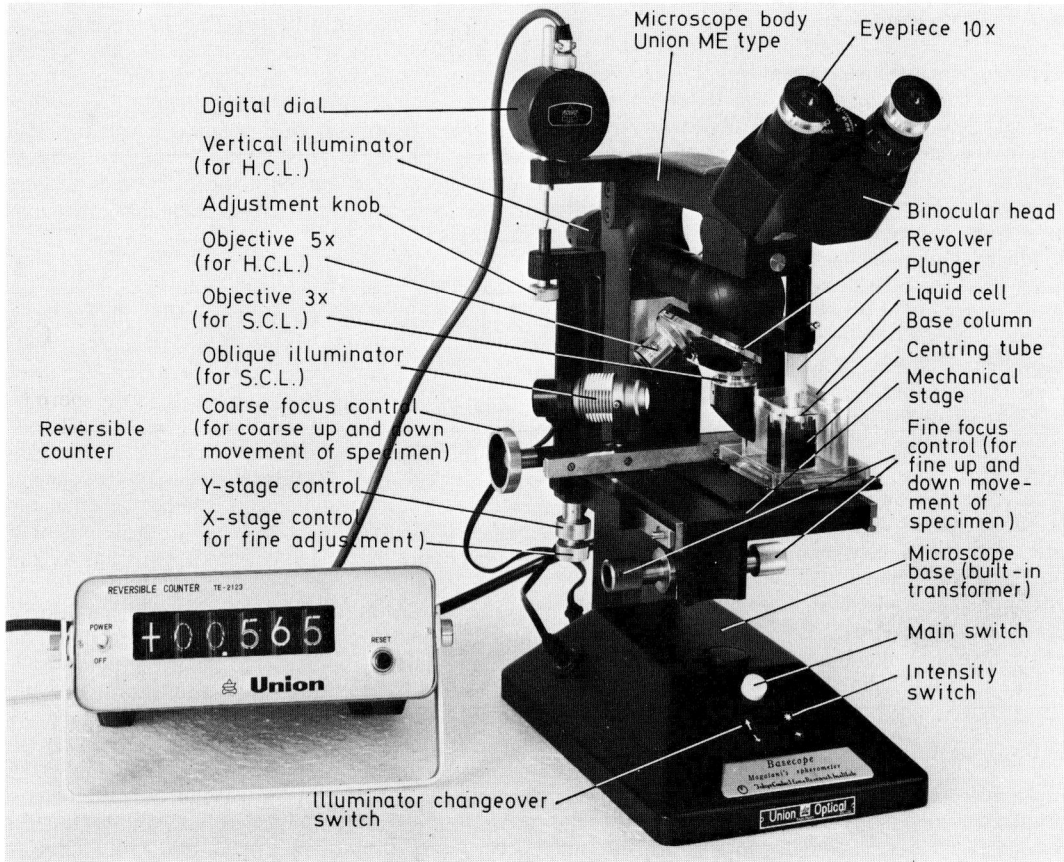

Digital dial

Vertical illuminator (for H.C.L.)

Adjustment knob

Objective 5x (for H.C.L.)

Objective 3x (for S.C.L.)

Oblique illuminator (for S.C.L.)

Coarse focus control (for coarse up and down movement of specimen)

Y-stage control

X-stage control for fine adjustment)

Reversible counter

Microscope body Union ME type

Eyepiece 10x

Binocular head
Revolver
Plunger
Liquid cell
Base column
Centring tube
Mechanical stage
Fine focus control (for fine up and down movement of specimen)
Microscope base (built-in transformer)
Main switch
Intensity switch

REVERSIBLE COUNTER TE-2123

POWER OFF

+00.565

RESET

≜ Union

Illuminator changeover switch

Figure 15.11–The Basecope, produced by Union Optical Co., is a precision instrument utilizing microspherometry to measure the back central optic radius. The primary sag is read off a digital counter and the radius determined from tables or from a graph (photograph by courtesy of Union Optical Co.)

radius of a spherical hydrogel contact lens in the hydrated state.

The lens rests on a support ring which determines the chord diameter and is centred in normal saline solution by four obliquely directed posts covered with soft plastics sleeves. A sagittal section of the lens is then viewed by the observer through an inclined, externally illuminated monocular microscope. A micrometer probe is now viewed, and adjusted vertically upwards through the support ring until contact is made with the back surface of the lens. The upward probe movement is continued until one or both sides of the lens are just perceptibly raised from the support ring. The probe movement necessary to lift the lens represents the sag for a known chord diameter, and the BCOR is directly read off the micrometer adjustment screw to an accuracy of ± 0.10 mm (Contact Lenses (Manufacturing) Ltd., 1975).

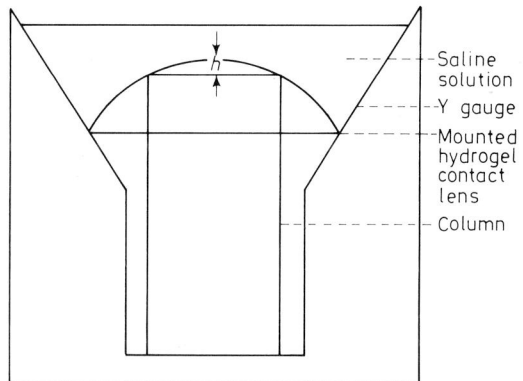

Saline solution
Y gauge
Mounted hydrogel contact lens
Column

Figure 15.12–The Cuvette centration device used to centre and mount the hydrogel lens in saline solution in the Basecope

The Wöhlk Microspherometer

This instrument is illustrated in *Figure 15.10*. Like the Wet Cell Radius Gauge it also determines the primary sag, but unlike other microspherometers it measures the back central optic radius of soft lenses in air.

The lens is removed from its storage solution and excess fluid is eliminated first by shaking and secondly by wiping the back surface with the finger. The lens is then placed, convex side up, onto the holding ring which locates a chord diameter of 10 mm. The upward motion of the central probe is observed through a magnifier from above. The back central optic radius is read in millimetres from a clock dial when the probe just contacts the back surface of the lens. The manufacturers (Wöhlk Contact Linsen, Kiel) stress that this initial point of contact is critical and the operator must therefore cease upward movement of the probe immediately contact occurs. Furthermore, the measurement should – in common with all measurements of soft lens parameters made in air – be made reasonably quickly. The instrument is calibrated against a concave quartz master sphere and with practice an accuracy of ±0.05 mm is claimed (Burns, 1975).

The Basecope

This instrument is produced in Japan by the Union Optical Company and is illustrated in *Figure 15.11*. The submerged lens is mounted, convex side up, on a 6 mm column, which locates the chord diameter with an accuracy of 0.50 μm (micrometres or microns), and is circumferentially supported by a Y-shaped transparent funnel, thus facilitating rapid and precise centration as illustrated in *Figure 15.12*. A sagittal section of the lens is seen reflected through a 45 degrees inclined mirror and viewed at ×30 magnification through a binocular microscope. The sag from the chord diameter to the lens vertex is now displayed in μm on a digital counter (*Figure 15.11*), compensation having been made for lens thickness.

The back central optic radius is now read off either from tables or from a graph, and an accuracy of ±0.015 to ±0.025 mm is claimed for this precision instrument (Nakijima *et al.*, 1974; Hirando, 1975).

Electronic Microspherometers

Electric circuit microspherometry utilizes the hydrogel property of conducting electricity in order to facilitate the critical point of contact between the palpating pin and the back surface of the lens (Forst, 1979; Laboratories Médicornéa, 1979; Chaston and Fatt, 1980).

The upward movement of the probe is monitored and displayed continuously on a digital readout and at the point of contact an electrical pathway is established between the support ring and the probe where a difference in potential is maintained. A signal is then relayed back to the measuring device which it blocks and the corresponding sag value appears on the readout display. Electronic microspherometers currently on the market include the B.C. Tronic (Médicornéa), the B.C.O.R. Electrogauge (Kelvin Lenses Ltd), the Rehder Gauge (The Rehder Development Co) and the S.M. 100 Softometer (Neitz Optical Co) (Chaston and Fatt, 1980).

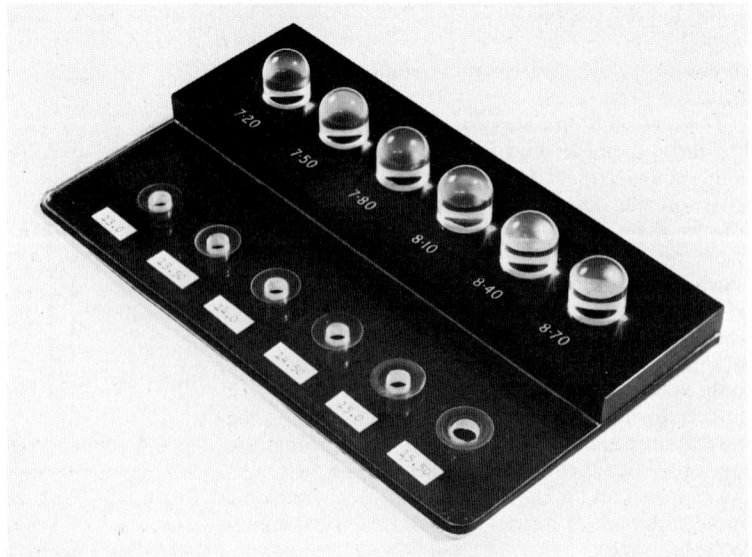

Figure 15.13–The Lensmaster, formerly produced by Contactalens Ltd., which uses optical gauging to determine the approximate back central optic radius in air, using the hemispheres at the back; and overall size using the circles engraved at the front, known as a comparator

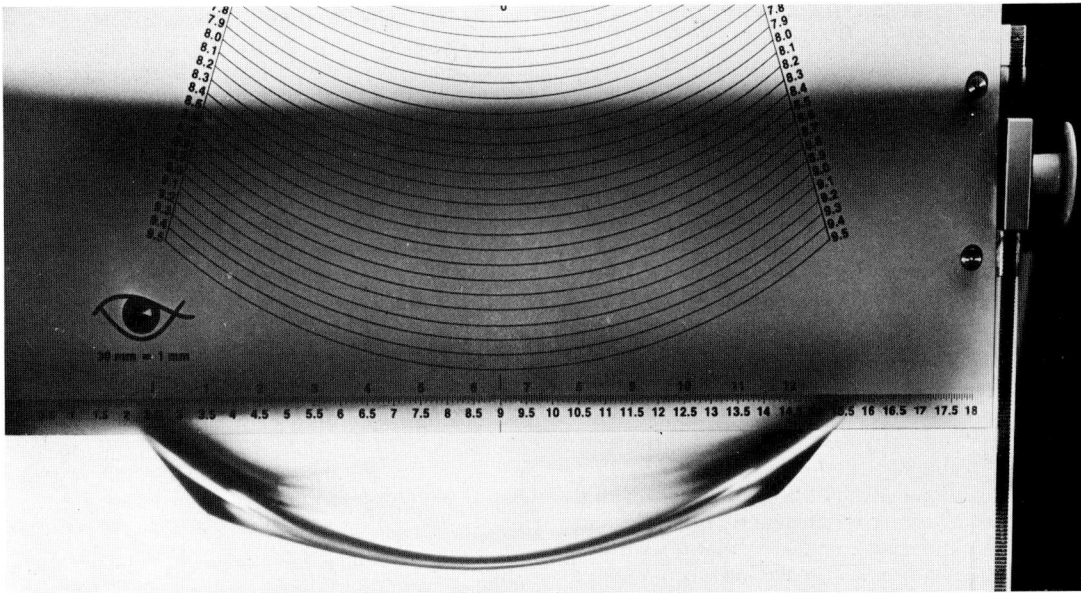

Figure 15.14–The image of the sagittal section of an immersed lens projected in the Söhnges System onto a screen containing annuli which may be adjusted vertically until alignment is achieved (photograph by courtesy of Söhnges Optik, and reproduced by kind permission of the National Eye Research Foundation)

OPTICAL GAUGING

Master Spheres

One of the simplest methods of obtaining an approximate value for the radius of a soft contact lens is to utilize master spheres and apply a system known as optical gauging. The lens, in the hydrated state, is placed with its convex face upwards onto one of a series of accurately made acrylic spheres of known radii. If the two surfaces are not aligned a bubble forms and its location determines the relative curvature of the hydrogel lens with respect to the master sphere. If the back central optic radius is steeper than the master sphere a bubble forms centrally, whereas a peripheral bubble indicates that the back surface of the lens is flatter than the test plate. The Lensmaster is an example of this type of system and is shown in *Figure 15.13*. This system is relatively inexpensive, is rapid and simple and has the advantage of allowing the checking to be done in air, but according to Harris, Hall and Oye (1973) only produces a reliability of ±0.30 mm. Hampson (1973) attributed inaccuracies to capillary attraction and also to stretching between the master spheres and the hydrogel material. For these reasons, assessment of the relative curvature should be made within a few seconds of placing the lens on the master sphere.

The Söhnges Control and Projection System

Söhnges (1974) projects the profile of a fluid-immersed lens onto a screen by means of a projector incorporating a high luminosity 24 volt/250 watt halogen bulb and a cooling system. The screen is engraved with horizontal and vertical linear millimetre scales and a series of annuli graded from 7.20 to 9.50 mm in 0.10 steps which may be adjusted vertically. The projection distance is approximately 1 m and is determined by calibrating the instrument against a known test plate. The profile of the lens is projected onto the graticules which are adjusted vertically until alignment is achieved (*Figure 15.14*).

Inaccuracies may occur with the Söhnges system due to an increase in the ambient temperature of the saline solution and also from eccentricity of projection. Loran (1974) claimed an error of measurement of −0.107 mm in measuring production lenses and a reliability of ±0.10 mm for this instrument.

MEASUREMENT OF PARAMETERS IN AIR

Lathe-cut hydrogel lenses are made in the hard state and are then smaller and steeper than in their final form. In the xerogel state parameters may be checked in air, using conventional instruments, to achieve a similar tolerance to hard lenses, as shown

Table 15.3–Manufacturer's Tolerances of Xerogel Parameters (Hydron (U.K.), 1975)

Parameter	Reliability
Back central optic radius	±0.04 mm
Back vertex power	±0.12 D
Centre thickness	±0.02 mm
Diameter	±0.05 mm

in *Tables 15.3* and *15.5*. After xerogel verification the lenses are rigorously sterilized, the assumption being made that a known and predetermined expansion factor may be applied to determine the hydrated parameters. Unfortunately, however, the hydrogel material does not possess plastic memory and if allowed to dry spontaneously in air does not normally contract in a regular manner because of differential hydration across the lens surface due to differences in lens thickness. If, however, the ambient humidity is monitored and slowly reduced in a controlled environment, then the lens may dehydrate without significant distortion and, indeed, limited modifications may be possible (Bier and Lowther, 1977).

Consequently, although xerogel lenses may be verified with a high degree of accuracy there is normally no way this tolerance may be checked once the lens is received by the practitioner in the hydrated state. It might therefore be argued that the accuracy claimed by the manufacturers is to some extent academic.

DIAMETERS

Diameters are important considerations in specifying, fitting and duplicating contact lenses and a tolerance of ±0.05 mm (Australian Draft Standards, 1975) to ±0.10 mm (American National Standards, 1972) is suggested for hard lenses. Soft contact lenses are often monocurve on one surface and bicurve on the opposite surface, and whilst verifying diameters it is important to examine the transition between adjacent radii which, in the author's experience, are sometimes sharp. If sharp transitions are present in soft semi-scleral contact lenses they may present a potential source of limbal indentation, corneal anoxia and abrasion.

The basic optic diameter is a significant parameter in determining the primary sag and hence the physical and physiological fit of the lens. A complete lens specification should perhaps include overall size and intermediate diameters. In practice, however, it is more convenient to specify the overall size which

for a given edge form and thickness varies directly with the basic optic diameter.

Ruben (1974) and Bailey (1975) suggest that diameters should be measured in a liquid, whilst Stone (1975) and Mandell (1974c) believe checking in air to be clinically adequate and certainly more convenient. It should be pointed out, however, that diameters measured in air may differ from those measured in liquid and account for apparent discrepancies between the laboratory and the practitioner if different measuring techniques are used. If diameters are measured in air it is normal to dry the lens which, in turn, is mounted on a plane surface such as a microscope slide. Initially, the lens size increases due to surface tension and adhesion between the lens and the glass mount (Bailey, 1975) followed by contraction on dehydration.

Band Magnifier

It is without doubt more convenient to check diameters and, indeed, all soft lens parameters in air using conventional instrumentation, and for measuring the overall size and intermediate diameters the band magnifier is recommended (Stone, 1975; Bailey, 1975).

The air-dried lens is mounted horizontally and orientating the axis of the instrument vertically the lens is measured against an external light source;

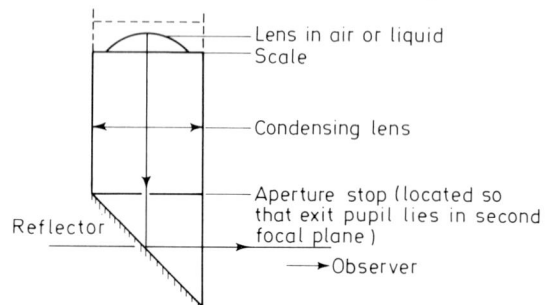

Figure 15.15–Modification of a band magnifier to determine the diameters of a hydrogel lens in a liquid or in air

with this technique one may expect an accuracy of approximately ±0.10 mm which is similar to that achieved for the diameters of hard lenses.

Bailey (1975) measures the transverse section of a liquid-immersed soft lens with a band magnifier placed in contact with the liquid cell wall which should be as thin as possible to reduce parallax errors. A microscope slide offers reasonable optical quality and is recommended for this purpose.

If a band magnifier is modified as illustrated in *Figure 15.15* it is possible to examine the transverse lens section either in air or liquid with the examiner's head in a normal, comfortable position. The scale and the lens plane almost coincide, and the

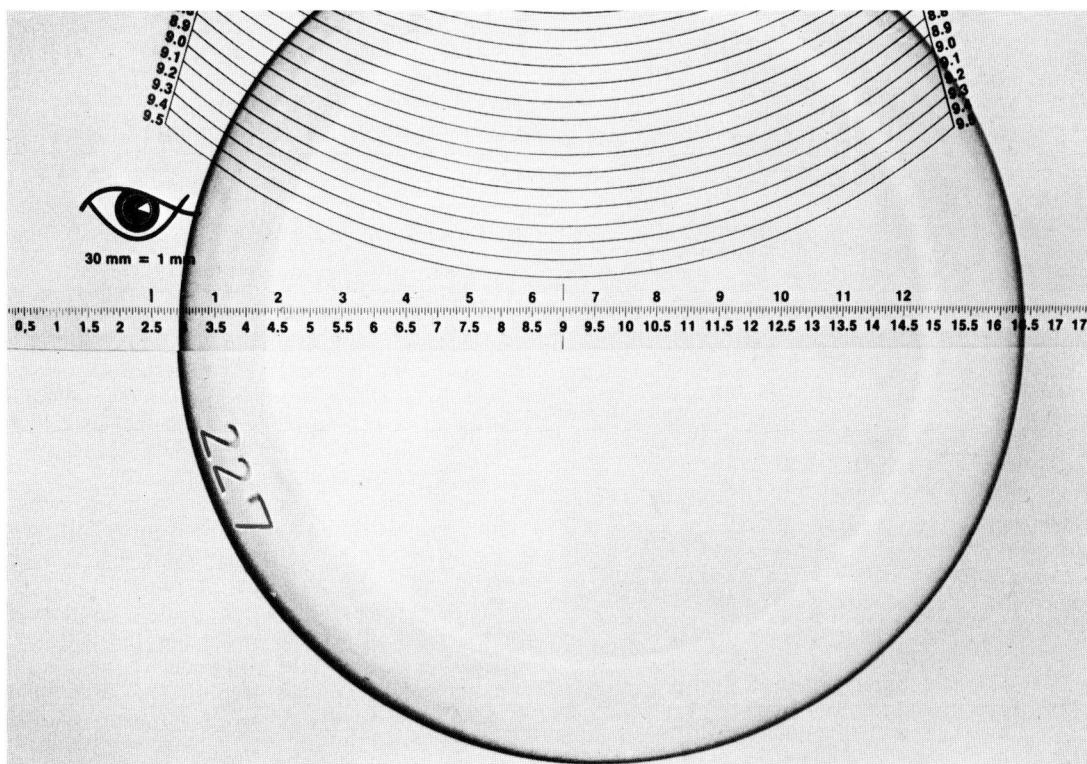

Figure 15.16–Projection of a transverse section of an immersed lens onto a linear scale to determine diameters (photograph by Söhnges Optik, and reproduced by kind permission of the National Eye Research Foundation)

telecentric principle may be incorporated by placing an aperture stop in the second focal plane of the lens thereby overcoming most of the objections previously mentioned.

Projection

The Söhnges system provides an efficient and reasonably accurate method of determining the back and front surface diameters and also the overall size of a liquid-submerged lens. Either a sagittal or transverse section may be projected as illustrated in *Figures 15.14* and *15.16* respectively and the pertinent diameters read off a millimetre scale previously calibrated against a test plate to determine the correct projection distance. Microfilm projectors may also be used, preferably suitably adapted to take a parallel optically flat surfaced cell containing the lens in saline solution. A millimetre scale, engraved on one surface of the cell against which the edges of the lens rest, is magnified along with the lens and thus the appropriate diameters may be read off on the receiving screen. This is an excellent system used by some of the lens manufacturers. An example of such a projection magnifier is shown in

Figure 15.17, but here the scale is printed on the screen.

Travelling Microscope

Ruben (1974) recommends the use of a travelling microscope to measure the overall size of a liquid-immersed soft lens, and although the reliability of this method is not stated one must assume it to be accurate.

V Gauge

The V gauge illustrated in *Figure 15.2* has been designed to hold the lens while the back vertex power in a liquid is determined, but could presumably be modified by incorporating a millimetre scale adjacent to the channel, from which the overall size could be quickly and conveniently read off.

Comparators

An example of a comparator is illustrated in *Figure 15.13* and comprises a series of translucent annuli

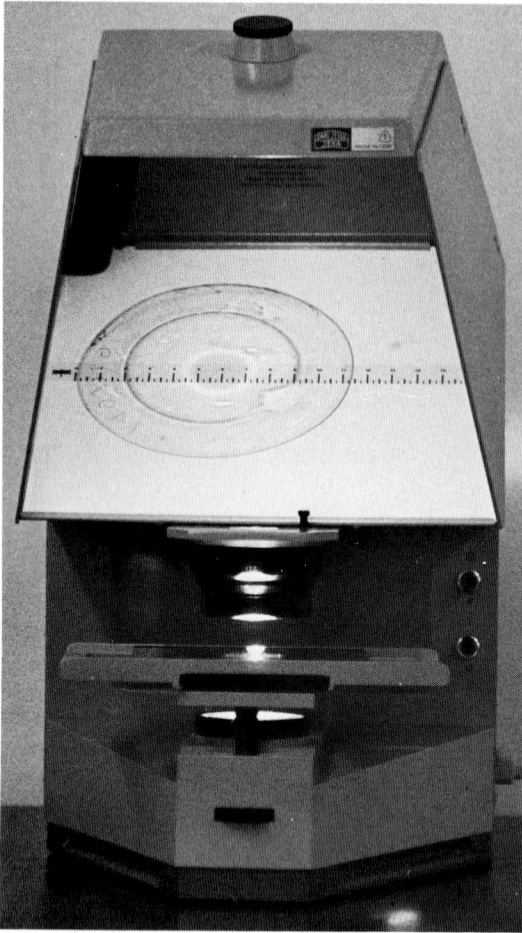

Figure 15.17–Zeiss projection magnifier DL2 showing projection of a soft lens (photograph reproduced by kind permission of Wöhlk-Contact-Lenses Ltd.)

inscribed in a translucent Perspex base. The air-dried lens is simply superimposed onto the test circle to which the overall size is compared. This method is quick and simple but it is not logical to expect an accuracy better than ±0.25 mm as the graduations are in 0.50 mm steps.

THICKNESS

The thickness of a hydrogel contact lens is a significant parameter which contributes to the oxygen diffusion, optical stability and durability of a lens, and Barradell (1975) suggests that soft lenses should be as thin as durability will permit. As one reduces thickness a hydrogel lens becomes fragile and more difficult to handle. Conversely, thinner lenses offer the advantages of greater oxygen transmissability, improved comfort and better centration. At the time of writing ultra-thin hydrogel lenses are becoming increasingly popular and those currently available are listed in *Table 15.4*.

The practitioner should be capable of examining the lenticulation and also measuring the thickness within reasonable limits, from the centre to the periphery. Due to the fragility and distensible nature of the hydrogel matrix, however, normal thickness measuring devices such as micrometers, verniers, or thickness gauges cannot be utilized, but instead indirect measurements which may employ reflected light, optical doubling or projection are relied on.

Radiuscope

The conventional radiuscope, which employs Drysdale's method to determine the radii of reflecting surfaces, may be used to measure lens thickness

Table 15.4–Ultra-thin Hydrogel Lenses

Lens	Manufacturer	Approximate centre thickness (mm)
Hydroflex S.D.	Wöhlk Contact Linsen	0.08
U Series Soflens	Bausch and Lomb Inc.	0.07
Hydromarc	Frontier Contact Lenses	0.06 to 0.07
Zero Six	Hydron Europe	0.06
Hydrocurve II/S.T.	Hydrocurve Soft Contact Lens Inc.	0.05
O Series Soflens	Bausch and Lomb Inc.	0.035
Membrane Lens	Membrane Lens Co.	0.01 to 0.02

by focusing the vertically travelling microscope first on the centre of one surface of the lens, and then on the centre of the other surface. Hartstein (1973) recommends the following procedure.

(1) Mount the lens, back surface down, on a master sphere with a steeper curvature than the lens being measured so that centre contact occurs.

(2) The target is first focused on the sphere and the dial gauge zeroed. This may be done with or without the lens in place.

(3) The radiuscope is now refocused on the front surface of the lens and the travel noted on the dial.

(4) Although not mentioned by Hartstein, if step (2) is carried out with the lens in place the apparent thickness should now be multiplied by the refractive index of the hydrogel material to obtain the real thickness. If step (2) is carried out without the lens in place, step (3) will give the real thickness directly.

The accuracy of this technique depends on the location and precise focusing of the two images of the radiuscope target and this process has been improved by employing a special holder known as a bisurfaced hydrogel lens platform (B.H.L.P.). This is essentially an aluminium cylinder, one half of which is highly polished and the other half dull. The lens is dried and mounted in air concave side upwards on the platform which fits over the lens holder part of the microscope. The radiuscope is first fixed on the polished half of the cylinder and then on the back surface of the lens by observing the target against the dull side of the holder (Paramore and Wechler, 1978; Wechler and Paramore, 1978).

The radiuscope has the dual advantage of air checking and also utilizing conventional instrumentation. The British Standard Tolerances for hydrated centre thickness is plus or minus 0.05 mm, and according to Paramore and Wechler (1978) and Wechler and Paramore (1978) the use of B.H.L.P. produced a repeatability range of 0.01 mm and reliability of 0.02 mm.

Pachometer

This is the method recommended by Ruben (1974) to give an approximate thickness of a hydrogel lens mounted on a scleral contact lens in saline solution. The apparent thickness of the lens is measured with the pachometry attachment of a Haag-Streit lamp, and whilst this technique is subject to errors, a reliability of ±0.02 mm is claimed. Although the thickness of a soft contact lens in both air and liquid is of theoretical interest it could be argued that it is the lens dimensions *in situ* which are significant, and these may alter with environmental variables such as osmolarity, pH, tears evaporation and temperature. Presumably the thickness of the lens could also be measured *in situ* using pachometry.

Projection

In addition to the annuli, and the horizontal millimetre scale, the screen of the Söhnges' system also incorporates a vertical millimetre scale which is adjusted to determine the edge and the centre thickness of the lens profile.

Electric Circuit Micrometry

Water-bearing hydrogels conduct electricity and this property has been utilized in a modified micrometer which it is claimed will measure the thickness of a hydrogel contact lens to an accuracy of ±0.003 mm (Fatt, 1977).

The probes which are made of plastics incorporate an electric wire cast into the centre line so that when the probes just make contact an electric circuit is completed. An ohm-meter is incorporated into the circuit so that when the probes either just contact each other, or the front and back surfaces of a hydrogel lens, a deflection is recorded on the needle. The probes are first brought into contact, the deflection noted and the instrument zeroed. The probes are next separated and a hydrogel lens is mounted convex side up on the lower support; the upper probe is now lowered until the ohm-meter needle is again deflected and the thickness read from the micrometer.

POWER

A possible limitation of hydrogel contact lenses is that the visual acuity with the contact lens may be less than the equivalent acuity obtained with spectacles or hard contact lenses. It is therefore important that the refraction is accurate, the lens is fully settled on the eye (to allow for ambient environmental factors) before an over-refraction is attempted and, finally, that the back vertex power of the lens has been accurately worked and verified.

FOCIMETRY

Liquid Cells

In measuring the back vertex power of a soft contact lens it is preferable that a projection focimeter is utilized to enhance the accuracy of the reading, and Nakijima *et al.* (1974) recommend mounting the lens in a liquid cell or cuvette and reading off the power of the resultant thick polymer-liquid lens on a projection focimeter.

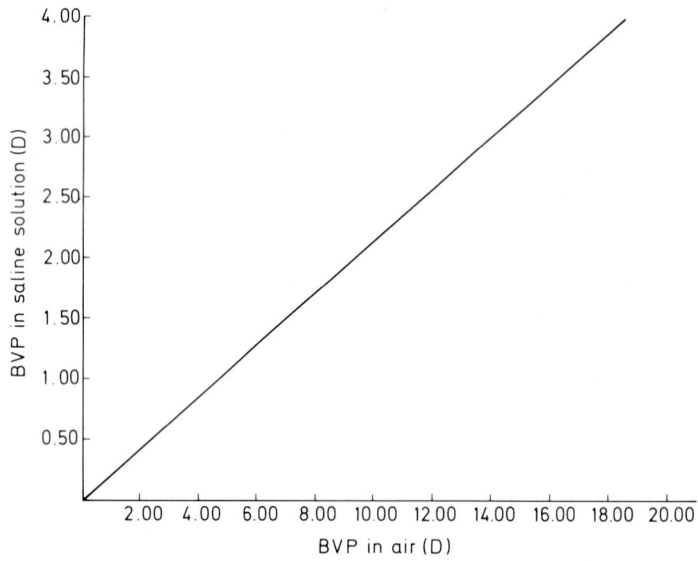

Figure 15.18–Conversion from back vertex power in liquid to back vertex power in air

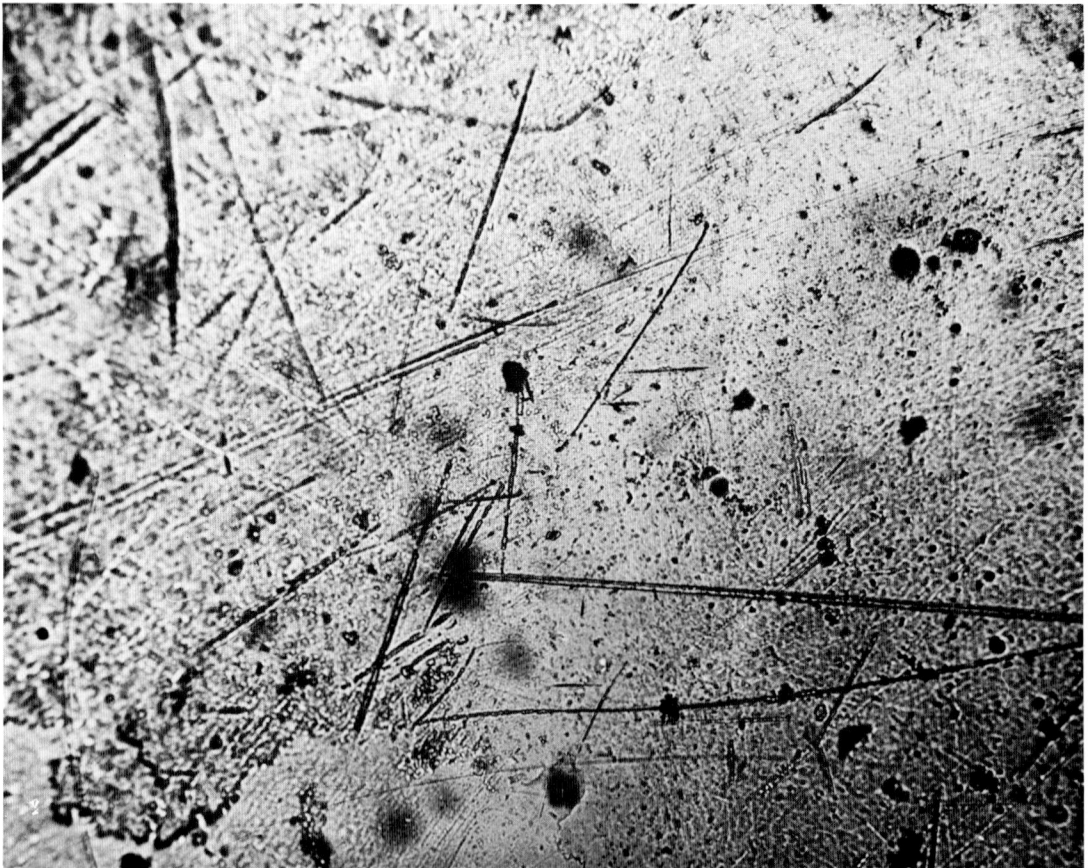

Figure 15.19–Polishing marks seen on a lathe-cut lens at ×40 magnification (reduced to three-quarters in reproduction)

Table 15.5–Potential Lesions of Hydrogel Surfaces

Lesion	Possible cause	Possible effect	Possible remedy
Tears, cracks and splits*	Mishandling or manufacturing defect	Accumulation of debris. Discomfort, abrasions and infection	Replacement lens
Linear indentations*	Polishing marks in manufacture	Accumulation of debris. Discomfort abrasions and infection	Replacement lens
Lens engraving	Inscribed in xerogel state	Accumulation of debris. Discomfort, abrasions and infection	Replacement lens although debris may be removed by surfactant cleaning followed by boiling, enzyme or oxidative cleaning
Foreign bodies	Airborne debris	Discomfort, lacrimation, abrasions and infection	Massage and irrigation with 0.9 per cent saline solution
Aerosol sprays	Make-up incorrectly applied	Discomfort and reduced wetting	Surfactant cleaning followed by boiling or oxidative cleaning. Replacement lens often necessary
Fungi (Filppi, Pfister and Hill, 1973)	Poor hygiene	Enzymatic degradation of material	Asepticization. Replacement lens often necessary
Microbes (Phillips, 1980)	Exogenous or endogenous aetiology	Infection	Surfactant cleaning followed by heat or chemical disinfection
Chemical binding	Incorrect or incompatible solution (for example, hard lens solution, eyedrops and medications	Eye irritation, chemosis, infection	Discontinue soft lens wear and seek medical treatment. If binding is due to protein deposits on lenses, clean lenses to remove deposits
Surface crazing and cracks (Bier and Lowther, 1977)	Hydrogel dehydration followed by stress. Incomplete polymerization or degradation of the material	Accumulation of debris and microbes. Discomfort, abrasion and infection	Replacement lens

*Most lenses carry a manufacturer's warranty against mechanical defects

Table 15.6—Potential Surface Films on Hydrogel Lenses

Lesion	Possible cause	Possible effect	Possible remedy
Tenacious milky film (Bausch and Lomb, 1974) which may appear green on phase contrast microscopy (see Figure 15.27)	Proteins deposited on the lens surface which may become denatured, especially if heat disinfected. May contain albumin, gammaglobulin, A1-lipoprotein, mucopolysaccharides, lipids and phospholipids. Predisposition to the build up of other inorganic materials (for example, chlorhexidine binding) and inactivation of anti-microbial additives	Impaired wettability, reduced contact lens acuity and reduced oxygen transmission. Red eye reaction, tarsal papillae (protein or giant cell conjunctivitis), mucous discharge, itching and increased lens movement	Non-denatured protein build up may be prevented by surfactant cleaning or treatment by electrical pull copolymers. Denatured proteins may be treated by broad spectrum proteolytic enzyme cleaners, bleaching (for example, chlorine), or hydrogen peroxide. Lipoprotein treated by lipase cleaners and phospholipids by phospholipase cleaners
Greasing	Meibomian secretions, sebaceous secretions or tear cholesterol	Intermittent blurring, reduced acuity and reduced oxygen transmission	Surfactant cleaning. Lipase and phospholipase cleaners

Table 15.7—Potential Discoloration of Hydrogel Lens Material

Lesion	Possible cause	Possible effect	Possible remedy
White spots (Ruben, 1976)	Tears calcium. Crystalline deposits from solutions prepared from non-purified water	Lens intolerance	Possible treatment with calcareous chelating agent such as EDTA or oxidation cleaners
Red spots (Loran, 1973)	Ferrous particles endogenously or exogenously induced. The ambient saline solution and also heat sterilization make them highly susceptible to corrosion	No known adverse effects to date, although the possibility of ocular siderosis must be considered	Probably replacement lens though possibly inhibited by ferrous chelating agents such as Desferrioxamine (CIBA), EDTA or oxidation cleaners
Green film (Bier and Lowther, 1977)	Accidental contamination with fluorescein	Discoloration of lens, and possibly exogenous infection by pathogenic microbes such as Pseudomonas auruginosa	Heat or boil in normal saline solution. If heavily stained then soak in Milton* for 15–30 minutes. Place in a vial containing sterile, normal saline solution and boil for 30 minutes. Transfer to a clean vial and fresh saline solution and repeat the boiling process (up to four times) until the pH returns to normal. Finally, rehydrate in appropriate solution
Red film (Hodd, 1975)	Accidental contamination with rose bengal	Discoloration of lens. Possible exogenous infection	Not normally removed by boiling
Yellow/brown discoloration (Stewart, 1978; Phillips, 1980)	Tobacco smoke. Aromatic compounds in tears. Chlorhexidine reaction especially with chlorinated cleaners	Reduced acuity, discomfort and possible infection	Boiling in saline solution followed by the use of strong oxidation cleaners

*Milton (Richardson-Merrell)

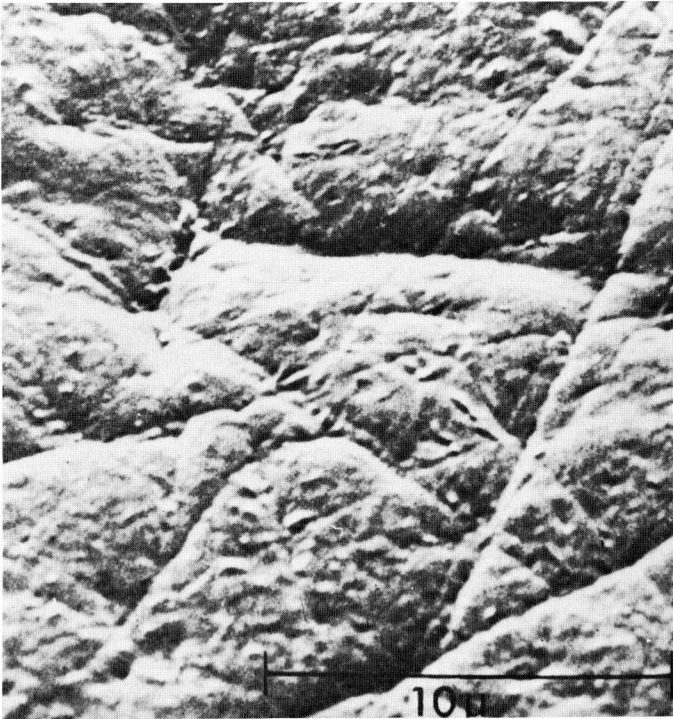

Figure 15.20–Electron micrograph showing the relatively rough appearance of a lathe-cut lens at ×3000 magnification. (Matas, Spencer and Hayes, 1972 and reproduced by kind permission of the American Medical Association)(reduced to three-quarters in reproduction)

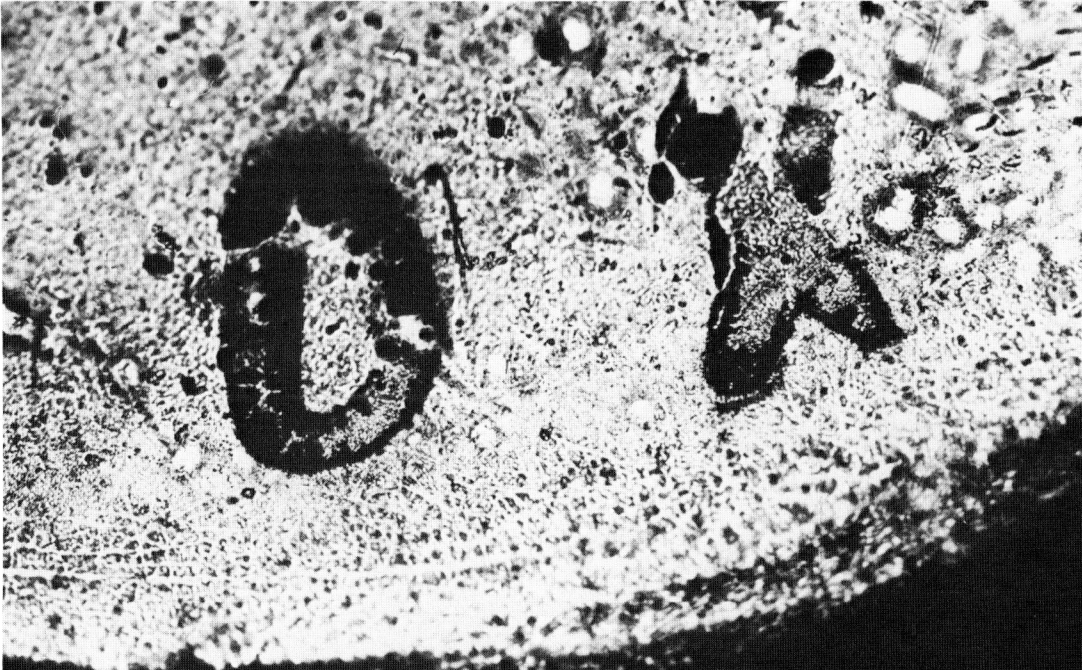

Figure 15.21–Appearance of lens engraving at ×40 magnification showing the accumulation of dirt and debris which may harbour pathogenic microbes (reduced to three-quarters in reproduction)

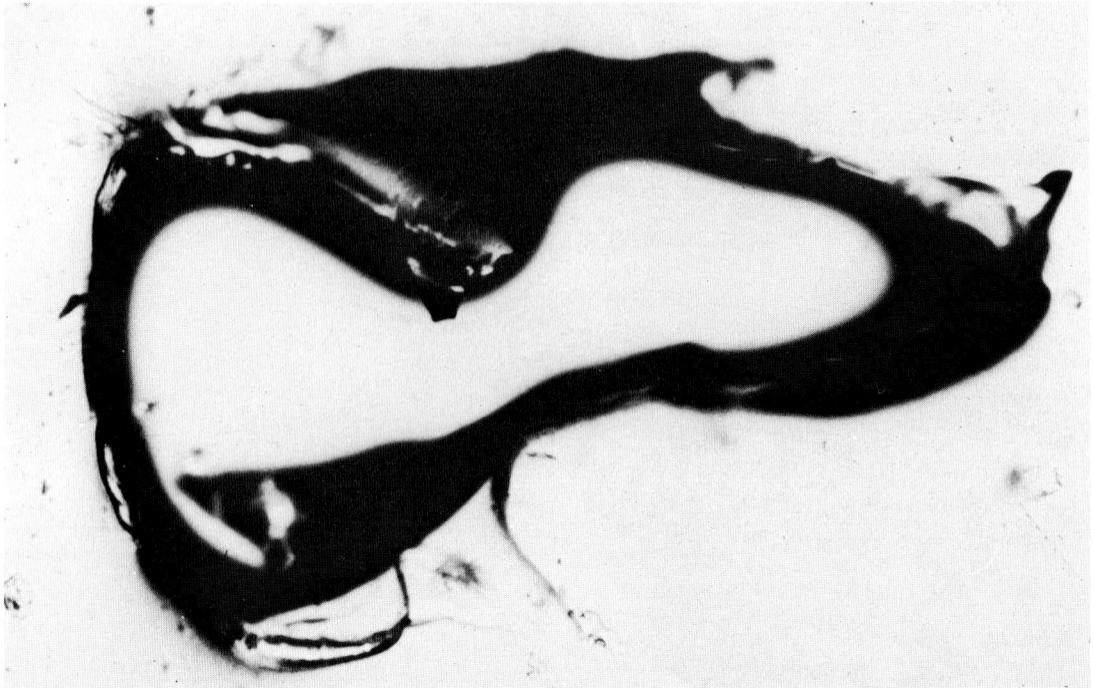

Figure 15.22–Appearance of a hole in the hydrogel matrix caused by a penetrating foreign body without ocular damage

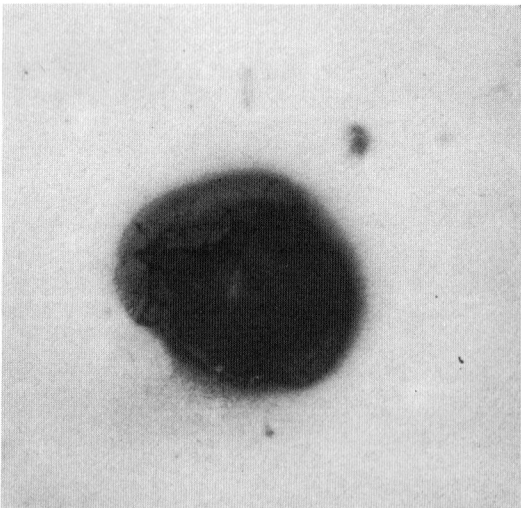

Figure 15.23–Contaminant embedded on the front surface of a semi-dehydrated hydrogel contact lens in contact with a saline solution droplet (original magnification ×40: same-size reproduction)

In order to determine the back vertex power in air of a lens measured in liquid a compensation factor, K, must be applied (Poster, 1971).

If n is the refractive index of air = 1.00
n' is the refractive index of the saline solution = 1.336
n'' is the refractive index of the hydrogel materials $\simeq$ 1.430
F_1 is the back vertex power in air
F_2 is the back vertex power in the liquid
Then $F_1 = F_2 K$
Where, approximately,

$$K = \frac{(n'' - n)}{(n'' - n')} = \frac{1.43 - 1.00}{1.43 - 1.336} = 4.57$$

Thus, the back vertex power measured through the liquid cell must be multiplied by the compensation factor. This may be more conveniently read off from tables or from a graph as illustrated in *Figure 15.18*. This means that the accuracy of focimetry must be improved by 457 per cent and the required sensitivity necessitates readings of 0.05 D. Thus, an error of 0.12 D in the focimeter reading would lead to an error of over 0.50 D in the actual lens power in air. Hampson (1973) also points out that surface distortions of the hydrogel lens may be masked by the ambient saline solution; furthermore pseudo-cylinders, prisms and other distortions may be introduced by the cell walls. In view of these limitations it is doubtful if liquid immersion offers substantial advantages for checking the power of soft contact lenses.

Air Checking

This has been recommended by Isen (1972), Gasset (1972), Hampson (1973), Ruben (1974), Mandell (1974a) and Stone (1975) for which a projection focimeter is recommended. There is a critical period of the first minute after removing the lens from the saline solution during which the reading should be taken. For 30 seconds this image is hazy (Isen, 1972) although shrinkage on dehydration does not substantially affect the readings for a period of 4 minutes (Mandell, 1974a). The focimeter scale is initially set to the expected reading (Stone, 1975), the lens carefully dried and placed convex side upward either on a reduced aperture focimeter or a conical contact lens holder, and the reading taken in air. With practice a reasonably clear image can usually be obtained with this method for which a

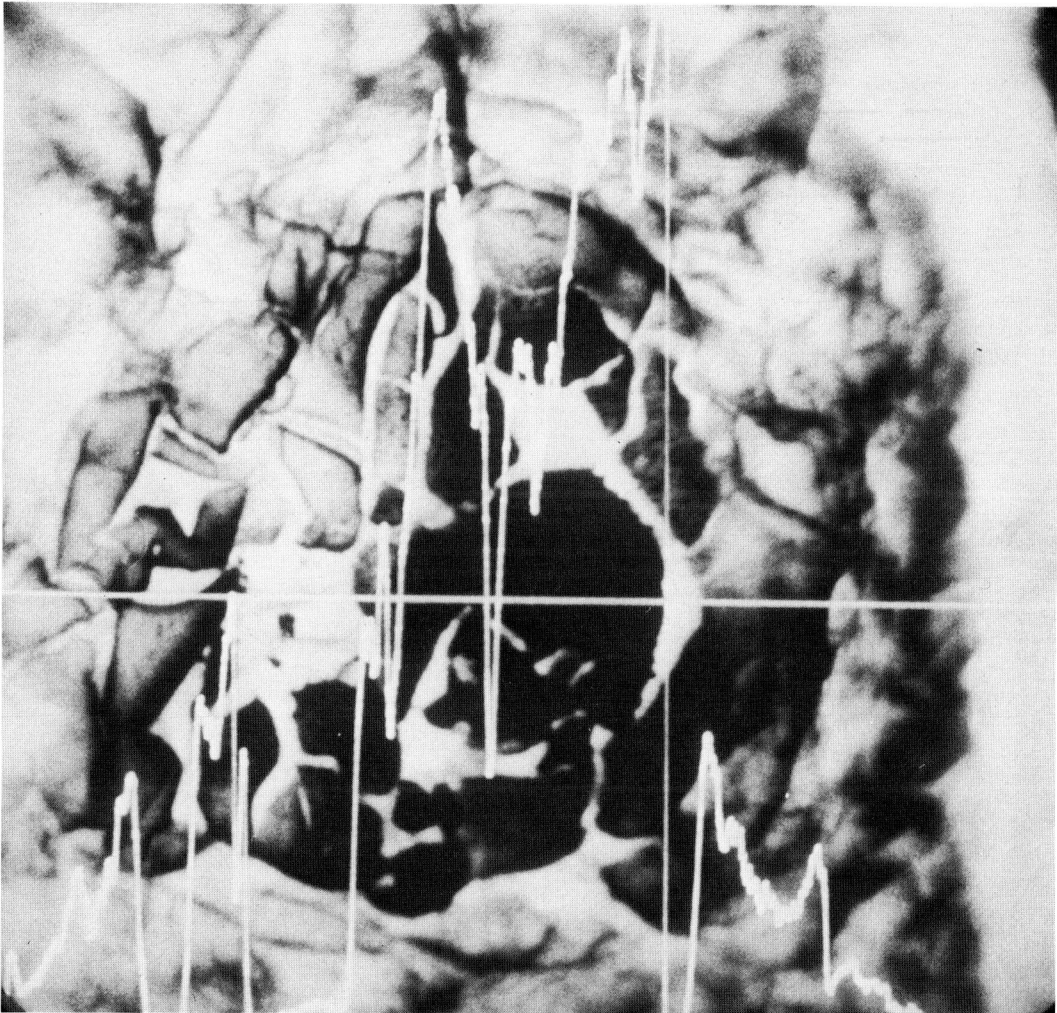

Figure 15.24–Electron microprobe analysis of the contaminant illustrated in Figure 15.22 which was coated with a thin layer of carbon to enhance conductivity of the electrons. The subsequent X-ray scan was superimposed on a ×300 electron image and shows strong iron radiation in the alpha (mean) component of the K band of the spectrum. A lens intense oxygen radiation was also present (Loran, 1973) (reduced to three-quarters in reproduction)

490

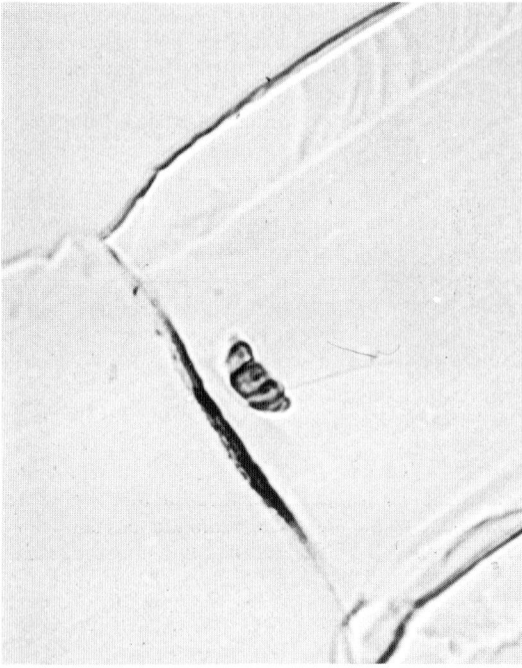

Figure 15.25–Sagittal section of a red spot which shows a deeply embedded ferrous particle of unknown aetiology. The location of the contaminant, however, suggests an endogenous aetiology possibly introduced during spincasting

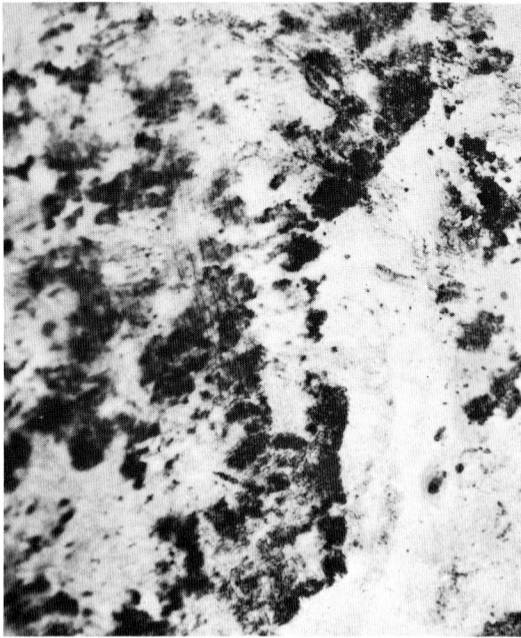

(a)

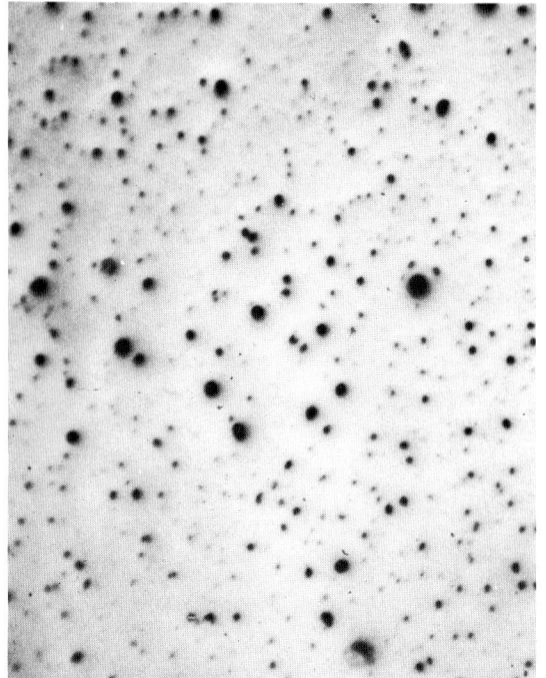

Figure 15.26–Hydrogel surface contaminated with hair rinse

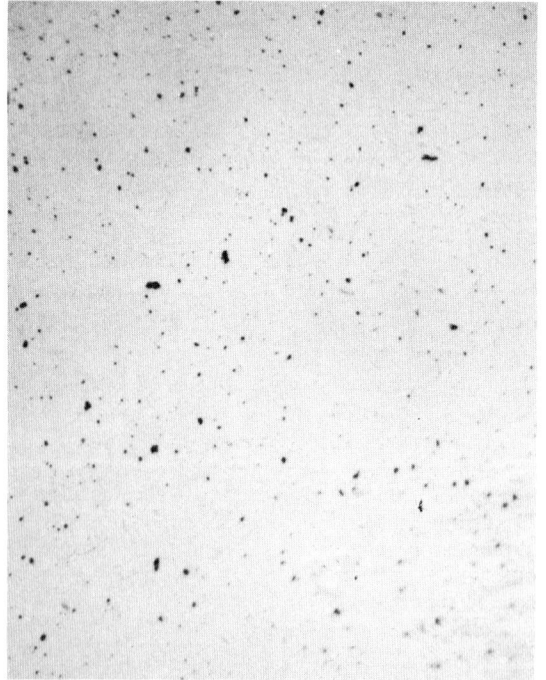

(b)

Figure 15.27–(a) Coagulated proteins on the surface of a hydrogel lens. (b) The same surface after treatment by a proteolytic enzyme cleaner

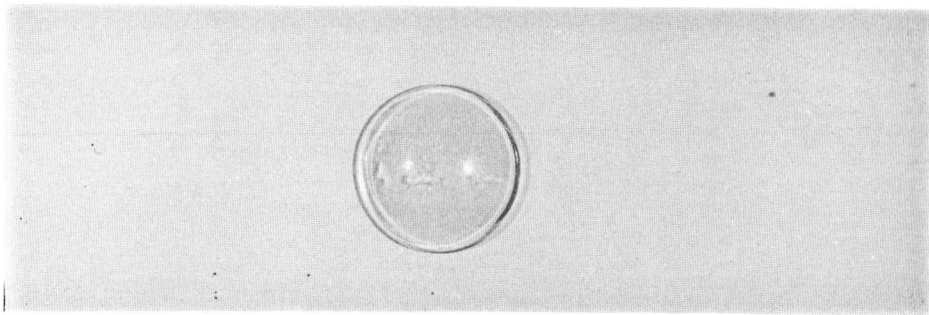

Figure 15.28–Lens mounted on a microscope slide, with white background, for air surface inspection

reliability of ±0.25 D is claimed (Harris, Hall and Oye, 1973).

SURFACE INSPECTION

Hydrogel contact lenses are inherently fragile, especially in the higher water content polymers recommended for extended wear (de Carle, 1972), and are also liable to exogenous and endogenous contamination, examples of which are given in *Tables 15.6* and *15.7*. It is generally accepted that continuous irrigation is an efficient method of removing debris and microorganisms, and this important function is performed in the conjunctival sac by the tears. If the irrigation interface (and this includes the cornea or the contact lens) presents an irregular surface resulting, for example, from scratches, crevices and other lesions, the surface may harbour microorganisms which collect and multiply away from the natural protective mechanisms (Tripathi and Ruben, 1972, 1973). It therefore follows that the importance of inspection of the surfaces and edges of hydrogel contact lenses both on and off the eye cannot be over-emphasized.

Light Microscopy

The surface area of a soft contact lens varies from approximately 140 to 200 mm^2 and clinically it is necessary to scan the hydrogel surface not only with reasonable speed but also to employ high magnification to critically evaluate suspect areas. In practice a range from ×5 to ×40 is adequate and the slit lamp biomicroscope performs the function admirably, although, if preferred, a separate stereomicroscope can be used.

When the lenses are inspected in air they should be shaken or blotted dry and examined under magnification, preferably on glass, against a white background. For this purpose the lens may be mounted on a microscope slide with a white adhesive background (*Figure 15.28*) or, alternatively, the test plate of the slit lamp may be modified

as shown in *Figure 15.29*. It should be pointed out, however, that if the test plate is mounted on the body of the slit lamp in the normal manner then the lens plane is displaced forward slightly from the focal plane of the microscope and the lens surface is permanently out of focus unless the microscope has an independent focusing control. It may therefore be necessary to hold the lens mount by hand which may be tilted and moved as necessary. By employing conventional variations in slit lamp illumination the lens surface may be examined and evaluated. Brandreth (1975) recommends that the examiner use moderate magnification with direct focal illumination, 'sclerotic scatter', to evaluate the edges, and parallelepiped illumination with moderate magnification for inspection of the lens surfaces.

If the practitioner wishes to employ even higher magnification, Brandreth also suggests modifying the slit lamp in the following manner. The lens is

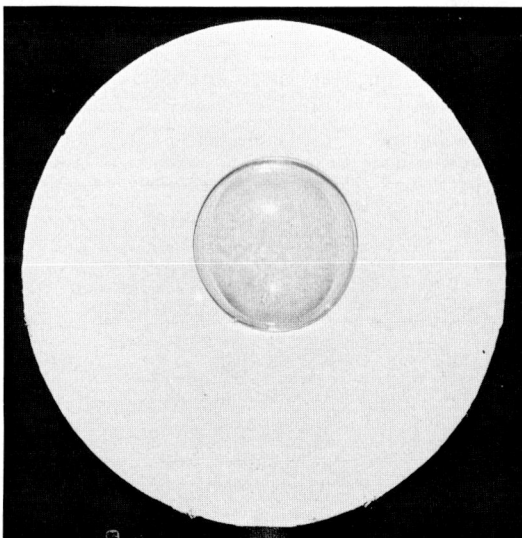

Figure 15.29–Lens mounted on a slit-lamp test plate (with white background) for air surface inspection

Table 15.8–Summary of the Reliability of Soft Lens Verification Methods

Parameter	Method of measurement	Reliability	Comparable hard corneal lens tolerance*
BCOR	Master spheres lens in air)	±0.30 mm Harris, Hall and Oye, 1973)	±0.02 mm
BCOR and FCOR	Sagometer (lens in liquid)	±0.10 mm (Contact Lenses (Manufacturing) Ltd., 1975)	±0.02 mm
BCOR	Sagometer (lens in liquid)	±0.02 mm (Nakijima *et al.*, 1974)	±0.02 mm
BCOR	Sagometer (lens in air)	±0.02 mm (Burns, 1975)	±0.02 mm
BCOR	Liquid immersed radiuscope	±0.02 mm (Nissel, 1975)	±0.02 mm
BCOR	Keratometer (lens in liquid)	±0.10 mm (Forst, 1974)	±0.02 mm
BVP	Focimeter (lens in air)	±0.50 D (Ruben, 1974)	±0.12 D (< 10.00 D)
BVP	Focimeter (lens in air)	±0.25 D (Harris, Hall and Oye, 1973)	±0.12 D (< 10.00 D)
BVP	Focimeter (lens in air)	±0.125 D Titmus Eurocon, 1974)	±0.12 D (< 10.00 D)
Overall size	Comparator (lens in air)	±0.10 mm (Harris, Hall and Oye, 1973)	±0.10 mm
Overall size and optic diameter	Band magnifier (lens in air)	Reliability not given (Mandell, 1974c)	±0.10 mm (OS) ±0.20 mm (BCOD)
Back central optic diameter	Band magnifier (lens in air)	±0.10 mm (Titmus Eurocon, 1974)	±0.20 mm
Overall size and back central optic diameter	Projection (lens in liquid)	Reliability not given (Söhnges, 1974)	±0.10 mm (OS) ±0.20 mm (BCOD)
Thickness	Vertical travelling microscope (lens in air)	±0.01 mm (Harris, Hall and Oye, 1973)	±0.02 mm
Thickness	Travelling microscope	±0.03 mm (Titmus Eurocon, 1974)	±0.02 mm
Thickness	Pachometer (lens in liquid)	±0.02 mm (Ruben, 1974)	±0.02 mm
Thickness	Electric micrometer	±0.003 mm (Fatt, 1977)	±0.02 mm

*British Standards Institution, 1978

mounted on a glass slide or held by hand in the region of the head-rest directly in the beam of light. The illuminating system is aligned with the axis of the microscope set opposite to each other at a zero reading, so that the contact lens is located between the light source and one of the microscope objectives. By moving the eyepiece, if necessary, a greatly magnified image may now be projected onto a convenient wall and examined for imperfections.

Degradation of the lens surfaces can and does occur in wear as *Figures 15.22* and *15.27* illustrate, and such lesions may not only interfere with vision or cause discomfort but may be extremely hazardous. It is therefore necessary for the practitioner to critically examine the lens surfaces each and every time the patient is seen for soft lens after-care. The practitioner would normally employ the slit lamp whilst the lenses are *in situ* to evaluate centration, lag and conjunctival disturbances. It is suggested that at the same time the lens surfaces should be examined. The lens should also be examined out of the eye as previously explained either using the slit lamp or a stereomicroscope.

ELECTRON OPTICS

Light microscopy is limited by the wavelength of light to a magnification of approximately ×1000 and a resolution from 100 to 200 nm which is considerably greater than is required clinically. In research, however, greater magnification may be necessary to make ultrastructural studies of the hydrogel polymer (Matas, Spencer and Hayes, 1972; Tripathi and Ruben, 1972, 1973; Filppi, Pfister and Hill, 1973; Loran, 1973; and Holden, Pain and Zantos, 1974).

If it is necessary to employ higher magnification, electron optics must be used, which is that branch of physics concerned with the projection of the electron beam. Electron microscopy permits 1000 times greater resolution than light microscopy so that magnification of up to ×100,000 may be achieved. The beam is focused directly onto a suitably sectioned specimen through electron lenses in transmission electron microscopy, or arranged to scan the specimen in scanning electron microscopy; the latter technique being recommended by Holden, Pain and Zantos (1974) for hydrogel contact lenses. The reflected electrons are then picked up by a suitable detector and finally the signal is amplified and is displayed on a cathode ray tube where the electron image may be photographed as a micrograph as shown in *Figures 15.20* and *15.24*.

It is also possible to identify some hydrogel contaminants by a technique known as electron microprobe analysis in which the electron probe scans a prepared specimen, which, subsequent to excitation, emits characteristic X-rays. The latter may then be analysed and identified by crystal spectrometry. An example of an X-ray scan superimposed on an electron image of ferrous contamination of a hydrogel lens is illustrated in *Figure 15.24*.

CONCLUSION

The verification of soft lens parameters is a relatively new problem, and although official recommended tolerances have recently been published, as shown in *Table 15.1* on page 472, some manufacturers are working to finer tolerances than those recommended. For example, Bausch and Lomb give the centre thickness of the hyper-thin lenses as 0.035 ± 0.005 mm.

Contact lenses may only be manufactured and prescribed as accurately as they may be checked, and in attempting to establish an acceptable system of tolerances for contact lens parameters it is necessary first to establish fitting criteria which should then be correlated with the cost of manufacture and also the reliability of available quality control instrumentation. The checking of soft lenses in air is more convenient and adequate for verification of most parameters, and where possible the practitioner obviously prefers to utilize conventional instruments. Port (1975, 1976), however, cites the use of holography (laser and ultrasound) to determine lens curvatures and is currently developing a system based on ultrasonics to measure soft lens parameters. Measurements of FCOR, BCOR, centre thickness, edge shape and water content are possible.

A summary of the probable reliability of present soft lens verification methods is given in *Tables 15.3* and *15.8*. From these figures it is suggested that for the present a tolerance of ±0.10 mm for radii, ±0.10 mm for diameters, ±0.25 mm for overall size, ±0.05 mm for thickness and ±0.25 D for power is reasonable and can be checked by the practitioner.

ACKNOWLEDGEMENTS

At the time of writing the quality control of hydrogel lenses is in its infancy and I am most grateful to be able to draw on the experience of colleagues and laboratories whose valued assistance is acknowledged in the references, under Personal Communication. Furthermore, many of the instruments for verifying soft contact lens dimensions are in the developmental stage and often not available for personal appraisal by the author. Consequently, I must thank the laboratories who supplied photographs of their instruments for publication, the American Medical Association for permission to reproduce *Figure 15.20*, and The National Eye Research Foundation for permission to reproduce *Figures 15.1, 15.14* and *15.16*. Finally, I should like to thank Dr C. N. French for programming the computer and producing the figures on which the graphs in *Figures 15.6* and *15.18* are based, and also Mrs I. George for the typing.

REFERENCES

Australian Draft Standards (1975). Standards Association of Australia, 30pp. P.O. Box 458, North Sydney, N.S.W. 2060

American National Standards Institute Inc. (1972). *Prescription requirements for first quality contact lenses,* pp. 20–80. American National Standards Institute, 1430 Broadway, New York 10018, U.S.A.

Bailey, N. J. (1975). 'Inspection of hydrogel lenses.' *Internat. Contact Lens Clin.* **2**(1), 42–48

Barradell, M. J. (1975). 'Re-appraisal of attitudes in prescribing soft lenses.' *Optician* **170**(4393), 20–26

Bausch and Lomb Ltd. (1973). Personal communication from J. Facletta

Bausch and Lomb Ltd. (1975). Personal communication from R. Myers

Bausch and Lomb Soflens Division (1977). *Soflens International Fitting Guide.* New York: Bausch and Lomb

Bennett, A. G. (1966). 'The calibration of keratometers.' *Optician* **151**, 317–321

Bier, N. and Lowther, G. E. (1977). *Contact Lens Correction,* p. 422. London and Boston: Butterworths

Brandreth, R. H. (1975). 'Biomicroscopic techniques for hydrogel lenses.' *Internat. Contact Lens Clin.* **2**(1), 33–41

British Standard 5562 (1978). *Specification for Contact Lenses.* London: British Standards Institution

British Standard 5321. Part III (1979). *Glossary of Terms Relating to Contact Lenses.* London: British Standard Institution

Burns, D. (1975). Personal communication

Chamarro Tormo, C. J. (1974). 'Las lentes de contacto flexibles, merced a un sencillo sistema optico, pueden ser medidas y controladas.' *J. Gaceta. Optica* **36**, 31–35

Chaston, J. (1973). 'A method of measuring the radius of curvature of a soft contact lens.' *Optician* **165**(4271), 8–12

Chaston, J. and Fatt, I. (1980). 'Survey of commercially available instruments for measuring the back radius of soft contact lenses.' *Optician* **18**(179), 19–44

Contact Lenses (Manufacturing) Ltd. (1975). 'The wet cell instruction sheet.' and also Personal communication

de Carle, J. (1972). 'Developing hydrophilic contact lenses for continuous wear.' *Contacto* **16**(1), 39–42

Driefus, M. (1968). 'A new hydrogel lens made from polyglycolmonomethacrylate.' *Augen Optik* **85**, 35–39

Emsley, H. H. (1963). 'The keratometer: measurement of concave surfaces.' *Optician* **146**, 161–168

Fatt, I. (1977). 'A simple electric device for measuring thickness and sagittal height of gel contact lenses.' *Optician* **173**(4474), 23–24

Filppi, J. A., Pfister, R. M. and Hill, R. M. (1973). 'Penetration of hydrophilic lenses by *Aspergillus fumagatus.*' *Am. J. Optom.* **50**, 553–557

Forst, G. (1974). 'New methods of measurement for controlling soft lens quality. *Contacto* **18**(6), 6–9

Forst, G. (1979). 'Profung der MeBgenauigkeit eines elektronischen Spharometers.' Sonderdruck aus der Fachzeitschrift. *Die Contactlinse,* Heft 5/1979. 13 Jahrgang

Gasset, A. R. (1972). 'The Griffin Naturalens: basic concepts and fitting techniques.' Chapter 12 in *Soft Contact Lens,* ed. by Gasset, A. R. and Kaufman, H. E. St. Louis, Missouri: Mosby

Gee, H. (1980). Personal communication

Harris, M. G., Hall, K. and Oye, R. (1973). 'The measurement and stability of hydrophilic lens dimensions.' *Am. J. Optom.* **50**, 546–552

Hartstein, J. (1973). *Questions and Answers on Contact Lens Practice,* 2nd ed., pp. 155–157. St. Louis, Missouri: Mosby

Hampson, R. (1973). 'Considerations in the checking and predictability of hydrophilic lenses.' *Optician* **165**(4283), 4–16

Hill, R. M. and Leighton, A. J. (1964). 'Physiological time courses associated with contact lenses – temperature.' *Am. J. Optom.* **41**, 3–9

Hirando, A. (1975). Personal communication

Hodd, F. A. B. (1975). Personal communication

Holden, B. A., Pain, P. and Zantos, S. (1974). 'Observations on scanning electron microscopy of hydrophilic contact lenses.' *Austral. J. Optom.* **57**, 100–106

Hydron Soft Lens Technical Report (1975), 2

Isen, A. A. (1972). 'The Bionite Naturalens.' Chapter 5 in Part III, The Griffin Laboratories Flexible Lens, in *Symposium on the Flexible Lens,* pp. 35–51. ed. by Bitonte, J. L. and Keates, R. H. St. Louis, Missouri, Mosby

Loran, D. F. C. (1973). 'Surface corrosion of hydrogel contact lenses.' *The Contact Lens* **4**(4), 3–10

Loran, D. F. C. (1974). 'The determination of hydrogel contact lens radii by projection.' *Ophthal. Optician* **14**, 980–985

Mandell, R. B. (1974a). 'Can gel lens power be measured accurately?' *Internat. Contact Lens Clin.* **1**(1), 36–37

Mandell, R. B. (1974b). *Contact Lens Practice: Hard and Flexible Lenses,* 2nd ed. Springfield Ill: Thomas

Mandell, R. B. (1974c). 'Lathe-cut hydrogel lenses.' *Internat. Contact Lens Clin.* **1**(1), 53–62

Masnick, K. B. and Holden, B. A. (1972). 'Studies of water content and parametric variations of hydrophilic contact lenses.' *Austral. J. Optom.* **55**, 481–487

Matas, B. R., Spencer, W. H. and Hayes, T. L. (1972). 'Scanning electron microscopy of hydrophilic contact lenses.' *Archs Ophthal.* **88**, 287–295

Nakijima, A., Shibata, H., Magatani, H., Hirano, A. and Terao, T. (1974). 'A method of soft contact lens measurement.' *J. Jap. Contact Lens Soc.* **16**, 123–131

Nissel, G. (1975). Personal communication

Paramore, J. E. and Wechsler, S. (1978). 'Reliability and repeatability study of a technique for measuring the centre thickness of a hydrogel lens.' *J. Am. optom. Ass.* **49**, 272–274

Pearson, R. M. (1980). 'Measurement of soft lens centre thickness.' *Optician* **18**(179), 32–43

Phillips, A. J. (1980). 'The cleaning of hydrogel contact lenses.' *Ophthal. Optom.* **20**(11), 375–388

Port, M. J. A. (1975). 'The radius measurements of hydrophilic contact lenses using ultrasonics.' M.Sc. Thesis, University of Aston in Birmingham

Port, M. J. A. (1976). 'New methods of measuring hydrophilic lenses.' *Ophthal. Optician* **16**, 1079–1082

Poster, M. G. (1971). 'Hydrated method of determining dioptric power of all hydrophilic lenses.' *J. Am. optom. Ass.* **43,** 287–299

Poster, M. G. and Skolnik, A. J. (1974). 'Effect of pH and tonicity change on some parameters of a soft lens (T.M.).' *J. Am. optom. Ass.* **45,** 311–314

Refojo, M. F. (1972). 'A critical review of properties and applications of soft hydrogel contact lenses.' *Surv. Ophthal.* **16,** 233–246

Ruben, M. (1973). 'Soft lenses 1.' *Optician* **166**(4296), 9–12, 15–16, 19–20

Ruben, M. (1974). 'Soft lenses: the physico-chemical characteristics.' *Contacto* **18**(5), 11–23

Ruben, M. (1976). 'Biochemical aspects of soft contact lenses.' *Optician* **172**(4462), 34–35

Söhnges Information (1974). Deutche Kontactlinsen Gamb. No. 9, Deutche Kontactlinsen GMBH, 8 München 2, Postfach 202207, W. Germany

Stewart, B. V. (1978). 'Soft contact lens discoloration and the use of tobacco.' *Internat. Contact Lens Clin.* **15**(6), 269–275

Stone, J. (1975). Personal communication

Tajiri, A. (1974). 'Measurement of the hydrogel lens with a radiuscope.' In *Symposium on Contact Lenses,* pp. 118–120. Japan: Toyo Contact Lens Company

Titmus Eurocon (1974). Information sheet of Titmus Eurocon Konactlinsen K. G., D–8750 Aschaffenburg, P. O. Box 74 Goldbacher Strasse 57, W. Germany

Tripathi, R. and Ruben, M. (1972/73). 'Degenerative changes in a soft hydrophilic contact lens.' *Ophthal. Res.* **4,** 185–192

Wechsler, S. and Paramore, J. (1978). 'Accuracy of manufacturers' stated centre thickness of hydrogel contact lenses.' *Am. J. Optom.* **55,** 677–680

Wichterle, O. and Lim, D. (1960). 'Hydrophilic gels for biological uses.' *Nature* **185,** 117–119

Chapter 16

After-care and Symptomatology

F. A. Burnett Hodd

Ideally, contact lenses should be undetectable in use, restore normal vision, permit unlimited wear and not produce harmful side-effects. After-care is the maintenance of these four criteria. It starts from the moment contact lenses are first placed on the eyes and continues for so long as they are retained and used. It covers the normal routine re-examination of the established contact lens wearer and his lenses, as well as emergency examinations and treatment, and the care of the new patient both during the adaptation period and during the initial contact lens trials.

After-care, therefore, is not only the constant concern of the practitioner or fitter who is initially providing lenses but also of any section of the health services to whom the contact lens wearer may appeal for advice. Be they opticians, optometrists, physicians, pharmacists, surgeons or nurses, all may be expected to display some knowledge of contact lens patient after-care. Even the laboratories where contact lenses and accessories are made are not without responsibility in this regard.

In 1964, the Contact Lens Society of Great Britain (now incorporated in The British Contact Lens Association) became aware of disquiet among the professions concerned, and appointed a small after-care committee of opticians and ophthalmologists from amongst its membership, who drew up a routine re-examination procedure of the established contact lens wearing patient which was subsequently recommended to members. Their recommendation will be followed in this chapter.

ROUTINE RE-EXAMINATION OF THE CONTACT LENS WEARING PATIENT

Two aspects arise: (1) general items common to all patients; and (2) special items for contact lens wearers.

Routine examination is for two purposes: first, to cover all aspects which would apply to a patient who does not wear contact lenses; and secondly, to cover those additional aspects peculiar to the wearing of these lenses. Neither must be allowed to outweigh the other. The time allowed for the routine re-examination of a contact lens wearing patient must, therefore, be longer than that allowed for a spectacle wearing patient.

The practitioner must be an ophthalmologist or an ophthalmic optician (optometrist) trained and experienced in contact lens work. It cannot be done by a dispensing optician. The practitioner should have access to the patient's previous records to permit evaluation of any changes observed.

When attending for a routine re-examination the patient should report wearing the lenses for a period long enough to generate any symptoms of which he may be complaining, unless instructed otherwise by the practitioner (*see* Section B, General Inspection with Lenses *In Situ* on page 499).

The first part of the examination – history and symptoms, general inspection and routine refraction with lenses *in situ*, inspection of the fit of the lenses and the removal and inspection of the lenses themselves – is designed to reveal defects in the performance of the lenses (Sections A to E). The second part of the examination is designed to reveal ocular changes induced by lens usage (pages 505–511) and includes both the detailed inspection of the eyes and adnexa with the slit lamp and ophthalmoscope, and of the optical characteristics of the eye with the keratometer, retinoscope and by subjective refraction (Sections F to J). Finally, normal supplementary diagnostic tests are performed (pages 505–511) and advice is given (Section L). Where modifications to the lenses are indicated in order to remedy a problem, then reference should be made to Chapters 22 and 23.

A. HISTORY AND SYMPTOMS

(1) General questions applicable to any patient.

(2) Contact lens wearing habits and limitations.

(3) Treatment arising from or bearing on contact lens use.

(4) Redness of the eyes, pain or discomfort.

(5) Variations in vision.

1. General Questions Applicable to any Patient

Over-concern on the part of the practitioner for contact lens problems could lead to important general ocular symptoms being overlooked. The initial questions should be those which one would direct to any patient. Symptoms of asthenopia, headaches, pain and difficulty in seeing should be sought, as well as the many points of detail which the practitioner needs to know concerning location, severity, duration and associated symptoms, frequency and date when first noticed. Visual symptoms, in particular, should be probed with care to decide whether or not they are associated with the use of the contact lenses (*see* page 498, Section A5). For example, a unilateral visual haze could be attributed to a dirty or damaged lens, to imperfect correction of the refractive error or to imperfect lens fitting, on the one hand, and not be particularly serious. On the other hand, it could be caused by disease of any of the ocular media, of the retinal vascular system or of the central nervous system which, if undetected, could have tragic consequences for the patient and be very serious.

While asking the patient these questions, the practitioner should be planning in his mind any special tests and inspections which he may wish to include in his examination to eliminate these possibilities (*see Summary of Symptomatology* on page 520). Although only passing reference is given in this book to ocular disease and its detection since the subject is beyond its terms of reference, the importance of carrying out tests to be reasonably sure of excluding disease in the routine examination of the contact lens wearing patient, as for any patient, must be emphasized.

2. Contact Lens Wearing Habits and Limitations

The period of daily use and, in parentheses, non-use in hours is recorded. Thus: *W.T. 16* = wearing time 16 hours daily; *W.T. (3)12* = lenses are put in 3 hours after rising and then worn continuously for 12 hours daily; *W.T. 7(½)7* = lenses are worn for 7 hours, then removed for half an hour and replaced for another 7-hour period daily. If the wearing time is not usually the same each day, this fact should be recorded, for example, *less week-ends*; or *3/12* / not used during the past 3 months; or *6 social – 5/7* = 6 hours for social use 5 days ago. Following this, a note is made of the period of time they have been worn that day, thus; *W.T. 16 now 6*. A careful inspection of an eye which has recently worn a contact lens usually shows some sign. Some reaction, therefore, is normal; but the amount depends on wearing habits, which must be ascertained and accurately recorded. This is particularly important during the adaptation period. Habits such as eye rubbing or excessive blinking should be corrected, after looking for their possible cause, as they may lead to loss of a lens by dislodging it from the eye or displacing it.

It should also be ascertained whether or not the wearing habits accord with the patients wishes. The week-end sportsman may be fully satisfied with 6 hours on Saturdays while the single-handed ocean sailor may, of necessity, require continuous day and night wear. Average individuals need 16 hours daily – enabling them to dispense with spectacles for all purposes other than rare emergencies – and this should be the minimum target. If the wearing habits fall below target or are changeable, the practitioner must plan to determine the reason. This is another point of particular importance during the adaptation period.

Inadequate wearing times may be due to a reduced incentive – the original motive may have become weakened by changed environment or circumstances – or to an incorrectly assessed incentive in the first place. A young person may have lenses to appease a relative, a journalist to gain information, a sportsman to gain a short-term success now passed – in each case with no personal desire to surmount the difficulties encountered. A frequent symptom in such cases is loss of ability to place the lenses on the eyes. Sympathetic questioning by the practitioner leading to advice to discontinue the use of contact lenses is gratefully accepted in such cases. Other patients exhibiting similar symptoms may be subconsciously seeking attention to disguise psychological difficulties, and a word with the patient's medical adviser may be helpful since psychiatric disorders have usually been manifested in other ways. The vast majority of patients, however, genuinely wish to succeed and, given adequate after-care, should do so. In the present state of our knowledge, all day wear is within the capability of all but a very small percentage of patients who need it.

3. Whether any Treatment Arising from or Bearing on Contact Lens Use has been Necessary

Anybody is liable to suffer ocular trauma or disease requiring medical treatment, and this information would be elicited in the course of the general questioning. There are some emergencies, however, which are side-effects from the use of contact lenses and which are not always recognized as such by general practitioners. Most doctors do refer the patient back to the contact lens practitioner when the medical treatment is completed and before contact lens use is resumed. The prescriber can then satisfy himself that the contact lens is both in perfect condition and perfectly fitted and that the patient is properly instructed in its re-use. But if this has not been done, and the practitioner has not elicited this history from the patient, there is a risk that sooner or later the emergency will arise again. Understandably, the patient may become alarmed and quite unnecessarily conclude that contact lens wear should cease entirely (see Pain on page 514). Careful questioning on any treatment which may have been necessary following the use of contact lenses is important.

A loss of tolerance to contact lenses can be a side-effect of medically prescribed drugs, pregnancy, oral contraceptives and menstrual disorders, emotional stress or general malaise (see Chapter 7, Volume 1). Frequently the symptom is associated with a bodily water retention problem and the patient is oedema prone (see 5b below). Medical advice may be required, or have already been sought, and this must be recorded.

4. Whether there is any History of Redness of the Eyes, Pain or Discomfort

In addition to redness of the eyes, pain or discomfort (see page 514), redness or swelling of the eyelids, photophobia or spectacle blur (see page 510, Section J1) may be mentioned. Few patients are reticent on these subjects: information on such symptoms, particularly if recurrent or persistent, is usually volunteered without prompting; if possible the details should be recorded using the patient's own words.

Questions must be directed towards determining the severity of the symptoms and whether or not they are secondary to the use of contact lenses – frequently they are – and deciding whether any special tests or change in the examination routine is necessary. For example, the symptoms described may so clearly point to switched lenses or damaged or dirty lenses that the practitioner will decide to check these points before proceeding further. It is

not beyond experience to discover that a patient is using two right lenses or even two superimposed lenses on the one eye. Probably the most striking example came from the late Clifford Hall (personal communication in Munich, 1963), one of whose patients, having lost three corneal lenses in the course of a year, had reverted to a former pair of scleral lenses only to discover, to his amazement, on removing the scleral lens from his eye that three corneal lenses were lying inside. Unbeknown to him, they had become lost beneath the upper eyelid and he was, in effect, simultaneously wearing four lenses on the same eye – and he was asymptomatic!

Questions must be directed to reveal possible causes of the symptoms which the patient describes (see Summary of Symptomatology on page 520). Causes likely to be associated with the use of contact lenses and their mechanism and correction, will be described later, but the practitioner must be ever mindful of possible pathological causes of redness of the eyes, photophobia, pain or discomfort other than due to the cause of contact lenses.

5. Whether any Variations in Vision have Occurred

The following possible causes of variations in vision should be borne in mind when the patient is questioned.

(a) Inadequate Pupil Coverage by the Optic of the Lens

Vision may vary as the eye moves, when the pupil is dilated for any reason, if the lens continually rides off centre or, for soft lenses in particular, if the lens surfaces distort in use. This form of visual variation is likely to fluctuate and to be immediate (see Sections B3 and C2 below).

(b) Corneal Oedema

The vision becomes hazy and distorted, there may be diffraction haloes round lights (c.f. glaucomatous haloes and crystalline lens haloes), photophobia, lacrimation and varying degrees of discomfort. These symptoms usually take several hours to develop and are associated with corneal anoxia due to poor lens venting (see pages 512–513). The visual haze and rainbow-coloured haloes are short-term symptoms which fade within half an hour of lens removal but the visual distortion and associated refractive effects are much more chronic (see Chapter 17): corrective measures are necessary. Proneness towards oedema varies greatly between patients, but is more intractable in patients with reduced tears output, or with bodily water retention problems.

(c) A Change in the Optical Correction with Contact Lenses

(*See* Sections H–J on pages 509–510).

(d) Dirty, Damaged or Inaccurate Lenses

(*See* Sections B2 and E below).

(e) Binocular Instability

(*See* Section C1 below).

(f) Discomfort

Discomfort from any cause leading to lagophthalmos or lacrimation and possibly associated with corneal and eyelid oedema (*see* Section B1 below).

(g) Disease

Disease involving any of the ocular media, the retina or the associated central nervous system.

(h) A Combination of any of the Above Factors

B. GENERAL INSPECTION WITH LENSES *IN SITU*

(1) Head and eyelid posture.
(2) Position, mobility and cleanliness of the tears and lenses.
(3) Fundus examination.

Contact lenses always induce trace changes of any eye on which they have been worn. Sometimes, the changes may be of clinical significance. Usually, they fade rapidly, but ideally they should not occur at all. To enable the practitioner to assess the importance of these induced changes, the patient is asked to report wearing the lenses, and it helps if the appointment is sufficiently late in the day for the changes to become fully developed. The only exceptions to this rule are when the patient has been obliged to discontinue wear for some special reason, such as loss or damage to the lens, ocular disability or the less obvious but equally important reason that the patient requires a prescription for spectacles.

One of the most readily evinced induced changes is in the spectacle refraction particularly following the use of hard lenses and, because it so frequently occurs, it renders a refractive measurement for a spectacle prescription very difficult (*see* pages 510–511, Sections J1 and 2). The recovery period may be anything from 24 hours to 2–3 months (*see* Chapter 17). The following should be noted.

1. Head and Eyelid Posture

Discomfort is sometimes avoided by the adoption of an abnormal head position. The 'chin in the air' pose of the inexperienced corneal lens wearer has been dubbed by Louis J. Girard (1964) 'the contact lens salute' and is an endeavour by the patient to see in the presence of a self-induced lagophthalmos. The edge of the upper eyelid is voluntarily lowered over the upper edge of the corneal lens to avoid impact between the two edges as the eye moves, or in blinking, or as the lens drops down after a blink. Another posture adopted to reduce the irritating edge contact is the retracted upper lid of the non-blinker, or there is an incomplete flick blink (Wilson, 1970) – the latter being the more difficult to detect (*see* SPEE Associated with Poor Blinking on page 516). To check that discomfort is caused by eyelid/lens edge contact the practitioner should lift or press the eyelid clear of the lens and ask the patient whether the discomfort is removed, then release the eyelid and confirm that the discomfort returns, first the upper then the lower lid. The edge of a scleral lens often causes discomfort as it passes the outer canthus on lateral eye excursions.

To correct discomfort when blinking the practitioner should seek for causes of extra sensitivity of the edges of the eyelids such as cysts or other abnormalities of the lid margins (*see* Section F5, and Benign Palpebral Diseases which may be Contraindications for Contact Lens Wear on page 519) and for causes of excessive movement of the lens, or from badly shaped or damaged lens edges (*see* pages 504–505 and Sections D and E). Sometimes it is an indication that the lens overall size must be increased by 1 mm (or more) or reduced by 0.5 mm to avoid excessive edge-to-edge contact. The thick bottom edge of a truncated prism ballasted lens may cause a similar irritation of the margin of the lower eyelid and, again, attention to the fit of the lens is indicated. Conversely, the thin top edge of a prismatic lens is unlikely to irritate the margin of the upper eyelid unless it is excessively sharp. A sharp edge or transition pressing on the cornea during blinking will also cause discomfort, as will a rough or dirty fenestration (*see* pages 515–516 and Sections E3 and E5).

2. Position, Mobility and Cleanliness of the Tears and Lenses

This inspection is a preliminary to refraction with the lenses *in situ* (*see* below). A fuller examination of the lenses *in situ* is carried out when inspecting the fit of the lenses (*see* page 503, Section D). If the position or mobility of the lenses is likely to interfere with the refractive measurement, the practitioner will be forewarned and must consider the need to refit. If the tears or lenses are not clean, he should now remove, wash and replace the lenses. Defects with the lenses still on the eye are easily seen by using an ophthalmoscope and/or, better still, a biomicroscope.

3. Fundus Examination

Examination of the fundus may be made at this point if the presence of the lenses *in situ* aids observation as, for instance, in a case of high myopia or gross corneal irregularity.

C. ROUTINE REFRACTION WITH LENSES *IN SITU*

(1) Routine refractive and oculomotor tests.

(2) Any imperfections which the patient may note in image quality.

1. Routine Refractive and Oculomotor Tests

Refraction with lenses *in situ* is sometimes called an 'over-refraction'. An accurate over-refraction and assessment of the binocular state must be made for comparison with that existing prior to the provision of the current contact lenses. The practitioner must have access to the previous notes and records if possible. Any inadequacy must be related to the patient's requirements and symptoms, and appropriate advice given. The inadequacy may be due to normal changes in the refraction of the eyes or to normal changes in the contact lenses such as distortion or lens flexure, or to limitations in the correction (cylinder, prism or tint) which a contact lens can give. Against this, contact lenses may give better binocular stability than do spectacles; this factor too should be assessed, as should the amplitude of accommodation, bearing in mind the effect of contact lenses on the onset of presbyopia (*see* Chapter 4, Volume 1).

Contact Lens Distortion

The material of a hard plastics contact lens is not as stable as a glass spectacle lens and after a period of use the curves may have flattened or, less likely, steepened slightly, or have become warped or been accidentally bent, so that the refractive effect of the lens on the eye may have changed. A soft contact lens is even less stable (*see* Lens Flexure below). The change in shape produced by distortion is similar on both surfaces and on a focimeter in air there is only a minimal, if any, change in lens power, but on the eye there is a significant change in the refractive effect. The refractive change at the front surface is nearly 3.2 times that at the back surface since the latter, when on the eye, has a plastics/tears interface, whereas the front surface has an air/plastics interface. The dioptric ratio is $(1-1.490)$ to $(1.490-1.336)$ or -0.490 to 0.154 which is approximately 3.2:1 (*see* Chapter 4, Volume 1). The practitioner must therefore conduct full refractive tests, first with the patient's own lenses on the eyes. Then, if he finds errors which he judges to be clinically significant but which could be due to contact lens distortion, he must repeat the refractive measurement with an accurate and well-fitting trial lens on the eye. A large library of sighted trial contact lenses is helpful. A lens which has become distorted should be replaced (though attempts to reform a hard lens which was originally cut from well annealed material, by gently boiling, are sometimes moderately successful as an expedient).

Lens Flexure

Large soft lenses are often fitted much flatter than the cornea. 'Iris diameter' (12.0 mm) and still smaller soft lenses, such as the Permalens, may be fitted steeper. As they settle and their back surface curves change to match the cornea, their effective power changes. Also, due to the presence of corneal astigmatism and because there may be uneven pressure from the eyelids, particularly as the eye is depressed for near vision, asymmetrical changes in lens power tend to occur. Furthermore, there are changes in the effective power of the lens as it dries on the eye, or if it rides off centre which, if the lens is aspheric, affects both sphere and cylinder. This behaviour of the soft lens in use is termed lens flexure. To the extent that the lens curvature is increased (steepened) there will be an increase in negative power; to the extent that the lens material is stretched (flattened) there will be a decrease in negative power. On balance the change is towards a negative power increase, and for high positive power lenses which are fairly thick centrally, the power change can be of significant extent (*see Table 4.11* in Chapter 4, Volume 1). Because it admits of mathematical analysis (*see* Addendum, page 523), the term lens flexure is sometimes confined to co-axial changes in curvature due to settling to a known spherical or toroidal surface. However, in clinical practice, the causes are more complex and the exact amount cannot be predicted but it is often clinically important. An over-refraction must therefore be carried out when the lenses have fully settled and after several weeks all day use in a variety of working conditions. To a much less extent lens flexure can also occur when very thin hard lenses are worn. Problems of soft lens flexure arise mostly during the fitting stage but can still be found during a routine re-examination (*see* Chapter 4, Volume 1, and Chapter 14).

Residual Astigmatism

Over-refraction, using a perfect trial lens, is particularly important when assessing the amount and clinical importance of residual astigmatism. Residual astigmatism may be defined as the astigmatism remaining when a bi-spherical contact lens is placed on the eye. Hard lenses behave differently from soft lenses.

Hard Lenses

Behind the hard contact lens *in situ* is a tears lens having a spherical front surface and a back surface matched to that of the cornea. The corneal astigmatism is thereby neutralized (*see* page 109, Chapter 4, Volume 1, and Chapter 18). The astigmatism neutralized is that of both the front and back surface of the cornea, that is, the total corneal astigmatism. Astigmatism remaining is therefore produced mainly at the crystalline lens either by a tilt with respect to the visual axis, displacement, or other lack of symmetry of either its refractive index or its surface curvatures. It is often stated that toricity of the retina is a contributory cause: this is wrong; astigmatism is a defect of the image-forming system and cannot be influenced by the shape of the screen on which the image is received.

Residual astigmatism with hard lenses is usually against-the-rule. The best spherical correction (assuming excessive negative power, or insufficient positive power has not been given) should give a blur in the horizontal direction (that is, horizontal lines look clear) for distance vision and (assuming the accommodation is minimal, that is, excessive positive power has not been introduced) should give

a blur in the vertical direction for near vision (both assumptions are usually valid). Although horizontal blurring for distance vision may lower the distance visual acuity, some vertical blurring for reading is often visually acceptable. This may explain why residual astigmatism does not, in many cases, produce symptoms in patients who do not require absolute perfection in distance vision. If the residual astigmatism is 0.75 D or less, the technical problems of correction may outweigh the clinical advantages. Large amounts, such as 4 or 5 dioptres, are strongly suggestive of dislocated crystalline lenses (for example, Marfan's syndrome).

Soft Lenses

Over-refraction with a perfect bi-spherical soft lens on the eye may also show astigmatism to which the term residual could be applied, but the cause is quite different. Unlike a hard lens the soft lens usually settles to match the front corneal surface and usually the tears lens is everywhere equally thin and of zero power. The refractive effect at the corneal front surface is now of a plastics corneal interface, and the total corneal astigmatism, which was formerly just corrected by a matching tears lens (n = 1.336), becomes over-corrected by a matching plastics lens (n = about 1.42) by approximately one-quarter. To this over-correction must be added an under-correction from a similarly matching flexure of the soft lens front surface which depends in amount on the lens thickness and on the induced change of curvature (Bennett, 1976) (*see* Chapter 4, Volume 1, pages 109 and 115). Furthermore, because the lens temperature on the eye is 12–14°C above normal room temperature there is some liquid loss – a partial dehydration – which causes a slight lens shrinkage and change in power both by increasing the refractive index and reducing the radii of curvature; the slight reduction in centre thickness has the effect of decreasing the power mainly in positive lenses. The amount of change depends on the initial water content of the plastics material and on the tears flow rate of the particular patient (Ford, 1974; 1976). On aggregate the astigmatism introduced into the soft lens approximately replaces the total corneal astigmatism.

If there is no corneal astigmatism then no residual astigmatism should be induced by these factors of lens flexure and partial dehydration, unless these occur asymmetrically. Usually, then, residual astigmatism occurring in these circumstances must be caused by a tilted or decentred crystalline lens or some other form of induced lens asymmetry or distortion. It is not uncommon.

In general, residual astigmatism with soft lenses is of the same order of magnitude as the total ocular astigmatism, but it can vary greatly from one patient to another.

The optical correction of residual astigmatism requires the use of one or two toroidal surfaces on the contact lens. This presents technical problems in that small toroidal surfaces are very difficult to manufacture in plastics material and it is difficult to stabilize the axis of a lens on the eye when fitting. The clinical need and the specification of toric contact lenses must therefore be very carefully assessed before they are manufactured and fitted (*see* Chapters 14, 18 and 22).

Limitations in the Optical Use of Contact Lenses

By comparison with spectacles the optical uses of contact lenses are limited. For example, plastics contact lenses cannot be used for selective absorption of ultra-violet or infra-red radiation as can glass spectacle lenses; prisms are limited to small base-down prescriptions (scleral lenses excepted), the problems of high astigmatism and presbyopia are technically more difficult to solve particularly with soft lenses, and the value of contact lenses in the field of industrial protection is barely explored.

Binocular Stability, Prismatic Corrections and Anisometropia

In other respects contact lenses offer important advantages (*see* Chapters 4 and 7, Volume 1) particularly in the maintenance of binocular stability. This arises from the fact that, unlike a spectacle lens, the contact lens moves with the eye and does not introduce oblique aberrations (astigmatism and coma) or prismatic effects (image displacement and chromatism) with eye movement. Also, being placed much closer to the principal plane of the eye than a spectacle lens, less change in image size is introduced by the optical correction. This means that the optical presentation more nearly approaches that of an emmetropic pair of eyes when contact lenses are worn than when spectacle lenses are worn; this results in improved binocular stability. Consequently, the need for small prismatic corrections is reduced; for example a patient who requires 3 dioptres of vertical prism or 5 dioptres of horizontal prism to maintain fusion when spectacles are worn, may have comfortable binocular vision with only 1.5 prism dioptres base-down in one eye or

without the horizontal prisms with contact lenses. Also, the aniseikonic and prismatic effects produced by the correction of high refractive error, including unilateral aphakia and both refractive and axial anisometropia, are greatly reduced. Unfortunately, it is not always realized by practitioners that disparity in retinal image size between two eyes of differing axial lengths may be compensated by an equivalent disparity in the spacing of the retinal receptors. As a result there are many anisometropes with only one eye corrected, living in the unhappy belief that their other eye is useless. The first time full and successful correction of 10 dioptres of myopic anisometropia with bilateral contact lenses is a common occurrence, and twice this amount has been satisfactorily corrected in adult patients: it is never too late to try. For anisometropic children and for unilateral aphakics of all ages the bilateral use of contact lenses is especially important. The main problem in fitting is in maintaining accurate centring of the heavier of the two lenses.

2. Any Imperfections which the Patient may Note in Image Quality

Despite a most careful over-refraction, a patient may read a line of test letters without error, yet comment that it is not seen clearly. As every refractionist knows, this is a possible sign of ocular disease, particularly if accompanied by foveal image distortion, or if the comment refers to one eye only, or is a recent development – a situation which merits investigation. To the contact lens practitioner, it is also a sign that the central optic portion of the lens is not fully covering the patient's pupil so that light from the peripheral optic zone is being refracted towards the macular area. If this is the cause, vision may be shown to improve by directing a light on to the eye to contract the pupil. Other possible causes include tears flowing over the lens thus distorting the image, or the lens itself may be distorting in the eye due to lens flexure, or the front surface of the lens may be greasy or scratched. The practitioner must be careful to distinguish between pathological and non-pathological causes. A helpful clue is that, in the latter case, the vision varies from moment to moment and is improved if an unfenestrated trial lens with a much larger central optic portion is placed on the eye. That such a lens may not be tolerated for regular use does not matter since it is here applied for diagnostic purposes only; but if a change in lens design is deemed necessary, care should be taken to ensure that the tears flow beneath the lens is not thereby restricted (*see* page 498, Section A5).

D. INSPECTION OF THE FIT OF THE LENSES

Hard Lenses

(1) Lens position and movement during normal gaze, blinking and eye movement.

(2) Fit of the optic – tight or loose areas and pupil coverage – with fluorescein and ultra-violet light and with the slit lamp and blue filter. The latter technique permits the causes of any corneal staining by the lens to be observed directly.

(3) Fit of the haptic: tight or loose areas and size, in all positions of gaze.

(4) Patency of channels or of fenestrations.

(5) Size, position, mobility and frothing of air bubbles beneath the lens.

Soft Lenses

(6) Lens position and movement during normal gaze, blinking and eye movement.

(7) Lens movement, especially speed of recentring if forcibly displaced.

(8) Image quality, by retinoscopy and by keratometry of the lens front surface (although measurements of the front surface curvature of the lens are only possible if its radius falls within the range of the keratometer).

(9) Lens contamination, if omitted at Section B2.

The inspection of the fit of the lenses is usually carried out with low magnification ($\times$ 3), but an ophthalmoscope or a biomicroscope permits more subtle fitting and contamination detail to be studied. Furthermore, the practitioner can relate fitting faults to epithelial stains or other induced changes in the cornea, conjunctiva or eyelids (see pages 513–520, Sections F and G, and SPEE on page 516). It is particularly important to study soft lenses in situ with the slit lamp in search of faults in surface or edge quality, bubbles or debris under the lens, and any limbal indentation caused by the lens edges which often shows up as a break in the blood column of one of the limbal or conjunctival vessels. Observation of engravings on both hard and soft lenses ensures that the lenses are worn in the correct eyes, and in the case of soft lenses that they are not inside out.

Criteria for assessing and correcting fitting faults of both hard and soft corneal and scleral lenses have been explained in earlier chapters and are equally applicable to after-care examinations and preliminary fittings. The procedure for lens modification and reconditioning – repolishing, repowering, reshaping edges or transitions, reducing diameters – are described in Chapters 22 and 23. Elaboration of the points listed above is not now necessary, but their separate importance is emphasized. At the after-care stage, the practitioner has the advantage of knowing the patient's reaction to prolonged use of the lenses. Any discomfort or deterioration in wearing or seeing ability, or the adoption of an unusual head posture, should alert the practitioner to the possibility of fitting faults. Ocular changes induced by the patient's own lenses, which may indicate the need to refit, will be considered when discussing the routine for inspection of the eye and adnexa (see pages 505–511 and Ocular Changes Induced by the Use of Contact Lenses on pages 512–520).

In general, a lens which does not produce untoward symptoms or cause ocular change is best left unaltered even though it may offend the practitioner's fitting philosophy.

E. REMOVAL AND INSPECTION OF LENSES

Points for inspection are as follows.

(1) Lenses are worn on the correct eyes.

(2) Soft lenses are not inside out.

(3) Contamination.

(4) Deterioration or damage.

(5) Lens parameters.

(6) Need for reconditioning or renewal.

Note: Excessive adhesion as a lens is removed suggests imperfect tears flow beneath the lens and the fit may be faulty or corneal oedema may be present. If corneal oedema is suspected tests for its presence should be conducted immediately the lenses have been removed, otherwise it may fade (*see* Sections A5*b* and F1*a*). A soft lens which is partially dehydrated may adhere to the eye, as may one which has inadvertently been soaked in a hypotonic solution or even distilled or tap water.

1. Lenses Worn on the Correct Eyes

Switched lenses are not uncommon. An unexpected refraction (page 500) may be suggestive. To assess the possibility the practitioner should allow for an introduced change in the powers both of the new liquid lenses (tears) and of the switched contact lenses. Checking the lens engraving (if present) *in situ* with the slit lamp is the quickest way to confirm if lenses are switched.

2. Soft Lenses not Inside Out

Most types of soft lenses tend to fit loosely if everted. The very thin lenses also tend to suffer in this way. Again, checking any engraving while the lens is on the eye, with the slit lamp, permits quick confirmation or otherwise of an everted lens.

3. Lens Contamination

Lens contamination is a frequent cause of discomfort. It may be a surface deposit, or due to chemical bonding by adsorption, especially by hydrophilic materials. It may be from air-borne chemical agents, cosmetics or dirt, or from *in vivo* secretions or metabolites and could become the site of pathogen development. Particles adhere more readily if the lens surface is scratched.

Lens 'greasing' is a common problem, particularly for hard lens wearers. Observation with the slit lamp at ×10 magnification, with the lens *in situ*, may show grease and mucus adherent to almost the entire front surface of the lens (*see Colour Plate XXVII*). Immediately after each blink the wetting action of the tears may momentarily improve the surface quality, but as drying occurs the tears form beads of moisture on the surface. This considerably impairs vision if it takes place in front of the pupil area. Frequently, with hard lenses, a ring of grease and mucus adheres to the front periphery of the lens, close to the edge. It is partly due to inadequate rubbing of the lens during the cleaning process, and once a build-up of such a deposit starts, it collects more debris following each blink, as can easily be seen with the slit lamp biomicroscope.

The remedy is thorough cleaning of the lens with a suitable cleaning solution. For PMMA lenses vigorous rubbing with 1 per cent Savlon (*I.C.I.*), or with Silvo (*Reckitt and Colman*), or even weak acetic acid (white spirit vinegar) may be required to get rid of stubborn deposits. Once clean the lens should be re-inserted and observed again with the biomicroscope to see if grease starts to accumulate after each blink, and if so where on the lens surface this occurs.

Scratches should be looked for as they readily pick up particles in the tears which then attract grease and mucus. If scratches are found the lens should be polished. Deposits near the edge may be encouraged to form by a thick blunt edge which may require tapering. As lenses age the problem seems to worsen, as not all scratches can be polished out, the only remedy then being a new pair of lenses. However, some patients are more prone to greasing than others, a high tears cholesterol level being related to a high cholesterol diet, and in some cases to the taking of diuretics and in others to certain stages of pregnancy (Young and Hill, 1973; Terry and Hill, 1975; Hill and Terry, 1976). In such patients the use of artificial tears drops or re-wetting solutions (*see* Chapter 3, Volume 1, pages 67 and 80) may help, but general medical attention to the underlying high cholesterol state – which is also evident in the blood – is desirable, and all patients manifesting this problem should be questioned about their state of health and the use of any medication.

In soft lens wearers the adherence of mucus to the lens has been shown to be associated with a low tears film break-up time (Koetting, 1976a and b) as well as to lens ageing. Again, the low break-up time of the tears film may be normal for the patient, but may be associated with some general underlying physical condition, such as treatment with certain drugs (*see* Chapter 7, Volume 1, pages 170, 179 and 180). Danker (1977) has suggested that oral vitamin A therapy may help to alleviate the basic faulty tears condition. Protein deposits on soft lenses are best removed by the use of an enzyme cleaner (*see* Chapter 3, Volume 1).

All contaminants may irritate the eye and cause abnormal secretory action and the further deposition of contaminants. Ocular allergy, sometimes noted after many months of asymptomatic soft lens use, may be a secondary reaction (*see* page 520). Contamination may be seen on a lens *in situ* (*see* Section B2) in the wet state as described above but it may be easier to see if, after removal, the lens surface is allowed to dry, especially in the case of hard lenses. Inspection can be carried out with the aid of a microscope (special devices and slit lamp attachments are available) but the author finds that a lens held up to the light of a naked tungsten filament lamp and viewed through a good quality ×10 magnifier can be given a quick check for all but the finest forms of surface contamination. A microfilm reader or similar projector is useful to demonstrate the defects to the patient. Soluble (or liquid) contaminants, such as incompatible wetting or soaking solutions, swimming pool disinfectants, absorbed atmospheric pollutants, etc., cannot be seen by visual inspection. Methods for chemically cleaning, disinfecting, sterilizing and re-soaking contact lenses are described in Chapter 3, Volume 1, in addition to those mentioned above.

4. Deterioration or Damage

Deterioration and damage, such as discoloration, surface cracks, edge chips, edge cracks, scratches, strains, warpage, wrinkling, polishing or grinding marks may be similarly inspected. With hard lenses, back surface scratches are more likely to cause discomfort than those on the front surface. A damaged lens can seldom be safely used but it has been observed that edge chips on soft lenses do not often cause discomfort.

5. Lens Parameters

The recording of lens parameters, especially with contact lens wearing patients who are new to the practitioner, is essential. The methods are fully described in Chapter 12, Volume 1, and Chapter 15. If the patient has complained of eyelid discomfort (*see* page 499), particular attention should be given to the design of the lens edge and transitions, and to any fenestrations.

6. Need for Reconditioning or Renewal

The methods for reconditioning lenses – repolishing, cleaning, disinfecting – or for modifying the lens design parameters are described in Chapter 3, Volume 1, and Chapters 22 and 23. If doubt exists on the efficacy of these measures, the lenses should be renewed.

F. SLIT LAMP MICROSCOPY

1. Using white light and broad beam or spot illumination the following corneal changes may be seen.
(*a*) Corneal oedema.
(*b*) Epithelial opacities and irregularities.
(*c*) Limbal vascular injection and proliferation of the limbal arcades.
(*d*) Stromal infiltration and striae.
(*e*) Stromal vascularization and scarring.
(*f*) Endothelial folds.
2. The depth of any lesions may be assessed using white light and narrow beam.
3. The state of the tears layer is inspected using cobalt filter, boosted full aperture beam and additional fluorescein.
4. Using cobalt filter and boosted broad beam, tissue staining is sought.
5. The remainder of the eye and adnexa may be examined.

Instrument Control

Although the cornea is readily accessible for examination, some of the more significant detail can be seen only under the high magnification given by a good stand slit lamp. The patient's eye must be steady, and the focus both of the illuminating beam and of the microscope must be accurately adjusted; in most modern instruments, they are coupled to a single positioning control of the joystick type. The practitioner sits opposite the patient and observes from the front with the illuminating beam set 45 degrees to the temporal side of the patient's eye. The patient must be comfortably seated, chin on rest and head gently but steadily in contact with the head-rest, and told to watch the fixation spot. The room is darkened. The dull beam from the fixation spot is directed from the front on to the eye not under inspection and focused (unless fixed) to compensate for the refractive error. If desired, the fixation beam may be angled later to bring peripheral parts of the eye into the frontal position. Using white light, the broad illuminating beam is directed on to the cornea and, with a magnification of about ×15, the anterior surface of the cornea is brought into focus. The beam is centred, then narrowed to check that it is also accurately focused (some instruments are pre-set by the manufacturer), and widened again. Thereafter, focusing is controlled with the joystick.

The anterior surface of the cornea, limbus, bulbar conjunctiva, eyelid margins and beyond, if necessary, are now scrutinized in a series of sweeps, moving first along the horizontal equator, then similarly with the eye depressed and the upper lid raised with the thumb to reveal the upper part of the cornea and adjoining structures; finally, with the eye slightly elevated, the lower part is seen. The focus is readjusted as necessary to permit successive inspection of all levels, from the tears layer through to the anterior part of the vitreous. This is observation by direct illumination. To inspect fine detail the magnification is increased maximally and the patient enjoined to keep quite still (some may need to hold their breath temporarily). To gauge the depth of detail the slit is narrowed and the illumination boosted to give an optical section which is then viewed with the illuminating and viewing systems set as far apart as possible.

It will be noticed that some of the delicate structures of the cornea or iris, for example, are seen more easily when they are just out of the beam – observation by indirect illumination. Indeed, it sometimes helps to oscillate from one to the other (illumination by oscillation) direct illumination to pick up the object, and indirect illumination to see detail which is otherwise flooded out of view. Dazzle to the observer can also be reduced by shortening the slit or by using a small round stop (spot illumination) to cut down the size of the brightly illuminated area which he sees, or by a polarizing filter or neutral density filter, if available, on the observing system of the instrument. It will also be noticed that, although some detail in the cornea is best seen against the unilluminated dark background of the pupil, other detail is best seen against the background of the illuminated iris or, to a less extent, the surface of the crystalline lens if these surfaces are deliberately brought under full illumination (this is the method of retro-illumination). The practised observer makes simultaneous use of all these methods, concentrating his attention more on the detail he is studying than on the mode of lighting.

Examination by diffuse illumination is also possible with those instruments having a diffusing screen which can be placed in the path of the illuminating beam. It is useful for general observation of the external eye at magnification of up to about ×10.

There are three other methods of illumination which require quite separate adjustment of the apparatus: illumination by sclerotic scatter; illumination by mire traverse; and illumination by specular reflection. For sclerotic scatter, the observer should focus on to the apex of the cornea using a broad beam, then uncouple the beam and, observing outside the microscope, move the beam only to the limbus and beyond, until the limbus, particularly on the opposite side, is seen to glow with light which has been totally internally reflected between the anterior and posterior corneal surfaces. Epithelial oedema may now be seen as a faint haze against the background of the unilluminated pupil (not to be confused with fluorescence from the crystalline lens). An area of central corneal oedema can be compared to a newsprint picture composed of a large number of tiny dots, and like the picture it is easier to recognize as a whole if seen without magnification, whereas the detail is best seen magnified. Thus, the cornea should then be observed through the microscope; faint corneal nebulae and non-staining epithelial changes which are quite unseen by direct illumination can often be picked out, as can the normal corneal nerves. This method should always be used by the contact lens practitioner.

To examine by mire traverse the practitioner should accurately focus a Purkinje image, using a full aperture beam either set off centre, or darkly (cobalt) filtered, to reduce glare to the patient, and slowly traverse the beam. If the reflecting surface (cornea or crystalline lens as required) is irregular, the size or shape of the image which it forms will be seen to change. This is useful information quickly gained. The Purkinje images are of the field lens of the illuminator, here used as a mire, and in a well adjusted system should be filled by an image of the lamp filament. Irregularities seen within the pupillary area will distort the ocular image and are significant. Traverses should be made with the patient's eye central, raised and depressed.

To examine in the zone of specular reflection, the observer should focus accurately on to a reflecting surface (anterior or posterior cornea or crystalline lens) then traverse the microscope only, away from the illuminating beam, to pick up the reflected beam. Within the bright reflected image (the zone of specular reflection) detail of the cellular mosaic of the anterior corneal epithelium, the more yellow posterior corneal endothelium or of the crystalline lens epithelium, as required, may be studied.

Abnormality of the endothelium is particularly significant. On the anterior cornea can be seen lipid and debris in the tears layer and any epithelial dimples. Dimples, incidentally, cast the most remarkable shadows by direct illumination on to the iris.

1. Corneal Changes Observed Using White Light and Broad Beam or Spot Illumination

(a) Corneal Oedema

To locate corneal oedema the observer should work in a completely darkened room and illuminate by sclerotic scatter. Boosted illumination helps. The field lens of the illuminator must be clean otherwise stray light scattered at the brilliantly illuminated lens surface may flood out the faint oedematous haze. (A camera flash makes photography of corneal oedema difficult for the same reason.) Delay in observation may cause the oedema to become too faint to see.

Many observers prefer to view the cornea with their naked eyes or through a binocular headband magnifier instead of through the microscope, directing the slit lamp as a focal illuminator. The observer then moves his head to locate a suspected central corneal haze by parallax against the background margin of the pupil. Parallax is less helpful if the suspected haze uniformly covers the entire pupil, as sometimes occurs after a large scleral lens or soft lens has been worn. The oedema is then more easily seen by viewing at right-angles to the beam; the haze then appears to be more dense and the view of the pupil through the haze becomes less clear. The unpractised observer should cross-check his observations on an oedema-free eye for comparison. Corneal oedema may also be seen by retro-illumination. The amount of corneal oedema may be measured in terms of the change in corneal thickness which it brings about (see Pachometry, Chapter 5, Volume 1). If oedema is present, endothelial folds and posterior stromal striate lines should be looked for (see (d) and (f)). A discussion on the aetiology and control of oedema is given on pages 512–514.

(b) Epithelial Opacities and Irregularities

Epithelial opacity associated with erosion or abrasion is often very faint prior to instilling fluorescein stain, and is best seen by retro-illumination or by oscillation, although sclerotic scatter is also helpful. Surface irregularities, especially if small, may be picked up by specular reflection from the overlying tears layer and are better seen if the tears layer is made to move by a blink. Larger surface irregularities and distortions are quickly located by mire traverse of the first and second Purkinje images. Epithelial erosion, abrasion and deformation induced by the use of contact lenses are discussed on pages 515–518.

(c) Conjunctival Injection and Proliferation of the Limbal Arcades

These relatively coarse details are easily seen and the precise method of illumination is not important, although indirect illumination assists observation of very fine new blood vessels in the cornea. To inspect the palpebral conjunctiva the eyelids must be everted (see Folliculosis and Follicular Conjunctivitis on page 519).

(d) Stromal Infiltration and Striae

Direct illumination with a small spot beam and high magnification or retro-illumination should be tried. A parallelepiped section is also useful.

(e) Stromal Vascularization and Scarring

If these are faint they may be seen as for Section 1(d), but normal direct illumination is usually adequate.

(f) Endothelial Folds

Endothelial folds are a complication of stromal oedema and may be obscured by the oedematous haze. They are best seen by direct spot illumination or by specular reflection.

The changes induced in the perilimbus and in the stroma and endothelium of the cornea are discussed on page 518.

2. Assessment of Depth of Lesions Using White Light and Narrow Beam

To be fully effective in judging the depth of a corneal lesion, inspection with the narrow beam requires a high magnification, a very steady patient's eye, boosted illumination and very accurate focusing of both the illuminating beam and the microscope, particularly if the lesion lies within the epithelium where most of the contact-lens-induced changes occur. The depth of opacities within this very thin epithelium has clinical significance but is exceeding-

ly difficult to judge. It is a test of the ability of the observer and the quality of the instrument. Direct illumination of the central area is used. The slit should be narrowed to that minimum which will give enough light (less than 0.20 mm) and the beam is set normal to the corneal surface. The boosted beam must not be accidentally widened since the dazzle is distressing to the patient. Observation is carried out from as wide an angle as possible; sometimes it helps to widen the angle still further by moving the beam slightly away from the normal. The corneal layers are parallel to the surface, and this procedure keeps the apparent thickness and width of the interface between layers to a minimum when seen in optical section (narrowing the beam yet further similarly reduces the apparent width of the interface seen).

Six layers can be identified: commencing from the anterior surface they are as follows.

(1) The tears layer which, if the patient is asked to blink, becomes mobile and glitters in the beam. The oily nature of the surface is well seen if the light is reduced and the beam widened slightly.

(2) The epithelium, which is normally transparent and is continuous with Bowman's layer.

(3) Bowman's layer is bounded by an anterior white band (the tears layer) and by a posterior white band (the front surface of the substantia propria) and is about 0.008 mm in thickness centrally but thicker peripherally.

(4) The substantia propria or stroma occupies most of the corneal thickness and has a granular structure which is most apparent when viewed from the direction of regular reflection and is thought to be due to the keratocytes.

(5) The posterior surface of the stroma is bounded by another structureless layer (Descemet's membrane) which is lined by endothelium.

(6) The endothelium.

The depth of the lesions is related to the structure in which they lie. Depth within the stroma can often be judged with fair accuracy under high magnification by the manner in which lesions have to be focused by the observer and by stereopsis with the binocular viewing system.

3. Tears Layer Inspection Using Cobalt Filter, Boosted Full Aperture Beam and Additional Fluorescein

One drop of fluorescein sodium (BP) solution is applied. The tears layer should fluoresce and be uniformly stained: if it does not fluoresce adequately, the solution is too strong, due to insufficient dilution by the tears – an indication of insufficiency of tears output (see Chapter 7, Volume 1, page 176).

Localized unstained areas of tears indicate a thinning of the layer due to 'dry' spots (breaks in the tears film – see *Colour Plate 'XXVb*) or to stretching over raised areas such as vesicles in the epithelial often associated with epithelial oedema. Arcuate epithelial waves are sometimes seen as dark bands under ultra-violet illumination for the same reason; so, too, is the corneal cone in keratoconus, while depressed areas such as dimples tend to hold fluorescein and to glow relatively brighter. Further indications of surface irregularity are seen as the tears surface reforms after blinking, and by observations of the quality of the bright first Purkinje image, which shows up small irregularities very well (*see* Mire Traverse on page 506). Sometimes the tears layer contains excess oil or is laden with debris.

4. Cobalt Filter and Boosted Broad Beam to Observe Tissue Staining

Areas of epithelial damage appear stained (*see* Mechanism of Corneal Staining on page 515), but holding stain and staining of the tears film layer should largely have disappeared. Rose bengal may also be applied if desired. Direct illumination is used to look for stained areas of the conjunctival and corneal epithelium and for adherent mucus.

5. Examination of the Remainder of the Eye and Adnexa Including Eversion of the Upper Lids

Special attention is given to both bulbar and palpebral disturbances such as injection or chemosis, to benign space occupying conditions such as pingueculae, pterygia, small lipomata, small marginal and other cysts of the eyelids, concretions and especially to conjunctival follicules and, of course, to any disease condition requiring medical advice.

G. OPHTHALMOSCOPY

(1) Examination from 20 cm (+5 dioptres).
(2) Close examination (+15 to +20 dioptres).
(3) General examination of the eye.

1. Examination from 20 cm (+5 dioptres)

Induced refractive effects can be observed, preferably from a distance of about 20 cm. The observer focuses on the cornea, when they are seen as light and dark shadows against the fundus reflex. Observation is not confined to the frontal position, and a much wider area of the cornea can be brought into view than by retinoscopy or by keratometry; indeed, the experienced practitioner may safely omit retinoscopy and keratometry for corneal inspection if ophthalmoscopy is to be used.

As in retinoscopy (*see* Section I2 on page 509) the dark shadows occur when the light rays, emerging from the patient's pupil towards the observer, are refracted away from the instrument sight hole: if the observer were now to move the instrument sideways to bring the sight hole into the path of the ray, the shadow area would brighten. For this reason small lateral head movements by the observer cause the light and dark shadows to move within the pupillary boundary. It must be emphasized that these shadow movements are purely refractive effects. They are not due to opacities; they are caused by local variations in refractive index or in surface shape of any of the refractive elements of the eye – cornea and crystalline lens. Shadow movement is quite distinct from the parallax movement caused by an opacity in the media, though both types of movement may be present together. Opacities can easily be seen in optical section, unlike refractive shadows. Indeed, by slit lamp biomicroscopy they are almost invisible. Sometimes a dull central shadow showing very little movement is seen following many years of daily hard lens wear; there are no associated slit lamp signs but it may be seen by retinoscopy (*see* Section I2(*b*), Central Shadow on page 510). It fades if contact lens use stops. The precise cause is not known but there is probably a deformation of the living epithelial cells. This certainly occurs in the epithelium of rabbit corneas, where contact lens pressure has caused a reduction in thickness of the epithelium as a whole, and shortening and widening of the basal epithelial cells (Greenberg and Hill, 1973; Hill and Greenberg, 1976). Where such a shadow is seen, refitting to avoid localized pressure areas should be considered.

2. Close Examination (+15 to +20 dioptres)

Inspection for changes in appearance is made from a very short distance. Epithelial dimples and arcuate waves can be seen from a short distance as light and dark structureless shadows. Sometimes spaces develop in the epithelium which do not stain and are probably intracellular epithelial vesicles. By ophthalmoscopy, they have the appearance of very small black dots and are best seen by retro-illumination by light scattered back from the optic disc. Careful focusing is necessary. They occur in the apical area of the cornea and do not produce symptoms; but, in the author's experience, they are a precursor to the overwear syndrome. When seen, the patient is always advised to reduce wear (*see* The

Over-wear Syndrome on page 514). They may be few in number or multitudinous, but they are never confluent. Gross corneal epithelial oedema, especially if of the 'steamy cornea' type, may be seen; as may corneal opacities, foreign bodies, infiltration or other non-transparent abnormalities which all show up as dark areas against the fundus background. Lesser degrees of corneal oedema are best detected during slit lamp microscopy (*see* Section F1(*a*) on page 506).

3. General Examination of the Eye

The remainder of the general ophthalmoscopic examination of the eye is now carried out if not done already with lenses *in situ*. If the surface of the cornea is irregular, the fundus view is distorted and observation is hampered. The optical quality of the corneal surface may be judged by this criterion, by observing the optic disc and moving from side to side to note any movement in the image – although sites for the cause of the aberration, other than that of the anterior cornea, are possible and should be sought. The ophthalmoscopic examination is then completed as for any patient.

H. KERATOMETRY

(1) Changes in measurements from the pre-contact lens findings.
(2) Irregular mire images.
(3) Curvature of the contact lens front surface *in situ*.

1. Changes in Measurements from the Pre-Contact Lens Findings

Ideally, the curvature of the cornea should not be changed by the use of a contact lens, but after hard lens use some induced change is frequently found. More than 1 dioptre, equivalent to a radius change of approximately 0.20 mm in any meridian, is excessive but, in the unlikely absence of other signs of corneal change, is not an important criterion. Soft lenses cause less change. Quite small changes in curvature of the front surface of the cornea have a marked effect on ocular refraction when the contact lenses are not worn, but are masked by the tears when the lenses are *in situ* (*see* page 500, Section C1). One dioptre of change in air becomes less than 0.12 D with the contact lens in place. The optical effect of these changes are discussed in Chapter 4, Volume 1, page 124, and their diurnal and long-term variations in Chapter 17.

2. Irregular Mire Images

Corneal irregularity shown by irregular mire images is of greater importance since it is likely to give disturbed vision; also, it is strongly suggestive of damage to the epithelium. The mire images appear ragged and the detail wavers after each blink as the tears layer reforms over the uneven corneal surface (*see* Mire Traverse on page 506).

3. Curvature of the Contact Lens Front Surface *in situ*

The curvature and regularity of the lens front surface, sometimes called 'over-K', measured with the lens *in situ*, is useful information in soft lens fitting and should have been taken at Section D8 (*see* page 503).

I. RETINOSCOPY (*see* also Chapter 17)

(1) Changes in measurements from the pre-contact lens findings.
(2) Irregular reflex characteristics.
(*a*) Arcuate epithelial waves and epithelial dimples.
(*b*) Central shadow.
(*c*) Gross irregularity of the reflex.
(3) Refraction with the lenses *in situ*.

1. Changes in Measurements from the Pre-Contact Lens Findings

Like keratometry, this is a quick method of assessing corneal changes induced by the use of contact lenses. No change is indicative of good fitting but the significance of change when found by retinoscopy cannot be judged on magnitude alone. The behaviour of the retinoscopic reflex (*see* Section 2(*c*) below) and the subjective refraction findings (*see* Section J below) are of greater value.

2. Irregular Reflex Characteristics

(*a*) Arcuate Epithelial Waves and Epithelial Dimples

Arcuate waves and dimples in the epithelium are readily seen within the pupillary area by retinoscopy, where they show at neutralization as dark shadows in an otherwise bright reflex. The light forming the retinoscopic reflex is deviated by the tilt of the corneal surface where the edge of the swollen or compressed area occurs and it does not enter the sight hole of the retinoscope. A simple surface tilt shows a dark area or band; a dimple is seen as a circular shadow with a small bright centre; an arcuate or linear depression or crest is seen as two long shadows, one on each side of a bright central band. A surface tilt of only a small part of 1 degree can be revealed by this method of examination, which is much more sensitive to corneal surface deformations than is slit lamp microscopy. Some observers have interpreted arcuate double shadows as duplicated edge indentations caused by periods of forced blinking following normal blinking; but when – as is usually the case – the two arcs are truly concentric, the author does not accept this explanation but feels that the appearance is due to an arcuate portion of swollen epithelium (*see* Arcuate Epithelial Waves on page 517).

(b) Central Shadow

This is the same central dulling of the reflex which can be observed by ophthalmoscopy (*see* page 508, Section G1). It is purely a surface refractive effect. It is not an opacity and cannot be detected by slit lamp microscopy (*see* Bedewing of the Corneal Epithelium on page 513).

(c) Gross Irregularity of the Reflex

If there is random tilting of the corneal surface by small surface undulations, patchy shadows appear in the retinoscope reflex whose movements cannot be neutralized and the behaviour of the retinoscopic reflex becomes grossly irregular. This cannot be detected by slit lamp microscopy but may be seen by ophthalmoscopy and probably gives rise to some spectacle blur (*see* Section J below). The absence of irregular reflex movements is a valuable and easy sign that the cornea has remained regular.

3. Refraction with the Lenses *in situ*

This is a standard method of detecting surface distortion of soft lenses when on the eye in the course of fitting and should have been carried out at Section D8 (*see* page 503 and Chapter 14). As already pointed out (*see* Section C1, Contact Lens Distortion, on page 500) over-refraction with a hard lens in place is most likely to show a change if the front surface of the contact lens has altered curvature. Changes of the back surface of the contact lens and of the cornea are largely masked by tears. Any other refractive change found would indicate an alteration in other media of the eye or a change of axial length.

J. SUBJECTIVE REFRACTION

(1) Assessment of spectacle blur.

(2) Prescribing for spectacles.

1. Assessment of Spectacle Blur

Any change from the pre-contact lens measurement in spectacle refraction and in visual acuity is noted. If the latter is not available, a comparison may be made with the visual acuity given with contact lenses *in situ*. Distortion of the corneal surface often gives a poor quality retinal image and the visual acuity is lowered, especially so if the surface of the epithelium has become very irregular (*see* Bedewing of the Corneal Epithelium on page 513). On other occasions, the distortion is sufficiently regular to be neutralized by changing the spectacle correction, and the visual acuity is unchanged. In either case the visual acuity with the pre-contact lens spectacle correction is reduced. This is known as spectacle blur.

A measure of the spectacle blur in terms of the amount of the induced refractive change and visual acuity change is a useful guide to the amount of corneal distortion which has occurred in the pupillary area. A change of not more than 1 dioptre and of about one line on the letter chart is usually considered acceptable. Nevertheless, even this amount of change can be embarrassing to a patient who wishes to use spectacles after wearing contact lenses, and the practitioner should hope to be well within this limit of tolerance. Soft contact lenses cause much less spectacle blur than do the hard ones, and, for the latter, absence of induced refractive change is a hallmark of good fitting.

2. Prescribing for Spectacles

Because of spectacle blur, patients frequently request a new spectacle prescription for use when contact lenses are removed. Unfortunately, the amount of refractive change induced by the use of contact lenses is rarely stable and it is very difficult to prescribe on the basis of measurements made when lenses are first removed, particularly when hard lenses have been worn.

If spectacle blur exceeds 1 dioptre, refitting, probably with soft lenses, is clinically necessary in any case and spectacle prescribing is deferred. For smaller amounts it is wiser to keep to the present spectacle prescription, if known, and to explain the reasons to the patient. If the present prescription is unknown or manifestly outdated so that a new prescription becomes inescapable, new measurements should be taken over a period of non-use of contact lenses if possible. This period should be long enough for reasonable stability to return, usually in excess of one week for hard lens wearers (*see* Chapter 17). If this is impossible a compromise prescription must be given, based on the refraction immediately after several hours of contact lens wear and that found some two to three days following discontinuation of wear. Usually the mean sphere and minimum cylinder provide an adequate correction, with the cylinder axis along the nearer of these two findings to 180 or 190 degrees.

K. SUPPLEMENTARY TESTS

Additional diagnostic tests, such as tonometry, examination of the visual fields, special oculomotor tests, etc., as for a patient with spectacles, may now be undertaken.

L. ADVICE TO THE PATIENT

The routine re-examination of the contact lens wearer is now concluded. Advice to the patient should now be given, and this must be based on the condition of the patient's eyes and lenses. Sometimes potentially serious corneal or other changes are seen (pages 512–519) of which the patient is unaware and he may be unwilling to take the advice given, particularly if it is a recommendation to discontinue or reduce lens wear, or to have new lenses fitted. In such cases, it may be advisable to suggest that a second unbiased opinion be sought.

In all cases the advice given should be noted on the record card, and if the patient chooses to ignore the advice he should be warned of the possible outcome. The importance of careful record keeping cannot be too greatly emphasized. If a patient has had an abrasion which requires medication as a prophylactic measure to prevent the risk of infection, the practitioner must be certain that the patient is not allergic to any drops or ointments which are recommended.

The usual chemotherapeutic agents used by ophthalmic opticians for prophylaxis are sodium sulphacetamide or propamidine (*see* Chapter 3, Volume 1) and both are well known to cause allergic reactions in some patients. If, after questioning the patient, there is any doubt about the possibility of allergy, the patient should either be left untreated and seen the following day, or, if an infection is suspected, should be referred to his general medical practitioner. Where a patient is recommended to use artificial tears for a dry eye giving persistent 3 and 9 o'clock staining, or hypertonic saline solution for corneal oedema associated with continuous wear soft lenses, or other drops for regular use, this should preferably be done by arrangement with the general medical practitioner.

RE-EXAMINATION DURING THE ADAPTATION PERIOD

The routine re-examination procedure for the established contact lens wearer may, in many respects, be used for the new wearer during the adaptation period.

Following the preliminary examination and assessment of fitting, lenses are prepared and issued to the patient, who is given full instructions in their care and use, including a wearing schedule as described in Chapters 7 and 8, Volume 1. The adaptation period then commences. The wearing schedule must be set to each patient's potential ability and so selected that progress will not be so slow and irksome that the patient becomes disinterested, nor so rapid that uncomfortable and even frightening side-effects arise. The author's usual procedure for wearers of both scleral and hard corneal lenses is to establish an initial tolerance of 3 hours under supervision during the fitting procedure and, when lenses are issued for use without supervision, to allow an increase of half an hour in wearing time each day thereafter. The initial period for those fitted with daily wear soft lenses is 6 hours with a daily increase of 1 hour thereafter. A re-examination is made 2 weeks later and again at the end of 4 weeks, when all-day wear may well have been achieved. Further examinations are conducted after 3 months and after 12 months when the patient is finally discharged. More visits are needed for those people having continuous or extended wear soft lenses. Thereafter, an annual routine re-examination is recommended. This is the procedure for a normally adapting patient, but considerable variations may have to be made in the light of the findings at each visit, and regular 3-monthly check-ups are recommended for those having continuous and extended wear soft lenses.

After-care checks at short intervals need not necessarily be as exhaustive as the routine detailed in this chapter, but in the opinion of the author, the minimum examination at any time must include at least the following: (1) history and symptoms; (2) refraction with lenses *in situ*; (3) lens removal and inspection; (4) slit lamp microscopy; and (5) ophthalmoscopy.

OCULAR CHANGES INDUCED BY THE USE OF CONTACT LENSES

The routine re-examination of the contact lens wearer, conducted with both care and candour, always reveals some degree of ocular change induced by lens use. These induced changes will now be considered. They will be taken in the order in which the routine re-examination of the eyes may be expected to reveal them and they will be related to symptoms and to lens performance. Also considered are certain ocular diseases and systemic disorders which may produce symptoms when contact lenses are worn.

CORNEAL OEDEMA

Aetiology

The presence of a contact lens on an eye limits both the flow of the tears over the cornea, and the normal exposure of the cornea to the atmosphere. The cooling effect of the surface evaporation of the tears is therefore reduced. The material from which the lens is made is a heat insulator and the effect is a rise in temperature of the tears (Hill and Leighton, 1965) with a reduction in their gas solubility. These factors combine to produce a corneal anoxia and the retention of metabolites and water within the tissues leading to corneal oedema, with all its ramifications of corneal curvature, thickness and refractive index changes as well as loss of transparency. The resultant effects on refraction and visual acuity are dealt with in Chapter 17, but have also been dealt with briefly on pages 506–510. Corneal sensitivity is also reduced (Millodot, 1976).

The mechanism of oedema associated with contact lens use is not proven but probably starts in the basal epithelial cells. The following account is taken from a paper by Wilson (1970).

'The basal epithelial cells presumably have the highest oxygen requirements as they are chiefly responsible for the metabolic activity of the epithelium, and particularly for active mitosis to occur. Early epithelial oedema is probably sited in these basal epithelial cells, so that oedema may be seen by sclerotic scatter technique without much observable surface epithelial change with the slit lamp. This basal cell oedema will lead to oedema of the more superficial cells which rely largely on the functional integrity of the basal cells for their viability and replacement. Stromal oedema will occur when the integrity of the basement membrane is breached, allowing fluid to pass passively into the stroma. Stromal oedema will then tend to increase because of the hydrophilic nature of the stromal tissue. The stromal oedema remains localized at first but will spread laterally and posteriorly as further areas of the epithelium become devitalized. Stromal oedema usually leads to symptoms of glare and photophobia before any effect on the visual acuity. In order to prove this concept, more accurate instrumentation is required to assess the relative thickness of the stromal and epithelial corneal elements. Higher magnification of slit lamp microscopy is also required to observe and to photograph corneal cross-sections, in order to localize the site of oedema.'

Corneal Oedema following Scleral Lens Wear

When a sealed scleral lens is worn, corneal oedema may occur within one hour or less. There are symptoms of hazy vision and photophobia and, later, diffraction haloes with discomfort and conjunctival injection, and the patient is obliged to remove the lenses. The visual reduction is known as veiling or Sattler's veil (Dallos, 1946). The oedema following scleral lens wear can be dense and is easily seen even when confined to the epithelium – evidence for this location may be seen by the stereopsis of the biomicroscope where small well-defined islands of clarity in the dense oedematous haze sometimes occur.

The oedema is a manifestation of corneal anoxia arising from inadequate tears flow beneath the lens, also termed (by Wilson) poor venting. Tears flow must be improved by channelling or fenestrating the lenses, or by using gas permeable corneal or soft lenses if other factors permit.

The tears exchange must be effective over the entire corneal area. Any area from which tears flow is barred, whether by obstruction by the lens material or by an air bubble, will develop oedema. The fact that the air bubble is renewed does not sustain the corneal metabolism. For example, if an annular bubble covers the limbal area so as to isolate a central tears pool, a central corneal oedema can rapidly develop, even though the air in the bubble is continually renewed through a fenestration. Conversely, an unfenestrated scleral lens with no air beneath it has been known to give all-day trouble-free wear because an accidental but nevertheless effective tears channel has been formed under a loosely fitted area of the haptic. As the eye is turned in all directions through 360 degrees, the air bubble should move through 360 degrees in the opposite direction; not only does this move air to all parts of the limbus but the bubble movement stirs the tears and prevents oedema. An air bubble locked in one position can, in time, produce an epithelial necrosis due to drying and calcification, with varying degrees of vascularization occurring in the area. Such incidents underline the fact that continued renewal of the tears over the entire corneal surface is essential for the maintenance of corneal normality.

Corneal Oedema following Corneal Lens Wear

The oedema associated with a corneal lens which restricts the tears flow over the apical area of the cornea is more difficult to recognize. It is usually restricted to the apical area of the epithelium unless it becomes severe, when the stroma may also be involved. There is nearly always eventual discomfort – a burning or hot sensation – and usually lacrimation and photophobia (Miller *et al.,* 1967). This leads to a mild orbicularis spasm which presses the lens on to the cornea and aggravates the condition. The patient notices a 'blue haze' and may liken vision to looking through bonfire smoke; and in the severe cases, there may be coloured haloes and reduced visual acuity. These symptoms are always indicative of oedema even if, on inspection, the oedema is apparently invisible.

Corneal oedema does not stain with fluorescein unless the oedematous epithelium has swollen to such an extent that it is abraded by the rubbing action of the lens, or unless the cells have swollen and ruptured. It is much less circumscribed than faint corneal scarring. The area may be a few square millimetres only and the shape may replicate that of the lens – round or truncated – or be irregular. It may fade and become invisible within minutes of lens removal. This early corneal oedema is best located by slit lamp microscopy (*see* Section F1(*a*), Corneal Oedema, on page 506) and the corneal surface irregularity which accompanies the later stages by ophthalmoscopy (*see* page 508, Section G1). The latter can also be seen by keratometry (*see* page 509, Section H2) and by retinoscopy (page 510, Section I2(*c*). The induced refractive changes are best assessed subjectively (*see* page 510, Section J1). The occurrence of corneal oedema is fairly normal in the early stages of adaptation especially if the eyelids tend to swell and exert extra pressure on the lens, thereby restricting tears flow. Incidence is related to lens weight and is more prevalent if the lenses are thick, prismatic or large.

Many observers are able to identify corneal oedema in about 50 per cent of all corneal lens wearers at some stage; since corneal thickness changes and the commonly found induced refractive changes are associated conditions, 50 per cent could well be an underestimate of its true frequency. With skill, it is possible to assess the efficiency of the tears flow beneath the lens, and therefore the correctness of this aspect of a corneal lens fitting, entirely on observation of corneal oedema without the use of fluorescein (Boyd, 1969).

To correct corneal oedema tears flow must be improved by either or all of the following: fenestration; attention to the lens fitting (*see* Chapter 11, Volume 1); or to the patient's blinking habits, particularly if non-blinking or flick-blinking is observed (*see* pages 499 and 516). Following fenestration, small irregular areas of oedema may still be observed when the fenestration hole(s) do not allow sufficient tears exchange. Refitting consideration should be given to reducing lens weight and size, to increasing lens mobility, possibly by using lid hitching techniques (Korb and Korb, 1974) (*see* Chapter 11, Volume 1, page 266) and to reducing eyelid sensation (page 499, Section B1). Alternatively, hydrophilic soft lenses may be substituted, or lenses of a more oxygen-permeable material.

Corneal Oedema following Soft Lens Wear

The incidence of corneal oedema at the corneal apex is greatly reduced if hydrophilic contact lenses are used, the high water content materials being the most effective. Since soft lenses are large, the oedema, should it occur, is not confined to the apical area but is diffused over the entire corneal surface and, because there is no clear periphery for comparison, the corneal haze is difficult to identify. In the opinion of the author this wide uniform distribution suggests that tears flow, although still restricted and insufficient, is through the hydrophilic lens material and not, as for hard corneal lenses, from the periphery. The tears layer is often abnormal having an uneven oily appearance, containing 'holes', or is laden with debris (page 507, Section F3). The oedema may be dense and involve the entire stroma; vertical striae (page 518) and endothelial folds may accompany it. It is most commonly caused by low water content materials and by thick positive lenses.

Sustained oedema from soft lens wear may eventually lead to proliferation of the limbal arcades and to a marginal keratitis (page 518). Apparent detachment of a central area of endothelium has been reported by Mackie (1975) after over-wear of soft lenses (*Colour Plate XXIb*). This condition resolved after 2 weeks without wear. However, the condition caused pronounced discomfort, a hazy cornea, poor vision and a red eye and is a warning against over-wear of soft lenses.

Bedewing of the Corneal Epithelium

The corneal epithelium near the limbus and within the palpebral aperture is sometimes seen as a cellular structure by indirect illumination in a normal eye. It is probably caused by over-exposure from inadequate blinking. From its appearance it is described as 'bedewing' and is a form of corneal oedema. There may be associated superficial punctate epithelial erosions (page 515) which stain with fluorescein.

A much more pronounced and irregular bedewing is sometimes seen in the central area of the cornea after it has been subjected to long periods of apical pressure from a hard lens which is fitted to give apical touch and is also too thick and heavy. The apical pressure breaks the lipid tears layer and exposes the epithelium to excessively serous tears, causing oedema and swelling which increases the apical pressure still more; evidence of the increased apical tightness can be seen in the fluorescein fitting picture. The surface irregularity is confirmed by mire traverse with the slit lamp or by inspection with the retinoscope and keratometer, and the spectacle visual acuity is often reduced by more than two lines. There is usually some punctate staining with fluorescein. This form of bedewing is not only an oedema but also a necrosis of the superficial epithelial cells, and it seems to be accompanied by a prolonged reduction in sensitivity. Spectacle blur is often the only symptom. Given complete rest from contact lens wear, the cornea reverts to normal but there is sometimes a permanent induced change in the corneal astigmatism of as much as 2 dioptres. Refitting with small, lightweight lenses or with soft lenses is essential. The central shadow seen by retinoscopy (page 510, I2(b)) may precede this condition.

The Over-wear Syndrome

The over-wear syndrome, often called by contact lens practitioners the '3 a.m. syndrome', is a gross sequel to corneal oedema in an unadapted eye following over-wear, and causes severe pain.

During adaptation, a patient may suddenly increase the daily wear period either through forgetting to remove the lenses (possibly because of a reduction in corneal and lid margin sensitivity, leading to increased comfort), or in an endeavour to catch up on a previous reduction in wearing time. The excess wear usually occurs late in the day, often in a hot dry atmosphere and possibly in conditions where the orbicularis muscles are partially contracted and the blink rate is reduced through straining to see in the semi-darkness of night driving or at a cinema. The patient may admit that the eyes feel tired, but there is no particular discomfort until 2 or 3 hours after the lenses are removed. Pain then develops, often increasing rapidly to agony, and

sleep becomes impossible; there is conjunctival injection, lacrimation, blepharospasm, photophobia and dense corneal oedema giving hazy vision. The frightened patient either panics and calls the practitioner or waits unhappily for dawn, when the symptoms begin slowly to ease. By midday there is a marked improvement and by the following morning only the memory remains, though corneal signs may still be detectable. Even though there is always a complete recovery, it is an experience which the patient never entirely forgets.

If patients disclose irregular wearing times, especially during the adaptation period, they should be warned of the over-wear syndrome, not only to reduce the risk but also to reassure them should it occur. It is not just the severity of the pain which worries them but the fear that they may have irreparably damaged their eyes. This fear is communicated to those around them, and it has been known for a patient to be admitted to hospital as a bed patient for 2 days' sedation following such an incident. The cornea becomes exceedingly sensitive to touch and the eye photophobic, so that a darkened room and the comforting reassurance that repair will be total and rapid, plus pain-killers such as aspirin and sedation to induce sleep all help. It is probable that the temporary use of a soft lens to protect the cornea would alleviate the symptoms. This is because the eyelids also become oedematous and the extra pressure and possibly irregular palpebral conjunctiva irritate the damaged corneal epithelium which can be protected by a soft lens.

Epithelial Changes Associated with the Over-wear Syndrome

The very fine dots seen with the ophthalmoscope (see page 508, Section G2) against the pale background of the optic disc, if very numerous, can usually (but not always) be picked out with the slit lamp by a combination of direct and retro-illumination, when they are seen to be tiny unstained white dots or flecks in the anterior layers of the epithelium. This is the appearance in the precursor stages; but if pain has developed, mingled with the fine dots are fairly bright well defined spots of stain. These are probably swollen or ruptured deeper epithelial cells into which the stain has penetrated. Dark discrete or coalesced spots may also be seen within the stained area. These are probably elevated areas of epithelium overlying swollen basal cells or oedematous intercellular spaces. Once located with × 15 magnification, abnormal areas may be inspected with × 30 or × 40 magnification.

The epithelium, at the height of the overwear syndrome, stains deeply and there is a definite central oedema; but when the patient is distressed and the cause is obvious, there is no point in applying the fluorescein test and certainly no case for the use of a slit lamp which only aggravates the extreme photophobia.

EPITHELIAL EROSION, ABRASION AND DEFORMATION

In addition to corneal oedema other signs of epithelial change are frequently seen during the routine re-examination of the contact-lens-wearing eye and their assessment is an important aspect of patient care. The commonest are erosions and abrasions occuring in possibly 50 per cent of hard lens cases – less for soft. They are most easily seen when stained.

Mechanism of Corneal Staining

A cobalt filter for ultra-violet illumination is incorporated in most slit lamps. It is used to produce a fluorescent glow from either free fluorescein or fluorescein stained tissues. It is important to distinguish between them. Free fluorescein appears as a well-delineated homogeneous pool and its size, shape and density are controlled by the size, shape and thickness of the space containing it. Free fluorescein within a tissue which does not readily wash away is sometimes referred to as a 'holding stain'. True staining occurs when the dye invades the cellular tissue and enters into chemical composition with it so that it assumes a granular or fine punctate appearance. It is probable that the fluorescein stain usually seen is a mixture of holding intercellular and combined intracellular stain. Interspersed with it are sometimes seen circumscribed unstained areas which look dark by contrast with the surrounding fluorescent glow. They are surface elevations in the epithelium and can be caused by swollen basal epithelial cells (Wilson, 1970).

Fluorescein has a particular affinity for damaged epithelial cellular tissues, which stain yellowish-green. Rose bengal stains the keratin of degenerate epithelial cells red. It also stains mucus similarly. It gives pronounced staining in corneal and conjunctival drying and is frequently used to diagnose kerato-conjunctivitis sicca. Norn (1964) advocates the use of a mixed stain of sodium fluorescein 1 per cent and bengal rose in normal saline solution. He states 'Fluorescein staining indicates epithelial degeneration. It may be seen on the cornea, the bulbar conjunctiva or the palpebral conjunctiva. This condition is hardly dangerous to the eye but, if the wearer has subjective troubles, often involving a reduced wearing time, we must modify the contact lens guided by the stain seen'. If rose bengal staining is suspected to be due to mucus, alcian blue 1 per cent, which stains mucus only, may be used as a following stain. Alcian blue must not be used in the presence of a deep corneal abrasion since it may give a lasting green-blue tattooing.

Superficial Punctate Epithelial Erosions (SPEE)

There are many types of epithelial erosion which occur when contact lenses have been worn. The commonest, occurring in fully 25 per cent of eyes, produces an area of very fine punctate stains sometimes confluent in places. These are erosions of the superficial epithelium caused by the rubbing action of scratches or deposits on the lens back surface, by a sharp transition, or by extraneous material such as dust getting between the lens and the cornea or by the edge of a clumsily inserted lens. They are asymptomatic or mildly irritative only and usually clear within a few hours. They may be exceedingly faint or, if new, fairly bright, and the damage can often also be seen unstained with white light by retro-illumination or sclerotic scatter.

Those caused by scratches or deposits on the lens back surface are related to the position of these faults in the lens and will be diffuse. That due to a sharp back surface transition is more arcuate in shape and so, to some extent, is the erosion from a clumsily inserted lens. If the exact cause is in doubt, the practitioner should re-check with the lens *in situ*. Fine SPEE covering the whole corneal area and associated with conjunctival injection (kerato-conjunctivitis) (*see Colour Plates XXVIII and XXIX*) and discomfort can be produced by chemical toxins such as unsuitable preservatives in wetting solutions. The true cause must be determined and corrected. Treatment to the eye is seldom necessary. If the superficial punctate erosions are mostly in the central area of the cornea, there is often an associated central epithelial oedema which has devitalized the cells (*see* Bedewing of the Corneal Epithelium on page 513).

The erosion due to dust should perhaps be termed a superficial punctate epithelial abrasion since it is usually not a repetitive rubbing but a number of scratches, each taking a new path across the cornea and leaving a trail of punctate stains termed a foreign body track, in the superficial epithelium. The path may be curved or straight and the scratches may be single or multiple, but they are always linear and – while the foreign body is present – painful to the patient. *Colour Plate II*, Volume 1, shows a typical foreign body stain. If severe, medications may be necessary (*see* Advice to the Patient on page 511, and Chapter 8, Volume 1).

SPEE Associated with Soft Lens Wear

The incidence of epithelial erosion from the rubbing action of scratches or deposits on the lens back surface, by sharp transitions, by dust or by the edge of a clumsily inserted lens is reduced if the lens itself is soft and yielding and the staining and discomfort is less frequent after the use of soft rather than of hard lenses. On the other hand, SPEE following soft lens wear frequently take longer to heal and give more persistent discomfort than erosions from hard lens wear, possibly because the primary cause is epithelial metabolic disorder rather than simple trauma. Erosions due to cell necrosis associated with corneal oedema are seen as a wide distribution of very fine punctate fluorescein or rose bengal stains and are not infrequent (*see* Corneal Oedema following Soft Lens Wear on page 513). If the edge of a soft lens leaves the cornea exposed, dead and damaged epithelial cells will stain with both fluorescein (*Colour Plate XXVa*) and rose bengal in an arcuate area where the lens periphery has exposed the cornea and there may be considerable discomfort. Refitting is necessary. Sometimes a coalescent film of fluorescein stain is seen which is not punctate and has the appearance of a surface deposit, like that seen on the front surface of a contaminated soft lens, but whether it is cellular, lacrimal or exogenous in origin is not known. It clears quickly after lens removal.

SPEE Associated with Poor Blinking

Surface drying of both conjunctiva and cornea and of the front surface of the contact lens follows incomplete or infrequent blinking (flick-blinking or non-blinking) and punctate staining, frequently confluent, occurs within the palpebral aperture in the areas which are not protected by either the lens or the eyelids – the 3 o'clock and 9 o'clock staining described by Mackie (1967). Pingueculae also may be present.

Another fault is squeeze-blinking. This may force the lens downward and press the upper edge of the lens on to the cornea to produce an arcuate area of punctate epithelial staining; but when the eyelid is lifted by the practitioner, the lens rides more centrally so that the stained area is seen beneath the peripheral zone of the lens parallel to the edge which caused it. If there is no squeeze-blinking, a stain in this position could be caused by a sharp transition. Squeeze-blinking may also cause the opposite edge of the lens to override the limbus to both deform and stain the conjunctiva there.

Blinking Exercises

If patients exhibit flick-blinking, non-blinking or squeeze-blinking, or 3 o'clock and 9 o'clock staining is observed, they should be instructed to improve their blinking, and exercises for this purpose have been devised. The patient is told to blink 20 times slowly and fully two or three times daily, keeping the eyes closed for a brief moment each time. The practitioner should explain to the patient that the lids must not be squeezed. To demonstrate this feature he should place the tip of the patient's forefinger at the outer canthus and get the patient to feel that the desirable full and total eyelid closure does not move the finger whereas a forcible squeeze-blink pulls the finger sideways. The practitioner should explain that the purpose of the full lid closure and slight moment of pause – long enough to utter the word 'pause' – is not only to wipe the lids over the lens but also to stimulate the upward roll of the eyeball (Bell's phenomenon) whereby the cornea is carried towards the openings of the lacrimal gland ducts and fresh tears at the upper fornix. This simple exercise helps to establish the habit of correct blinking and is an important aid to comfort. Causes for the arrested blinking, such as uncomfortably positioned or poorly shaped lens edges, should be corrected. Frequently, there is an associated corneal oedema.

Deep Epithelial Abrasion

Sometimes a foreign body penetrates the epithelium and moves very little, giving a larger epithelial stain which is often surrounded by a white ring of infiltration and tags of epithelium; there is pain and conjunctival injection. Urgent removal of the foreign body, if still present, and medical treatment is necessary. Neglect could lead to corneal ulceration and scarring. A small foreign body will, if it protrudes from the cornea, cause considerable lid irritation after the lens has been removed from the eye. Sometimes a deep epithelial stain will lie over a larger area of diffusion of fluorescein into the anterior layers of the stroma, where it is seen as a structureless haze with indefinite boundary; presumably, Bowman's layer has been penetrated by the large fluorescein molecules at this point. A deep epithelial abrasion may be caused by a patient inadvisedly wearing a cracked corneal lens when the discontinuity of the surface at the crack has sheared off the epithelial surface. If deep, this can be almost as painful as the over-wear syndrome. There is bright epithelial staining and fluorescein may be seen in the anterior chamber.

Recurrent Epithelial Erosion
(see Colour Plate XXVb)

If a small area of full-thickness epithelium has been traumatically stripped from the cornea, the regenerated epithelium sometimes becomes detached as a contact lens is removed or as the eyelids are opened after prolonged closure. There may be a sudden severe pain for which treatment is necessary. The incident can recur, and the resumption of contact lens wear should be delayed for several months. On resumption, the area must be inspected with care following the first few periods of re-use for any signs of further detachment.

Healed erosions from which small areas of regenerated corneal epithelium may spontaneously detach, may show a narrow line or spot of brilliant stain where fluorescein is lodged beneath or within the adjacent basal epithelial cells. Bowman's layer from which the cells have detached will not stain but any local damaged cells will. Medical treatment is necessary. Several months' rest from contact lens wear may be advised.

Epithelial Deformations

Surface Irregularity

Surface irregularity of the corneal epithelium has already been explained. Its detection, corrrection and avoidance is an important aspect of after-care. Identification may be by slit lamp microscopy, ophthalmoscopy, keratometry or retinoscopy (*see* Sections F1(*b*), G1, H2 and I2 respectively). Its significance in the production of spectacle blur and in the prescribing of spectacles has been discussed in Sections J1 and 2 on page 510 and in Chapter 17. Other surface deformations – epithelial dimples, rings and waves – are less significant because they recover very rapidly, but they should be corrected by modifying the lens fitting if possible.

Epithelial Dimples

A small bubble trapped beneath a contact lens is, in effect, a smooth foreign body. The smaller the bubble the more resistant it is to deformation, and it will quickly indent the less resistant surface of the corneal epithelium, producing a small circular dimple. More frequently a cluster of tiny bubbles, or froth, forms to produce a mosaic of indentations (*see Colour Plate IV*, Volume 1). They occur in areas where the lens arcs clear of the cornea to form a closed retrolental tears pool. Sometimes the indentations are oval or linear in shape and radially arranged. If they overlap the pupillary area, there is visual interference (termed 'dimple veil') when the lens is removed. After lens removal, the indentations and the mild discomfort and conjunctival injection which may accompany them fade rapidly. They hold fluorescein but also may exhibit true SPEE stains. Attention to the lens fitting is required (*see* Chapters 9, 10 and 11, Volume 1, and Chapter 14). They may occur with any form of contact lens and are not intrinsically harmful.

Epithelial Rings

Rapid dimpling and recovery is an indication that the surface of the epithelium has plastic properties. If a corneal lens becomes completely static on a cornea for a long period and is then removed, an impression of the lens on the cornea may be found where the lens has been. It is rare for a lens to be sufficiently static for this to occur but, if an impression is taken of the eye, the indentation is sufficient to leave a clearly discernible ring on a cast of the cornea. An indentation of the full thickness of the cornea has been observed. Bron and Tripathi (1970) have shown that if the cornea is rubbed through the eyelids a net-like pattern is produced in the epithelium, which they have suggested is due to ridges on the surface of Bowman's membrane.

A more serious condition is that of the epithelial ring seen in patients complaining of pain from soft lens wear. It is shown in *Colour Plate XXIa*. The ring does not stain and lies slightly proud of the epithelial surface. Its location can change from week to week; it can expand or contract. It probably represents a collection of inflammatory cells. This condition continues for months and the eye is painful and red. There is no associated iritis but a stromal keratitis may develop (Mackie, 1978). It should not be confused with the endothelial ring (*Colour Plate XXIb*) which also follows soft lens wear and is described on page 519. Discontinuation of lens wear is imperative in both cases, until the condition has resolved, and ophthalmological supervision of treatment is essential.

Arcuate Epithelial Waves

Not only is the epithelium compressible but it will also swell. After a corneal lens has been removed from the eye, epithelial swelling is frequently found in the region previously covered by the peripheral part of the lens. When a lens has been riding high on the cornea, arcuate swelling occurs inferiorly; if the lens has ridden low, it occurs superiorly. These are regions where the peripheral part of the lens has stood away from the cornea. The tendency for these corneal surface deformations to develop varies greatly from one patient to another, but it is usually bilateral. They fade quickly when the lens is removed and appear to be harmless. Whether these swellings should be ascribed to epithelial oedema, as explained by Wilson (1970), or to a mechanical bunching of the epithelium at the periphery of a compressed area is not clear; but since they occur frequently in a region in which corneal oedema is rarely seen, the latter hypothesis seems the most acceptable. Epithelial proliferation of this nature may be seen with the slit lamp in cases of keratoconus immediately surrounding the cone when the latter has been subjected to pressure by a contact lens, but the milder bunching postulated here has not been so positively identified. Similar linear swellings may be seen in non-contact-lens wearers where the lid margins have rested against the cornea.

CHANGES IN THE CORNEAL STROMA, LIMBUS AND ENDOTHELIUM

Corneal oedema and changes in the corneal epithelium are the normal accompaniment of a contact lens wear and should present no hazard, given good routine case management and adequate hygiene during the adaptation period and thereafter. The epithelial surfaces of the eye can withstand most contact lens trauma, they regenerate rapidly and heal perfectly (*see* Chapter 2, Volume 1). When lenses are removed the eye recovers totally and quickly (but *see* Corneal Oedema following Soft Lens Wear on page 513, and SPEE Associated with Soft Lens Wear on page 516).

If, however, the epithelial surfaces are breached a true keratopathy with associated ocular responses can quickly develop and the condition is immediately more serious. Healing is slower, it is seldom perfect and there are always disagreeable symptoms. Medical supervision is essential. Subsequent refitting from a different lens form, or even a prolonged rest from contact lens wear, may be necessary (*see* Advice to the Patient on page 511).

The management of keratopathy is not within the terms of reference of this textbook but the early detection of the premonitory symptoms and signs associated with contact lens use is. Although already covered in the routine re-examination (*see* page 507, Section F1(*c*) to (*f*)) the following notes are added by way of emphasis.

Conjunctival Injection, Proliferation of the Limbal Arcades and Stromal Vascularization

Conjunctival injection associated with contact lens use can follow from eyelid margin irritation (*see* page 449, Section B1, Head and Eyelid Posture), oedema, and, of course, from any corneal irritation, but it is most likely to occur if a predisposing benign palpebral disease (*see below*) is already present. Both bulbar and palpebral conjunctiva may be affected.

Limbal vascular injection, proliferation of the limbal arcades and stromal vascularization are successively more serious sequelae of corneal irritation and/or disturbed corneal metabolism (*see Colour Plate VII*, Volume 1). They may all be seen by direct illumination, though old corneal 'ghost' vessels in which there is no blood flow (not to be confused with the corneal nerves) show well by retro-illumination or by sclerotic scatter. The primary cause induced by contact lens wear is restriction of the tears flow over the cornea, producing anoxia which causes oedema and leads eventually to a compensating increase in the blood supply. The ocular area involved is greater when scleral lenses or soft lenses are worn than with corneal lenses, consequently the final sequel of stromal vascularization is rarely found with corneal lenses. Refitting is essential (*see* Chapters 9, 10 and 11, Volume 1, and Chapter 14).

Stromal Infiltration and Striae

Stromal infiltration by leucocytes is a natural response to infection but may also be seen when the limbal vessels have been continuously engorged for a long period of time, as, for example, in association with 3 and 9 o'clock staining with corneal lens wear, and continuous slight oedema with soft lenses (*see* page 513). The infiltration is a precursor to vascularization and is visible as a stromal haze. In the experience of the author it is liable to occur approximately 1 mm internal to the superior limbus as an arcuate band in the area where the upper lid margin bears on the cornea through a soft lens. It has been termed (by Wilson, 1974, in a case report) a marginal keratitis. Recovery is slow. Areas of infiltration may also surround a deep epithelial abrasion (*see* page 516) which reaches down to the basal layers. The presence of infiltration of the stroma may be seen with the slit lamp. *Colour Plate XIX* shows a typical appearance. Its presence should indicate urgent attention to the fit of the lenses or possible discontinuation of lens wear. If infection is suspected medical advice must be sought.

Small, circular patches or nebulae, about 1 mm in diameter or less, sometimes occur in the superficial stroma along with diffuse punctate epithelial erosions and conjunctival injection. Only the epithelial erosions stain with fluorescein. The patient complains of mild discomfort and a red eye, and possibly a slight drop in visual acuity. The condition is like nummular keratitis and occasionally follows overwear of a soft lens, or occurs following a long period of wear of a soft lens during which there has been a mild degree of corneal oedema but the patient has been symptom-free. Removal of the contact lenses results in the disappearance of the small nebulae within 2–3 days, but the superficial epithelial erosions may not completely heal for up to 2 months, during which time the lenses should not be worn. The condition is shown in *Colour Plate XXII*.

Corneal striae are probably in the posterior stroma, or at the level of Descemet's membrane. They are always vertical or almost so. According to Sturrock (1973) glassy striae ocur in 85 per cent of normal subjects, the incidence being greater with age. They are fine translucent white streaks, rather like corneal nerve fibres when seen with the slit lamp by either direct or retro-illumination as shown in *Colour Plate XXX*. They appear almost as if etched and are easily missed. In soft lens wearers their presence is usually associated with oedema, they then disappear if digital pressure is applied to the globe (Kerns, 1974). It is thought that generalized corneal swelling associated with soft lens wear leads to a swelling of the cornea posteriorly into the anterior chamber thereby causing the back surface of the cornea to fold or buckle (Wechsler, 1974).

Stromal Vascularization and Scarring

Encroachment of limbal vascularization into the stroma of the cornea may occur as a result of limbal drying (for example, at 3 and 9 o'clock, *Colour Plate VII*, Volume 1) or following prolonged oedema associated with soft lens wear (*Colour Plate XXXI*), or even due to dessication of the cornea caused by an immobile bubble under a scleral lens. In all cases it is a natural 'defence mechanism' reaction, but requires attention to the fit of the lenses and medication to reduce vascularization. Stromal scarring and thinning may follow central oedema, ulceration, folds, keratoconus and all forms of keratitis.

Endothelial Folds

Obvious horizontal arcuate folds of the endothelium at the corneal apex have been seen in the presence of a dense stromal haze in an oedema-prone male patient following 6 hours use of medium water content (39 per cent hydrated w/v) soft lenses. Folds did not occur with high water content (68 per cent) material but 8 hours only was the maximum wear period which could be achieved in comfort. It is possible that the striate corneal lines first described by Sarver (1971) are of this character (*see Colour Plate XXX*).

Changes in the corneal endothelium may be observed and photographed by the technique of specular microscopy (Sherrard, 1977), provided that the corneal stroma is not oedematous. In the United States, the FDA has recommended that this technique is carried out in investigations on wearers of 'continuous' or 'extended' wear soft lenses. However, this technique requires applanation of the cornea, which may itself cause slight damage to the cornea, so that a newer slit lamp photographic technique developed by Holden and Zantos (1977) may well supersede it. They have reported the formation of transient endothelial blebs as a result of contact lens wear, observed by this method.

An acute phenomenon following soft lens wear is the appearance of an endothelial ring, as shown in *Colour Plate XXIb*. The endothelium surrounding the ring is bedewed and there is a fusiform swelling where the endothelium is apparently absent. Apparent endothelial restoration occurs within 48 hours, very much as in the case of traumatic posterior annular keratopathy (Forstot and Gasset, 1974).

BENIGN PALPEBRAL DISEASES WHICH MAY BE CONTRA-INDICATIONS FOR CONTACT LENS WEAR

The contra-indications for contact lens wearing have been dealt with in Chapter 7, Volume 1. The following benign ocular diseases are now mentioned since they do not immediately cause symptoms when lenses are first used in most cases and are frequently overlooked until the after-care stage is reached, which can be embarrassing to both patient and practitioner.

Folliculosis and Follicular Conjunctivitis

Folliculosis, a non-inflammatory condition of unknown aetiology affecting mainly the lower eyelid; and follicular conjunctivitis, which is probably viral in origin and occurs on both eyelids, especially in the angles, are chronic infections which are very difficult to cure and usually cause no trouble either to practitioner or patient – until, that is, contact lenses are worn.

Unless the eyelids are everted to permit inspection of the palpebral surface of the conjunctiva, the presence of follicles will probably not have been detected in a spectacle wearer; but every time the wearer of a hard contact lens rubs the edge of the lens against them by blinking or turning the eye, pain ensues followed by palpebral injection, a sensation of burning with photophobia and a tendency for the eyes to close.

The symptoms may be alleviated by using very small, thin lenses and sometimes by treatment designed to reduce the irritability of the follicles, but fitting is always difficult. Sometimes the symptoms are mild in the early stages of the adaptation period, and difficulty is not experienced until the wearing time has increased to beyond 8 hours per day. Then the follicles become sensitive and there is a fairly sharp reduction to 3 hours or less, which is difficult to reverse. A complete rest from contact lens wear for 6 months or longer may bring success. Alternatively, the patient may be refitted with soft lenses. The yielding edge of the soft material causes less mechanical irritation to the follicles and many hard lens failures have been successfully refitted in this way (Hodd, 1973). Allansmith et al. (1977), however, have described a form of giant papillary conjunctivitis, in which follicular formation of the tarsal conjunctiva, mucous discomfort and wearing difficulties develop in successful soft lens wearers (Colour Plate XX). This appears to be an allergic type reaction which may disappear on lens cleaning or replacement, indicating deposits on the lens as the antigen. The affected eyelid develops slight ptosis due to its swollen state and drags the soft lens upwards so that poor and variable vision may be the first complaint. Mackie (1977) has also described this condition, as well as a number of others caused by soft lens wear.

Serous Cysts of the Glands of Moll

Small serous cysts on the posterior margin of the lid, seldom bigger than1 millimetre in diameter, normal-ly disappear without treatment within a few weeks. They are entirely non-inflammatory and cause no comment or discomfort until a corneal lens is worn. Curiously, even when they are situated on a part of the eyelid remote from the position of the corneal lens, the patient is still aware of their presence. Treatment designed to break them by puncture or pressure may help, but thermal cautery is a more permanent cure. The discomfort is a soreness or irritation which, unlike a corneal irritation, is readily localized by the patient.

Hay Fever and Nasal Catarrh

Hay fever and nasal catarrh produce an over-secretion of nasal mucus with oedema of the mucosa and may involve the conjunctiva similarly. When this occurs the presence of a contact lens may become intolerable. Hay fever sufferers should be warned of the possible occurrence of symptoms during early summer when high pollen counts are recorded.

Other Diseases of the Eyelids

Other non-inflammatory space-occupying pathology of the eyelids such as sebaceous cysts, benign melanomata and chalasia seldom cause symptoms, but inflammatory conditions such as blepharitis, unless very mild, and hordeola do. Appropriate medical treatment should be advised.

In recent years the lens of first choice in the presence of any space occupying, non-inflammatory pathology of the eyelids or of the conjunctiva is the soft lens, provided that regular and complete after-care checks are carried out.

Table 16.1–Summary of Symptomatology

Presenting symptoms	Principal clinical considerations	Page No. and section or paragraph
(A) Poor vision		
(1) Constant	(a) Ocular disease	497, A1; 498, A5(g); 502, C2
	(b) Refraction with lenses in situ	499, A5(c); 500, C1; 502, C2; 510, I3
	(c) Incorrect lens power	503, E1 & 2; 504, E5
	(d) Switched lenses	503, E1
	(e) Residual astigmatism	502, C1
	(f) Loss of lens or displaced lens	498 and see E5, page 504

Table 16.1 (*cont.*)–Summary of Symptomatology

Presenting symptoms	Principal clinical considerations	Page No. and section or paragraph
(2) Variable	(a) Back or front optic small	498, A5(a); 503, D2
	(b) Lens too mobile or eccentric	500, B2; 502, C2
	(c) Lens dirty or damaged	498, A5(d); 500, B2; 504, E3
	(d) Binocular instability	499, A5(e); 500, C1
	(e) Lens distortion or flexure	504, 523, C1; 500
	(f) Discomfort giving lacrimation	499, A5(f); 502, C2; 504, E3
	(g) Poorly fitted soft lens	520, 500, C1; 503, D6, 7 & 8
(3) Deteriorates in use	(a) Corneal oedema	498, A5(b); 506, 512, 513
	(b) Refraction with lenses *in situ*	500, C1; 502, C2
	(c) Frothing	503, D5; 517
	(d) Tears insufficient, too oily or mucous	499, A5(d); 500, B2; 504, E3; 507, F3
(4) Sudden loss	(a) Ocular disease	497, A1; 499, A5(g)
	(b) Displaced or lost lens	498, A4
	(c) Lacrimation especially from a foreign body	515
(5) Spectacle blur	(a) Induced corneal irregularity	510, J1
	(b) Corneal oedema	498, A5(b); 506, 512, 513
(6) Photophobia	(a) Corneal oedema	498, A5(b); 512, 513
	(b) Ocular disease	498, A4; 520

(B) Pain

(1) Sudden onset and rapid recovery	(a) Foreign body beneath lens	515
	(b) Incompatible soaking or wetting solution	504, E3; 515
	(c) Other exogenous irritants	504, E3
(2) Sudden onset and persistent	(a) Deep epithelial abrasion	507, F2 & 4; 516
	(b) Foreign body embedded in cornea	507, F2 & 4; 516
	(c) Damaged lens	504, E4; 516
	(d Recurrent epithelial erosion	517
	(e) Acute ocular pathology	497, A1; 498; A3; 498, A4
(3) Gradual onset and persistent	(a) Epithelial ring	517
(4) Severe, a few hours after removal	(a) Over-wear syndrome	514
(5) Asthenopia	(a) Ametropia	500, C1
	(b) Oculomotor disorder	500 & 502, C1
	(c) Uncorrected presbyopia	500, C1; Chapter 19

(C) Discomfort

(1) Burning sensation and lacrimation	(a) Corneal erosion (SPEE) or abrasion	511, 515, 516
	(b) Corneal drying	507, F3; 516
	(c) Excess pressure of lens on cornea	503, D2; 514, 515
	(b) Lens dirty or damaged	497, A1; 500, B2; 504, E3; 504, E4
	(e) Chemical contamination of the lens	504, E3; 515
	(f) Back central optic too large in a corneal lens	502, C2; 503, D2
	(g) Lens too static	503, D1 and D7; 517

Table 16.1 (*cont.*)–Summary of Symptomatology

Presenting symptoms	Principal clinical considerations	Page No. and section or paragraph
	(*h*) Hay fever, nasal catarrh	520
	(*i*) Folliculosis	519
	(*j*) Allergy to soft lens storage solution	515
	(*c*), (*f*) and (*g*) are often associated with corneal oedema which, in turn, is associated with insufficient tears exchange beneath the lens.)	*see* A3(*a*), (*d*); and 5(*b*); page 498
(2) When blinking	(*a*) Lens edge shape poor or standing too clear of cornea	499, B1; 503, D1, 3, 5, 6, 27; 504 E4 and 5
	(*b*) Lens too mobile or too low	503, D1 to 9
	(*c*) Eyelid disease	508, F5; 519, 520
	(*d*) Lenses switched if fittings differ	503, E1
	(*e*) Lens edge or transition too sharp	499, B1; 504, E5; 515
	(*f*) Foreign body protruding from cornea	516
	(*g*) Folliculosis	519
(D) Red eye	As for (B) and (C) above	
(E) Lens management		
(1) Loss of ability to place lens on eye	(*a*) Reduced incentive	497, A2; 498, A3
	(*b*) Development of pathology including psychopathology	497, A2
	(*c*) Result of (A) to (D) above	*see* (A) to (D) above
(2) Loss of ability to remove lens	(*a*) As E1 but less frequently found	
	(*b*) Dehydrating or hypotonic hydrophilic lens	504
(3) Loss of tolerance	(*a*) Oedema prone	498, A3; 498, A5(*b*)
	(*b*) Palpebral disease, especially folliculosis	519
	(*c*) Result of (A) to (D) above	*see* (A) to (D) above
(4) Dirty lens	(*a*) Scratched lens	504, E3
	(*b*) Excess mucus in tears	507, F3
	(*c*) Dry eye	504, E3; 507, F3; 516
	(*d*) Conjunctivitis	498, A4; 516, 518
	(*e*) Catarrh	520
	(*f*) Poor blinking	499, B1; 516
	(*g*) Poor hygiene	500, B2; 504, E3
(5) Loss of lens from eye	(*a*) Lens too small	503, D1 to 3, 6 and 7
	(*b*) Lens edge too thick	499, B1; 504, E5
	(*c*) Lens too heavy	504, E5
	(*d*) Patient behaviour	497
	(*e*) Not patient's lens	504, E5
	(*f*) Lens fitted flat	503, D1, 2, 3, 6, 7 and 8
	(*g*) Rough lens surface	504
	(*h*) Soft lens dehydrated or inside out	503, D6 to 9; 503, E2

The above summary is for guidance only. It is not intended to be exhaustive. Nevertheless, the clinical considerations touch on most of the techniques both of initial contact lens fitting and of general ocular and refractive examination. Actions to be taken under the heading Principal Clinical Considerations require knowledge and experience, not only of the whole of the techniques, facilities and equipment described in this book but also of the general studies of which they are a part and from which they are derived. Action detail is too interrelated to be usefully tabulated. Practical experience is essential to its mastery.

It is frequently asserted that, while the provision and fitting of contact lenses is the province of the specialist practitioner, after-care should be the province of the general ocular practitioner. It is also asserted that fitting may be referred to a skilled fitter by a responsible practitioner provided that the patient is referred back at the conclusion of fitting (General Optical Council, Notice to Opticians, N15, 1977). To the author, it appears that these frequently heard assertions are made more in an endeavour to satisfy the prestige of those who make them than in the interests of patient protection. Fitting and after-care are not separable operations for separated operators. After-care to fitting is as a bloom to a plant – neither can flourish without the other.

ADDENDUM ON SOFT LENS FLEXURE
by M. W. Ford

Many people have been baffled initially by the statement that both positive and negative hydrophilic lenses acquire additional negative power if their surface radii are shortened by applying them to a cornea having a steeper radius of curvature than the back surface of the lens. (This is the method of fitting used for the vast majority of soft contact lenses – see Chapter 14.)

The statement appears to be illogical as it implies that the front surface radius shortens appreciably less than the back surface radius. That this differential change in radii does, in fact, occur has been established by Bennett (1976) and explained with the pellucidity which is now expected of him.

The explanation depends on the acceptance of two assumptions, the first of which is already widely accepted, particularly in the case of lenses having a water content of 40 per cent or more, and the second of which is supported by a mathematical analysis by Wichterle (1967) of the forces and resultant stresses involved when a hydrogel lens is not in its relaxed state. The two basic assumptions are: (1) that the back surface of the lens assumes the contour of the cornea; and (2) that there is no significant redistribution of lens substance during flexure.

From these assumptions it follows that: (a) the centre thickness and the volume of the lens remain unchanged; and (b) the front surface of the lens remains spherical if the cornea is spherical.

Although it can be argued that none of the above assumptions is absolutely correct, mathematical considerations show that the errors introduced by their acceptance are of an insignificant order (Wichterle, 1967; Bennett, 1970, 1976).

In order to assist calculation a positive lens of knife-edge form is taken as an example, but the same arguments can be applied to a lens of any specified edge thickness.

Example 1: A lens has BOR 9.50 mm, 0S 14.50 mm, BVP +6.00 D, $n = 1.44$. This lens must have t_c 0.616 mm and front optic radius 8.599 mm to give a knife edge (Jalie, 1974) (*see Figure 16.1*).

The volume of this lens can be calculated, as explained by Bennett (1976), by subtracting the volume of the spherical cap bounded by the back surface from the volume of the spherical cap bounded by the front surface. Now, volume of spherical cap = $\pi/3 \, (3r - s) \, s^2$ where r = radius and s = sag.

For the unstressed lens defined above, the volumes are thus:

Front spherical cap	= 361.113 mm³
Back spherical cap	= 297.379 mm³
Volume of lens, thus	= 63.734 mm³

If this lens is applied to a spherical cornea of radius 8.00 mm, the semi-diameter, y (7.25 mm) is reduced to some new value y' and since the BCOR is assumed to equal the corneal radius, the sag s_2' of the new back surface, can be calculated, as therefore can the volume. Because (for a knife-edge lens), $s_1' = s_2' + t_c$ and the semi-diameter y' is common to both front and back surfaces (*see Figure 16.1*), the new front surface radius r_1' is readily obtainable from the general expression relating radius to sag and semi-diameter, namely,

$$(r = \frac{y^2 + s^2}{2s}).$$

The volume of the new front surface spherical cap can also be readily calculated.

The value of y' must be found iteratively, the correct value being the one which gives the flexed lens the same volume as the unstressed lens. In Example 1 $y' = 6.9$ mm, $r'_1 = 7.496$ mm, BVP = +5.21 D, showing a power change of –0.79 D.

After steepening the volumes become:

Front spherical cap	= 391.951 mm³
Back spherical cap	= 328.217 mm³
Flexed lens (= that of unstressed lens)	
	63.734 mm³

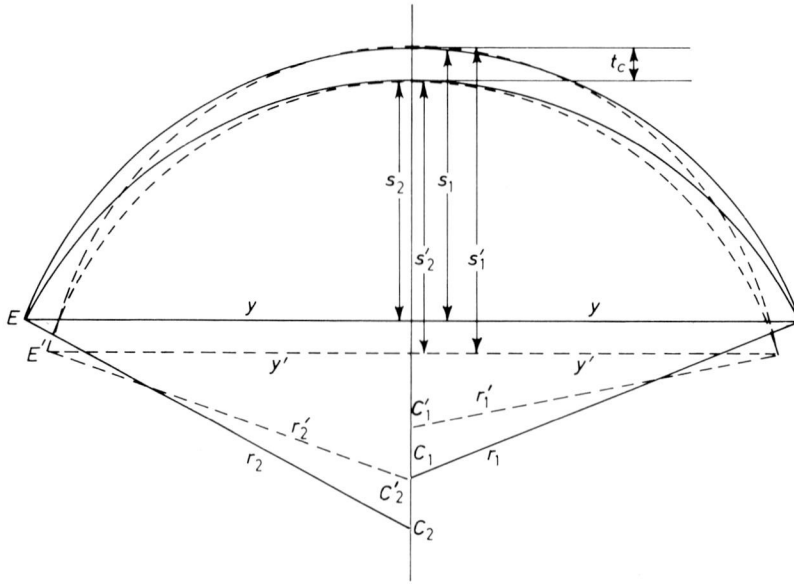

Figure 16.1–Steepening of a positive soft lens with knife edge: solid line before steepening and broken line after steepening. Before steepening: edge E, centres of curvature of front and back surfaces C_1 and C_2 with their radii of curvature r_1 and r_2 and sagitta s_1 and s_2 respectively, and semi-diameter y. After steepening these become: E', C_1', C_2', r_1', r_2', s_1', s_2' and y' respectively. Centre thickness t_c is the same before and after steepening

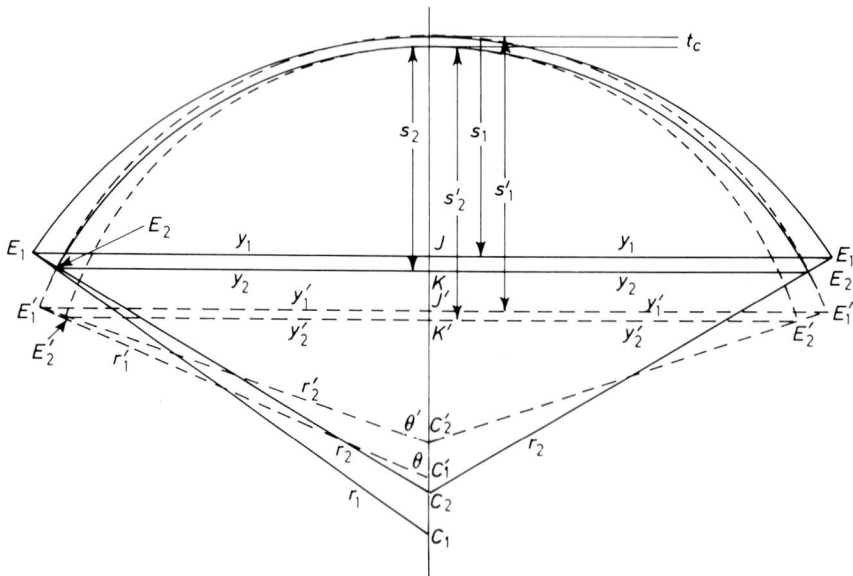

Figure 16.2–Steepening of a negative soft lens: solid line before steepening and broken line after steepening. Before steepening: front and back surface edges E_1 and E_2 with semi-diameters y_1 and y_2 intersecting the primary axis at J and K and subtending an angle θ at C_2. After steepening these become: E_1', E_2', y_1', y_2', J', K', and θ' at C_2' respectively. Other symbols are as in Figure 16.1

From the above it can be seen that whereas the BCOR has shortened by 1.5 mm (from 9.5 to 8.0 mm) the front optic radius has shortened by only 1.103 mm. If both radii had shortened by 1.5 mm the volume of the lens would have increased to:

Front spherical cap	= 490.939 mm^3
Back spherical cap	= 328.217 mm^3
Volume of lens, thus	= 167.722 mm^3(!),

and the centre thickness would have increased to 1.483 mm!

Clearly, if the front surface radius steepened more than the BCOR, both volume and centre thickness would increase to an even more ridiculous extent.

The differential change in radii which does occur can be envisaged by going back to FLOM fitting (*see* Chapter 10, Volume 1) and thinking of the effect on sag when shortening the radius. For a given change of radius the sag is altered more when the radius is steep than when it is flat (*see* Appendix C, Volume 1).

Because the front surface radius of a positive contact lens is shorter than that of the back surface, the front radius must alter substantially less than the back optic radius if the volume and thickness of the lens are to remain the same.

The values used in calculating the above example and another example using a steeper cornea are listed below in case they may be of interest. Linear values are in mm, the volumes of the front and back spherical caps, V_1 and V_2 respectively and the volume of the lens, V, are in mm^3. Back vertex powers (BVP) are used throughout. The power changes shown below agree with the findings of Bennett (1976) as shown in *Table 4.10*, Chapter 4, Volume 1, page 111.

Parameter	Unstressed	Flexed	Change
t_c	0.616	0.616	Nil
BCOR	9.50	8.00	1.50
y	7.25	6.90	0.35
BVP	+6.00	+5.21	−0.79
r_1	8.599	7.496	1.103
s_1	3.975	4.570	0.595
s_2	3.361	3.954	0.593
V_1	361.113	391.951	30.838
V_2	297.379	328.217	30.838
V	63.734	63.734	Nil

Example 2: BCOR 8.00 mm, OS 12.00 mm, BVP +10.00 D, $n = 1.44$, t_c 0.7028 mm, FOR 6.984 mm.

t_c	0.7028	0.7028	Nil
BCOR	8.00	7.00	1.00
y	6.00	5.792	0.208
BVP	+10.00	+9.059	−0.941
r_1	6.984	6.333	0.651
s_1	3.409	3.771	0.362
s_2	2.708	3.069	0.361
V_1	213.564	226.862	13.298
V_2	163.565	176.863	13.298
V	49.9989	49.9989	Nil

Negative lenses are treated in much the same way, except that edge thickness must be taken into account, and so it is necessary for the convenience of calculation to make one further assumption. It is assumed that the lens has a conical edge, with the apex of the cone at C_2 (*see Figure 16.2*). The edge E_1E_2 is therefore normal to the back surface and it is assumed that E_1E_2 and its relationship to the back surface remain unchanged after flexure.

The volume of the lens is the volume of the front spherical cap plus the volume of the frustum of the cone bounded by E_1E_2, minus the volume of the back spherical cap. (Volume of frustum of cone = $\pi/3$ (y_1^2 . JC$_2$) − (y_2^2 . KC$_2$) and $\theta = \sin^{-1} y_2/r_2$ (Bennett, 1976)).

Hydrophilic lenses acquire additional positive power if they are flattened. The change of power due to flexure =

$$\frac{-(n-1)}{(n)} t_c \left(\frac{1}{(r^1_2 2)} - \frac{1}{r_2 2} \right)$$

(n = refractive index and other symbols are as in *Figure 16.1.*)

It is evident from the above formula that the change of power due to flexure is dependent on refractive index, centre thickness and the degree of bending and is independent of the original BVP (Bennett, 1976).

ACKNOWLEDGEMENT

I am indebted to several colleagues who have made helpful suggestions in the preparation of this chapter and in particular to Miss Janet Stone, Mr M. S. Wilson and Mr I. A. Mackie.

REFERENCES

Allansmith, M. R., Korb, D. R., Greiner, J. V., Henriquez, A. S., Simon, M. A. and Finnemore, V. M. (1977). 'Giant papillary conjunctivitis in contact lens wearers.' *Am. J. Ophthal.* **83**, 697–708

Bennett, A. G. (1970). 'Variable and progressive power lenses: 1.' *Optician* **160**, 421–427

Bennett, A. G. (1976). 'Power changes in soft contact lenses due to bending.' *Ophthal. Optician* **16**, 939–945

Boyd, H. H. (1969). 'Enlightened concepts in contact lens medical practice.' *Highlts Ophthal.* **12**, 140–163

Bron, A. J. and Tripathi, R. C. (1970). 'The anterior corneal mosaic.' *Br. J. physiol. Optics* **25**, 8–13

Dallos, J. (1946). 'Sattler's veil.' *Br. J. Ophthal.* **30**, 607–613

Danker, F. (1977). Personal communication to one of the editors (Janet Stone)

Ford, M. W. (1974). 'Changes in hydrophilic lenses when placed on an eye.' Paper read at the joint International Congress of The Contact Lens Society and The National Eye Research Foundation. Montreux, Switzerland

Ford, M. W. (1976). 'Computation of the back vertex powers of hydrophilic lenses.' Paper read at the Interdisciplinary Conference on Contact Lenses, Department of Ophthalmic Optics and Visual Science, The City University, London

Forstot, S. L. and Gasset, A. R. (1974). 'Transient traumatic posterior annular keratopathy of Payrau.' *Archs Ophthal.* **92**, 527–528

General Optical Council (1977). *Notice for the Guidance of the Profession (Notice N. 15)*, p. 21

Girard, L. J. (1964). *Corneal Contact Lenses*. St. Louis, Missouri: Mosby

Greenberg, M. H. and Hill, R. M. (1973). 'The physiology of contact lens imprints.' *Am. J. Optom.* **50**, 699–702

Hill, R. M. and Greenberg, M. H. (1976). 'The pressure response to contact lenses.' *Contact Lens Forum* July, 49–51

Hill, R. M. and Leighton, A. J. (1965). 'Temperature changes of human cornea and tears under a contact lens.' *Am. J. Optom.* **42**, 9–16, 71–77, 584–588

Hill, R. M. and Terry, J. E. (1976). 'Human tear cholesterol levels.' *Archs Ophthal. (Paris)* **36**, 155–160

Hodd, F. A. B. (1973). 'The use of hydrophilic contact lenses for hard lens problem cases.' *Optician* **166**(4304), 16, 18, 20, 27, 33

Holden, B. A. and Zantos, S. (1977). 'Australians discover endothelial bleb.' Report in *Optician* **174**(4513), 15–16

Kerns, R. L. (1974). 'A study of striae observed in the cornea from contact lens wear.' *Am. J. Optom.* **51**, 998–1004

Koetting, R. A. (1976a). 'Tear film break-up time as a factor in hydrogel lens coating – a preliminary study.' *Contacto* **20**(3), 20–23

Koetting, R. A. (1976b). 'Predicting soft lens surface problems.' *Contact Lens Forum* October, 18–21

Korb, D. R. and Korb, J. E. (1974). 'Fitting to achieve a normal blinking and lid action.' *Internat. Contact Lens Clin.* **1**(3), 57–70

Mackie, I. A. (1967). 'Lesions at the corneal limbus at 3 o'clock and 9 o'clock in association with the wearing of contact lenses.' In *Contact Lenses, XXth International Congress of Ophthalmology Symposium*, pp. 66–73. Munich–Feldafing, August 13th, 1966, ed. by Dabiezes, O. H., Laue, H., Schlossman, A. and Halberg, G. P. Basel and New York: Karger

Mackie, I. A. (1975). Paper read to Scandinavian Contact Lens Society, May, Oslo, Norway

Mackie, I. A. (1977). 'Complications of soft lenses.' Paper read at Summer Clinical Conference of the British Contact Lens Association, April, 1977, Torquay, Devon

Mackie, I. A. (1978). Personal communication

Miller, D., Wolf, E., Geer, S. and Vassallo, V. (1967). 'Glare sensitivity related to use of contact lenses.' *Archs Ophthal.* **78**, 448–450

Millodot, M. (1976). 'Effect of the length of wear of contact lenses on corneal sensitivity.' *Acta Ophthal.* **54**, 721–730

Norn, M. S. (1964). 'Vital staining in practice using a mixed stain and alcian blue.' *Br. J. physiol. Optics* **21**, 293–298

Sarver, M. D. (1971). 'Striate corneal lines among patients wearing hydrophilic contact lenses.' *Am. J. Optom.* **48**, 762–763

Sherrard, E. S. (1977). 'Specular microscopy of the corneal endothelium.' *Ophthal. Optician* **17**, 709–710, 712–713

Sturrock, G. (1973). 'Glassy corneal striae.' *V. Graefe's Archs für Klin. Exp. Ophthal.* **188**, 245–252

Terry, J. E. and Hill, R. M. (1975). 'Cholesterol: blood and tears.' *J. Am. optom. Ass.* **46**, 1171–1174

Wechsler, S. (1974). 'Striate corneal lines.' *Am. J. Optom.* **51**, 852–856

Wilson, M. S. (1970). 'Corneal oedema from corneal contact lens wear, its causes and treatment.' *Trans. ophthal. Soc. U.K.* **90**, 31–45

Wilson, M. S. (1974). Cited by Hodd, F. A. B. (1974). 'A clinical comparison of soft lens materials currently in use in the U.K.' *Optician* **168**(4342), 13, 15–17, 20

Chapter 17

Refractive Changes After Wearing Contact Lenses

R. H. Rengstorff

Through many studies and clinical observations a great deal is known about the effects of polymethyl methacrylate (PMMA) corneal lenses since they became popular over 25 years ago. Far less is known about the effects of lenses made from some of the new materials, for example, hydrogels, especially effects that may occur after wearing such lenses more than 1 year. Hydrogel lenses do cause refractive changes during the adaptation period, but comparisons between PMMA and the newer lens materials are difficult to make without further study.

What is known about refractive changes after wearing PMMA contact lenses will be reviewed from the following aspects.

(1) Temporal variables.
(2) Changes in corneal curvature.
(3) Relationship between changes in refraction and changes in corneal curvature.

TEMPORAL VARIABLES

Some contact lens wearers experience blurred vision when they temporarily remove their lenses and wear spectacles (*see* page 510, Chapter 16). According to many early reports in the 1950's, the blur generally lasts from minutes to hours. This is particularly common during the adaptation period and can be attributed to temporary corneal distortion and epithelial oedema. Another type of blurred and variable vision occurs among persons adapted to contact lenses when they resort to wearing their spectacles. This may persist for many weeks and is caused by refractive changes (Rengstorff, 1965a).

Knowledge of these changes is important. From a practical point of view, refractive changes affect the practitioner's ability to prescribe satisfactory spectacle lenses. From a theoretical point of view,

refractive changes may be controlled for therapeutic purposes such as reducing or eliminating certain refractive conditions. Basic to these considerations are the findings that refractive changes follow orderly and specific patterns. One such pattern refers to short-term changes (circadian variations), occurring from day to day as the individual normally wears contact lenses. Another pattern refers to long-term changes (withdrawal variations), occurring for days and weeks after wearing is discontinued.

Both short-term and long-term changes occur after wearing contact lenses for at least 1 year. During adaptation to contact lenses there is usually an increase of about 0.50 D more myopia (Carney, 1975a), but little information is available about refractive changes when lenses are worn for less than 1 year. Therefore, most of the material in this chapter pertains to individuals who have worn contact lenses 1 year or longer.

Another consideration is the method of determining refractive error. After removal of contact lenses, many long-term habitual wearers respond poorly to subjective testing, and they cannot discriminate lens changes as can persons who do not wear contact lenses. This may persist for many days after they remove their contact lenses (Rengstorff, 1965a, 1966). Arner (1970) likened the subjective testing of some of these individuals 'to examining a bilateral amblyope with metamorphopsia and low intelligence'. The best method to determine refractive error is by careful subjective testing and not by retinoscopic measurements which are in many cases unreliable when corneal distortion is present (Rengstorff, 1965a) (*see* page 509, Chapter 16). A recommended procedure to determine refractive error is to monocularly blur vision with a lens +2.00 D over the retinoscopic or other objective measurement and reduce the lens power in 0.50 D steps until the subject can read 6/12 (20/40) letters. Additional reductions in 0.25 D steps are made until he attains the best visual acuity with the minimum of concave lens. Cross-cylinder and astigmatic chart testing are used to measure astigmatism.

SHORT-TERM CHANGES (CIRCADIAN VARIATIONS)

Overnight: Myopia Decreases While Lenses Are Not Worn

Contact lens wearers frequently describe improved unaided visual acuity after arising in the morning. Saks (1966) reported this occurrence and other studies (Rengstorff, 1970a, b) confirmed the improvements, showing them to be caused by a measurable decrease in myopia. The improvements occurred among myopic men, aged 20–27 years, who had worn contact lenses 12 hours or more daily for at least 1 year. All individuals showed consistent overnight decreases in myopia ranging from 0.25 to 1.50 D. Changes were smaller when contact lenses were not worn all waking hours.

Astigmatism Increases Slightly Overnight While Lenses Are Not Worn

Subjective tests for astigmatism on 10 habitual contact lens wearers at 11 p.m. and 7 a.m. revealed a slight trend towards increased with-the-rule astigmatism overnight. This occurred in about two-thirds of the tests (Rengstorff, 1971c).

Sleeping With Contact Lenses Increases Myopia

Wearing lenses during sleep did not consistently decrease myopia; in fact, there was a slight trend towards increased myopia (Rengstorff, 1970b). After wearing lenses overnight, 6 of 10 eyes had increased myopia. When these men did not wear lenses overnight all had decreased myopia.

Diurnal: Myopia Increases During the First 8 Hours That Lenses Are Worn

Individuals who do not wear contact lenses show no evidence of daily (diurnal) variations in refractive error. However, there is a specific diurnal pattern of changes among individuals who wear contact lenses (Rengstorff, 1970c). This pattern of changes is illustrated in *Figure 17.1*, based on habitual wearers,

men between the ages of 19 and 26 years, who removed their lenses at specific times during the day for refractive tests. Myopia can be seen to increase from 0 to 8 hours and decrease slightly from 8 to 16 hours, followed by further overnight decreases in myopia when lenses are not worn. The mean change from 0 to 8 hours was almost 1.00 D; the decrease in myopia from 8 to 16 hours was approximately 0.25 D.

Measurements of myopia at the same time on different days showed considerable variation. This lack of consistency (that is, over 0.50 D) is not remarkable since contact lens wearers frequently lack discrimination in subjective tests following the removal of their lenses. The reliability problem was common to all subjects; nevertheless, a diurnal pattern was obvious. The pattern was evident in both averages and in single measurements.

Diurnal increases in myopia appear to be directly related to the daily wearing time and the number of years that contact lenses have been worn. The average diurnal increase in myopia for individuals who wore lenses for 6 months was less than 0.75 D, compared to about 1.50 D increase for those who wore lenses for more than 3 years. Wearing lenses all waking hours was associated with diurnal increases in myopia over 1.00 D, but individuals who wore contact lenses only 12–14 hours a day had diurnal increases of less than 1.00 D.

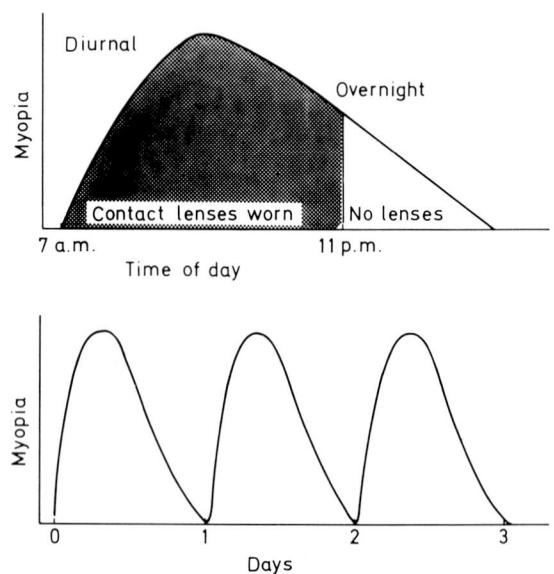

Figure 17.1–(Upper graph): Circadian changes in ametropia when contact lenses are worn during the day and removed overnight during sleep. (Lower graph): Circadian changes in ametropia for 3 consecutive days

Astigmatism Varies During the Hours That Lenses Are Worn

Repeated diurnal measurements of 8 habitual wearers of contact lenses have failed to reveal any conclusive pattern of changes in astigmatism such as those found for myopia. The responses of the subjects were not as critical as those of non-wearers, but some of the variance may be attributed to irregular astigmatism and the difficulties these subjects had in discriminating small lens changes (Rengstorff, 1971c).

LONG-TERM CHANGES (WITHDRAWAL VARIATIONS)

Days After Removing Contact Lenses: Myopia Decreases For About 3 Days (1–14 Days), and Then Begins to Increase

There is considerable evidence of refractive variations for many days after contact lenses are removed (Rengstorff, 1965a), and these variations follow a specific pattern. Measurements for myopia in 68 habitual wearers of contact lenses revealed a transitory reduction in myopia (Rengstorff, 1967). These results are illustrated in *Figure 17.2*. The average individual had decreases in myopia up to 1.32 D for 3 days, followed by increases until 21 days. Some

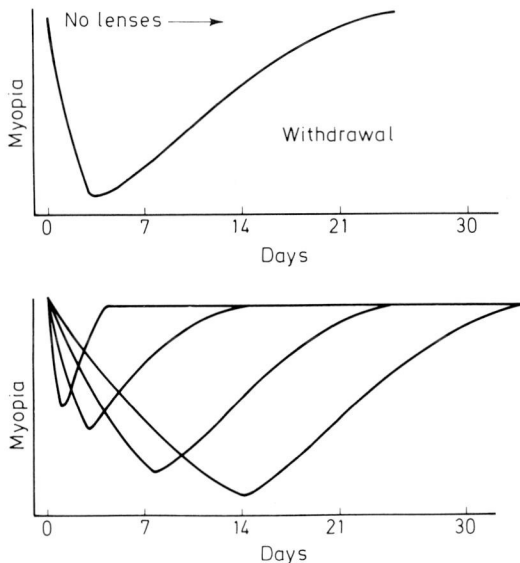

individuals showed progressive decreases in myopia for 1, 3, 7 or 14 days. A 7.50 D decrease in myopia is described in an individual case. The extent and duration of the after effects were found to be directly related to the daily wearing time and the number of years that contact lenses had been worn (Rengstorff, 1968b).

Myopia Measurements Are Relatively Stable 3 Weeks After Removing Contact Lenses

Variations in myopia stop or become very small in most cases after 3 weeks without contact lenses (Rengstorff, 1965a; Harris, Blevins and Heiden, 1973).

Astigmatism Increases After Removing Contact Lenses

There is a strong trend towards increased with-the-rule astigmatism associated with the withdrawal pattern (Rengstorff, 1965c; Pratt-Johnson and Warner, 1965). The average increase was 0.45 D for 64 subjects who had worn lenses for 6 months to 6 years. The astigmatism increased from 0 to 3 days after removing the lenses. From the third to the forty-eighth day, no significant variation was apparent (Rengstorff, 1968b). Hartstein (1965, 1967) found 2.50–6.00 D of with-the-rule astigmatism in 27 patients who had worn their contact lenses from 2 to 6 years without difficulties.

PRESCRIBING SPECTACLE LENSES

How to determine a satisfactory spectacle lens prescription for an habitual wearer of contact lenses is a difficult clinical problem. Results from the studies cited should be helpful in making this determination. It can be seen in *Figures 17.1* and *17.2* that a considerable range of possible spectacle prescriptions depend on when measurements are taken. Arner (1970) and Barradell (1972) have considered the diurnal and long-term refractive variations in their recommendations for prescribing spectacles to contact lens wearers. The relative stability of ametropia measurements after 21 days has, unfortunately, led some practitioners to insist that their patients stop wearing contact lenses for 21 days or more before they prescribe spectacles. Such treatment is rarely necessary; it can be very inconvenient for the patient to experience these withdrawal effects, often without any suitable spectacles. It is also recommended not to advise patients with severe corneal distortion to stop wearing contact lenses

Figure 17.2–(Upper graph): Withdrawal changes in ametropia at specific times after the removal of contact lenses. (Lower graph): Individual examples of myopia changes between test days

suddenly after many years because of a potential exacerbating effect (Rengstorff, 1975).

Corneal damage can be minimized and refractive variations can be reduced to obtain a suitable spectacle lens prescription by recommending that patients gradually reduce their wearing time. The practical requirement to provide the best possible all-round spectacle prescription is probably best accomplished by prescribing for the maximum amount of myopia, which is found after contact lenses have been worn for 8 hours (*see Figure 17.1*). The least satisfactory approach occurs when prescriptions are based on measurements taken hours or days after removing the lenses (*see Figure 17.2*) because this is when myopia is temporarily decreased.

MYOPIA CONTROL

The literature contains several suggestions that myopia may be controlled by the wearing of contact lenses. Neill (1962), reporting on cases since 1946, found that while contact lenses were worn the development of myopia was inhibited. Rengstorff (1967) has reviewed the period 1956–1966 when there were many conflicting reports on the subject of myopia control (Bier, 1956; Morrison, 1956, 1958; Dickinson, 1957; Steele, 1959; Black, 1960; Treissman, 1960; Barksdale, 1960; Fonda, 1962; Boyd, 1962; Nolan, 1964; Black-Kelly and Butler, 1964; Jessen, 1964; de Carle, 1965; Mandell, 1965; Enoch, 1965; Hodd, 1965; Saks, 1966). There are still conflicting views on this subject but now more reports acknowledge the short-term and long-term effects and the unstable state of myopia during the 3-week period following the removal of contact lenses (Black-Kelly and Butler, 1971; Grosvenor, 1972; Stone, 1973). After removing contact lenses for more than 3 weeks, Rengstorff (1965b) reported that the average change was 0.60 D less myopia in a study of 55 eyes. Kemmetmuller (1972) found that patients wearing contact lenses show a significantly slower progress of their refraction than those of the same age-group who wear spectacles. Stone (1973) is conducting a longitudinal study to determine how contact lenses affect changes in myopia in children. Her tentative conclusions from reviewing data gathered on over 100 children suggest that after wearing contact lenses for 2 years, myopia in growing children appears to stabilize, although it increases up to that time. Over a period of 4 years the rate of of increase of myopia may be expected to be slowed down by 0.75–1.00 D (Stone and Powell-Cullingford, 1974). Black-Kelly (1975) has described myopia control using atropine in conjunction with wearing contact lenses.

CORNEAL CURVATURE

The anterior corneal surface is the predominant refracting surface of the eye and it has been reported frequently that corneal contact lenses cause a change in corneal curvature. Because of this close association between corneal curvature and refractive changes, a brief discussion of changes in corneal curvature is included in this chapter. Similar to the preceding discussion on refractive changes, both short-term and long-term changes in corneal curvature apply to individuals who usually wear lenses all waking hours for at least 1 year (Rengstorff, 1971a). When lenses are worn less than all waking hours, the magnitude of the changes is reduced significantly. Furthermore, the effects appear directly related to the number of years contact lenses are worn. This information has proved useful to optometrists in the management of patients who wear contact lenses.

During adaptation to contact lenses the corneal curvature steepens about 0.50–1.00 D* (Pratt-Johnson and Warner, 1965; Miller, 1968; Hazlett, 1969; Manchester, 1970; Masnick, 1971; Farris *et al.*, 1971; Westerhout, 1971; Berman, 1972; Carney, 1975b) and this steepening gradually decreases during the first year (Rengstorff, 1969b; Grosvenor, 1972; Hill, 1975).

SHORT-TERM CHANGES (CIRCADIAN VARIATIONS)

Overnight Corneal Curvature Flattens While the Lenses Are Not Worn

A conspicuous finding in testing habitual wearers for consecutive days was a flattening of the cornea (about 0.75 D), which occurred overnight when the contact lenses were not worn (Rengstorff, 1968a, 1971b). The horizontal curvature was consistently flatter in the morning than on the previous evening, but when the vertical curvature was measured only a slight trend toward flattening was evident.

Sleeping With Contact Lenses Steepens Corneal Curvature

Tests of habitual wearers showed that wearing contact lenses during sleep causes steepened curva-

---

*Curvature changes are expressed in approximately equivalent dioptre effects for convenience in relating changes to ametropia. Further elaboration on curvature/refractive power appears on page 532.

ture (about 0.50 D) of both the horizontal and vertical principal meridians of the cornea (Rengstorff, 1971d).

When contact lenses are prescribed, patients are usually advised not to wear them during sleep because of possible corneal damage. However, there have been many reports describing patients who have worn their lenses not only during sleep but continuously for months and even many years without ever removing them (Levey, 1964; Rengstorff, 1965a; Allen, 1968). How these individuals can do this without experiencing any harm to the eyes, or discomfort, is not completely understood, but evidence indicates that tolerance must be built up gradually. A frequent consequence of wearing contact lenses during sleep, particularly with new wearers, is superficial corneal damage and considerable discomfort. Some months after wearing contact lenses every day, these individuals can often tolerate the lenses during and after short naps and sleeping. However, such tolerance is rapidly lost when the lenses are not worn for a few days. It appears, therefore, that the more completely the patient adapts to wearing contact lenses and the more consistently he wears them, the smaller the risk of corneal damage will be from wearing the lenses when sleeping.

Diurnal: Corneal Curvature Steepens During the First 8 Hours That Lenses Are Worn

The measurements of corneal curvature at the same time on different days showed some variations; nevertheless, a diurnal pattern was obvious in both averages and single measurements found in 5 habitual wearers who were tested before inserting their lenses and at intervals after wearing them. Mean horizontal curvature steepened an equivalent 0.71 D, 0.84 D and 0.55 D after 4, 8 and 16 hours of wear; mean vertical curvature steepened an equivalent 0.52 D, 0.50 D and 0.38 D at the same time (Rengstorff, 1971b). These findings suggest that the fit of contact lenses changes during the day. The magnitude of this pattern appears to be directly related to the number of years contact lenses have been worn and the amount of daily wearing time. Similar tests on non-wearers confirmed the generally held assumption that the corneal curvature of non-wearers is stable (Rengstorff, 1972), or so small that it challenges the reliability of keratometer measurements (Grosvenor, 1972).

Consistent astigmatic changes are not a part of the circadian pattern. Meridional differences in corneal curvature may vary considerably and even appear as irregular astigmatism.

LONG-TERM CHANGES (WITHDRAWAL VARIATIONS)

Days After Removing Contact Lenses

Some individuals showed progressive flattening for 1, 3 or 7 days.

A specific pattern of variations in corneal curvature occurs following the withdrawal of contact lenses from individuals who have habitually worn lenses at least 1 year (Rengstorff, 1969a). Group data on over 100 eyes of men aged 18–26 years showed progressive corneal flattening (about 0.75 D) of both the vertical and horizontal meridians for 1 and 3 days, respectively, followed by corneal steepening to the forty-eighth day of the test period. Some individuals showed progressive flattening for 1, 3 or 7 days. The most common changes in astigmatism were increases in with-the-rule astigmatism from 0 to 3 days.

Insertion of contact lenses, after not wearing them for 2 or more weeks, caused corneal steepening (Rengstorff, 1969a; Ong and Bowling, 1972). After wearing lenses again for 60–90 days, removing lenses for many days caused less corneal curvature variations than they did the first time they were removed, after wearing them at least 1 year.

The extent and duration of changes in corneal curvature were found to be directly related to the number of years contact lenses had been worn. The variations were less for individuals with reduced wearing time than for subjects who wore lenses all their waking hours.

Corneal Curvature is Relatively Stable 3 Weeks After Removing Contact Lenses

Many of the early observations in the 1960's suggested that the cornea reverted to its former curvature after lenses were removed for varying periods of time. However, a study of 64 subjects (Rengstorff, 1969a) indicated that the cornea did not revert to its former curvature after lenses had been removed for more than 30 days. In most cases variations in corneal curvature have stopped or become very small after 3 weeks without contact lenses. At that time the cornea is somewhat flatter (0.50–0.75 D) than before wearing contact lenses and there is an increase in with-the-rule astigmatism.

Although information has been obtained by studying certain time variables, the whole field of corneal changes still remains tremendously complex. The problem may be approached by eliminating other variables, specifically, physical factors such as contact lens specifications and physiological mechanisms which may affect corneal curvature.

CONTACT LENS DESIGN

From the preceding discussion it is obvious that there are a number of significant time variables which influence changes in corneal curvature. Failure to eliminate these variables is likely to invalidate research in this area. Such is the case in many conflicting reports that attribute changes in corneal curvature to the design of the contact lens. A review of these changes (Rengstorff, 1969a) includes the possibility that flattening of the cornea is associated with flat-fitting, lenses and steepening of the cornea is associated with steep-fitting lenses. However, Goldberg (1965) did not find changes in corneal curvature related to the fitting technique or to the design of the contact lens. In the Sarver and Harris (1967) study, no significant difference in changes in corneal curvature was found between one group of subjects fitted with small lenses 0.37 D 'steeper than K' and another group fitted with large lenses 'on K'. Rengstorff (1973) measured the corneas of 81 long-term wearers immediately after removal of their contact lenses and only one cornea had increased in curvature. In that study, most lenses were fitted 'flat' or 'on K' and only 10 eyes were fitted 'steep'. Another study was made to determine whether steep fitting lenses cause steeper corneal curvature (Hill and Rengstorff, 1974). Since only slightly more than half the corneas became steeper, one cannot conclude that steep-fitting base curves will steepen the corneal curvature. Both studies eliminated the withdrawal variable, since measurements were taken immediately after removal; however, the diurnal variable was not eliminated and it probably influenced the results.

Finally, there are physiological mechanisms which may affect corneal curvature (Rengstorff *et al.,* 1974). It has been shown that structural changes in the cornea can have circadian and long-range effects. The mechanism for these changes is unknown; however, every anatomical change has a chemical basis and it is possible that a return to a normal environment may play a role in the corneal curvature and refractive variation.

RELATIONSHIP BETWEEN CHANGES IN REFRACTION AND CHANGES IN CORNEAL CURVATURE

Myopia is frequently reduced by wearing contact lenses. Study has shown that these refractive changes are not solely attributable to changes in corneal curvature, as measured with an ophthalmometer.

Myopia and changes in corneal curvature during a period of weeks after the removal of contact lenses have been analysed (Rengstorff, 1969c). Group data for more than 100 eyes show a certain agreement between myopia and changes in corneal curvature. This can also be seen in some individual cases where there is good agreement either throughout the test period, after the first day, or after the third day. However, it has also been shown that individual data give conflicting results and lack of agreement occurred more frequently than agreement. The quantitative differences cannot be attributed to the ophthalmometric conversion. The changes between test days were frequently in opposite direction. Many examples show differences up to 4.00 D. These contradictory findings restrict the generality suggested by group similarities and point out that the process of changes in myopia following the removal of contact lenses cannot be attributed solely to changes in corneal curvature. It is more likely that changes in myopia are functionally related to a number of variables besides anterior corneal curvature.

Throughout this chapter the corneal curvature is expressed in dioptres rather than in radius of curvature, and it is well recognized that clinical determination of corneal dioptric power is determined arbitrarily. It is a result of a conversion of the instrument by the manufacturer whereby each corneal radius is assigned a specific refractive power based on an average refractive index. Stone (1973), for example, found the discrepancy between the Gambs and the Bausch and Lomb ophthalmometers was about 0.15 D. Determination of the actual corneal refractive power requires precise knowledge of the refractive index, corneal thickness, and curvature of the anterior and posterior corneal surfaces. The effects of altering these variables have been studied (Rengstorff and Arner, 1971). Some optical changes of the eye caused by contact lenses are discussed on pages 124–125 in Chapter 4, Volume 1.

The effects of changes in parameters other than anterior corneal curvature may serve to explain the variance between keratometric changes and refractive changes associated with wearing contact lenses. An analysis has shown how refractive changes may be influenced by changes in other corneal parameters as well as a change in anterior chamber length. These changes may occur either individually or collectively and the net effect on the total refraction of the eye will be the algebraic sum of the individual variations. For example, reduction of refractive power (myopia) may occur by: (1) flattening of anterior corneal curvature; (2) steepening of posterior corneal curvature; (3) increased index of refraction; (4) decreased corneal thickness; and (5) depressing the cornea and reducing axial length.

REFERENCES

Allen, M. J. (1968). 'Contact lenses, six months continuous wear.' *J. Am. optom. Ass.* **39**, 231–233

Arner, R. S. (1970). 'Prescribing new contact lenses or spectacles for the existing contact lens wearer.' *J. Am. optom. Ass.* **41**, 253–256

Barksdale, C. B. (1960). 'The attrition and control of myopia in some selected cases.' *Contacto* **4**(8), 349–366

Barradell, M. J. (1972). 'Spectacles for contact lens wearers.' *Ophthal. Optician* **12**, 763–768

Berman, M. R. (1972). 'Central corneal curvature and wearing time during contact lens adaptation.' *Optom. Wkly* **63**(6), 27–30

Bier, N. (1956). 'A study of the cornea in relation to contact lens practice.' *Am. J. Optom.* **33**, 291–304

Black, C. J. (1960). 'Ocular, anatomical and physiological changes due to contact lenses.' *Ill. med. J.* **118**, 279–281

Black-Kelly, T. S. B. (1975). 'The clinical arrest of myopia.' *Optician* **169**(4387), 13–23, (Part 1); **169**(4388), 8–11, (Part 2); **170**(4389), 4–8, 35, (Part 3)

Black-Kelly, T. S. B. and Butler, D. (1964). 'Preliminary report on corneal lenses in relation to myopia.' *Br. J. physiol. Optics* **21**, 175–186

Black-Kelly, T. S. B. and Butler, D. (1971). 'The present position of contact lenses in relation to myopia.' *Br. J. physiol. Optics* **26**, 33–48

Boyd, H. H. (1962). 'One thousand consecutive contact lens cases.' *Northwest med. J.* **61**, 933–936

Carney, L. G. (1975a). 'Refractive error and visual acuity changes during contact lens wear.' *The Contact Lens* **5**(3 and 4), 28–34

Carney, L. G. (1975b). 'The basis for corneal shape change during contact lens wear.' *Am. J. Optom.* **52**, 445–454

de Carle, J. (1965). In an abstract of a lecture on 'Contact lenses and myopia.' *Optician* **150**, 467

Dickinson, F. (1957). 'The value of microlenses in progressive myopia.' *Optician* **133**, 263–264

Enoch, J. M. (1965). Discussion of papers dealing with plans for contact lens research in myopia; lecture delivered at First International Conference on Myopia. Printed as a separate publication. Chicago: Professional Press

Farris, R., Linsy, Kubota, Z. and Mishima, S. (1971). 'Epithelial decompensation with corneal contact lens wear.' *Archs Ophthal.* **85**, 651–660

Fonda, D. (1962). 'Complications of contact lens wearing.' *Southern med. J.* **55**, 126–128

Goldberg, J. B. (1965). 'A commentary on corneal curvature and refraction changes observed among twenty contact lens patients.' Paper read at Am. Acad. of Optom., Section on Contact Lenses, Chicago, Dec., 1965

Grosvenor, T. P. (1972). *Contact Lens Theory and Practice.* Chicago: Professional Press

Harris, M. G., Blevins, R. J. and Heiden, S. (1973). 'Evaluation of procedures for the management of spectacle blur.' *Am. J. Optom.* **50**, 293–298

Hartstein, J. (1965). 'Corneal warping due to contact lenses.' *Am. J. Ophthal.* **60**, 1103–1104

Hartstein, J. (1967). 'Astigmatism induced by corneal contact lenses.' In *Current Concepts in Ophthalmology*, pp. 207–210. ed. by Becker, B. *et al.* St. Louis, Missouri: Mosby

Hazlett, R. D. (1969). 'Central circular clouding.' *J. Am. optom. Ass.* **40**, 268–275

Hill, J. F. (1975). 'A comparison of refractive and keratometric changes during adaptation to flexible and non-flexible contact lenses.' *J. Am. optom. Ass.* **46**, 290–294

Hill, J. F. and Rengstorff, R. H. (1974). 'Relationship between steeply fitted contact lens base curve and corneal curvature changes.' *Am. J. Optom.* **51**, 340–342

Hodd, F. A. B. (1965). 'Changes in corneal shape induced by the use of alignment fitted corneal lenses.' *Contacto* **9**(3), 18–24

Jessen, G. N. (1964). 'Contact lenses as a therapeutic device.' *Am. J. Optom.* **41**, 429–435

Kemmetmuller, H. (1972). 'Results of contact lens correction in myopia compared with spectacle correction.' *Klin. Mbl. Augenheilk.* **160**(1), 75–83

Levey, E. M. (1964). 'A case history of two years continuous wearing of contact lenses, followed by six months of non-continuous wearing.' *Am. J. Optom.* **41**, 703–718

Manchester, P. T. (1970). 'Hydration of the cornea.' *Trans. Am. Ophthal. Soc.* **68**, 425–461

Mandell, R. B. (1965). *Contact Lens Practice: Basic and Advanced*, Springfield, Illinois: Thomas

Masnick, K. (1971). 'A preliminary investigation into the effects of corneal lenses on central corneal thickness and curvature.' *Austral. J. Optom.* **54**, 87–98

Miller, D. (1968). 'Contact-lens-induced corneal curvature and thickness changes.' *Archs Ophthal.* **80**, 420–432

Morrison, R. J. (1956). 'Contact lenses and the progression of myopia.' *J. Am. optom. Assoc.* **28**, 711–713

Morrison, R. J. (1958). 'Observations on contact lenses and the progression of myopia.' *Contacto* **2**(1), 20–25

Neill, J. C. (1962). 'Contact Lenses and Myopia.' In *Transactions of the International Ophthalmic Optical Congress, 1961*, pp. 191–198. New York: Hafner

Nolan, J. (1964). 'Progress of myopia and contact lenses.' *Contacto* **8**(1), 25–26

Ong, J. and Bowling, R. (1972). 'Effect of contact lens on cornea and lid on a 10-year wearer.' *Am. J. Optom.* **49**, 932–935

Pratt-Johnson, J. A. and Warner, D. M. (1965). 'Contact lenses and corneal curvature changes.' *Am. J. Ophthal.* **60**, 852–855

Rengstorff, R. H. (1965a). 'The Fort Dix report.' *Am. J. Optom.* **42**, 156–163

Rengstorff, R. H. (1965b). 'Contact lens application and myopia research in the US Army.' *Optom. Wkly* **56**(10), 34–35

Rengstorff, R. H. (1965c). 'Contact curvature and astigmatic changes subsequent to contact lens wear.' *J. Am. optom. Ass.* **36**, 996–1000

Rengstorff, R. H. (1966). 'A study of the visual acuity loss after contact lens wear.' *Am. J. Optom.* **43**, 431–440

Rengstorff, R. H. (1967). 'Variations in myopia measurements: an after-effect observed with habitual wearers of contact lenses.' *Am. J. Optom.* **44**, 149–161

Rengstorff, R. H. (1968a). 'An investigation of overnight changes in corneal curvature.' *J. Am. optom. Ass.* **39**, 262–265

Rengstorff, R. H. (1968b). 'Contact lenses and after effects: some temporal factors which influence myopia and astigmatism variations.' *Am. J. Optom.* **45**, 364–373

Rengstorff, R. H. (1969a). 'Variations in corneal curvature measurements: An after-effect observed with habitual wearers of contact lenses.' *Am. J. Optom.* **46**, 45–51

Rengstorff, R. H. (1969b). 'Studies of corneal curvature changes after wearing contact lenses.' *J. Am. optom. Ass.* **40**, 298–299

Rengstorff, R. H. (1969c). 'Relationship between myopia and corneal curvature changes after wearing contact lenses.' *Am. J. Optom.* **46**, 357–362

Rengstorff, R. H. (1970a). 'Overnight decreases in myopia.' *Sth Afr. Optometrist* **27**(16), 18–22

Rengstorff, R. H. (1970b). 'Overnight myopia changes induced by contact lenses.' *J. Am. optom. Ass.* **41**(3), 249–252

Rengstorff, R. H. (1970c). 'Diurnal variations in myopia measurements after wearing contact lenses.' *Am. J. Optom.* **47**, 812–815

Rengstorff, R. H. (1971a). 'Corneal curvature: patterns of change after wearing contact lenses.' *J. Am. optom. Ass.* **42**, 264

Rengstorff, R. H. (1971b). 'Diurnal variations in corneal curvature after wearing of contact lenses.' *Am. J. Optom.* **48**, 239–244

Rengstorff, R. H. (1971c). 'Variations in astigmatism overnight and during the day after wearing contact lenses.' *Am. J. Optom.* **48**, 810–813

Rengstorff, R. H. (1971d). 'Wearing contact lenses during sleep: corneal curvature changes.' *Am. J. Optom.* **48**, 1034–1037

Rengstorff, R. H. (1972). 'Diurnal constancy of corneal curvature.' *Am. J. Optom.* **49**, 1002–1005

Rengstorff, R. H. (1973). 'The relationship between contact lens base curve and corneal curvature.' *J. Am. optom. Ass.* **44**, 291–293

Rengstorff, R. H. (1975). 'Prevention and treatment of corneal damage after wearing contact lenses.' *J. Am. optom. Ass.* **46**, 277–278

Rengstorff, R. H. and Arner, R. S. (1971). 'Refractive changes in the cornea: mathematical considerations.' *Am. J. Optom.* **48**, 913–918

Rengstorff, R. H., Hill, R. M., Petrali, J. P. and Sim, V. M. (1974). 'Critical oxygen requirement of the corneal epithelium as indicated by succinic dehydrogenase reactivity.' *Am. J. Optom.* **51**, 331–339

Saks, S. J. (1966). 'Fluctuations in refractive state in adapting and long-term contact lens wearers.' *J. Am. optom. Ass.* **37**, 229–238

Sarver, M. D. and Harris, M. G. (1967). 'Corneal lenses and 'spectacle blur'.' *Am. J. Optom.* **44**, 316–318

Steele, E. (1959). 'Observations on the fitting of corneal contact lenses.' *Am. J. Optom.* **36**, 194–199

Stone, Janet (1973). 'Contact lens wear in the young myope.' *Br. J. physiol. Optics* **28**, 90–134

Stone, Janet and Powell-Cullingford, G. (1974). 'Myopia control after contact lens wear.' *Br. J. physiol. Optics* **29**, 93–108

Treissman, H. (1960). 'The role of corneal microlenses in ophthalmic practice.' *Trans. ophthal. Soc. U.K.* **80**, 25–37

Westerhout, D. (1971). 'A clinical survey or oedema, its signs, symptoms and incidence.' *Contact Lens* **3**(2), 3–25

Chapter 18

Toric Contact Lens Fitting

D. Westerhout

Toric forms of contact lenses have been in use for many years; and now that laboratories are prepared to devote more time and resources to the manufacture of such lens forms, they are being used more widely in a greater number of cases. But very little information is to be found on them in existing textbooks, and even more recent literature does not cover the subject very comprehensively.

It appears that many practitioners attempting to fit a patient in whom it seems a toric lens might be of value are reluctant to actually use one, partly due to their lack of experience of such lenses as well as the acknowledged difficulty in having them manufactured accurately and the high cost involved.

There is no doubt that the accurate manufacture of a contact lens incorporating a toroidal optical surface is extremely difficult. This difficulty is more than doubled if two toroidal optical surfaces are used, and the problems become still greater if other toroidal surfaces are involved as in, for example, the case of a bi-toric corneal lens with a multi-curved toroidal periphery.

Manufacturing costs of such a lens are related to the difficulty of production, and are therefore linked to the number of toroidal surfaces used in the final construction of the lens.

PART I: TORIC CORNEAL LENS FITTING

INDICATIONS FOR THE USE OF TORIC CONTACT LENSES

The main uses of toric lenses are as follows.

(1) To improve the vision in cases where a lens employing spherical front and back central optic radii is unable to provide adequate refractive correction.

(2) To improve the physical fit in cases where a lens with a spherical back central optic radius (BCOR) and spherical peripheral radii fails to provide an adequate physical fit. The terms spherical BCOR and spherical peripheral radii include, in this context, any lens of any construction whether it be aspherical, conoidal or using any non-spherical curves, provided that the BCOR specifications are the same in two meridians at right-angles to one another and the peripheral construction has the same specification in meridians mutually at right-angles.

These two main uses of toroidal surfaces on contact lenses are usually distinct, and a lens is normally employed for either a physical or an optical reason. There are occasions on which the two types of use overlap – notably, when the front surface of a contact lens has to be made toroidal to correct the astigmatism induced when a lens with a toroidal back central optic portion is worn on a cornea in order to produce a good physical fit. This is known as a compensated bi-toric contact lens.

FORMS OF TORIC LENS

There are seven main varieties of toric corneal lens available to the practitioner, as follows.

(1) With toroidal back central optic portions and toroidal peripheral zones.

(2) With toroidal back central optic portions and spherical peripheral zones.

(3) With spherical back central optic portions and toroidal peripheral zones.

(4) to (7) Each of the first three varieties can be produced with or without a toroidal front optic surface, as can a lens with a spherical back central optic portion and spherical peripheral zone.

There might be said to be a subdivision of such a classification, as follows.

A lens which has a toroidal back central optic portion and a toroidal front surface may be said to be of bi-toric construction. If the principal meridians of the toroidal front and back surfaces are not parallel then the lens is of oblique bi-toric construction.

With respect to toric contact lenses, British Standard 3521 (1979) states that a toroidal surface should be specified by the radii of curvature in its two principal meridians, the radius in the flatter meridian being written above a line and the radius in the steeper meridian below it (as in *Figure 18.1*). Where it is necessary to specify the orientation, the direction of the flatter meridian in standard axis notation should be written after the longer radius, prefixed by the letter m to denote meridian. The abbreviation Tor may be used with BS to denote back surface, FS to denote front surface, COP for central optic portion and POZ for peripheral optic zone so as to indicate which surface is toroidal.

It is obviously better to avoid some of the loose terminology used to describe toric forms of lenses and use only the correct, full descriptions with the accepted nomenclature laid down in British Standard 3521:1979.

Lenses with Toroidal Back Central Optic Portions and Toroidal Peripheral Zones

This type of lens is generally used in attempting to obtain a good physical fit on a cornea which is too astigmatic to allow a good fit with a lens having a spherical BCOR and spherical peripheral radii.

Although corneal lenses in general may be successfully fitted with either apical clearance or apical contact, it is generally more satisfactory to fit lenses with toroidal back central optic portions in or near alignment. Fitting in alignment may be difficult to define, and many practitioners differ in their interpretation of this term. Fitting in alignment is often held to mean fitting with a BCOR of the same radius as the corneal radius in its flattest meridian as found by keratometer (or K reading, as it is often termed). This may be a reasonably accurate interpretation in cases in which the cornea to be fitted is almost spherical; but 'fitting on flattest K' is unlikely to represent alignment in medium or high degrees of corneal astigmatism. Alignment, to some practitioners, may mean a situation in which the lens fitted shows no apical clearance with fluorescein, but if the BCOR is decreased or the back central optic diameter is increased by clinically significant amounts, then the fluorescein picture would change to one of apical clearance (Westerhout, 1969).

Since the lens form under discussion is made with a toroidal back central optic portion to fit the contour of an astigmatic cornea, it may be seen that there is sound reasoning in trying to match the BCOR* to the corneal radii. This generally means fitting on or near the keratometer reading in each meridian. Such a lens usually gives a good physical fit in close alignment, especially if the peripheral toroidal curves are fitted with similar consideration to the difference in peripheral radii of the corneal principal meridians.

Such a lens frequently gives a physical fit, as denoted by the fluorescein pattern, similar to that seen with a well fitted spherical lens in alignment to a cornea devoid of clinically significant astigmatism. However, a lens in such close alignment is sometimes likely to create physiological problems. A lens with both spherical BCOR and peripheral radii fitted to an eye with a clinically significant degree of corneal astigmatism does have an inbuilt advantage in that the slight looseness in the meridian of steepest corneal curvature helps the lens to rock slightly on the flattest corneal curve, thus aiding the interchange of tears across the cornea behind the lens. Indeed, this rocking motion tends to act as a pump; and it is interesting to watch the flow of tears behind such a lens with a slit lamp biomicroscope – especially as the lens moves with and between blinks.

Conversely, it may happen that a spherical lens closely fitted to a spherical cornea, or an astigmatic cornea fitted with a lens utilizing toroidal back central and peripheral curves, may give a poor liquid interchange, and it may be necessary to aid the maintenance of normal corneal metabolism by using a slightly modified lens form.

In the case of the closely aligning toric lens, the following possibilities exist.

(1) The use of a toroidal back central optic portion fitted slightly flatter (longer radii) than the corneal radii. Either or both radii may be made flatter, and it is common for the steeper radius of the pair to be fitted a little flatter than the appropriate corneal radius to assist the interchange of tears.

(2) The use of spherical peripheral radii with a toroidal back central optic portion. These peripheral radii may be chosen to give a conventional clearance and fit along the meridian of the flattest corneal curve (*see* Chapter 11, Volume 1). This tends to produce a looser peripheral fit in the meridian at right-angles which may aid the flow of tears behind the lens, especially if the cornea has astigmatism 'with-the-rule'. In such cases, the peripheral clearance is greater in the vertical meridian – which is

---

*BCOR indicates back central optic radius for a spherical surface, and back central optic radii for a toroidal surface.

probably the most helpful position if the lacrimal flow behind the lens is to be improved. This method also simplifies the lens production and reduces its cost.

In the production of lenses with both toroidal back central and peripheral curves, it is not uncommon for a laboratory to cut and polish the peripheral radii so that they do not lie along the same meridians as the corresponding BCOR – that is, the flatter peripheral radius does not lie along the same meridian as the flatter BCOR. This results in a lens which appears to have a markedly elliptical or oval back central optic portion (*Figure 18.1*). A properly

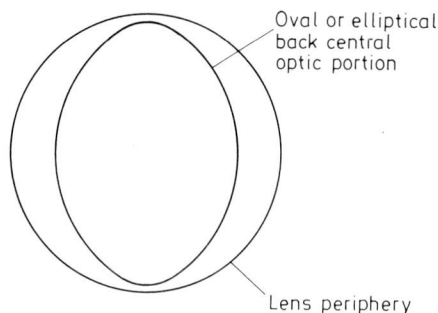

Figure 18.1–The radii of the toroidal peripheral zone incorrectly worked at right-angles to the corresponding BCOR, that is

C2 Toric/8.00:6.50/8.00:9.50
        7.50   8.50

instead of

C2 Toric/8.00:6.50/8.50:9.50
        7.50   8.00

made lens with a toroidal back central optic portion and toroidal peripheral curves which differ by the same amount from the corresponding BCOR has a similar appearance to a lens with a spherical BCOR and spherical peripheral radii. In both cases, the transition between the back central optic portion and the peripheral zone is circular, or almost so.

(3) The toroidal peripheral zone may be made substantially flatter in relation to the BCOR than might normally be used for a spherical lens.

(4) The back central optic diameter and/or the overall size may be kept as small as is consistent with adequate visual acuity and comfort.

(5) The lens may be fenestrated. With a toroidal back central optic portion, a central 0.5 mm hole is often found to be most effective.

Lenses with both toroidal back central and peripheral curves are much easier to fit if keratometer readings are available, and still easier if the practitioner has a fitting set of such lenses. Such

fitting sets are not commonly used by practitioners, possibly because of their high cost. Many practitioners have, however, accumulated a series of prescription lenses which have had to be rejected when new replacement lenses have been prescribed. Such lenses are very useful, both for fitting and refraction purposes.

An example of the type of physical fitting one might derive from keratometer readings is shown below, related to two different types of peripheral fit used for reasonably spherical corneas.

Example 1:
Spherical cornea, keratometer reading 8.00 mm

Practitioner A might prescribe:
C2/8.00:6.50/9.00:9.50

Practitioner B might prescribe:
C4/8.00:6.50/8.50:7.50/9.00:8.50/9.50:9.50

Toric cornea, keratometer readings
8.00 mm along 180
7.50 mm along 90

Using the same approach to the physical fitting as they would use for spherical corneas:

Practitioner A might prescribe:
C2 Toric/8.00:6.50/9.00:9.50
           7.50   8.50

Practitioner B might prescribe:
C4 Toric/8.00:6.50/8.50:7.50/9.00:8.50/9.50:9.50
           7.50   8.00   8.50   9.00

The refraction of such an eye wearing a lens with either an 8.00 mm BCOR or 8.00 mm × 7.50 mm BCOR is very different with the two types of correction. This is dealt with on page 524.

In the event of keratometer readings not being available in the case of a toric cornea, such as that considered in *Example 1*, the lens could be fitted by observing conventional lenses having spherical back surface curves.

An experienced or skilful practitioner observing only the flatter meridian would probably find that an 8.00 mm BCOR combined with his favoured peripheral fit would fit very well along that particular meridian. By observing the degree of flatness in the vertical meridian and/or by consideration of the spectacle astigmatism and degree of residual astigmatism, it is possible to estimate the required fit in the vertical meridian with a fair degree of accuracy. Fitting in this way usually produces a sufficiently good physical fit, but may make it difficult to quantitatively predict the refractive effect of the lens. A more precise method of prescribing by consideration of the spectacle refraction and the use of spherical trial lenses is shown on page 546.

Since corneal lenses with both spherical BCOR and peripheral radii are often used successfully on corneas with a medium to high degree of astigmatism, it is important to decide what degree of astigmatism should indicate the use of toroidal back central optic portions. In general, it may be said that these should only be used when a lens with a spherical BCOR cannot be made to fit successfully. It is rare to find that toroidal back central optic portions are necessary unless the difference in the corneal radii, as measured with a keratometer, exceeds 0.5 mm.

A great deal depends on factors other than corneal astigmatism. Lid positions and tension are important. In a case of high corneal astigmatism, with-the-rule, and a low, loose lower lid, a toroidal back central optic portion may be needed to obtain a good physical fit and centration. But a similar eye with a firm, high lower lid may well be successfully fitted using a lens with spherical back surface curves.

Consideration should also be given to the likely moulding effect of a spherical lens on a toroidal cornea. The undesirable difficulties which may occur with spectacle blur and variations in visual acuity and refractive error (see Chapters 16 and 17) if the wearing of the contact lens has to be ceased for any reason, must be carefully weighed against the advantages of fitting a spherical lens. When such a lens is fitted, the post-wear refractive error should be carefully monitored at all after-care visits, and modification to the fit carried out if gross changes occur.

The majority of cases of corneal astigmatism are found with the steeper corneal curve in the vertical (with-the-rule). If an attempt is made to fit such an eye with a spherical BCOR, the lens often drops low on the cornea, causing physical discomfort and/or poor vision. Such an example is illustrated in *Colour Plate XXXII*. If the same eye is fitted using a lens with toroidal back central and peripheral curves, then the physical fit and centration are usually much improved (*Colour Plate XXXIII*).

Sometimes, with such astigmatism, it is found that a lens with a spherical BCOR is lifted high on the cornea by the top lid. This may give a reasonable standard of steady vision but can cause physiological problems through its immobility and tendency to cause a stagnant pool of tears just below the upper limbus.

A fitting set of lenses with both toroidal back central and peripheral curves is extremely valuable, as already mentioned. Even a limited set can be of great value. A suggestion for a minimum set is one covering the range 7.5 × 7.00 mm to 8.5 × 8.0 mm BCOR in 0.1 mm increments in both meridians.

The peripheral radii may be chosen to reflect the type of peripheral fit usually preferred by the practitioner concerned. Each meridian is considered separately, and the peripheral fittings in the two principal meridians are selected to provide the same difference between back central and peripheral radii most commonly used by the practitioner in fitting spherical corneas.

Since the cutting and polishing of each pair of peripheral radii on a toroidal surface is such a complicated and costly process it may be as well to choose the simplest possible form of peripheral fit preferred. If the practitioner normally uses a tri-curve periphery, that is, a tetra-curve lens, when using only spherical back surface radii, he may well find some advantage in using a simpler, less sophisticated lens with one pair of toroidal peripheral curves only, that is, bi-curve lens in each principal meridian.

Since such a fitting set is extremely useful for refraction purposes as well as for observation of the fluorescein pattern, the back central optic diameters should be between 6.5 and 7.0 mm and the overall size about 9.0–9.5 mm.

Lenses with Toroidal Back Central Optic Portions and Spherical Peripheral Zones

As already mentioned, it can be useful to use spherical peripheral radii with the intention of improving the circulation of tears beneath these lenses. However, when this is done, it is possible that the lens may become less stable with regard to resisting rotation. A fully toroidal peripheral zone may assist in preventing excessive lens rotation, and this can be helpful if it is necessary to hold the lens in a non-rotating position to correct residual astigmatism or to correctly position a bifocal segment.

One difficulty that may arise with the use of a toroidal back central optic portion and a spherical front surface, is that there is a variation of edge thickness, which may give rise to discomfort. The use of spherical peripheral radii makes it easier for the laboratory to produce a more uniform edge thickness, and this may be of some slight physical advantage in certain cases.

It is often said that toric lenses cannot be adjusted, but this is not correct. If, for example, a lens with toroidal back central and peripheral curves provides too little tears flow behind the lens, it is possible to re-cut or polish the peripheral radii to spherical form using a radius or radii identical to those used for the original flatter meridian. The radii can also be made flatter than the original flatter radius or radii. The steeper peripheral radii may also be made only a little flatter, but not as much as the flatter meridian.

PART I: TORIC CORNEAL LENS FITTING

Table 18.1–Fitting Set of Toroidal Back Surface Corneal Lenses, but with Two Final Spherical Peripheral Curves

Toroidal BCOR (mm)	:	BCOD (mm)	Toroidal BP$_1$OR (mm)	:	BP$_1$OD (mm)	Spherical BP$_2$OR (mm)	:	BP$_2$OD (mm)	Spherical BP$_3$OR (mm)	:	OS (mm)
7.00 × 7.60	:	7.00/	7.55 × 8.30	:	7.80/	8.70	:	8.60/	9.30	:	9.00
7.10 × 7.70			7.70 × 8.45			8.90			9.60		
7.20 × 7.80			7.80 × 8.55			9.00			9.90		
7.30 × 7.90			7.95 × 8.70			9.20			10.10		
7.40 × 8.00			8.10 × 8.80			9.40			10.30		
7.50 × 8.10			8.20 × 8.95			9.60			10.50		
7.60 × 8.20			8.30 × 9.05			9.80			10.70		
7.70 × 8.30			8.45 × 9.25			10.00			11.00		
7.80 × 8.40			8.55 × 9.30			10.20			11.30		
7.90 × 8.50			8.70 × 9.50			10.30			11.50		
8.00 × 8.60			8.80 × 9.60			10.50			11.80		
7.00 × 8.00			7.55 × 8.80			9.10			9.90		
7.10 × 8.10			7.70 × 8.95			9.30			10.10		
7.20 × 8.20			7.80 × 9.05			9.50			10.30		
7.30 × 8.30			7.95 × 9.25			9.60			10.50		
7.40 × 8.40			8.10 × 9.30			9.80			10.80		
7.50 × 8.50			8.20 × 9.50			10.00			11.00		
7.60 × 8.60			8.30 × 9.60			10.30			11.30		
7.70 × 8.70			8.45 × 9.80			10.50			11.60		

BVP of all lenses: plano on flattest meridian

In theory, if a lens with an all-toroidal back surface rotates, then the steeper peripheral radii may come to rest along the flatter corneal meridian. In this position, they are far too tight and may cause corneal abrasions or disturbance. This is seldom seen as a problem in practice; but if encountered, it may provide an indication for the use of spherical peripheral radii.

The back surface specification of a useful fitting set having the first back peripheral curve toroidal, as well as the back central optic portion, but with the two most peripheral curves being spherical, is given in *Table 18.1*. Some practitioners may prefer the latter two curves to be even flatter to encourage tears interchange.

Lenses with Spherical Back Central Optic Portions and Toroidal Peripheral Zones

These lenses are frequently used as a means of attempting to improve the physical fit of a lens on an astigmatic cornea without the optical complications inherent in the use of lenses with toroidal back central optic portions.

Since the BCOR of such a lens has to align as well as possible with a toric cornea, these lenses are usually fitted fairly small and centrally rather

steeper than the flatter corneal meridian. Many practitioners favour fitting steeper than the flatter keratometer reading by about one-third of the difference between the keratometer readings. Back central optic diameters are usually around 6.5 mm, with a commonly encountered range of between 6.0 and 7.0 mm. Overall sizes tend to be between 8.5 and 9.5 mm.

The toroidal peripheral zones are chosen in much the same way as when fitting lenses with all-toroidal back surface curves. The practitioner, however, is using a spherical BCOR and is able to observe his fitting set lenses on the cornea with fluorescein. Observing the peripheral fit along the flatter corneal meridian, he can then choose an appropriate radius or radii for the steeper peripheral meridian by consideration of the keratometer reading and/or the fluorescein pattern.

A typical case might be as follows.

K readings: 8.00 mm along 180
                7.40 mm along 90
BCOR chosen: 7.80 mm

Consider the philosophies of peripheral fitting by *practitioners A* and *B* in *Example 1* (page 537).

Both *A* and *B* might find that a fitting lens with a BCOR of 7.90 mm gives good alignment and peripheral fit in the 180 meridian.

If the optimum BCOD and OS were chosen to be 6.5 mm and 9.5 mm respectively, the final specifications might be as follows.

Practitioner A
C2/7.80:6.50/8.90:9.50
　　　　　　　8.30

Practitioner B:
C4/7.80:6.50/8.40:7.50/8.90:8.50/9.40:9.50
　　　　　　　7.80　　　8.30　　　8.80

These lenses have an elliptical back central optic portion of the shape illustrated in *Figure 18.1*.

This type of lens can be very useful in certain cases where a fully spherical lens is not adequate; but the toroidal peripheral zones are, at best, only an attempt at a compromise. Such lenses frequently rotate sufficiently to cause difficulty in stabilizing a correction for residual astigmatism or for keeping a bifocal addition in the correct position. They often rotate more than lenses with all-toroidal back surface curves; and the steeper peripheral radii occasionally end up in close proximity to the flatter corneal meridian, thus causing slight corneal abuse. This occurs more often than in a lens utilizing a fully toroidal back surface.

It is comparatively easy to see if the lens is rotating much by observing the peripheral fit with fluorescein, but the inexperienced practitioner may find it helpful to have the steeper peripheral meridian marked with two dots, one at each edge of the lens. Two dots are much more useful than one for this purpose. Temporary dots may be put on with a waterproof fibre pen.

OPTICAL CONSIDERATIONS OF TOROIDAL BACK CENTRAL OPTIC PORTIONS

It is important that the fundamentals of the optics of contact lenses are understood if some of the complications of toroidal optic surfaces on corneal lenses are to be appreciated.

To help understand and perform some of the calculations needed in toric lens work the reader is referred to Chapter 4, Volume 1, particularly page 121, and also to *Optics of Contact Lenses* by A. G. Bennett (1966) and *Optical Tables for Contact Lens Work* by J. L. Francis (1968), now included in Chapter 4. This topic is therefore covered here in somewhat abbreviated form and consists mainly of the different approaches to the problems concerned.

The most useful basis for the consideration of toric corneas and lenses is Gullstrand's Schematic Eye (No. 1, Exact).

The refractive indices used in this Eye are:

Cornea	1.376
Tears	1.336
Aqueous	1.336

The refractive index of the contact lens plastics material, polymethyl methacrylate, is 1.49.

The tears lens does not, therefore, fully neutralize the refractive effect of the front surface of the cornea, as some imagine, but only 0.336/0.376 (approximately nine-tenths) of its power.

Considered in relation to contact lenses, this does not adversely affect the prescribing of a lens with a spherical back central optic radius as any necessary correction may be worked on the front optic surface of the lens, but it does mean that only nine-tenths of the front surface corneal astigmatism is corrected by the tears lens.

The back surface of the cornea is seldom considered as relevant to contact lens work, but it should be considered if all the optical complications of contact lens prescribing are to be appreciated.

It is difficult to know whether or not the back surface of the cornea follows the same trends in contour and shape as its front surface, but on the evidence available it seems reasonable to assume that there is at least a similarity.

If the back corneal surface does follow the same curve as the front surface, then the astigmatism created by the back surface is opposite in effect to that of the front surface. This can be seen in an example using Gullstrand's Schematic Eye (No. 1, Exact) and assuming a certain degree of corneal astigmatism (Bennett, 1966; Westerhout, 1969).

Assuming corneal astigmatism, with-the-rule, of 5 per cent on the front surface and a similar contour on the back surface:

Front corneal surface

Vertical radius of curvature = 7.70 mm
Horizontal radius of curvature = 7.70 mm + 5 per cent = 8.085 mm

This is equivalent to

$$\frac{1000(1.376 - 1)}{7.70} - \frac{1000(1.376 - 1)}{8.085} \text{ D}$$
astigmatism with-the-rule = 2.35 D　　　　　(1)

Corneal astigmatism measured with a keratometer calibrated for a nominal refractive index of 1.3375 is:

$$\frac{1000(1.3375 - 1)}{7.70} - \frac{1000(1.3375 - 1)}{8.085} \text{ D}$$
astigmatism with-the-rule = 2.08 D
= approximately nine-tenths of (1) ....(3)

Back corneal surface
Vertical radius of curvature = 6.80 mm
Horizontal radius of curvature = 6.80 mm + 5 per cent = 7.14 mm
This is equivalent to

$$\frac{1000(1.336 - 1.376)}{6.80} - \frac{1000(1.336 - 1.376)}{7.14} \text{ D}$$

astigmatism against-the-rule = 0.28 D   (2)

Note that (1) + (2) = 2.07 D
= (approximately) keratometer reading, 2.08 D   (3)

The tears then neutralize all but one-tenth of the front surface corneal astigmatism; and this is likely to be corrected by the back surface corneal astigmatism, which may be about equal to approximately one-tenth of the front surface astigmatism and opposite in effect.

The index of calibration of the keratometer (1.3375) is chosen to take this effect of the corneal back surface into account, in order to give the user a guide to the total refractive effect of the cornea.

In contact lens practice, this refractive index is very helpful because it is so close to that of the tears (1.336). Thus, the corneal astigmatism measured with the keratometer should be almost completely corrected by the liquid lens between the cornea and contact lens.

Expected Residual Astigmatism

If the practitioner measures a degree of corneal astigmatism which is very different from the cylinder element in the most accurate spectacle prescription, then a certain amount of residual astigmatism may be expected. The degree of this residual astigmatism should, in theory, be equal to the difference between the corneal astigmatism and spectacle astigmatism (provided that the vertex distance is allowed for). It is difficult, however, to think of an aspect of visual optics in which theory and practice are so far divorced. It is common to find an estimated residual astigmatism of over 1.00 D by calculation, only to discover that the actual residual astigmatism measured by refraction over a corneal lens is no more than 0.25–0.50 D.

Many examples of the lack of correlation between calculated and measured residual astigmatism can be quoted, and it has been estimated that in no more than 38 per cent of eyes do the two closely approximate (Fairmaid, 1967).

This is due, in part, to the fact that the estimated residual error is based on measurement of corneal astigmatism over a small area of the corneal surface, whereas the refractive effect of the cornea is also influenced by other areas of the surface lying outside the chord lengths used by the keratometer.

The amount of residual astigmatism is also based on two measurements of astigmatism – one taken from spectacle refraction of the eye and the other taken from a refraction over a contact lens. These measurements are almost invariably fully or partly subjective, and are thus hardly scientifically measured quantities. It may well be that closer correlation between estimated and actual residual astigmatism would be found if the calculations were based on objective measurements of refraction with and without the lens in place. Retinoscope or eye refractometer measurements could be used, or perhaps a combination of both types.

Unfortunately, the term 'residual astigmatism' is often used loosely and is frequently confused with induced astigmatism or corneal astigmatism. Residual astigmatism has been variously defined (Goldberg, 1964) but maybe said to be the astigmatic component of a lens required to fully correct an eye wearing a spherical powered contact lens with a spherical back optic radius. However, it is not quite as simple as this since the degree and axis of residual astigmatism varies with different lenses. If the parameters of the lens *in situ* for refraction are changed, then the measured residual astigmatism is also likely to alter. In particular, changing the back central optic diameter, overall size, amount of prism, back central optic radius, thickness, and position on the cornea are likely to have a noticeable effect on the measured residual astigmatism.

When stating the degree of residual error, therefore, it is as well to state the specification of the lens through which the astigmatism has been measured.

Residual astigmatism is probably most commonly anatomical, the site of which may be in the cornea, crystalline lens or retina. The effect may be due to irregularities in the surfaces of these structures, irregularities in the refractive index of the transparent media of the cornea and/or crystalline lens, or due to obliquity of one or more of the surfaces to the direction of the incident light.

Residual astigmatism measured over a lens having a spherical BCOR may also be induced by the following.

(1) An irregular tears film caused by a tilted or poorly centred lens.

(2) The obliquity of a tilted lens to the incident light.

(3) Irregular refractive index of the liquid lens caused by stagnation or partial evaporation of the tears liquid.

(4) Warping of a lens due to bad handling, or even under the influence of heavy lid pressure. The effects of the latter are discussed on page 555 and in Chapter 4, Volume 1.

There are other factors which individually or collectively may have an influence on residual astigmatism (Goldberg, 1964), but the most important aspect of this subject is its clinical significance and correction, which is dealt with on page 544.

Refraction with Toroidal Back Central Optic Portions

The main purpose of fitting such a lens is to obtain a good physical fit in cases of high or medium astigmatism. Unfortunately, its use is complicated by the introduction of induced astigmatism.

Induced astigmatism, in this context, may be taken as the astigmatic effect created in the contact-lens/tears-liquid system by the toroidal back central optic portion bounding two surfaces of different refractive index – 1.49 and 1.336 (Westerhout, 1969).

Induced astigmatism is introduced into the system every time toroidal back central optic surfaces are used and, despite all the methods of attempting to reduce its effect, it remains one of the biggest problems to be overcome with this form of lens. It is due only to the lens/tears boundary, as the following example shows.

Example 2

Spectacle Rx: –2.00/–3.00 × 180

Keratometry: 8.20 mm along 180
7.70 mm along 90

An afocal corneal lens of BCOR 8.20 mm might be inserted and a refraction of –2.00 DS found with this lens *in situ*. (The back surface of the tears neutralizes the front and back surface corneal astigmatism.)

If, however, the lens is changed to one having a toroidal back central optic portion to align with the cornea, the power of the system combining the lens BCOR and tears liquid is as follows.

In the vertical meridian

Lens back surface: $\dfrac{1000(1 - 1.49)}{+7.70}$ = –63.64 D

Tears front surface: $\dfrac{1000(1.336 - 1)}{+7.70}$ = +43.64 D

Total power in vertical meridian   = –20.00 D

In the horizontal meridian

Lens back surface: $\dfrac{1000(1 - 1.49)}{-8.20}$ = –59.76 D

Tears front surface: $\dfrac{1000(1.336 - 1)}{+8.20}$ = +40.98 D

Total power in horizontal meridian   = –18.78 D

Total effect of lens/tears surface =
–18.78 DS with –1.22 DC × 180

The back surface of the tears remains unchanged in its effect.

Thus, if the front surface of the contact lens remains spherical, a spectacle lens of +1.22 DC × 180 is needed in front of the contact lens to fully correct the eye.

It is possible for this +1.22 DC × 180 to be added to the front surface of the contact lens; but this addition, although easy to calculate and prescribe, is often very difficult to fabricate in the laboratory and its effect in practice is not always as anticipated.

It is worth noting at this point that *Example 2* deals with the most commonly encountered type of case – namely, corneal and spectacle astigmatism with-the-rule. The induced astigmatism is, however, against-the-rule (positive cylinder axis horizontal), which is of the same form that the majority of residual astigmatism takes.

It is often thought that the induced astigmatism created by using a toroidal back central optic surface on an eye with corneal astigmatism and residual astigmatism will fortuitously cancel out the residual astigmatism. In practice, however, this is most unlikely to occur in more than a few cases. Indeed, the induced astigmatism usually exaggerates the effect of the residual astigmatism.

Very occasionally, however, an example of induced and residual astigmatism cancelling out one another is encountered, as in the following case met in practice.

Keratometry:

R.E. 8.03 mm along 147, 7.65 mm along 57
L.E. 8.07 mm along 27, 7.57 mm along 117

Residual astigmatism over spherical lenses:
R.E. –1.00 DC × 130
L.E. –1.25 DC × 45

Calculated induced astigmatism with aligned toroidal back optic:
R.E. –1.00 DC × 147
L.E. –1.27 DC × 27
that is, this virtually cancels out the residual error.

Actual total residual error measured over lenses with toroidal back central optic portions:

R.E.   –0.25 DC × 75
L.E.   plano

In the calculation of induced astigmatism, it is not necessary to go to the trouble of calculating the surface powers for plastics and tears separately. It is quicker to use the appropriate radii considered with the change in refractive effect travelling from plastics to tears.

that is, power of lens/tears boundary

$$= \frac{1000(1.336 - 1.49)}{r}$$

$$= \frac{-1000(0.154)}{r}$$

$$= \frac{-154}{r}$$

where r = radius in mm.

By subtracting the values found of $-154/r$ for one principal meridian from the other, the value for the induced astigmatism may be obtained directly.

Appendix B, *Table I*, Volume 1, on page 309, gives surface powers for a refractive index difference of 0.154, and astigmatic differences can be obtained directly from *Appendix B, Table VIII*, page 327, making the calculations in *Example 2* unnecessary.

In *Example 2* it is useful to consider the power of the final bi-toric lens in steps:

Power meridians shown relative to back central optic meridians

Spherical front surface – giving –2.00 D on 8.20 mm BCOR

Back surface lens astigmatism

$$= \frac{1000(1 - 1.49)}{8.20} - \frac{1000(1 - 1.49)}{7.70}$$

$$= -3.88 \text{ DC} \times 180$$

$$= -5.88\text{D on } 7.70 \text{ mm BCOR}$$

This is shown diagrammatically in *Figure 18.2a*.

Lens after adding +1.22 DC × 180 to front surface (*Figure 18.2b*).

Powers are –2.00D on 8.20 mm BCOR
and –4.66D on 7.70 mm BCOR

(In practice, +1.25 DC would be added.)

In this example, the lens described should give a reasonable visual acuity with very little residual error.

It is frequently thought that a bi-toric lens should not rotate at all, or certainly not more than a few

degrees (Capelli, 1964). It is also felt by many practitioners that such a lens, when it does rotate, creates a visually disturbing, constantly changing cylindrical correction before the eye. In fact, however, in the type of case given in this example, the correction for induced astigmatism is only necessary because the toroidal back central optic portion creates the induced astigmatism along its principal meridians. With such a lens, made with a spherical front surface, the axis of the induced astigmatism depends only on the position of the principal meridians of the back central optic portion before the eye. With the lens under discussion, if it rotates until the 8.20 mm BCOR lies along the 45 meridian, then the axis of the +1.22 DC is also required along this meridian. If, therefore, the front surface cylinder power is ground on to the lens in the correct meridian relative to the principal meridians of the back central optic portion, then it does not matter if the lens does rotate as the lens carries its correction for induced astigmatism with it when it moves away from its intended position. This is worth remembering when correcting an eye with a bi-toric lens containing a front surface cylinder for the correction of induced astigmatism only, that is, a compensated bi-toric contact lens.

It may well be that many practitioners believe, due to their experiences when refracting over lenses with toroidal back central optic surfaces and spherical front surface, that bi-toric lenses must not rotate. When refracting over such a lens, the cylinder addition is frequently found to fluctuate in axis with the lens rotation. This gives the impression that the lens must not be permitted to rotate, but this does not matter once the correction for induced astigmatism is ground on the front of the lens in the appropriate meridian as the correcting cylinder then rotates with the surface inducing the astigmatism.

Most eyes, however, do have some residual astigmatism. Therefore, while going to the trouble of having a front surface cylinder ground on to the lens to make it bi-toric, it is good practice in certain cases to incorporate a correction for residual astigmatism (*see* calculations on page 548). When this is done, however, the lens must not rotate more than a few degrees as the axis of correction for the residual astigmatism remains fixed in relation to the eye. This limitation on rotation is important, for when residual astigmatism is of a low degree, from the clinical standpoint, then it is not worthwhile incorporating its correction with that for the induced astigmatism.

For residual astigmatism of 0.50 D or more, if the patient can obtain a good visual acuity without its correction, it is probably not worthwhile adding a front surface cylinder to correct more than the calculated induced astigmatic error. If, however, the

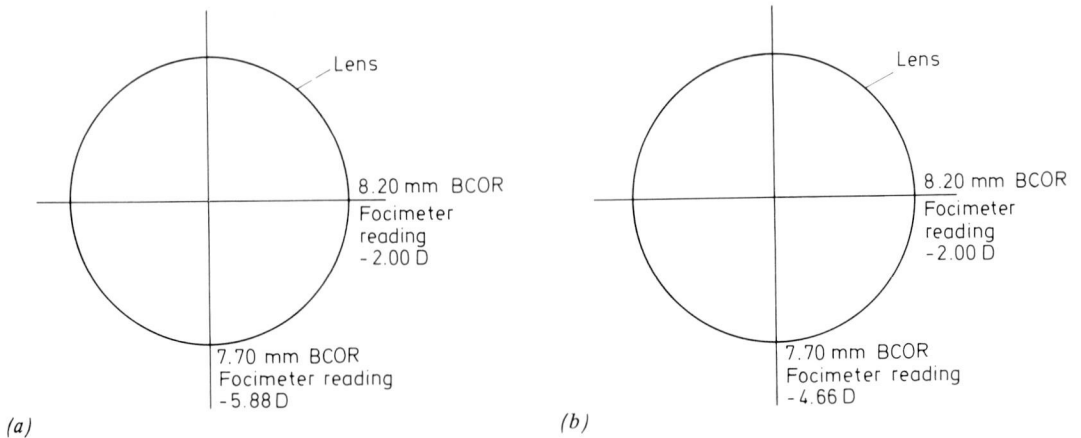

Figure 18.2–(a) Focimeter readings of a toric lens with BCOR 8.20 × 7.70 mm and BVP –2.00 D along the flatter meridian. (b) Focimeter readings of the same lens shown in (a) with +1.22 DC × 180 added to the front surface

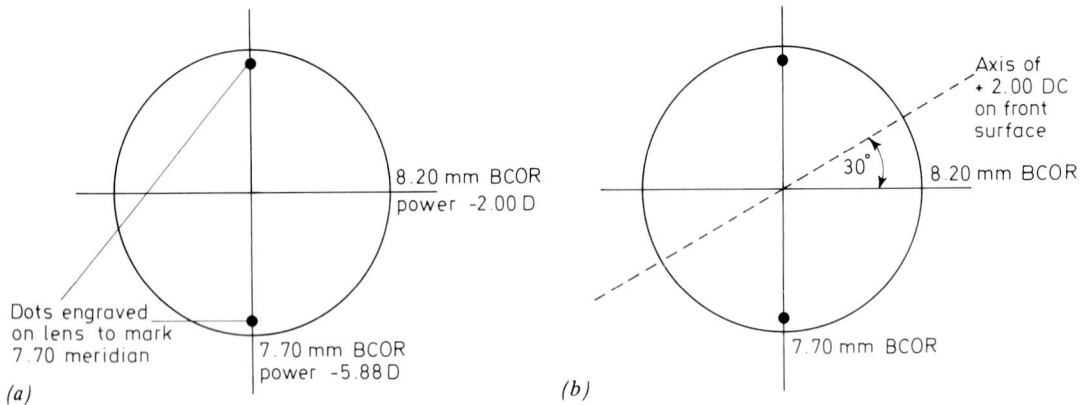

Figure 18.3–(a) Instructions to laboratory. Step 1: spherical front surface. (b) Instructions to laboratory. Step 2: add +2.00 DC × 30

residual astigmatism is clinically significant, then it is worth incorporating provided that lens rotation can be kept to a minimum (*Colour Plates XXXIV and XXXV*).

Probably the easiest method of estimating the significance of the induced and residual astigmatic errors is not by calculation but by the use of a fitting set of lenses with toroidal back central optic portions, as mentioned previously. Frequently, a discrepancy is found between the estimated and actual effects. If the refraction over such a lens reveals an astigmatic component not more than 0.50 D different from the calculated induced astigmatism, then it is almost certainly not worth while adding more than a correction for the latter to the front surface of the lens. A great deal also depends on the amount of rotation of the toroidal back

surface of the trial lens used. If such trial lenses are not available, it is reasonable to expect lenses with a small difference between the principal back optic radii to rotate more than lenses with a large difference.

The value of trial fitting lenses with toroidal back central optic surfaces cannot be over-estimated and, almost invariably, it is found that the best visual results are obtained where they have been used. They certainly help to obviate the need for resolving obliquely crossed cylinders, which frequently needs to be done in calculating the powers required.

For example, in the case just considered, a refraction is performed over the BCOR 8.20 mm × 7.70 mm (with a spherical front surface giving –2.00 D along the 8.20 mm meridian):

Refraction +2.00 DC × 30

The lens does not rotate more than a few degrees and, thus, the full cylinder effect is desired on the front surface.

It may be best to order the lens by sketching the requirements as shown in *Figure 18.3a and b.*

It may also be useful to calculate the resolved effect and give the laboratory the final focimeter reading and axis expected. Laboratories often seem to have difficulty in working this out and it must not be forgotten that some contact lens technicians are not familiar with standard notation and the transposition of sphero-cylinders. An unambiguous order is therefore very helpful.

It is important to have clear marks on the lenses to denote the position of one of the principal meridians of the back surface. These marks should be permanent as they provide a check on the amount of rotation with the lens *in situ* and also provide an axis of orientation about which the accuracy of the powers and axes of the surfaces produced by the laboratory can be checked.

Some laboratories mark the axis with dots of paintlike material which is luminescent under ultra-violet illumination. These are not as good as permanent marks as they are removed when a front surface cylinder is added. The best marking is a pair of engraved dots along the steepest (shortest) back surface meridian. This is the thicker meridian near the periphery and usually has ample substance for such engraving. The small pits fill with fluorescein, and during examination with ultra-violet illumination they thus provide an easily visible reference meridian.

Calculation of the salient points in bi-toric corneal lens work follows in the form of examples.

Example A

Calculating the back vertex power of a bi-toric lens

Spectacle refraction (vertex distance ignored):
–2.00/–3.00 × 180

Keratometer reading: 8.10 mm, 41.62 D along 180
7.60 mm, 44.37 along 90

A contour, multi-curve or similar trial lens is placed on the cornea and the fit is examined along the flattest corneal curve (horizontal). The peripheral fit is examined in this meridian only to select the appropriate peripheral radii.

Having chosen an appropriate spherical lens to fit this meridian – say, for example, C2/8.10:6.50/8.70:9.00/–2.00 D – then a refraction with this lens *in situ* is carried out.

Spectacle refraction and visual acuity with contact lens: plano, 6/6 (no residual astigmatism).

Rx along 180 meridian: C2/8.10:6.5048.70:9.00/–2.00 D

This lens is approximately in alignment with the horizontal meridian, and from the keratometer reading the BCOR 7.60 mm might be chosen to fit the vertical meridian.

The front surface of the tears lens has radii of: 8.10 mm in the horizontal, 7.60 mm in the vertical.

Knowing this, the power of the front surface of the tears lens is calculated from its refractive index (1.336). Thus (*see* Appendix B, *Table V,* Volume 1),

$$F = \frac{(1.336 - 1)1000}{r}$$

Tears: dioptric value of 7.60 mm radius = +44.21 D
Tears: dioptric value of 8.10 mm radius = +41.48 D
Therefore, tears lens front surface astigmatism = +2.73 D

The steeper meridian is more positive in power by this amount. Therefore, total lens power required in the vertical meridian is:

–2.00 D + (–2.73 D) = –4.73 D.

Final Rx of lens:

BCOR 8.10 m 180, –2.00 D
BCOR 7.60 m 90, –4.75 D

Since the principal meridians of the front and back toroidal surfaces have the same orientation the full specification of the lens is as follows.

C2 Parallel bi-toric/8.10 m 180:6.50/8.70:9.00
                           7.60   8.20

–2.00/–2.75 × 180

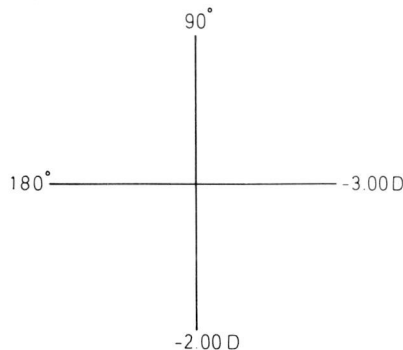

Figure 18.4

Example B
If refraction with the 8.10 mm –2.00 D lens used in *Example A* had been: plano/–1.00 × 90 then power along flattest meridian (180) = –3.00 D.
Required meridional powers with 8.10 mm BCOR are as shown in *Figure 18.4.*

Consider the steepest meridian (as in *Example 1*) with BCOR 7.60 m 90:

Converting radii to dioptres ($n = 1.336$)

7.60 mm	=	+44.21 D
8.10	=	+41.48
Difference	=	+2.73 D

Refraction along 90 with 8.10 mm BCOR = -2.00 D (*see* above).
Along this meridian, the liquid lens is more positive by +2.73 D
Therefore, additional BVP required along 90 = -2.73 D

Therefore, required power along 90 = -4.73 D

Full Rx = 8.10 m 180, -3.00 D
       7.60 m 90, -4.73 D

In *Examples A* and *B*, the powers specified are the back vertex powers of the bi-toric lens in the appropriate meridians. These are the powers read by the laboratory when checking the lens on a focimeter if the image quality is good enough.

Example C
Keratometer readings not known.
    Bi-toric specification based on spectacle Rx and trial corneal lenses with spherical BCOR.
    As in previous examples, the flattest meridian is fitted in a conventional manner with a spherical BCOR and a refraction is performed with such a lens *in situ*.

Spectacle Rx = $-2.00/-3.00 \times 45$.

Flattest meridian (45)
BCOR of trial contact lens used = 7.70 mm (power -2.00 DS)
Spectacle addition over this trial lens = -1.00 DS (no residual astigmatism)
Total required power with 7.70 mm BCOR = -3.00 DS
Therefore, liquid lens power = +1.00 D
But liquid lens front surface power of the 7.70 mm meridian ($n = 1.336$) = +43.64 D
Therefore, liquid lens back surface power (+1.00 D -43.64 D) = -42.64 D
Therefore, radius of back surface of liquid lens ($n = 1.336$) = 7.88 mm

This is the same as the corneal radius. Therefore, BCOR chosen to align with flattest corneal radius for a bi-toric lens might thus be 7.90 mm.
Rx in this 45 meridian: 7.90 mm, -2.00 D.

Steepest meridian (135)
Flattest meridian of 7.88 mm radius has a power of 42.64 D for $n = 1.336$. Spectacle Rx indicates

corneal astigmatism (no residual astigmatism detected) corrected by -3.00 DC $\times$ 45, which has all been corrected by the liquid lens.
Thus, the 135 meridian must be steeper than the 45 meridian by approximately this amount, and the back surface of the liquid lens has a power along 135 = -42.64 D -3.00 D = -45.64 D
Therefore, liquid lens radius along 135 = 7.36 mm ($n = 1.336$)
and corneal radius = 7.36 mm

BCOR chosen for alignment along 135 meridian might thus be 7.35 mm.
Power required for correction of refractive error in this meridian is power required along 45 meridian plus power of liquid lens cylinder

  = -2.00 D $+(-3.00$ D) = -5.00 D

Therefore, Rx for steepest meridian (7.35 mm) = -5.00 D
Complete lens Rx with BCOR and back vertex powers in the meridians appropriate to the radii is:

   7.90 m 45, -2.00 D
   7.35 m 135, -5.00 D

If residual astigmatism had been found when refracting with the original 7.70 mm BCOR -2.00 DS lens *in situ*, an allowance would merely have to be made for this when calculating the corneal astigmatism.
    If the refraction over this lens had been $-1.00/-1.00 \times 45$, then clearly -1.00 D of the -3.00 DC $\times$ 45 spectacle Rx would not have been due to corneal astigmatism, and thus the correction for corneal astigmatism would have been estimated at -2.00 DC $\times$ 45.
    Thus, the 135 meridian would be steeper than the 45 meridian by 2.00 D and its power would be

  +42.64 D + 2.00 D = +44.64 D

Therefore, radius of 135 meridian = 7.53 mm.
    If residual astigmatism is measured in negative cylinder form and has its axis parallel to the negative cylinder axis in the spectacle Rx, then the estimated corneal astigmatism is reduced by the amount of the residual astigmatism. If the residual negative cylinder axis is perpendicular to the negative cylinder axis in the spectacle Rx, then the estimated corneal astigmatism is increased by the amount of the residual astigmatism. Unfortunately, the calculations involved are not always quite as simple as those shown above. It is rare, for example, for the axis of the residual astigmatism to correspond exactly with one of the principal meridians of curvature of the cornea. This means that resolution of obliquely crossed cylinders is frequently necessary before completing the calculations. It is also

rare for the estimated corneal astigmatism, as in the last example, to agree with the corneal astigmatism found with the keratometer. In clinical practice, it is unusual for residual astigmatism, measured by refraction through a spherical corneal lens, to equal that expected from consideration of the spectacle correction and keratometer readings.

The calculations so far have not considered the effect of vertex distance, which must be taken into account if this distance is great or if the refractive power in either meridian exceeds 3.00 D.

It is frequently useful, in considering bi-toric lenses, to draw a representation of meridional powers to ensure that simple errors in confusing axes and meridians are not made. A slightly more complicated example is now shown, in which the BCOR of the toric lens do not exactly agree with the principal corneal radii, and the axes of the spectacle refraction do not correspond with the principal meridians of corneal curvature.

Example D
Spectacle Rx = −4.50/−3.50 × 180
Vertex distance = 14 mm
Ocular refraction = −4.23 DC × 90, −7.19 DC × 180
Ocular astigmatism = −2.96 DC × 180
Meridional powers (ocular refraction) are shown in *Figure 18.5.*

Keratometer reading: 8.50 mm along 20
                       8.05 mm along 110

BCOR chosen for the toroidal back surface of the lens:
  8.45 mm on 20
  8.10 mm on 110

Surface powers of tears lens given by

$$F = \frac{(1.336 - 1)1000}{r}$$

Power of back surface of tears lens (taken from keratometer radii)
  = −39.53 D along 20,
  −41.74 D along 110

Front surface power of tears lens (taken from lens BCOR)
  = +39.76 D along 20,
  +41.48 D along 110

Tears lens total power
  = +0.23 D along 20,
  −0.26 D along 110
  = +0.23/−0.49 × 20

Back vertex power required on bi-toric lens to correct ametropia
  = ocular refraction − power of tears lens

Back vertex power with:
BCOR 8.45 mm on 20
        8.10 mm on 110
        = −7.19/+2.96 × 90
           −(+0.23/−0.49 × 20)
        = −7.42/+2.96 × 90 with
           +0.49 × 20

These oblique cylinders must be resolved (*see* Stokes' Construction: Stokes, 1883) (*Figure 18.6*).

Sphere/cylinder effect of resolved cylinders =
  +0.41/+2.62 × 86½

Total back vertex power of bi-toric lens =
  −7.01/+2.62 × 86½

This type of lens specification is very interesting but difficult for the laboratory to interpret and convert to lens fabrication specifications.

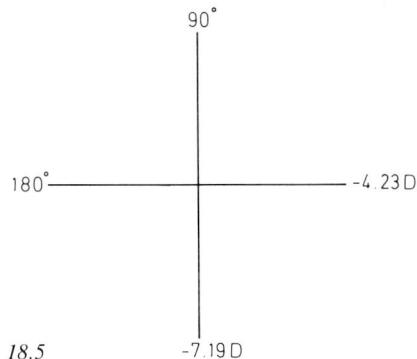

Figure 18.5

This prescription for a lens involves the principal meridians of the back central optic portion oblique to the principal meridians of the back vertex power (an oblique bi-toric contact lens). The greatest use of such a specification is to allow the laboratory to mount the final bi-toric lens on a focimeter with the toroidal back central optic surface orientated along the appropriate axes in order to check the focimeter readings against the back vertex power ordered.

In the case of *Example D*, there are three different pairs of principal meridians relative to the horizontal meridian. The toroidal back central optic portion has principal meridians at 20 and 110, the back vertex power at 86½ and 176½ and those of the toroidal front surface are different again – all this on a thin piece of plastics with an optic diameter of between 6.00 mm and 7.50 mm. It should not be difficult to understand the problems involved in both making and checking such lenses.

Stokes' Construction

This is an excellent method of resolving two cylinders F_1 and F_2, with an angle between their axes of $\propto$, into an equivalent sphere/cylinder power (*Figure 18.6*).

A parallelogram is constructed with the two sides OA_1 and OA_2 proportional to F_1 and F_2, with the angle between them $2\propto$.

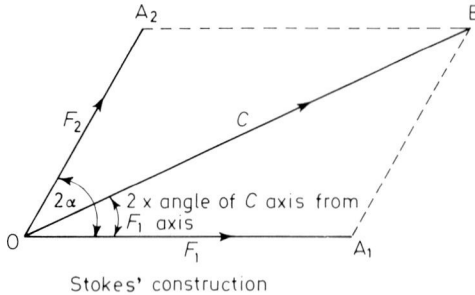

Stokes' construction

Figure 18.6

The parallelogram is completed and the resultant OB drawn. This is proportional to the resultant cylinder C. The angle between OB and OA_1 being twice the angle between the axis of C and that of F_1, where

    S = equivalent sphere
    C = equivalent cylinder
    S = ½ $(F_1 + F_2 - C)$

Another approach to the calculation of the final power of bi-toric lenses is shown in *Example E*.

Example E

In this example, all measurements and quantities are rounded off to clinically significant amounts.

Keratometer reading:
    7.65 mm, 44.12 D along 90
    8.16 mm, 41.37 D along 180
Spherical trial lens (BCOR 8.15 mm) placed on cornea, BVP = –2.25 DS
Refraction through lens = –1.50/–1.00 × 180
Thus, total power through 8.15 mm BCOR lens = –3.75/–1.00 × 180
BCOR 8.15 mm × 7.65 mm used for final lens
These radii give induced astigmatism = –1.25 × 180
Therefore, cylinder power to be placed on front surface of lens = +0.25 × 180   (a)
And sphere power required = –3.75 D   (b)
Cylindrical effect of back surface of lens (measured in air) = –4.00 × 180   (c)
Thus, final total power of lens = (a) + (b) + (c) = –3.75/–3.75 × 180

It is also possible to calculate the power of a bi-toric lens by considering a theoretical emmetropic cornea (Capelli, 1964).

Example F

Keratometer reading:
    7.42 mm, 45.50 D along 90
    7.94 mm, 42.50 D along 180
Corneal power = +42.50/+3.00 × 180
Ocular refraction = –3.00/–1.50 × 180
Thus, theoretical corneal power to produce emmetropia = +39.50/+1.50 × 180
Back surface power of lens (BCOR 7.95 mm × 7.40 mm) plastics/tears boundary (relative n = 0.154) = –19.37/–1.44 × 180
Therefore, required front surface power of lens = +58.87/+2.94 × 180
Back surface power of lens in air (BCOR 7.95 mm × 7.40 mm) = –61.64/–4.58 × 180
And final total lens power = –2.75/–1.62 × 180

Toroidal Front Surfaces Combined with Spherical Back Central Optic Portions

Residual astigmatism frequently needs to be corrected in cases where the patient is fitted well, physically, with a lens utilizing a spherical back central optic portion. Such a lens therefore requires a toroidal front surface but must not be allowed to rotate sufficiently to cause the changing cylinder effect to give rise to visual discomfort.

Rotation is normally prevented by the use of prism ballast or by the use of truncation to align with the lower or upper lids or both.

Prism ballast is most commonly used and the lens is prescribed in the normal manner with the addition of between one and three prism dioptres. When ordering the lens, some practitioners assume that the weight or prism ballast orientates the lens in a certain fixed position on the cornea and order the cylinder axis orientated to this expected position.

Alternatively, the lens can be made without the front cylinder but with the position of the prism base marked with a small permanent dot. The spherical power is calculated to give the necessary cylinder in positive form. A refraction is performed over the lens *in situ* and the average position of the dot in normal, common directions of gaze is estimated. The laboratory is then asked to add the residual refractive error – expressed in positive cylinder form – to the front of the lens, using the dot position as a point of reference for the cylinder axis.

It is important to realize that it is the angular position of the dot on the lens that is significant and not the position of the dot on the cornea. This is illustrated in *Figures 18.7* and *18.8*.

It is difficult accurately to assess the position of the dot on the lens. One of the best methods is to photograph the lens on the cornea in the desired direction of gaze and enlarge the photographs, or project slides on to a screen where they can be superimposed on a protractor and the angle measured easily and accurately. These photographs are easily taken through slit lamp biomicroscopes with photographic attachments.

The illustrations in this chapter were taken from transparencies obtained in this manner.

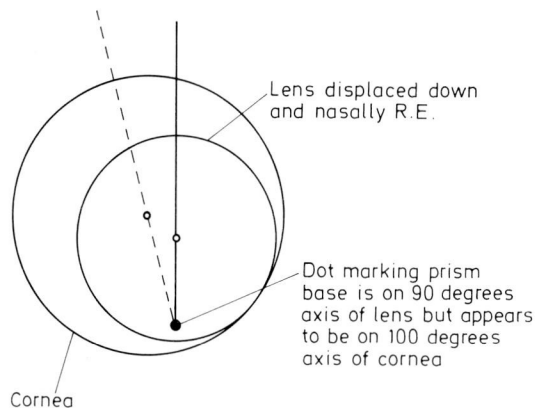

Figure 18.7–The importance of the position of the prism base-apex line is indicated relative to the lens when the latter is off centre. The position of the prism base relative to the cornea is irrelevant

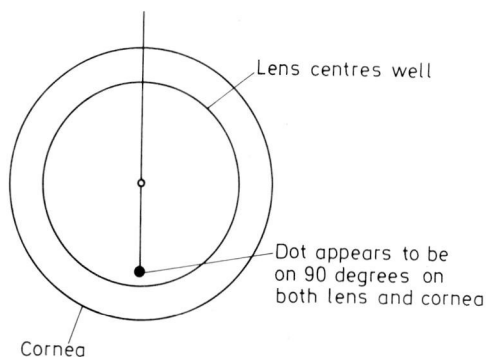

Figure 18.8–If the lens centres well then the prism base-apex line is at the same angle with respect to either the lens or cornea

This type of photograph can be useful for assessing the angle of eyelid contact with the lens and for measuring the eye if an appropriate scale is photographed. A lens of known overall size *in situ* acts as a useful unit on which to base measurements.

The most commonly used method of assessing the axis taken up by the prism base-apex line is to place a trial frame before the eye and hold a transparent

ruler through the dot and through the middle of the lens. Alternatively, a transparent plastics disc or afocal trial case lens, with a diagonal line finely drawn upon it, can be placed in the frame and rotated until the line passes through the dot and contact lens centre. The angles are read from the trial frame protractor.

It must not be forgotten that it is impossible to add a negative front surface cylinder to the lens without transposing to positive cylinder form and altering the sphere power. Only positive cylinders, therefore, should be prescribed.

If it is intended to use a prism ballasted lens with a toroidal front surface, it is important when refracting to use a trial lens with almost identical specifications to the lens to be prescribed. BCOR, BCOD and OS should be the same, if possible. The trial lens should also contain the appropriate amount of prism, if such a lens is available. It is common to measure different degrees of residual astigmatism with lenses of different specifications, as the following case record shows.

Mrs R. C. (left eye)
Keratometer reading: 8.03 mm along 180
$\qquad\qquad\qquad\qquad\quad$ 7.86 mm along 90

Spectacle refraction: –5.00/–0.50 × 95

Rx over trial lens,
C4/8.00:6.50/8.50:7.50/9.00:8.50/9.50:9.50/–2.00 D
$\quad$ = –2.50/–1.50 × 95, V.A. = 6/6

Prescription lens made up to the following:
C4/8.00:6.50/8.50:7.50/9.00:8.50/9.50:9.50/–6.00 D
with 1△ base down
Refraction with this lens = +1.00/–0.50 × 75, V.A. = 6/6

Refraction with
C4/8.00:7.00/8.50:7.80/9.00:8.60/9.50:9.50/–5.00 D
= +0.25/–1.50 × 100, V.A. = 6/6 (no prism ballast used).

Ideally, the contact lens with which to measure residual astigmatism should be worn for a few hours for several consecutive days and refraction carried out on each occasion. The measured degree and axis of astigmatism is often found to change significantly during this period.

A fitting set of prism ballasted lenses is very useful in order to assess likely prism position. If the position of the prism appears stable and predictable, then a lens can often be made up straight away with both prism and front toroidal surface, missing out the intermediate stage.

It is difficult to predict the final position of the prism base and the effect of the nasal rise of the lower lid. This latter has been estimated at 10–15 degrees (Fairmaid, 1967), while the former has been quoted as being 20 degrees displacement nasally (Goldberg, 1964) and 10 degrees nasally (Westerhout, 1971a). The differences in these figures may be accounted for by the fact that the authorities quoted used different lens designs, sizes, thicknesses and degrees of prism ballast.

One of the disadvantages of fitting a prism ballasted lens with a spherical front surface and subsequently adding a front cylinder is that the altered lighter lens may well take up an entirely different position on the cornea – especially if a positive cylinder is added with its axis horizontal, thus thinning the upper and lower edges. The influence of the lids may well be altered.

The average positions of the prism base and wide variations from the normal are shown in *Colour Plates XXXVI* to *XXXIX*.

It will be seen from the variations shown in *Colour Plates XXXVIII* and *XXXIX* that it is unwise to place too much reliance on the expected positions of the prism base unless a trial prism ballasted lens has been observed after several hours of use.

If the patient has an occupation involving unusual positions of gaze, the prism base position should also be observed with the eyes held in an appropriate direction. If the direction of gaze influences the dot position greatly, consideration must be given to this fact in prescribing the cylinder axis on the lens.

When asking the laboratory to add a front cylinder at a certain axis, it is worth drawing a sketch showing the corrected position of the axis with the dot at 6 o'clock (or down along 90). If, for example, the dot marking the ballast position is found to settle at 100 and the required cylinder axis is at 120, the axis is ordered at 110 with the dot at 6 o'clock (along 90).

It should be mentioned that a lens which is physically comfortable before the cylinder is added to the front surface frequently becomes uncomfortable after the addition of the toroidal surface. This is usually because the addition of a cylinder has materially altered the edge finish and this may not have been reworked and repolished sufficiently. Since the upper edge of a prism ballasted lens is very thin, it may well be worthwhile ordering the original lens about 0.2 mm larger in overall size to allow for re-edging after the cylinder is added. This same suggestion remains valid even if the lens is not prism ballasted.

A common laboratory error is to mark the dot some way off the position of the prism base. This does not matter greatly provided that the cylinder axis is prescribed relative to the dot, which should remain visible so that the added cylinder axis can be checked.

CHECKING HARD TORIC LENSES

Although covered in Chapter 12, Volume 1, a brief resumé of verification techniques for hard toric lenses is appropriate here, with elaboration of certain points. Many of the parameters of toric lenses are checked as for spherical lenses. Overall size and thickness are measured in the conventional way, not forgetting that truncated lenses need to have their overall size dimensions measured along the major and minor axes, and the edge finish in the truncated area should be checked to ensure that it is satisfactory. Similarly, lenses with spherical back central optic portions and toroidal peripheral zones, or vice versa, should have both diameters of the back central optic portion measured. Lenses with toroidal back central optic portions and toroidal peripheral zones may also appear to have slightly oval back central optic portions, if the difference between the two BCOR is very large, or the difference between BCOR and peripheral radius in one meridian is different from that in the other meridian.

Toroidal back central optic surfaces are usually measured on a radiuscope, and it is useful to remember that on most instruments the line in focus is at right-angles to the meridian whose radius is being measured when the target image is formed at the centre of curvature. (In order to locate the meridians accurately, the lens must be rotated until one of the target lines is sharply in focus.) This is probably the reason why the dots marking the required meridian are so often found at right-angles to their correct position. The dots are also often found 5–15 degrees off the true meridian, even if the meridian approximates to the required one. This may well be due to the fact that it is difficult to mount a lens on a radiuscope lens holder in such a way as to facilitate the exact marking of the meridians. It is better for the laboratory to mark the lens directly, with respect to the axis of the holding device, while the lens is mounted for cutting and polishing the BCOR. Unfortunately, few laboratories have such efficient methods of cutting and polishing toroidal surfaces and some still resort to a hand-held flexed lens (that is, one in which the lens is physically distorted, or bent, to give the required astigmatic surface: it is then cut to a spherical curvature and, when the pressure on the lens is released, it slowly returns to its original state and assumes an equal but opposite astigmatic surface to that produced by the bending).

It is difficult for the checking to be done with the meridian-identification dots at an exactly set position on the radiuscope lens holder. If the lens has a toroidal back central optic portion, the best procedure is to measure the radii on a radiuscope and check the meridians of the radii relative to the dots by mounting the lens on a keratometer. There are many methods of mounting the lens. A simple one, shown in *Figure 18.9*, is to place the lens on a 45 degree reflecting prism. The lens is then adjusted until the dots appear horizontal. This can be done by marking permanent lines on the prism, which

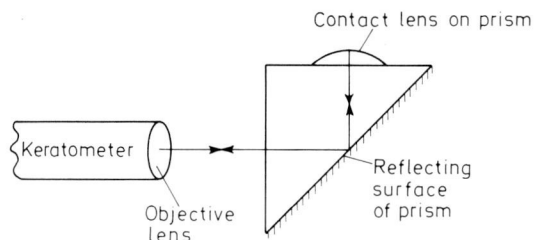

Figure 18.9–The use of a 45 degree reflecting prism to position a contact lens in order to measure its BCOR and principal meridians with a keratometer

remain horizontal with the prism in position. The keratometer is racked forward to focus the lens and dots while the lens is being adjusted. The instrument is then moved back to focus on the mire images, and the radii and their axes are read off on the keratometer protractor scale. With the magnification provided by the keratometer and the use of its accurate protractor scale, far greater accuracy can be achieved than with the radiuscope alone. Even a rotation test using a crossed line chart does not provide a high degree of accuracy.

One difficulty which is hard to overcome is that on a small lens the dots themselves subtend quite a large angle.

The keratometer and prism mount are also useful for checking the actual cylinder power added to the front surface of a lens. The lens point of reference (dot or dots) is mounted in a set position, which is checked by focusing on the lens surface. The front surface radii and axes of their meridians are then measured with the lens mounted on water to prevent reflections from the back surface. The radii are then converted to dioptric power using a refractive index of 1.49. (The dioptric scale on the keratometer cannot be used.) This is an excellent way of measuring the added cylinder. The focimeter is very useful for checking toric corneal lenses, but it does have several disadvantages. The main disadvantage is that the focimeter images are rarely perfectly clear and are usually considerably off centre due to the prisms often used. If the lens is bi-toric, the relatively small front surface cylinder is completely dwarfed by the invariably much larger back surface cylinder, which does not need be checked since it is automatically created by the toroidal back central

optic surface. It is also difficult to mount the reference points in a precise position on the focimeter.

It is common to find discrepancies between front cylinder measurements taken with the keratometer and focimeter. If there is a discrepancy, it is often found that the keratometer reading is more compatible with the result obtained from refraction with the lens *in situ*.

Some examples found in clinical practice serve to illustrate this point. To simplify the examples, the peripheral radii are not specified.

Miss M. (left eye)
All lenses of OS 9.50 mm and BCOD 7.00 mm
Spectacle refraction: –1.00/–2.00 × 80
Trial lens: 8.00 mm BCOR, –2.00 D, Add. = –1.25 × 85
Lens ordered: 8.00 mm BCOR, –2.00 D 1△ (base dotted)
Rx with this lens: +0.50/–2.00 × 85, dot on 85
This power added as –1.50/+2.00 × 175 to the front surface.
(*Note:* it would have been more satisfactory to order –3.25 D in the first place).

After addition
Rx with lens: plano/–0.50 × 85
Focimeter reading: (dot at 6 o'clock) –3.50/–2.00 × 85
Front surface cylinder checked on keratometer (dot at 6 o'clock): –1.40 × 90.

Frequently, the most baffling results are obtained where no measurements seem compatible. In such cases, the focimeter images are frequently found to be of poor quality.

Mrs L.
All lenses of OS 8.50 mm and BCOD 6.50 mm

Spectacle refraction: R.E. –3.50/–0.50 × 25
L.E. –4.00/–0.50 × 170

Keratometer reading: R.E. 7.02 mm along 170
6.81 mm along 80
L.E. 7.02 mm along 180
6.78 mm along 90

Trial lens
R. 7.00 mm BCOR, –3.00 D 1△ (base dotted). Add. = +0.75/–1.25 × 75, dot on 120
L. 7.00 mm BCOR, –3.00 D 1△ (base dotted). Add. = plano/–1.50 × 100, dot on 100

Lenses ordered
R. 7.00 mm BCOR, –2.25/–1.25 × 45, 1△ base at 6 o'clock (along 90)
L. 7.00 mm BCOR, –3.00/–1.50 × 90, 1△ base at 6 o'clock (along 90)

Lenses checked on focimeter with prism base dots at 6 o'clock
R. –2.25/–1.50 × 45
L. –3.50/–1.50 × 90

Refraction with lenses *in situ*
R. +0.25/–1.00 × 105, dot at 100
L. +0.75/–1.50 × 115, dot at 100

Front surface cylinders checked on keratometer with dots at 6 o'clock (along 90)
R. –1.62 × 45
L. –1.12 × 90

It is relatively rare to find an oblique bi-toric lens with clear focimeter images and so the keratometer cylinder measurements can be very helpful.

It may be said that, in checking toric lenses, the focimeter readings are a useful guide but should not be relied upon too fully. They are useful to relate to the refractive effect upon the eye. Apparently identical lenses, as measured with the focimeter, may give entirely different effects on the eye; but in such cases, the keratometer or radiuscope readings usually reveal differences in front surface cylinder and optical quality.

Frequently, the cylinder added to the front surface of a lens is inaccurate and, if the lens has enough substance, one feels inclined to ask the laboratory, rather than reworking the cylinder to repolish the surface to a spherical power so that the refraction can be checked with the lens *in situ* once again. This process is often unsuccessful for, frequently, the polishing appears to follow the contour of the cylinder, and the intermediate stage is an irregular and undetermined toricity. Since many lenses with front surface cylinders also have prism ballast, it is very difficult to remount the lens on the polishing tools without producing irregularity.

TRUNCATION AND DOUBLE TRUNCATION

Truncation of corneal lenses has long been used as a method of attempting to secure freedom from rotation in stabilizing bifocal and toroidal front surface lenses. It is generally found associated with prism ballast, and the combination of both methods is frequently very effective.

The usual method with truncated prism ballasted lenses is to prescribe the lens in the normal way with the addition of the front surface cylinder at the correct angle relative to the estimated or observed position of the prism base. The relationship of the lower lid to the edge of the lens is observed and a truncation is then cut to align with the lower lid (*Colour Plate XL* and *Figures 18.10* and *18.11*).

In *Figures 18.10* and *18.11*, the lower lid chord makes an angle of 5 degrees to the horizontal at its contact with the lens, and the truncation might well be cut at that angle. The lower edge is thick at the truncation, and thus the lens is unlikely to slip below

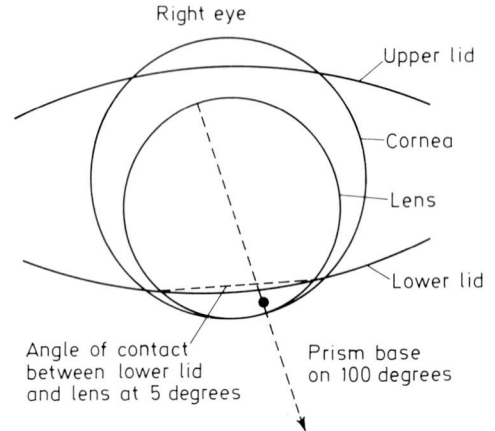

Figure 18.10–The position of contact between a prism ballasted corneal lens and the lower lid margin

the lower lid and tends to be influenced by it. If the nasal rise of the lower lid during blinking is excessive, then, in the case illustrated, the angled truncation may cause the lens to rise too much nasally. A truncation at 10 degrees may be more effective in these circumstances.

Much depends on the position of the lower lid. Clearly, if the lower lid is situated well below the lower limbus, or even below the average position of the lens, it cannot be depended on to give a great deal of stable support for the lens. This type of truncation works mainly by the support given by the lower lid between blinks. Knowledge of the patient's occupation is also important in these cases as it obviously influences the lid/lens relationship. A clerical worker, with his visual axes depressed throughout much of the day, needs to be examined with the eyes in this position and the lid angles and their influence assessed. Some degree of support from the lower lid can almost certainly be counted on with the patient looking down; but unfortunately, the resultant position of the lens may be entirely different from that taken up in distance vision. This is probably one of the reasons why some patients wearing a high correction for residual astigmatism which is stabilized by prism and/or truncation complain that either distance or near vision is poor in comparison with the other. It is not always, as one supposes, a mere over or under correction of the basic refractive error. In addition there are other problems encountered during close work by wearers of toric or non-toric lenses (Stone, 1967).

Prism ballasted lenses, with or without truncation, are not always as physically comfortable as non-prism lenses. Fortunately, therefore, it is possible to use truncation or double truncation to stabilize a lens without the use of a prism. Such truncations often work extremely well even if the lower lid position is very low and well below the limbus. This type of lens relies on the effect of blinking on the truncations and is not required to rest almost constantly on the lower lid.

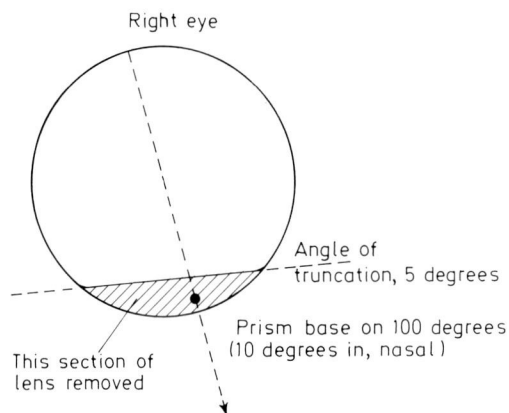

Figure 18.11–The lens shown in Figure 18.10 has been truncated to enable the lower edge of the lens to align with the lower lid margin

Very little interest appears to exist in double truncation but, if fully exploited, it can give better comfort and visual acuity than the more common forms of stabilization.

Large lenses, and prism ballasted lenses in particular, are heavy and therefore tend to locate low on the cornea. Lenses also tend to be made thicker by the laboratories if they contain a cylinder correction.

It is a natural inclination to attempt to prescribe double truncated lenses as large as possible due to the loss of so much of the vertical dimension. This is a mistake. The lenses are usually found to work best if prescribed in alignment or with slight apical clearance and with the horizontal overall size about 0.5 mm larger than would normally be used for a conventional lens. The most common horizontal overall sizes are between 8.80 and 9.70 mm and the vertical overall sizes between 7.50 and 8.50 mm, depending on the palpebral aperture size and pupil diameter. The vertical overall size should be as small as possible consistent with good visual acuity, and considering possible use for night driving. The greater the discrepancy between horizontal and

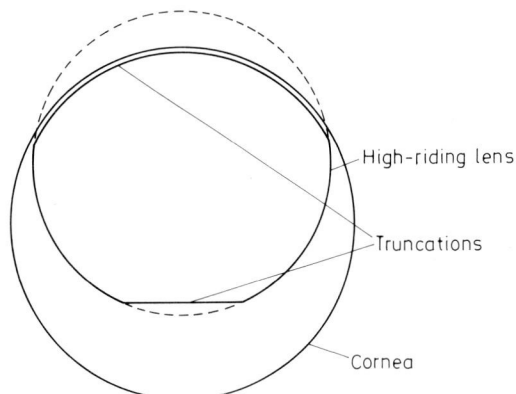

Figure 18.12–The upper truncation of a high riding lens cut to run parallel with the upper limbus. This type of truncation also assists a bifocal corneal lens to rise adequately for near vision

vertical overall sizes the better, since this gives a greater truncated chord length on which the lids can act.

The BCOD of this lens design is usually between 6.50 and 7.20 mm, and edge thickness needs to be carefully controlled. Edge thickness depends on the size and power of the lens, and so the final edge finish may have to be carefully modified by a good technician. The general principle is that the edge finish must permit the lid to slide over it comfortably while still influencing the truncated edge and aligning it.

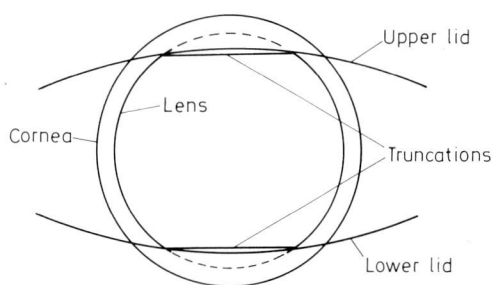

Figure 18.13–The correct positions for double truncations to permit upper and lower edges of the lenses to align with the lid margins

It would appear that an edge thickness of about 0.15–0.20 mm for the non-truncated edge is helpful, with the truncated area in the region of 0.17–0.25 mm thick. Much depends on the degree and axis of the front surface cylinder. The vertical edges tend to be thinner with the addition of a positive cylinder axis horizontal. The peak of the edge is best arranged to fall nearer the front surface of the lens on the truncated area, and the edge does not need to be as blunt as in bifocal truncation.

The longer axis of the double truncated lens almost invariably aligns with the flattest corneal meridian, which is usually nearly horizontal. If this is down and nasal (that is, at 170 in the right eye), then the effect is counteracted by the tendency for the lower lid to rise nasally. Fairmaid (1967) states that he has never observed a truncated lens stabilized downward nasally and that most lenses, when settled, stabilize within a degree or two of the horizontal.

The upper lid influences the lens when blinking and assists in aligning it. The lens rises with the upper lid after the downward movement of the blink and may rotate up and nasally during that movement. It may have been noticed that most corneal lenses tend to resist sliding far over the upper limbus on to the conjunctiva. The upper junction of cornea and conjunctiva and the irregular thickness of tissue at the limbus tend to act as stabilizing factors if the lens rises this far on blinking. Even if it does not rise on blinking the lens tends to rise on the cornea on depression of the visual axis, as during clerical work, and this may assist with stabilization. There may be a case for cutting the upper truncation on a line using a radius equal to that of half the corneal diameter. This may well be appropriate if the lens locates high and is almost constantly under the top lid, so that the truncation lines up with the limbus as shown in *Figure 18.12*.

Truncations are, however, usually most effective if cut straight, parallel and horizontal with only the corners rounded off. This rounding off should only be a smoothing and should not result in an oval lens. In many cases, it seems unnecessary to cut the truncations to correspond with the lid angles; and unless the nasal rise of the lower lid is excessive, it is best to cut the truncations horizontal – especially if

the practitioner has little experience in judging the effect of lids upon truncations. It is foolish, however, to ignore wide departures from normal lid orientation, and especially so if the front surface cylinder is high.

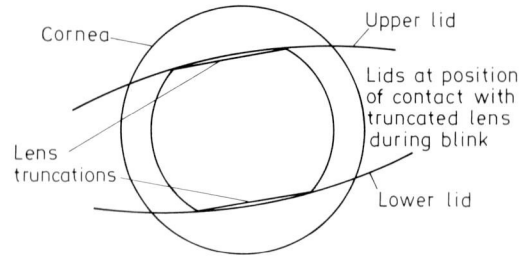

Figure 18.15–The same right eye as in Figure 18.14 during the act of blinking. Note that during a blink the angle of lid margin contact with the lens is different from that expected from the relaxed position. The truncation is cut accordingly

A lens which is overlapped by one or both of the eyelids in normal use can be converted to an interpalpebral design by double truncation (*Figure 18.13*).

A small interpalpebral lens in its round state can also be double truncated to produce an effective control of rotation; but when calculating the angles at which the truncations must be cut, it is worth considering the angles of the lids at the moment when they just contact the lens during a blink. The lid angle, relative to the horizontal, may be found to change considerably in comparison with the non-blinking state (*Colour Plates XLI* and *XLII*, and *Figures 18.14* and *18.15*).

PHYSIOLOGICAL PROBLEMS

The use of toric forms of lens often produces severe physiological problems. The use of a toroidal back central optic portion to align the cornea closely, or of a prism ballasted lens can often produce excessive oedema during the adaptive stage.

Westerhout (1971b) found that in a group of cases fitted with toroidal back central optic portions the incidence of oedema after 2 weeks of adaptation rose from an expected 38 per cent with spherical back surfaces to 83 per cent with the toroidal forms. Westerhout also found that if prism ballasted lenses were to be exchanged for non-prism ballasted lenses after 2 weeks adaptation, the incidence of oedema was as high as 92 per cent after a further 2 weeks of adaptation, compared with an expected incidence of approximately 20 per cent with non-ballasted lenses at that stage.

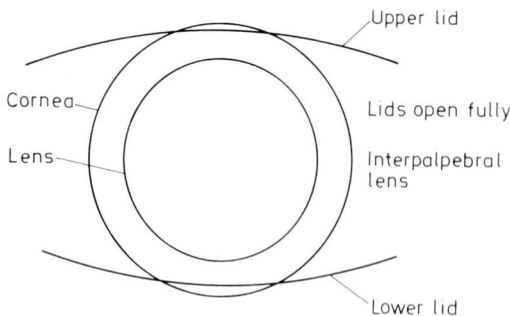

Figure 18.14–An interpalpebral lens shown on a right eye with the lids in a relaxed, fully open position prior to blinking

The same survey indicated that if a patient suffering from oedema with prism ballasted lenses were to be refitted with double truncated lenses without prisms then 80 per cent of these eyes would lose their oedema after 4 more days of wearing.

Clearly, the use of toric forms of corneal lens can be made difficult for other than optical considerations.

The author has found that although central fenestration of 0.5 mm can be helpful physiologically (*see* page 278, Chapter 11, Volume 1), it is usually better to employ one or more fenestrations of 0.2–0.3 mm in the mid-periphery of the lens. Central fenestrations tend to cause visual disturbances, possibly from tears fluid passing through the holes and cascading down the front of the lens in front of the pupil.

Mid-peripheral fenestrations are usually better visually, and if a lens stabilizes well, such as that in *Colour Plate XXXIV*, then it is possible to place the fenestrations beside the pupil area without much risk of their covering the pupil region.

As is well known, fenestrations can produce additional adhesion to the cornea in alignment fitted lenses (because of the additional tears meniscus created between lens and cornea) and tend to work best in central clearance fittings.

Hard Gas Permeable Materials

The relief of oedema, in cases such as those referred to in preceding paragraphs, is often made considerably easier by using hard, gas permeable materials.

The author has found materials such as the hard, gas permeable CLP-2A (du Pont) extremely helpful in overcoming oedema without using fenestration or modifying the lens fitting. This material is capable of giving an equivalent oxygen performance of 7.8 per cent when made with a central thickness of 0.12 (Hill, 1975). This figure is comparable with the findings of Fatt, Freeman and Lin (1974) who estimated that during sleep the cornea receives between 7 and 8 per cent oxygen. The writer has found that in tests on a patient using two lenses with toroidal back central optic portions, one of orthodox PMMA and one of a gas permeable material, the degree of oedema produced with the latter material was negligible compared with that produced by the former. These tests were repeated on several patients who were experiencing severe oedema symptoms with toroidal BCOR being used on each eye. One lens was then replaced using the gas permeable material and this gave a remarkable reduction of both subjective symptoms and signs. In one case a patient who could not attain more than 4 hours comfortable wear with orthodox lenses was

able to wear lenses of a gas permeable type for constant use within a few days.

Numerous types of hard gas permeable materials are now available for use.

FLEXING OF HARD CORNEAL LENSES

Many practitioners will have noticed that visual acuity with very thin lenses is often variable and poor. Refraction over these lenses can be very unreliable and most practitioners will have noticed the irregular retinoscopic reflexes through such lenses.

There is no doubt that very thin lenses flex with lid movement and pressure and the warping effect induces an astigmatic component in the system. Harris and Chu (1972) investigated 10 cases and found that corneal lenses with a central thickness of less than 0.13 mm flexed toroidally on a toroidal cornea and changed the residual astigmatism in a predictable fashion. They reasoned, therefore, that residual astigmatism could be altered by changing the central thickness of the corneal lens (*see* Volume 1, Chapter 4, page 111). They produced ingenious graphs showing how much change in residual astigmatism could be produced, for a given change in central thickness, for a known toricity.

For example, on a cornea having 4 D of astigmatism with-the-rule, changing the central thickness from 0.15 to 0.08 induces a 1.25 D cylinder, with-the-rule, which would cancel out 1.25 D of residual astigmatism against-the-rule (if the latter were present with the thicker lens).

This is very useful and certainly a thin lens can be used to reduce residual astigmatism when the residual astigmatism with a thick lens and corneal astigmatism are in opposite directions, which is the usual case. Unfortunately, many cases of residual astigmatism occur with fairly spherical corneas.

Westerhout (1976a) investigated 24 cases of 'thin' corneal lens wearers and found that there was very little relationship between lens flexure and corneal astigmatism and that there was no evidence of the highest changes in flexure occurring with the highest corneal astigmatism.

It is, however, worth trying much thinner lenses if the conditions are right (*see* Chapter 4, Volume 1).

PART II: TORIC SOFT LENSES

Soft contact lenses have made a very big impact on contact lens practice since their introduction by Wichterle and Lim (1960). The unique form of the soft lens material has enabled a large number of difficult cases to be fitted, many of whom had failed to wear well-made hard corneal lenses. It would appear that one of the reasons for the very large proportion of soft lenses fitted in the last few years is because many of these are fitted to hard corneal lens wearers who have only been partially successful and who have therefore been refitted with soft lenses.

Soft contact lenses have also found a wide use in unusual circumstances such as in military environments (Westerhout, 1977) and in therapeutic conditions, but throughout many years of their use it has always been held, until fairly recently, that a contra-indication for soft lenses is the presence of significant astigmatism. Attempts were made to overcome these difficulties and Westerhout (1973) reports investigating the correction of astigmatism with a hard lens worn in combination with a soft lens.

It is clear that a soft flexible material tends to follow the curvature of the underlying cornea and thus any corneal astigmatism tends to be transferred through the lens material. In the early years of the development of soft lenses, various ideas for overcoming the problems of astigmatism were postulated and detailed results were described involving the use of thick lenses to reduce the amount of corneal astigmatism transferred to the front surface of the soft lens. It is obvious, however, that attempts to use a thick soft lens may well result in poor physiological performance as thickness is undoubtedly a most significant factor in successful long-term use of soft contact lenses (Hill and Jeppe, 1975). Numerous manufacturers of soft contact lenses have made extremely optimistic, perhaps irresponsible, claims of their lenses being able to correct, satisfactorily, astigmatism of between 1 and 2 D. Only rarely is this achieved, and in reality, most experienced practitioners are now well aware that the most helpful indication of the likely residual astigmatism found while wearing a spherical soft contact lens is the ocular astigmatism determined from an accurate subjective spectacle refraction of the eye.

The optimistic and misleading claims of the ability of a spherical soft lens to correct astigmatism has resulted in a very large number of soft contact lens wearers who are only partially successful and who basically wear their lenses for social use without really adequate visual acuity. In the initial euphoria of early soft lens wearing, when their great comfort is so much enjoyed by the wearer, the limitations of visual acuity are often not noticed, but after a relatively short period these patients become aware of the fact that their visual acuity is poorer than with their spectacles, particularly for near vision.

It is ironic that one of the reasons why this limitation is noticed is due to the absence of spectacle blur following the removal of the majority of soft lenses. Most hard contact lens wearers suffer from some degree of spectacle blur and often report that their spectacle visual acuity is worse than with their contact lenses. They are unaware of the spectacle blur effect and compare their spectacle visual acuity, on contact lens removal, with their contact lens visual acuity before removal.

Now that there is such a large number of soft contact lens wearers, and this appears to be an increasing proportion of contact lens wearers fitted, it is clear that more and more patients are going to need a correction for the residual astigmatic errors present when the soft lens is being worn.

As soft contact lenses became more viable, several workers began experimenting with toric forms of soft lens in the early 1970's. Strachan (1975) describes early development work on toric lenses in 1972 as does Hirst (1975). Much of the earlier development of toric soft lenses took place in Australia and New Zealand. Useful forms of toric soft lens have only become available in Great Britain since 1975 but from that time onwards, there has been development in many countries.

INDICATIONS

Due to the complexity and expense of manufacturing toric forms of soft lens, most practitioners are inclined to prescribe them only when it is absolutely necessary. Obviously, orthodox hard corneal lenses are able to cope with a large variety of astigmatic problems but in many instances the patient may be unable to wear such a lens with sufficient comfort.

However, if a soft lens is preferred by a practitioner, or patient, for physical reasons and the resultant residual astigmatism is significant, then a toric soft lens should at least be considered, even if subsequently rejected on the grounds of cost or the difficulty of manufacturing the complex lens design required.

There are other obvious indications for a spherical soft lens such as the classic case in which the patient manifests a spherical spectacle refraction, but has appreciable corneal astigmatism. In this instance it is clear that the use of a spherical hard corneal lens would result in a correction for residual astigmatism being necessary, whereas a spherical soft lens immediately provides an adequate correction.

The incidence of astigmatism in a sample of ametropes is of interest, as it gives some indication of the likely requirement for toric soft lenses. The author reviewed a group of 500 consecutive eyes examined in practice, excluding only post-operative conditions, and found the percentage incidence of spectacle astigmatism to be as follows.

Astigmatism (in D)

0–0.50   0.75–1.00 1.25–2.00 2.25–3.00 Over 3.00

Percentage incidence

| 36 | 40 | 13 | 9 | 2 |

Holden and Garner (1976), in discussing the criteria for the prescribing of toric lenses, gave a statistical analysis showing that 45 per cent of the population required a cylindrical correction of up to 0.75 D and 25 per cent of the population required a correction of 1.00 D or more.

FORMS OF TORIC SOFT LENS

Some of the most common types of toric soft lens fitting have already been discussed briefly in Chapter 14. A more comprehensive discussion of this form of lens now follows.

Westerhout (1976b) has described 12 different forms of toric soft lens, the principal categories being as follows.

(1) Toroidal back surface with a spherical front surface.

(2) Toroidal back surface with toroidal front surface (bi-toric).

(3) Spherical back surface with toroidal front surface.

It should be noted that the toroidal back surface can be prescribed without any other form of stabilization save that of the back surface toricity, but that all three varieties of lens described above can be stabilized with either prism ballast or truncation, or a combination of both prism ballast and truncation.

(4) Another variety of lens utilizes what is termed dynamic stabilization (Fanti, 1975) in which the upper and lower portions of the front surface of the lens are chamfered (*Figure 18.16*) to allow the action of the lids, moving over the thickened and chamfered portions during blinking, to orientate the lens.

(5) A combination of a hard lens on top of a soft lens could be construed as a method of correcting astigmatism with a soft contact lens (Westerhout, 1973).

PRINCIPLES OF FITTING

If an accurate spectacle refraction indicates a degree of astigmatism similar to that found with keratometry, then it is clear that the astigmatic error is mostly corneal. If, therefore, it is possible to prescribe accurately a lens with a toroidal back surface, to align with the corneal curvatures in each meridian, then the back surface of the lens may wrap itself sufficiently precisely onto the cornea to enable the front spherical surface of the lens to remain spherical. In this instance it is assumed that the spherical front surface of the contact lens corrects the ametropia and the toroidal back surface of the lens corrects the astigmatism. This is the principle now used by many practitioners. The optical considerations are little different from those encountered when using hard corneal lenses, as the total optical effect of the tears film in contact with the front surface of the cornea remains as it would be in using a toroidal back surface hard lens. However, the toroidal back surface of the soft lens in contact with the tears film is somewhat different as its refractive index is different from that of a hard lens. The refractive indices of soft lens materials vary considerably and although they are closer to that of the tears, than PMMA, there is still sufficient difference in most cases to leave an induced astigmatic effect at this soft lens/tears interface.

The same principle applies as has already been dealt with in the section dealing with corneal lenses on page 542. Even if the toroidal back surface soft lens aligns exactly with the toric cornea there is still some induced astigmatism despite the front surface of the lens remaining spherical. Hence, many of the principles employed by some clinicians appear to be based on a false premise. However, by making the back surface of a soft lens less toroidal than the cornea, when it flexes to match the cornea, the front surface of the lens also becomes slightly toroidal. Thus, with care and careful calculation, the undercorrection of the astigmatism by the front surface of the soft lens can be made to neutralize (or largely so) the overcorrection by the back surface.

Other faulty considerations apply to the assumption that if a soft lens wraps itself onto the cornea in close alignment, any change in the back surface radius gives rise to an almost equal change in the front surface radius. Most of these assumptions (Strachan, 1973; Baron, 1975) do not appear to have been supported by theoretically correct arguments.

Bennett (1976) has, however, produced a mathematical method of calculating the power changes expected when a soft lens flexes (*see* Chapter 4, Volume 1, page 110; and Ford's Addendum to Chapter 16, page 523. Bennett's results indicate that the power changes are likely to be much greater in magnitude and even different in sign to those predicted by the use of the 'wrap factor' (Strachan, 1973).

If it is assumed that the principal meridians of the toroidal back surface of the contact lens align with the principal meridians of the cornea, then it can readily be seen that this method of correction is only applicable in the absence of any significant lenticular or residual astigmatism. It must also be assumed that the lens will orientate accurately in the correct meridian, as it is rarely found that toroidal back surfaces align accurately without additional methods of stabilization such as prisms or truncation.

If there is a significant difference between the spectacle refraction cylinder and the keratometric cylinder then, clearly residual astigmatism will result and a straightforward toroidal back surface and spherical front surface is inadequate. In this case a bi-toric soft lens can be prescribed in which the toroidal back surface corrects the corneal astigmatism and the toroidal front surface corrects the lenticular or residual astigmatism together with any induced astigmatism. Such a lens is extremely difficult to manufacture accurately, especially if the residual astigmatism is at an axis different from the principal meridians of the cornea. If the axis of the residual astigmatism corresponds to one of the corneal principal meridians then the lens may not be too complex, but as this is not often encountered the lens becomes extremely complicated, especially if it is inclined to rotate despite methods used to stabilize it.

In some cases, where the residual astigmatism and the corneal astigmatism have parallel axes, it is possible to order the toroidal back surface radii so that they are not the same as the corneal radii. As described for the correction of corneal astigmatism above, this results in the lens wrapping itself around the cornea in such a way that the increased or decreased astigmatic effect from the back surface of the lens is transferred through the flexible material to induce front surface astigmatism on the contact lens. By careful selection this may be made to correct any residual error. This is clearly impossible to achieve if the residual astigmatism is at a different axis from that of the cornea.

Spherical Back Surfaces

A spherical back surface is normally employed with a toroidal front surface to correct a variety of types of residual astigmatism found by refraction while a spherical soft contact lens is being worn. If such a lens can be made to stabilize precisely with an accurately made toroidal front surface, it may be utilized to correct any form of regular astigmatism. It does not matter whether the astigmatism is totally corneal, residual (lenticular), or induced, provided the front surface of the lens corrects the astigmatism found by refraction over a spherical lens. This is clearly a great advantage over the other more complex forms of lens all of which have a limited application.

Stabilization

All forms of astigmatic soft lens need to be stabilized to prevent unnecessary rotation. It has already been stated that even a fairly toroidal back surface, without other forms of stabilization, is unlikely to prove satisfactory. With many years of experience of stabilizing hard corneal lenses it is only natural for practitioners and laboratories to turn to the existing methods which are well-known and tried.

The Use of Prism Ballast

The use of prism ballast is well-known in stabilizing toric forms of lens but it does have certain disadvantages when applied to soft lens designs. Since many forms of soft lens are relatively thick in comparison to hard lenses, and are made larger than the corneal diameter, the additional thickness brought about by the use of a prism can be a problem with regard to oxygen permeability. The additional thickness can also cause physical discomfort in patients with sensitive lids, but a great deal depends on the position of the lids relative to the edge of the contact lens. Fortunately, the thicker edge in the region of the prism base can be thinned during the manufacturing stage without neutralizing the effect of the prism ballast. The thickest portion of the lens is also usually situated underneath the lower lid.

One of the difficulties which arises with the use of prism ballast is that if it is going to be prescribed monocularly it may well cause vertical prismatic effects which may make the patient uncomfortable. This then requires the use of a similar prism for the other eye. Although this is not a serious difficulty if that eye is also to wear a contact lens, it can be an inconvenience if the other eye is emmetropic. Fortunately, however, prism ballast does not often given rise to binocular problems (Gasson, 1977) (*see* page 453).

The principle of the use of prism ballast is to balance the forces acting on the lens in order to stabilize it. The effect of the centre of gravity being displaced away from the geometric centre helps to rotate the lens around the geometric centre and it is very important, therefore, that the lens be fairly free-moving. A tight lens will not move freely and be influenced by the prism ballast, and such lenses are to be avoided. A reasonably loose, free-moving lens is important if the prism ballast is to work satisfactorily.

Truncation

Truncation has already been described in the section dealing with corneal lenses and is a very well tried and successful method of stabilizing lenses. Many practitioners (Strachan, 1975; Garner and Holden, 1976) advocate the use of double truncation although Fanti (1975) has described the difficulties that apply when truncation is utilized. Whereas double truncation is preferred by some practitioners for most of their cases, other practitioners (Davy, 1976; Hodd, 1976) appear to prefer single truncation. It is certainly true that a proportion of patients are less comfortable with a single or double truncated soft lens than they are with a non-truncated lens. The author's first experience of truncation occurred inadvertently when, in the earlier days of 1970, numerous damaged or torn soft lenses were partly truncated in an attempt to repair them and make them useful for wear. These truncated regions usually stabilized when situated at an angle parallel with that of one of the lid margins.

These earlier, accidentally truncated soft lenses were not prism ballasted and yet appeared to stabilize well and there is no doubt that many lenses do stabilize satisfactorily in this way. A great deal depends on the lid tension, position and angle, and in truncating a lens, consideration to these details must be given.

One of the greatest difficulties with truncations is the instability which can occur when truncation is used with oblique cylinders. The uneven thickness produced by oblique cylinders can make the lens very difficult to stabilize successfully.

Dynamic Stabilization

This ingenious method of stabilization developed by Fanti (1975) utilizes a similar principle to truncation in that lid action is made use of to stabilize the lenses. In this instance, however, Fanti has been able to retain the comfortable, round shape of the lens and, in effect, has moved his truncated action areas within the periphery of the lens to form what he terms dynamic stabilization areas. *Figure 18.16* shows the construction of such a lens. In this particular method, movement of the eyes or lids results in pressure being applied superiorly and inferiorly to help stabilize the lens. This has a very wide application and as it avoids the complications of truncation and prism ballast it appears to be a practical method in many instances. The complexity of the lens, however, requires that it also be made reasonably large (about 15 mm) and this large size combined with its greater thickness can produce physiological problems, especially if the refractive errors are low and the central thickness is greater than desirable. The author feels that as this lens is made of HEMA, with low oxygen permeability (Hill and Jeppe, 1976), its ingenious design could be better utilized without physiological complications

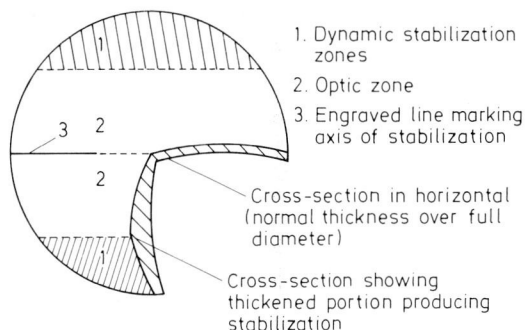

1. Dynamic stabilization zones
2. Optic zone
3. Engraved line marking axis of stabilization

Cross-section in horizontal (normal thickness over full diameter)

Cross-section showing thickened portion producing stabilization

Figure 18.16–Weicon-T lens showing the form and position of the dynamic stabilization zones. This diagram shows a plano lens with a cylinder of –3.00 D × 180, worked on as +3.00 D × 90

by using other more oxygen permeable materials (Westerhout, 1977).

Its disadvantages are that since most eyes have with-the-rule astigmatism, this means that the thickest portions of the lens are at the top and bottom which can cause the lids to rotate the lens 90 degrees off axis; also in lenses of 15 mm overall size, only negative powers are available with cylinders of up to 4 D (*see* page 457).

PRINCIPLES OF CORRECTION

It is clear that to produce a stable ocular correction for the astigmatic eye, the lens must align closely over the central cornea in front of the pupil. It is important that the lens does not flex more than the anticipated amount in this vital central, optical area as it is well known that flexing of a contact lens produces a power change. Although this is no great problem if the power of the final lens is similar to the trial, spherical lens, it can be a problem with a final toric lens, as the meridional powers are different. For lenses incorporating cylinders of up to 2.50 D it is possible to have cylindrical errors of 0.50–0.75 D induced by the flexure of the lens.

The lens must provide the correct power while it is *in situ*.

The lens must stabilize effectively to prevent the rotation of the meridional powers away from their correct meridians.

Alignment

To achieve what has been referred to in the previous section, certain factors must be taken into account.

The material of which the lens is made is of vital importance. Some materials are very much softer and more flexible than others, thus allowing closer moulding to the corneal shape. Other materials are

Table 18.2–Residual Refractive Error Induced by Mislocation of Toric Lenses of Various Cylindrical Powers

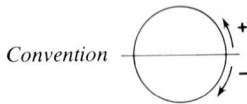

Convention — ⊕
1. Axes in standard axis notation
2. Anti-clockwise is +ve, clockwise –ve

Example:
(i) –2.00 × 180 required refractive correction
(ii) –2.00 × 170 obtained, that is, –10 degrees mislocation
(iii) Residual cyl. axis is +40 degrees
(iv) Residual sph. cyl. power is +0.35/–0.69
(v) Expected residual error +0.35/–0.69 × 40

Mislocation (degrees)	*–1.00*	*–2.00 (×2)*
5	+0.08/–0.16 × 42.5	+0.17/–0.34 × 42.5
10	+0.17/–0.34 × 40	+0.35/–0.69 × 40
15	+0.26/–0.52 × 37.5	+0.52/–1.04 × 37.5
20	+0.34/–0.69 × 35	+0.68/–1.37 × 35
25	+0.43/–0.85 × 32.5	+0.85/–1.69 × 32.5
30	+0.50/–1.00 × 30	+1.00/–2.00 × 30
35	+0.57/–1.14 × 27.5	+1.14/–2.29 × 27.5
40	+0.64/–1.28 × 25	+1.29/–2.57 × 25
45	+0.71/–1.42 × 22.5	+1.41/–2.83 × 22.5
50	+0.76/–1.53 × 20	+1.53/–3.06 × 20
55	+0.82/–1.64 × 17.5	+1.64/–3.28 × 17.5
60	+0.87/–1.73 × 15	+1.73/–3.46 × 15
65	+0.90/–1.82 × 12.5	+1.81/–3.63 × 12.5
70	+0.94/–1.88 × 10	+1.88/–3.76 × 10
75	+0.96/–1.93 × 7.5	+1.93/–3.85 × 7.5
80	+0.98/–1.97 × 5	+1.97/–3.94 × 5
85	+0.99/–1.99 × 2.5	+1.99/–3.98 × 2.5
90	+1.00/–2.00 × 180	+2.00/–4.00 × 180

Reproduced by kind permission of Holden and Frauenfelder (1973)

more elastic and springy in action and this can make a lens somewhat erratic in its alignment, especially if the lens is a little steep in relation to corneal curvature.

The overall size of the lens is clearly relevant as this parameter determines to some degree how stable the lens will be in centration and thus also in alignment.

The relationship of the BCOR of the soft lens to the corneal shape is very important in achieving alignment. In general, flat fitting lenses tend to give better alignment than steep fitting lenses. If the lens is inclined to give apical corneal clearance, there tends to be a springing backwards and forwards of the soft lens on and off the corneal apex during the act of blinking.

The central thickness and variations in thickness of the lens greatly influence alignment. Variations in thickness such as occur with the use of prisms or lenticular forms are therefore clearly important.

Effect of Lens Rotation

It is surprising how much induced cylindrical error is produced when a lens does not stabilize satisfactorily and rotates. Holden and Frauenfelder (1973) have produced a table indicating the degree of error induced when a lens rotates (*Table 18.2*). If the correction requires –2.00 DC × 180, the table reveals that a mislocation of the axis by 10 degrees results in a cylindrical error of –0.69 D × 40. A 20 degree movement gives a cylindrical error of –1.37 D × 35 and a 25 degree rotation gives a cylindrical error of –1.65 D × 32.5. These errors are considerable, but use can be made of this table in assessing the amount of rotation of the lens (provided that the lens is well made) by carrying out an accurate refraction with the lens *in situ*. The cylindrical error thus determined can then be related to the induced error in the table to show the degree of lens rotation. *Table 14.29* is a similar table covering cylinders of up to 6.00 D, but giving only four possible angular values for mislocation of the cylinder axis (*see* Chapter 14, page 452).

PRESCRIBING AND FITTING OF TORIC SOFT LENSES

Spherical Back Surface Combined with Toroidal Front Surface Utilizing Prism Ballast Stabilization and/or Truncation

In this category may be included lenses having a non-toroidal back surface which is not truly spherical. This would include lenses having aspheric back surfaces, as are commonly used in Australia and New Zealand (Hirst, 1975). (Some details of these lenses are given on page 456 in Chapter 14.) Such lenses may be fitted with or without truncation. For this reason it maywell be worthwhile ordering the lens with prism ballast, but without truncation, as the truncation can easily be added later either in single or double form.

Since there are different options available in the use of this lens, and the lens can be adjusted after manufacture, it is more constructive and avoids repetition to consider the two approaches involved separately. These follow under (1) and (2).

(1) The Use of a Spherical Back Surface and Toroidal Front Surface Combined with Truncation but Without Prism Ballast

Hirst (1975) has stated that it has been shown clinically that if the position of the truncation can be judged accurately while the trial lens is on the eye, prism ballasting may not be necessary or, if necessary, a small amount of prism (no more than $1\triangle$) need be used to give the correct location.

In the fitting of this lens it is suggested that a single truncated, non-toric, non-ballasted trial lens should be utilized, and fitted using the same principles as those the practitioner would normally use with an orthodox spherical, soft lens (Hirst, 1975). It is not suggested that the practitioner change his normal principles of soft lens fitting because the lens fitted is in a truncated form. It is, as always, helpful if the prescription of the spherical trial lens is as near as possible to that of the final prescription lens.

In the selection of the overall size of the truncated soft lens it is generally found that the major axis is up to 0.5 mm larger than a conventional, round, soft lens fitting in the same eye. The minor axis perpendicular to the truncation is between 1.0 and 1.5 mm shorter than the longer axis. The author

finds that it is seldom necessary to make these lenses with more than a 1.5 mm truncation and finds that the average overall size is 14 mm × 12.5 mm.

A careful refraction is carried out over the single truncated or circular, soft trial lens after the lens has settled for a period in excess of half an hour. In general terms, the longer the lens has settled on the eye before refraction, the more accurate the results are likely to be.

Axis Rotation

When the truncated lens is carefully observed on the eye, it may be seen that the truncation has swung nasally 5 degrees or more from the horizontal axis. If a rotational movement is noted its extent should be measured and the prescribing of the cylinder axis in the final lens will have to be modified to compensate for this rotation. There is, of course, no need to describe the rotational swing to the laboratory provided this rotation is provided for in the final prescription.

Example: The refraction over a plano prescription trial lens is found to be –3.00/–1.50 × 180. During the fitting, the right truncation locates at approximately 10 degrees instead of the expected 180 degrees position. Thus, the prescription ordered from the laboratory should read: –3.00/–1.50 × 170. This, of course, means that with the lens *in situ*, the truncation will rotate to a position along approximately 10 degrees, thus rotating the cylinder axis to approximately its correct position at 180 degrees.

If the final lens is made up accurately to the practitioner's satisfaction and yet is found to rotate in an unpredictable fashion, evident by direct observation and over-refraction, it may be possible to modify the truncation on the lens to attempt to bring it to its correct orientation.

The angle of the truncation relative to the cylinder axis can be modified by cutting the lens with scissors

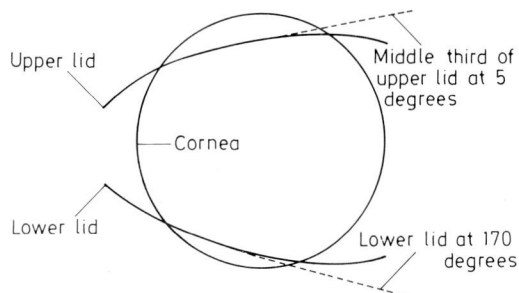

Figure 18.17–Relationship of upper and lower lid angles to the cornea

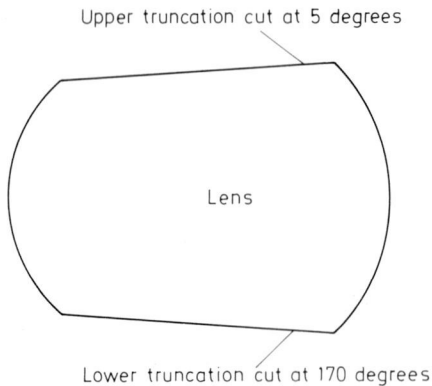

Figure 18.18–Truncations cut on a soft lens to fit the eye illustrated in Figure 18.17

in its wet state, dehydrating the lens and repolishing the newly truncated area with a soft lens polishing paste whilst in its dry state and then rehydrating the lens. The author has found this a very satisfactory way in which to deal with the problem.

If the single truncation, despite modification, proves to be unsatisfactory, then the lens can be double truncated by removing between 1.0 and 1.5 mm in the superior region. Before this is done, however, a careful observation of the lid angle of the middle third of the upper and lower lids should be made as this information may well be utilized in cutting the truncations. *Figures 18.17* and *18.18* illustrate this point.

Unlike the utilization of truncation for bifocal fitting, where it is normally necessary that the truncation be cut square so as to rest on the lower lid, this is not the case with toric soft lenses. Indeed, as the lower lid margin is generally found to lie near to or above the position of the lower limbus, and if the lens were forced to ride above this position by being constantly in contact with the margin of the lower lid, the patient could well suffer from irritation caused by the truncation.

The author finds that in the majority of cases it is better if the truncated area rests on the conjunctiva below the lower limbus even if this is well below the position of the lower lid margin.

With these points in mind it must be said that the use of truncation in soft lens fitting is totally different from that used in hard corneal lens fitting. Indeed it can be observed that only in pronounced vertical movements of the eyes do the lid margins actually have any direct contact with the truncated edge or edges. This point is illustrated in *Figure 18.19*.

For this reason observation of the angle of the middle third of the lower lid may be better noted

with the eyes looking up and noting the lid angle at the point of expected contact with the truncation. The upper lid angle is then noted whilst looking down using the same principle.

The exact method by which the lids act on the soft lens truncations is not fully understood. Possibly the action of the palpebral orbicularis muscle fibres which run parallel to the lid margins have a similar effect on truncated soft lenses as do the lid margins on truncated hard lenses.

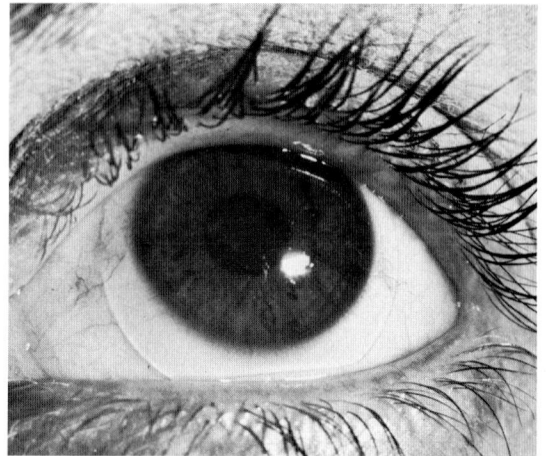

Figure 18.19–This is a prism ballast, single truncated, soft lens with a spherical back surface and toroidal front surface. The lower truncation has been cut at the angle of the middle third of the lower lid, but it can be seen how far below the lower limbus it is situated. In this photograph the patient had to look up in order to bring the truncation near the lower lid. The lid margin may thus only have a limited effect on the truncation

If, as stated by Hirst (1975), the lens is still found to be unsatisfactory due to rotational movement, the lens may be re-ordered with the addition of prisms of between $1\triangle$ and $1\frac{1}{2}\triangle$.

Since rotation of toric lenses is the main problem encountered in this form of prescribing it would seem that the majority of practitioners are currently using a combination of both prism ballast and truncation for the initial prescription lens.

(2) Spherical Back Surface with Toroidal Front Surface Combined with Prism Ballast and Truncation

It should be noted that as it is frequently desirable, with such complex and expensive lenses, to order lenses capable of modification, it may be better for the novice practitioner to order the lenses with prism ballast but without truncation. If the truncation is then required subsequently, it can be added in the manner already described.

It is clearly extremely helpful, in this type of case, to use a prism ballasted, non-toric, non-truncated lens to make the observations for the final fitting.

The initial fitting of the trial lens should be done as if fitting an orthodox soft spherical lens with no provision made for the fact that the lens would be made truncated or with a toroidal front surface. It is highly desirable that marks are made on the contact lens to indicate the position of the prism base, and when the lens is settled for at least half an hour the position of the prism base is noted. If the lens is to be prescribed in truncated form then the angle of the middle third of the lower eyelid should be noted relative to the position of the prism base. The truncation is then ordered to be cut at this angle.

A careful refraction is then carried out and the final prescription written, making allowance for the position of the prism base. It should be unnecessary to state the position of the prism base provided that this is done.

Example: If the prescription is R.E. −1.00/−2.00 × 10 and the prism base is found to locate at 280 degrees, the lens is then ordered with the cylinder axis at 180 degrees with the prism base at 270 degrees. When the lens is in position on the eye the prism base will rotate 10 degrees up nasally, from 270 to 280 degrees, thus allowing the cylinder axis to return to its correct position at 10 degrees. It is generally found more satisfactory and less confusing to order the prism base at the 6 o'clock (270 degrees) position.

Toroidal Back Surface Lenses, Stabilized by One or Two Truncations

Such a lens may be made with or without a toroidal front surface to correct lenticular or induced astigmatism. The somewhat complex calculations involved in prescribing these lenses are generally left to the laboratory, especially as different materials are used in the manufacture and the refractive index of these materials varies considerably. The principle of fitting is as follows.

The practitioner fits the patient with the flattest spherical trial lens that will remain stable on the eye. The stability and centration should be at least as good as that found with an orthodox spherical soft lens to be fitted to the same eye. The patient is then carefully refracted after the lens has settled for at least half an hour, followed by keratometric readings taken from the front surface of the contact lens *in situ*. The angle of the middle third of the lower

and upper lids is estimated, relative to the horizontal, as these will be used for the cutting of the truncations.

When the final lens arrives from the laboratory and has been checked for accuracy, it is inserted and allowed to settle. If it is found to rotate, judged by over-refraction and observation, then the truncation can be added, if this has not already been done. If no truncation has been used, any additional nasal swing of the prism base can be compensated for by cutting a truncation along the angle of the middle third of the lower lid. This should be done with the prism base at the correct position to obtain orientation of the cylinder at the required axis. In the above example the truncation would be cut with the prism base at 280 degrees.

Once the truncation is cut, however, it is often found that the influence of the lids is not as expected and the truncation may not orientate parallel to the lower lid. Any such additional rotation may sometimes be compensated for by cutting a second truncation at a different angle to attempt to re-orientate the lens. This principle is illustrated in *Figures 18.20, 18.21* and *18.22.*

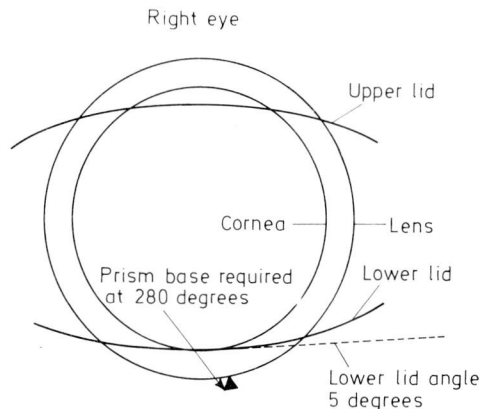

Figure 18.20–With the lower lid angle at 5 degrees, the lower truncation would be cut initially at 5 degrees to allow the prism base to position at 280 degrees thus allowing the cylinder to take up the correct axis

The techniques described in (1) and (2) above appear to be satisfactory methods of correcting astigmatic errors, especially as the relationship of lenticular to corneal astigmatism is irrelevant with such lenses. The lens is simply stabilized and the front surface cylinder added to correct the overall cylindrical refractive effect.

If, however, the lenses are uncomfortable and the patient proves to be intolerant to the use of prisms, with or without truncation, then other methods of correction may have to be found.

Another type of toric lens incorporating a front toroidal surface with a spherical back surface is that utilizing dynamic stabilization, but this is dealt with separately on page 565. A description of those techniques which make use of a toroidal back surface now follows.

From the above results the laboratory then calculates the back surface toricity to correct the astigmatism. Garner and Holden (1976) recommend the double truncation of such lenses for stabilization, but it may be worthwhile, in view of the complexity of the lens to initially order the lens with a single lower truncation, with the upper truncation to be added later if the lens is not sufficiently stable. If the lens is double truncated the average size is between 11.5 mm × 13 mm and 12 mm × 14 mm. As can be seen, each truncation is normally in the region of 1 mm.

Unfortunately, due to their complex design, these lenses are frequently found to be very unstable and need to be made rather large in order to work satisfactorily. As toroidal surfaces are always difficult to work on a very thin lens, the combination of a thick lens in a large size may prove to be physiologically unsatisfactory. Very often such lenses prove to be unstable optically, but if the lens is held in a stable position on the cornea with the fingers, good visual acuity may be obtained. As soon as the support of the fingers is removed, however, the lens may rotate and provide poor and unstable acuity. The visual acuity is most likely to be satisfactory if the lens has only to correct corneal astigmatism, and least likely to be satisfactory if the lens has to correct

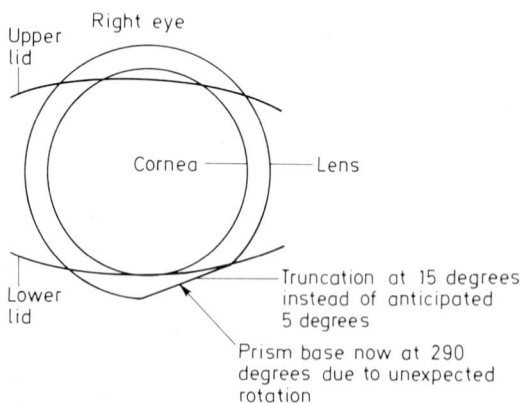

Figure 18.22–The faulty lens positioning (see Figure 18.21) maybe corrected in some cases by cutting a new truncation. Here the new truncation is cut at an angle of 15 degrees, with the prism base at 280 degrees. If the truncation has more influence than the prism, the truncation may orientate in the same position as in Figure 18.21, thus allowing the prism base to settle in its correct position at 280 degrees with the truncation at 15 degrees

more than this. If the lens is made in bi-toric form then, clearly, its complexity is a major problem if it cannot be stabilized to prevent rotation.

Back Surface Toroidal Lenses Without Prism or Truncation

Once again this form of lens can be made with or without a toroidal front surface to correct residual or induced astigmatism and, due to the wide variety of materials used and the variations in refractive index, most laboratories prefer the practitioner to supply basic information for the calculation of the toroidal back surfaces. These are suitably cut in the dehydrated state to allow for the increase in radii and lowering of refractive index with hydration.

Mathematical formulae for these calculations have been presented (Garner and Holden, 1976) but despite this, most laboratories prefer to work with basic information, rather than be told by the practitioner, what radii to use on the lens. For the fitting of this type of lens the laboratories require to be given accurate keratometric readings and an accurate refraction. The corneal diameter is also carefully measured. The lens is made up by the laboratory with a toroidal back surface to correct corneal astigmatism, without the use of truncation or prism. If the ocular astigmatism is different from the corneal astigmatism then the laboratory will make a bi-toric lens to correct the residual astigmatism. As, however, in this instance the residual astigmatism has only been calculated rather than

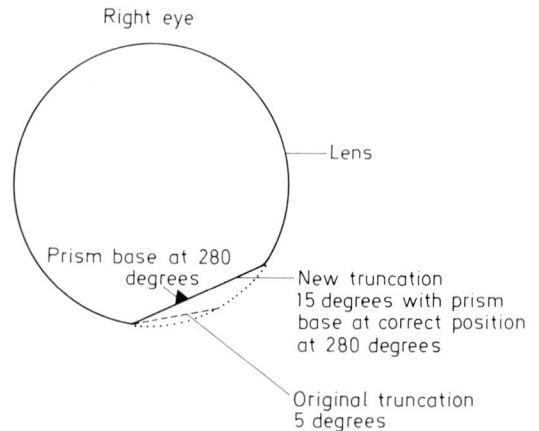

Figure 18.21–The prism base of the lens illustrated in Figure 18.20 unexpectedly rotates a further 10 degrees nasally. The cylinder is now 10 degrees off axis. This may sometimes be corrected as shown in Figure 18.22

determined *in situ*, errors may arise, as mentioned in the section dealing with hard, corneal, toric lenses. The great difficulty with this type of lens, as with the previous variety, is that with toroidal back surfaces it is almost impossible to check the lenses accurately. Optimistic attempts have been made to do this, and claims have been made that lenses can be checked very accurately by keratometric methods involving the suspension of the lens in a saline solution bath. Some authorities, however, are somewhat unhappy with the accuracy of this method, even with a spherical surface, and the task of measuring a toric soft lens becomes even more difficult.

This type of lens, without additional stabilization, usually produces poor results. The lens frequently rotates between 10 and 30 degrees (usually excyclorotation) with resultant poor and variable acuity. Most practitioners are familiar with the fact that lenses which give poor but stable acuity are more acceptable than those which give moments of clear vision followed by moments of poor vision as the lens rotates.

When the lens rotates it also flexes differently in the different meridians, and this also produces fluctuations in the effective power on the eye. If the lens rotates in an unpredictable fashion then it can be truncated by the practitioner in the manner already described. Either one or two truncations can be added, and this is frequently sufficient to stabilize the lens enough to give satisfactory vision.

Back Surface Toroidal Lenses with Prism Ballast

Lenses of this type have been made to prescription by several laboratories and are also manufactured under the trade name Hydroflex/m-T. The latter lens, as described in Chapter 14, on page 450, has been designed by the German laboratory of Wöhlk, and consists of a toroidal back surface which is stabilized on the eye by means of prism ballast of approximately $1\frac{1}{2}\triangle$. The lens is designed for use in cases of corneal astigmatism only, although it is possible to modify the back surface toricity to cope with residual astigmatism, provided the axis of the residual astigmatism is similar to that of the corneal astigmatism. Such lenses can be made in a full range of powers from −20.00 to +20.00 D with cylinders from 0.75 to 6.00 D. With this form of lens, as with most of those having toroidal back surfaces, special fitting lenses are not necessary. When ordering the final lens the laboratory may either be given the necessary information to design it to correct the manifest astigmatism, or the practitioner can work out the back surface radii required from *Table 14.28*

(*see* Chapter 14, page 452) which is the method preferred by the laboratory. In the former case the laboratory requires accurate corneal radii and meridians, the exact refraction of the eye, with the cylinder expressed in negative cylinder form and the specification of the orthodox Hydroflex/m lens giving the best physical fit in as large an overall size as possible. Wöhlk claim that in approximately 70 per cent of cases the desired result can be achieved with the very first pair of lenses, although Hodd (1976) reports that the success rate appears to be somewhat lower than this. As is common with all forms of toroidal back surface soft lens, considerable skill and experience is required in fitting these lenses.

Laboratories can, or should, be able to make their lenses with any marks requested by the practitioner, and the Hydroflex/m-T is provided with two small marks at the edge. These are only visible using magnification. The base of the prism lies at an angle of 90 degrees to an imaginary line drawn between these two marks, the latter normally being expected to lie along the 180 degree meridian. If this is not the case in the final prescription lens the amount of divergence from the 180 degrees meridian should be determined and the laboratory should be notified of this divergence. The lens is then remade, taking this variation into account, so that, although the markings of the second lens do not lie along 180 degrees, its cylinder axis should locate correctly. The author has experimented with numerous lenses made with toroidal back surfaces and prism, and one of the difficulties of such lenses is that they are almost invariably rather thick, which often leads to poor physiological results. Within the overall size range available for Hydroflex/m lenses the Hydroflex/m-T lens is fitted as large and flat as possible (average overall size of 13.0 mm). By so doing it is inclined to give a somewhat better physiological result than larger more steeply fitted lenses; also because the lenses are reasonably thin. A Hydroflex/m-T lens of −3.00 D with a 1.5△ prism and an overall size of 12.5 mm would have a central thickness of 0.2 mm. Unfortunately, as is well-known, some of the smaller soft lenses can give considerable discomfort in the conjunctival region adjacent to the limbus and also on the lid margins, which may offset their other physiological advantages.

Paradoxically, these very small, thin toric lenses often give very unstable results due to their thinness. The larger, thicker toric lenses are generally reasonably stable due to their thickness and give fairly good visual acuity; whereas the image quality obtained by the patient wearing a thin toroidal back surface lens is often poor, and the visual acuity is sometimes reduced in spite of a spectacle overcorrection.

Despite these problems, however, which are common to most forms of toric soft lens, the lenses are well made and provide a logical way of dealing with some of the problems of corneal astigmatism. As with so many of these forms of lens, it is important that the refraction over the spherical trial lens be performed with a lens as near to the final prescription as possible.

These lenses can be fitted as large as 13.5 mm overall size although the majority are in the region of 12.5 mm. As the toroidal back surface is the primary form of stabilization, the greater the corneal astigmatism the more likely the lens is to stabilize. Unfortunately, however, the higher the corneal astigmatism, the smaller the degree of rotation the patient will tolerate optically. It is obviously necessary for the spectacle refraction cylinder and keratometer cylinder to be almost identical for accurate results. Skilful changing of the prescription of the toroidal back surface can also give an induced front surface cylinder to correct residual astigmatism. Hodd (1976) found that with the use of the Hydroflex/m-T lens for the correction of corneal astigmatism, fair to good visual acuity was obtained in 19 out of 40 lenses made for 24 eyes. With the same type of lens used for the correction of lenticular astigmatism he reported only obtaining fair to good visual acuity in 3 cases out of 15 lenses made for 10 eyes. Hodd also reported that in a group of 14 cases, for which this lens was indicated, only 1 was able to achieve constant wearing time with visual acuity equivalent to that of spectacles.

The lens appears to work somewhat better in the hyperopic eye than in the myopic eye and this may well be due to the increased thickness and thus more stable lens form. Possibly for this very reason Wöhlk also make a larger, prism ballasted and truncated toroidal back surface lens which is slightly thicker and more stable. It is known as the Hydroflex-TS lens and is fully described in Chapter 14, on page 453. It is often necessary to use a vertical prism in both eyes if lenses are to be equally comfortable and in order to prevent an induced vertical heterophoria. Gasson (1977), however, finds that it is often possible to omit the prism if the contralateral eye can be fitted with a non-toroidal lens.

Dynamic Stabilization

This technique (Fanti, 1975) has been used to considerable advantage as the lens design is not stabilized by gravity or adhesion but, as explained on page 559 and in Chapter 14, by the kinetic forces associated with blinking. The lens is made by Titmus Eurocon under the name Weicon-T. The Aoflex toric lens is a similar lens made by American Optical Co.

There are two segments, one each at the top and bottom of the lens, as illustrated in *Figures 14.42* and *18.16*. The remaining central portion of the front surface is toroidal. The dynamic stabilization axis (known as the DS axis) is symmetrical to these two zones and passes through both the optical and geometric centres of the lens. The method in which the lens is inserted is not important since the action of the lids during blinking stabilizes the lens very quickly. *Figure 18.16* and *Colour Plate XLIII* indicate that the action of the lids on the superior and inferior lens chamfers are inclined to stabilize the lens with the DS axis approximately horizontal.

Even if such a lens is put into the the eye with the DS axis vertical, the lens will normally rotate within 30 seconds to bring it to its stable axis position. Advantages of this type of lens are that the lens is very smooth and round in shape which gives the patient a very good reaction initially, comparable to that of orthodox soft spherical lenses. The lens is, however, fitted very large (15 mm) and, as it is necessary for it to be thick enough to permit chamfering, it is often unsatisfactory where the refractive error is lower than –3.00 D. The laboratory now usually declines to make lenses where the spherical ametropia is positive or less than –3.00 D, unless a smaller overall size can be employed.

Due to the unique nature of the lens it is necessary that the lens be fitted with a fitting set of lenses with the dynamic stabilization periphery. The fitting lenses are spherical and are marked with the DS axis (*see Colour Plate XLIII*). Due to the large size of the lens (*see Figure 14.43*) it is fitted approximately 1.2 mm flatter than the mean of the principal corneal radii and it is recommended that such a lens be fitted a little tighter than the simple spherical form. In general, the fit can be considered optimum if the lens centres satisfactorily and shows minimal movement with blinking. The author usually fits these lenses as tight as possible consistent with finding no indentation of the conjunctiva underneath the extreme periphery of the lens when the lens is gently moved with digital pressure.

A diagnostic fitting set, as outlined in *Table 14.34*, page 455, is normally in steps of 0.2 mm radius, ranging in BCOR from 8.2 to 9.4 mm. Most diagnostic lenses are made in –3.00 D power with an overall size of 15 mm.

The author has found this lens design extremely satisfactory for the correction of astigmatic errors in myopes of over 3.00 D and if careful selection of the right patient is made, the success rate should be very high. The visual acuity is almost invariably extremely good with very little rotation. Lenses which orientate with the DS axis more than 20 degrees from the horizontal should be considered with suspicion as the lens may not be stable in its final form. Frequently, if fitting lenses are found to rotate in an unsatisfactory manner, the difficulty can be overcome and stabilized by fitting a slightly tighter lens. If, however, the lens design is to be tightened, consideration must be given to the possible adverse physiological effects. (Poor physiological results occurred with some high positive experimental lenses made for the author with cylinders of up to −7.00 D. The focimeter images with these lenses were comparable with those of orthodox spectacle lenses, so the optical quality was very good.)

The prescribing of the final cylinder is relative to the DS axis which is assumed to be on the horizontal for the purposes of prescribing. Thus, if the cylindrical error, during over-refraction, is found to be at an axis of 45 degrees and the DS axis is at an angle of 10 degrees, then the final prescription lens must be ordered with the cylindrical axis at 35 degrees. When the lens rotates to its correct DS axis of 10 degrees on the eye, the cylindrical component will rotate to its true position of 45 degrees.

Indications for this lens include both corneal and residual astigmatism, or combinations of the above. The real advantages of this form of lens are its ability to stabilize reliably and the ability to prescribe both for corneal and residual astigmatism.

Contra-indications to this type of lens are unstable positioning on the eye with whatever fitting is attempted and any unusual lid action or closure. It is also contra-indicated in irregular astigmatism.

The use of the Weicon-T lens is made considerably easier if the practitioner has a reliable and accurate method of measuring the axis of the dynamic stabilization region. The trial lenses are engraved with a broken line along this axis, but it is often extremely difficult to view this line in the eye (*Colour Plate XLIII*). The author normally measures this angle by placing before the eye a plano glass trial lens with an engraved line across the middle of the lens. This is aligned with the engraved line on the Weicon-T lens and the angle is read on a trial frame. However, it is often extremely difficult to see the engraved lines clearly through the plano trial lens. The patient is then best observed with a slit lamp biomicroscope using low magnification. Although there is limited depth of focus the microscope can be racked back and forth slightly to easily align the trial lens axes. The axis of the spectacle trial lens can then be read off on the trial frame.

An even better method involves the use of a special biomicroscope eyepiece containing a graticule ruled as a protractor, on which the DS axis of the Weicon-T lens can be read off directly. Another method described by Fanti (1975) is to use a slit lamp microscope with a measuring graticule which is connected to a protractor fixed on the outside of the eyepiece of the instrument. The measuring graticule is then turned to correspond with the angle of the DS axis seen through the microscope and the axis can then be read on the protractor.

A further excellent method of measuring the angle of the DS axis accurately is to use an ophthalmometer employing the Javal principle with the doubling device in only one meridian. If such an instrument is focused onto the engraved DS reference line, the observer will generally detect the doubled image of the lens and the DS axis line. If the instrument is rotated, as for normal axis determination, until the two images coincide and can be superimposed, then only one line will be visible. The axis of the DS line can now be read off on the ophthalmometer.

It is extremely useful to observe what happens to the soft trial lens when the patient blinks in different directions of gaze. Frequently, the lens remains stable, but if the patient looks down and blinks the lens may rotate 10 degrees or more. If this recurs when the test is repeated it may be taken as a contra-indication, especially if the astigmatism is high and if the patient's work involves a lot of looking down such as carrying out clerical tasks.

It is worthy of note that any lens which is found to rotate more than 10 degrees will almost certainly be unsatisfactory in its final form. Obviously, a great deal depends on the power of the cylinder to be incorporated on the front surface. Wearers of high cylinders are clearly not able to tolerate much rotation. Greater rotation can be tolerated by the wearer of a low cylinder.

The reliability of stabilization of the Weicon-T lens is also dependent on the degree of myopia present in the correction. From *Figures 14.42* and *18.16*, illustrating the form and principle of the lens, it will be seen that the more myopic the patient the thicker the peripheral region will be, thus giving greater stabilization by permitting better chamfering at the top and bottom of the lens. Tests by the author indicate that a lens of approximately −3.00 D will stabilize on the eye in approximately 5–10 minutes, but may still then rotate by some 5–7 degrees. A lens of as high as −10.00 D will stabilize almost immediately and will often remain almost immobile in terms of rotation.

However, the DS axis of the final lens may differ from that of the spherical trial lens due to the effect on edge thickness of the front surface cylinder and its axis (*see* pages 559 and 568).

Irregular Astigmatism

None of the previously mentioned forms of soft lens is capable of being used to correct irregular astigmatism. Conventionally, astigmatic errors of this nature are corrected with hard lenses but in some severe types of irregular astigmatism, such as that encountered in moderate or advanced keratoconus, some patients are physically unable to wear such lenses satisfactorily. One solution to this problem would be the use of an advanced design in which the periphery of the lens were soft and flexible and the central region over the pupil would remain rigid. Attempts have been made to produce this form of lens for many years but so far they have been unsatisfactory.

Westerhout (1973) has described a means of overcoming this problem by fitting the eye conventionally with a soft lens so as to provide an artificial cornea over which an orthodox hard lens can then be fitted, as shown in *Colour Plate LIX*. Naturally enough, in severe keratoconus, the fitting of the soft lens can produce certain difficulties but most lathe-cut lenses can be made sufficiently steep to deal with this problem.

Once a suitable soft lens has been fitted and is found capable of being worn comfortably for daily use, the front surface of the soft lens is then measured with a keratometer, and forms an artificial cornea to which the hard lens is then fitted. Gas permeable hard corneal lenses are preferable to PMMA lenses for this purpose.

Westerhout (1973) has recommended that the soft lens used should be of fairly high negative power in order that its front surface radii are lengthened so as to approach more closely the average, normal fitting range of hard lenses. The 'combination lens' has been used very successfully in a large number of cases of irregular astigmatism and keratoconus and will continue to be a viable proposition, although it may well be replaced by a lens with a soft periphery and central hard region. It has been reported to the author that the Japanese have now taken this combination a stage further by cutting a recess on the front surface of the soft lens to retain the hard lens. The author has not seen this technique described but difficulties can be visualized, with the edges of the hard lens damaging the soft lens material at the periphery of the recess. The author has also experimented with the prospect of cementing corneal lenses onto soft lenses but the results so far have not been satisfactory.

Checking Soft Toric Lenses

The methods of checking soft lenses are covered in Chapter 15 and need not be further elaborated here. The special features of lenses with toroidal surfaces apply as much to soft lenses as hard lenses and the approach to verification is similar (*see* page 284). Because of the relative fragility of the soft lens

material it is important to look for areas of damage to the lens where axis markings or other engravings have been made. These areas are also more likely to become contaminated during use.

Variations in Astigmatism

Unfortunately the prescribing of toric soft lenses is made more complex by the fact that the astigmatism may vary with different directions of gaze. These changes are mainly due to the varying effects of the lids in different positions of gaze.

Westerhout (1976) has reported variations in the degree and axis of astigmatism in transferring the gaze from distance to near. He reported 1 patient who manifested a residual cylinder of $-2.50\,D \times 165$ for distance and $-4.00\,D \times 150$ for near. Analysis of 40 eyes revealed that the change in astigmatism on looking down varied from a shift towards with-the-rule astigmatism of a maximum of 1.25 D (mean 0.72 D) to a shift towards against-the-rule astigmatism of a maximum of 0.50 D (mean 0.29 D).

Clearly these problems are additional complications in the use of toric forms of soft lens. It should also be noted that even if accurate trial lenses are used for the fitting of soft toric lenses, the stabilization may well be different when the edge and centre thickness vary in the final lens form. A notable example of this is in the use of the Weicon-T lens where, if the trial lens is found to stabilize accurately and the prescription lens is made up with a high cylinder correction for astigmatism against-the-rule, the reduction of the thickness in the stabilization areas, in the vertical meridian, may considerably affect the lens stabilization because adequate chamfering of the lens may be difficult to achieve. Results may be still worse if the axis of the front surface cylinder is oblique. In this case the edges may vary enormously in thickness and may have a profound effect on the rotation of the lens. Similar variations with oblique cylinders on lenses with toroidal back surfaces can also produce unreliable and unpredictable rotational effects.

All toric soft lenses are difficult to manufacture and the material used in manufacture is, therefore, very important. Laboratory technicians find that some soft lens blanks in their hard form can be cut and polished with far more accuracy than others and these better materials are therefore clearly worth using when manufacturing such complicated lenses. Oxygen permeability is, however, a factor to consider as such lenses are thicker than normal. The ideal material for toric soft lens manufacture is, therefore, a material of high oxygen permeability, great flexibility and ease of accurate cutting and polishing.

SUMMARY

It has been requested that a brief and simplified summary of the appropriate types of toric lens fittings be included at the end of this chapter. Over-simplification is never desirable in a clinical subject, but the brief notes below may be of assistance to some.

TORIC HARD CORNEAL LENS FITTINGS

The required initial information is as follows.
(1) An accurate subjective spectacle refraction.
(2) An accurate keratometric reading with radii, powers and axes.

In the following discussion the term 'compatible' means that a comparison of the cylinder elements in the refraction and keratometric readings reveals a discrepancy of 0.75 D or less. It is clearly up to the clinician to decide whether or not a residual cylinder of 1.00 D or greater, is going to be acceptable to his patient. 'Compatible axes' means axes which are similar, and it is clear that patients may well be able to tolerate the visual limitations of axes varying by larger angular discrepancies with low cylinders than they would with high cylinders. In general, compatible, in this context, means approximately plus or minus 10 degrees.

Principal Clinical Indications

(1) The refraction cylinder is compatible with the keratometric cylinder. Here a spherical corneal lens can be used if the amount of toricity is small enough to permit its fitting.
(2) The refraction and keratometric cylinders are compatible but highly toroidal. Here a toroidal back surface may be required physically, in a lens of compensated bi-toric form.
(3) The refraction cylinder is not compatible with the keratometric cylinder which may be very small. This will give residual astigmatism with a spherical lens and may thus require a stabilized lens with toroidal front surface.
(4) The keratometric cylinder is high with the refraction cylinder not compatible, but axes are similar. Here a parallel bi-toric lens maybe found useful.
(5) The keratometric cylinder is high, but the refraction cylinder axes are not compatible. Here an oblique bi-toric lens may be required.

(6) The keratometric cylinder is high, but the refraction cylinder is higher, such that the residual astigmatism with a spherical lens is cancelled out by the cylinder induced by a toric back surface. This occurs when the ocular astigmatism is about 50 per cent greater than the corneal astigmatism and the axes are similar. Here a toric back surface with a spherical front surface may suffice.

TORIC SOFT LENS FITTINGS

(1) Low refraction cylinder. A spherical soft lens is indicated no matter whether or not the keratometric cylinder is high or low.
(2) A high refraction cylinder, but the keratometric cylinder is low. In this case a toroidal front surface is indicated or, if axes are compatible, the more complex toroidal back surface to induce a toroidal front surface. Either form must be stabilized by prism ballast and/or truncation.
(3) A high refraction cylinder compatible with keratometric cylinder in power and axes. Here a toroidal front surface, or a toroidal back surface to correct corneal astigmatism, may prove successful. Stabilization in some form is likely to be necessary.
(4) A high refraction cylinder with keratometric cylinder at different axes. A toroidal front surface lens is the only lens likely to succeed, although an oblique bi-toric lens could be attempted, as, in theory, it is the better proposition but is extremely difficult to make. Either type would need to be stabilized.
(5) A high refraction cylinder and high keratometric cylinder, although not compatible. If the axes are compatible then a parallel bi-toric lens may suffice, although a toroidal front surface is simpler and easier to prescribe and manufacture. If the axes are not compatible, fit as in (4) above.
(6) A high refraction cylinder, but a high keratometric cylinder not compatible and with different axes. Here an oblique bi-toric soft lens may prove successful, although a toroidal front surface lens is preferable. Again stabilization is likely to be necessary.

ACKNOWLEDGEMENTS

I am indebted to my father, Mr N. E. Westerhout, for all the line drawings in Part I and also to Mrs V. Campbell for the line drawings in Part II. I am also grateful to the many laboratory technicians who have so skilfully made complex forms of toric contact lens for me.

REFERENCES

Baron, H. (1975). 'Some remarks on the correction of astigmatic eyes by means of soft contact lenses.' *Contacto* **19**(6), 4–8

Bennett, A. G. (1966). *Optics of Contact Lenses*, 4th ed. London: Association of Dispensing Opticians

Bennett, A. G. (1976). 'Power changes in soft contact lenses due to bending.' *Ophthal. Optician* **16**, 939–945

British Standard 5562. (1978). *Specification for Contact Lenses – BS 5562:1978*. London: British Standards Institution

British Standard 3521. (1979). *Glossary of Terms Relating to Ophthalmic Lenses and Spectacle Frames – BS 3521:1979. Part 3. Glossary of Terms Relating to Contact Lenses*. London: British Standards Institution

Cappelli, Q. A. (1964). 'Determining final power of bitoric lenses.' *Br. J. physiol. Optics* **21**, 256–263

Davy, M. W. (1976). 'Success for toric soft lenses.' Letter in *Optician* **172**(4451), 33

Fairmaid, J. A. (1967). 'The correction of residual astigmatism with double truncated front surface toric corneal lenses.' *Ophthal. Optician* **7**, 1046–1050

Fanti, P. (1975). 'The fitting of a soft toroidal contact lens.' *Optician* **169**(4376), 8–9, 13, 15–16

Fatt, I., Freeman, R. D. and Lin, D. (1974). 'Oxygen tension distributions in the cornea: A re-examination.' *Exper. Eye Res.* **18**, 357–365

Francis, J. L. (1968). *Optical Tables for Contact Lens Work*. London: Hatton Press (now incorporated in Chapter 4, Volume 1 of this work)

Gasson, A. P. (1977). 'Back surface toric soft lenses.' *Optician* **174**(4491), 6–7, 9, 11

Goldberg, J. B. (1964). 'The correction of residual astigmatism with corneal contact lenses.' *Br. J. physiol. Optics* **21**, 169–174

Gullstrand, A. (1924). Appendices II and IV in *Helmholtz's Treatise on Physiological Optics, Vol. I*, ed. by Southall, J. P. C. New York: Optical Society of America (reprinted by Dover Publications, New York, 1962)

Harris, M. G. and Chu, C. S. (1972). 'The effects of contact lens thickness and corneal toricity on lens flexure and residual astigmatism.' *Am. J. Optom.* **49**, 304–307

Hill, R. M. (1975). 'Can you teach an old ("rigid") lens new tricks?' *Austral J. Optom.* **58**, 322–325

Hill, R. M. and Jeppe, W. H. (1975). 'Hydrogels: is a pump still necessary?' *Internat. contact lens Clin.* **2**(4), 27–29

Hirst, G. (1975). Personal communication

Hodd, N. F. B. (1976). 'Clinical appraisal of toric soft lenses.' *Optician* **172**(4445), 8, 11, 13

Holden, B. A. and Frauenfelder, G. (1973). 'The principles and practice of correcting astigmatism with soft contact lenses.' *Austral. J. Optom.* **58**, 279–299

Stokes, G. G. (1883). *Mathematical and Physical Papers, Vol. 2*, pp. 172–175. Cambridge: Cambridge University Press

Stone, J. (1967). 'Near vision difficulties in non-presbyopic corneal lens wearers.' *Contact Lens* **1**(2), 14–16, 24–25

Strachan, J. P. F. (1973). 'Some principles of the optics of hydrophilic lenses and geometrical optics applied to flexible lenses.' *Austral. J. Optom* **56**, 25–33

Strachan, J. P. F. (1975). 'Correction of astigmatism with hydrophilic lenses.' *Optician* **170**(4402), 8–11

Westerhout, D. I. (1969). 'Clinical observations in fitting bi-toric and toric forms of corneal lenses.' *Contact Lens* **2**(3), 5–6, 8–9

Westerhout, D. I. (1971a). 'The first toric back optic multifocal corneal lens.' *Br. J. physiol. Optics* **26**, 143–149

Westerhout, D. I. (1971b). 'A clinical survey of oedema, its signs, symptoms and incidence.' *Contact Lens* **3**(2), 3–14, 18–22, 24–25

Westerhout, D. I. (1973). ' "The combination lens" and therapeutic uses of soft lenses.' *Contact Lens* **4**(5), 3–10, 12, 16–18, 20, 22

Westerhout, D. I. (1976a). 'Contact lenses: corneal, residual and induced astigmatism.' *Internat contact Lens Clin.* **3**(3), 52–61

Westerhout, D. I. (1976b). Lecture to Maryland Optometric Association, June 1976, University of Maryland

Westerhout, D. I. (1977). 'A rationale for the use and further development of a continuously worn contact lens for the military.' Awaiting publication in *Military Medicine*, U.S.A.

Wichterle, O. and Lim, D. (1960). 'Hydrophilic gels for biological use.' *Nature* **185**, 117–118

Chapter 19

Bifocal and Multifocal Contact Lenses

J. T. de Carle

INTRODUCTION AND HISTORY

The presbyopic patient presents a problem to all contact lens practitioners and it is important to discuss this problem with the patient at the initial visit. Such patients may be fitted with single vision contact lenses, corrected for distance, and wear a pair of additional glasses for near vision (this correction could be made up in the form of plano distance bifocal spectacles), or they may be fitted with bifocal or trifocal contact lenses. Possibly the biggest problem occurs with early presbyopes who are just becoming aware of the fact that they are experiencing difficulty with near vision and have only been wearing single vision spectacles or contact lenses. It is sometimes difficult to convince such patients that it is necessary to change from single vision spectacle lenses to single vision contact lenses plus spectacles, or to bifocal contact lenses. In these cases, it may be preferable to fit them with contact lenses with +0.50 D added to aid near vision, at the same time explaining that presbyopia happens to everybody and that these changes occur whether or not they have contact lenses; also that reading spectacles in addition to the contact lenses will be needed after a short time, or bifocal contact lenses.

A number of practitioners have given a single vision distance contact lens to the dominant eye and a single vision near contact lens to the non-dominant eye. Although this technique, known as 'monovision' is becoming increasingly popular patients should be selected with care and the slight loss of stereopsis taken into account.

Generally, patients who would be considered suitable for single vision lenses should be suitable for bifocals. But care must be taken with neurotic patients who might just pass suitability tests for single vision lenses but would prove unsuitable for the more complicated bifocal lenses.

The first reference to bifocal contact lenses is credited to Feinbloom of New York, who showed diagrams of bifocal and trifocal segments in the optic portion of scleral contact lenses in a patent specification in 1938 (*Figure 19.1*). F. A. Williamson-Noble (1951), a British ophthalmologist, mentioned his own work on bifocal contact lenses when he gave the presidential address to the Contact Lens Society in 1950. He had become interested in the possibility of these lenses after seeing a patient aged 71 years who could read small print easily, both with and without a +2.25 D near addition. Slight lens opacities had made the crystalline lens, in effect, bifocal and it occurred to him that something similar might be possible with a contact lens. A lens was made with a central portion 2.00 D more convex than the remainder of the front surface (*Figure 19.2*). This lens was tried on his own eye but at first did not work in the way he had hoped. However, he found that if he kept his eye open for some time the print gradually became clearer. This was felt to be due to the front surface of the lens becoming dry and then allowing the near addition to have its proper effect; also that an accumulation of tears liquid around the small near addition prevented the lens from working properly. It was therefore suggested that a fused bifocal would probably be the answer.

De Carle (1959) considered these experiments in 1957 and, because of the difficulties involved in making a fused bifocal, decided that a similar effect could be achieved by putting the bifocal surface on the back of the lens so that the partial neutralization effect of the tears would be constant. De Carle also reversed the positions of the near and distance portions so that there was now a small distance portion in the centre (*Figure 19.3*). Provided that the distance portion was small (2.00 to 4.00 mm was usual), the fact that the back central curve was much steeper than the cornea did not create problems.

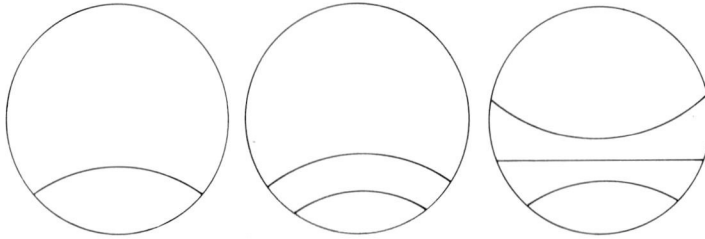

Figure 19.1–Bifocal and trifocal constructions in the optic portion of scleral lenses as suggested by Feinbloom (1938)

(Large distance portions, particularly with the higher near additions, were found not to be practical as a bubble or bubbles would form between the lens and the eye.) In this type of concentric bifocal lens, the patient looked through both the distance and near portions at the same time.

The de Carle bifocal may best be visualized as a near vision contact lens with a small portion in the centre of the back surface, ground and polished to a much steeper radius for distance vision use. This creates a positive tears lens between the central portion of the lens and the cornea. The power difference in air between the distance portion and

the near portion is just over three times the near addition actually required (see Chapter 4, Volume 1): for example

Distance Rx +2.00 D
Near addition +2.50 D
Distance BCOR 6.92 mm
Near BCOR 7.80 mm
Distance BVP of lens in air −3.50 D
Near BVP of lens in air +4.50 D

To some extent most multicurve corneal lenses act as back surface bifocals, for the BVP through the periphery of the lens is more positive, or less negative, than through the central portion, due to the back surface peripheral flattening.

In 1957–1958, Wesley and Jessen of Chicago (Jessen, 1960) were also working on a concentric bifocal lens with a central distance portion. One difference between their bifocal and the de Carle bifocal was that the bifocal surface was worked on to the front surface. A second difference was that the distance portion was larger (Figure 19.4). The Wesley–Jessen bifocal had the same power difference in air between the distance and near portions as the near addition actually required. As the difference in radii on a de Carle bifocal is three times greater than that on a Wesley–Jessen bifocal, the manufacturing problems are slightly less as there is

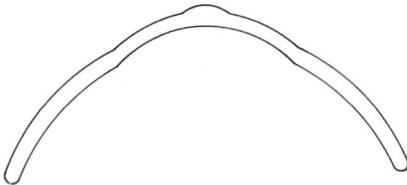

Figure 19.2–Bifocal scleral lens suggested by Williamson-Noble (1950) with a small convex central near portion on the front surface

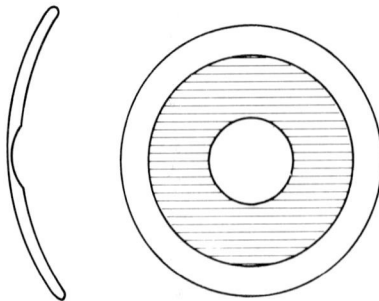

Figure 19.3–De Carle concentric back surface bifocal (1957) with a 2.0–4.0 mm central distance portion surrounded by the near portion used as a bearing surface

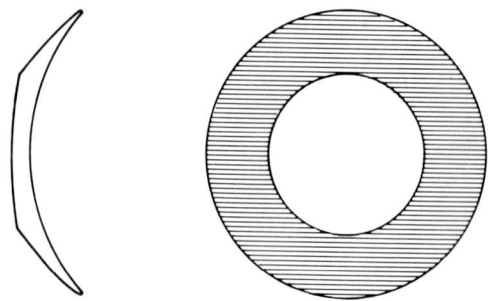

Figure 19.4–Wesley-Jessen concentric bifocal (1957–58) with a relatively flat distance portion on the front surface surrounded by a more convex near portion

less tendency for the two curves to blend together when being polished. Also, any errors of this nature are two-thirds eliminated by the tears liquid on the de Carle bifocal.

The main effect of the difference in sizes of the distance portions of these two lenses conveniently illustrates the two ways in which bifocal contact lenses work. The average distance portion diameter of the de Carle bifocal is 3.00 mm and the lens is fitted so that this completely covers the pupil with only a small amount of movement. The distance portion diameter is determined by the pupil size so that approximately the same amount of light enters the eye through the distance portion as the near portion. This is the 'bivision' principle. When viewing distant objects, there is a sharp image from the distance portion and, superimposed over it, a very blurred image from the near portion, and vice versa when the patient reads or does close work. This has the advantage that the patient does not have to hold his reading matter in any particular position to read. The main disadvantage is that the vision is not as sharp because of the side-effects from the superimposed images, although this is not as bad

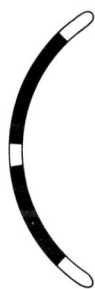

Figure 19.5–Cross-section of a pin-hole contact lens with opaque areas of the lens shown in black

as might be expected and has proved to be quite acceptable to many patients. The Wesley–Jessen bifocal originally had a 6.00 mm distance portion, but this was later reduced slightly to 5.00 mm to increase the near portion. The near portion on this lens can only cover the pupil by movement of the lens – the 'alternating vision' principle. This normally occurs by the patient looking down to read and the lens being pushed upwards by the lower lid. The advantage is sharper image formation with less visual side-effects – the disadvantage being that some lower lids are very loose, so that the lens tends to slide between the lid and the eye and is therefore not pushed upwards sufficiently. These lenses are often fitted slightly looser than average to allow them to move up easily. This can have the disadvantage that the near portion may partly cover the pupil immediately after a blink – probably for a second or less, but enough to be very disturbing to the patient.

The tendency over the past 18 years has been to concentrate on the alternating vision principle, trying to eliminate the disadvantages. A combination of the two principles is possible and, in fact, is present with most bifocal fitting to some degree.

Pin-hole lenses have been suggested as a means of giving a presbyopic patient clear vision from distance to a normal near working position (Freeman, 1952). This can be easily achieved with contact lenses, half the normal near addition being added to the distance prescription (*Figure 19.5*). The diameter of the aperture is between 1.00 and 2.00 mm, according to the near addition: the higher the near addition the smaller the aperture needs to be to achieve an acceptable degree of vision by reducing the size of the blur circles. Unfortunately, this cannot be done without a number of disadvantages as follows.

(1) Considerable loss of light. A 1.00 mm aperture is the equivalent of a very dark-tinted spectacle lens.

(2) Reduced field of view; this could be as little as 15 degrees, depending on the depth of the anterior chamber; that is, the distance of the lens from the eye's entrance pupil.

(3) Poor cosmetic appearance.

(4) A lens with a minimum of movement is essential. This is often difficult to achieve without sacrificing comfort and upsetting corneal metabolism.

Wesley (1962) developed a very unusual and ingenious lens, utilizing the chromatic aberration of the eye: red light being brought to a focus beyond blue. The near portion of his lens was of a blue or violet plastics material and the distance portion was tinted red. Simply by using different colours, the dioptric difference on the eye, between the distance and the near portions can be varied. The greater the difference between the two main wavelengths of light transmitted the greater the dioptric difference.

When non-tinted plastics material is used for the distance portion, of the wavelengths this transmits, the eye is most sensitive to 550 nm. With blue plastics used for the near portion, the wavelength of maximum transmission is 486 nm. This gives an effective near vision addition of 0.45 D. By using red plastics of approximately 656 nm maximum transmission for distance instead of clear plastics, this can be increased to 0.85 D.

Even greater dioptric differences can be obtained by using violet at 400 nm and red at 700 nm, but these lenses are darker and rather impractical for use indoors. This idea of varying the colour used for the two portions, instead of the curvature, works in the same way as the red and green duochrome test used by many refractionists.

The lenses can be made to any design, such as concentric or prism ballasted. It is obvious that their use would be mainly for early presbyopes. If it were possible to surface tint one portion of an existing bifocal successfully, it should be possible to increase the effective near addition by about 0.50 D. This could be very useful if an early presbyope who had had bifocals a year or so needed a slight increase in the near addition.

The dioptric difference obtained with these lenses is only apparent on the eye. If a single vision lens is tinted in this way, it will not alter the focimeter reading.

In 1967, Wesley announced another ingenious lens to achieve a bifocal effect (Plastic Contact Lens Company, 1970). Essentially, it has a small central distance portion with a plurality of light-transmitting apertures in the opaque remainder (*Figure 19.6*).

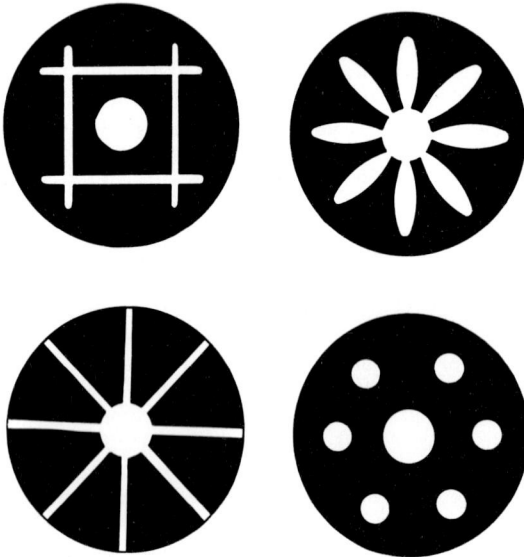

Figure 19.6–Multiple aperture lenses for distance and near vision use suggested by Wesley in 1967

This corrected one of the major objections to pin-hole lenses, namely, the restricted field of view. Many different patterns of apertures have been tried, the average width of the slits being 0.8 mm. The central transparent portion has been made as large as 3.00 mm. The distance correction is the same as would be prescribed for a single vision distance lens, the near vision focus being achieved by the reduced blur circles from the peripheral apertures.

A further type of bifocal lens was suggested by McKay Taylor (1962) and consisted of a small lens placed on top of a contact lens *in situ* (*Figure 19.7*). The lens was held in place by the surface tension of the tears and was made with a single back surface curve slightly flatter than the front radius of the carrier lens to allow a certain amount of movement of the additive lens. When the parent lens was a corneal contact lens, it was necessary to flatten the peripheral curve of the front surface slightly to prevent the additive lens from sliding off entirely. The combined weight caused the corneal lens to rotate in the same way as a prism ballasted lens. When the patient wished to see only in the distance, he removed the small additive lens with a suction holder.

From about 1960, bifocal contact lenses resembling spectacle bifocals became increasingly popular. The segment shapes were mostly very similar to their spectacle lens counterparts. Nearly all the lenses were prevented from rotating and kept in their correct position by the use of a prism which settled base-down. *Figure 19.8* shows two of the first of these lenses, both worked on the front surface. *Figure 19.9* shows a decentred de Carle bifocal incorporating prism and with the distance portion decentred upwards relative to the base of the prism. *Figure 19.10* shows some solid bifocal lenses designed by Hodd (1967) that are theoretically excellent visually but extremely difficult to make in practice. In fact, all these lenses and variations of them appear to suffer from some disadvantages. Because the two front surface curves are so similar, front surface bifocals are very difficult to make to ensure a sharp focimeter image right up to the

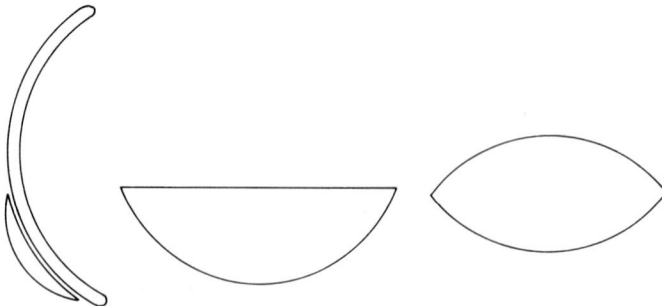

Figure 19.7–McKay Taylor additive bifocal. A small supplementary additional lens is placed on top of the carrier lens in situ. Two suggested shapes for additive lenses are shown on the right of a cross-section through carrier and additive lens (left)

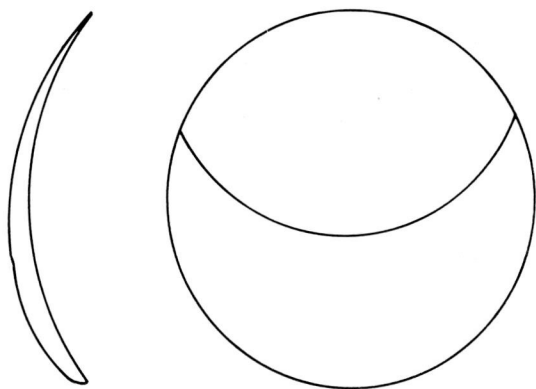

(a)

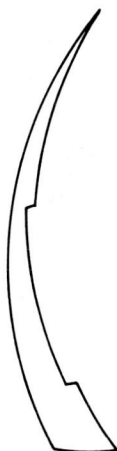

(a)

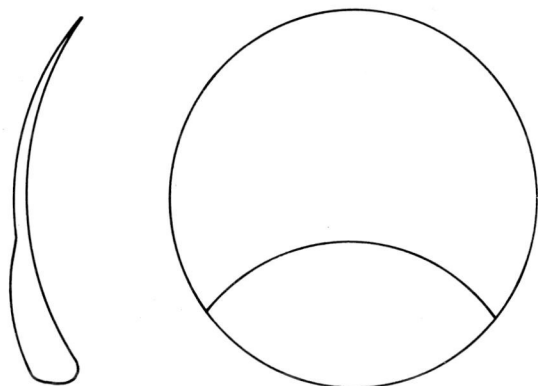

(b)

Figure 19.8–Two early suggested front surface solid prism ballasted bifocals

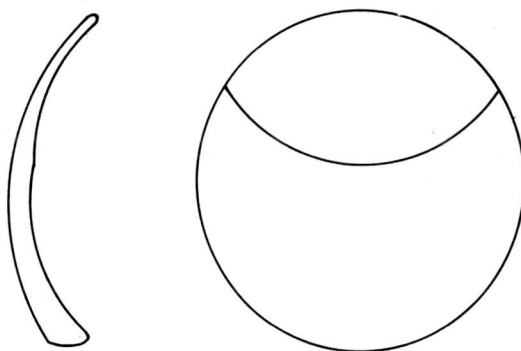

(b)

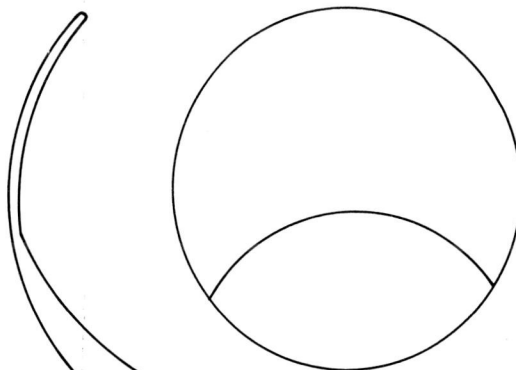

(c)

Figure 19.9–De Carle concentric bifocal incorporating prism ballast and with the distance portion de-centred upwards relative to the base of the prism

Figure 19.10–Some solid bifocal contact lenses suggested by Hodd (1967). (a) With recessed near portion on the back surface. (b) An upcurve prism ballasted back surface bifocal. (c) A downcurve prism ballasted back surface bifocal

transition, with no blending of the two curves at all. Nevertheless, some excellent lenses of this type have been made. The main difficulty is that vision is not always as definite as with single vision lenses. This is probably for the reason given by Williamson-Noble in 1950, that is, the accumulation of tears liquid prevents the bifocal form working properly. Back surface bifocals do not have this disadvantage, but the type shown in *Figure 19.8* must either have a small distance portion to avoid bubbles becoming trapped or be fitted so that the radius on the back surface for the near portion is flatter than the cornea. This results in the transition touching the cornea, which could cause corneal abrasion. Corneal abrasion from the edge of the recessed portion of the lens shown in *Figure 19.10a* could be a problem, the segment needing to be recessed as the radius of curvature of the near portion has to be flatter than the distance portion. Blending is undesirable as it creates an area of blurred vision.

Mandell (1966) was commissioned by a laboratory (Kontur Kontact) to design a prism ballast bifocal to try and eliminate the problems encountered with earlier front surface bifocals.

The result is the Mandell 'No-Jump' bifocal, and it is probably the most successful of the front surface bifocals.

The making of this lens is an example of contact lens manufacturing technique at its finest. The near portion is cut into the front surface so that there is a slight 'ledge' between the distance portion and the near portion (similar to a semi-visible centre controlled spectacle bifocal, but on the front surface). The amount of this ledge increases towards the edge of the lens and is absent in the centre (*Figure 19.11*). This ledge does not appear to cause irritation of the upper lid.

Monocentric fused bifocals should give an equal performance and have the advantage that the front surface can, within reason, be repolished or have a small power change carried out. Due to the very

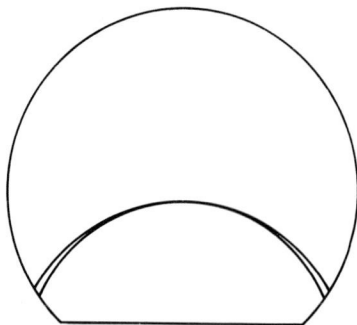

Figure 19.12–(a) Fused 'no-jump' bifocal (cross-section). (b) Inserted segment fused bifocal (Ysoptic Laboratories) with a double back optic surface to help locate the lens with the desired optic portion in front of the pupil

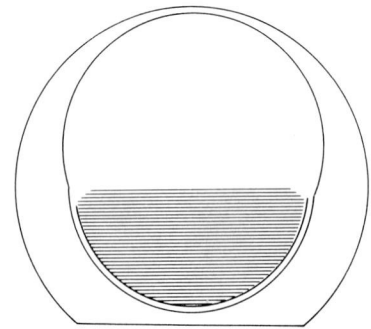

(a)

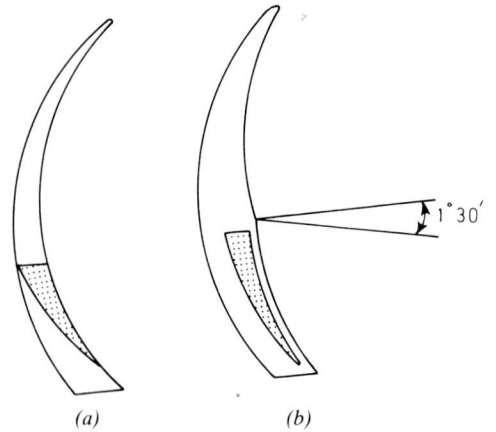

(b)

Figure 19.13–(a) Front view of the Ysoptic inserted fused bifocal. (b) Ysoptic measuring lens for determining segment height

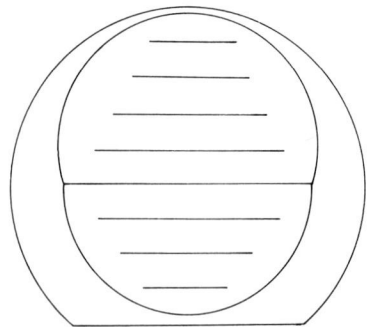

Figure 19.11–Mandell 'no-jump' front surface bifocal lens

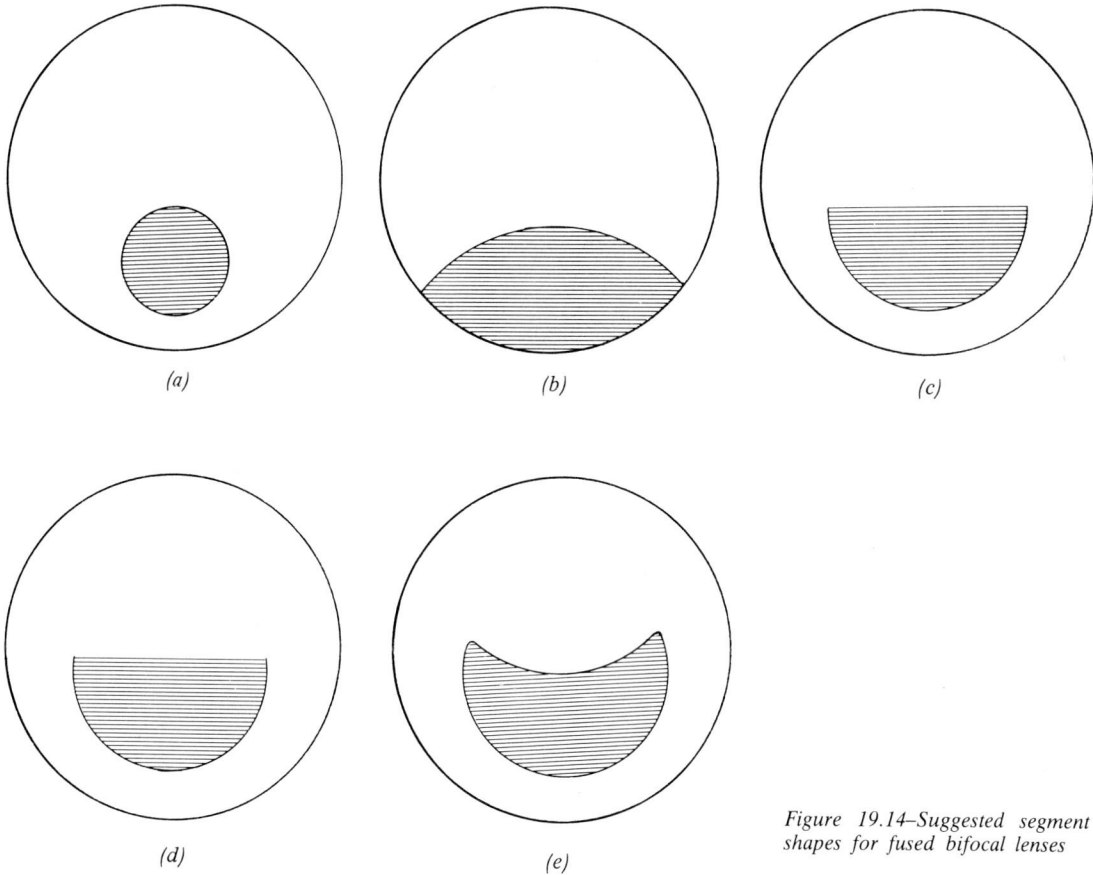

Figure 19.14–Suggested segment shapes for fused bifocal lenses

precise nature of the front surface of the Mandell bifocal, repolishing is not advised.

A bifocal with an inserted segment of a higher refractive index, or a fused bifocal (Camp, 1966), would overcome the objections to the back and front surface solid bifocals. The French company of Ysoptic have made an inserted segment type of lens (Guilbert, 1969a and b). This lens has a unique back surface. The distance and near portions have the same radius but are set at a slight angle to each other so that the lens can rock on the cornea. This is intended to anchor the lens more firmly for distance or near use (*Figure 19.12b*). Ysoptic also make a bifocal measuring lens (*Figure 19.13*), for determining segment heights. Fused bifocals, on the other hand, are nearly always made so that the segment is worked from the back surface and can be made slightly thinner than lenses with an inserted segment. Their construction and manufacture has been described by Bryant (1973).

A variety of segment shapes can be made, the usual ones being shown in *Figure 19.14*. The first segment has the disadvantage that near vision becomes blurred if the lens slips slightly to one side. The second segment largely overcomes this problem, but the optical centre of the near portion is a greater distance from the optical centre of the distance portion so that a 'jump' is created as the visual axis passes from one portion to the other. The third segment is theoretically monocentric so that there should be no 'jump', and the width of the segment is therefore exactly twice the height. This sometimes limits the height of the segment as an increase in size would increase the thickness, which might be undesirable in negative lenses. The fourth segment is a good compromise, not theoretically monocentric but the 'jump' is so slight that it is no problem in practice. The fifth segment is also monocentric, the aim of the up-curved top of the segment being to ensure that the centre of the segment top is always in the same position in relation to the pupil if the lens swings slightly in a pendulum manner on the eye (Goldberg, 1969). Theoretically, the radius of curvature of the top of the segment should be the same as half the overall lens size. The disadvantage of this type of segment is the possibility of slight peripheral blur at the sides when using distance vision.

The portion of the edge just below the segment is of extreme importance. It is this part of the lens that is pushed upwards by the lower lid when the patient looks down to read. Positive lenses obviously create the biggest problem of how to increase the lower edge thickness without increasing the overall thickness and weight more than is absolutely essential.

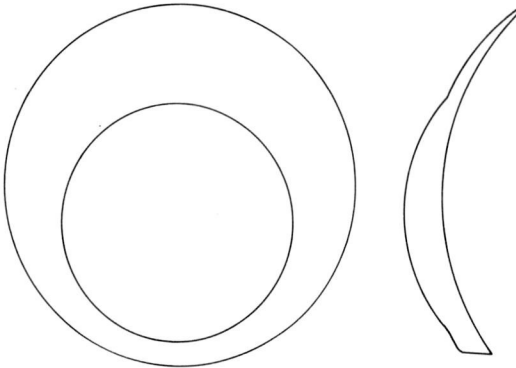

Figure 19.15–Positive lens with a prism ballasted convex carrier peripheral portion and decentred downwards with respect to the base of the prism. Such a lens has a sufficiently thick lower edge to rest on the lower lid without being excessively heavy and may therefore be made in bifocal form

Unless the patient has a very tight lower lid, most positive lenses are better made in a decentred convex carrier lenticular form (*Figure 19.15*). This keeps the weight down but increases the lower edge thickness.

The greater the prism the poorer the focimeter image. However, in many cases, this would appear to be preferable to the alternatives of either a very thick lens or a lens which does not ride up when the patient is reading because the lens slips under the lower lid. For the same reason, no lower edge thinning should be attempted except on very high negative lenses. This gives an edge similar to the one shown in *Figure 19.16*, which would seem to be a highly undesirable edge to those who have studied edge forms for single vision lenses (Shanks, 1966). In practice, it is found that – provided that this unusual edge does not continue right around the lens and there is a normal corneal lens edge at the top – the lens is perfectly comfortable to wear and, when inserted, quickly rotates to the correct position.

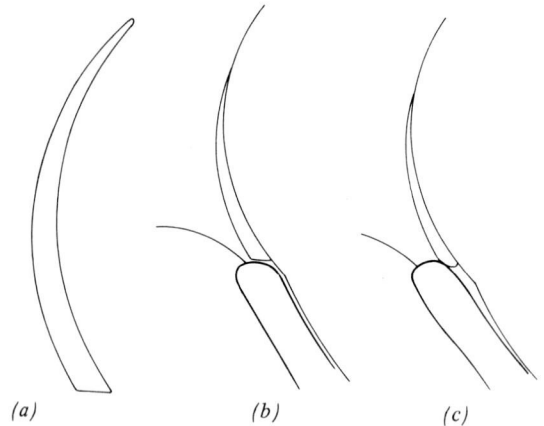

Figure 19.16–(a) Diagrammatic representation of the ideal inferior edge shape in a prism ballasted lens to be made in bifocal form. (b) The 'square' edge shown in (a) rests on the lower lid (shown in cross-section) and moves upwards and downwards on the cornea as the eye is depressed or elevated. (c) Excessive rounding of the inferior edge enables the lens to pass behind the lower lid and the near portion may not then move in front of the pupil on depression of the gaze

The practitioner new to prism ballasted bifocals usually visualizes them moving as illustrated in *Figure 19.17*. On closer examination, it can be seen that this is not normally possible. A lens of 8.00 mm overall size on an 11.50 mm diameter cornea can move approximately 4.00 mm, allowing for the fact that it is on a curved surface. However, if the pupil diameter is 4.00 mm, an average size for a presbyopic patient, it will be seen that the pupil can only be covered entirely by the distance or near portions if the lens has moved from the extreme lower area of the cornea to the extreme upper area; also, that there is no room on this lens for peripheral and intermediate curves so that a situation of completely alternating vision is only possible when the pupil is very small. For most patients, we must accept the fact that there will be a combination of 'alternating vision' and 'bivision'.

Figure 19.18 shows a larger lens where the upper edge of the near portion coincides with the lower edge of the pupil. However, the lens is only able to move vertically by 2.00 mm, and on a 4.00 mm pupil this means that only half the pupil area is covered by the near portion when the patient looks down for near vision.

In *Figure 19.19*, the top of the near portion covers 1.00 mm of the 4.00 mm pupil when the lens is in the low position. When the lens rises by 2.00 mm, the near portion covers 3.00 mm of the 4.00 mm pupil. It can be shown mathematically that when this lens

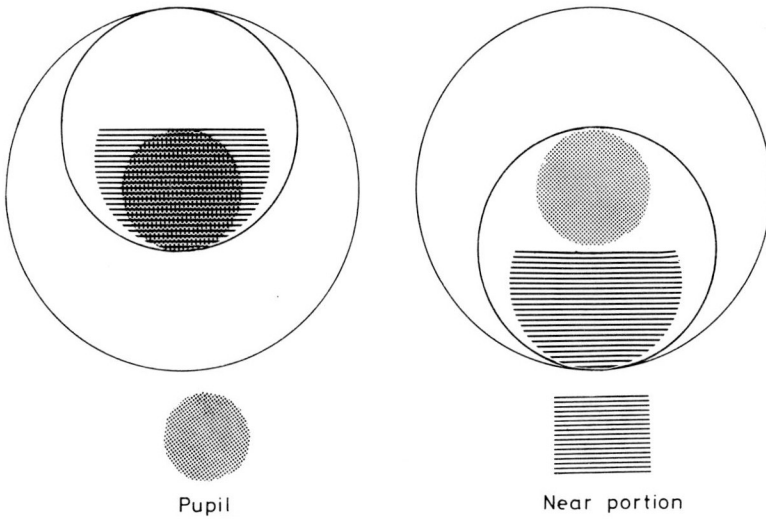

Pupil

Near portion

Figure 19.17–The theoretical ideal for a bifocal contact lens where the entire distance portion is centred before the pupil for distance vision (right) and the entire near portion centred for close work (left)

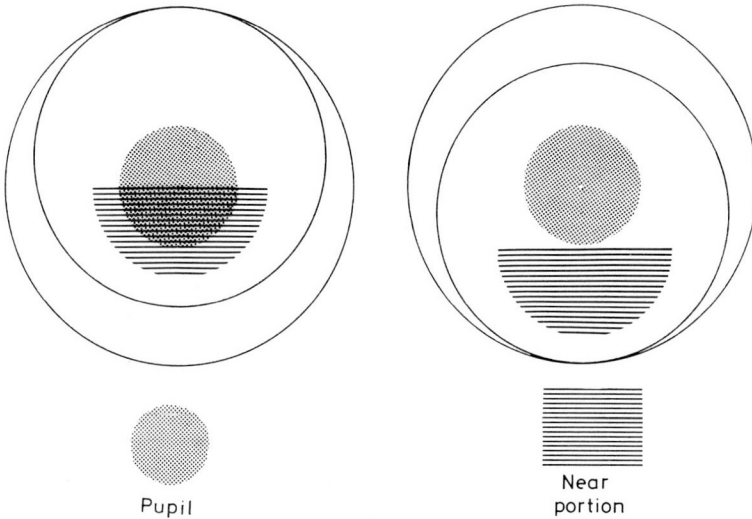

Pupil

Near portion

Figure 19.18–In practice, a lens made with the top of the near portion level with the bottom of the pupil (right) usually only covers half of the pupil when the gaze is depressed (left)

is in the position for maximum distance vision, 80 per cent of the pupil area is covered by the distance portion of the lens. Similarly, when the lens is in the near position, 80 per cent of the pupil area is covered by the near portion. This is the method of fitting preferred by the author.

Prism ballasted bifocals can be truncated, but this does not necessarily keep them in their correct position. In fact, some lenses of this type have occasionally rotated through 180 degrees showing no tendency to return to the normal position. One advantage of a truncation is to increase the area of edge to be raised by the lower lid, but edge thickness and shape are probably of greater importance. The truncation should preferably not be straight but slightly curved to match the radius of curvature of

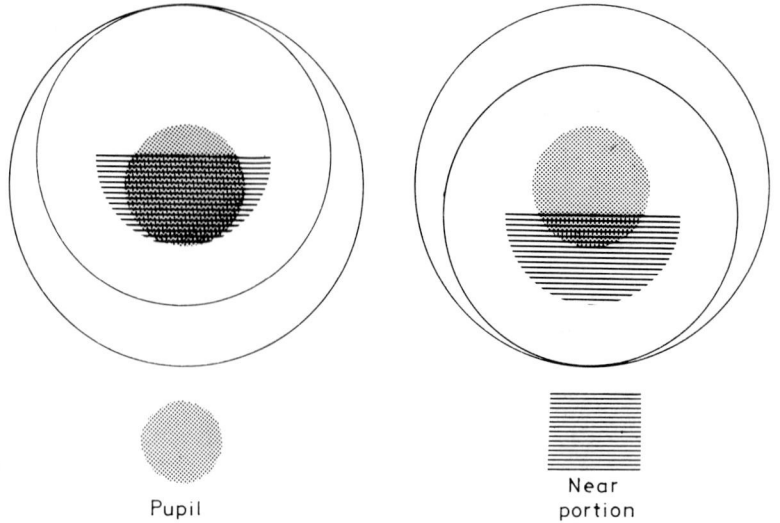

Figure 19.19–A compromise is usually found to be the ideal so that 80 per cent of the pupil area is covered by the distance portion of the lens during distance vision (right) and a similar proportion is covered by the segment during near vision (left)

Pupil

Near portion

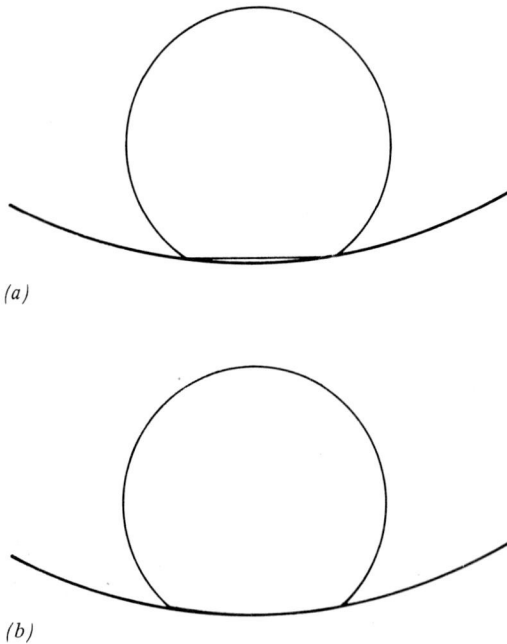

(a)

(b)

Figure 19.20–The lower edge of a truncated prism ballasted lens should not be straight as shown in (a) but curved to match the line of the lower lid as shown in (b)

the lower lid (*Figure 19.20*). Examination of photographs of the eye has shown this radius to be between 15.0 and 21.0 mm. A radius of 18.0 mm is a good average.

Lenses may be stabilized by other means (Gates, Ewell and Remba, 1961), the principal methods are as follows.

(1) An oval lens or a double truncation. The BCOR should be approximately the same as the keratometer reading at 180 degrees if it is intended to keep the long axis horizontal. It must be remembered that there is a strong tendency for the long axis of the lens to settle along the meridian of the cornea with a similar curvature and for this reason the method is unsuitable in cases of oblique or 'against-the-rule' astigmatism.

(2) A spherical BCOR combined with toroidal peripheral curves on the back surface (only appropriate for toroidal corneas).

(3) A small metal weight embedded in the plastics near the edge, which should rotate to the 6 o'clock position.

(1), (2) and (3) all lose the advantage of the prism ballasted lens for bifocals, namely, increased thickness at the lower edge to enable the lower lid to raise the lens. Methods (1) and (2) also have the disadvantage that the lenses can fit in two positions at 180 degrees to each other, so that a bifocal near portion would be correct in one position but upside down in the other.

CHOICE OF BIFOCAL TYPE

The patient's occupation is a very important consideration which should help to determine whether or not to supply him with bifocal and trifocal contact lenses and also the type of lens. This is an area where the practitioner's skill and experience is invaluable. It is important that the practitioner realizes that there is no one design of bifocal or trifocal lens that is ideal for every single patient. This point has been elaborated by Hodd (1974) who has published some case histories illustrating the use of different types of bifocal lens, which he also describes. By the correct choice of the type of lens, a very high percentage of patients should be successfully fitted. It is important to question the patient carefully regarding his near and intermediate distance visual requirements and, if necessary, give a demonstration of these requirements. These should fall into one of the following categories.

Good Distance Vision Essential (for flying, driving, etc.)

Good peripheral vision will also be essential, so the concentric type bifocal should not be fitted to these patients. A prism ballasted bifocal should give the best results; and to ensure that the near portion does not ride up or rotate on the eye when the patient is using distance vision, slightly more prism ballast should be given and the near portion should possibly be fitted slightly lower than average. This latter situation is not possible if the patient insists on very good near vision.

Very Good Near Vision Required for Long Periods of Time

In these cases, the largest possible near portion on a prism ballasted bifocal should be supplied and fitted as high as possible without interfering with the distance vision. Alternatively, a concentric back surface bifocal with a small distance portion may be used.

Good Intermediate Vision at, or Slightly Below, Eye Level

Musicians are examples of this type of patient. One approach is to make the near portion suitably powered for the intermediate distance. However, there are very few patients who are satisfied with poor near vision, trifocals are therefore the lenses of choice in these cases (see page 588).

Good Intermediate Vision Required Above Eye Level

An example of this type of patient is a chemist with bottles on high shelves to be seen continuously throughout the day. In this case, a trifocal with the intermediate portion above the distance portion would be the lens of choice.

Good Near Vision Required Above Eye Level

Usually, a concentric bifocal is the most satisfactory lens, particularly if it tends to settle below the central position on the cornea.

Lenses Required Mainly for Social Reasons

In such cases, long-sustained critical near vision is not usually carried out with the bifocal contact lenses. Possibly, nothing more critical than reading a menu or theatre programme is required. This can usually be achieved with a concentric bifocal. However, if the patient is a keen bridge player, trifocal lenses might be the best answer.

Two anatomical features are of importance with bifocal contact lenses that are of lesser importance with single vision lenses. These are the pupil diameter and the position and tightness of the lower lid. The pupil diameter may be a very important factor if it fluctuates very considerably between bright and dark conditions. This particularly applies when considering concentric bifocals. It has sometimes been stated that patients with small pupils are unsuitable for bifocal contact lenses; but back surface concentric bifocals with distance segments as small as 1.50 mm have been successfully fitted. The larger the pupil diameter the greater the difficulty in fitting prism ballasted bifocals because the possibility of achieving good alternating vision becomes harder and some degree of bivision has to be accepted.

The lower lid should be carefully examined, particularly if prism ballasted bifocals are being considered. The lower lid is essential to raise the lens when the patient lowers his eyes for near vision. A very loose lower lid or a lower lid below the limbus may be unable to do this sufficiently to obtain enough vertical movement of the lens. In such cases, a concentric bifocal fitted on the bivision principle will probably be the lens of choice.

FITTING PROCEDURES

BACK SURFACE CONCENTRIC BIFOCALS

These lenses must be fitted so that they centre well with the minimum amount of movement that is acceptable to the patient and practitioner. This can be done by fitting the lenses larger, steeper or thinner than usual. All three methods could result in an uncomfortable lens, so considerable care is required by the practitioner. Such lenses often need to be fenestrated. A lens that rides up very slightly is preferable to one that settles slightly below centre. A low fitting lens makes near vision difficult, although patients may be able to read quite well if they hold the reading matter above eye level (*Figure 19.21*).

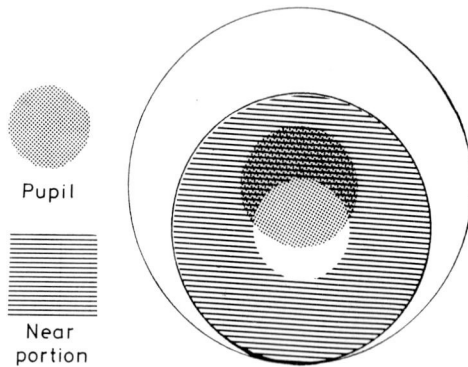

Figure 19.21–A low fitting concentric bifocal interferes with good distance vision and makes near vision difficult unless looking above eye level

Table 19.1–Recommended Diameter of the Distance Portion in Concentric Bifocals Related to the Pupil Diameter

Pupil diameter (mm)	Distance portion diameter (mm)	Pupil diameter (mm)	Distance portion diameter (mm)
4.5	3.20	3.2	2.25
4.4	3.10	3.1	2.20
4.3	3.05	3.0	2.10
4.2	2.95	2.9	2.05
4.1	2.90	2.8	2.00
4.0	2.80	2.7	1.90
3.9	2.75	2.6	1.85
3.8	2.70	2.5	1.75
3.7	2.60	2.4	1.70
3.6	2.55	2.3	1.65
3.5	2.45	2.2	1.55
3.4	2.40	2.1	1.50
3.3	2.30	2.0	1.45

The diameter of the distance portion is mainly dependent upon the pupil diameter. One method is to measure the pupil in low illumination and order the distance portion according to *Table 19.1*. The pupil is difficult to measure with a scale, however, in low illumination (although ultra-violet illumination is useful as the crystalline lens fluoresces). The most accurate method is by photography. A scale – preferably divided into 0.1 mm graduations – is held in approximately the same plane as the iris and photographed, using a flash gun. The pupil does not contract until immediately after the flash has taken

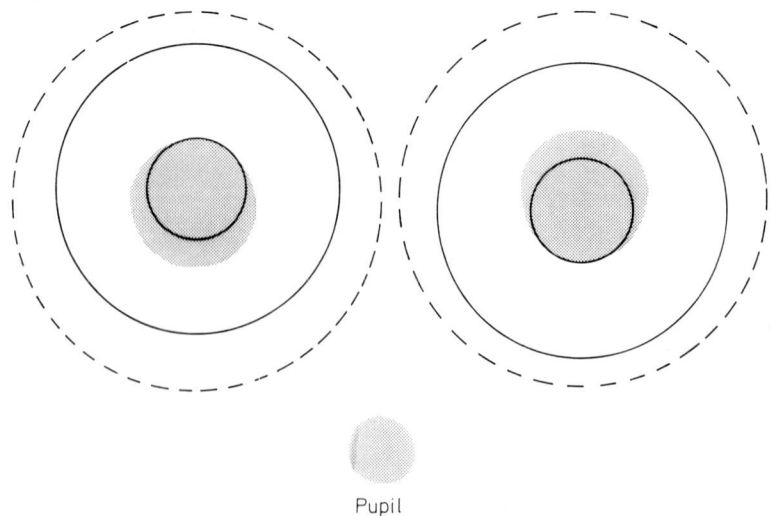

Figure 19.22–A well-fitting concentric bifocal can move up to 1.0 mm and still have all the distance portion in front of the pupil (shaded)

Pupil

place. Another method is to measure the pupil diameter when a bright light is shone into the patient's eye and order the distance portion of the same diameter. Where both methods are used, some practitioners order a distance portion diameter half way between the two diameters indicated. A laboratory can usually slightly reduce the diameter of the distance portion on the finished lens, if necessary, but cannot increase the diameter satisfactorily. *Figure 19.22* shows how a well-fitted lens can move approximately 1.00 mm and still have all the distance portion over the pupil and the same percentage of the pupil area covered by the near portion.

Trial lenses with different sized distance portions are preferable as an added check on these calculations. However, with the advent of other types of bifocal, back surface bifocals are now seldom fitted, so the outlay on a fitting set may not be considered justified. Nevertheless, these lenses can be very useful when the prism ballasted type has been found unsatisfactory because of a very loose lower lid.

The distance portion diameter can also be varied according to the patient's visual requirements. For example, a woman who needs bifocals only so that she can see to read a menu or a theatre programme can be given a larger distance portion than a person who needs to read small print for long periods of time.

FRONT SURFACE CONCENTRIC BIFOCALS

The BCOR is determined by the flattest keratometer reading. If the BCOR is flatter than this, the lens may have a tendency to ride slightly high on the cornea so that the distance portion is displaced upwards. Conversely, if the BCOR is made steeper the lens may tend to remain in a central position, and for near vision the patient will have difficulty in getting the lens to move in order to use the near portion.

The BCOD should be as large as possible, but at the same time, the intermediate and peripheral curves must be sufficiently flat to allow a moderate amount of lens movement. The overall size is usually increased to 0.30 mm larger than a single vision lens, and the thickness is approximately 0.05 mm thicker than the equivalent single vision lens except with higher powered negative lenses. Most positive lenses should be made in a lenticular form to prevent very thin edges as the lower lid must move the lens slightly upwards when the patient is looking at a near object. Bronstein (1959) recommends putting an empirical 1.00 D of additional positive power on the near addition. This is presumably to compensate for a slight negative tears lens on

the front surface (*see* page 122, Chapter 4, Volume 1).

The diameter of the distance portion must be carefully measured. If the distance portion is too large, the lens will not be able to move sufficiently to allow the patient to look through the near portion. If the distance portion diameter is too small, the patient will have a noticeable blur surrounding distant objects and this becomes aggravating when the lens moves during blinking. The diameter of the distance portion should not be smaller than the pupil size in a normal artificially lit room. If the pupil is larger than 5 mm, it is preferable to fit these lenses by the bivision method; but with smaller pupils, they are normally always fitted using the alternating vision principle.

An alternative method of arriving at the distance portion diameter is to measure the distance from the bottom edge of the lens to the bottom edge of the pupil, then double this value and subtract it from the overall size of the lens. For example, if the bottom edge of the lens is 2.50 mm from the lower edge of the pupil, the number doubled equals 5.00 mm and subtracted from a trial lens of 9.50 mm overall size it gives a distance portion diameter of 4.50 mm.

PRISM BALLASTED BIFOCALS

The fitting requirements are the same whether the lens is a front surface, back surface or fused bifocal. In addition to all the information required when ordering a single vision lens the practitioner needs to calculate the following.

(1) Near addition.
(2) Size and shape of segment.
(3) Height of segment above the lower edge of the lens.
(4) Amount of prism ballast and thickness of the lower edge.
(5) Vertical overall size.

These are examined in detail below.

Near Addition

This varies according to the type of lens being ordered. When Wesley and Jessen (Jessen, 1960) introduced their front surface concentric bifocal, they also suggested that the near addition should be made 1.00 D stronger than that actually required. Some practitioners have continued this practice with solid front surface prism bifocals but the majority claim it is unnecessary. With solid back surface bifocals of every design, it is necessary to allow for the fact that the tears neutralize just over two-thirds of the difference in power between the two areas.

For example, to achieve a near addition of 2.50 D, the dioptric difference in air between the distance and the near portions needs to be approximately 8.00 D. For fused bifocals, the near addition should definitely be no stronger than that which would be ordered for spectacle bifocals.

Size and Shape of Segment

The segment should normally be the largest possible without increasing the thickness. However, there is no point in having a segment that is so large that it extends beyond the back central optic diameter or is cut into by the lower edge of the lens. This particularly applies to fused bifocals, where the vertical dimension of the segment should not be made greater than the height of the top of the segment above the bottom of the lens. Occasionally, it is necessary to increase the thickness of a lens slightly to obtain a sufficiently large segment. This particularly applies to fused bifocals and could occur, for example, with the combination of a large pupil, a high near addition, and myopia (that is, with a flat-top segment and the thickest part of the segment coinciding with the thinnest part of a negative lens). *Table 19.2* gives the minimum

moves with the eye, many of the criteria that are used to determine the size and shape of spectacle bifocal segments do not apply to contact lens bifocals. For instance, whether a book-keeper can see books on both sides of the desk will depend as much on whether the lenses are stable and remain over the pupil area as on the segment width. It is interesting to note that patients complain far less about seeing the segment when they walk, go up stairs, etc., than those with bifocal spectacles. The author's preference is for flat-top fused segments, the particular dimensions being calculated for every case.

Table 19.2–Minimum Central Thicknesses Recommended for Fused Bifocals According to Segment Width (or Diameter) and Near Addition

Reading addition (D)	Minimum central thickness (mm) Segment widths (mm)					
	5.00	5.50	6.00	6.50	7.00	7.50
+1.50	0.12	0.14	0.17	0.20	0.23	0.28
+1.75	0.14	0.16	0.19	0.23	0.27	0.32
+2.00	0.16	0.18	0.22	0.26	0.31	0.37
+2.25	0.17	0.20	0.25	0.29	0.35	0.42
+2.50	0.19	0.23	0.27	0.33	0.40	0.47
+2.75	0.21	0.25	0.30	0.36	0.44	0.52
+3.00	0.22	0.27	0.33	0.40	0.48	0.57

thicknesses advised by one manufacturer of fused bifocals for certain segment widths and near additions. If this table is used in conjunction with *Table 19.3*, it may easily be determined if a particular reading addition and segment width are possible without increasing the central thickness.

The segment shape is usually determined by the type of lens which the practitioner has decided is likely to give the best performance. As the lens

Table 19.3–Minimum Central Thicknesses for Prism Ballasted Lenses of 9.00 mm Overall Size According to Back Vertex Power (and Prism Ballast in Negative Powered Lenses)

Positive lenses, 9.00 mm overall size all 1½△ prism ballast		Negative lenses, 9.00 mm overall size		
BVP (D)	Central thickness (mm)	BVP (D)	Central thickness (mm)	Prism (△)
0.00	0.32			
+0.50	0.34	−0.50	0.31	1½
+1.00	0.35	−1.00	0.30	1½
+1.00	0.35	−1.00	0.30	1½
+1.50	0.36	−1.50	0.29	1½
+2.00	0.37	−2.00	0.27	1½
+2.50	0.39	−2.50	0.26	1½
+3.00	0.40	−3.00	0.25	1½
+3.50	0.41	−3.50	0.24	1½
+4.00	0.42	−4.00	0.25	2
+4.50	0.44	−4.50	0.25	2
+5.00	0.45	−5.00	0.24	2
+5.50	0.46	−5.50	0.23	2
+6.00	0.47	−6.00	0.22	2
+6.50	0.49	−6.50	0.25	2½
+7.00	0.50	−7.00	0.24	2½
+7.50	0.51	−7.50	0.23	2½
+8.00	0.52	−8.00	0.22	2½
+8.50	0.54	−8.50	0.25	3
+9.00	0.55	−9.00	0.24	3
+9.50	0.56	−9.50	0.23	3
+10.00	0.57	−10.00	0.22	3
+10.50	0.59	−10.50	0.25	3½
+11.00	0.60	−11.00	0.24	3½
+11.50	0.61	−11.50	0.23	3½
+12.00	0.62	−12.00	0.22	3½
+12.50	0.64	−12.50	0.25	4
+13.00	0.65	−13.00	0.24	4
+13.50	0.66	−13.50	0.23	4
+14.00	0.67	−14.00	0.22	4

Height of Segment Above the Lower Edge of the Lens

The height of the segment can be stated in two ways: (1) in relation to the centre of the lens (with a truncated lens this is taken as that of the round lens prior to truncation); (2) as the height above the lower edge of the finished lens. The author strongly recommends the second method.

The higher the segment without having any noticeable effect on the distance vision the better. In this way, the amount by which the lens has to rise to allow good near vision is reduced. It has been found, in practice, that the top of the segment can be

one of the most important factors in the successful fitting of prism ballasted bifocals and an accuracy of 0.10 mm is desirable. Photography is the most accurate method. An ordinary camera with an auxiliary lens may be used at 25–35 cm from the eye, with a scale divided into 0.10 mm divisions placed close to the eye. It is important that this is held at the same distance from the camera as the pupil and iris. The photograph is taken in ordinary room illumination with a flashlight. As the pupil contracts after the photograph has been taken, the normal pupil diameter may be measured. The main disadvantage is waiting for the film to be developed.

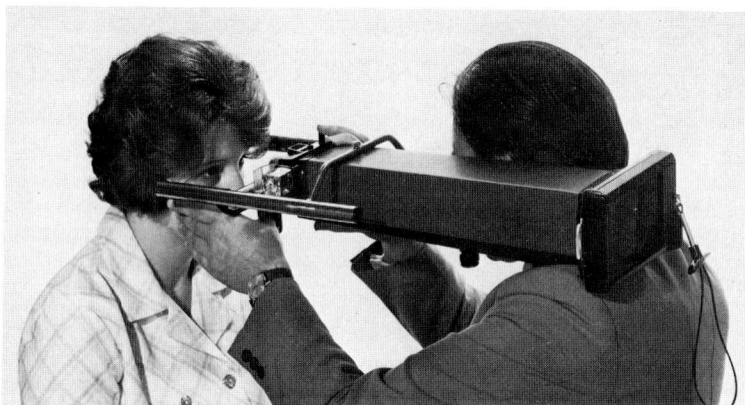

Figure 19.23–Camera designed by the writer for photography of the external eye (photograph by kind permission of Contactasol Ltd)

one-quarter of the pupil diameter above the lower edge of the pupil without causing visual annoyance. In other words, if the pupil diameter is 4.00 mm, the top of the segment can be 1.00 mm above the bottom of the pupil when the patient is looking straight ahead (see Colour Plate XLIV).

It is therefore necessary to measure the distance from the lower lid to the bottom of the pupil and then add one-quarter of the pupil diameter. When the lower lid is below the limbus, a prism ballasted lens – not necessarily a bifocal but one of approximately the correct thickness – should be placed on the eye so that the practitioner may observe the lowest point that the lower edge reaches. The position of the lower edge in relation to the edge of the iris should be noted to aid this measurement. Due to the added weight of a prism ballasted lens, and the fact that a tight lens is unlikely to move sufficiently for a satisfactory visual result, prism ballasted lenses normally rest on the lower lid if this is on or above the limbus. However, it is not very easy to measure this with a scale as the eye does not keep still. An accuracy of 0.50 mm is as much as can normally be attained. The height of the segment is

Ideally, to obtain the measurements most accurately, it should then be projected on to a screen. The author has had a Polaroid camera specially made so that it takes a photograph of the eye five times the normal size (Figure 19.23). Special devices have had to be made to ensure that the eye is exactly the correct distance from the camera lens when the photograph is taken; even an error of 1.00 mm would make an appreciable difference in the measurements.

Bifocal trial lenses are an excellent method of assessing the segment height as well as other factors. However, unless an extremely large trial set is available, estimation is needed in deciding the segment height. The use of trial lenses also enables a subjective visual check on the segment height to be carried out. The rule of the segment top being one-quarter of the pupil diameter above the bottom of the pupil must not be followed too rigidly, and the segment height may be varied by pushing the lens upwards with the lower lid. If the vision with the trial lens is reasonably good, the patient should be able to make valuable comments on the effect of the near portion on his distance vision. An assistant may be able to hold a trial spectacle lens in front of the eye to see if this improves the distance visual acuity. In most cases, the segment may be lowered by pulling down the lower lid. It is essential for the practitioner to be able to see the top of the segment, and this may be done by marking the top line with instant drying waterproof ink or a grease pencil. The entire segment area may also be coloured in with waterproof ink, which has the advantage of permitting the patient to notice a colour change, as soon as the visual axis enters the segment area, thus checking the segment position. This is particularly useful if the trial lens segment is of insufficient power (or even when a single vision trial lens – without a segment – is used). A fluorescent mark may also be used. One advantage of fused bifocals is that the whole segment may be made slightly fluorescent (Bier, 1965), although an ultra-violet lamp is needed to show it up (*see Colour Plate XLV*). The top of flat-top fused bifocal segments can also be seen quite easily with an ophthalmoscope or slit lamp. It has been suggested that a scale placed in the focal plane of the eyepiece of a slit lamp biomicroscope would be a useful way of determining the segment height. Such graticule eyepieces are available as accessories to most slit lamp biomicroscopes.

If in doubt, it is best to err on the high side when ordering the segment height – but not excessively so if the patient is not to notice any deleterious effect on his distance vision. The segment may usually be lowered by removing material from the bottom of the lens (that is, by truncating the lens) but plastics material cannot be added to raise the segment. The segment height may be as small as 2.50 mm above the lower edge, if the lower lid is tight and high above the lower limbus, or as big as 5.00 mm on a large eye with a loose or low lower lid. Giving an average in every case will result in many failures.

Amount of Prism Ballast and Thickness of the Lower Edge

This can usually be left to the laboratory. *Table 19.3* gives details of average centre thicknesses and prisms. These may need to be modified, for example, if ordering negative lenses for a patient where there is a considerable prescription difference between the two eyes. The prism must normally be the same for the two lenses.

Advocates of small, thin single vision lenses must modify their techniques when fitting bifocals. The extra thickness often helps to keep the lens from riding up every time the patient blinks, which can be so annoying visually; but unnecessary thickness beyond this point usually reduces the comfort.

Vertical Overall Size

The factors determining the vertical overall size are quite different from those that determine the overall size of a single vision lens. The main factor is that the lens must be able to move vertically by not less than half the pupil diameter. This is to enable the lens to rise upwards from the position where the segment covers one-quarter of the pupil diameter to covering three-quarters of the pupil diameter. If the lens has more movement than this, it may be considered excessive. If there is less movement than this, the patient will have near vision difficulty. Trial lenses can also be a help in assessing the vertical overall size.

ADJUSTING PRISM BALLASTED BIFOCAL LENSES

A number of adjustments are possible to these lenses; despite the most accurate measurements, it is often necessary to adjust them to obtain the best possible results. The following are the most common problems and the adjustments that will usually correct them.

Good Distance Vision with Poor Near Vision

Assuming that the reason is not an incorrect prescription, it is usually due to the near portion not sufficiently covering the pupil when the patient looks downwards. This may be caused by one of the following.

(1) If the lens is unable to move up sufficiently when the patient's gaze is directed downwards. The adjustment in this case would be to remove material from the top of the lens in order to reduce the vertical overall size to allow the lens to ride up higher or, if the lens is not moving up to the upper limbus, to flatten the back surface intermediate and peripheral curves at the upper part of the lens. It is not essential – and, in fact, is often inadvisable – to flatten these curves all the way round the lens. By carefully masking the lower portion of the lens on the back surface with thin tape and then holding the lens on to the appropriate tool of the adjustment kit, it is possible to flatten the curves only at the top of the back surface of the lens. Sometimes, a reduction in both overall size and flattening of the curves is needed.

(2) If the near portion rises too high when the patient looks down, the patient will look partly through the near portion and partly through the area below the lens (*Figure 19.24*). This tends to happen particularly if the patient's lower lid is well above

the lower limbus. In this condition, it is important to have as little non-optical area below the near portion as possible. The method of rectification is to remove material from the bottom of the lens, but not so much that the lower edge actually cuts into the near portion. This is usually done by a slightly curved truncation, and it is recommended that no more than 0.50 mm is removed before trying out the lens again. If necessary, more can be removed; but if too much material is removed, a new lens will have to be ordered, so it is better to do a little at a time.

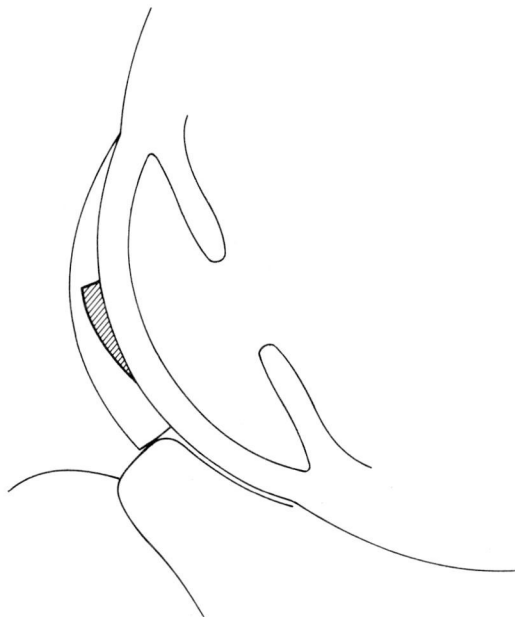

Figure 19.24–A fused bifocal which rises too high on depression of gaze causes the patient to look through the distance portion below the segment as well as partly through the segment

The vertical size of the near portion is often no greater than the pupil diameter, and sometimes smaller. It is very important that this is positioned as closely as possible over the pupil area when the patient looks down in his normal position for near work. A difference of 0.50 mm up or down can often make a great deal of difference. As the horizontal size is often considerably larger than the pupil diameter, a little movement laterally is usually of small consequence visually. It is also surprising that it is often possible for the lens to twist considerably on the cornea and for the patient still to obtain good vision. The critical factor seems to be how much of the pupil area is covered by the near portion when it is required to see at near.

Good Near Vision with Poor Distance Vision

This is almost certainly caused by the near portion being too high and covering too large an area of the pupil. First, it is important to determine whether this is due to the near portion height being too great or to the lens settling above the lower lid when the gaze is directed straight ahead. If it is the former, the only adjustment possible is to remove material from the lower edge so that if the lens continues to rest on the lower lid the segment height will be lowered by the same amount that is removed from the lower edge of the lens. If it is the latter, there is no one answer. High-riding single vision lenses will often settle higher still if the intermediate and peripheral curves on the back surface are flattened, and a steeper lens is often required to achieve better centration. This may apply to bifocals; but generally, the increased weight due to the prism helps the lens to settle low so that flattening the intermediate and peripheral curves may have the desired effect.

If not, re-ordering a lens with an increased prism is indicated.

Poor Vision Due to Excessive Lens Movement

Thinning the edge on the front surface, being careful not to reduce the lower edge thickness, may help. However, it is nearly always necessary to order a larger lens by at least 0.50 mm. (The overall size canalways be reduced later, if necessary.)

General Discomfort

It would be wrong to assume that a prism ballasted bifocal is far more uncomfortable than a normal single vision lens. The intermediate and peripheral back surface curves should be adjusted in the usual way, if necessary; but care must be taken to ensure that the BCOD is not reduced. It is always advisable to make several small adjustments – trying the lens on the eye in between – rather than one large adjustment.

SCLERAL BIFOCAL LENSES

All the forms of corneal lens bifocals are possible with scleral lenses. The type recommended by the author is an upcurved near portion worked on the back surface. This design has been suggested by Hodd (1967) for corneal lenses but has the disadvantage that the back surface may be unacceptable in contact with the cornea. However, as the back optic surface of a scleral lens clears the cornea, this does not apply; and there is a major advantage in that the lens can be made in distance form first. The BCOR should be up to 0.25 mm steeper than would normally be ordered but with the usual apical clearance, so some slight limbal touch can be expected. The lens can be adjusted, if necessary, and a line then marked on the front optic surface one-quarter of the pupil diameter above the lower pupil margin. The lens is returned to the laboratory for a second BCOR to be cut and polished, decentred inferiorly (*Figure 19.25*). For example:

BCOR 8.00 mm
Near add. +2.25 D
2nd BOR 9.05 mm

This will ease the limbal touch considerably. The lens should be fitted and allowed to settle before any further adjustments are considered. Adjustments to aid the comfort of the lens at this stage may affect the visual performance.

If the lens is not being raised sufficiently for the patient to obtain good near vision when the direction of gaze is lowered, the vertical size should be reduced by removing material from the upper edge. Not more than 1.00 mm should be removed at a time. Increasing the inferior limbal clearance may also help slightly.

If the near portion is too high and affecting the distance vision, removal of material from the lower edge should help to lower the lens slightly. Care must be taken, because if too much material is removed it is possible for the lower edge to rise above the lower lid on an upward gaze and to hold the lower lid down when looking normally again. Removing material from the lower back haptic surface or increasing the superior limbal clearance should also help to lower the lens slightly.

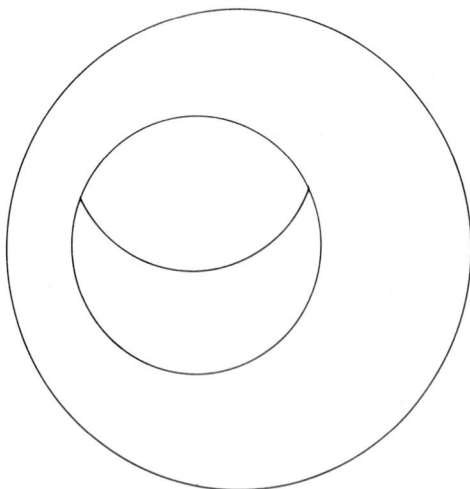

Figure 19.25–Upcurve back surface solid bifocal scleral lens

TRIFOCAL CONTACT LENSES

The first multifocal contact lens, to the author's knowledge, was made by accident. In 1958, Jessen, of America, suggested that it should be possible to make and fit a concentric back surface bifocal by fitting a single vision corneal lens corrected to the patient's near vision and then setting this up on a lathe and cutting a small steep central curve on the back surface. This necessitated removing approximately 0.01–0.02 mm of material, which was extremely difficult. Polishing this area was even more difficult. When the final lenses were checked, it was found that the focimeter target remained in focus over a range of 8 D, although fainter than normal. By blending the two curves together, a multifocal lens had inadvertently been produced with a range of focus from infinity to about 25 cm. Unfortunately, the side-effects experienced with this lens were so great that it was not a practical proposition.

In 1974, Wesley, of America, suggested a new lens that was almost identical in concept to the one described above, that had been made accidentally 16 years before. The idea had been forgotten and by strange coincidence, was re-invented by Dr Jessen's partner, Newton K. Wesley. The new lenses should succeed where others failed because of new methods of manufacture. This lens is the result of research into fitting using the P.E.K. method (*see* Chapter 5 in Volume 1).

In 1959, Jessen (personal communication) produced a lens which was a combination of a back surface concentric bifocal and a front surface concentric bifocal. By making the diameter of the distance portion on the back surface smaller than the distance portion on the front surface, a trifocal effect was achieved.

Söhnges (1962, 1963) developed a blended multifocal lens on the front surface consisting of a small central distance portion and concentric rings 0.50 mm wide, each ring 0.50 D more positive in power than the one before it, so that the positive addition increased gradually towards the edge of the lens.

The problem with any type of blended multifocal lens, or varifocal lens, must be that the majority of the light entering the pupil has passed through an optical area that is not correctly focused for the distance in use. There is a sharp image with a blurred image superimposed over it. This also happens with the de Carle concentric back surface bifocal, but to a lesser extent, and the patient usually learns to accept the side-effects and ignore them. The greater the varifocal effect the greater the side-effects. The brain can ignore the side-effects to some extent (the fact that we are not normally aware of our blind spot in monocular vision is proof of

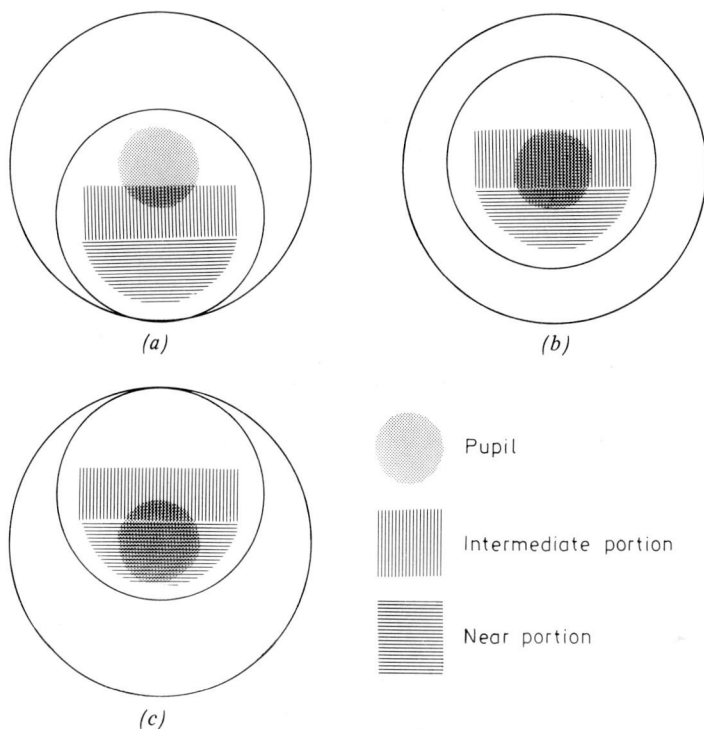

(a)

(b)

(c)

Pupil

Intermediate portion

Near portion

Figure 19.26–A flat-top fused tri-focal. (a) In the distance position. (b) In the intermediate position. (c) In the near position

that) but patients are unable to adapt if the side-effects are too obvious.

These comments also apply to a much more recent development of the back surface bifocal, the Presbycon lens, developed by Compucon Contact Lens Laboratory in the United States. It is a corneal lens having an entirely aspherical back surface with three possible variations of that asphericity. The peripheral flattening of the back surface provides a continuously variable near addition. Due to the rapid degree of flattening the posterior apical radius of the lens is fitted some 0.20–0.25 mm steeper than the flattest corneal keratometer reading (El Hage, 1976). To provide maximum near addition the greatest degree of peripheral flattening, or asphericity must be used, and this can result in too mobile a lens even though fitted centrally steeper than the cornea. In general, results with the lens are reported to be good, and it has even been used to relieve symptoms of near esophoria and esotropia in young patients (El Hage and Cook, 1976).

From the author's experience, it is preferable, for good vision, for the area in front of the pupil to be at least 60 per cent of one power so that using a combination of alternating vision and bivision, a trifocal lens should be possible in many cases,

particularly if the pupil diameter is not greater than 4.00 mm. Experience with flat-top fused trifocal lenses has shown that the patient is not normally aware of looking through a particular area of the lens and that objects from infinity to approximately 25 cm from the eye may all be perfectly in focus. *Figure 19.26a* shows a trifocal lens in the distance position, *Figure 19.26b* the same lens in the intermediate position, and *Figure 19.26c* in the near position. Close examination of the diagrams makes it obvious that there is very little latitude for error with this type of lens. Unless the pupil is very small (approximately 2.00 mm), the top of the segment must cover approximately 40 per cent of the area of the cornea when in the distance position (slightly higher than when fitting a bifocal lens). The depth of the intermediate segment must be at least half the pupil diameter. As 2.00 mm is the greatest depth that is practical, it can be seen that 4.00 mm is theoretically the upper limit for the pupil diameter with trifocal lenses.

Trifocals, as shown in *Figure 19.26*, are made by using two different plastics with the refractive index of the intermediate segment half way between that of the near segment and the remainder of the lens. The segments need to be kept small so that the

Table 19.4–Basic Fused Bifocal Fitting Set
(All values in mm)

BCOR	BCOD	BP₁OR	OS	
7.20	7.00	7.80	8.80	BP_2OR: 12.25
7.35	7.00	7.95	8.90	All lenses round
7.50	7.00	8.10	9.00	Segment on datum
7.65	7.25	8.35	9.10	Suggested Rx: Distance plano
7.80	7.25	8.50	9.20	Near addition +2.50 D
7.95	7.25	8.65	9.30	Prism: 2△ base-down
8.10	7.50	8.90	9.40	Upper edge as thin as possible
8.25	7.50	9.05	9.50	Lower edge as shown in *Figure 19.16a*
8.40	7.50	9.20	9.60	

Table 19.5–Additional Truncated Fused Bifocal Fitting Set
(All values in mm)

BCOR	BCOD	BP₁OR	Horizontal OS	Truncation	
7.20	7.00	7.80	9.00	0.70	BP_2OR: 12.25
7.35	7.00	7.95	9.10	0.75	Radius of truncation 18.00 mm as
7.50	7.00	8.10	9.20	0.80	shown in *Figure 19.20b*
7.65	7.25	8.35	9.30	0.85	Segment on datum before truncation
7.80	7.25	8.50	9.40	0.90	Suggested Rx: Distance plano
7.95	7.25	8.65	9.50	0.95	Near addition +2.50 D
8.10	7.50	8.90	9.60	1.00	Prism: 2△ base-down
8.25	7.50	9.05	9.70	1.05	Upper edge as thin as possible
8.40	7.50	9.20	9.80	1.10	Lower edge as shown in *Figure 19.16a*

thickness of the segment is minimal, otherwise annoying reflections occur from the tops of the intermediate and near segments. The trifocal effect can also be achieved by cutting two different curves on the segment. This reduces the areas likely to give reflections from two to one, and will probably be the lens of choice in the future when a multifocal effect is required. Lenses of this type are being made by Neefe in America.

Trifocals with an intermediate portion near the upper part of the lens are unusual but possible in the fused form (*Figure 19.27*). They would be useful for chemists, librarians, etc., who need to look at objects above eye level and in the intermediate distance range.

BIFOCAL SOFT LENSES

With the growing interest in hydrophilic lenses and the solution of many of the earlier fitting problems, attention is now being turned to the possibility of making these lenses in bifocal and multifocal forms.

The author has fitted several pairs of concentric front surface bifocals based on the Permalens and in the majority of cases good distance and near vision was obtained. The patients were all highly motivated, being mostly actors. Thus, these lenses may not be suitable for all presbyopes. Ideally, a

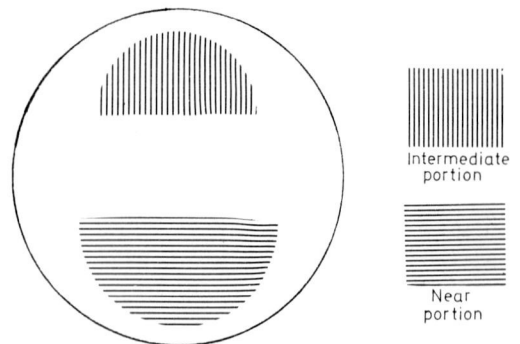

Figure 19.27–Fused trifocal with an upper intermediate portion and lower near portion

hydrophilic fused bifocal would probably prove to be the best lens as it has been in most cases with hard lenses. The technical problems of making such a lens are very considerable as the material used for the near segment would need to have a higher refractive index but must swell by exactly the same amount as the main lens material.

At the time of writing, hydrophilic bifocal lenses have been introduced by two laboratories in the United Kingdom.

Madden Contact Lenses manufacture a lens designed by Randolph Layman, and made from Flexsol 43 per cent water content material, prism ballasted and truncated. The suggested overall size is 2.0 mm larger than the visible iris diameter. As the top of the segment cannot be seen when the lens is on the eye two small indicator lines, 1.50 mm in length, have been engraved on the lens to enable the practitioner to locate it. The bifocal surface is worked onto the front surface and is therefore of 'solid' design.

An alternative lens design is made by Focus Contact Lens Laboratories. This is a concentric type bifocal worked onto the front surface of the lens. The diameter of the distance portion is normally 3.5 mm. The manufacturers suggest an overall size of 13.0 mm and the BCOR 0.75 mm more than the flattest keratometer reading. This lens therefore works on the 'bivision' principle.

The possible problems with the prism ballasted type of lens in hydrophilic form are the difficulties in keeping the lens from becoming excessively thick and heavy. Also, that whilst vertical movement is normally required for this type of lens to function properly hydrophilic lenses are usually more comfortable and successful when this movement is minimal.

With concentric bifocal hydrophilic lenses the most likely problems will be the same as those experienced with the de Carle bifocal lens described earlier (see pages 572 and 582). However, the greater size should aid centration and minimize movement, and so reduce the unwanted side-effects.

FITTING SETS

The most useful fitting set is a set of fused bifocals (*Table 19.4*). The top of the segment shows very clearly, which helps considerably in judging the correct segment height and the correct amount of lens movement. If necessary the lens may then be ordered in another form, for example, the two lenses shown in *Figure 19.14d and e*. It is suggested that the basic fitting set should consist of round lenses only, but truncated lenses are sometimes required for patients with high lower lids, and a second set of truncated lenses would certainly be very useful, as shown in *Table 19.5*.

REFERENCES

Bier, N. (1965). 'Prescribing for presbyopia with contact lenses.' *Ophthal. Optician* **5**, 439–454

Bronstein, L. (1959). 'Bicon lenses.' *C.L.A.O. Papers* **1**, 13–20

Bryant, P. G. (1973). 'Construction and manufacture of a fused bifocal lens.' *Ophthal. Optician* **13**, 1052–1056

El Hage, S. G. (1976). 'Clinical evaluation of the Presbycon aspheric contact lens.' *Internat. Contact Lens Clin.* **3**(2), 65–74

El Hage, S. G. and Cook, J. L. (1976). 'The effect of the aspheric Presbycon contact lenses on esophoric patients.' *Internat. contact Lens Clin.* **3**(4), 42–47

Feinbloom, W. (1938). United States Patent 2,129,305. Application 21 August, patented 6 September, 1938

Freeman, E. (1952). 'Pinhole contact lenses.' *Am. J. Optom.* **29**, 347–352

Gates, H., Ewell, D. G. and Remba, M. J. (1961). 'Bifocal contact lenses.' *Ophthal. Optician* **1**, 1045–1053

Goldberg, J. B. (1969). 'A comprehensive method for fitting monocentric crescent bifocal contact lenses.' *Optom Wkly* **60**, 24–26

Guilbert, J. (1969a). *Biaptal Bifocal Lenses.* News Bulletin, Laboratories Ysoptic, Paris

Guilbert, J. (1969b). 'La lentille bifocale.' Paper read at The Contact Lens Society's World Congress, Eastbourne

Hodd, F. A. B. (1967). 'Bifocal and multifocal contact lenses.' Presidential address to The Contact Lens Society in *Transactions of The Contact Lens Society 1967–70*, pp. 1–20. Also published (1969). 'A design study of bifocal corneal contact lenses.' *Ophthal. Optician* **9**, 450–454, 467–469, 588–592, 597–560, 644–648, 651–653, 700–702; and published as a monograph with the same title by The British Optical Association

Hodd, F. A. B. (1974). 'Bifocal contact lens practice.' *Ophthal. Optician* **14**, 315–320, 325–326, 378–380, 385–388; and published as a monograph with the same title by The British Optical Association

Jessen, G. N. (1958). Personal communication

Jessen, G. N. (1960). 'Bifocal contact lenses.' *Br. J. physiol. Optics* **17**, 217–221

Mandell, R. B. (1966). *No-Jump Bifocal.* Technical memorandum, Kontur Kontact Lens Co. Inc., U.S.A.

Plastic Contact Lens Co. (1970). British Patent 1,178,211. Application 20 April, 1967, patented 21 January, 1970

Shanks, K. R. (1966). 'Subjective comparison of corneal lens edges.' *Br. J. physiol. Optics* **23**, 55–58

Söhnges, W. P. (1962). 'Multifocal micro-pupil lens.' *Contacto* **6**, 156–159

Söhnges, W. P. (1963). British Patent 939,016. Patented 9 October, 1963

Taylor, C. McKay (1962). 'The McKay Taylor additive bifocal.' *Optician* **143**, 585–587

Wesley, N. K. (1962). Personal communication

Williamson-Noble, F. A. (1951). 'Contact lenses – what of the future?' *Br. J. physiol. Optics.* **8**, 244–246

Chapter 20

Impression Scleral Lens Fitting for Special and Pathological Conditions

P. J. Marriott

In spite of the great progress in hard corneal and hydrophilic lens design and fitting techniques, there are still many conditions which can only be satisfactorily fitted with scleral lenses. Many of these are pathological conditions and need constant frequent ophthalmological supervision. They are therefore mostly seen and fitted in hospital contact lens departments. Knowledge of their fitting, however, is essential for the full understanding of the uses of contact lenses and many cases may eventually be seen by the practitioner in private practice. Further, more practitioners are likely to be involved in the fitting of contact lenses within the hospital eye service as the use of such lenses for special conditions increases.

The basic principles of scleral lens fitting apply just the same to pathological conditions as to healthy eyes (*see* Chapter 9, Volume 1). The fitting process, however, is usually considerably more prolonged, and frequent modifications may be needed to maintain the correct fit as the ocular condition changes.

Basically, as with all contact lens fitting, the aim is to achieve a final result that will interfere as little as possible with the tears flow and, consequently, the metabolism of the eye.

KERATOCONUS

Keratoconus is a condition which presents many and varied fitting problems. In the early stages, when the cone is fairly symmetrical, and the corneal irregularity shown by the keratometer is clinically insignificant from the fitting point of view, it can be corrected quite adequately with corneal lenses (*see* Chapter 24, page 661). Even when corneal lenses can no longer be satisfactorily fitted, and scleral lenses have to be used, at first it presents no great problem, as the fitting is the same as for a steep but fairly regular cornea. It is in the later stages, when the cone becomes very steep, irregular, misplaced and tilted, that the fitting difficulties arise.

The cone can assume various shapes, as shown in *Figure 20.1*, from a regular steep central portion (*a*), or a 'pip' (*b*), to a tilted form (*c*).

This type of corneal condition can only be fitted satisfactorily with impression lenses that parallel or align the corneal contours. When the condition has reached this stage, it is impossible to even remotely align these surfaces with single or multiple co-axial spherical curves, as has often been advocated.

For maximum wearing time the lenses should be fenestrated. A minimum clearance alignment or parallel fit is in most cases absolutely essential. Although it has been recommended that central hard touch on the cone should be employed to prevent progression of the condition, this is impossible in many cases as the cone is extremely sensitive and touch is not tolerated. Touch can also cause rubbing on the cone, leading to scarring and perhaps even perforation. Too much central clearance can also lead to disastrous results, as this may cause negative pressure, and the cone may be literally sucked into the optic portion of the lens.

Minimum clearance over the central 8–9 mm of the cornea, giving a fluorescein picture similar to that of a corneal lens alignment fit, but with the weight of the optic portion supported by the haptic portion, is the ideal result (*Figure 20.2*).

The impression of the eye to be fitted is done in the conventional manner as described in Chapter 9, Volume 1. Special conical shaped impression shells may be needed in order to clear very steep cones (*Figure 20.3*).

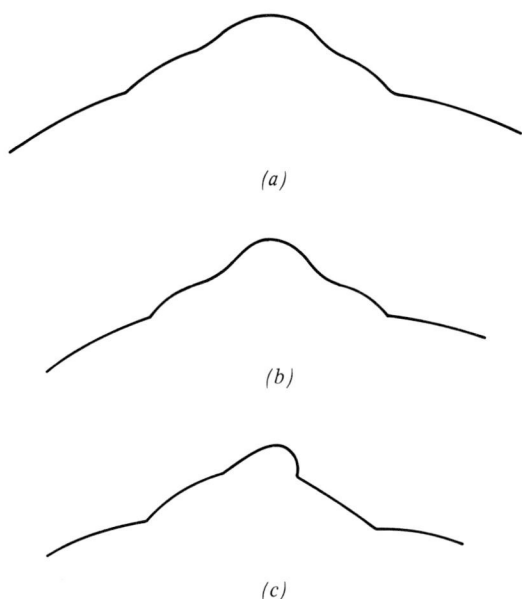

Figure 20.1–Keratoconus showing (a) regular steep central cone, (b) 'pip' cone, and (c) tilted cone

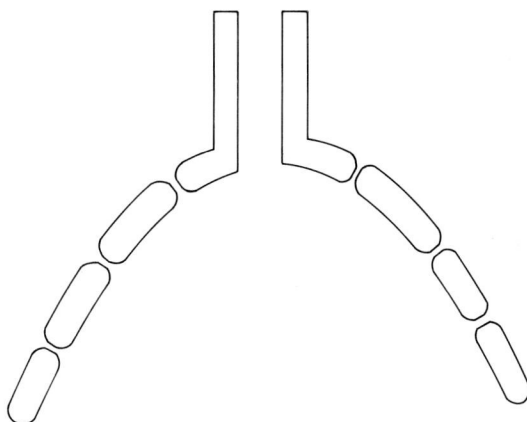

Figure 20.3–Cross-section of conical-shaped impression shell used for advanced cases of keratoconus

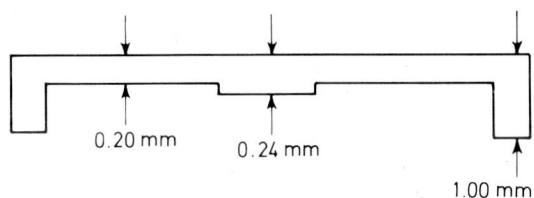

Figure 20.4–Cross-section of laminate used in the manufacture of shells from casts of keratoconic corneas showing the variation of thickness necessary

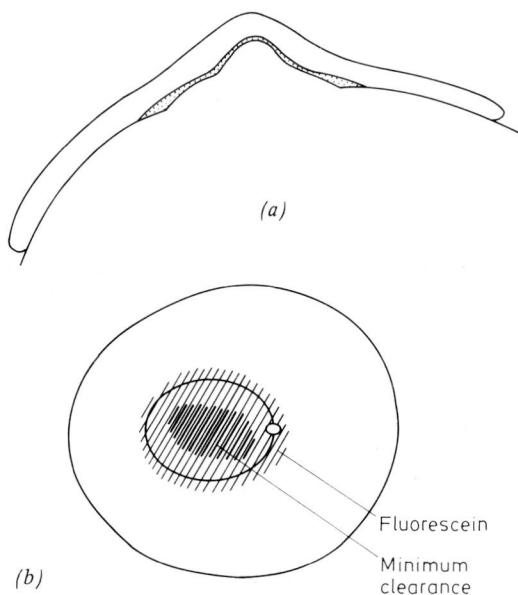

Figure 20.2–The ideal fitting in keratoconus with minimal central clearance shown (a) in cross-section and (b) as viewed under ultra-violet light with fluorescein

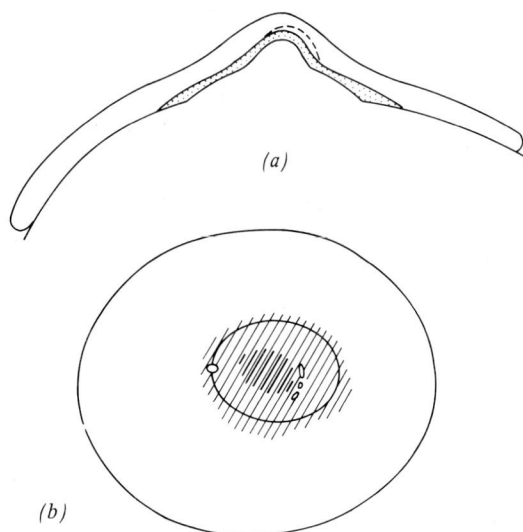

Figure 20.5–(a) Cross-sectional representation of the fitting of a keratoconic shell with the dotted line indicating the area ground out if a spherical BCOR is attempted. (b) Fluorescein picture if a spherical BCOR is attempted, showing the bubbles often introduced

The parallel alignment fit is obtained either by hand grinding of the shell, or by using acrylic laminates on the cast. In advanced cases of keratoconus the use of a laminate on the cast is the only useful method of obtaining this critical clearance, as it is often impossible to find tools small enough to grind into such steep curves.

When using laminates, it must be remembered that the cone is almost invariably compressed during the impression taking, and allowance must be made for this by using a laminate of even thickness, or perhaps one that is thicker in the centre than at the periphery (*Figure 20.4*).

When the shell has been fitted and the correct clearance obtained, difficulties frequently arise if an attempt is made to work a back central optic portion. The alignment over the cone is spoiled, causing bubbles around the base of the cone, and touch on one side of the cone on the slightest version movement. In *Figure 20.5a* the dotted line shows the effect on the alignment of working a back central optic radius, and in *Figure 20.5b* the resulting fluorescein picture is shown.

In these cases, the back surface of the optic is simply highly polished, and no attempt is made to work a true spherical curve. The visual acuity is often very good. It is, in any case, impossible to work a good test-plate surface with very steep diamond impregnated tools of 3–4 mm radius. The diameter of the tool is so small, that when a surface is ground on with these tools, the lens rocks and creates a very wavy surface.

When a lens without a true back central optic radius is used, a front surface of known radius (and power) is cut on the shell. A refraction is then done with the 'lens' *in situ*. The front surface is then re-cut to a different radius in order to give the desired correction, in terms of front surface power change.

The fitting of a lens to a keratoconic eye is often never really finished. Because of changes in the corneal surface, frequent rechecks and modifications may be needed.

CORNEAL GRAFTS

The fitting of scleral lenses to patients who have had corneal grafts may be considered as a follow-on from surgery. The use of scleral shells as splints and immediately following surgery has been fully described by Ruben (1975).

This section is concerned with fitting and controlling the curvatures of the graft after the sutures have been removed and the graft is sound. Steep curvatures and high astigmatism are frequent occurrences in penetrating grafts, and the graft is often proud in one sector, or perhaps all round its circumference.

The fitting of this condition with scleral lenses can give very good visual results, but it is very critical and must be regularly monitored and adjusted, and needs frequent ophthalmological assessment.

The reasons for fitting scleral lenses for this condition are basically three-fold: (1) visual; (2) to establish a more regular corneal contour; and (3) comfort – when proud edges of the graft would otherwise cause considerable discomfort on blinking.

In many cases the grafts exhibit a considerable amount of astigmatism, perhaps as much as 3 mm difference in radius between the principal meridians, and the astigmatism is very irregular.

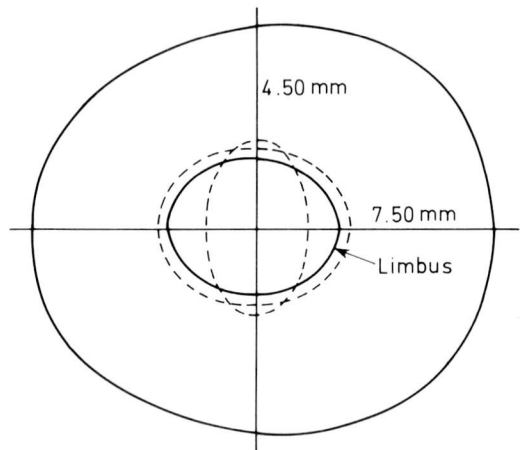

Figure 20.6–With-the-rule astigmatism, the curvature of the principal meridians as shown. A spherical back central optic would produce a vertically oval shaped back central optic portion as shown

These are best fitted in the first instance by using parallel minimum clearance, with no worked back optic surface. In fact, with astigmatism of such a high degree, and perhaps with proud edges to the graft, it is impossible to obtain anything like a satisfactory fit with a spherical back central optic portion. A toroidal back central optic is also generally impossible as the principal meridians of the astigmatic graft are frequently not at right-angles to each other.

Consideration is now given to what would happen if an attempt were made to fit a spherical back central optic portion to two cases of high astigmatism with raised sectors, either combined together in the same eye, or in two eyes each exhibiting one of these conditions.

First, in the case of astigmatism: the back central portion of the shell made from the impression would have more or less the same curves as the cornea. In *Figure 20.6* the corneal radii are shown as 7.5 mm in the horizontal and 4.5 mm in the vertical. The shell would also have these measurements. If a spherical back central optic were attempted, even with a compromise curve of, say, 6.00 mm radius, the resultant back central optic portion would be a vertical oval, as illustrated, and this is nothing like the alignment required.

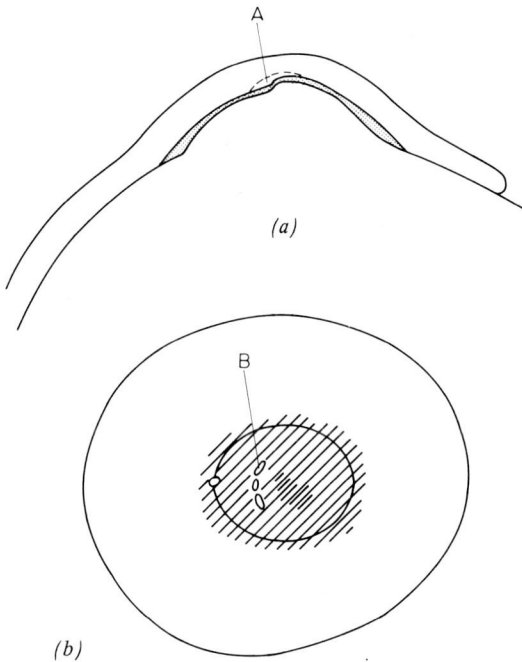

(a)

(b)

Figure 20.7–(a) Diagrammatic cross-sectional representation of a raised sector of corneal graft. A spherical back optic portion, indicated by the dotted line, would cause excessive central clearance at A. (b) Fluorescein picture of (a) showing the central bubble(s) introduced at B with a spherical back optic portion

Secondly, when there is a raised sector of the graft (*Figure 20.7*): this can easily be paralleled, especially if a laminate is used on the cast. If a spherical back optic portion were to be put on, too much clearance would be caused at A (*Figure 20.7a*) resulting in frothing or a continuous bubble at B (*Figure 20.7b*).

This is exactly the same result as that which occurs when a spherical back central optic portion is worked in cases of advanced keratoconus.

FITTING PROCEDURE

An impression is made of the eye, and a shell prepared in the usual way. The impression must be of a high quality, and the limits of the graft and the

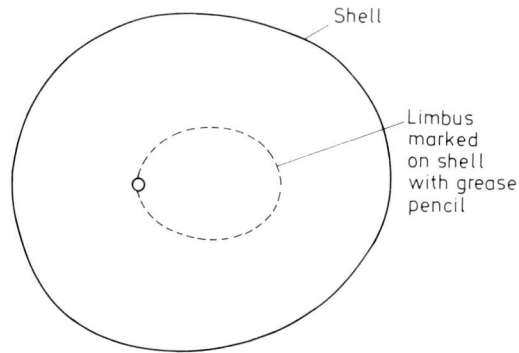

Figure 20.8–The limbus position is marked on the front of the shell with a grease pencil

limbus clearly visible. These features should also be clearly discernible on the shell when it has been pressed over the cast.

The shell is then tried on the eye and marked for fenestration (*see* Chapter 10, Volume 1, page 251). When fenestrated it is again tried on the eye, and fluorescein instilled in order to check the accuracy of the impression. There should, at this stage, be complete alignment of the sclera, host cornea and graft. If not, the shell is adjusted until this condition obtains. If this is not possible, a new impression is taken.

The limbus position is then marked on the front of the shell with a grease pencil before removing the shell from the eye (*Figure 20.8*).

The original cast must be retained for making any future shells, so a duplicate cast is now made. The

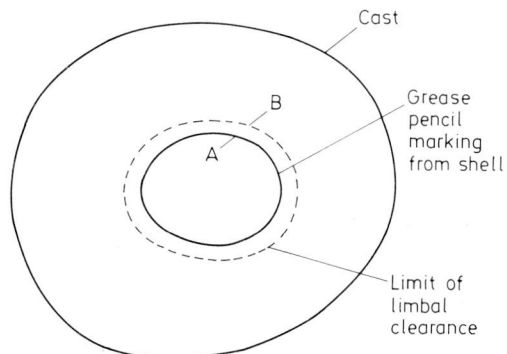

Figure 20.9–A duplicate cast is made from the first shell. The line of the limbus, drawn on the back surface of the first shell with grease pencil will be marked on the duplicate cast. A second, outer line, is then drawn indicating the limits of the limbal clearance

limbal markings are copied, again with a grease pencil, on the back surface of the shell. A cast is then made of the shell with a mixture of dental stone which is thinner than usual. When this has set, the shell is removed from the cast, and it will be seen that the limbal markings on the back surface of the shell have been transferred to the cast A (*Figure 20.9*).

Another line B, (*Figure 20.9*) is drawn on the cast indicating the limit of the limbal clearance. A laminate, of thickness 0.20 mm, is then stuck on to the cast as described in Chapter 9, Volume 1, page 234. *Figure 20.10* shows this.

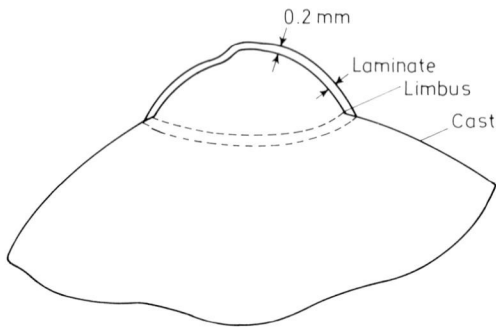

Figure 20.10–A laminate of 0.20 mm thickness is stuck to the corneal area of the duplicate cast and cut to the line of limbal clearance

A new shell is now pressed over the combination of laminate and cast, and the whole back surface is lightly but highly polished. This shell should give an accurate, parallel or alignment minimum clearance fit over the entire irregular cornea.

The clearance between the lens and the cornea must be very small indeed – theoretically and ideally just the thickness of the tears layer, but this is not practical. The use of the conventional ultra-violet lamp for assessing the fit with fluorescein is not critical enough, as this will often give the appearance of complete touch centrally even though there is a good tears flow between the lens and cornea. The slit lamp should be used and this should show a good flow of tears over the cornea and through the fenestration hole even though the ultra-violet lamp appears to indicate considerable touch.

When this critical clearance has been achieved, a front optic surface is cut on the shell. The shell is placed on the eye, a refraction is done, and the front surface is re-cut to give the best visual acuity, as explained on page 594.

This very close fit over the graft and host cornea creates a certain amount of even pressure on the graft, and tends to mould it into a more regular shape. Obviously, with a fitting as critical as this, frequent ophthalmological and fitting observations must be made. There must be no movement of the lens on normal version movements, which could cause rubbing and perhaps epithelial damage to the cornea.

Variations in the visual acuity are a good indication that the lens is settling too close to the cornea, in which case the tears lens is excluded and the visual acuity decreases.

At this stage there is always some residual astigmatism which must be corrected with spectacles, as it is not worthwhile working a toroidal front surface on the shell.

This type of fit is maintained, often by frequent adjustments, for perhaps several months, until the graft begins to become more regular. Then the clearance can gradually be increased, and a spherical back optic surface incorporated.

With close fitting lenses such as these, the pressure must be evenly distributed. Small central areas of touch on the graft, apart from being uncomfortable, could be disastrous.

If it proves necessary to work a spherical back central optic portion while the graft is still highly astigmatic or proud, either for visual or moulding reasons, bubbles may be introduced along the raised edge of the graft, or at the extremities of the steeper corneal meridian (*Figures 20.6* and *20.7*). This can sometimes be alleviated by introducing extra fenestrations (0.5 mm in diameter) over the areas of excessive clearance.

By this method of fitting, which is prolonged and sometimes tedious both for the patient and practitioner, good results can often be obtained. Irregular astigmatism with corneal radius differences of 2 mm or more, by keratometry, may gradually be reduced to a fairly regular astigmatism of 0.50 mm difference in keratometer readings, by which time a normal regular fitting procedure can be used.

RAISED CORNEAL SCARS

Raised corneal scars result from penetrating injuries. Probably the most frequent causes are traffic accidents, and childrens' play accidents (bows and arrows, etc.).

Exactly the same difficulties and fitting problems exist as with grafts with raised edges.
In *Figure 20.11*, a raised corneal scar is shown as viewed from the front (*a*), and below (*b*). If the scar is very proud, the working of a spherical back central optic portion will have exactly the same effect as with a tilted graft, that is, a bubble or frothing along one or both sides of the scar (*Figure 20.12*).

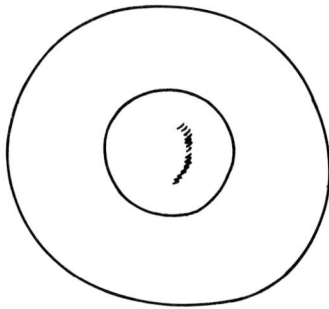

(a)

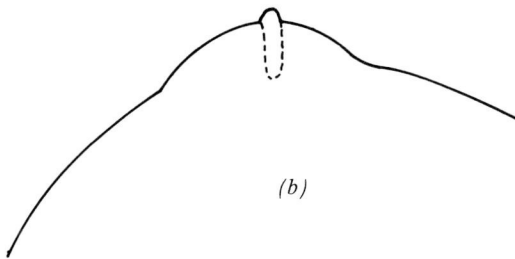

(b)

Figure 20.11–A raised corneal scar shown (a) from the front and (b) from below

APHAKIA

It is not intended to discuss the optical problems of contact lenses and aphakia – these are adequately covered in Chapter 4, Volume 1. This section deals solely with the fitting procedure with impression scleral lenses. Whilst more aphakic patients are now being successfully fitted with corneal and hydrophilic lenses, it must be remembered that the majority of aphakic patients are elderly, for whom both corneal and hydrophilic lenses present handling problems. Modern surgical techniques result in greatly improved corneal regularity after cataract extraction, with little astigmatism, enabling corneal and hydrophilic lenses to be used. However, there still remain those eyes that have presented surgical complications which result in very irregular corneas. These must be fitted with scleral lenses.

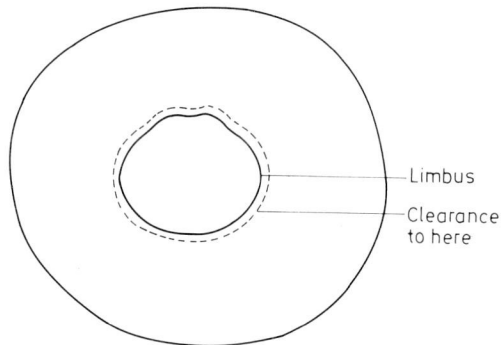

Figure 20.13–Superior extension of the (dotted) line of limbal clearance above an aphakic's cornea to follow the new slope of the limbus

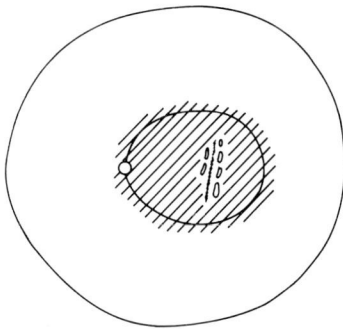

Figure 20.12–A spherical back optic portion ground on to an impression of the cornea in Figure 20.11 will produce a bubble or frothing along one or both sides of the scar

If this condition is fitted with minimum clearance and alignment, with slight touch over the scar, it can have the effect of smoothing out the scar, and reducing the proudness. Frequent modifications may be necessary, but in the long term successful results can be obtained.

As in all scleral lens fitting, the same criteria of correct central clearance and adequate limbal clearance apply. The clearance over the limbus, and the clearance of limbal scars, is very important. The limbus can assume varied shapes after cataract surgery, and may deviate considerably from its original reasonable symmetry. The clearance of these irregularities can only be achieved by hand-grinding or using a laminate on the cast (*Figure 20.13*).

In *Figure 20.13* the upper limbus is shown distorted, and must be cleared as indicated by the dotted line.

In general, aphakic eyes seem to be 'softer' than normal eyes, in that the lens settles much more. Therefore, more corneal clearance must be given initially. If a laminate is used it must be thicker than that used for non-pathological eyes – usually 0.26 mm at the periphery and 0.24 mm centrally.

The shell is pressed from a special disc of polymethyl methacrylate which is 1.5 mm thick in the centre and 1.00 mm thick at the periphery (*Figure 20.14*).

This allows enough material to work a high positive powered correction after the shell has been fitted. However, both haptic and optic portions of the lens must be kept as thin as possible to avoid

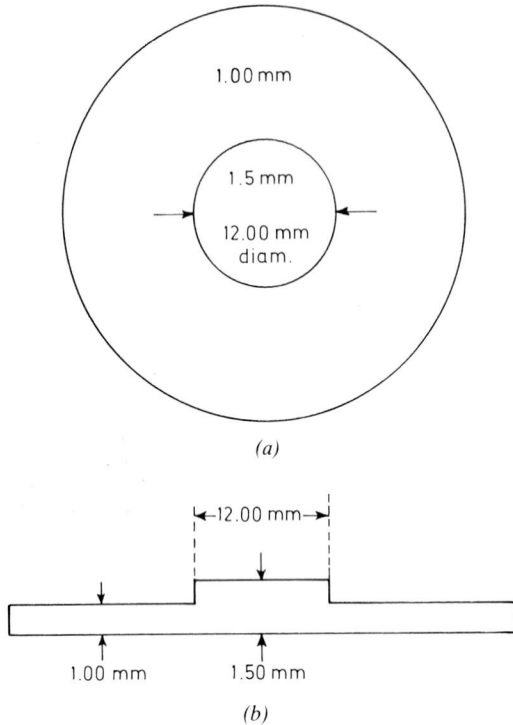

(a)

(b)

Figure 20.14–Frontal (a) and cross-sectional appearance (b) of polymethyl methacrylate disc necessary for the pressing of aphakic shells to allow sufficient central thickness for the high positive powered corrections necessary

sagging of the lens due to weight and from upper lid pressure. This is helped by using a BCOR as steep as possible (consistent with good fitting) as this adds positive power to the tears lens thereby reducing the contact lens power and enabling a thinner optic portion to be used.

PTOSIS

The problems and difficulties associated with correcting ptosis with a scleral lens are multitudinous. Many methods have been in use for a long time, each successful in certain cases. More research

needs to be done to correlate particular types of ptosis with the types of fitting found to be most successful in their correction. There are opposing factors which make the task very difficult. It is a relatively simple matter to make a lens which will raise the upper lid, for example, by fitting a ledge to the lens on which the lid rests. This quite successfully raises the lid and gives a reasonably good cosmetic appearance. However, the weight of the lid generally pushes the lens down, completely spoiling the fit. When this happens another ledge can be fitted to rest on the lower lid in an endeavour to stop the lens sagging. In this situation the patient is unable to blink at all. This results in drying and smearing of the front surface of the lens, causing poor visual acuity and a 'glassy' appearance. The 'pumping' action of blinking, which is essential to provide good tears flow behind the lens, is absent, thereby impairing the corneal metabolism.

Several methods of correcting ptosis with scleral lenses will now be described, with an attempt at an assessment of the relative merits of each. Unfortunately, this can only be a rough guide, because even after considerable experience of these cases, the practitioner may have to change methods and techniques when the one originally thought to be best, fails.

THICK SHELLS

A plain shell or lens of 2.50 mm or 3.00 mm thickness, instead of the normal 0.8 mm, may be used in mild cases, and can give excellent results. The edges are, of course, thinned down to normal thickness. If the shell is inserted, marked up,

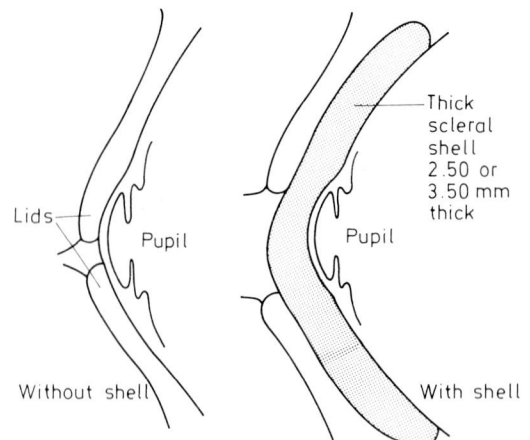

Figure 20.15–The effect of a thick lens or shell, shown in cross-section, in holding the lids apart in ptosis

removed and fenestrated, it can then be re-inserted, fluorescein instilled, and the alignment checked as described in Chapter 9, Volume 1. There is frequently some central clearance caused by 'bridging' over the cast when shells of this description are pressed out. The corneal and limbal clearance are arranged in the usual way. This method can produce good functional results, and has the advantage that blinking, even if incomplete, will keep the front surface of the lens clean, and provide a reasonable tears flow behind the lens. It does, however, give the eye a somewhat bulbous appearance, as the lower lid is pushed out and down (*Figure 20.15*).

The lower portion of the lens can be thinned down to compensate for this as shown in *Figure 20.16*.

If the upper lid is not sufficiently raised by using a thick shell, it can sometimes be improved by hollowing out the upper and lower surfaces of the shell (*Figure 20.17*).

In theory the upper tarsal plate should lie along this surface and thereby the lid is raised, but in practice this is not always achieved.

This method is perhaps the best first approach to fitting ptosis cases. If successful, apart from thinning down portions of the lens as required, it involves little more than a normal scleral lens fitting. It has the advantage of allowing normal blinking, good tears exchange, power and fitting changes and reproducibility.

It also has the advantage that if it is not successful, the technique can be changed by using props or ledges thus doing further work on the same shell.

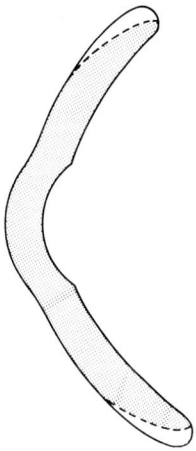

Figure 20.16–The edges of the thick lens shown in Figure 20.15 may be thinned down as shown by the dotted lines to reduce the bulbous and glassy appearance of the eye and the pushing down of the lower lid

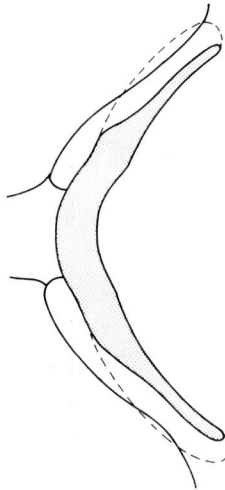

Figure 20.17–If the thick lens shown in Figure 20.15 does not raise the lids sufficiently it can sometimes be improved by hollowing out the upper and lower front surface of the shell as shown

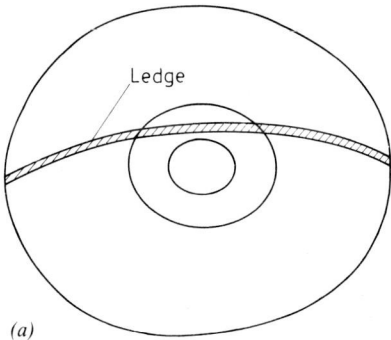

(a)

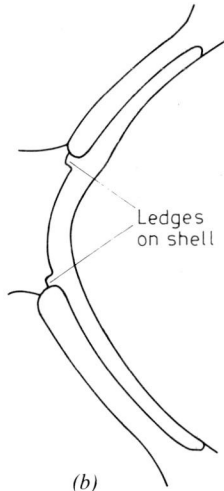

(b)

Figure 20.18–The use of props or ledges in ptosis to hold the lids apart. A single ledge is shown from the front in (a) and two ledges in cross-section in (b)

PROPS OR LEDGES

The fitting of props or ledges on to a scleral lens was probably the first method of correcting ptosis with contact lenses (*Figure 20.18*).

The shell is fitted in the normal way, and the front surface worked. The position of the ledge is determined by lifting up the top lid to the correct height, and then marking the position of the lid margin on the lens with a grease pencil. At this stage a wax ledge may be built on, to determine ledge shape and size. When this is correct, a similar acrylic ledge is fashioned and cemented on to the lens. The weight of the upper lid frequently pushes the lens downwards and another ledge is necessary to rest on the lower lid in an endeavour to prevent the lens from sagging.

When this has been done, the shell is inserted, and the lid placed on the ledge. The shell is invariably displaced downwards, causing a large inferior bubble (*Figure 20.21*).

This should be left alone at this stage. If the lens can be tolerated, the patient is instructed to wear it, if possible, for up to 3-hour stretches, daily for a week. This sometimes allows the lens to settle and the lid to become more flaccid and exert less pressure. Sometimes, following surgical attempts to cure the ptosis, the lid is stiff and very rigid – this is the extreme case. At the other end of the scale, in elderly patients and cases of ocular myopathy, the lid is much looser and tends to exert less pressure on the lens after a few weeks of use.

If the lens is wearable, functional and permits goods tears exchange, but a static bubble persists

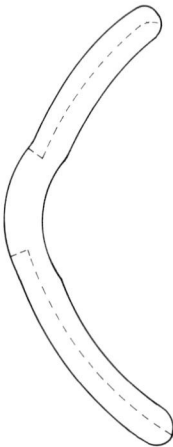

Figure 20.19–A thick shell may be ground out, as shown by the dotted line in cross-section, to create a ledge or ledges suitable for retaining the lids in ptosis cases

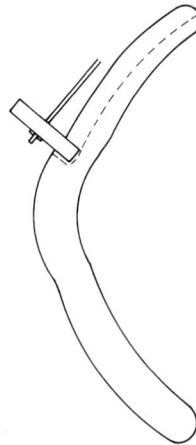

Figure 20.20–The ledges shown in Figure 20.19 are created by using a carborundum grinding wheel as shown

Apart from this, other disadvantages of this method are as follows.

(1) Once the ledges are in place no adjustment can be made to the front surface of the lens should the power need to be altered.

(2) Replacement of a lost or broken lens is impossible, and refitting is therefore necessary.

The same result as a ledge can usually be achieved with a thick shell of about 3.5 mm thickness.

If the fitting procedure is commenced with a 'thick shell' which has failed, been 'hollowed' (*Figure 20.17*) and still not been successful, this shell can be transformed from one with a 'hollowed out' superior portion, to one with a ledge, or ledges, by grinding the shell as shown by the dotted lines in *Figure 20.19*.

The advantage of making ledges in this manner is that the front surface can be worked *after* the shell is fitted and seen to be functioning correctly.

The shell is ground with a carborundum wheel to leave a ledge, which is then highly polished (*Figure 20.20*).

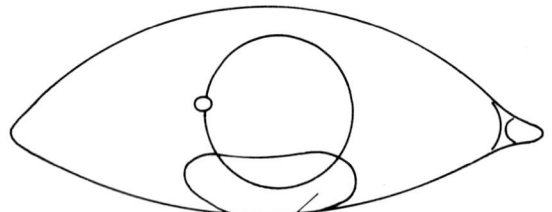

Large inferior bubble

Figure 20.21–The effect of a superior ledge only is to displace the lens downwards creating a large inferior bubble

inferiorly, there is the danger of causing drying of the cornea beneath the immobile bubble. Also cosmetically it is very poor, giving a very glassy appearance. This can occasionally be eliminated by 'settling' the lower haptic portion of the lens and, in effect, tilting the whole lens. This is done by

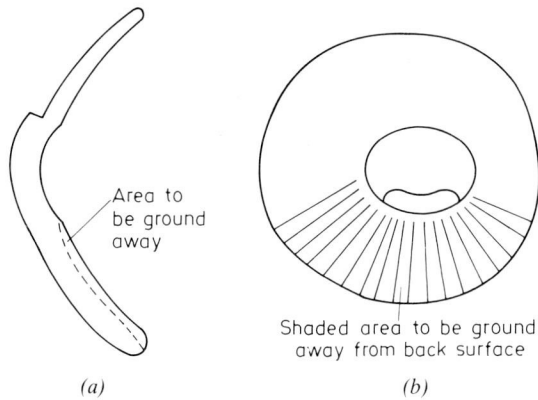

Figure 20.22–The bubble shown in Figure 20.21 can often be reduced and the cosmetic appearance improved by an inferior haptic grindout as shown (a) in cross-section, and (b) from the front

grinding out the lower back haptic surface to the dotted line in *Figure 20.22a*, and over the hatched area in *Figure 20.22b*.

SOLID LID PROPS IN OCULAR MYOPATHY

This type of scleral lens for ptosis can be very successfully used in cases of ocular myopathy when the lid tension is not very strong. The prop or ledge is formed on a shell of 1.5 mm thickness by cutting right through it to make a ledge (*Figure 20.23*), as described by its originator, Trodd (1971).

Such an appliance is of value where the eye movement is limited by myopathy. Its uses in eyes with normal excursions has not yet been fully assessed.

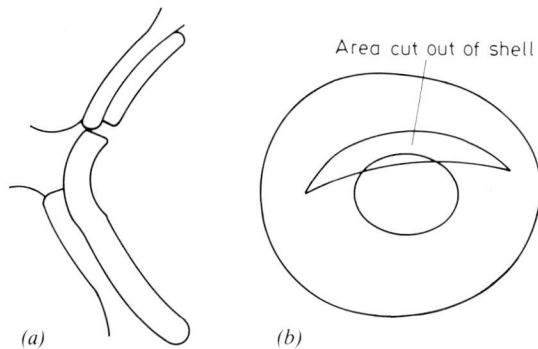

Figure 20.23–Ocular myopathy. A prop or ledge is formed by cutting right through the shell to make a ledge shown (a) in cross-section and (b) from the front

BULLOUS KERATOPATHY

Hard scleral lenses are used in cases of bullous keratopathy for two main reasons: (1) to alleviate symptoms; and (2) to decrease the corneal oedema.

The alleviation of pain and discomfort is more important than the reduction of oedema, according to Ruben (1975) who has fully discussed the ophthalmological implications of the disease, and the reasons for fitting contact lenses.

As far as the actual fitting is concerned, this is fairly straightforward. The object is to obtain constant compression of the cornea over at least the central two-thirds of its area. A very close parallel fit is therefore necessary. The lens must be as close to the cornea as possible without obliterating the tears flow. Good limbal clearance must be maintained at all times. The fit needs to be modified frequently as the disease passes through its various phases. In fact, the same technique of fitting is used as for eccentric grafts, etc., (page 594) and the same, but much more frequent controls of the fitting must be maintained.

COSMETIC SCLERAL LENSES

This section is concerned solely with contact lens prostheses as such; that is, those which can rightly be called contact lens fitting. It does not deal with full prostheses as fitted after enucleation, or with the fitting of very small microphthalmic eyes. It does include the fitting of unsightly, but relatively normal-sized eyes – conditions such as total or partial aniridia, unsightly corneal scarring and the occasional unsightly mature cataractous eye.

The lenses may be sighted or unsighted.

Cases of large iridectomies resulting from trauma, penetrating wounds or surgery are fitted with a normal-sighted scleral lens incorporating an artificial iris, which improves the cosmetic appearance and usually improves the visual acuity by reducing glare and aberrations. These cases sometimes require considerable skill and ingenuity to place the pupillary area in such a position as to give good visual acuity, but at the same time avoid any appearance of a squint. For example, *Figure 20.24* shows an eye with an iridectomy, where the remaining iris is indicated by the hatched area. In order to give a good cosmetic result and avoid the appearance of a squint, the sighted pupil may have to be placed as shown in the diagram, leaving a part of the remaining iris encroaching on the pupillary area of the lens. Obtaining a good cosmetic and a good visual result in such cases can be very exacting.

Ideally, for fitting reasons, these lenses should be made from the original shell, and the cosmetic portion built up on to it. However, this does sometimes produce a rather 'flat' appearance with little corneal thickness and no anterior chamber effect. The procedure is as follows.

An impression is made of the eye, from which is produced a normal clear shell. This is fitted in the usual manner. If a sighted prosthesis is required, the shell is completed with a back and front optic, giving

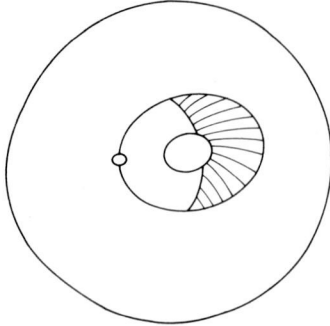

Figure 20.24–Large iridectomy with the remaining pupil shown on the nasal side. The pupil must be placed where shown, that is, exposing some of the remaining iris, in order to avoid the appearance of a squint

the correct prescription. If an artificial pupil is to be made, that is, a complete prosthesis for a blind eye, then an optically worked front surface is obviously unnecessary.

When the fitting has been completed, the patient is issued with the clear shell. This is worn until all the necessary modifications to the back surface have been made to ensure comfortable all-day wear. It is absolutely necessary that this is done with a clear shell, through which the fluorescein picture can be checked, because when the final prosthesis has been made, it is obviously quite impossible to check the fit with the opaque lens on the eye.

Subsequently, when the clear shell or lens can be worn for suitably long periods, the cosmetic lens is made. There are two main ways in which this can be done: (1) by copying the clear shell and making the prosthesis with dental acrylic; or by (2) building up the prosthesis on to the existing clear shell.

Copying

A cast is made of the original clear lens, and the full or partial prosthesis is made by preparing and making a lens of dental acrylic to include the iris and scleral pattern which is formed over the cast. This method gives good cosmetic results for the matching of the iris and sclera, but it can produce problems.

In theory, if a cast is made of a lens and another lens is pressed or moulded over this cast, an exact copy should result. Unfortunately, in practice, this frequently does not happen. The fit of the copy is often quite different from the original, no matter how skilled the technician may be. The difference can occur through faulty casting, poor pressing or moulding of the lens over the cast, but probably chiefly from errors introduced during cleaning and polishing of the back surface. It must be remembered that a difference of ± 0.05 mm central clearance can completely spoil the fit of the lens (*see* FLOM Fitting, Chapter 10, Volume 1).

Another problem which sometimes arises with this method is severe conjunctival injection caused by free monomers left by incorrect curing of the acrylic. This, of course, should not happen when these are made by a highly skilled technician.

Clear Shell

The best method is to use the existing clear lens or shell and build up the prosthesis on to it. This is done by thinning down the original lens or shell, and then building it up again to its original thickness with dental acrylic (*Figure 20.25*).

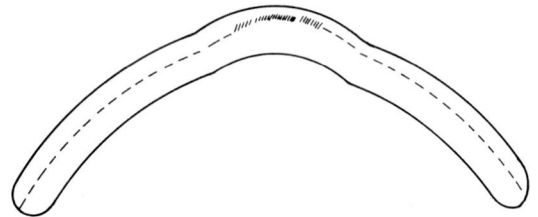

Figure 20.25–A clear shell is thinned, the prosthesis formed on the front surface as shown by the dotted line, and the thickness then built up again using liquid dental acrylic

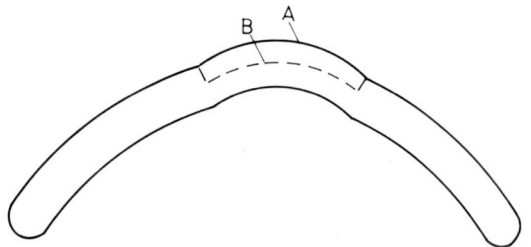

Figure 20.26–In the case of an artificial iris the appearance of an anterior chamber may be created by grinding out the corneal zone, inserting the painted iris and pupil disc (shown by the dotted line), and then inserting a clear disc

This can be done with a full or partial prosthesis. For a partial prosthesis, that is, an artificial iris, Mr R. Wilson, Chief Technician in Charge of Prosthetics, Contact Lens Department, Moorfields Eye Hospital, London, has devised a technique which gives a good appearance of an anterior chamber and avoids the 'flat' appearance associated with just a painted iris (Ruben and Wilson, 1975).

The corneal zone AB (*Figure 20.26*) is ground away and the area recessed to receive the painted iris and pupil disc, over the dotted line B. A clear disc is then inserted to bring the lens back to its original thickness. Thus, the iris and pupil are on the dotted line B and the lens between A and B is clear, giving the appearance of an anterior chamber. This method of making contact lenses avoids the possible changes in fitting which can occur when copying the original, and also lessens the possibility of conjunctival injection from free monomers.

The principles outlined in this chapter should allow the specialist contact lens practitioner to develop other special techniques of fitting appropriate to the eye condition encountered.

REFERENCES

Ruben, M. (1975). 'Special diseases.' In *Contact Lens Practice: Visual, Therapeutic and Prosthetic,* pp. 278–313, ed. by Ruben, M. London: Baillière and Tindall

Ruben, M. and Wilson, R. (1975). 'Cosmetic and prosthetic appliances.' Chapter 15 In *Contact Lens Practice: Visual, Therapeutic and Prosthetic,* pp. 343–352, ed. by Ruben, M. London: Baillière and Tindall

Trodd, T. C. (1971). 'Ptosis props in ocular myopathy.' *Contact Lens* **3**(4), 3–5

Chapter 21

The Use of Soft Lenses in Ocular Pathology

D. Westerhout

Both scleral and corneal lenses have, for many years, been used in the presence of ocular pathology for the treatment as well as the optical correction of eyes in this category. It is, perhaps, wrong to deal specifically, in this chapter, with the use of soft lenses alone as a certain amount of duplication could be avoided if each ocular condition were discussed with the indications and contra-indications for the different forms of lenses available.

As, however, there is a tendency to categorize lenses into hard and soft types it may be more helpful to describe the uses and value of soft lenses in both therapeutic and optical treatment of ocular pathology.

For the pathological eye the soft lens may be utilized in two ways.

(1) Therapeutic use as in the treatment of indolent ulcers.

(2) Optical use such as in the treatment of post-operative aphakia to provide adequate visual acuity.

There is clearly a large overlap in many cases, where the lens is used for both therapeutic and optical reasons.

The therapeutic use of soft lenses is expanding constantly, depending on the preparedness of the ophthalmologist or ophthalmic optician (optometrist) to experiment with these forms of lens in the patient's best interests. In dealing with ocular pathology in this chapter, no attempt will be made to describe in detail the conditions themselves, as these may readily be obtained from ophthalmological textbooks.

In numerous cases, the soft contact lens is used therapeutically as a means of bandaging the cornea to protect it from abnormalities of the lid or lack of tears. Many conditions of the cornea are really only painful due to the lid action on the corneal nerve endings, and if the area is protected with a suitable soft lens bandage, the physical discomfort may be considerably reduced or removed altogether.

A soft lens bandage can be used instead of medical or surgical procedures such as tarsorrhaphy, especially if the patient is unhappy about the cosmetic appearance of tarsorrhaphy and it is thought that the soft lens bandage is as likely to be effective. Soft lens bandages and shells can also be utilized to separate inflamed areas of bulbar and palpebral conjunctiva to prevent adhesions such as those found during acute inflammatory conditions and burns.

Some varieties of soft contact lens can be satisfactorily used in dry eye conditions in an attempt to keep the cornea wet, although this is not as satisfactory in every case as might be imagined. It will readily be seen that with the principles outlined above the application of soft lens bandage therapy can be very wide indeed and thus it is best discussed by dealing with individual examples of ocular conditions.

BULLOUS KERATOPATHY

This condition of chronic oedema of the cornea can be extremely painful, and the main aim of the contact lens is to alleviate the symptoms of pain, epiphora, photophobia and blepharospasm, and also to reduce the chronic oedema. In the author's experience in almost all cases the pain can be considerably reduced or removed but the reduction of oedema is somewhat more difficult to attain. Ruben (1975) has described the compression of a large area of the cornea with a contact lens as a means of creating an anterior water barrier and reducing oedema, and this is one of the main purposes for which a compression hard or soft contact lens is used in the treatment of this condition (*see* also Chapter 20, page 601).

The soft contact lens relieves the discomfort by the simple expedient of separating the painful bullae from the lid. Some pain may persist due to the epithelial swelling causing a stretching of the nerve endings. The greater reservoir of fluid in the large soft lens can also permit a rapid rate of evaporation from the new anterior surface, thus possibly decreasing the flow of water into the cornea. A relative dehydration of the cornea can be achieved by the use of 5 per cent saline solution therapy which, giving a reservoir of hypertonic saline solution in the lens, tends to dehydrate the cornea, thus reducing oedema. Hypertonic saline solution had been used for many years before the development of soft lenses but the therapy does not work effectively without a soft lens to act as a reservoir for the solution. Repeated instillation permits the ion concentration in the fluid contained in the lens to reach a level similar to that of hypertonic saline solution. The resultant osmotic pressure gradient is sufficient to detergesce the cornea in some cases.

Some practitioners prefer to prescribe the prophylactic use of chloramphenicol drops, 0.5 per cent made without preservative, for the first week of bandage wear (Leibowitz and Rosenthal, 1971). The use of Diamox (*Lederle*) and similar diuretic drugs is also helpful with or without the hypertonic saline solution therapy.

The majority of cases seen by the author have been secondary to cataract surgery, and some of these cases in a mild form have responded so well that the condition has been completely cured by the use of a soft lens bandage.

Occasionally, the author has seen severe oedema of the cornea, which was diagnosed as bullous keratopathy, disappear on the use of a soft lens bandage never to reappear again, even when the use of the bandage was removed within a few weeks. These cases have occurred in the presence of low intra-ocular pressure.

Liebowitz and Rosenthal (1971), in observations using the Bausch and Lomb Soflens, reported no improvement in the signs observed (*see Colour Plate XLVI*). This was, of course, despite the improvement in the relief of discomfort. The author has found that the use of high water content lenses (for example, Sauflon PW) is considerably more effective than low water content lenses in some of these conditions and there has certainly been an improvement in some of the signs, especially when combined with the use of the hypertonic saline solution

therapy. It appears necessary to instil 5 per cent saline at approximately one or two hourly intervals to produce a continuous beneficial effect on the oedema.

Unfortunately, the visual acuity is often extremely poor in bullous keratopathy due to the presence of other pathology.

It is very important to attempt to limit the movement of the soft lens on the eye and this is best done by using a large, semi-scleral soft lens. Since daily removal by a clumsy patient will often make the eye extremely painful and negate much of the benefit that has been gained, the use of a continuously worn bandage (other than for those who can easily remove the bandage) is to be preferred. Provided that lenses of low water content material are made sufficiently thin (Hill and Jeppe, 1976; Westerhout, 1977) or are made of a very high water content material (for example, Sauflon PW or Permalens) there appears to be very little risk in comparison with that associated with the daily use of these lenses.

Even with continuous wear lenses, they should be removed at least weekly and sterilized and cleaned carefully to remove foreign bodies such as mucus or dead cells. Any protein or other deposits adhering to the lens surface should also be removed.

Unfortunately, although such a lens is extremely effective in reducing pain, the patient almost always becomes totally dependent on the use of the bandage lens and occasionally the initial progress is not maintained. Vascularization is inclined to increase and a drop in visual acuity is often noticed after a period. The eye often becomes infected in the later stages of the condition and the overall prognosis over a long period is not all that good. Some of the patients respond very well to the therapy and improve sufficiently to be able to cease the use of the bandage eventually, and go on to using more conventional medical therapy such as the use of glycerine and saline solution drops.

The author has found that in the early stages of the condition, treatment with the soft lens bandage sometimes improves the acuity from as low as 6/60, to 6/9. This is probably due to the restoration of a reasonably smooth regular anterior refracting surface. In a patient who handles the bandages skilfully, normal daily wearing of the bandage is often recommended, but if the bullae rupture and cause severe discomfort, then continuous wear may be indicated. This painful rupture of the bullae has often been found to occur at night when the lens has not been worn.

The bandage can also be used to good effect in the treatment of keratopathy of uncertain classification and unknown aetiology (*see Colour Plate XLVII*).

Naturally enough, as in all cases of continuous

wear of a contact lens, the corneal condition should be checked regularly with a slit lamp microscope.

Compared with the often-used alternative of tarsorrhaphy, the continuous or daily wear contact lens provides the ophthalmologist and optometrist with a clear view of the eye for observation over a period. The use of a conjunctival flap is also a commonly used successful alternative treatment.

The fitting of the soft lens bandage is often difficult and it can be helpful to take keratometric readings from the non-affected eye to give some guidance as to the required fitting. In general, larger lenses perform better than small ones and the author finds most lenses used for this condition have an overall size in the region of 14.0–14.5 mm (*see Colour Plate XLVIII*). Central thickness should not exceed 0.10 mm.

Accuracy of fit is important as it is essential to avoid excessive movement of the lens but, at the same time, too tight a lens can result in vascularization of the stroma (Ruben, 1971). Neovascularization is not always a serious problem in these cases provided it is limited to the peripheral cornea. In some cases the vascularization produces an improvement in the keratopathy and its symptoms, thus allowing therapy with a soft lens to be discontinued.

Subsequent infection and ulceration from fungus or herpes are not uncommon in the later stages. Unfortunately, especially with the continuously worn bandage, protein contamination is often a serious problem and the soft lens may become incapable of being cleaned and thus need replacement (*see Colour Plate XLIX*).

SYMBLEPHARON

Symblepharon is the adhesion of the palpebral conjunctiva to the bulbar conjunctiva. It results from a variety of causes such as burns, and inflammatory conditions such as the Stevens–Johnson syndrome (*see page 609*). Symblepharon in its severe form may reduce normal blinking, and secondary corneal conditions may result as a consequence of the exposure keratitis.

The therapeutic use of soft contact lenses in this condition takes two different forms.

(1) The lenses can be used to prevent the formation of symblepharon if inserted within a few hours of the burn. It is desirable that hospitals should have soft contact lenses in their casualty departments for the immediate treatment of burns.

(2) The contact lenses can be used to keep the cornea in a moist state.

In the event of irregularity or scarring the soft lens is somewhat limited in improving visual acuity compared with the effectiveness of hard lenses.

This condition has frequently been very successfully treated with an annular ring cut from a scleral lens; but soft contact lenses with a flat radius and large overall size are also very effective. The soft lens must of necessity be made large (15–20 mm) to prevent adhesions forming or reforming, and due to the large overall size it is important that the lens is made of an adequately gas-permeable material. High water content materials are desirable although less permeable materials can be used if they are made in very thin form. If the lens is made too thin or too soft it may buckle and not hold its shape. In this case it may wrinkle up in the eye and permit the formation of adhesions and also cause discomfort. Obviously, continuous use is necessary and local and systemic steroids are often given to discourage vascularization.

NEUROPARALYTIC AND NEUROTROPHIC CONDITIONS

Secondary corneal disease frequently results from lesions of the fifth cranial nerve. As is well known, the fifth nerve has a trophic effect with regard to the cornea, and lesions to this nerve frequently result in insensitivity. This also adversely affects the tears secretion and blink reflex. The epithelium becomes dry and areas of necrosis eventually occur. The corneal state is thus very vulnerable to infection and very often these areas of necrosis eventually become infected, with severe corneal ulceration. Most of the patients seen by the author have previously been treated by tarsorrhaphy, the initial cause being the result of brain surgery. As the patient was bedridden in each case, a soft lens worn as a bandage for continuous use proved very satisfactory. If, as frequently happens, the patient is hospitalized, the nursing staff can readily irrigate the continuously worn lens at regular intervals to ensure that the lens, and thus the cornea, is kept wet.

Ruben (1975) prefers the static fitting scleral lens with adequate limbal clearance. Daily wear only of this appliance is advised. Obvious possible complications resulting from the use of an unfenestrated scleral lens would be vascularization and scarring. The author has found that the continuous use of soft lens bandages has been very effective with the lenses being removed every 5–10 days for complete cleaning and sterilization before being re-inserted. The eye should be irrigated with sterile saline solution before the bandage is re-inserted, as debris and mucus may well accumulate on the eye's surface whilst the lens is removed. If it is not irrigated regularly the periphery of the soft lens begins to dry out and stand away from the conjunctiva, thus causing irritation and possible fracture of the lens.

EXPOSURE KERATITIS

In this condition, which often results from lid dysfunction after lesions of the seventh cranial nerve, the cornea becomes extremely dry despite a normal tears secretion (*see Colour Plate L*). Many cases are the result of brain surgery and involve some degree of facial paralysis. As in the last category of case, the soft contact lens is used purely to provide protection for the eye, but as the tears secretion is usually normal, irrigation is not so vital as in the neuroparalytic and neurotrophic conditions. If these patients are viewed during the hours of sleep, a drying of the lens surface through non-closure of the lids is frequently noticed, but the author has been interested to find that an upward rotation of the eye still appears to take place despite the other complications, and this partially protects the lens and eye from drying. The treatment decided on by the ophthalmologist greatly depends on the overall general prognosis.

KERATOCONUS

Keratoconus, in which the central cornea becomes progressively steeper in curvature, is one of the oldest forms of corneal pathology to be treated with contact lenses. There appears to be a hereditary factor in this condition and the vast majority of keratoconus patients also appear to suffer from allergies. Ruben (1975) reports that at least 50 per cent of keratoconus patients suffer from vernal catarrh. It may well be this irritation which causes the eye rubbing so common in this condition. The rapid changes in the anterior segment are – as described by Ruben (1975) – as follows.

(1) A thinning of the corneas, one eye almost always being more advanced than the other.

(2) The keratometry readings are steep with high irregular astigmatism.

(3) The stroma shows deep striate scarring and, later, tears in Descemet's membrane can be seen.

(4) The epithelium can show stains with fluorescein even without contact lens wearing.

(5) The epithelium frequently shows a superficial mosaic pattern with fluorescein.

(6) Tears in Bowman's and Descemet's membranes can lead to sudden oedema of the cornea with or without contact lens wearing.

(7) Vascularization of the cornea can occur especially after long use of scleral lenses.

It is the author's experience that nearly all wearers of scleral lenses in this condition show pronounced vascularization of the cornea.

(8) Fleischer's ring occurs as an annular or broken concentric yellowish-brown ring seen with direct white light by biomicroscopy. The line shows up as black when illuminated with blue light.

(9) The cornea may rupture in extreme cases, especially after trauma.

(10) The whole anterior segment is possibly involved.

(11) The condition is often associated with other diseases such as vernal catarrh, conjunctivitis, neurodermatitis and metabolic disturbances.

The condition usually begins in puberty but frequently appears to level off at the age of 25–35 years. The earliest detectable signs are generally found at a refractive examination when the practitioner finds it difficult to achieve satisfactory visual acuity with confusing cylindrical readings. The usual diagnosis is based on very steep keratometer findings combined with irregular astigmatism particularly noticeable as a swirling, irregular retinoscopy reflex and the slit lamp signs of a thin cornea at the apex and Fleischer's ring.

From the contact lens practitioner's point of view, patients suffering from keratoconus are excellent candidates for contact lens wear, due to their high motivation; as no form of spectacle lens can really give them adequate acuity. It is impossible to cure the condition with the aid of contact lenses, but it has long been held that the use of contact lenses may prevent or retard its progression. In the past the main use for contact lenses has been to correct the vision and give adequate acuity. In some really advanced cases only a scleral lens can be used with satisfactory results but in the early and medium stages the use of a corneal lens can provide excellent acuity and comfort (*see* Chapters 20 and 24).

In early keratoconus soft contact lenses can give a reasonable visual acuity without the use of additional spectacles for correction of the astigmatic component. In the author's experience, up to one-third of the astigmatism may be corrected by the soft lens which, if it is reasonably thick, also makes the astigmatism more regular, thus making an overcorrection more effective, if used. In the progressive stage, however, a soft contact lens proves inadequate and hard forms of lens must be used. The use of corneal lenses is usually satisfactory, although, as the cornea becomes more steeply curved, fittings become complicated and unstable. Lenses on steep corneas are very frequently excessively mobile and easily lost. Even a scleral lens can be difficult to fit in these conditions due to the high degree of irregularity and the difficulty in controlling bubbles if the lens is made in fenestrated form. If the bubble is extremely difficult to control then techniques such as those developed by Marriot (1968) will have to be used (*see* Chapter 9, Volume 1, and Chapter 20). The author has found that in some of these advanced cases no amount of work on a scleral lens can avoid visual interference by the bubble, but the use of a very small, thin, soft lens worn underneath the scleral lens can be a very satisfactory means of moving the bubble out of the central area (Westerhout, 1975) (*see Colour Plate LI*).

If a scleral lens proves unsatisfactory and the orthodox corneal lens is impossible to fit, then a 'combination lens' consisting of a hard lens and a soft lens can be used (Westerhout, 1973). The author has used these lenses on a large number of occasions and has found them extremely useful in overcoming serious problems with other forms of lens (*see* page 614). If, however, the practitioner is prepared to persevere with advanced, multi-curved designs of corneal lens using back central optic diameters as small as 4–5 mm, such a lens is often very satisfactory.

PTERYGIUM

Pterygium is hardly an example of the treatment of corneal pathology, but it is frequently necessary or desirable to fit contact lenses to a patient with a considerable growth of pterygium onto the cornea. Some of these cases are patients who may have successfully worn corneal lenses for many years before the edge of the lens begins to cause irritation by its contact with the enlarging pterygium.

Surgery is sometimes resorted to before lenses are fitted, or to remove a pterygium which is beginning to cause discomfort in a previously successful wearer. Unfortunately, in addition to the commonly seen re-growth of the pterygium, the tissues often become extraordinarily sensitive after surgery and corneal lenses are often not tolerated, although very small lenses of 8.0 mm overall size, or less, may be of value.

Soft lenses are of great value after excision, or if the lens is to be fitted over the pterygium. The use of a small soft lens is, however, of limited application as the edge may irritate the sensitive tissue left post-operatively and if fitted over a pterygium it may lift, thus allowing the edge to dry out, risking damage to the lens and possible irritation. The author finds larger lenses of 14–15 mm overall size are more applicable in both types of case. The edge of the lens should reach well beyond the limbus to cover a large proportion of the affected areas (*see Colour Plate LII*).

INDOLENT CORNEAL ULCERS

Patients with indolent corneal ulcers probably constitute one of the largest groups of patients who are treated with soft contact lenses for therapeutic purposes.

Many of these patients are treated for a long period before soft lens therapy is considered, and since herpes simplex keratitis appears to be one of the most common causes of this condition, many patients will have undergone some degree of therapy with idoxuridine. It is normally considered appropriate to use soft lens treatment only for cases where the corneal ulcers are sterile. This form of therapy is well known and has been prescribed for many years (Gasset and Kaufman, 1970; Liebowitz and Rosenthal, 1971; Westerhout, 1973 and Ruben, 1975).

A wide variety of clinical pictures exists but the general picture is one of an area of chronic erosion exposing Bowman's membrane and often some stroma. Previous medical treatment often indicates that the epithelium appears unable to grow across the crater area. In most cases prior therapy has resulted in intermittent and temporary healing, particularly in the herpes infections when recurrent attacks occur with consequential epithelial loss and further infection. Later in the progress of the condition secondary stromal involvement occurs, further reducing visual acuity.

Treatment is sometimes initiated by the total denudation of the corneal epithelium after topical application of proparacaine (Leibowitz and Rosenthal, 1971) or local debridement of the ulcer at its margins and cleaning of the crater (Ruben, 1975). The eroded area will often then heal. The slit lamp picture usually indicates that the epithelium appears to grow under the bandage from the periphery of the crater inwards.

Liebowitz and Rosenthal (1971) indicate that the soft lens bandage can be fitted without recourse to keratometry. Keratometry, of course, is usually impossible on an ulcerated eye but the author finds that a very useful indication of the likely fitting is obtained by keratometry on the other eye. It is normally considered necessary to clean the edges of the ulceration to remove the necrotic and hyperplastic tissue, but on numerous occasions the author has had to fit patients where this was not possible. The results seem to be equally satisfactory provided that the bandage lens is removed regularly and cleaned thoroughly, and the eye itself irrigated to remove loose debris.

Most of the earlier work involving the treatment of corneal ulceration with soft lenses related to the use of large, HEMA-type contact lenses which were not particularly thin and although these appeared to produce good results it is now found that large, high water content lenses such as Sauflon PW, used continuously, produce better results. It seems generally better to leave the lens *in situ* for the first week, whilst watching the condition carefully with a slit lamp microscope, as premature removal of the bandage can be dangerous by disturbing the vulnerable area during early healing. Most practitioners appear to prefer to use the bandage in conjunction with chloramphenicol drops, made up without preservative (Liebowitz and Rosenthal, 1971; Westerhout, 1973) although it is felt that low quantities of preservatives (Ruben, 1975) may be satisfactory.

It is especially interesting to observe the growth of the epithelium underneath the bandage lens as it appears to grow initially on the posterior surface of the bandage, forming a bridge across the crater. This is not always the case but has been described by Liebowitz and Rosenthal (1971). It is disappointing that so many of these cases seen are frequently the result of the prescribing of steroids for viral infections of the cornea which might well have been satisfactorily treated by other means (Westerhout, 1973) (see Colour Plate LIII).

Another fairly common cause of peripheral ulceration is that seen in conditions associated with rheumatoid arthritis, as shown in *Colour Plate LIV*. The soft contact lens used as a bandage appears to produce the desired result by means of shielding the ulcerated area from irritation, due to blinking, and from a variety of noxious environmental stimuli. It is important, however, that since the regenerating tissue requires a fairly high level of oxygen, the material used for the bandage lens should either be a high water content material, adequately permeable to oxygen, or else a very thin conventional soft lens should be used which also allows sufficient permeability to oxygen (Hill and Jeppe, 1976). One of the most difficult aspects of this form of treatment is to know when the bandage should be removed from the eye, after healing appears complete. Westerhout (1973) feels that the corneal surface should appear as regular as possible before the use of the bandage is discontinued, and not merely show the absence of staining with fluorescein.

It is not uncommon to find ulceration recurring with severe results (even to the extent of corneal perforation and loss of aqueous) after the bandage has been discontinued for a matter of a few days (Westerhout, 1973) (see Colour Plates LV and LVI). Frequently, the corneal surface seems to have healed reasonably well, but the appearance of dry spots, between blinking, and slight irregularity are suspicious signs suggesting that the bandage use should be continued for a longer period.

Despite the complications of this form of treatment it is found to work extremely well in the majority of patients (Liebowitz and Rosenthal, 1971) and there is frequently no other method of treatment available for some of these severe chronic conditions. At the time when soft lens bandage therapy is commenced the condition has frequently progressed to the stage where tarsorrhaphy or enucleation has been considered (see Colour Plate LVII). The author has seen several cases in this category where enucleation has been seriously considered but which, after several months of soft lens bandage treatment, have resulted in the healing of the cornea with useful vision.

One serious problem with the use of the bandage soft lens in cases of ulceration is the fact that severe contamination of the lens frequently results. It is not uncommon for a lens to become completely contaminated beyond reclamation within 1–2 weeks, and this is clearly an economic consideration which cannot be ignored. Although the use of continuous wear bandages is usually desirable in the early stages of the treatment there is no reason why, when the cornea has largely healed, a normal, conventional daily wear lens cannot be used which is removed at night. This form of lens, as it can be cleaned satisfactorily, is very often much more economic during the later stages of treatment.

OCULAR PEMPHIGOID

This progressive primary degeneration which, in its chronic state, usually affects senile eye tissue, often produces corneal complications similar to those seen in the Stevens–Johnson syndrome (see below).

Some patients suffering from this condition are also affected by rheumatoid arthritis (Ruben, 1975) which may also present a difficulty since the patient may be unable to handle soft lenses satisfactorily. The causes and prognosis of the condition are well described in the ophthalmological textbooks, and the main task of the contact lens practitioner is to protect the cornea and keep it wet, especially if lid surgery is undertaken to overcome entropion.

Unfortunately, keeping the cornea wet is only a partial solution to the problem. Ruben (1975) has pointed out that, although devices such as spectacles with manual or electronic fluid injection are worthy of consideration, solutions without the necessary lipid or protein concentrations will eventually produce epithelial oedema and necrosis. Unhappily, therefore, no matter whether or not the contact lens used is hard or soft the prognosis is poor and the disease normally remains progressive and results in blindness.

STEVENS–JOHNSON SYNDROME

The Stevens–Johnson syndrome is most commonly found in young persons between the ages of 6 and 15 years although older patients are seen. The ocular effects are usually corneal with conjunctival scarring, ankyloblepharon and symblepharon. In some cases the eyes are wet, but dry eyes are also commonly found.

Unfortunately, the tears are seldom normal and due to an absence of normal levels of lipid and proteins the corneal and conjunctival epithelial layers are severely affected. For many years scleral lenses have been used in this condition either in a full form or fitted as an annular ring. Often the scleral lens ring is utilized after the surgical division of symblepharon.

This condition frequently responds well to medical and contact lens treatment although antibiotic and wetting drops are almost invariably required.

The use of soft contact lenses is somewhat limited by the fact that the eye condition is frequently dry and in this instance constant irrigation is required either by the patient or, if dryness is severe, by using some form of mechanical apparatus.

DRY EYES

In the wide variety of conditions resulting from a deficiency of tears, a hydrophilic contact lens can be useful. Unfortunately, as has been pointed out by Ruben (1975), in these conditions the tears, as well as being deficient, may also be abnormal in their chemical composition. A scleral-type lens can be used to keep the available tears in contact with the eye and soft contact lenses may also be used in these conditions. However, in the experience of the author, the corneas eventually become sclerosed and vascularized and the soft lens bandage is usually eventually worn purely as a means of reducing discomfort.

In a large number of these cases the lens becomes severely contaminated with protein and other deposits, and requires frequent replacement. Occlusion of the lower puncti and the use of artificial tears may be of value (Ruben, 1975) but many opthalmologists prefer to treat these dry-eyed patients medically with a combination of acetylcysteine, 10 per cent, and wetting agents.

POST-OPERATIVE APHAKIA

Contact lens practitioners have for a long time been familiar with the optical treatment of post-operative aphakia with contact lenses. The well-known advantages of contact lenses over conventional spectacles have been dealt with elsewhere in this book (*see* Chapter 4, Volume 1) and in the majority of cases, orthodox corneal lenses prove very satisfactory for the treatment of this condition whether it be binocular or monocular.

One of the common indications for the use of soft contact lenses is in the non-tolerance of a hard form of lens. Since most post-operative aphakic patients are relatively insensitive in the corneal region, it is not often necessary to use a soft contact lens. Despite the great success of corneal lenses for aphakia there are some patients, however, who are unable to satisfactorily tolerate hard lenses, and soft contact lenses can be used to advantage in these cases.

The decreased sensitivity of the cornea is not the advantage it may seem, since infections and abrasions may be relatively severe before the patient is aware of difficulties. Trophic disorders of the cornea may occur but these may be secondary to anomalies of the tears secretions or blink rate (Ruben, 1975). Since soft lenses have very little abrasive action on the cornea compared to corneal lenses their use for aphakia is recommended.

Referral for the fitting of contact lenses occurs as early as 2–3 weeks after surgery in the case of some surgeons and as long as 6 months in the case of others. Contact lenses are contra-indicated if there is continuing inflammation of the eye, or the presence of suture material which may interfere with the physical fitting of the lens. Loose sutures should be removed before contact lenses are fitted. Due to their large size, soft contact lenses can frequently be made to centre very well compared with the likely sagging effect of a high positive-powered hard lens. This sag, of course, produces a prism base-down effect which is especially troublesome in unilateral aphakia.

The decision to fit soft contact lenses, however, depends greatly on the surgical technique used. Some surgical techniques result in a high degree of astigmatism against-the-rule and it is not uncommon to find, even a year after surgery, that two or more dioptres of such astigmatism are still in evidence. Astigmatism of medium to high degree is a well-known contra-indication to the use of orthodox spherical soft lenses, but good surgical techniques resulting in a regular cornea and a round pupil often permit the fitting of a soft contact lens, should this be desirable.

The handling of soft contact lenses by aphakic patients is, however, a matter of some concern, particularly by those who are senile and may have difficulty in physically manipulating the lens. They may find it is difficult to remove or insert the lens without fairly rough handling of the eye. This can result in conjunctival tears, episcleritis, and more seriously in a retinal detachment, or vitreous in the anterior chamber, and the ability of the patient to handle a contact lens of this nature must therefore be considered carefully prior to fitting.

Even if the surgical technique has resulted in

fairly considerable corneal astigmatism the soft contact lens is well worth fitting if there are difficulties with the tolerance of hard lenses. Since the majority of difficulties resulting from the use of spectacles in aphakia are due to the very high powered lens situated some distance from the corneal surface, it is a very considerable improvement to fit a spherical soft lens to the cornea and prescribe the small residual correction in spectacle form. The use of spectacles over a soft contact lens is also useful in the event of troublesome aniseikonia and to provide a near addition.

Occasionally, however, it is disappointing to note that the visual acuity obtained with a soft contact lens, even with an over-correction in spectacle form, cannot equal that obtained with a hard lens. This is especially noticeable if a soft lens with a lenticular front surface is utilized on an eye with a displaced pupil. The incident light, falling obliquely on the front surface of the lens, creates oblique astigmatism which may vary with eye movement. Re-designing the form of the lens may sometimes help, but in certain instances it remains difficult to achieve a satisfactory standard of visual acuity with a soft lens.

Of equal importance is the difficulty that some patients encounter when finding variations in their visual acuity whilst doing close work compared with distance vision. Westerhout (1976) has reported on variations in the residual astigmatism noted in the primary position of gaze compared with that measured looking down for close work. The lens frequently flexes in this near working position and this can induce changes in the astigmatism which can be troublesome.

CONTINUOUS WEAR LENSES IN APHAKIA

It is not uncommon for the aphakic patient to wear a lens continuously without serious changes in corneal integrity. The author has found that the cornea is generally far less prone to initial, adaptive oedema than in the case of the non-aphakic corneal lens wearer. Aphakic patients have frequently worn soft contact lenses for very long periods of time without removal and this can be of considerable assistance to elderly patients who find difficulty in handling the lens. Due to the thickness of the lens, however, the oxygen transport through it is poor (Hill and Jeppe, 1976) and this is not totally satisfactory, therefore, unless the lens is made of a high water content material such as Sauflon PW. More recently, Kersley (1976) has described the fitting of a continuous wear Sauflon PW lens immediately after the conclusion of surgery.

Perhaps, however, the most valuable application of the continuous wear aphakic lens is its use in the infant aphakic. The author has fitted several infants, all congenital, bilateral cataract sufferers who have had surgery on both eyes and in each case the use of a continuous wear aphakic lens has been apparently satisfactory. One of the great difficulties in these cases is to know whether or not the patient should be fully-corrected or over-corrected. Ruben (1975) states that over-correction in early infancy is probably preferable to avoid foveal suppression for near. Naturally enough, the lens will require to have its power changed as the child grows older and the eye length increases. Unfortunately, the problem is not as simple as straightforward optical correction of the eyes, the difficulties of functional optical correction being intimately related to cerebral visual perception as discussed by Ruben (1975), who has also pointed out the considerable advantages achieved by the removal of cataract by aspiration. This technique, leaving a normal central pupil, is very much better suited to adequate optical correction with contact lenses.

Unfortunately, some babies are very difficult to fit with lenses as they are able to rub even a well-fitting soft lens from the eye. General anaesthesia is not always required for the fitting of such lenses but very often a much better assessment of the physical fitting can be achieved if such anaesthesia is used.

The continuous use of a soft lens for post-operative aphakia has proved successful for several years (Westerhout, 1973; Kersley, 1976). When the lens is fitted at operation, or shortly afterwards, consideration of the keratometer readings and likely changes in corneal curvature must be made. Kersley (1976) reported that an average corneal flattening of 0.4 mm in radius was seen on the first post-operative day and this gradually returned to normal after 6 months.

The author finds it helpful to take keratometer readings of both eyes before surgery, if possible, as this gives some idea of the likely measurements after surgery and in the following months.

When lenses are being fitted at operation it is often difficult to do keratometry accurately. If the patient is supine there is no reason why the keratometer should not be used on a mobile table with a 45 degree angled mirror to view the cornea, the instrument being positioned to one side of the patient. Ellis (1977) has described the use of an adaptor which allows a keratometer to be used vertically, from above the patient, by attaching it to the stand of an operating microscope. This sounds an admirable solution to the problem.

Many aphakes have been fitted with Sauflon PW lenses but there is often some advantage in using these lenses with overall sizes slightly larger than the standard 13.5 mm, although a great deal depends on the surgical technique used and also the site of the incision. Ruben (1975) has pointed out the dangers of contact lenses used in the presence of a large filtering cicatrix.

The author's experience supports the view of Kersley (1976) that the high water content lenses, such as Sauflon PW, should be fitted approximately 0.4 mm flatter than the flattest keratometer reading when fitted in an overall size of 13.5 mm. This applies at operation and in the first few weeks after surgery. It is often necessary to change the lens and obtain the fitting and prescription again some 6–10 weeks after the initial fitting. Even at this stage it is worth having a second identical lens made which can be exchanged for the original after 1–4 weeks. The original is then cleaned to remove protein and other contamination and the lenses continue to be alternated whilst one lens is being cleaned.

Unfortunately, it is difficult to duplicate the high water content lenses exactly. The swell factor of materials such as Sauflon PW is very high and somewhat variable, and it is very difficult to manufacture lenses to exact specifications. Even lenses which appear to be the correct prescription are often found to perform inadequately and need to be replaced. This also applies, but to a lesser extent, to the lower water content materials.

It is clear that the composition of tears varies in different individuals (Hathaway and Lowther, 1976) and analysis by the author of the progress of 300 consecutively fitted soft lens patients indicates a strong predisposition on the part of some patients to severe contamination, despite the use of regular cleaning regimens.

It appears that the molecular diameter of some proteins is almost equal to that of the pore (void) size of the soft lens materials. Much of the protein does not, therefore, enter the lens materials and is thus readily removed from the surface by cleaning agents such as non-ionic surfactants and the enzyme papain (see Chapter 3, Volume 1). Some of the smaller molecules do, however, enter the pores of the material and gradually build an internal deposit which is not readily removed. It is thought that the enzyme papain will not penetrate materials such as HEMA and remove proteins which have penetrated the surface.

Many lenses, therefore, become internally contaminated despite regular cleaning, and surface deposits also form which cannot then be removed. Much more work needs to be done in the field of the analysis of deposits and methods of removing them. Some substances which are believed to have a larger molecular size than the pore size of the material are still able to enter. Fluorescein is one example and substances in this category may be small enough in one dimension to enter the pores although their other dimensions appear too large to do so. Thus, entry of contaminating molecules depends on their shape as well as their size.

The correct insertion of a continuous wear lens is of greater importance than a daily wear lens. It is essential that the lens is first cleaned and sterilized, and it is preferable that the lens then be kept in sterile saline solution for a period to reduce any initial reaction to chemicals used in cleaning. As is well known, the term 'sterilize', as applied to soft lenses, is a misnomer unless the lens has been autoclaved (Litvin, 1977), and all that can really be hoped for is that the lens inserted is not contaminated with pathogenic microorganisms.

Cleaning alone is very important and recent tests conducted to test a locally made soft lens cleaner used by the author are of interest. Lenses were contaminated with ocular pathogens in large numbers (approximately 10^6/ml of contaminating solution). The lens surfaces were merely rubbed with the surfactant cleaning solution and then rinsed. Subsequent tests revealed that 99 per cent of contamination had been removed from the lens.

It is worth irrigating the eye before inserting a lens to remove any foreign bodies which might prove harmful under a continuously worn lens. The author then usually places the lens directly onto the cornea. If air bubbles are seen, which is quite common, then the patient squeezes his lids together tightly and this is usually sufficient to remove them. If squeezing the lids is insufficient then the lens can be moved with the fingertips in order to evacuate the bubbles. If bubbles still cannot be removed, the lens is removed and the patient asked to lean forward until the head is horizontal. The back surface of the lens is then filled with as much sterile saline solution as it will hold and the lens is placed directly on to the cornea and the excess solution escapes, usually leaving the lens in position with no bubble. The procedure is rather similar to placing a sealed scleral lens on the eye.

Other practitioners (for example, Kerr, 1976) often prefer placing the lens onto the temporal bulbar conjunctiva and smoothing out any bubbles in this position. The patient then looks in the direction of the lens to centre it on the cornea. Since, however, the sclera is much flatter than the cornea, one is more liable to find bubbles under the lens if it is placed on the conjunctiva.

It is worthwhile attempting to instruct the patient in the handling of an orthodox soft lens preferably using a tougher material such as HEMA. If the case is unilateral then the other non-operated eye should be used for instruction. There is considerable advantage in the instruction of these patients, or members of their family, so that in the event of any subsequent ocular emergency where immediate ophthalmological or optometric help may not be available, the lens may be removed.

Unfortunately, however, the contamination of the aphakic lens due to proteins is very much worse than that of thinner lenses. The author has seen several aphakic patients who contaminate their lenses beyond reclamation in 1–2 months of continuous wearing (*see Colour Plate XLIX*). Improved cleaning compounds such as Monoclens (*Sauflon*), Reno-gel (*Alcon*), Hexaclean (*Barnes-Hind*) and the use of enzymes such as papain (Hydrocare or Soflens cleaning tablets – *Allergan*) are now making it easier to clean some of these lenses.

THE USE OF DRUGS WITH SOFT LENSES

One of the advantages of soft lenses is the possibility of treating glaucoma with isotonic 2 per cent pilocarpine. The lens may be soaked for approximately 1 hour in a pilocarpine solution, which appears to control the intra-ocular pressure very well for a period of approximately 12 hours wearing time. Some lenses become badly discoloured with a dark brown stain if they are used with epinephrine which is used in glaucoma therapy.

The use of drugs after surgery is important as these may strongly influence the effects of the contact lens. Many patients initially consult a practitioner fairly soon after surgery and whilst still using local antibiotic cover or steroid therapy. Premature fitting in this instance will frequently result in fairly severe corneal oedema, far worse than would have been encountered had steroids not been utilized.

It is considered unsafe to use commercially prepared drugs with a soft lens on the eye. The preservatives, such as benzalkanium chloride, which are commonly used, are thought to become concentrated in the lens material and may possibly reach dangerous levels. The drugs should thus be made up without preservatives or the lens removed, if possible, before the drug is instilled and left out for 15 minutes thereafter.

Idoxuridine (IDU) can be used with the lens in place and the lens may be soaked in a solution before application.

In many cases standard collyria have been used with a soft lens in place without any apparent ill effects. These collyria have included antibiotics, mydriatics, corticosteroids and IDU. It may be that with the drug being instilled 3 or 4 times each day, the tears are able to wash out much of the preservative and reduce the concentration.

FILARIASIS

Filariasis, a relatively uncommon condition resulting from nematodes, is a condition in which the eye can frequently become extremely painful. This is normally due to corneal involvement and the author has found that considerable relief and comfort can be afforded by the wearing of a soft lens used as a corneal bandage. The pain without a corneal bandage can be very severe indeed, and it appears that it is frequently impossible for the patient to manage without a bandage (Westerhout, 1973). In this instance it is probable that the bandage is acting purely as a mechanical protection for the corneal epithelial layer.

PENETRATING CORNEAL WOUNDS

Liebowitz (1972) has described the use of a hydrophilic contact lens as a means of sealing a corneal laceration. Soft lenses appear to be relatively effective as a splint and a temporary seal, provided that cases are selected for the small size of the laceration, good apposition in the alignment of the wound edges, and absence of incarceration or prolapse of the uvea and crystalline lens. Since it is a very much simpler procedure than suturing with very fine sutures, or other alternative methods, this technique has been recommended, especially as the outcome is not prejudiced if initially unsuccessful. The lens supporting the laceration may be removed easily and adhesives or direct suturing employed if required. The use of the soft lens bandage in this instance also permits direct vision of the wound edges at the time of repair and afterwards and also requires far less skill than the suturing of a wound by a highly skilled ophthalmologist.

KERATOPLASTY

Ruben (1975) has described the use of soft contact lenses in keratoplasty as a protective membrane immediately following surgery in an attempt to compress or mould the graft or to re-align partially everted grafts. They can also be used to treat graft rejection and in the long term to give the best visual acuity and maintain binocular vision.

When keratoplasty is carried out, the surgeon, anticipating the gradual change in curvature of the grafted cornea, attempts to give a result which will eventually restore the refraction to near emmetropia and give nearly normal keratometry readings. To this end many types of contact lens splints have been designed in attempting to mould the cornea. Soft lens splints can be utilized and left in position for several weeks without adversely affecting the metabolism of the corneal graft. Splinting can also be utilized until the curvatures of the graft are consistent with a good acuity with contact or spectacle lenses (Ruben, 1975).

Due to the unusual shape of the grafted cornea, in most cases a bicurve lens is necessary for a satisfactory splint. If low water content lenses such as those made of the HEMA materials are used, then thin, small lenses should be utilized of not much larger than 12–12.5 mm overall size. With much higher water content lenses, overall sizes of up to 15 mm can be utilized provided that they are also thin to permit normal corneal metabolism to be maintained. 'Combination lenses' (*see below*) can also be used successfully.

ALBINISM

For many years the ocular effects of congenital albinism have been treated with various forms of contact lens. Most of the attention has been devoted to an attempt to limit the amount of light entering the eye, usually by utilizing a tinted lens or an occluding lens with a 3–4 mm optically worked pupil. Unfortunately, however, the visual results are seldom encouraging and this may well be due to the fact that the albino eye is unable to form satisfactory retinal images because of light scattered through the anterior uvea. It also appears that during the developmental period, abnormalities of the foveal region may occur. The inability of the neurological sensory receptors to function at a high level of integration will limit achievement of good acuity in the developmental period and can lead to permanent loss of vision at a perceptual level (Ruben, 1975). Thus, the purely mechanical correction of this light scatter may produce only very limited improvement in visual acuity. It is also likely that an abnormality of the retinal pigment is a contributory factor to the severe visual limitations which occur. In the past, the fitting of a cosmetically occluding lens was usually accomplished by utilizing a scleral lens or a large corneal lens. Both of these types of lens are extremely difficult to fit in this form. Often the patient is able to tolerate a perfectly fitting lens in transparent material but subsequently finds the occluding cosmetic lens uncomfortable.

Fortunately, today, the fitting is considerably simplified by the utilization of soft contact lenses which can be accurately made containing a hand-painted iris pattern with a clear pupil. The pupil in these lenses should normally not be made smaller than approximately 3.5 mm and due to difficulties in colour matching these lenses are generally better made simultaneously for both eyes.

Although such lenses are very much easier to fit and much more satisfactory than the larger scleral design with their limited wearing time, the nature of the pigmented material used to make the 'iris pattern' is such that oxygen permeability through the lens is somewhat limited and the tears pump between lens and eye becomes of vital importance (Hill and Jeppe, 1976). This is not necessarily a great disadvantage as the pump normally permits sufficient oxygen to reach the cornea.

In general, however, too much should not be expected of occluding lenses used for patients suffering from albinism.

'COMBINATION LENSES'

Corneal pathology or trauma such as is found in advanced keratoconus, or corneal scarring due to penetrating wounds, can cause severe irregular astigmatism which is not correctable by spectacles or orthodox soft lenses. Usually, it is possible to use hard lenses in this type of case provided that scarring is not severe. Unfortunately, however, hard contact lenses are often not tolerated by a patient despite the motivation given by their great improvement of the visual acuity.

Westerhout (1973) has described a method by which the 'combination lens' may be fitted to such a patient. In this technique the cornea and surrounding tissues are treated as they would normally be treated for the fitting of an orthodox soft contact lens. The lens is usually fitted relatively large, to achieve stability, and keratometer readings are then taken from the front of the soft lens *in situ*. These keratometric findings are then utilized to allow the practitioner to fit a hard corneal lens on top of the soft lens to overcome the effects of the irregular astigmatism. For keratoconus the soft lens is usually supplied as a fairly high negative lens so as to provide a flatter front surface to which a steeper and therefore less mobile corneal lens can be fitted. In other cases a low positive soft lens (of about +4.00 D) is found to be more suitable. The fact that the combination hard lens is able to fit on the soft contact lens rather than on the naked cornea enables much greater comfort to be achieved than would be the case on the cornea itself and these results have been extremely helpful in a large number of cases. Fortunately, as the soft lens still permits the pump action to be maintained, the hard corneal lens may be fitted substantially tighter on the soft lens than it would be on the cornea. This technique is particularly helpful in cases of advanced keratoconus (*see also*

Chapter 18, page 567, and *Colour Plates LVIII* and *LIX*. The hard lens is usually best fitted using a gas-permeable material.

THE USE OF SOFT LENSES WITH SCLERAL LENSES

Westerhout (1975) has described a method by which scleral lens fitting may be improved and simplified by the use of soft lenses. It is based on the technique developed by Marriott (1968) whereby a highly irregular eye may be accurately fitted with a scleral lens by covering the plaster cast, made from an eye impression, with a laminate to provide the correct amount of clearance over the entire cornea and limbus.

The latter method is usually successful but is somewhat time consuming and requires a considerable amount of technical skill.

The method Westerhout (1975) has described involves the eye being fitted with a large, tight-fitting, soft lens of negative power which allows the practitioner to take an eye impression directly over the soft lens resting on the cornea. A cast is then taken from the impression. As the cast now represents the anterior surface of the globe with a layer of soft lens on the cornea, a scleral lens shell can be pressed directly from this cast and will normally provide adequate and gradually increasing corneal clearance from centre to limbus (due to the negative soft lens) (*see Colour Plates LX and LXI*).

This method permits the very much more rapid fitting of scleral lenses to irregular eyes and also has the effect of permitting covering and thus protection of the cornea whilst the impression-taking is being carried out. This can also be of benefit in areas of the world where optometrists are not permitted to use topical anaesthetics for impression-taking. Certainly very little subsequent corneal staining, if any, is seen when this method is used. Covering the cornea with a soft lens during tonometry may also be of value for protective purposes.

The control of the bubble in fitting a scleral lens to a highly irregular eye is also found to be extremely difficult on occasions. In some instances, no matter what technique is utilized, the bubble control becomes difficult. Westerhout (1975) has described the use of a small (almost corneal diameter) high water content, soft lens fitted underneath the scleral lens which is then ground out to permit a slightly larger than normal corneal clearance. The use of the soft lens underneath the scleral lens can, in some cases, considerably reduce the size of the troublesome bubble and may be found satisfactory, particularly in cases of high or advanced keratoconus (*see Colour Plate LI*).

CONTINUOUSLY WORN SOFT LENSES

In a large proportion of pathological cases for whom soft lenses are indicated, the continuously worn lens is often the best form to be considered. The continuous use of any form of contact lens must be regarded with some degree of suspicion, as there is obviously an increased risk of vascularization of the cornea (Westerhout, 1973). In many of the pathological cases seen, however, the risk of trauma to the eye during an attempt by the patient to remove the lens, is much more serious than the slight risk of complications following continuous use. One of the important aspects to consider when recommending continuous use is to know whether the patient can satisfactorily handle the lens in case of necessity. Where serious and painful conditions of the cornea exist it may well be better to encourage continuous use for at least 2–4 weeks before attempting to teach the patient to remove the lens. Even then it is generally better to attempt to learn the handling technique utilizing the non-affected eye if possible.

In many cases, however, it is better that, as soon as possible, the bandage is worn by day and removed during the hours of sleep. This is only safe if the patient can handle it satisfactorily. Quite obviously, sterilization of lenses is absolutely vital for patients who are suffering from a pathological corneal condition, and this fact should be stressed to patients when instructing them.

It is particularly important that the lens should be very thoroughly cleaned mechanically as the contamination of lenses by protein and other materials seems very much more common in the pathological eye than in the normal eye. Adequate mechanical cleaning is frequently difficult to achieve and it may well be necessary for the patient to visit the practice from time to time in order that the practitioner himself can service the lenses with chemical cleaning methods to ensure adequate cleanliness. It is probably fair to say that in serious cases of corneal infection or ulceration, bandages should be used for a period and then discarded and replaced. The main difficulty with this recommendation is the considerable cost of such treatment, and much more attention must be devoted towards adequate sterilization and cleaning of these soft lens bandages. At present, part of the difficulty with cleaning is due to the fact that most cleaning agents are designed for, and are therefore more effective with, low water content HEMA lenses, which are less often used for continuous wear. It is easy to criticize the use of the soft lens bandage as a therapy in view of the complications and difficulties, such as vascularization, that may be encountered (Ruben, 1976). It is important, however, always to look at the therapy in the context of what alternatives are available. In comparison with alternatives, such as tarsorrhaphy or enucleation, bandages are of great value even if only to achieve an extension of the useful life of the eye for several years. In many cases, however, the soft lens permits an almost total cure when no other therapy proves effective. A great deal of work is now being directed at the utilization of continuous wear lenses for cosmetic as well as for pathological conditions. In the past it has been thought that the most important parameters of soft, continuous wear designs are those of the lens overall size and water content. Recent work (Hill and Jeppe, 1976; Westerhout, 1977) has indicated, however, that the central thickness of a lens is of vital importance, thinner lenses being more gas permeable. It also appears that thin lenses contaminate more slowly than thick lenses and this is also of importance in the treatment of pathological conditions.

There has been a considerable improvement in the chemical treatment of contaminated lenses over the last few years and some of the procedures, such as the use of enzymes and oxidizing agents, have been of very great value in renovating lenses which have apparently been beyond reclamation. Despite this, however, some of these soft lens bandages degenerate rapidly and some contamination is found to resist all attempts at removal.

It would appear that the ideal material for a continous wear lens is one in which the pore (void) size is relatively small, preferably smaller than 0.4 nm and in which the material will withstand continual cleaning and sterilization procedures. Currently, the contamination seems to result mainly from naturally occurring proteins in the tears,

penetrating the lens and contaminating it. It is significant that some of the early morning oedema symptoms which sometimes occur in the initial stages of adaptation to continuously worn lenses, begin to recur when the lenses become contaminated. Thus, contamination must either reduce the oxygen permeability or upset the tears pump under the lens, until it can be cleaned effectively again. Fatt and Morris (1977) have shown that contamination has little effect on oxygen transmissibility, so it seems likely that the water content and fit of the lens are affected. It is possible that steepening occurs and this could cause oedema symptoms.

Some patients who wear soft contact lenses continuously, eventually develop a follicular conjunctivitis which is usually most severe in the upper palpebral conjunctiva. This is usually seen in patients who have some protein contamination on their lenses (see Chapter 16, page 520).

In view of the nature of the condition and the fact that the lens contamination is frequently caused by albumin, lysozyme, immunoglobulin, betaglobulin and alphaglobulin occurring in the tears, it is likely that the follicular condition is caused by an allergic type response to protein on the lenses.

Even if the lenses are removed the condition may linger on for months and treatment with steroids may be necessary. The condition is also seen in some daily wear soft contact lens patients, suffering from lens contamination.

The condition is more common in those with an allergic background and lens cleaning is of even greater importance for patients in this category.

REFERENCES

Ellis, P. (1977). 'The use of permanent wear contact lenses on young aphakic children.' Contact Lens J. 5(8), 23–26

Fatt, I. and Morris, J. A. (1977). 'Oxygen transmissibility changes of gel contact lens during wear.' Optician 174(4505), 17–20

Gasset, A. R. and Kaufman, H. E. (1970). 'Therapeutic uses of soft lenses.' Am. J. Ophthal. 69, 252–259

Hathaway, R. and Lowther, G. E. (1976). 'Appearance of hydrophilic lens deposits as related to chemical etiology.' Internat. contact Lens Clin. 3(3), 27–35

Hill, R. M. and Jeppe, W. H. (1976). 'Hydrogels: is a pump still necessary?' Internat. contact Lens Clin. 2(4), 27–29

Kerr, C. (1976). 'A fitting regime for Sauflon 85 per cent in aphakia.' Optician 171(4427), 9

Kersley, H. J. (1976). 'The use of a "continuous wear" hydrophilic lens in aphakia, fitted at operation.' Contact Lens J. 5(6), 13, 16–17

Liebowitz, H. M. (1972). 'Hydrophilic contact lenses in corneal disease: IV. Penetrating corneal wounds.' Archs Ophthal. 88, 602–606

Liebowitz, H. M. and Rosenthal, P. (1971). 'Hydrophilic contact lenses in corneal disease: I. Superficial, sterile, indolent ulcers.' Archs Opthal. 85, 163–166

Litvin, M. W. (1977). 'The incidence of eye infections with contact lenses.' Optician 174(4496), 11–14

Marriott, P. J. (1968). 'The construction of impression haptic lenses.' Contact Lens 1, 3, 8–10, 12, 14

Ruben, M. (1971). 'Soft lenses.' Trans. ophthal. Soc. U.K. 91, 59–74

Ruben, M. (1975). Contact Lens Practice: Visual, Therapeutic and Prosthetic, London: Baillière and Tindall

Ruben, M. (1976). 'The factors necessary for constant wearing of contact lenses.' Optician 172(4453), 19, 27, 30, 33

Westerhout, D. I. (1973). ' The "combination lens" and therapeutic uses of soft lenses.' Contact Lens 4(5), 3–10, 12, 16–18, 20, 22

Westerhout, D. I. (1975). 'The use of soft lenses in the fitting of haptic lenses.' Optician 169(4363), 13, 16

Westerhout, D. I. (1976). 'Contact lenses: corneal, residual and induced astigmatism.' Internat. contact Lens Clin. 3(3), 52–61

Westerhout, D. I. (1977). 'A rationale for the use and further development of a continuously worn contact lens for the military.' Awaiting publication in Military Medicine, U.S.A.

Chapter 22

Contact Lens Manufacture

E. J. D. Proctor

This chapter aims at giving the clinician and student a brief outline of manufacturing procedures. It in no way claims to be comprehensive for there are now many advanced and sophisticated techniques used in mass production of both hard and soft lenses which herein are mentioned only briefly. Scleral lenses will not be discussed because with the advent of soft lenses their usage is further declining and for those cases for which they are indicated the impression technique seems to offer better results. This latter procedure, which is mainly carried out by the clinician is dealt with in Chapter 9, Volume 1, which deals fully with the making of the lens from the stage of the eye impression. Some more complicated scleral lens manufacturing techniques are covered in Chapter 20.

The two main methods of manufacturing contact lenses are: (1) moulding; and (2) generating.

MOULDING

Moulding can be by casting, compression or injection. Spin-casting is used for mass production of soft lenses, while compression and injection moulding are largely used for mass production of hard corneal lenses.

Bausch and Lomb in the United States have refined the Czechoslovakian spin-casting technique to produce soft lenses. This procedure involves spinning a mould, at a computer-controlled speed, into which the mixture of monomers is injected. The centripetal force causes the mixture to climb the wall of the mould to form into the required shape, the polymerization and spinning takes place simultaneously. The method is described in Chapter 14, page 430 and Chapter 15, and *Figures 14.23* and *14.24* show diagrammatically the form of the mould and the resultant shapes of some lens back surfaces.

The formed dehydrated lens has to be edged before being hydrated and released from its mould. This is a technique which is extremely suitable for mass production of soft spherical lenses. Its disadvantages are as follows.

(1) It is extremely expensive to set up the laboratory and therefore a large production is essential for it to be viable. This means that the available lens parameters are very restricted.

(2) The technique cannot be used for individual prescriptions such as soft toric lenses, which may soon become routine fitting for the practitioner.

Further details and other lens properties are discussed in Chapter 14.

In a compression moulding technique developed by Kelvin in the United Kingdom for production of hard lenses separate steel tools for front and back surfaces are made. Under controlled conditions of heat and pressure both front and back curves are produced simultaneously on a disc of PMMA inserted between the tools.

On removal from the pressing jig the surface finished lens has to be cut to the required overall size and edged. This procedure requires a very large number of tools to obtain all the various possible combinations of parameters. It has the advantage that lenses can be made both quickly and fairly cheaply because it requires less skilled labour than for lathe-cut lenses. The expense and expertise are introduced when making the steel tools. It is a good technique for producing a continuous curve lens, but it does have the following disadvantages.

(1) Because of the cost of tooling the available range of parameters is limited. For example, only one BCOD can usually be obtained with any one given radial edge lift.

(2) If manufacturing conditions are not carefully controlled it can introduce stress into the lens

material and this can cause the lens curvature to change after manufacture and during usage. This is particularly the case with thin lenses.

(3) For the same reason as (2) above, poor optics and hence poor power readings are easily produced.

Another moulding technique for hard lens production, developed by Wöhlk of West Germany, involves placing powdered PMMA in the concavity of a Pyrosil mould to which is clamped a quartz-glass convex die. This is slowly moved through an oven at 200°C for three-quarters of an hour, after which the surface-finished lens is removed from the separated mould. The lens is then cut to the required size and

out as the procedures are described, otherwise it is to be assumed that the same techniques apply to both.

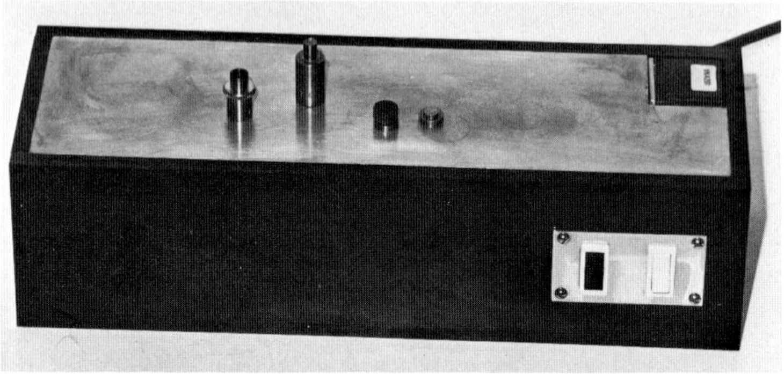

CUTTING BACK SURFACES

A PMMA (or soft lens) blank is mounted on a heated stepped steel button (*Figures 22.1* and *22.2*) with the aid of a thin layer of bees wax to hold it approximately central. When the button is cool it is placed in the collett of a heavy based high precision micro-lathe (*Figure 22.3*) and the diameter of the

Figure 22.1–Hot plate for heating steel buttons and chucks

edged. A similar technique using stainless steel moulds and dies is used by Silor in France. This procedure has one big advantage over the compression technique in that it does not introduce any strain. However, there are disadvantages, as follows.

(1) As with compressed lenses the cost of tooling reduces the available range of parameters.

(2) There are difficulties preventing impurities, such as specks of dust, from entering the powdered PMMA and thus the matrix of the finished lens.

GENERATING

Generating is the technique favoured by most small to medium laboratories as well as most of the large ones throughout the world. For this reason it is the technique on which the author has concentrated in this chapter. This procedure does not lend itself to mass production as readily as the moulding techniques, the emphasis being on individual prescription work. The method of manufacture is basically the same for soft lenses as it is for hard corneal lenses; in fact, it is the main method of manufacturing soft lenses throughout the world. Any difference between hard and soft lens fabrication will be pointed

blank is reduced to 0.10 mm or 0.15 mm above the final overall size of the required prescription lens (*Figure 22.4*). The next operation is to cut the required BCOR. This is done with a diamond-tipped tool which ensures that an extremely high surface finish is achieved prior to polishing (*Figure 22.5*). Material is first removed from the centre and, in increasingly wider sweeps, eventually from across the entire surface of the blank, thus covering the whole diameter. The last few cuts remove a thickness of 0.005–0.02 mm; the speed at which the diamond traverses the surface during these final cuts is very much slower in order to produce a smoother

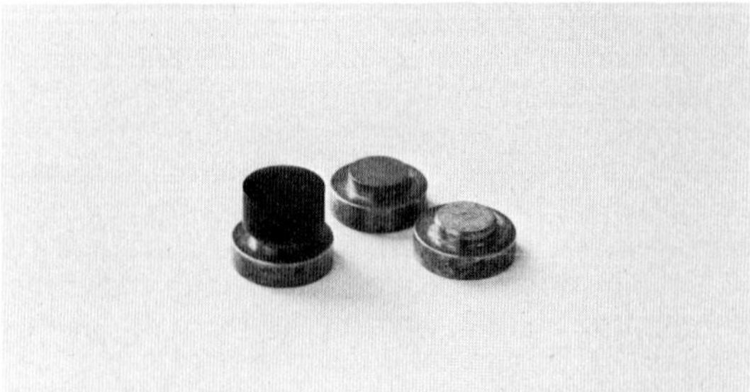

Figure 22.2–Stepped steel buttons, one mounted with a PMMA blank

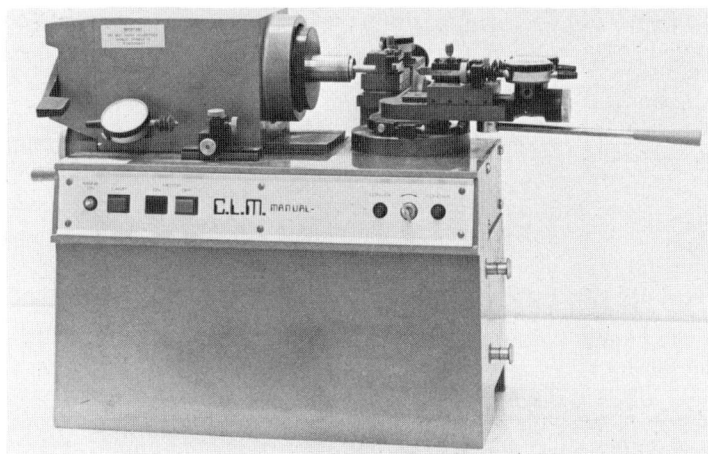

Figure 22.3–High precision lathe set for cutting front surfaces

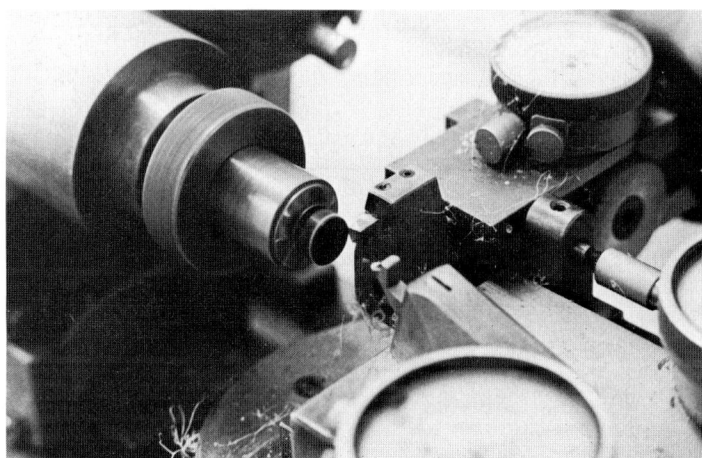

Figure 22.4–Reducing the diameter of the blank

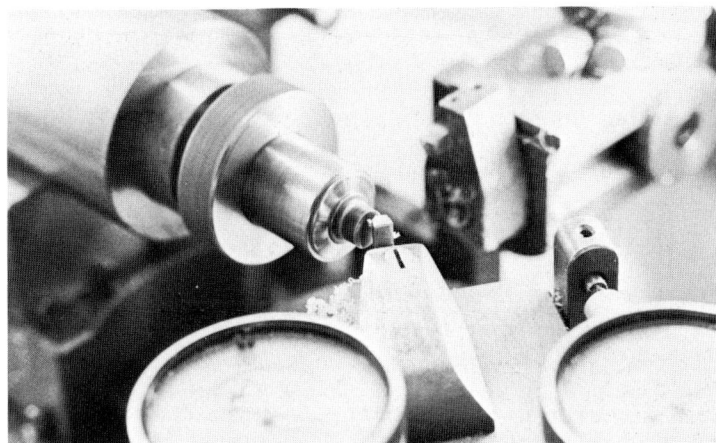

Figure 22.5–Cutting the back central optic radius. The material removed is termed 'swarf'

finished surface. The cutting finishes in the centre of the lens, the collett holding the blank is wound back from the diamond, and the extreme knife-edge of the blank blunted with a blade or grinding stone. If the last-named procedure is not done the edge of the blank digs into the wax polisher in the next phase of work.

POLISHING BACK SURFACES

The steel button with semi-finished blank attached is removed from the collett and the blank and button separated; this helps to release any strain which has been introduced during cutting. After removing wax from the base of the blank, using paraffin in an ultrasonic cleaner, it is mounted on a clean steel button using double-sided sticky tape. For hard lenses a wax polisher is then cut on the lathe to the required radius (*Figure 22.6*) and a spiral groove (*Figure 22.7*) or series of circular grooves made in its surface to aid the distribution of the polish. The blank is polished on an automatic polisher (*Figures*

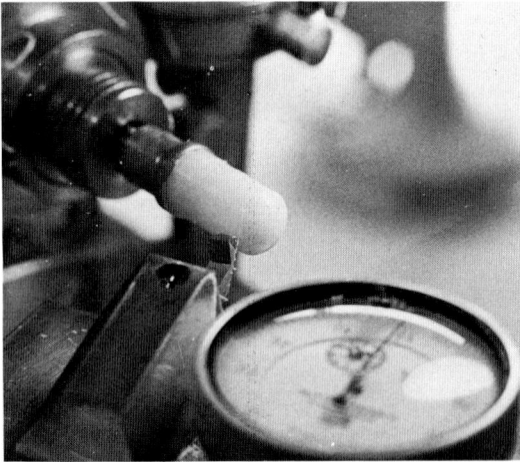

Figure 22.8–Polishing the back surface using automatic back surface polishing machines. Detail is shown in Figure 22.9

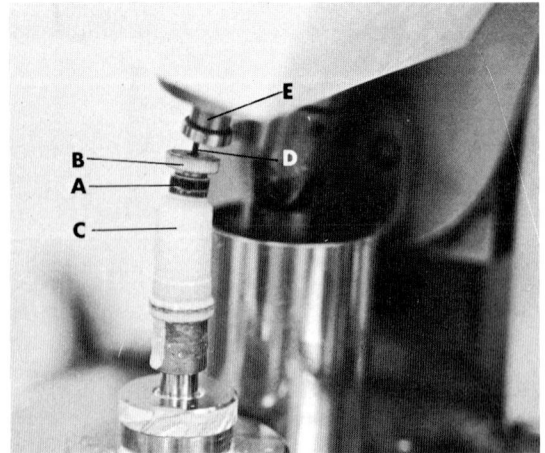

Figure 22.6–Cutting the back surface wax polishing tool

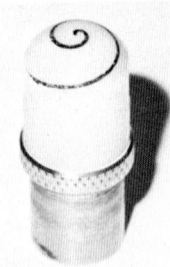

Figure 22.7–Spiral groove in wax polishing tool. Ink has been run into the groove for illustration purposes

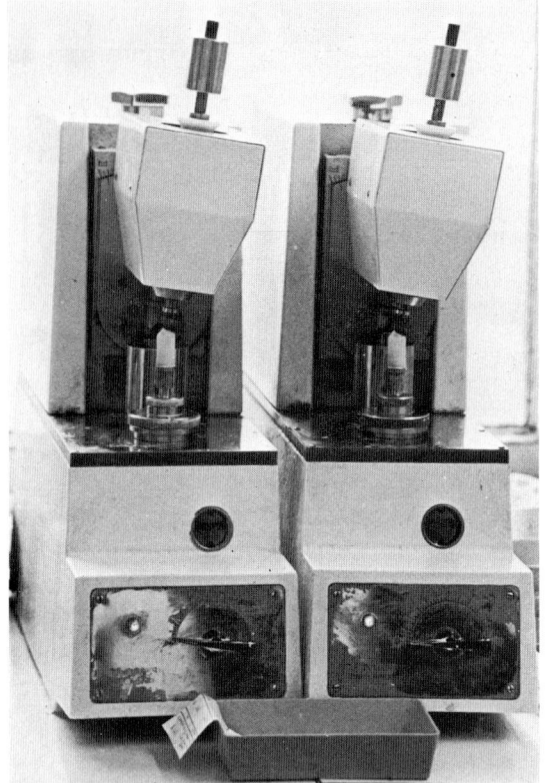

Figure 22.9–Close-up of polishing the back surface. The blank (A) mounted on its steel button (B) being polished on the wax tool (C). The steel button is held and rotated by a steel pin (D) held in the head (E) of the polisher

PERIPHERAL CURVES

The next stage is to generate the secondary and peripheral curves using fine diamond-coated tools (*Figure 22.11*, right-hand side) which give a high degree of accuracy. With hard lenses, water or paraffin is used as a lubricant. The BCOD and peripheral diameters are measured using a band measuring magnifier (*Figure 22.12*) and a skilled

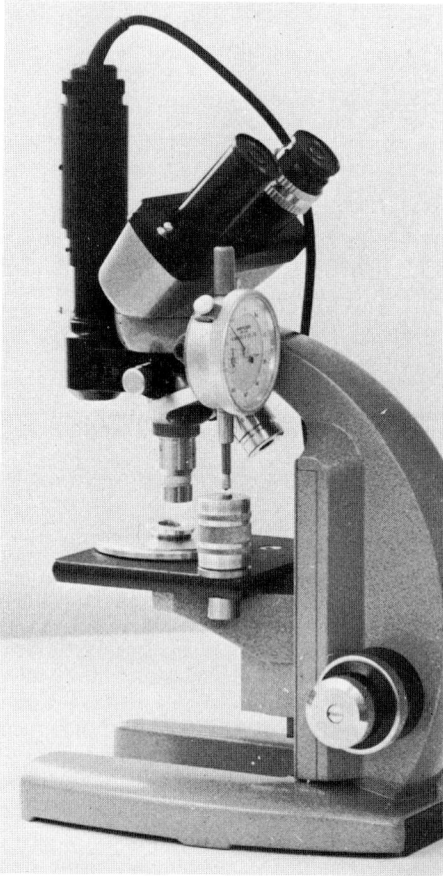

Figure 22.11–Set of chucks. From left to right; two edging chucks (convex and concave tips); hollow and solid front surface chucks; unmounted and mounted stepped buttons; diamond impregnated generating tool. Radius of curvature is engraved on each tool where appropriate

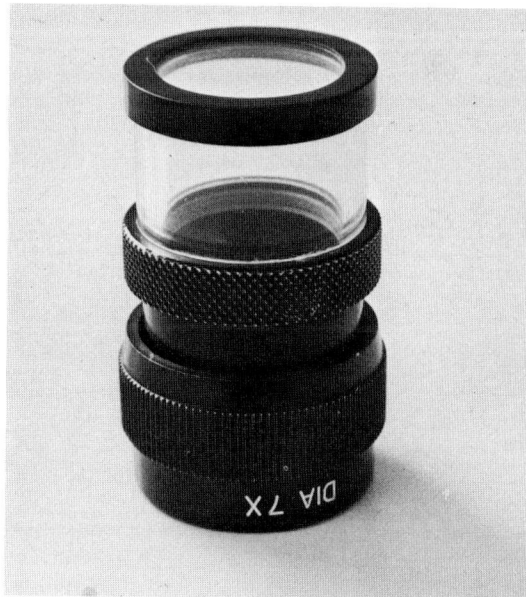

Figure 22.10–Radiuscope set for checking the back central optic radius

22.8 and 22.9) using a double rotation technique; the movements involved are as follows.

(1) The wax polisher rotates clockwise on a vertical spindle.

(2) The angled steel pin describes an anti-clockwise movement.

(3) The head oscillates from side to side.

(4) The blank rotates due to friction.

The polish for hard lenses is concentrated Silvo (*Reckitt and Colman*), most of the surplus ammonia having been drained off. For gas permeable materials, such as CAB, Polycon and Boston, an ammonia-free polish is used (X-Pal, Alox-PG, Alumina, dissolved in water or silicone oil).

The finish of the surface is checked using a high powered loupe ($\times 10$), and the radius checked on a radiuscope (*Figure 22.10*) to an accuracy exceeding 0.01 mm. The radius can be adjusted by polishing for longer periods and recutting the wax polisher to make any necessary allowances.

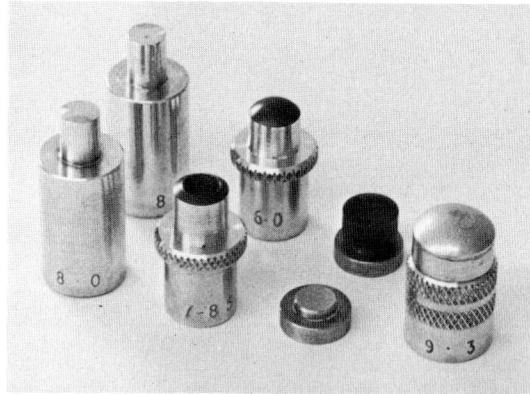

Figure 22.12–Band measuring magnifier. The upper surface has a scale engraved on it in 0.1 mm divisions

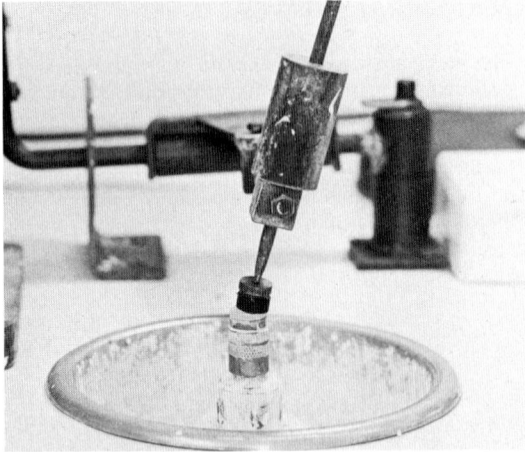

Figure 22.13–Generating back peripheral curves

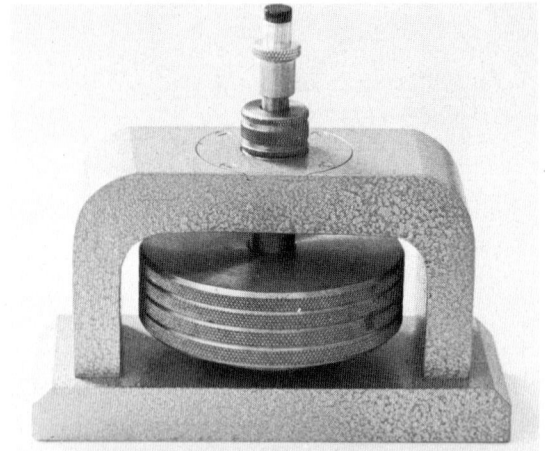

Figure 22.14–Blank mounted on a front surface chuck on a centring device

technician can control the diameters to within ±0.05 mm. These peripheral curves are generated on the semi-finished blank (*Figure 22.13*). This technique ensures that the peripheral curve exactly matches the diamond tool. Some laboratories grind these curves after generating the front curves, using a suction holder to grip the lens. If the lens is to be as thin as it should be, the latter procedure allows it to flex and flatten slightly under the pressure of grinding and polishing, and the result is a peripheral curve that becomes steeper than required once the pressure is removed, and which may also be distorted.

Once the peripheral curves have been generated many laboratories polish them using a tape-covered polisher (instead of a wax tool) on a double rotation polishing machine. If the practitioner asks for them to be well blended some laboratories merely over-run the polishing, thus blurring the transitions, not, in fact, removing the apices of the transitions. This results in a back surface with relatively sharp transitions which are more prone to causing phy-

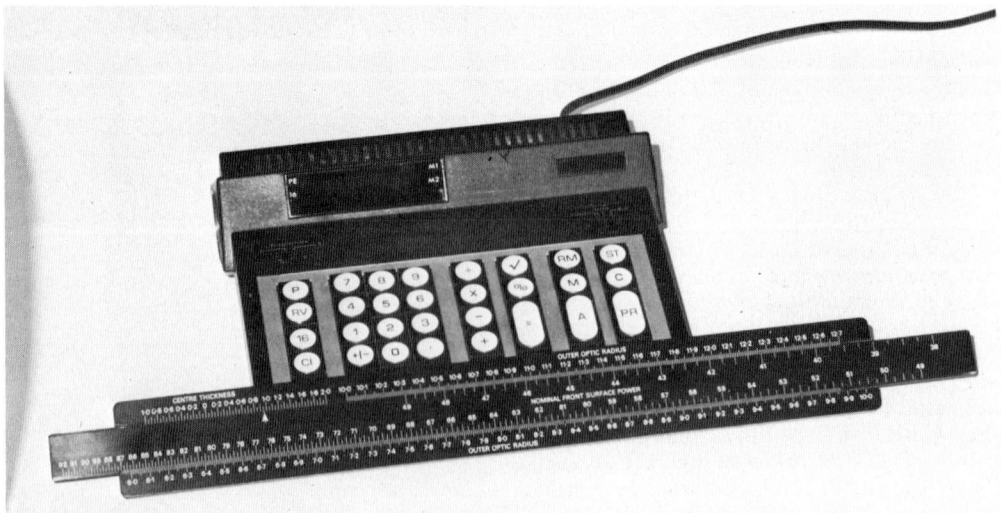

Figure 22.15–Contact lens slide-rule in front of a programmable calculator

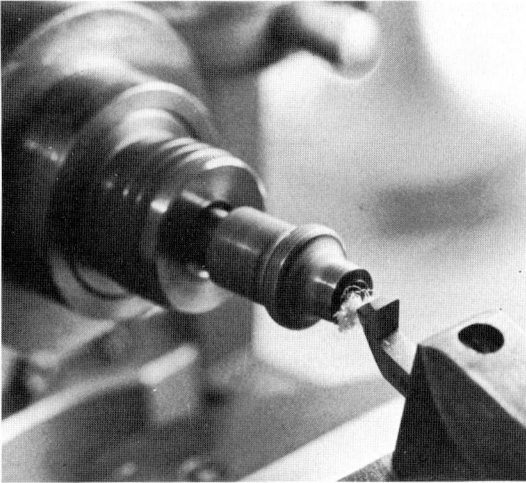

Figure 22.16–Cutting the front surface

siological problems since they cause an effectively 'tight' fitting periphery to the lens (*see* Chapter 11, Volume 1). Thus, poor tears exchange under the lens may result, and turbulence of the tears resulting in bubbles with consequent dimpling of the corneal epithelium.

The author feels that the correct procedure is to leave the peripheral curves unpolished until the very last stage of production, when polishing, blending and edging can be done accurately in one stage. This has the advantage that the surface of the peripheral zone, which is the bearing surface in the next stage of production, will not sustain any permanent damage in the following procedures, whereas if it is fully polished and blended, fine scratches may develop during the next stages and such scratches are likely to go unnoticed and hence unrectified by the laboratory.

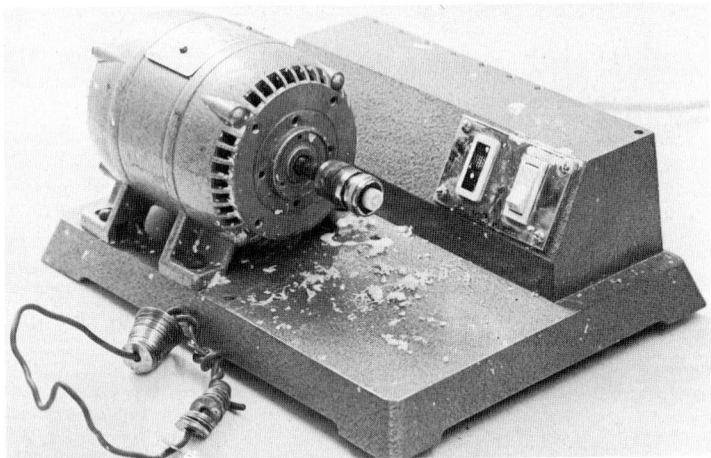

Figure 22.17–Front surface wax polisher mounted for cutting. Also shown are male templates threaded on flex in the foreground

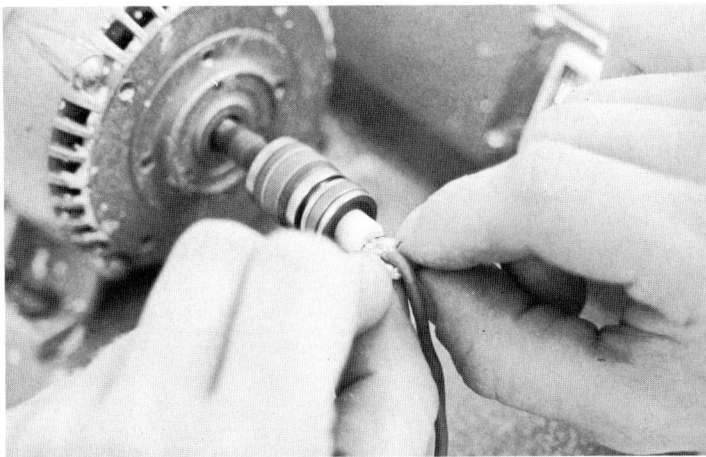

Figure 22.18–Close-up of cutting front surface wax polishing tool using a male template

CUTTING FRONT SURFACES

The blank is removed from the stepped button, cleaned and the centre thickness recorded. It is then mounted by its back surface on a hot hollow chuck (*Figure 22.11*) using wax as an adhesive (normally a solid chuck is used for soft and gas permeable materials; this is necessary with soft materials because the forces that are introduced during the cutting and polishing may cause the optic portion of the lens to drop if a hollow chuck is used). The blank is centred on a vertical spindle or special rotating centring device as shown in *Figure 22.14* by watching the reflected image of a strip light seen in the rotating back surface edge adjacent to the chuck, and not the flat top. The front surface power required is calculated using a special slide-rule or a programmable calculator (*Figure 22.15*) and hence the front optic radius determined. The hollow chuck is placed on the taper of the front surface lathe and the front optic radius is cut using a diamond tool, the

blank being reduced to the required centre thickness in the process (*Figure 22.16*). At this stage any lenticulation of positive powered lenses has to be carried out. With hard positive lenses it is usual to put on a 'negative' front surface carrier curve such as a −10.00 D or −15.00 D curve (that is, to give the peripheral zone this power) which will facilitate lid attachment and thus assist greatly in stabilizing the lens; or alternatively, a front surface carrier curve which is parallel with the back peripheral surface (*see* Chapter 11, Volume 1, page 266). The determination of these curves is made easier if a cross-section of the lens is drawn out to scale (*see* Chapter 4, Volume 1, page 136).

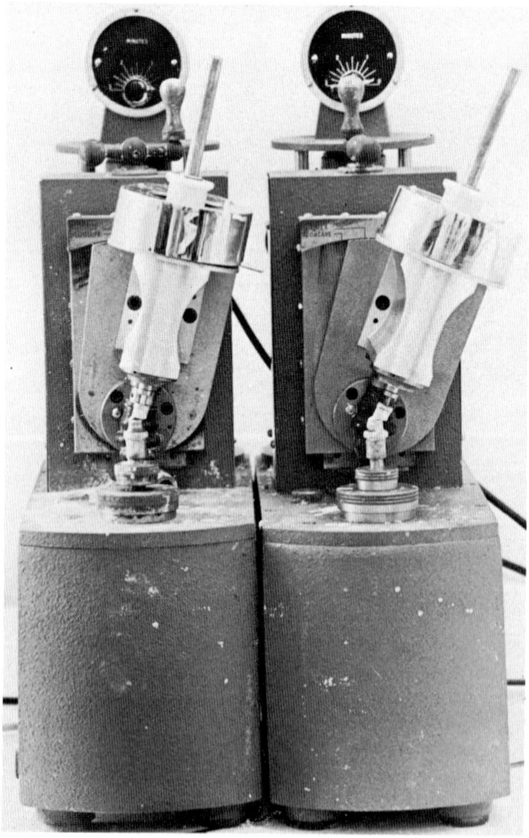

POLISHING FRONT SURFACES

Finally, the lenticulation on a positive lens is polished while the lens is still on the lathe. For hard lenses this is done by hand use of a chamois leather impregnated with Silvo. The lens and hollow chuck are then removed from the lathe. A front surface wax polisher is cut using steel male gauges to obtain the correct radius (*Figure 22.17* and *22.18*). The sharp edge of the wax polisher is now removed and a small central recess made to retain the polishing liquid. For hard lenses the front optic is then polished on the double rotation polishing machine (*Figure 22.19*) using this small wax polisher and Silvo (*Figure 22.20*). The movements executed during this polishing process are the same as those for back surface polishing (*see* page 621).

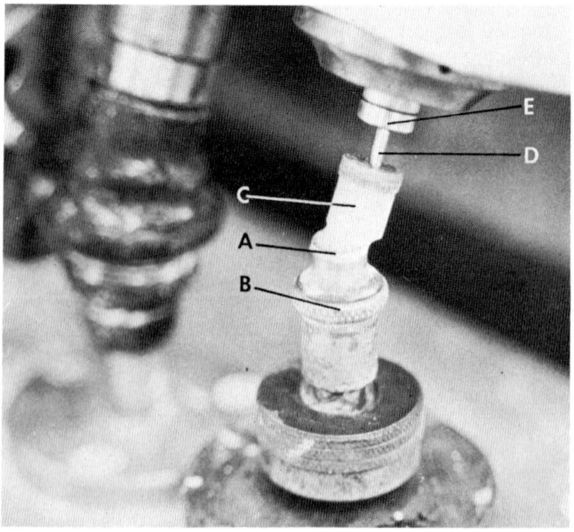

Figure 22.19–Polishing the front surface using automatic front surface polishing machines. Detail is shown in Figure 22.20

Figure 22.20–Close-up of polishing the front surface. The blank (A) mounted on its steel button (B) being polished on the wax tool (C). The steel button is held and rotated by a steel pin (D) held in the head (E) of the polisher

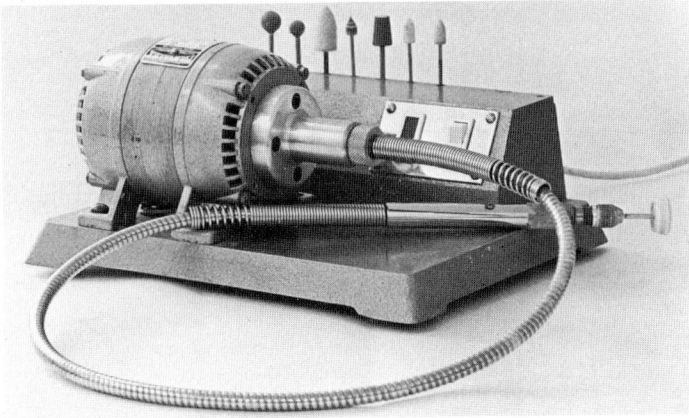

Figure 22.21–A flexible drive unit with a felt wheel mounted in the chuck

With negative lenses the optic is polished before lenticulating; this is because it is difficult to control the power accurately once the front periphery of the lens has been removed (*see* Power Adjustments, page 634). It is usually better to lenticulate negative lenses by hand so that a gradually changing curve can be formed ending in the correct edge thickness. This is done by removing material with a razor blade while the lens, which is still mounted on the hollow chuck, is rotating on the vertical spindle of the edging bench. It requires a skilled and experienced technician to be able to judge the correct thickness across the peripheral surface. This lenticulation is then polished with a felt wheel in a flexible drive (*Figure 22.21*) while the lens rotates on the vertical spindle (*Figure 22.22*).

While polishing the front optic, the power of the lens could, if necessary, be altered by several

dioptres, although the greater the shift in power the poorer the focimeter reading is likely to be (*see* Power Adjustments, page 634).

The edge of a soft lens is formed and polished on the lathe while the lens is mounted on the front surface chuck. It is necessary to do so at this stage

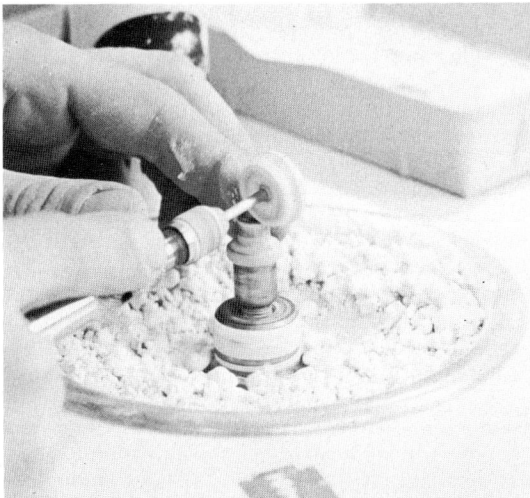

Figure 22.22–Polishing the 'cut-down' on a negative lenticular lens, using the felt wheel in the flexible drive handpiece

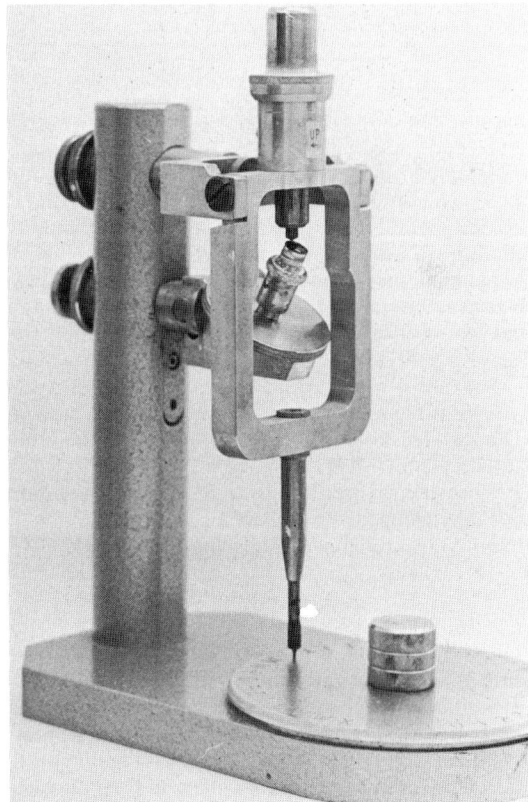

Figure 22.23–Engraving the front surface of a lens using the pantograph system

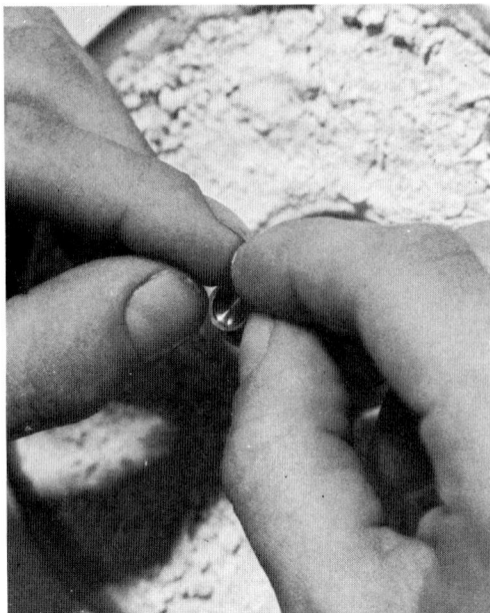

Figure 22.24–Centring a lens on an edging chuck using forefingers and thumbs

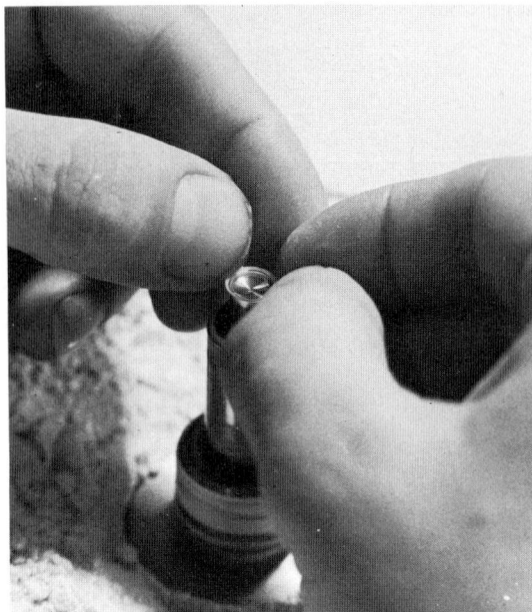

Figure 22.25–Centring a lens on an edging chuck: the reflections from the back surface must remain stationary as the lens rotates

because the dehydrated soft lens material is fragile and needs adequate support to stop it chipping.

After polishing the front surface, and while the lens is still on the chuck, any necessary engraving is carried out (*Figure 22.23*). Engraving is usually confined to hard lenses because of the possibility of weakening the structure of a soft lens and also because the risk of mucoprotein binding to the uneven surface would be increased (although the engraving of a hard lens also attracts grease).

The lens is removed from the chuck and the wax cleaned off in an ultrasonic bath containing paraffin. The hard lens is now ready for edging, and polishing and blending of its peripheral curves, while the soft lens has to be hydrated in 0.9 per cent saline solution and later cleaned in a hypertonic wetting solution to remove any remaining polishing compound.

EDGE SHAPING

Edging, polishing and blending are the most difficult procedures in making a hard lens, and the success or otherwise of the lens is largely decided at this point.

The dry lens is mounted with wax on a hot chuck, the concave surface being uppermost. The hot chuck is then transferred to a rotating vertical spindle, and centring, which should be extremely accurate so as not to offset the lens, is achieved by steadying the rotating lens between the thumb and index finger of both hands (*Figures 22.24* and *22.25*). If the reflection of an overhead spotlight or striplight from the rotating surface is seen to be steady then the lens is centred correctly. It is then left to cool so that the wax sets with the lens correctly centred.

Any reduction of overall size and shaping of the edge is done by arching a razor blade around the rotating lens, starting on the back surface and working onto the lower front surface (*Figure 22.26a, b* and *c*). Care has to be taken not to cut into the peripheral curve on the back surface and to hold the razor blade so that it trails against the edge, that is, with its edge facing in the direction of travel to avoid nicking the edge. The shape and thickness are checked by observing the edge with a high powered loupe ($\times 10$) and the overall size is measured using a micrometer gauge (*Figures 22.27* and *22.28*). The edge surface is smoothed off using a conical-shaped carborundum stone which is rolled around the rotating edge of the lens (*Figure 22.29a–e*). The edge surface is again inspected before polishing.

As a practitioner, the author feels the ideal edge shape for a hard lens is as in *Figure 22.30*; this type of edge will not be damaged so easily from handling as one with its apex towards the back of the lens. The final edge shape will be influenced to a certain extent by the peripheral curves and hence the thickness of material available.

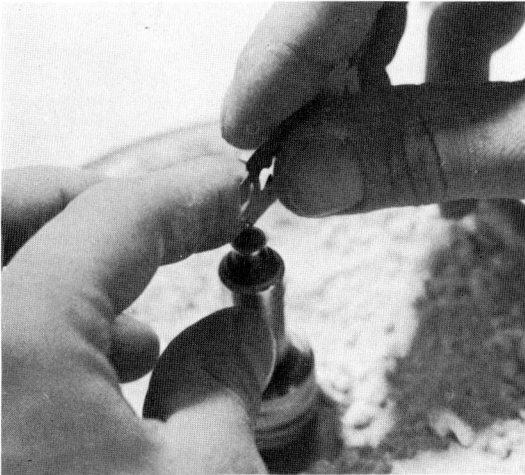

(a)

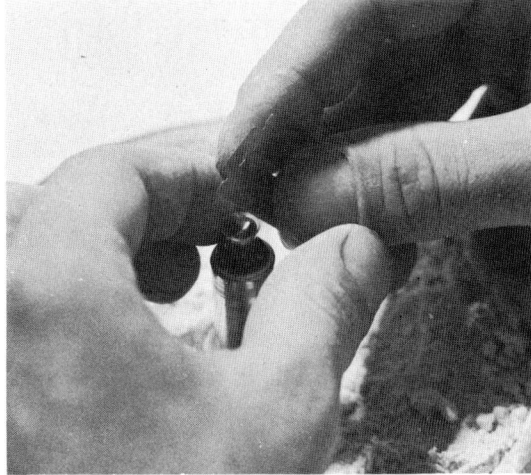

(b)

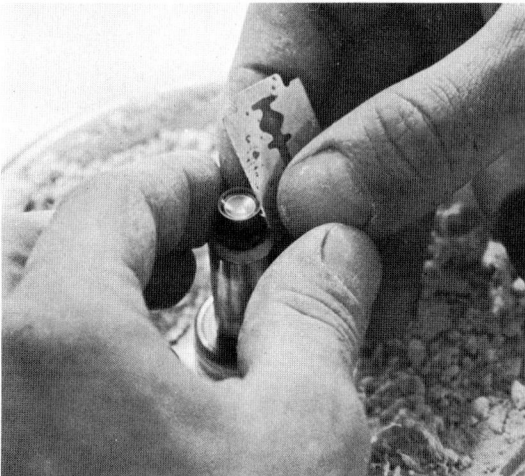

(c)

Figure 22.26–Reducing overall size and edge shaping with a razor blade: (a), (b) and (c) show successive positions of the trailing cutting edge of the blade

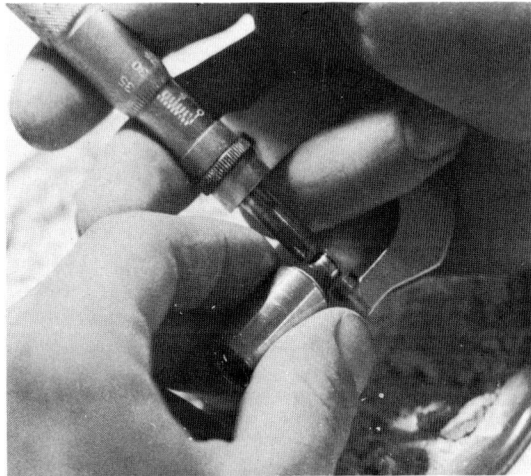

Figure 22.27–Checking the overall size with a micrometer gauge

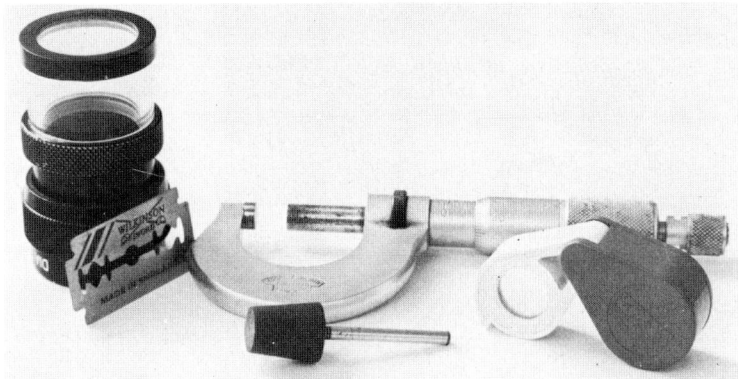

Figure 22.28–Tools for edging and checking. From left to right; band measuring magnifier, razor blade, micrometer gauge, conical carborundum tool, ×10 loupe

628

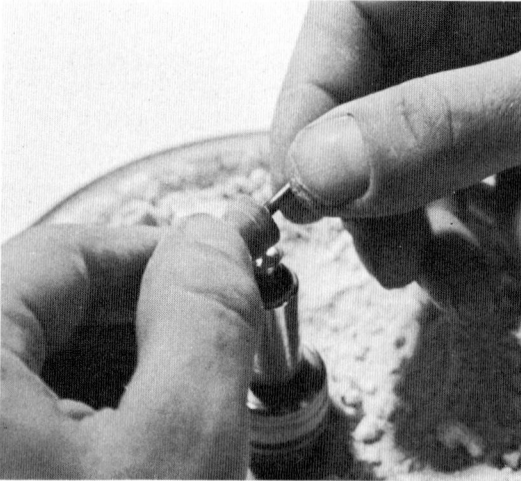

(a)

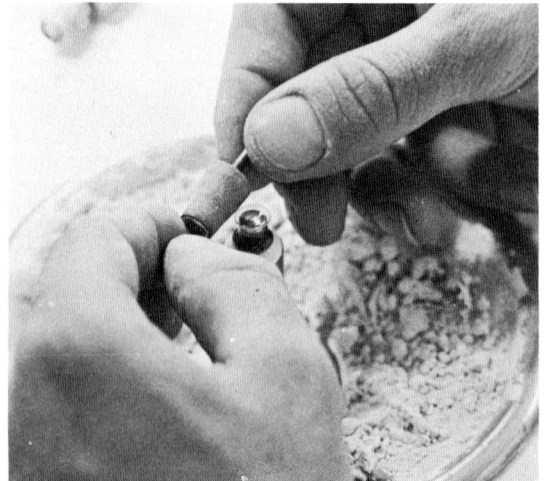

(d)

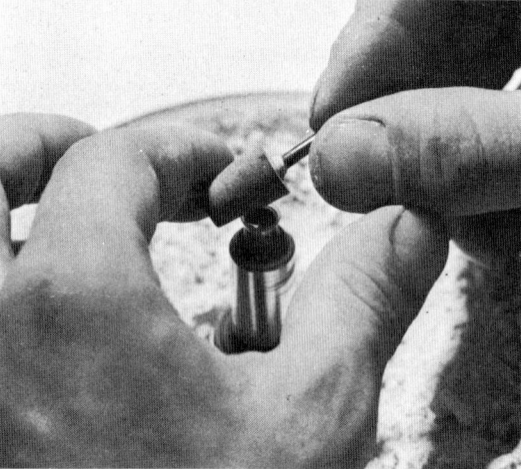

(b)

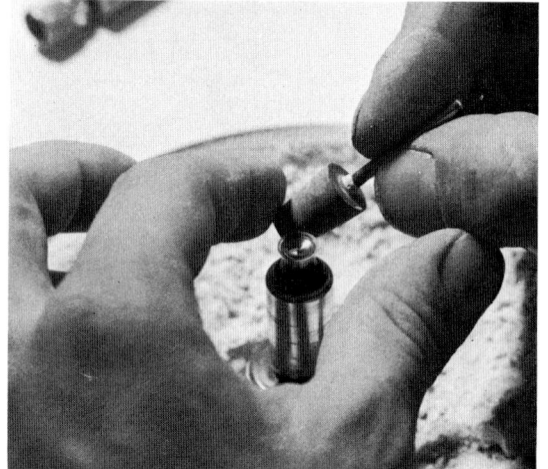

(e)

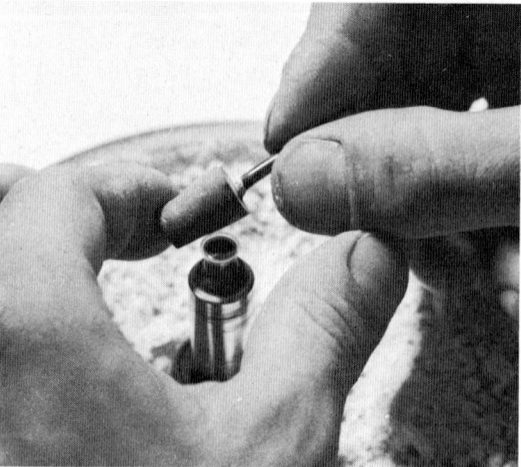

(c)

Figure 22.29–Shaping and smoothing the edge with a conical carborundum stone. The stone is carefully 'rolled' around the lens edge: (a)–(e) show successive positions of the conical tool

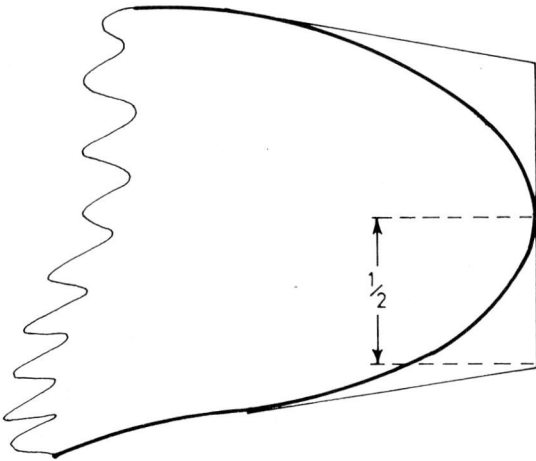

Figure 22.30–The author's ideal edge shape shown in cross-section

POLISHING AND BLENDING PERIPHERAL CURVES

The peripheral curves are now ready to be blended and polished. With the lens still mounted on the edging chuck so that it is held firmly by the wax and will not flex, the apices of the transitions are removed. This is done with wax tools, each cut to the required radius, usually one-third to midway between the two adjacent curves. The wax tool is mounted on the vertical spindle and the lens/edging-chuck combination is allowed to rotate and at the same time is oscillated to and fro on top of the polishing tool (*Figure 22.31*). The lens is periodically inspected using a ×10 loupe, and when all the transitions have been blended (to whatever degree has been requested by the practitioner) all the remaining peripheral curves are polished and blended using a progression of felt tools (*Figure 22.32*) so as to obtain a gradual and continuing flow of curves. Thus, as near as is possible, a continuous curve lens is then produced but with the advantage that the original curves are known and can thus be altered at a later stage if modification becomes necessary.

EDGE POLISHING

Finally, the edge has to be polished. With the lens still on the edging chuck and placed back on the taper of a vertical spindle with the concave side uppermost, this is done by wrapping a chamois leather around the index finger and a forwards and backwards movement is made across the top of the lens edge, the chamois leather being soaked in Silvo (*Figure 22.33*). The ball of the finger is then rolled around and under the edge of the lens as shown in *Figure 22.34a–d*. These two procedures remove material from the inner or more central part of the edge of the lens to the apex of the edge. When the inner or back edge of the lens is fully polished the

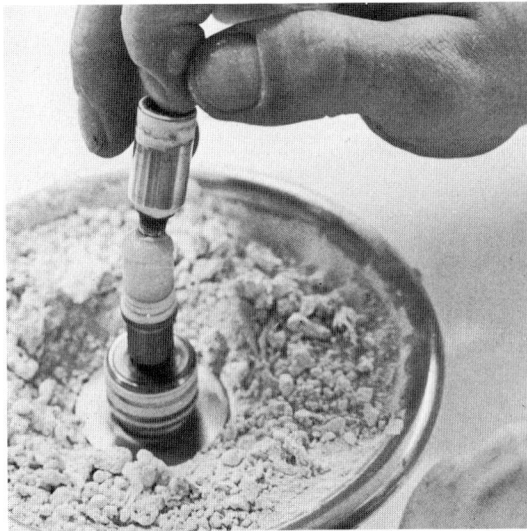

Figure 22.31–Blending transitions by removing their apices on a wax tool

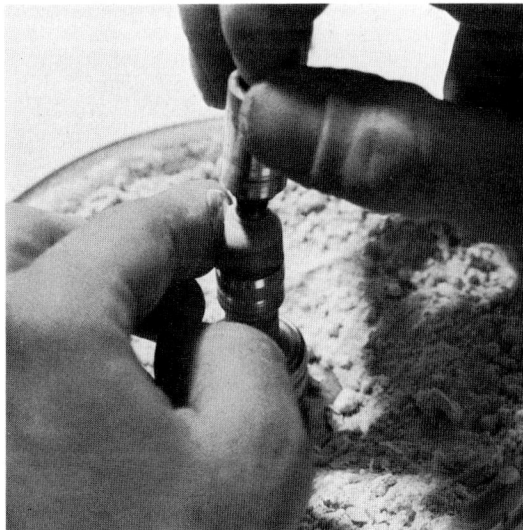

Figure 22.32–Blending of transitions and polishing of peripheral curves may be done with felt tools in this manner

630

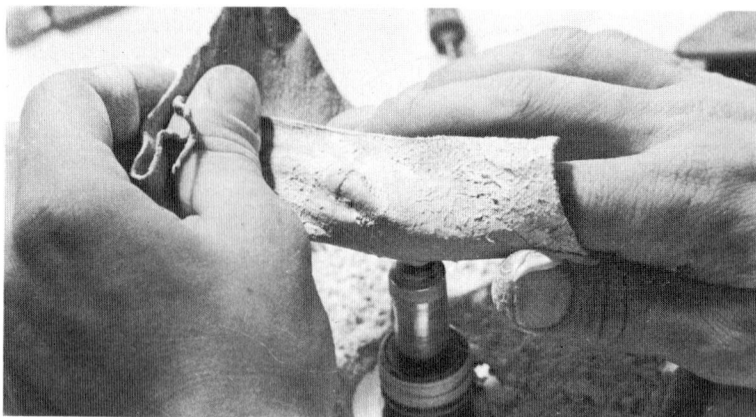

Figure 22.33–Starting to polish the edge of a corneal lens with a Silvo-soaked chamois leather moving the finger forwards and backwards across the lens edge with its back surface uppermost

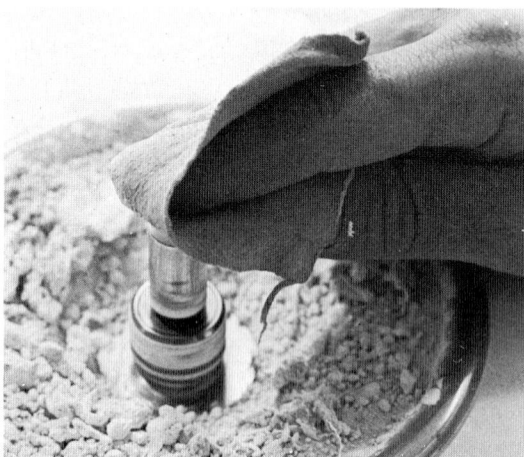

(a)

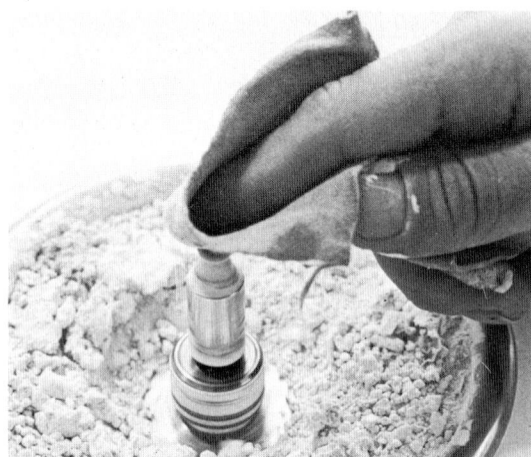

(b)

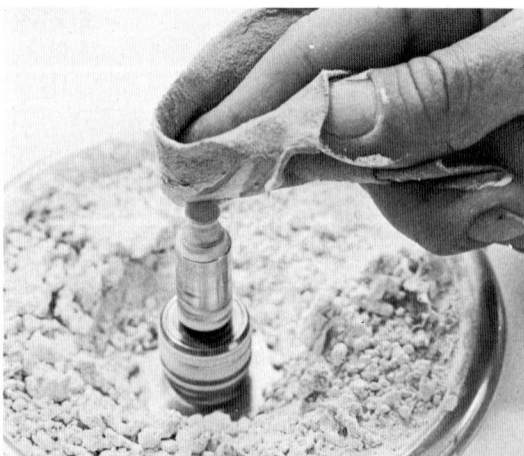

(c)

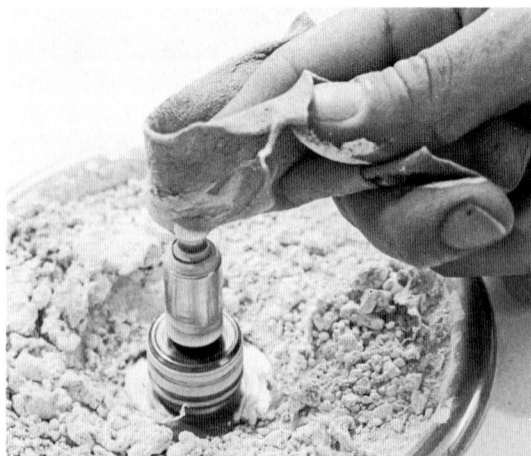

(d)

Figure 22.34–Polishing the edge of a lens – concave surface uppermost. The chamois leather is rolled over the edge of the lens on the ball of the finger as shown in the successive photographs (a)–(d)

lens is cleaned and remounted the other way round on a convex edging chuck. The outer or front edge of the lens is polished in a similar manner (*Figure 22.35a–d*). The lens is removed from the edging chuck and cleaned in paraffin. Some laboratories use a series of hollow cone tools of varying angles to shape and polish the edge (*see* Chapter 23). These rotate on a vertical spindle and the edge shape and polish is produced by running the lens inside each tool for a specific time. Alternatively, many laboratories use an automatic edge polisher. The lens is held by a suction cup and rotated on a revolving sponge containing Silvo. While neither procedure gives the best results, the latter technique usually means that the edge is polished, but not correctly shaped; thus, the lens may have a polished square edge. The edge may also be polished by hand on a rotating chamois or velveteen-covered drum chuck,

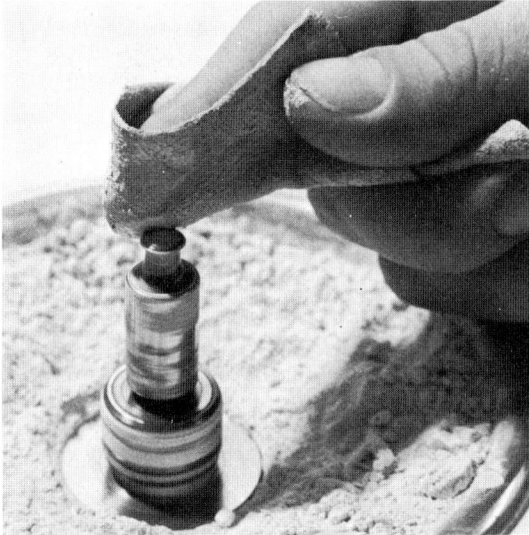

(a)

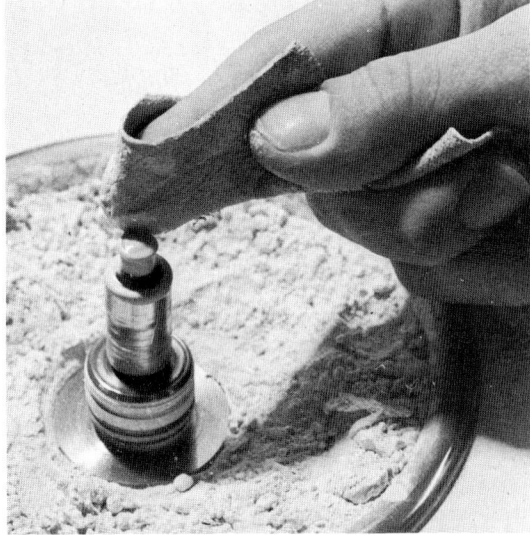

(b)

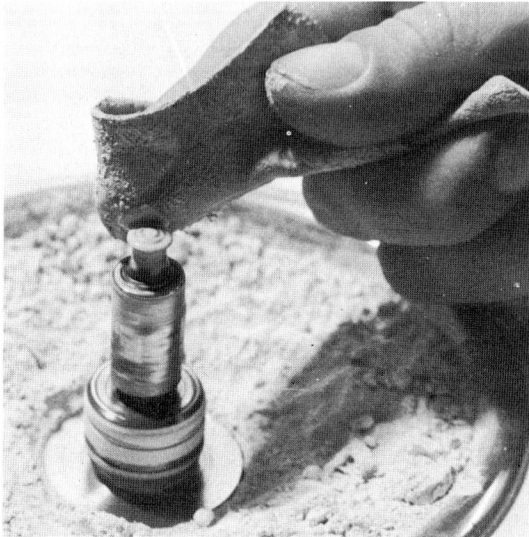

(c)

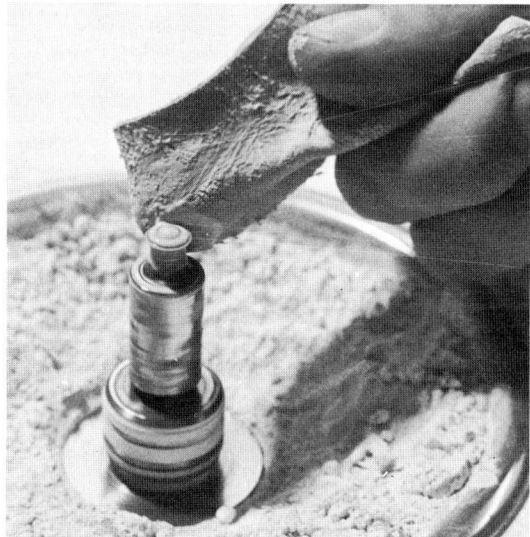

(d)

Figure 22.35–Polishing the edge of a lens, convex surface uppermost. Again the chamois leather is rolled over the edge of the lens as shown in the successive pictures (a)–(d)

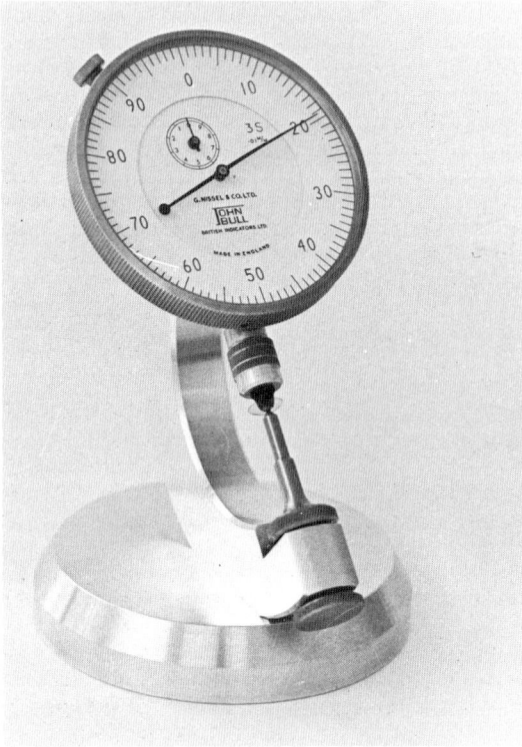

Figure 22.36–Checking centre thickness using a dial gauge marked with 0.01 mm divisions

the lens being held on some type of suction device and rotated by hand with first the concave and then the convex surface facing the direction of rotation of the drum. This is followed by apical polishing of the edge with the lens rotated parallel to the edge of the drum. There seems to be no better way of shaping and polishing the edge of a lens than by the hand of a skilled technician. Unlike a machine, he is able to observe the lens constantly and make allowances for the different thickness of individual prescription lenses.

The finished lens is dried, inspected for surface blemishes and finally its specification is checked. Thickness checking is shown in *Figure 22.36*.

SOFT LENS FABRICATION

Lathe-cut soft lenses are produced in an almost identical manner to hard lenses. The variations, other than those already mentioned, are few but important.

Because the lens is formed in the dehydrated state any error in tolerance will be increased by a multiple of the linear expansion ratio. Thus, an environment which will cause the lens to start to hydrate before completion of its fabrication has to be avoided. Contrary to popular belief, this does not usually mean excessive environmental humidity control. However, extremes of humidity and temperature will have an effect on manufacture just as they do with hard lens fabrication. Of course, it does mean

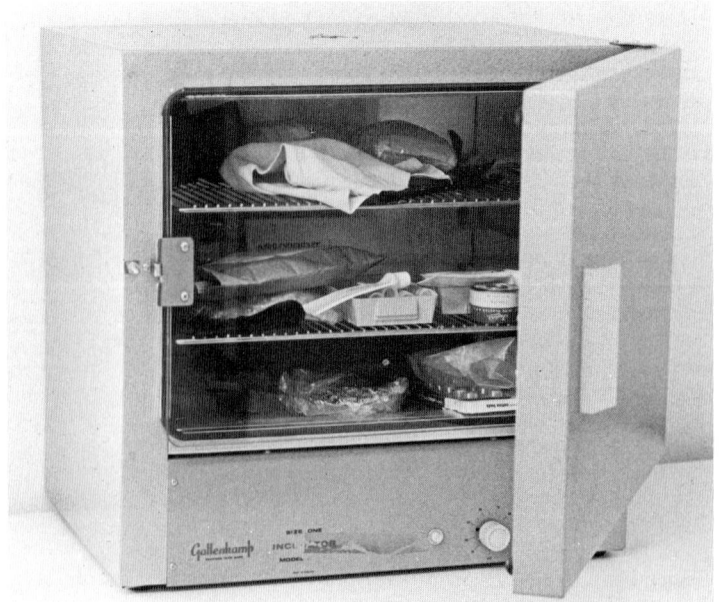

Figure 22.37–An incubator for storing soft lens blanks and related materials

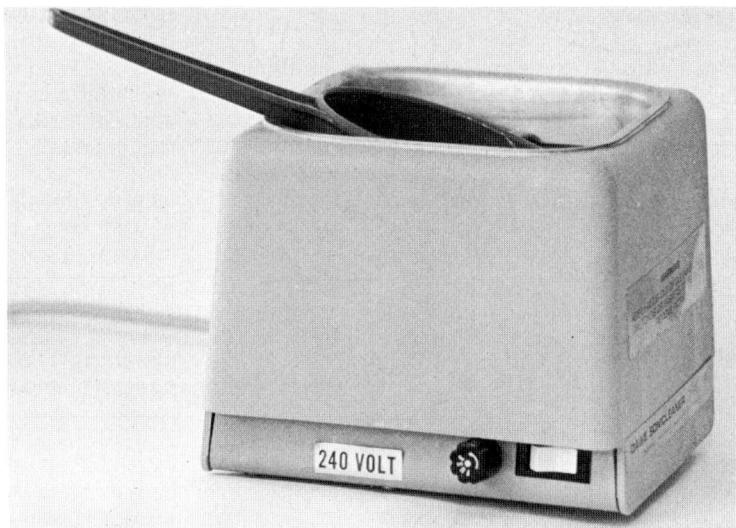

Figure 22.38–An ultrasonic cleaner for removing wax and grease from tools and lenses

that all materials that come into direct contact with the lens must be completely free from moisture, and this is achieved by storing such articles as polish, polishing tape, chamois leathers, cotton wool and so on, in an incubator (*Figure 22.37*), and only removing small quantities at the time they are required for use in the laboratory. The polish has to be free of all water and thus a grease based medium has been developed. Additionally, if there is a pause in manufacture, the lens blank should be sealed in an air-tight tube which has previously been stored in the incubator. The technicians must take great care not to breathe over the lens nor to touch the surface with their skin. If any of these precautions are not taken the surface starts to hydrate prematurely and, besides affecting the final hydrated parameters, the surface finish is poor resulting in areas which may be relatively hydrophobic. Equally, dust has to be kept to an absolute minimum so that the surface finish is perfect.

The dehydrated lens has to be cleaned in an ultrasonic bath of paraffin (*Figure 22.38*) and is then hydrated in sterile normal (0.9 per cent) saline solution. The hydration time varies with the type of polymer. Many of the HEMA materials, once fabricated, have to be boiled in saline solution, then boiled in a diluted alkaline solution and finally boiled in normal saline solution – the whole process is aimed at removing any residual monomers which may be toxic to the ocular tissue. With most of the higher water content lenses such as lenses manufactured from Duragel materials and the Sauflon range (made from PMMA and VP), this procedure is not necessary as the residual monomer content is insignificantly small and this quantity will be removed during the autoclaving stage. Following

hydration the lens should be checked. *Figure 22.39* shows a wet cell radiuscope. Other items used for checking are described in Chapter 15.

Practitioners are also reminded of the effect of *average* lens thickness on oxygen transmissibility and hence corneal metabolism both at the time of lens ordering as checking (*see* Addendum).

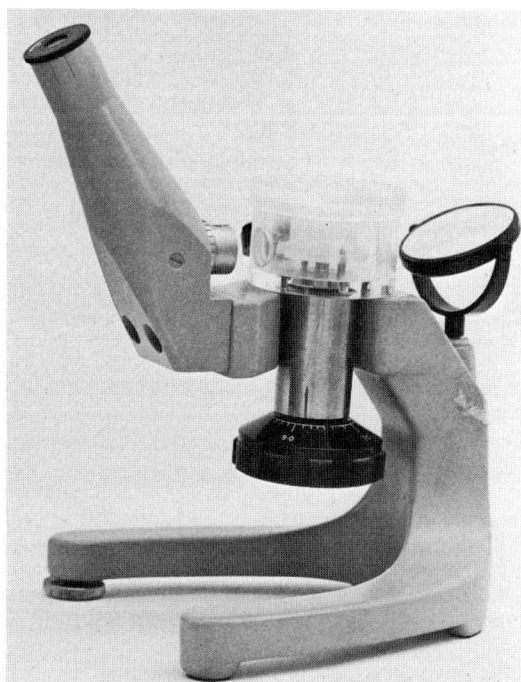

Figure 22.39–A wet-cell radiuscope for checking soft lens radii

Sterilization

The only satisfactory way of sterilizing a soft lens is by autoclaving (*Figure 22.40*). Asepticization by chemicals or boiling is not, in the present day, an acceptable procedure as there may be a significant time delay before the lens is actually used, and microorganisms may survive simple disinfection by forming spores. Besides being in the patient's best interest it should be remembered that it is also in the practitioner's best interest, for it is he who is in the litigation front line.

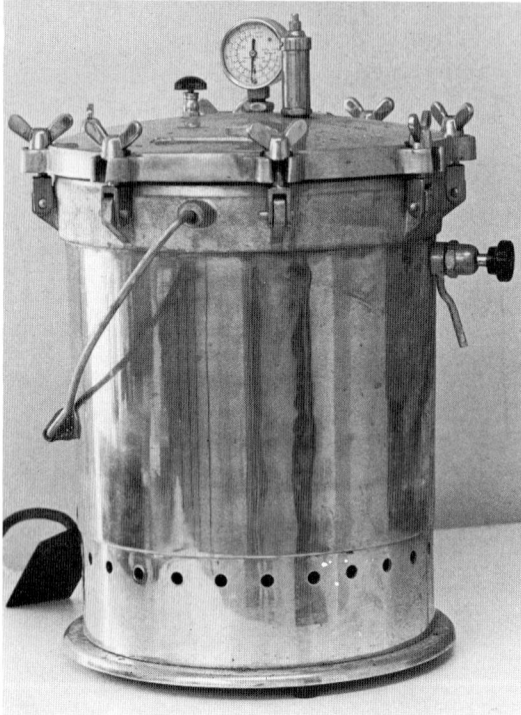

Figure 22.40–A very basic and inexpensive autoclave

The autoclave is thus an essential tool, not only for the laboratory, but also for the practitioner (Litvin, 1977). A few words of advice on its usage are therefore appropriate.

(1) Isotonic saline solution should always be used, never solutions containing preservatives.

(2) Ensure that the bottles are only three-quarters full, thereby avoiding a build-up of excess pressure which will force off the caps.

(3) The caps must be screwed on tightly and ideally held with a 'sterile' shrink-sealing band.

(4) The practitioner must ensure that the lens material will not be damaged by the high temperature of autoclaving.

POWER ADJUSTMENTS TO HARD LENSES BY THE LABORATORY

When the lens is being fabricated the power can be adjusted at the polishing stage, subject to certain requirements. On a lenticulated positive lens it is almost impossible to add plus power without ending up with a double optic, whereas adding minus power is very much easier. The reason for this is the relative difficulty in removing material at varying rates from the different areas of the optic, all of which is necessary to bring about these power changes. *Figure 22.41* shows a lenticulated positive lens in cross-section. In the case of adding positive power, material has to be removed from the periphery of the optic and it can be seen from *Figure 22.41a* that the lenticulation prevents a proper sweep across the lens surface. This means the polisher cannot even out the bands which are formed when the removal of material from this area has taken place. However, when adding negative power the majority of material is removed from the centre of the lens with hardly any from the periphery

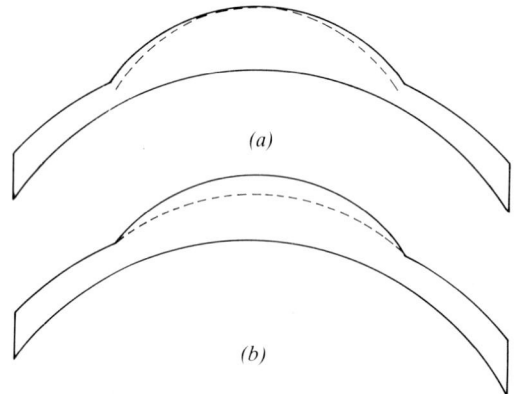

Figure 22.41–Power adjustments to positive lenticulated lenses. The broken lines represent areas where material is removed. (a) Adding plus power. (b) Adding minus power

of the optic as shown in *Figure 22.41b*. Thus, the bands which have formed can be blended into one another to produce a single optic.

With a negative lens the power can be altered either by adding positive or negative power provided that the lens has not been lenticulated and that there is sufficient thickness of material at the removal regions. *Figure 22.42a* and *b* shows the areas where material has to be removed. Once a negative lens has been lenticulated it is difficult to adjust its power accurately because the polishing button drops over the edge of the optic and, again, it becomes difficult to blend the polishing bands into one another.

The alteration of a patient's hard lens involves the above difficulties, but if the lens is thin in the centre, as with negative lenses, it is extremely difficult to re-centre the lens correctly on the hollow chuck. With a lens which is so thin, no pressure can be used to re-centre it on the hollow chuck without causing distortion. If this happens the lens is held in this distorted manner and the distortion or irregularity polished off the front surface, only to find on releasing the lens from the chuck that it relaxes back to an equal but opposite distortion of the front surface and hence a resultant poor power reading. The use of a polishing drum (see Chapter 23) for power modification has similar inherent problems and its use frequently results in a poor power reading. The real answer to this problem lies with the practitioner. First and foremost he should have good quality diagnostic fitting lenses with a comprehensive range of powers. Secondly, if the lens

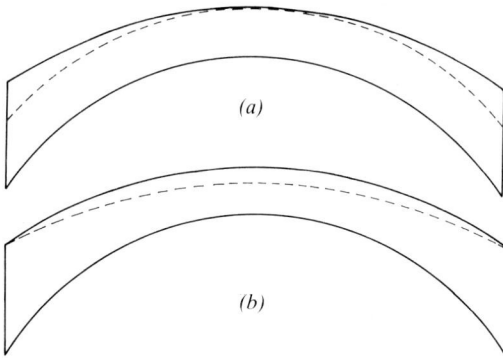

Figure 22.42–Power adjustments to negative lenses. The broken lines represent areas where material is removed. (a) Adding plus power. (b) Adding minus power

requires a power alteration it is usually better to order a new one, the old lens adding to the practitioner's fitting set of prescription lenses. Practitioner modifications are best restricted to altering the overall size, edge shape, optic diameters and peripheral curves; interfering with the optic, front or back, does not result in a good lens.

TORIC LENSES

Concave and convex toroidal surfaces can be produced by crimping, polishing or generating.

Crimping

To produce a toroidal back surface a concave spherical surface is first cut and polished with its radius midway between the required radii. The

blank is cut with a central thickness of approximately 0.20 mm and a diameter of 0.20 mm above its final requirement. An outer stepped rim at the base of the blank is formed on which to apply the pressure during crimping. The blank is placed concave surface uppermost in the small crimping tool (*Figure 22.43*) which applies pressure at four points on the

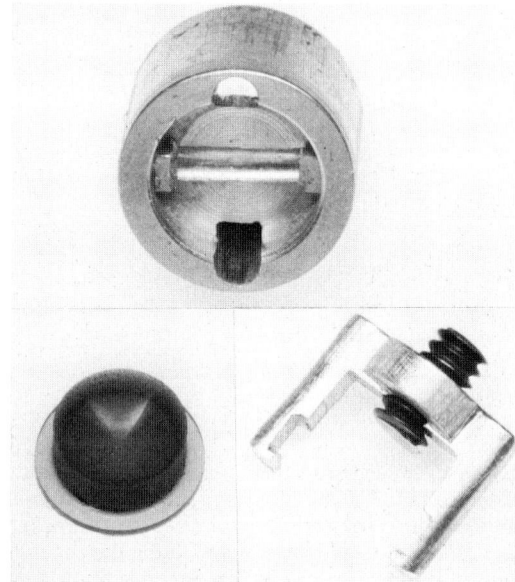

Figure 22.43–A simple crimping tool showing its three component parts, and a lens blank with an outer stepped rim, in place for crimping

stepped rim – two points along the one meridian to flatten the radius and the other two points at right-angles to steepen the radius. The amount of toricity is then produced by altering the pressure until the required difference between the radii is achieved. The toroidal surface thus produced is then checked on the radiuscope. The blank, still held in the crimping tool, is then re-cut on the lathe to produce a spherical curve midway between the required radii. After polishing, the blank is released from the crimping tool and forms into a toroidal surface.

A similar procedure is used to produce a toroidal front surface. However, it is necessary to cut a curve on the back of the blank before crimping, although this does not require polishing. This back curve is necessary to reduce the amount of pressure required to flex the lens. Once the toroidal front surface is completed the final back surface has to be produced. At the same time any prism necessary for stabilizing the lens has to be incorporated, as well as reducing the blank to the required thickness of the finished lens.

Polishing

This involves creating a toroidal surface by hand polishing and is usually confined to the front surface of the lens. The lens has to be finished on both surfaces and mounted on a hollow chuck. A positive cylinder is then polished on using a felt wheel which

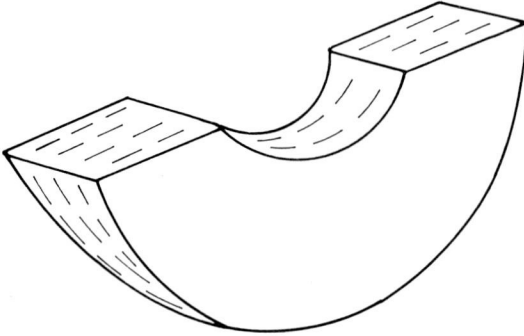

Figure 22.44–Half a felt tool with central cut-out for hand polishing a toroidal front surface

has been cut across its diameter and a radius cut out of its centre, giving the appearance of a female cutting gauge shown in *Figure 22.44*. An allowance has to be made initially when working the spherical power as some negative sphere is added at the same time as the positive cylinder. It requires an extremely skilled technician to obtain an acceptable result.

Generating

To obtain a toroidal concave surface a spherical curve is first cut on the blank. The toroidal curve is then generated by attaching a toric wheel to the polishing machine by means of a spindle. A fork, which holds the arms on which the blank is mounted, maintains the arms at right-angles to the spindle of the toric wheel. The whole unit then rotates together while the oscillating head of the polisher moves the blank across the axis of the toric wheel (*Figure 22.45*).

The toric wheels are usually cut from brass (*Figure 22.46*), and emery is used as an abrasive. For the more popular toric radii, diamond-coated toric wheels may be used. A wax toric wheel, which is cut in a similar manner to the brass wheel, is used for polishing (*Figure 22.47*).

The cutting of brass and wax toric wheels involves the use of a special toric lathe. The radius is cut at right-angles to the spindle axis which is displaced by the required difference between the two radii (*Figure 22.48*).

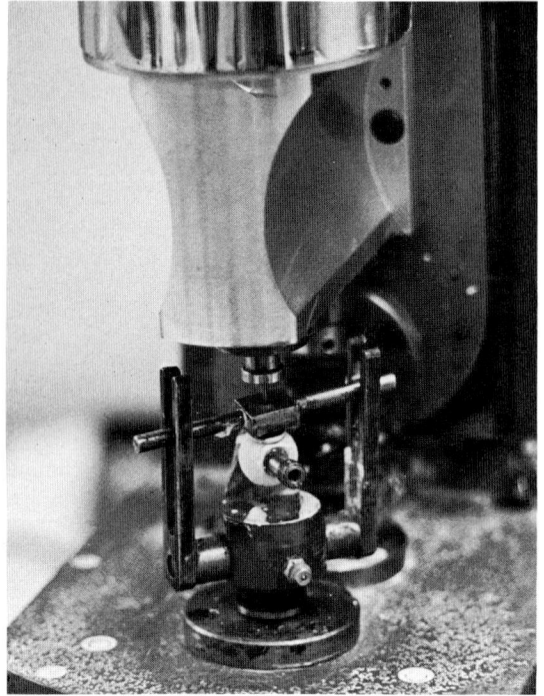

Figure 22.45–Close-up of a back surface toric polisher

Once the central curves have been generated any number of toric peripheral curves may be formed.

Generating convex toroidal surfaces poses a greater problem. To cut them on the toric lathe requires a special chuck for each lens because of the many possible combinations of power and thickness for each prescription lens. An alternative is to place the blank in the mould used for making the wax wheels. The hot wax is poured around the blank, so that the blank becomes integral with the wax wheel.

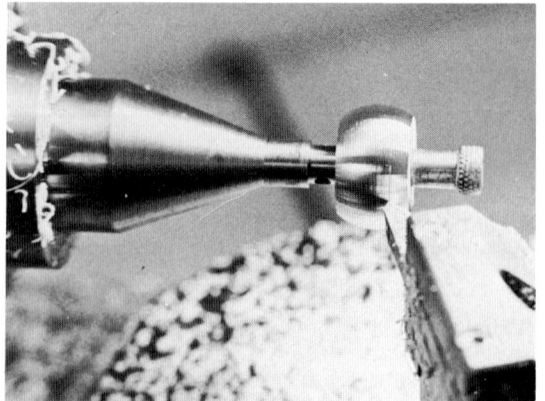

Figure 22.46–Cutting a back surface toric brass generator

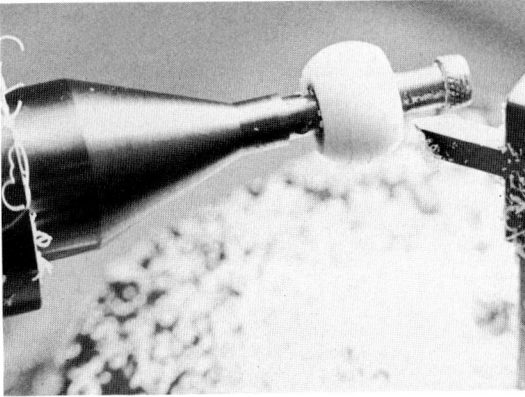

Figure 22.47–Cutting a back surface toric wax polisher

for toric soft lens production where, especially with the high water content materials, very steep radii have to be generated in the dehydrated state. These are usually too steep to cut on the toric lathe and so an extremely wide range of toric wheels, which have to be specially manufactured, are necessary, thus making the procedure very costly. Its one disadvantage is that in hard lens production it introduces strain into the lens. This does not happen with soft lenses as all strain is released on hydration.

Polishing gives varied results because it is very dependent on the skill of the technician. Its use is generally restricted to negative and low positive powered lenses, for with lenticulated positive lenses it is difficult to polish the periphery of the optic.

Generating is most definitely the best method of producing toroidal back surface hard lenses.

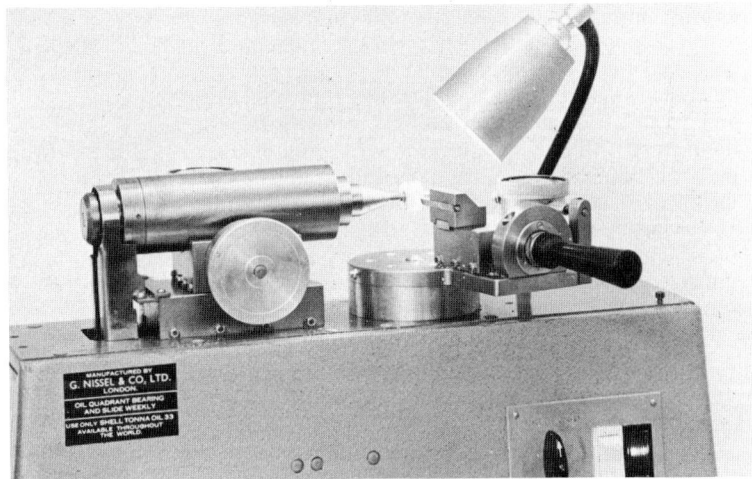

Figure 22.48–A toric lathe with wax tool in place for cutting

The wheel/blank combination is then cut to the required toricity on the toric lathe and polished using a small front surface wax polisher. This wax polisher, which is mounted on the rocker arm, has previously been moulded to the cut toroidal surface. In effect the small wax polisher takes the place of the blank on the polishing machine.

In this procedure, as with crimping front surfaces, the back surface has to be cut after the front surface has been completed.

Advantages and Disadvantages of Toric Techniques

Crimping has the advantage that a laboratory can produce a wide range of toroidal surfaces without the expense of a toric lathe. It is particularly useful

PRISMS

A prism may be incorporated into the lens either to correct a vertical extra-ocular muscle imbalance or more usually to stabilize the lens, that is, to stop it rotating on the eye.

The prism is introduced when the last surface, usually the front, is cut. Either a special hollow chuck or a prism adaptor, on which a standard front surface chuck may sit, is used for this purpose (*Figure 22.49*). The prism chuck has its face cut at an angle corresponding to the apical angle of the prism. The prism adaptor has an outer male taper which has a different axial centre line to that of its inner female taper. Thus, any standard chuck which sits on the adaptor is angled by the same amount as the apical angle of the required prism.

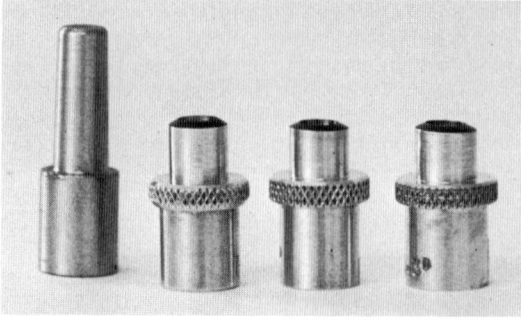

Figure 22.49–From left to right; 1½△ prism adaptor; standard hollow chuck; hollow chuck with 1½△ prism; hollow chuck with 3△ prism

WAX POLISHERS

Back and front surface polishers are made with dental or paraffin wax and magnesium carbonate, the latter acting as a very fine abrasive. Such wax polishers, their chucks, and the blocks in which they are made, are shown in *Figures 22.50* and *22.51*. In hot climates larger quantities of magnesium carbonate are required to prevent the wax from softening.

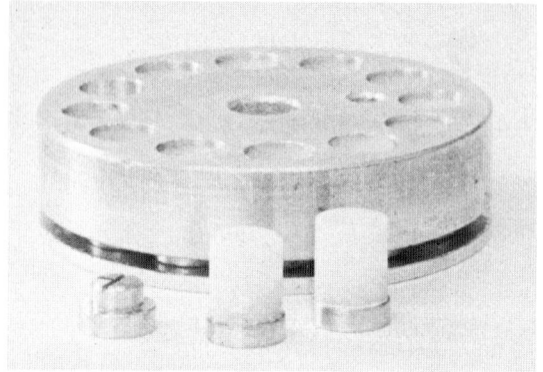

Figure 22.51–Block and chucks for casting front surface wax polishers: a basic chuck and a cut and uncut wax tool are shown in front of the block for making twelve wax tools

It is preferable to use a prism adaptor rather than a prism chuck; for after polishing the front surface, which is done with the standard chuck still mounted on the adaptor, the chuck should be placed back in the lathe without the adaptor. The lens is then recut and because it contains a prism only materials from the high spot (that is, the thickest part of the prism base at the lens edge) is removed. Thus, the thickness of the base of the prism is reduced, producing a lens with a good edge thickness all round but still containing the necessary ballast to stabilize it. The reduced base is then polished on a vertical spindle using a felt wheel in a flexible drive.

After cleaning the chuck and casting blocks in paraffin, they are heated to approximately 85°C and the molten mixture of wax and magnesium carbonate, which is at approximately 125°C, is poured into the blocks. The blocks are then banged several times on a solid surface to release any air bubbles. After cooling slightly the wax contracts and the blocks need to be topped up with additional wax.

When the wax is cold the chucks can be forced out of the casting blocks with the aid of a dowel. The back surface polishers are cut on the lathe while the front surface polishers are cut using steel male gauges.

TRUNCATING

Truncating is usually carried out to help stabilize a toric or bifocal lens and is nearly always combined with prism ballast. Most frequently it involves only the lower edge. The edge is removed using an emery board (*Figure 22.52*) or a diamond impregnated tool. It is polished with a felt wheel rotating in a flexible drive (*Figure 22.53*), while the lens is mounted on a chuck, the corners of the truncation are rounded to minimize discomfort to the lower lid.

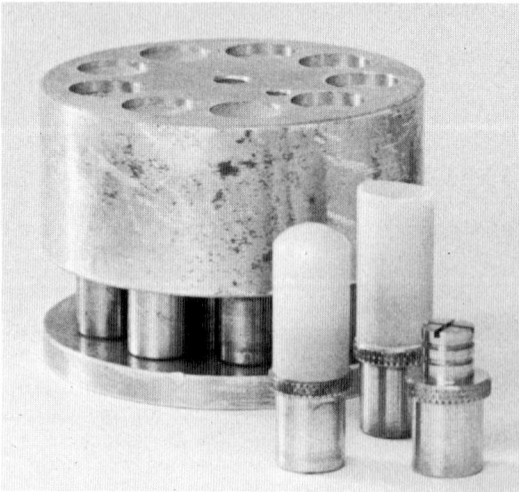

Figure 22.50–Block and chucks for casting back surface wax polishers: from left to right are the block for making nine wax tools, a finished tool with radius cut on, and uncut wax tool and basic chuck for taking a wax polishing tool

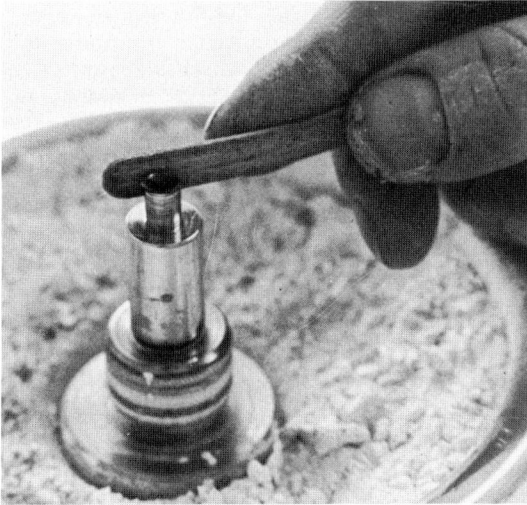

Figure 22.52–Truncating a lens with an emery board using the (stationary) vertical spindle as a base

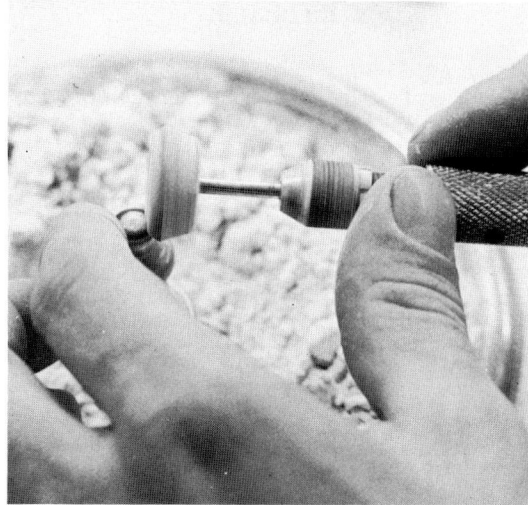

Figure 22.53–Polishing a truncation with a felt wheel driven by a flexible drive

With a bifocal, the edge is left fairly square to assist in raising the lens, by support on the lower lid margin, when the gaze is depressed.

ANNEALING

PMMA blanks are made from cast sheet, cast block or rod turned from cast block. All casting introduces strain which needs to be released from the material to ensure consistent results in hard lens fabrication. This is done by annealing which involves heating the material to a temperature of between 140 and 150°C for a short period and slowly returning it to room temperature. This does not cause any difficulty when done to thin sheet material but with thick material the temperature has to be low enough to prevent depolymerization of the surface but heated long enough to ensure the centre of the block reaches at least 130°C. Annealing is usually carried out by the supplier of the blanks.

FENESTRATION

Fenestration involves forming a hole, typically 0.20–0.30 mm diameter, with a vertical drill while the lens is mounted convex surface uppermost on a chuck containing a small depression (or hole) which receives the penetrating drill. Both sides of the fenestration must be countersunk and polished. This is best done with a sharpened boxwood stick which is rotated in a circular fashion in the opposite direction to the vertical spindle on which the chuck and lens is rotating. To polish and countersink the

back surface of the fenestration the lens is placed on a concave chuck with the fenestration hole at its centre. The lens may be held in place by wax or double-sided sticky tape, avoiding the central depression (or hole) in the chuck. The central part of the fenestration may be polished by running the lens up and down a length of Silvo-soaked cotton, threaded through the fenestration hole.

Note: Fenestrating, to aid tears exchange, only works successfully on a steep fitting lens; if the lens is an alignment or flat fit the fenestration merely creates another tears meniscus between it and the cornea which reduces the mobility of the lens and thus tends to aggravate any corneal oedema. Additionally, if the fenestration is small enough to minimize any interference with vision it usually quickly becomes blocked with mucoproteins – thus losing its usefulness and adding a site in which to harbour pathogens. Conversely, if the fenestration is large enough to prevent blockage then the vision may be greatly interfered with.

The author feels that if a corneal lens requires fenestrating then there is something basically wrong with the fit of that lens or the tears flow and these should be attended to rather than introducing a fenestration. Oedema problems can now be ellevi- ated much more successfully in hard lens patients by using one of the range of gas permeable materials (*see* Addendum).

Fenestration of corneal and scleral lenses is also dealt with on pages 655 and 658, respectively, of Chapter 23.

BIFOCALS

Bifocals may be fused or solid in the hard lens form, but can only be made solid in a soft lens construction at the present time. Of recent years the most frequently fitted hard lens bifocals have been the

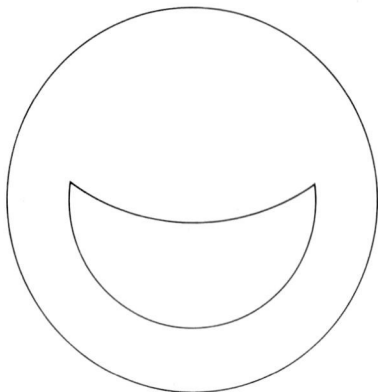

Figure 22.54–Crescent fused bifocal lens

D-shaped and, more recently still, the crescent-shaped fused bifocals (*Figure 22.54*). The last two years have seen the appearance of soft lens bifocals; these are constructed in the dehydrated state in exactly the same manner as the hard solid bifocals.

FUSED BIFOCALS

The fused bifocal blank (*Figure 22.55*) is made by fusing together two pieces of PMMA with different refractive indices, in an oven at high temperature. This is a similar process to constructing a fused bifocal spectacle lens. The segment is fused on the

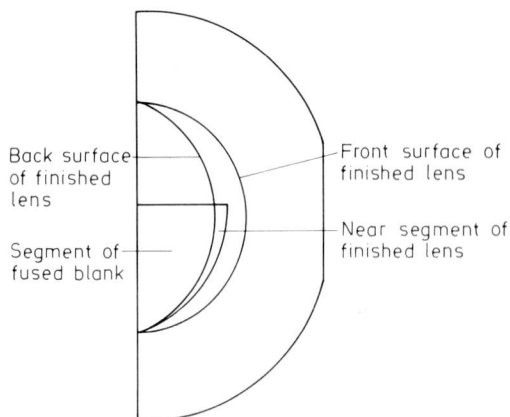

Back surface of finished lens

Front surface of finished lens

Near segment of finished lens

Segment of fused blank

Figure 22.55–Crescent fused bifocal blank in cross-section

back surface of the blank, the different powers of the near additions being obtained by varying the radius of the segment interface. Thus, for any given BCOR with any given near addition an appropriate segment radius is cut into the blank and the matching segment inserted into this cavity. Therefore, for any given blank there is a fixed BCOR and near addition. Consequently, a comprehensive stock of blanks is required to cover all possible combinations of BCOR and near additions (*see* Chapter 4, Volume 1, page 123), as well as the range of tints.

The fabrication of a fused bifocal lens is much the same as for a single vision lens. Greater care has to be taken in centring the lens on its mount, and in calibrating and cutting the thickness in order to avoid the segment breaking through the lens onto the front surface. A prism and truncation are usually needed to stabilize the fit and quite often the optic is displaced upwards. Displacement of the optic requires the initial diameter of the blank to be cut oversize by an amount slightly above the required displacement. The back peripheral curves are then generated. The lens is displaced on its button by the required amount and the diameter recut to 0.20 mm above the finally required overall size to allow for edging. The front surface is then cut in the normal manner.

SOLID BIFOCALS

Solid bifocals may be crescent, downcurve or concentric-shaped. All of these have the segment worked on the front surface.

Crescent or Upcurve-shaped

This is constructed by cutting a lens incorporating a large prism (*Figure 22.56*). The front surface is polished and then replaced on the lathe with a lower powered prism adaptor. The base of the prism is then removed by cutting a steeper front surface curve corresponding to the near power of the lens. This produces a crescent-shaped segment which is then polished.

Downcurve or Arc-shaped

This is constructed by the reverse approach to the crescent-shaped segment (*Figure 22.57*). That is, the lens is cut to a much thicker substance and with a small prism. The front surface radius is such that it produces the required near portion power. After polishing the front surface, the lens, still mounted, is placed on a higher powered prism adaptor and is

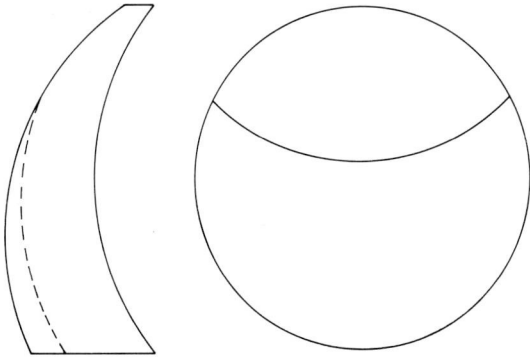

Figure 22.56–Crescent or upcurve solid bifocal lens. The broken lines represent the area where material has been removed to create the near segment on the front surface. Cross-section and front views are shown

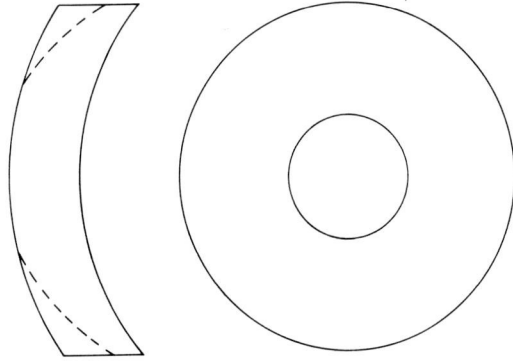

Figure 22.58–Concentric solid bifocal lens. The broken lines represent the area where material has been removed to create the near portion on the front surface. Cross-section and front views are shown

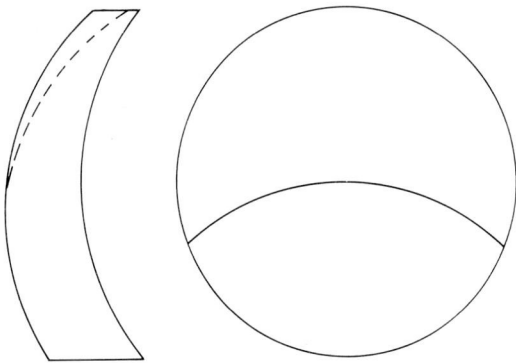

Figure 22.57–Downcurve or arc solid bifocal lens. The broken lines represent the area where material has been removed to create the distance portion on the front surface. Cross-section and front views are shown

recut using a flatter radius corresponding to the distance power. This produces an arc-shaped or downcurve segment, ballasted with a prism. The segment is then polished.

Concentric-shaped

These do not contain a prism as they are often used for simultaneous vision or 'bivision' through both distance and near portions. If used for successive vision or 'alternating vision' any rotation on the eye is not important. The centre is sighted for distance vision and the main outer lens for near. Although in theory it could be reversed, in practice there are difficulties in constructing the junction properly because of the change from steeper to flatter radius; also, with a distance negative prescription the edge

of the lens could be unduly thick. The lens is cut, with the front radius for distance vision, and polished; the periphery of the lens is cut down with a steeper radius corresponding to the near prescription (*Figure 22.58*). This cut-down is taken into the centre of the lens far enough to produce the required central segment diameter, and is then polished.

The difficulty in fabricating a solid bifocal lens is in obtaining a sharp transition between the distance and near segments. During the process of polishing the second radius there is inevitably some blending of the junction of the near and distance portions and hence an area of visual confusion may be produced for the patient, although this blending may be sufficient to provide a progressive power lens.

PRACTITIONERS' ORDERS

Laboratories quite frequently have to refer back to a practitioner about an order which has been received with either insufficient or total lack of instructions. For example, a tint is omitted; there may be no instructions as to whether a lenticulation is required with a positive lens; no position given for a fenestration; no amount, angle or location (top or bottom) of a truncation given. Impossible or extremely complex orders may be received. For example, a practitioner may specify, with a positive lens, a centre thickness which is too thin for a given front optic diameter or overall size; or the almost impossible order for an oblique bi-toric lens – almost impossible, that is, if a good power reading and accurate axes are wanted.

If a negative lens is requested to be made extremely thin in the centre (less than 0.10 mm), the

Table 22.1–Hard Lens Tints

Code number	Description	Code number	Description
⋆200	Light yellow	⋆2092	Bright green
⋆300	Amber	2219-1	Pale amber
⋆400	Bright red	2240-1	Dark green
⋆401	Bright cherry red	2240-2	Light green
⋆512	Light brownish-grey	2240-3	Medium green
⋆600	Bright medium green	2241-1	Ruby red
⋆603	Bright green	2241-2	Medium pale pink
⋆700	Pale blue	2241-3	Pale pink
⋆703	Medium blue	2241-4	Very dark ruby red
⋆911	Very pale grey	2241-5	Dark pink
⋆912	Pale grey	2242-2	Pale lavender
⋆962	Very dark grey	2285	Dark brown
⋆999	Dark grey	2285-1	Light brown
1077	Very dark blue	2285-2	Medium brown
1077-1	Light blue	6077	Dark grey
1077-2	Dark blue	6610-1	Medium grey
1077-3	Medium blue	6610-2	Extreme pale grey
⋆2002	Bright light green	⋆⋆9042	Very light brownish-grey
⋆2045	Bright light blue	⋆⋆9043	Light brownish-grey
⋆2069	Very light blue	⋆10910	Violet
⋆2082	Very pale green		

Commercial grade polymethyl methacrylate (I.C.I.) is available in those tints marked with an asterisk. Other tints are the American 'De Luxe' material. Double asterisk indicates CQ or clinical quality material.

lens will have to be fabricated on a solid chuck so that the centre of the lens is properly supported and will not drop during the cutting and polishing stages. This means that the power cannot be assessed and adjusted as the polishing proceeds, any adjustments having to be made after the lens has been removed from its initial mounting. Hence, poor power readings may result (*see* Power Adjustments, page 634).

A little thought by the practitioner before putting pen to paper would save both the practitioner and laboratory a lot of time and annoyance. Chapter 4, Volume 1, covers the calculations and/or drawing to scale necessary to determine adequate thicknesses to permit lenses to be made.

To help in the choice of hard lens thickness, lenticulations and tints the practitioner is referred to *Table 22.1* and to Chapter 11, Volume 1.

CONCLUSION

Some of the procedures described in this chapter may not be followed by the majority of laboratories. A few laboratories, for reasons of their own even argue against them. There are of course many variations possible in making a lens, but if constant observation by skilled personnel is the order of the day then the quality is usually high. Unfortunately,

quality does not always come cheaply and if a laboratory is operating on a large scale and using all of the above procedures, then the cost of lenses must naturally be higher than from a laboratory using a production line of part-time semi-skilled technicians – a situation regrettably seen in some present-day laboratories.

At one time, soft lenses looked as though they might cause the demise of the smaller specialist laboratories. However, with the advent of toric soft and gas permeable lenses it appears that their individual expertise is what is needed and many will, legislation permitting, weather the storm – all to the good of the patient and the practitioner.

BRITISH AND AMERICAN APPROVED NAMES FOR CONTACT LENS MATERIALS

Any new 'drug' licensed in the United Kingdom must have a British Approved Name (BAN). There is a high degree of international co-operation in establishing approved names and the BAN is usually the same as the United States Approved Name (USAN) and the International Non-proprietary Name (INN).

The USA approved names are already adopted for contact lens materials. Names employ a characteristic suffix of which two are currently in use:

Table 22.2–Published USAN's Contact Lens Materials

Name	Type	Manufacturer	Trade name
Bufilcon A	HEMA	Burton Parsons	Meso-lens
Cabufocon A	CAB	Danker-Wöhlk	
Crofilcon A	HEMA	Corneal Sciences	
Dimefilcon A	HEMA	Calcon Labs.	Gelflex
Droxafilcon A	HEMA	Ophthalmos, Inc.	Hydralens
Etafilcon A	HEMA	Frontier c/l	Hydro-marc
Hefilcon A	HEMA	Automated Optics	PHP
Lidofilcon A	Vinyl	CLM	Sauflon 70
Lidofilcon B			Sauflon 85
Mafilcon A	HEMA	N & N/Menicon	
Ocufilcon A	HEMA	Urocon Int.	Tresoft/Urosoft
Phemfilcon A	HEMA	Wesley/Jessen	Durasoft/Phemecol
Polymacon	HEMA	Bausch and Lomb	Soflens
Porofocon A	CAB	Rynco Scientific	Rx-56
Porofocon B	CAB	Soft Lenses, Inc.	CAB-Curve
Silafocon A	PMMA/Silicone	Syntex	Polycon
Tetrafilcon A	HEMA	UCO Optics	Aquaflex/Aosoft
Vifilcon A	HEMA	Warner Lambert	Softcon

Filcon, applied to hydrophilic type materials making no distinction between HEMA-based and other materials.

Focon, applied to CAB materials.

Names also have a letter suffix A, B, C etc., which is used to indicate the same polymer from different manufacturers. It has also been used in the case of Lidofilcon (Sauflon) to indicate different content of two materials from the same manufacturer. Sauflon 70 is Lidofilcon A and Sauflon 85 is Lidofilcon B.

No direct reference is made to water content in any USAN. A new letter suffix would be applied to a new formulation of an existing material.

The naming system is not totally consistent since the first material in the hydrophilic group (the Hydron/B & L material) has the name Polymacon omitting the suffix and letter, and the Danker-Wöhlk CAB material has a USAN (Cabufocon A) different from the two other named CAB materials (Porofocon A and B). The reason for these anomalies is unknown.

ADDENDUM

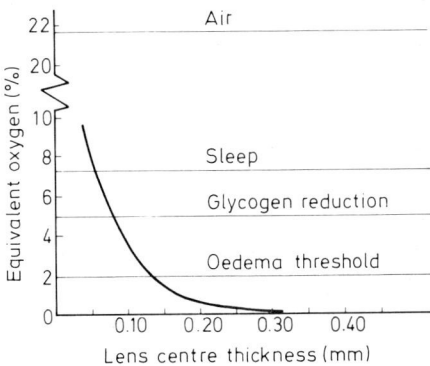

Figure 22.59–Equivalent O_2 transmission vs lens centre thickness for HEMA (after Hill, R. M., 1975)

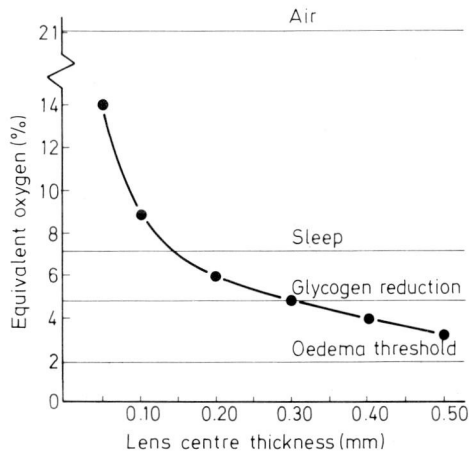

Figure 22.60–Equivalent O_2 transmission vs lens centre thickness for Boston material (after Loshaek, S. and Hill, R. M., 1977)

Table 22.3–Comparison of Lower Wetting Angle and Gas Permeable Lens Materials

Material	Manufacturer	Known constituents	Approximate oxygen permeability at $20°C$ (DK)	Comments
Alberta	Corneal Science	PMMA Silicone	14.00	Relatively new material at time of writing. Comments probably apply as for Boston material
Boston	Polymer Tech.	PMMA 55% Silicone 45%	12.3	Higher oxygen permeability than many other gas permeable materials but more fragile and easily abraded. Avoid PVA-containing solutions
BP Flex	Gasflex	Modified PMMA	Negligible	Treat like PMMA. Lower wetting angle
CAB	Various	Moulded or lathe cut	Range 4.3–6.0	Large hydration–dehydration changes. Easily warps and abrades. Difficult to modify
Calgary	Corneal Science	PMMA 50% CAB 40% Silicone 10%	4.5	Stable. Avoid PVA-containing solutions
Menicon O_2	Menicon-Toyo	PMMA Silicone	5.1	Good clinical results although limited parameters only available. Special surface or cleaning treatment prevents modification. Use 'O$_2$-solution'
Paraflex Paragon 18	Paragon	Modified PMMA	Negligible	Treat like PMMA. Lower wetting angle
Polycon	Syntex	PMMA 65% Silicone 35%	5.0	Greater rigidity than many other gas permeable materials. Limited range of parameters from main producer
SR Range	Duragel	Water active silicone	Range 7.9–14.3	Some difficulties found in manufacture. Little clinical information available

Note: It should be emphasized that because of the relative newness of some of these materials only limited comments on their various properties have been made. Practitioners are referred to laboratory and current journal literature for recent information.

ACKNOWLEDGMENTS

I am indebted to Mr Phillip Downs, my technical director, and to Mr W. Spencer of Moorfields Eye Hospital laboratory for their advice and help; also I am indebted to Mrs Sheila Lawes for typing the manuscript.

REFERENCES

Hill, R. M. (1975). 'Hydrogel lens design: the thick and thin of it.' In *Proc. 2nd National Symposium on Soft Contact Lenses*, pp. 51–56. Chicago: Prefessional Press
Litvin, M. W. (1977). 'The incidence of eye infections with contact lenses.' *Optician* **174**(4496), 11–14
Loshaek, S. and Hill, R. M. (1977). 'Oxygen permeability measurements: correlation between living-eye and electrode-chamber measurements.' *Internat. Contact Lens Clin.* **4** (6), 26–29

BIBLIOGRAPHY

Bryant, P. G. (1973). 'Construction and manufacture of a fused bifocal lens.' *Ophthal. Optician* **13**, 1052–1056
Cordrey, P. (1973). 'Technical and economic effects of contact lens production methods.' *Ophthal. Optician* **13**, 230–236
Crundall, E. J. (1977). 'Spun to curve.' *Optician* **173**(4483), 15–16, 19–20, 23, 28
Haynes, P. R. (1965). 'Modification Procedures.' Chapter 14 in *Contact Lens Practice: Basic and Advanced*, 1st ed., pp. 252–280, ed. by Mandell, R. B. Springfield, Illinois: Thomas
Hicks, M. (1975). 'More than a million.' *Optician* **170**(4407), 18–26
Hodd, F. A. B. (1974). 'Bifocal contact lens practice.' *Ophthal. Optician* **13**, 315–320, 325–326, 378–380, 385–388
Inman, D. R. (1974). 'Peripheral design of toric corneal lenses.' *Optician* **167**(4318), 13–17
Nissel, G. (1975). 'Manufacturing Techniques.' Chapter 14 in *Contact Lens Practice: Visual, Therapeutic and Prosthetic*, pp. 314–342, ed. by Ruben, M. London: Baillière and Tindall
Phillips, A. J. (1970). 'Alterations in curvature of the finished corneal lens.' *Ophthal. Optician* **9**, 980–986, 1043–1054, 1100–1110
Shanks, K. R. (1966). 'Subjective comparison of corneal lens edges.' *Br. J. physiol. Optics* **23**, 55–58

Chapter 23

Modification Procedures

A. J. Phillips

THE IMPORTANCE OF THE PRACTITIONER BEING ABLE TO CARRY OUT MODIFICATIONS

Nowadays, when modifications can be carried out relatively quickly and cheaply by laboratories, it is often difficult to impress on students, and even qualified practitioners, the following reasons why the contact lens practitioner should be able to carry out his own modifications.

(1) There is no interruption to the patient's wearing schedule and no necessity for extra visits.

(2) Often, only the practitioner knows exactly what is desired and it may be difficult to describe to the laboratory just what is required. (This is particularly so with scleral lenses.)

(3) Modifications can be done in increasing stages, with the effect of the modifications on the patient noted at each stage. Laboratories either have to do the full modifications in one step, or the patient is required to make many unnecessary visits and to be without lenses for several days.

(4) Subsequent modifications may become apparent and can be done immediately.

(5) Practitioners who carry out modifications are better able to evaluate lenses which have been made or which have to be modified by a laboratory.

Against these advantages must be set the cost of the equipment involved. However, much of this cost can be redeemed, not only from tax relief but also on the savings of doing the modification oneself. It is important to remember also that patients are more satisfied because they do not have to be without their lenses. Further, most of the equipment, especially the more expensive items, will last a lifetime.

The following section lists the equipment which can be used for contact lens modification. It should be emphasized that many of these are alternatives and are discussed as such.

MODIFICATION EQUIPMENT FOR CORNEAL LENSES

Corneal Lens Holders

Glass Tube and Double-sided Adhesive Tape

This is one of the simplest and cheapest forms of corneal lens holder.

A glass tube of about 6 mm in diameter, with rounded ends, has a small strip of double-sided adhesive tape stretched over one end on to which the lens is lightly pressed. An inverted glass tube from a dropper bottle is ideal.

This holder has the disadvantages that tape adhesive may stick to the lens when removed for checking and that the tape may need replacing if polishing liquid gets between the lens and tape.

Modified Scleral Lens Holder

The simplest form of corneal lens holder consists of an ordinary scleral lens suction holder which has been cut down and thinned on a rotating rough grinding stone to an internal diameter of about 7.5 mm and an edge thickness of about 0.5 mm (*Figures 23.1* and *23.2*). A corneal lens holder may also be used with a hollow plastics tube in the stem to give support (Haynes, 1965). These holders are best used filled with water.

They have the disadvantage that they cannot be allowed to rotate between the fingers and may therefore occasionally cause oval optic portions – when polishing peripheral curves, for instance – or possibly occasional lens scratches. They can, however, be rotated manually.

Figure 23.1–Corneal lens holders. (a) Cross-section of a scleral lens suction holder with the dotted line indicating the reduced size suitable for holding corneal lenses. (b) Cross-section of the end of a corneal lens suction holder mounted on a Perspex or nylon rod. (c) Cross-section of a double-ended suction holder. The lower shaded portion is removable and reversible having a flat end and a concave end for holding back and front surfaces of corneal lenses, respectively

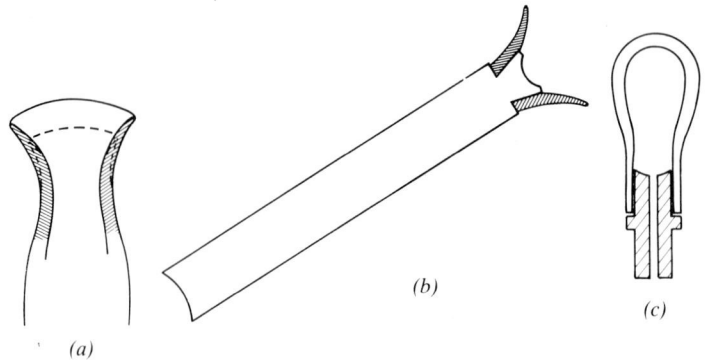

(a)

(b)

(c)

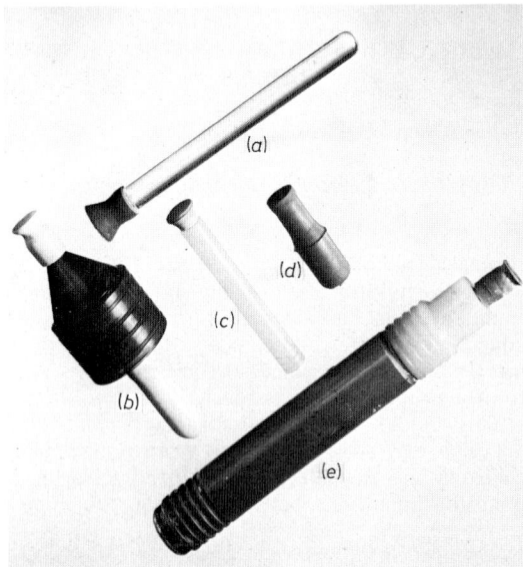

Figure 23.2–Corneal lens holders. (a) Corneal lens suction holder cup mounted on a Perspex handle. (b) Spinner (Belgravia Optical Co. Ltd.). (c) Corneal lens suction holder cup mounted on a nylon handle. (d) Modified scleral lens suction holder. (e) Spinner

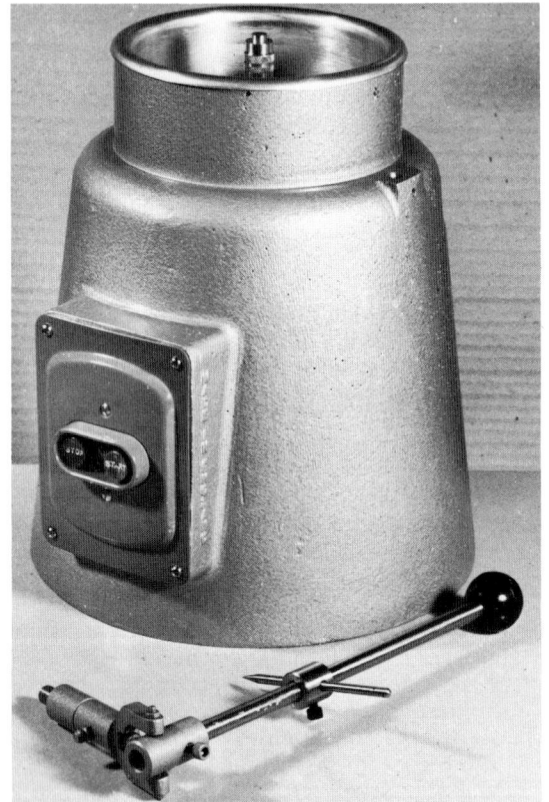

Figure 23.3–Vertical spindle or 'Office Modification Unit' (G. Nissel & Co.)

Modified Corneal Suction Holder

This design, as used by Shick in America and sometimes known by his name, is shown in *Figures 23.1* and *23.2*. The end of a corneal lens suction holder is placed over a short nylon or Perspex rod cut as shown. Again, best used with the open end full of water, this type gives good control and spins easily with one finger resting lightly on the upper end.

Spinner

A more efficient version of the previous holder, the spinner consists of a rotatable spindle with a corneal suction holder at the end, mounted in a handle (*Figure 23.2*). The lens can rotate freely on the end of the spindle while the handle is held still.

Double-ended Suction Holder

This type of suction holder has a reversible end, one end for attachment to convex surfaces and the other for concave surfaces. As this is the only type of lens holder, apart from those using adhesive tape, which will attach to the back surface of a corneal lens, it finds particular application in the alteration of lens power and removal of front surface abrasions (*see* page 655). A cross-section is shown in *Figure 23.1*.

All suction holder ends have the disadvantage that the lens may flex, particularly with thinner lenses, so that the curves will be produced slightly steeper than desired, or slightly distorted.

Double-sided Adhesive Tape

Double-sided adhesive tape, of about 7 mm in width is ideal as a corneal lens holder.

Verticle Spindle or Office Modification Unit (*Figure 23.3*)

A speed of between 500 and 1500 rev/min is required – ideally, variable over this range, especially in the slower region. Models with clockwise or anti-clockwise rotation may be obtained, as preferred.

This is the most expensive single item of all modification equipment.

Ideally, the unit should be mounted in a bench with the taper slightly above the level of the bench. This enables the operator: (1) to rest his elbows on the table top and to thus steady his hands; and (2) to roll the cutting blade and smoothing tools around the edge of the lens when shaping the edge or reducing the overall size.

Spindle Lens Chuck or Edging Chuck

This lens chuck (*Figure 23.4*), used for edge and overall size modifications, should be carefully chosen so that its taper fits the practitioner's own vertical spindle (for example, standard or 0-morse tapers). It is preferable to have a chuck the stem of which is not too short or too thick. Approximately 6 mm wide and 2 cm long enables easy holding by the stem.

The same chuck may also be used for holding lenses for peripheral curve modification of the back surface. The lens is stuck on to the chuck with wax or double-sided adhesive tape. As the lens is held rigid on the tool there should be no flexing of the

lens during polishing, although if the stem is very narrow the periphery of a large corneal lens may still flex.

Adhesive Wax and Bunsen Burner

Adhesive wax, obtainable in stick form, is necessary to attach the lens to the spindle lens chuck. A bunsen burner is used to melt the wax. Alternatively, a compressed butane burner may be used, or even a spirit burner. More sophisticated electric heaters are also available to heat the metal chucks (*see Figure 22.1*, Chapter 22).

Centring Devices

Centring devices are used where double-sided adhesive tape is used on the spindle lens chuck instead of beeswax, and where the lens must be accurately centred when it is placed on the chuck.

The lens is placed in the well of the device. The centring part is carefully lowered on to the lens and

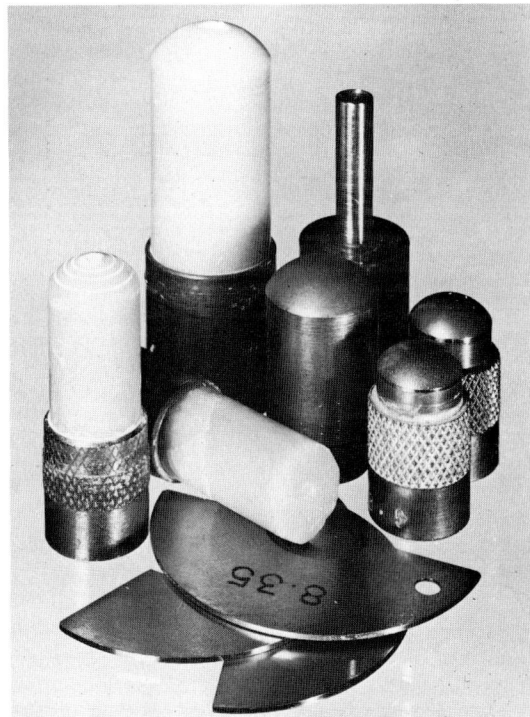

Figure 23.4–From left to right – Rear: large wax tool and spindle lens holder (or edging chuck). Centre: small wax tools, cut and uncut, and large and small diamond impregnated brass tools. Front: female gauges

slowly rotated to centre the lens within the well and is then withdrawn.

These devices do not, in general, give such accurate lens centration as that carried out by hand, as described below.

Wax Polishing Tools

These tools are made up by the practitioner with molten wax poured into moulds and allowed to set hard. They are used for accurate polishing to a specific radius (*Figure 23.4*). Instructions for the manufacture of the tools are given by the laboratory supplying them. Alternatively, the tools may be made up by the laboratory. Further details are given in Chapter 22 on page 638, and *Figure 22.50* and *Figure 22.51* show the blocks and chucks used for making back and front surface wax polishers, together with cut and uncut finished wax tools. Normally, only convex curves are cut on these tools by practitioners doing their own modifications. Front surface wax polishers (concave) are used almost exclusively by laboratories.

Female Gauges

Female gauges are necessary to cut the wax tools to the required radius (*Figure 23.4*). Stainless steel gauges are the most accurate and long-lasting. Ideally, a razor blade should be used to cut the wax cylinder to approximately the correct radius, and the female gauge should be used only for final 'truing up' in order to prevent excessive wear on the gauge.

Metal or Plastics Tools and Adhesive Tape

Adhesive cloth tape 'sticking plaster' of the 'zinc oxide' type is stretched over a suitable tool, and this cloth surface is used for polishing lens peripheries– an allowance of approximately 0.2 mm (depending on the tape used) being made for the thickness of the tape. This can be used as an alternative to the wax polishing tools mentioned above. The practitioner using brass or plastics tools of this type must check with the manufacturing laboratory whether or not an allowance for an average tape thickness has been made when constructing the tool.

This method has the advantage that it is not normally necessary to put on a separate transitional curve as with the wax tools. For this reason, it is the one favoured by most laboratories for peripheral curves. 'Cloth polishing' has the one serious drawback that the accuracy of curves polished by this method cannot be guaranteed.

Wax tools may be used instead of the metal or plastics tools, the tape being stretched over the suitably cut wax curve.

Tools may also be covered in muslin, stretched taut and held in place with a rubber band.

Polishing Liquids

The polishing liquid used most frequently for PMMA lenses is the metal polish Silvo. The container should be allowed to stand for 2 or 3 days, after which most of the excess clear fluid is poured off. This is in order to give a more suitable, slightly thicker polishing fluid.

For most gas permeable lens materials the ammonia in Silvo acts as a solvent and this polish should not therefore be used. Polishes such as Alox–PG (*Carium Chemical Co.*) may be more appropriate but individual material manufacturers should be consulted first.

Paraffin Oil

Ordinary paraffin oil (kerosene) is used to remove any wax that remains attached to a lens after removal from a chuck. It may also be used as a lubricant with diamond impregnated tools when putting on the major part of a corneal lens peripheral curve prior to final polishing, or grinding out the back optic surface of a scleral lens. Being slightly more viscous than water, it prevents such deep scratches (though grinding is slightly slower), enabling the final polishing to be done more quickly.

Paraffin oil, water, and polishing liquids are best used in 250 ml wash bottles with jet dispensers or 'sprays'. They may possibly be more economically applied with a large artist's paint brush from a bowl, especially where they are being used frequently and evaporation causes no problems – though, where applicable, fire hazards must be considered.

Razor and Scalpel Blades

Single-edge ('safety') razor blades and scalpel blades, straight and curved, are useful for certain modifications (*see* page 651). Alternatively, a thicker square-edged cutter may be used.

Carborundum Tool for Overall Size Reduction

This consists of an internally tapering cone, which is held in a Jacobs' chuck (*Figure 23.5*). It is used for reduction in lens size. It has the disadvantage that, if the lens is not placed centrally in the hollow, stock will be removed unequally (Haynes, 1959). Also, with lenses incorporating prism, there is a tendency for more material to be removed from the thinner lens edge than the thicker edge.

Before use, the tool should be soaked well in water.

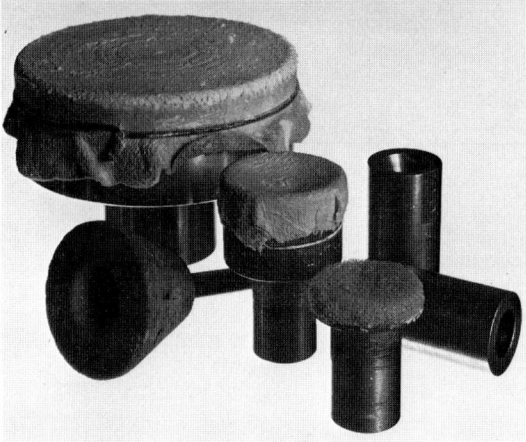

Figure 23.5–From left to right – Rear: large polishing drum. Centre: carborundum tool for reduction of overall size, small polishing drum, and Conlish tools. Front: flat plate sponge chuck

Assorted Carborundum or Diamond Impregnated Burrs

These are used for final edge shaping (*Figure 23.6*). Very fine emery paper may also be used.

Polishing Cloth

This very soft cloth (for example, 'Selvyt' cloth) is used for adding small amounts of power to lenses. Suitable cloth may be obtained from any contact lens laboratory at little cost, or ordinary velveteen material may be purchased.

Flat Plate and Sponge or Drum Chucks

These chucks (*Figure 23.5*) are used on a vertical spindle for adding positive and negative power to lenses, removing surface scratches, and for edge polishing. The drum chuck consists of a hollow chuck over which a piece of chamois leather or similar material has been stretched and held in place with a rubber band or wire. The flat plate chuck consists of a chuck with an upper flat portion to which is attached a thin piece of sponge rubber or moleskin.

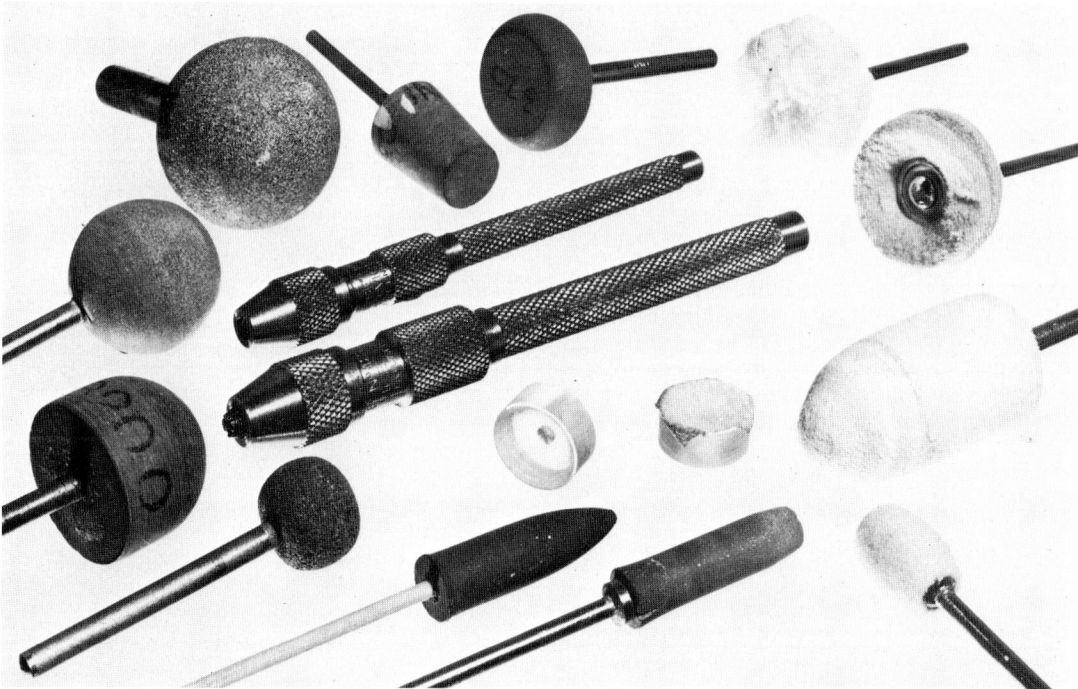

Figure 23.6–Assorted grinding tools and polishing buffs. Top centre: large and small pin-vice holders for drills. Lower centre: corneal lens buttons with one surface cut for use as scleral lens runners. Left button shows guide hole on rear surface and right button has double-sided adhesive tape on concave surface

Chamois Leather

A large piece of chamois leather 15 × 15 cm often forms a useful backing to the polishing cloth mentioned above, and is sometimes used as an alternative.

A smaller piece of thinner chamois leather may be used for edge polishing while the lens is still mounted on the spindle lens chuck as shown in *Figures 22.33–22.35*. Alternatively, a small piece of sponge rubber may be used.

Conlish Tools (from CONical and poLISH)

These are a series of hollow cone tools of varying angles which are used on a vertical spindle (*Figure 23.5*).

Lined with adhesive cloth tape, they are used for shaping lens edges. The lens is mounted, for instance, on a glass tube and the edge is polished for a specific number of seconds on each tool. Generally, a slower speed vertical spindle appears preferable (100–500 rev/min). Although used successfully by certain laboratories, often as diamond impregnated tools, they are not very popular with practitioners in the United Kingdom. Further details can be found in most American textbooks on this subject and in the original paper on this method by Cepero (1959).

Drills

Drills of diameters from 0.10 to 0.30 mm mounted in hand drill (or pin-vice) holders are used to fenestrate corneal lenses. *Figure 23.6* shows pin-vice holders.

A dental countersink rose, as fine as possible (size 0 or 1), is necessary for countersinking fenestrations. Several finely sharpened boxwood sticks are also needed for hand polishing the countersink, or may be used for complete countersinking if the lens is mounted on a suitable chuck on a vertical spindle.

For scleral lenses the following additional tools are required.

Scleral Lens Runners

Scleral lens runners are attached to the front optic surface of lenses by means of broad (12 mm) double-sided sticky tape on the concave runner surface. They are used with a pencil or ball-point pen tip in the guide hole on the upper flat surface to control the lens on wax or diamond tools (*Figure 23.6*).

Runners can be obtained from laboratories; or a corneal lens blank may be used, with the concave surface cut but not polished and a small central guide hole drilled a short way into the flat surface.

Rough Grinding Stone and Buff

These are used respectively for reducing lens overall sizes and edge polishing (*Figure 23.7*). The grinding stone is not an essential since a file and emery paper serve the same function, though more slowly; or a 25 mm carborundum ball may be used (*Figure 23.6* top left).

Horizontal Spindle with Jacob's Chuck Fitting or Flexible Drive (*Figure 23.7*)

This is necessary for holding many of the tools used for back haptic surface modifications and in fenestrating. A Jacob's chuck attachment may also be

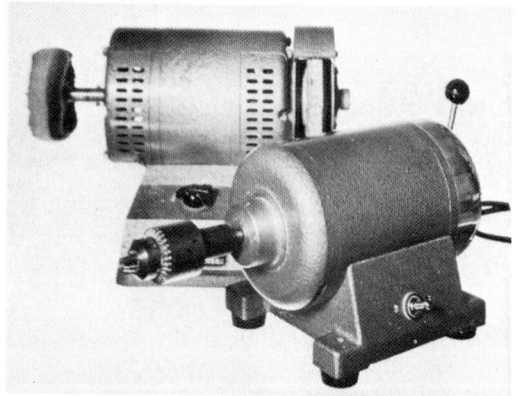

Figure 23.7–Grinding stone and buff (rear), and variable speed horizontal spindle with Jacob's chuck fitting (front). A flexible drive may be attached to the right-hand end of the grinding stone and buff motor

obtained for the vertical spindle. Alternatively, some practitioners prefer to use a small motor with flexible drive attachment, which should have a foot operated speed control to allow both hands freedom for lens and tool manipulation (*see Figure 22.21*).

Grinding Balls and Polishing Buffs

A selection of grinding balls and polishing buffs of various sizes and shapes are necessary (*Figure 23.6*).

Tripoli or Buffite Polishing Compound

One or more polishing compounds are preferred by many practitioners for use with polishing buffs. The initial polishing after grinding is carried out more quickly with these compounds, but with some danger of burning the plastics. Final polishing is best carried out with Silvo or similar compounds.

Diamond Impregnated Brass Tools

Used with or without a runner, back optic and spherical transition grind-outs are performed by means of these tools (*Figure 23.4*). Tools or radii commonly used by the practitioner for transitional curves are usefully obtained. A basic set includes the radii 7.80, 8.00, 8.20, 8.40, 8.60, 8.90, 10.00 and 11.00 mm.

Large Wax Tools

These are used for polishing spherical transitions (*Figure 23.4*).

Drills and Dental Burrs

Drills of 0.50 mm, 0.75 mm and 1.00 mm in diameter may be required for making fenestration holes in scleral lenses. Slightly larger round or flame-shaped dental burrs may be used for counter-sinking, or even a larger drill may be used.

CORNEAL LENS MODIFICATIONS

REDUCING THE OVERALL SIZE OF A LENS

Reduction of the overall size of a lens may be carried out for any of the following reasons.

(1) To relieve corneal oedema by exposing more of the cornea to a normal atmosphere.

(2) To reduce excessive edge clearance which may be causing discomfort, or causing visual interference due to bubbles getting under the edge during blinking. These bubbles frequently get under the lower edge of a high riding lens and can readily be seen with the slit lamp. They cause reflections and may result in dimpling of the corneal epithelium. Excessive edge clearance can also cause the lens to become misplaced easily or even ejected from the eye. It may also be partially responsible for drying of the 3 and 9 o'clock areas of the cornea which then stain with fluorescein when this is applied.

(3) To reduce edge thickness of a high negative lens, which can cause discomfort, and if the upper lid is tight and grips the lens after a blink, the lens may ride too high. Alternatively, a thick edge may cause a loose lid to knock the lens down after each blink. Thick edges also encourage 3 and 9 o'clock stain as does excess edge clearance by holding the eyelids away from these areas of the eye during blinking, thereby preventing proper wetting.

(4) To reduce the weight of a lens, thereby encouraging it not to ride so low on the cornea.

The lens overall size is first checked on a magnifying gauge or V-gauge, and the amount to be removed is noted. A spindle lens holder is now heated at its upper end with a bunsen burner for a few seconds, old wax polishing compound being removed with a tissue.

Directing the bunsen flame on to the top of the chuck, the end of the adhesive wax stick is touched on the upper end of the chuck stem so that one small drop of the wax is left in the concavity. Too much wax here causes it to spread over the underside of the lens when placed on the stem, often making the edge difficult to modify as well as making it difficult to check and clean.

While the wax is still soft (reheat for a second, if necessary), the lens with convex side down is placed on the chuck as near centrally as possible. Setting the spindle in motion will show that the lens is not yet exactly centred about the spindle axis of rotation. Cutting it now would give a non-circular lens. The next step, therefore, is to centre the lens.

For this, the wax on the chuck, if not still soft, must be softened without burning the lens. The safest way of doing this is shown in *Figure 23.8*. Holding the inverted chuck by the stem, the base of the chuck is held in the lower part of the bunsen burner flame until the stem begins to get too hot to hold. It is now placed firmly on the spindle, and the spindle is set in motion. One finger of each hand is immediately but very carefully touched on the lens – one on the side, and the other on the opposite top edge (*Figure 23.9*). This is done until an object (such as a strip light) mirrored by the concave surface of the lens appears perfectly stationary as the lens rotates. Two smooth round wooden rods may be used as an alternative to the fingers. The lens is now perfectly centred. (Centration will be difficult in those lenses incorporating a prism.)

Carefully holding the chuck as near vertically as possible, the base is held under running cold water to cool it. Care should be taken not to allow water to enter the spindle recess in the base and not to knock the lens off the chuck.

The lens is then replaced on the spindle, which is set in motion. A single-edge razor blade or hard, carborundum impregnated rubber tool is carefully brought into contact with the lens edge in line with the centre, with its cutting edge vertical and very slightly trailing to the direction of rotation of the lens edge. The lens overall size is now reduced.

Every few seconds, the overall size of the lens is checked, and cutting is ceased about 0.20–0.30 mm above the final required overall size to allow for the edging.

The lens is now edged as described below.

Unfortunately, many laboratories – even those using automated edging techniques – only produce good edges on about two-thirds of their lenses. Edging and re-edging therefore becomes the most desirable modification to be able to carry out oneself at the present time.

The lens is mounted on a spindle lens chuck, as described above. The edge of the lens is then examined by the Plasticine and binocular microscope (or slit lamp) method described in Chapter 12, Volume 1, and the points to be altered are noted.

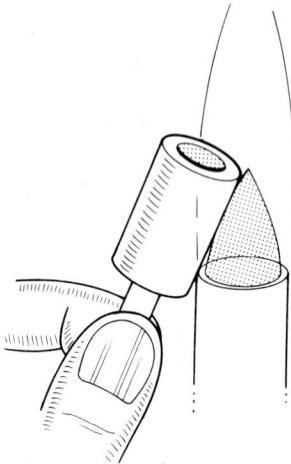

Figure 23.8–Heating the spindle lens chuck. The chuck is held by the stem and the base placed in the lower part of the bunsen burner flame

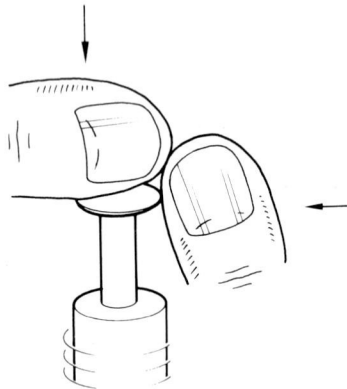

Figure 23.9–Centring the lens. While the adhesive wax is still soft, the lens is centred on the edging chuck by gently touching the top edge with one thumb and the side edge with the other (c.f. Figures 22.24 and 22.25)

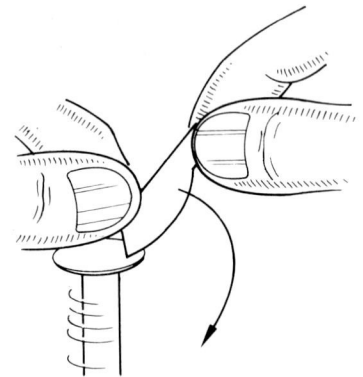

Figure 23.10–Shaping the edge. The blade or cutter is arching around the lens working from the back surface to just over the mid-edge, and then again from the front surface to slightly over the mid-edge position

EDGING AND RE-EDGING

When the overall size is reduced a lens must be re-edged. Otherwise it may be done if a small chip has accidentally been removed from a lens, and re-rounding that portion of the edge, although making the lens slightly 'truncated' saves having to order a new lens. This is an easy remedy for such slightly damaged lenses. Lenses with thin edges are easily damaged at the edge, for example, positive lenses (unless made lenticular) and the upper edge of a prism ballasted lens, and in all these cases, re-edging may become necessary to restore a comfortable fit. Occasionally, a replacement lens has a different edge from its original and from the lens in the other eye, and it needs reshaping to make it comfortable to wear. Edges which indent the cornea or conjunctiva and cause epithelial damage should always be well-rounded.

A thick square-edged cutter or large curved scalpel blade with the tip removed (*Figure 23.10*) is used for cutting and shaping, though some practitioners prefer a single straight-edged razor blade. This is preferably held gently against the rotating lens by the first finger and thumb of both hands, as shown. A little practice and regular checking of the edge profile soon shows how much to remove from the lens, but the following points may be of assistance.

First, cutting should start either on the back or front surface of the lens, working round the outside of the edge and slightly over to the opposite surface.

Secondly, when cutting on the front surface, care should be taken not to cut more than 0.5–1.0 mm in from the lens edge as scratches caused by the blade can be difficult to remove. Similarly, when cutting on the back surface edge, care should be taken not to scratch any peripheral curve.

Thirdly, if the lens has yet to have a peripheral curve put on, the edge must be shaped as in *Figure 23.11a* with a very rounded rear edge to allow for the material which will be removed when polishing on the peripheral curve (*Figure 23.11b*).

Farnum (1959) has stressed the importance of matching left and right lens edge thicknesses for optimum patient comfort.

These points having been carried out and the edge shaped to the practitioner's satisfaction, any sharp points, for example, those at the junction between the peripheral curve and edge curve, and scratches must be removed. This is carried out by means of a hard rubber burr, preferably cylindrical or conical in shape and impregnated with carborundum or diamond. The burr is carefully rolled around the edge a few times in the same manner as the cutting blade (*see Figure 22.29a–e*).

Inspection should show the lens edge now ready for polishing and with a profile as in *Figure 23.11c*.

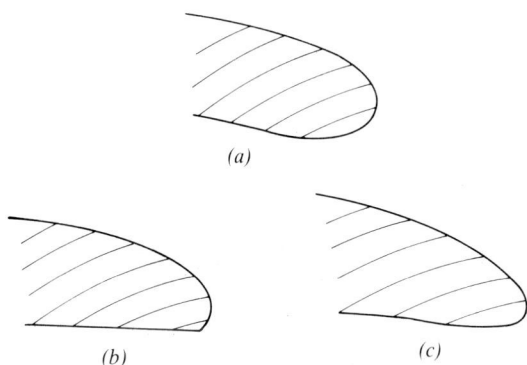

Figure 23.11–Corneal lens edge profiles. (a) Profile or initial monocurve lens prior to the addition of peripheral curves. (b) The same lens after the addition of a small peripheral curve (no edge treatment). (c) The final edge profile

This is most easily done by means of a piece of thin chamois leather and Silvo polish, the leather either being wrapped around a finger or folded double and the folded edge used. Polishing should be done for several minutes until a high polish is obtained (*see page 629 in Chapter 22*).

To remove the lens from the chuck, it is given a light flick with the finger on the front surface and it comes away easily. Any adhesive wax remaining on the front lens surface can be removed by wetting the surface with paraffin and rubbing gently with the finger, when the wax will slowly dissolve.

Some manufacturers produce edge contours by means of a rag wheel buff. While this is not so easily variable for each lens, it does have the advantage of

speed and can be usefully employed when razor-cutting the edge. For preference, a sewn rag wheel buff should be used, since this has plenty of body, and it should be only lightly applied with buffing compound. Ideally, the lens should be mounted on a spinner-type holder for regular polishing, as recommended by Haynes (1959), but is held lightly against the edge of the rotating buff, hardly penetrating the fibres, and, if not mounted on a spinner, slowly and evenly rotated, arching the holder and lens round the full edge curve. A final minute or so is spent polishing with Silvo, using a piece of chamois leather. This gives a highly polished well-shaped edge curve.

The edge may also be polished (or the overall size reduced) on a drum tool or flat sponge pad. The lens, mounted by its front surface, is pressed lightly into the drum surface perpendicular to the direction of rotation. It is now arched around the edge profile, parallel to the direction of drum travel, the lens being rotated all the while. this is then repeated with the lens mounted on its back surface.

REDUCTION OF THE BACK CENTRAL OPTIC DIAMETER, ALTERATION OF PERIPHERAL RADII, ADDITION OF NEW CURVES AND TRANSITION BLENDING

All these modifications are normally carried out to improve tears flow under the lens, as a remedy for corneal oedema. Transition blending may be necessary to remove sharp transitions causing arcuate epithelial damage seen with fluorescein staining. Flattening of peripheral curves can remedy the epithelial damage caused by too steep a peripheral curve which digs into the cornea as the lens moves. All sharp transitions can cause breaking up of any bubbles which may get beneath a lens, thereby causing dimpling.

A wax tool, free from cracks and air bubbles, is first cut to the required radius by means of a razor blade and a female gauge of the correct radius. This is held vertically and stationary on the centre of the wax tool rotating on a spindle. If stainless steel tools are used, it is best to incline them very slightly towards the operator initially and gradually approach the true vertical as the wax tool is cut to the correct radius. This avoids the gauge 'skidding' and damaging the wax tool.

Two or three small circular grooves are then cut in the surface of the wax with a pin point while the tool is rotating (*Figure 23.4*). These grooves aid in retaining the polish on the tool surface and in preventing the lens adhering to the tool by suction. They also prevent surface waves forming, due to build-up of polish on the tool, during polishing. One small identation cut in the very centre of the tool aids positioning of the female gauge during final cutting. The female gauge is then retouched on the wax tool to smooth off the surface of the grooves. Alternatively, tape or cloth-covered tools may be used.

The lens is then placed on one of the corneal holders or edging chuck as described earlier. A few drops of polishing liquid are applied to the rotating wax tool and the lens is slowly oscillated either backwards and forwards from near the edge to near the centre of the tool or across one side of the tool, being slowly rotated at the same time. Too fast a movement results in the periphery being scratched. Polishing liquid should be applied to the tool every 5–10 seconds to prevent the surface drying and scratching the lens.

Depending on the adjustment being done, the lens should be taken off its holder every so often to see the effect of the polishing. Blending transitions and alteration of a peripheral curve by a small amount may only take 2 or 3 seconds; a small peripheral curve or reduction of the back central optic diameter takes a little longer; and putting on a complete peripheral curve may take several minutes.

Measurement of the back central optic diameter is best carried out by means of a scale and magnifier. With a very narrow peripheral curve, however, the width may be impossible to measure. Such curves are best judged by means of a slit lamp or other high-powered magnifier, or by optical projection. The degree of blending may also be judged by inspecting the reflection of a strip light from the back of the lens surface using a × 8 loupe.

Approximate measurement of curves is facilitated by coating the lens back surface with a waterproof 'instant drying' ink. This is removed in the areas where the lens is being polished and makes the curve easily seen, though it is not necessarily sufficiently accurate for measurements to be made from it. When blending transitions, this becomes extremely useful. It may also be used as a gross test for checking the accuracy of a peripheral curve. The periphery is marked with ink and the lens is touched briefly on a wax tool of the correct radius. If the peripheral radius is accurate, ink will be removed over the whole width of the curve.

ALTERATION OF POWER

Addition of Negative Power

Addition of negative power becomes necessary as the refractive error changes, particularly in children, keratoconic patients and those with senile nuclear sclerosis of the crystalline lens. Any other marked change in refraction should lead to further investigation in case of lens warpage, gross changes in the corneal curvature occasioned by the fit of the lens, gross changes in the crystalline lens due to pathological conditions, or changes in the retina also due to pathological conditions. It should be noted that lens warpage often occurs when patients accidentally squeeze their lenses in the screw cap of the soaking case. The power on a focimeter may then appear satisfactory, but this distortion of the surfaces can be seen with a radiuscope or keratometer. Usually, an irregular, hazy line where the lens has been bent is visible if it is held up to the light.

This is considered by some practitioners to be a much easier modification than increasing positive power. For this reason, most practitioners tend to err on the positive side when ordering lenses.

The simplest method of carrying out this modification is by means of a 15 cm square of soft, clean, moistened polishing cloth spread over a similar-sized piece of chamois leather or moleskin laid on a smooth flat surface. A small amount of polishing fluid is spread in a circle on the cloth, using a finger. The dry back surface of the lens is then positioned, preferably, on a suitable lens holder, or on the tip of either the first or second finger. This is then placed on the polishing cloth in the circle of polish. Circular movements of about 5–8 cm in diameter are then described by the hand, exerting only a light pressure on the lens and taking great care not to tilt the lens holder or finger. After every six complete circular movements, the direction of rotation should be reversed to counteract the effect of any slight tilting, which will either cause distortion or give cylindrical power. Depending on the pressure on the lens, approximately twelve rotations are needed for every –0.25 D increase; and when nearing the end of a power alteration, the pressure on the lens must be gradually lessened to almost zero. Even when adding more than –0.25 D, the power must be checked frequently, not only to check on the progress of the power alteration but also because this will ensure that the lens is rotated to a different position on the finger, again to counter any distortion effects.

A more accurate method of adding negative power is by the use of a 10 cm drum chuck as described by Isen (1959). The lens is mounted on a holder by its back surface and placed near the edge of the rotating chuck, normally being tilted to about 20 degrees to the horizontal (*Figure 23.12a*). The drum 'skin' should be kept continually moist with polishing fluid and the lens kept slowly rotating, using both hands. Pressure on the lens should be just sufficient to contour the drum material to the lens shape. Excessive pressure will cause vibration of the lens and holder.

Addition of Positive Power

A drum chuck is also used for this modification, except that the lens is placed at or near the centre of the drum. Since the drum speed of rotation is zero at its centre, more lens material is removed from the lens edge and, consequently, positive power is added. Provided the chamois surface is kept moist with Silvo, the addition of positive power is straightforward; and as long as the lens is gently rotated, no cylindrical effect is introduced.

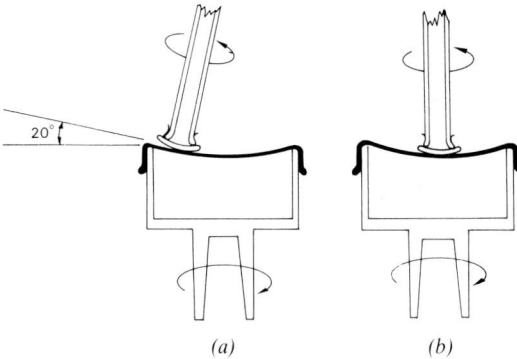

(a)   (b)

Figure 23.12–The use of a drum chuck for power alterations (cross-sections). (a) Addition of negative power. The lens is held near the drum edge at approximately 20 degrees to the horizontal. The lens is slowly rotated in either the same or the opposite direction to drum movement. (b) Addition of positive power. The lens is held vertically close to the drum centre and again slowly rotated

With conditions as for the addition of negative power, the lens is slowly moved in a small circle of about 3 or 4 mm or less around the drum centre, in either the same or opposite direction to that of drum rotation (*Figure 23.12b*). This avoids the small 'pip' sometimes obtained in the centre of the lens if it is held stationary at the drum centre, where there is no polishing action.

In adding positive power, occasionally a 'haze' may apear round the targets of the focimeter when checking the lens power. If this occurs, the diameter of the circle that the lens is being moved in should be increased to about 8 or 9 mm. This gives a more even polishing over the whole front surface and should add neither positive nor negative power. If this does not remove the 'haze', an alternative method is to add about +0.12 D too much positive power and then remove this by adding –0.12 D.

Either of these two latter methods may also be used for removing superficial front surface scratches.

FENESTRATION

If corneal oedema occurs, central fenestration holes – up to five in number – may help to encourage tears flow, but only if the lens is fitted apically well clear of the cornea; otherwise each hole can provide an additional meniscus of tears between lens and cornea – discouraging tears flow but aiding lens centration and reducing movement. Occasionally, holes may be drilled near the edge in one sector of a lens to lighten the weight there, that is, the reverse of a prism ballast.

A typical diameter is 0.20–0.30 mm (0.01″).

The lens is placed on the tip of the forefinger and after marking the position of the holes with a waterproof fibre pen, it is drilled from the front by hand, using a pin-vice. This is easier from the front surface and keeps the drill at the correct angle, perpendicular to the convex surface. The pin-vice should be rotated slowly and without pressure as excessive pressure may break the fine drill or crack the lens. To minimize the risk of the drill slipping and scratching the front surface of the lens, it should protrude as little as possible from the pin-vice. Also, the hole can be drilled through sticky tape stuck to the front surface of the lens.

The edges of the hole must now be countersunk on both sides. This is achieved by gently rotating a dental burr, size 0 or 1, anti-clockwise in the fenestration. Only a touch is needed, and it is quite easy to see the countersunk effect when using a suitable binocular magnifier.

Finally, the hole is carefully polished by hand using a finely sharpened boxwood stick and a trace of Silvo polishing fluid with as rapid a rotation as possible. Several changes of sticks may be needed in order to maintain a sharpened point. For larger fenestrations, a fine-pointed felt buff in a spindle may be used for a few seconds. Final careful inspection is a necessity.

Alternatively, the lens may be mounted, using a double-sided adhesive tape, on to first a convex chuck, and then a concave chuck so that the fenestration hole is positioned over a small central depression in each chuck. As the chuck rotates on the vertical spindle, a drop of Silvo is applied in the hole, and a boxwood stick – sharpened to a suitably angled point – is gently held in the fenestration hole. The boxwood stick is slowly rotated in a small circle in the opposite direction to the spindle rotation. this both countersinks and gives a fine polish (Mackie, 1968). If necessary, the inner part of the fenestration may be polished by running the hole up and down a length of Silvo-covered cotton.

A fenestrating machine available to the practitioner is shown in *Figure 23.13*.

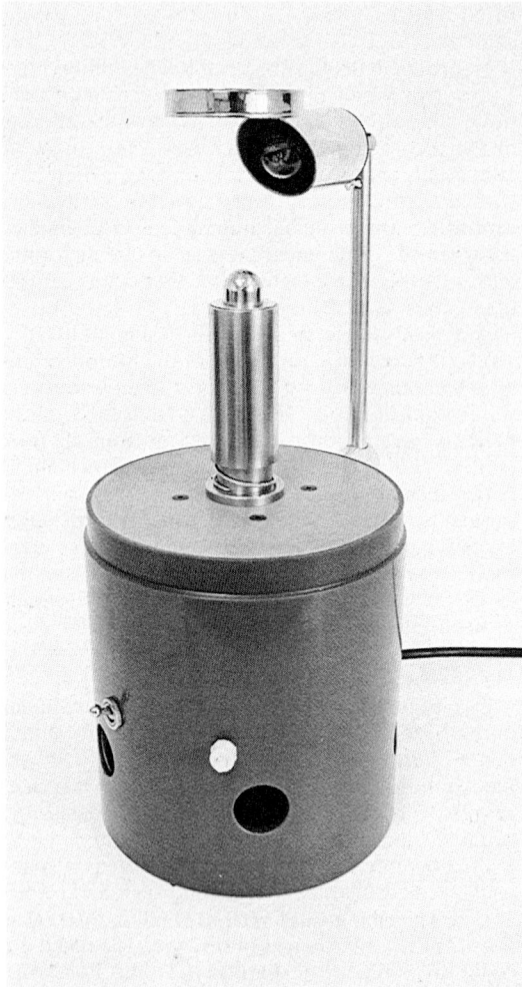

Figure 23.13–Fenestrating machine developed for the practitioner and suitable for both corneal and scleral lenses (photograph by courtesy of Focus Contact Lens Laboratory Ltd.)

TRUNCATION

Truncation may be necessary if an existing truncation does not line up correctly with the eyelid margin, or if the edge of a lens is slightly damaged in one place. Sometimes a round, prism ballast lens must be truncated to assist it to locate correctly if a front surface cylinder is present, or an already truncated bifocal lens must be truncated more to lower the segment height when the latter interferes with distance vision.

The most important factor to bear in mind before truncating a lens is the final edge thickness of the truncation (Haynes, 1959, 1965). For instance, it is useless to truncate a high-powered negative lens with minimal centre thickness as the edge thickness of the truncated portion may be too thin for easy modification and will be easily damaged.

The desired portion is first marked with a suitable marking agent, such as one of the 'instant drying' inks. Lens stock is then removed with either a pin-file, a hand manipulated abrasive stone or a rotating fine abrasive wheel, the lens being held between the fingers. The edge is then contoured, using a pin-file or fine emery paper. Polishing should be carried out using a rag-wheel buff, a drum chuck or a foam rubber pad. The part of the lens not being modified may be protected by adhesive tape. The lens may also be truncated by the edge being held firmly against the material of a rotating drum chuck and the edge shape rounded as previously described. It should also be stressed that in some instances the truncated edge may need to be kept relatively flat to align the lid margin.

SCLERAL LENS MODIFICATION

A general reduction in overall size is indicated when a lens remains stationary as the eye moves behind it; that is, the lens appears a 'steep fit'. Localized reductions of the size may be made if, for example, the lower haptic portion is too big for the lower fornix, or if the nasal haptic is pushed onto the nasal corneal limbus when the eye looks inwards. Sometimes the temporal haptic catches at the outer canthus but this is more often because that portion of the haptic is too small rather than too large.

A lens may be made horizontally oval if a horizontal oval fluorescein pool shows against-the-rule astigmatism with edge stand off at nasal and temporal edges and edge blanching at upper and lower edges. Making the vertical meridian smaller effectively flattens it in that meridian allowing it to settle but mid-temporal and mid-nasal back haptic grinding out may also be necessary. A vertical oval lens for with-the-rule astigmatism is not normally satisfactory cosmetically unless the palpebral aperture is particularly small.

Reducing an equal amount from all round the lens edge, in the case of a regular preformed lens, is carried out by simply rubbing the lens against a piece of medium-grade sandpaper placed on a flat surface. Care must be taken to maintain an even pressure around the whole lens edge.

Localized or overall reductions in lens size may be carried out by means of either a rotating grinding stone or an ordinary hand file.

The definition of back haptic size assumes sharp edges to the back lens surface. Thus, when reducing a lens to a specific back haptic size, provided that only minimal material is removed during the final edge shaping, little, if any, allowance need be made for plastics removed during this latter process.

EDGING

Edging is necessary when overall size reductions have been carried out; if the edge has been damaged; or if haptic modifications have altered the edge shape.

A stone grinding ball of 1 inch in diameter, previously soaked in water and held in a horizontal spindle, may be used for the rounding of both front and back haptic edge surfaces. Alternatively, an ordinary small hand file, followed by fine emery paper, may be used for the front surface. A large rounded rubber tool impregnated with diamond or carborundum may be used for the back surface.

Polishing is easily carried out, using a rag-wheel buff. The lens edge should be held vertically and approximately in line with the rotating buff to polish the back edge surface. The lens should be held lightly and continually rotated during polishing to prevent burning of the plastics. This also prevents a ridge of plastics building up on the back edge. Great care should be taken to check that this does not happen, and final examination must ascertain that there is no such ridge. The final edge should be of a blunt, rounded form.

Alternatively, the lens may be edged and polished by tools held in a flexible drive, as explained on page 228, Chapter 9, Volume 1.

BACK OPTIC GRIND-OUT

This is done to increase the clearance of the back optic portion from the cornea. A steeper radius may be required if heavy central touch exists with a large annular bubble at the limbus. A flatter back optic radius is indicated if central corneal touch and mid-peripheral corneal or limbal touch occur together. It must be borne in mind that changing the BOR alters the power of the contact lens and liquid lens (see Chapter 4, Volume 1). Where possible the BOR should therefore be kept the same.

The central optic thickness is measured and a central waterproof mark is made on the front surface at this point. A 'runner' is attached to the centre of the front surface of the optic with double-sided adhesive tape. A diamond impregnated brass tool of the desired radius is placed on a vertical spindle, which is then set in motion. Using paraffin or water as the lubricating agent, the optic

portion of the lens is ground out, using a pencil point or similar object in the runner guide hole, the lens being moved slowly backwards and forwards across one side of the head of the diamond tool. The lens should be allowed to rotate freely and lubricant should be used as necessary to prevent the tool surface drying out. The lens should be removed at frequent intervals to check the rate of reduction in central thickness. Final grinding is best performed with paraffin as the lubricating agent. Being slightly more viscous than water, it allows the tool less possibility of abrading the surface and thereby facilitates final polishing.

The increased viscosity slows the rate of grinding out, however. Paraffin is inconvenient with fenestrated lenses as it tends to leak through the fenestration, occasionally dissolving the adhesive, and causing the runner to become detached from the lens. About 0.02 mm thickness should be allowed for final polishing of the optic. This is carried out in exactly the same way as for corneal lenses – retaining the lens on the runner and using either a wax, tape or cloth covered tool of the correct radius with Silvo polish (see page 654).

TRANSITIONAL GRIND-OUT OR EXTENSION

This is done if the transitions are sharp and cause frothing of the bubble, if limbal touch occurs or where there is insufficient clearance beyond the limbus, as indicated by the extent of the fluorescein pool.

This is carried out as described under Optic Grind-out above but using the large-size diamond impregnated tool, the only other difference being that widths of transition are normally taken rather than thickness removed, and the final polishing is carried out using a large wax tool or felt ball.

A transitional grind-out is normally necessary after an optic grind-out owing to the reduction in width of the transitional curve(s) caused by the central grind-out. (A fenestration will similarly need re-countersinking and polishing when a transitional or optic grind-out has been performed.)

A transitional grind-out is best carried out after the optic has been polished to facilitate measurement of the transition width. Alternatively, the area may be marked with ink to show the border between the transition and optic portions during grinding. (Paraffin cannot be used as a lubricant if it dissolves the inks used.)

Polishing the rough ground transition extends its width slightly. This becomes important when extending a transition well into the optic, and especially when making a double curve optic.

LOCALIZED HAPTIC AND TRANSITION GRIND-OUTS

This is done in regions where the haptic or transition touch the eye heavily, as evidenced by blanching of the conjunctival blood vessels. The latter may be seen more easily if a little digital pressure is applied to the lens. Also, if the optic gives too much clearance from the cornea the whole back haptic surface may be ground out to settle the lens. More substance should be removed from near the transition region to maintain the same curvature and give the most effective settling.

One of the most common modifications needed is a temporal haptic grind-out near the transition to permit the lens to settle and move slightly nasally. This is indicated when a large temporal static bubble occurs at the limbus accompanied by nasal corneal touch from the optic. A slight reduction in nasal haptic size may also be needed to permit the nasal shift of the lens.

The area to be ground is first marked on the back surface (or front, according to preference) with a suitable quick-drying ink or grease pencil. For the beginner, it is useful to measure the average thickness of the area to be ground out – at several noted points in the area if this is large. This can be checked during the grind-out to determine the amount of material removed; and in a larger area, to check that the material is being removed evenly. If necessary, the optic may be protected with a small piece of Plasticine (Bier, 1957) or adhesive tape pressed firmly into the optic area.

The grind-out is performed with a spherical, cigar-shaped or wheel-shaped stone, the size of which depends on the size of the area to be ground

out. This is held in a Jacob's chuck on a horizontal spindle, and it should be kept moist throughout the operation. In order to prevent deep scratches in the haptic portion, the lens should be kept continually moving back and forth slightly, until the ink over the area (if on the back surface) is removed. Surplus lens material and polish should be regularly removed with a tissue. The haptic thickness should be checked before continuing.

The rough area may now be smoothed, if necessary, with a rotating hard rubber burr. Polishing may be carried out with a felt buff and polishing compound or, more slowly, with a soft mop buff and Silvo. Final polishing with a soft mop and Silvo is always preferable as it gives a better finish. To save time, this may be omitted until the lens has been checked on the eye and has been found to fit satisfactorily.

Examination under magnification will show areas which have not been polished completely. Forknall (1953) has shown that for equal haptic settling, relatively more plastics must be removed from near the transition than from the peripheral haptic.

FENESTRATION

Most scleral lenses are fenestrated to permit tears flow and oxygen exchange behind the lens. If a fenestration hole becomes covered by the upper lid regularly, or otherwise blocked as by loose conjunctival tissue or mucus, then a further hole or holes may be required within the palpebral aperture.

The position having been determined, as explained in Chapters 9 and 10, Volume 1, the fenestration hole is made as follows.

With a 0.50 or 0.75 mm drill (typically), a hole is drilled normal to the surface to minimize its length. Care should be taken not to slip with the drill and scratch the optic surface. The drill should be held in a pin-vice so that a minimum length of drill protrudes. This gives greater control over exact positioning. Alternatively, the drill may be held in a Jacob's chuck on a horizontal spindle, which lessens the risk of the drill or lens slipping and scratching the optic surface, and the lens 'fed' on to the drill.

A flame-shaped dental burr is then turned anti-clockwise (to give a finer cut) in the hole to countersink (*Figure 23.14*). A few turns initially with a 1.50 or 2.00 mm drill can be used to speed up the process of countersinking. Countersinking should be continued equally on both sides of the lens until examination under ×50 magnification shows the two countersinks are almost meeting. Funnel shaping is essential to create an even tears flow and prevent turbulence likely to remove epithelium from the corneal surface.

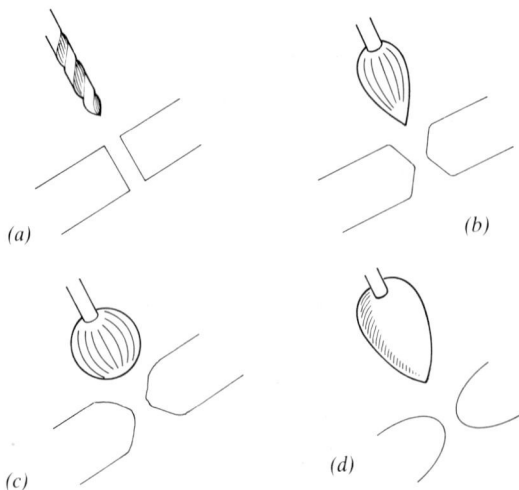

Figure 23.14–The four stages of fenestrating a scleral lens

A slightly larger spherical dental burr is then used, as before, to taper the outer edges of the countersinking.

The countersinks are then polished at low speed, to avoid burning, using a pointed soft felt burr soaked in Silvo, until a high polish is obtained.

Inspection under ×50 magnification should show a fenestration polished all the way through and with tapered edges as shown in *Figure 23.14*. Any remaining polishing residue may be removed with a tapered stick (for example, a toothpick), tissue, or bristle.

CHANNELLING

Channelling is an alternative to fenestration, and may be indicated if the limbal region is very irregular and the introduction of a bubble would lead to frothing, or if the limbal conjunctiva is very loose and blocks the fenestrations. (A loose conjunctiva may also block a channel.)

Although sometimes not so successful as fenestration, it may become a necessity under certain conditions. Various uses and designs of channel have been discussed by McKay Taylor (1969).

The channel is cut in exactly the same way as a local haptic grind-out, along a specific line or curve, and, where possible, using a sharp-edged wheel-shaped grinding tool. This is usually cut from the upper temporal lens edge into the mid-transition, though an inferior channel and/or other channels may also become necessary. The channel should occupy about half the lens thickness and have well blended edges to prevent conjunctival abuse.

Fluorescein examination should show a clear channel from the lens edge into the optic portion.

An alternative method, using either the cast of an eye impression or of a preformed lens, is to glue a suitable piece of nylon on to the cast along the desired line of the channel. A shell then made from the cast has a channel pressed into the plastics to the desired depth. The slightly raised area on the front of the finished lens is not noticed subjectively. The advantage of this method is that it enables the shell to be pressed from thinner sheet initially than for a lens where a channel is to be ground into the haptic portion.

POWER ALTERATIONS

Power alterations must be made if the refraction changes or if a change in BOR is carried out for fitting purposes. Other points to note are mentioned in connection with corneal lens power changes (*see* page 654).

These are normally carried out by the laboratory as the front surface must be recut each time. Minor

front surface alterations may be made on a drum, as for corneal lenses (*see* page 655).

Practitioners should bear in mind that an optic grind-out, by reducing the thickness of the optic portion, will effectively add a small amount of negative power to the lens. In order to prevent unnecessary modification, +0.25 to +0.50 D should be added to the power required if a back optic grind-outs are likely to become necessary (*see* Chapter 4, Volume 1).

SPATULATION

Spatulation should rarely be necessary but is indicated if an area of the haptic portion stands clear of the eye, and to settle the rest of the haptic by back haptic grinding out would not be feasible due to too thin a lens – or lack of time to carry out the tedious grinding.

Loose haptic areas may be removed by means of spatulation (Obrig, 1942; Bier, 1957). A cast is made of the lens, and the loose area is marked on the back surface of the lens and on the cast. Material is then scraped off the cast in this area. A spatula is heated to approximately 70°C for lenses cut from solid plastics and 60°C for impression lenses (Bier, 1957) and pressed on the front lens surface over the loose area, the cast being held in position against the back surface of the lens.

Tight areas may also be removed in an opposite manner by taking a cast of the front lens surface. Spatulation is best performed on thin lenses, that is thinner than approximately 0.75 mm. Too great a rise in temperature of the lens is not desirable as residual monomer may be released, which is toxic to the eye (Estevez, 1967).

PLASTICS BUILD-UP

Again, plastics build-up should not be necessary but it is an alternative to spatulation.

This method of building up the back lens surface, as described by Bier (1957), is no longer recommended as the new material added is likely to be toxic to the eye (Estevez and Ridley, 1966).

MODIFICATION OF CELLULOSE ACETATE (CAB) LENSES

CAB lenses may be modified with the same tools as conventional PMMA lenses. However, as CAB is softer than PMMA, material is removed more quickly and care should be taken not to proceed too fast during all cutting, grinding, and polishing actions. Similarly, the lens surface scratches more easily unless handled carefully. Polishes such as tin oxide and water should be used and not those containing solvents, such as Silvo (Danker, 1977).

MODIFICATION OF OTHER NEW HARD LENS MATERIALS SUCH AS THOSE WITH LOWERED WETTING ANGLES

Apart from BP-flex (*Burton Parsons*) which is known to be PMMA with a second methacrylic component, and which has a lowered wetting angle and very slightly improved oxygen transmission, new materials should not be polished with Silvo without instructions from the manufacturers. It must be remembered that not only may polishing compounds react with lens materials, but also the very actions of grinding and polishing may upset the chemical nature of the material, releasing toxic products. Thus, manufacturers' instructions should always be sought before modifications to lenses of new materials are made.

MODIFICATION OF SOFT CONTACT LENSES

As a general rule, it may be taken that the majority of laboratories will not modify finished (that is, hydrated) soft lenses and, further, that many soft lenses do not lend themselves to modification, particularly those of high water content.

Cordrey (1975) states that certain lenses may be modified by soaking them in distilled water, to effectively remove saline from the lens prior to dehydration. Failure to remove the saline content will cause irregularity of lens shape on dehydration. Regularity in shape may also be aided by allowing the dehydration to take place on a former of the same curvature as the lens back surface. After dehydration, edge curves may be added using a suitable oil-based polishing compound, fenestrations performed as described above, edge shape modified, cylinders added to front or back surface, lenticulation performed, etc., either by the practitioner or more usually by the laboratory.

Bailey (1975) recommends that all soft lenses entering the practitioners' office be engraved with a suitable code number to aid later identification. Bailey recommends that the lenses are partly dehydrated on a soft lens 'optical gauge' or brass tool, the curvature of which approximates to that of the lens back surface. Because soft lenses become increasingly brittle with extended drying time it is recommended that etching is done no more than one hour after dehydration commences. Engraving is performed using a fine-pointed instrument or small high-speed drill and viewed under a stereomicroscope. Bailey reports no increased incidence of lens tearing around the engraving but practitioners must obviously be aware of the increased risk of lens breakage, particularly with higher water content lenses.

Westerhout has discussed truncation of soft lenses by the practitioner on pages 558 and 561 in Chapter 18.

CONCLUSION

Practitioners are advised to obtain a selection of reject lenses on which to practise modifications. The majority of modifications may be accurately carried out with only a little practice, but practitioners are urged to maintain their own standards to at least those that they would expect from their laboratory.

REFERENCES

Bailey, N. J. (1975). 'Soft contact lens identification.' *J. Am. optom. Ass.* **46**, 1177–1178

Bier, N. (1957). *Contact Lens Routine and Practice*, 2nd ed. London: Butterworths

Cepero, G. (1959). 'Conical and concentric polishing.' *Contacto* **3**, 28–34

Cordrey, P. (1975). Personal communication

Danker, F. (1977). 'Progress with cellulose acetate butyrate contact lenses.' *Ophthal. Optician* **17**, 828–829

Estevez, J. M. J. (1967). 'Poly(methyl methacrylate) for use in contact lenses.' *Contact Lens* **1**(3), 19–21, 26

Estevez, J. M. J. and Ridley, F. (1966). 'Safety requirements for contact lens materials: and their manipulation and use.' *Am. J. Ophthal.* **62**, 132–139

Farnum, F. E. (1959). 'Refinements in contact lens adjustments to increase wearing time.' *Am. J. Optom.* **36**, 382–384

Forknall, A. J. (1953). 'Conversion of sealed to ventilated contact lenses.' *Optician* **125**, 327–330, 356–358

Haynes, P. R. (1959). 'Modification of contact lenses.' In *Encyclopaedia of Contact Lens Practice* **22**, 1–97. Ed. by Haynes, P. R. South Bend, Indiana: International Optics Publishing Corporation

Haynes, P. R. (1965). 'Modification procedures.' In *Contact Lens Practice, Basic and Advanced,* ed. by Mandell, R. B. Springfield, Illinois: Thomas

Isen, A. (1959). 'Spherical power changes in contact lenses.' In *Encyclopaedia of Contact Lens Practice* **22**, 72–74. Ed. by Haynes, P. R. South Bend, Indiana: International Optics Publishing Corporation

Mackie, I. A. (1968). Lecture to The Contact Lens Society

Obrig, T. E. (1942). *Contact Lenses.* Philadelphia: Chilton

Taylor, C. McKay (1969). 'The S-bend and other channelled haptic lenses.' *Ophthal. Optician* **9**, 1256–1258

Chapter 24

Special Types of Contact Lenses and Their Uses

Janet Stone

The majority of contact lenses are supplied as an alternative to spectacles. But there are also contact lenses which fall into quite a different category. These may afford the only possible type of refractive correction for a patient, or may protect the eyes or improve their appearance in a way which is impossible with spectacles. Other types of contact lens are used to diagnose abnormal ocular conditions or to give therapeutic aid in certain cases. And there are yet more types which have other special uses.

These special or less usual types of contact lens will now be considered.

CONTACT LENSES IN PATHOLOGICAL CASES

It is not intended to describe here in detail the pathological or abnormal conditions in which contact lenses may be fitted. Reference to any textbook of ocular disease will give the aetiology, signs, symptoms and treatment of these conditions. The uses of impression scleral lenses and soft lenses for such pathological conditions have been fully dealt with in Chapters 20 and 21 respectively. To avoid duplication, only a brief mention of the fitting of these types of lenses is given in this chapter which largely includes information additional to that found elsewhere in this book. The information which follows gives only those details which are pertinent to the fitting of contact lenses.

KERATOCONUS

Keratoconus is a classic example of a case in which an irregular corneal front surface causes poor vision which cannot be adequately improved with spectacles. The regular front surface of a contact lens, by

replacing the irregular corneal surface, frequently allows excellent vision to be restored.

In the early stages of the condition, corneal lenses are the ideal form of correction; but in advanced keratoconus, scleral lenses must be fitted as corneal lenses rarely remain *in situ*.

Because of the displacement of the apex of the cone (usually down and in) relative to the pupil, there is a common problem in all methods of fitting keratoconus. This is to make the back optic portion of the lens, which tends to centre itself on the apex of the cone, sufficiently large to cover the pupil area without introducing bubbles or leading to a stagnant pool of tears opposite the pupil.

Reference to *Figure 24.1* will show the difficulties which the practitioner has to overcome.

Conventional fitting methods, in which the back surface of the lens contours the cornea, would lead to too small a back central optic diameter being fitted and consequent visual dissatisfaction. All methods of fitting are, therefore, something of a compromise.

Corneal Lenses

Corneal lenses are most satisfactory in the early stages of keratoconus. Any rapid increase of astigmatism should lead the practitioner to suspect keratoconus. Its presence may be verified by observation of the corneal profile against the lower lid as the patient looks down and the upper lid is raised. In keratometry, the readings are usually very steep and may fall outside the normal range of the instrument. It is almost always impossible to properly align the mires in order to determine the principal meridians of the cornea. A placido disc or hand keratoscope may help in confirming the condition, when an appearance similar to that in *Figure 24.2* is seen. The central rings are much displaced with respect to the pupil and their spacing is very close, whilst peripheral rings are more normally spaced.

Where keratometer readings are within the range of the instrument, this in itself is an indication that the condition is in its early stages.

Retinoscopy may show a swirling reflex, and the reflex from the apical zone may be separated from the reflex from the rest of the pupillary area by a shadow.

Several techniques of fitting corneal lenses for keratoconus have been described and they are now being used in conjunction with hydrophilic lenses (*see* 'Combination Lenses', Chapter 21, page 614).

Flat Fitting

Clifford Hall (1963) has advocated fitting a large flat lens. The overall size recommended is between 9.50 and 11.50 mm and has a back peripheral zone 0.50–1.00 mm wide. The aim is to distribute the weight evenly over as large an area of the cornea as possible.

A lens is inserted which is flatter than the cone, having a fairly normal back central optic radius between 7.00 and 8.00 mm. This is initially left to settle for about 20 minutes, when the fit is examined. During this period, the lens – which at first may stand away from the lower cornea and is only held in place by the upper lid – gradually settles as the soft cornea is moulded to a flatter curve. The flattest lens which is acceptable and is reasonably stable on blinking and eye movement is used as a basis for determining the required power. Clifford Hall found that the larger the diameter the lower the negative power required, due to the compression of the cornea shortening the eye and giving a reduction in myopia.

After several weeks or months, patients may accept an even flatter lens with more reduction in negative power. Good tolerance of these lenses is reported, with minimal corneal abrasion and very few losses of lenses.

Alignment Fitting (*Figure 24.3*)

This method is only visually satisfactory if the cone is centrally situated about the visual axis – which is very rare. The back surface of the corneal lens is of multi-curve construction and the back central optic may have to be as steep as 3.00 mm in radius, although the method is more satisfactory in early keratoconus when back central optic radii of 6.00–7.00 mm are used. This method has been advocated

by Moss (1959) and by Chiquiar Arias (1963a). Fitting sets are necessary; and since the required power is of the order of –15.00 D or more, the steeper lenses must be small if edge thickness is to be kept to a reasonable amount. Lenses as small as 7.00 mm overall size have been satisfactorily fitted. In certain cases, it may be necessary to prescribe additional negative spectacles (also incorporating any cylindrical element) to prevent the edge thickness of the corneal lens becoming too great.

With small lenses, the alignment is limited to the conical area of the cornea so that the total amount of back peripheral flattening may only be as much as 1.00–1.50 mm. However, the peripheral zone of larger lenses aligns with an area of normal cornea and may have to be 3.00 mm or more flatter than the back central optic.

It is essential for practitioners to be able to do their own modifications. It is rarely possible to achieve an entirely satisfactory fit from a fitting set lens, which should therefore only be used as a basis for judging the lens to be ordered on the understanding that alterations in curvature are likely to be necessary – if not at first, then certainly later as the cornea alters in shape.

Steep Fitting

When an alignment fit is attempted on a cornea having a decentred conus, the back optic portion must be made sufficiently large to cover the pupil area. This may result in a steep fit or in apical and transitional touch, as described below.

Generally speaking, a steep fit is not desirable as it encourages steepening of the conus. Oedema may also result, due to stagnation of the tears trapped by the central portion of the lens. A sequel to this may be nebular opacification of the central cornea, owing to persistent imbibation of water in that region.

Three-Point Touch Fitting

The alternative to a steep fit is one which gives light apical touch as well as peripheral alignment, so that in at least one meridian (usually the horizontal) the lens is touching the cornea in three places. The lens may stand away from the lower cornea slightly, but this facilitates tears exchange. *Figures 24.4* and *24.5* show the fit, depicted in section, and fluorescein pattern. The latter shows the central touch and almost annular mid-peripheral touch.

Of all the methods of fitting corneal lenses in keratoconus, this now seems to be the most favoured. The weight of the lens is fairly well distributed on a relatively normal part of the cornea.

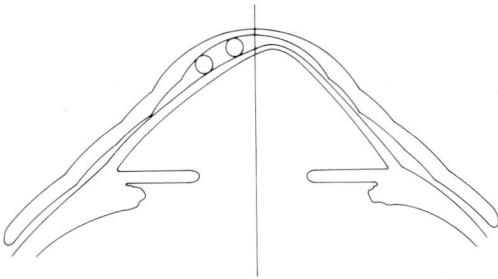

Figure 24.1–Cross-section of a scleral contact lens on a conical cornea, with the apex of the cone decentred. Bubbles are shown trapped between the optic and cornea (c.f. Figure 20.5, Chapter 20)

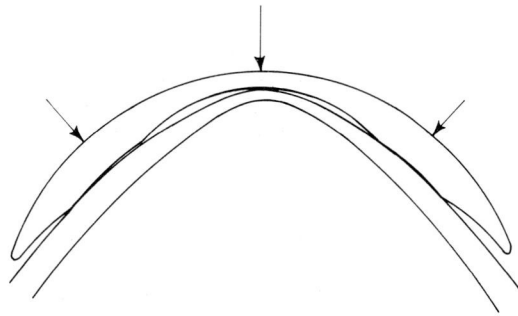

Figure 24.4–A cross-section to show 'three-point touch' of a corneal lens on the horizontal meridian of a conical cornea (areas of touch are arrowed)

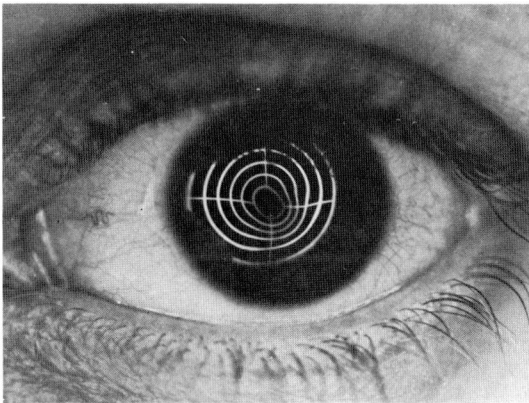

Figure 24.2–A typical keratoscope image formed by a conical cornea

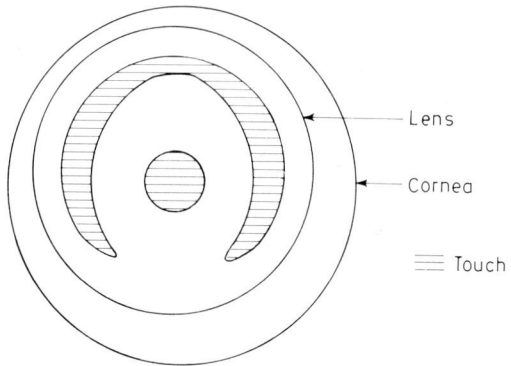

Figure 24.5–A typical fluorescein picture showing 'three-point touch' of a corneal lens in keratoconus

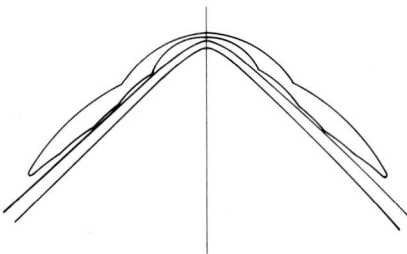

Figure 24.3–Alignment fitting of a conical cornea using a multi-curve corneal lens

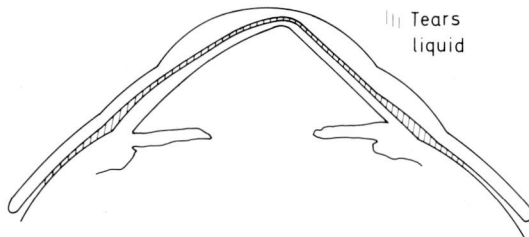

Figure 24.6–The optic portion of a scleral lens constructed so as to align a keratoconic cornea (c.f. Figure 20.2, Chapter 20)

The light central touch seems to prevent advancement of the cone without causing abrasion. The method represents a compromise alignment technique, allowing a sufficiently large back central optic portion to prevent visual problems.

Most lenses fitted in this way are large enough to extend over a normal area of cornea and are between 9.00 and 10.00 mm in overall size, with a 6.00–7.00 mm back central optic diameter. Back central optic radii typically fall between 6.00 and 7.00 mm, the radius being determined by fluorescein pattern assisted by light pressure to simulate lid pressure. A pressure rod may be used, as described by Chiquiar Arias (1963b).

The peripheral fit may be determined with trial lenses; and since this area of cornea is of fairly normal curvature, radii between 8.00 and 9.00 mm may be required to align with the cornea. One or two curves may be needed with a further flatter curve to give sufficient edge clearance.

Chiquiar Arias *et al.* (1959) have described a technique of using very small lenses to obtain the central fit and fitting rings to obtain the peripheral fit; but these are difficult to handle and the likelihood of corneal abrasion is high, so they have not been widely adopted.

Scleral Lenses

These are the lenses of choice in advanced keratoconus because they stay in place and are less likely than corneal lenses to cause abrasions of the greatly protruding cone. Unfortunately, they do slightly increase the apparent protrusion of the eye, due to their thickness.

To allow tears exchange, they should be fitted either fenestrated or channelled. However, fenestrations – because they purposely introduce a bubble beneath the optic – may be contra-indicated as the bubble frequently breaks up and may froth or cause small bubbles to collect in front of the pupil area (*Figure 24.1*). Channelled lenses can inadvertently cause similar problems, so a sealed minimum clearance lens may have to be resorted to if other methods fail, although McKay Taylor's (1969) design of an S-bend channel in the upper and lower haptic portion has been found to relieve frothing in fenestrated lenses.

The haptic portion may be fitted by preformed or impression techniques and the back optic specification may be determined by similar methods. It is advisable to carry out only one impression on each eye at any session, owing to the fragility of the cornea. FLOM (Fenestrated Lenses for Optic Measurement), having three or four back surface curves, have been described by Bier (1957) but are difficult to use satisfactorily as they do not centre on

the apex of the cone. A similar type of optic portion results when the manufacturer (or practitioner) grinds a number of curves on to the back optic portion of the shell corresponding to the eye impression, and these curves generally allow a better fit as they can be centred with respect to the cone apex. This is done to give the best possible alignment with the cornea and yet allow a sufficiently large back central optic diameter. The practitioner must decide whether to fit with apical touch or apical clearance, and ophthalmological advice is desirable. Clifford Hall found apical touch to be disastrous in some cases; but, on the other hand, apical clearance may encourage advancement of the cone – particularly if the clearance of the apex is greater than at the limbus. For this reason, adequate limbal clearance should be ensured. However, if the back optic truly aligns but just clears the cornea (*Figure 24.6*), the even thickness of tears fluid allows pressure to be evenly distributed over the cornea and should prevent advancement of the cone.

This even clearance is probably best achieved by the use of a laminate cemented to a cast of the eye impression and a scleral shell pressed over both cast and laminate. Full details of the fitting technique are given in Chapter 9, Volume 1, and in Chapter 20.

As settling of the lens takes place over a period of time, light apical touch may develop. It is probable that this is only harmful if the lens is not stable on the eye, when an abrasive action of the lens on the apex of the cone may result. The weight of the lens should be borne by the sclera. If it is transferred to the apex of the cone, it could obviously have unfortunate effects – whereas a very light touch may act as a support to the cone and prevent further advancement.

Great skill is required in fitting these lenses. A practitioner should be able to distinguish between a potentially harmful and a harmless apical touch. The fitting of such eyes can be very rewarding as the visual improvement is so remarkable.

Flush-fitting scleral lenses (*see* page 687) have been used following keratoplasty – particularly for keratoconus when the graft has become tilted – in an attempt to straighten the graft and also improve its transparency.

PTOSIS

When the upper lid droops, a scleral contact lens may be fitted to act as a crutch in order to raise the upper lid sufficiently to expose the pupil area. There are a number of ways in which this may be achieved. Full details are given in Chapter 20, page 598, but a brief résumé is included here for the sake of completeness.

Thick Scleral Lenses

A very thick scleral lens may be sufficient to hold the lids apart enough for the patient to see. The upper part of the scleral lens may be made thicker than the rest of the lens – a thickness of 1.50–2.00 mm being necessary (*see Figures 20.15, 20.16 and 20.17*).

Stepped-up Lenses

Bier (1960a) has described a scleral lens, as illustrated in *Figure 24.7a* which has a step aligned with the desired position of the upper lid margin and on

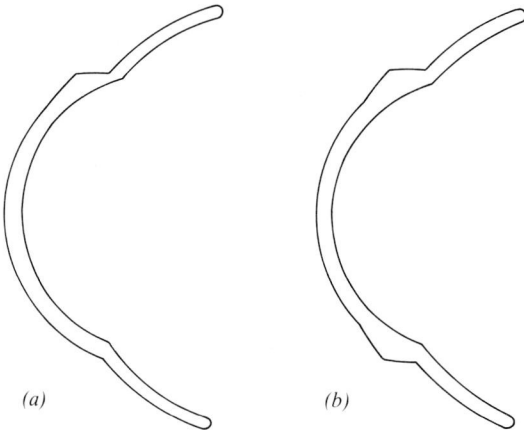

(a) *(b)*

Figure 24.7–(a) Cross-section of a ptosis crutch scleral lens designed to hold up the upper lid. (b) A similar lens designed to hold both lids apart (c.f. Figures 20.19–20.22, Chapter 20)

which the lid rests. However, the elevation of the upper lid may also pull up the lower lid or cause the lens to rotate, so a similar step in line with the lower lid may be required to hold this lid down (*Figure 24.7b*).

Lenses with a Projecting Shelf

Another method which has been used with success is to attach to the scleral lens a projecting shelf which fits into the marginal sulcus of the upper lid, thereby holding it up. Such a lens is depicted in *Figures 24.8a and b*.

As with the stepped lens, a lower shelf may also be required to hold the lower lid down and/or prevent lens rotation.

A minimum amount of cement should be used in attaching the shelf to the lens as there is reason to

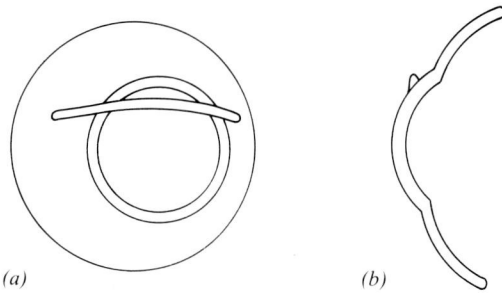

(a) *(b)*

Figure 24.8–(a) Front view of a scleral lens with a projecting shelf to act as a ptosis crutch. (b) Cross-section of this lens (c.f. Figure 20.18, Chapter 20)

believe that the cement may be toxic to the ocular tissues (Estevez, 1967).

The best cosmetic results are achieved in all cases if the lids are not held too widely apart. In unilateral ptosis, this minimizes the difference in appearance during blinking, when only the lids of the normal eye are able to close.

Those lenses which prevent blinking frequently rub the upper limbus region, as Bell's phenomenon occurs at each intended blink and the eye rotates upwards. This has, in some cases, resulted in blood vessel infiltration into the cornea from the upper limbus region.

PROSTHETIC LENSES AND SHELLS (*see Colour Plate III*, Volume 1)

Prosthetic lenses and shells are used to improve the appearance of eyes disfigured by injury or disease, or in cases of large-angle squints. In such cases, the psychological benefits to the patient are frequently remarkable and justify the time and effort expended by the practitioner in achieving a good cosmetic result. Iris colour changes may be effected for actors and others wishing to change the colour of their eyes.

Soft lenses are now the lens of choice, but scleral lenses or shells are essential where the sclera is to be covered or where a squint is to be masked. Corneal or soft lenses should be adequate if a corneal scar is to be covered, provided that a satisfactory fit can be achieved. This is an alternative to tattooing to prevent scattered light disturbing visual acuity. In polycoria (multiple pupils), a suitable patterned 'iris' incorporated in the contact lens may be used to mask out the unwanted pupils. Scleral and soft lenses having an area of the optic portion blacked out have been used with success for eyes with subluxated crystalline lenses, the clear optic portion being positioned in front of the pupil area containing the crystalline lens. Most prosthetic lenses or shells are provided for one eye to make the appearance simulate that of the other eye.

A satisfactory cosmetic effect may be achieved by using a shell, in which case the central pupil aperture is left unworked and usually consists of black plastics material. The size of the 'pupil' is made slightly larger than the normal pupil of the good eye so that when the latter pupil dilates the difference in size is less pronounced. This is also done with sighted lenses. The forward position of the effective entrance pupil means that it must be larger to allow in the same amount of light as the other eye.

In all cases, a satisfactory fit must first be achieved with a clear lens or shell which, in the case of a scleral lens, must be allowed to settle so that all necessary modifications have been made before a final prosthetic lens or shell is duplicated from it (*see* Chapter 20, page 602). If it is not necessary to sight the shell, a flush-fitting scleral shell is ideal, and only the front optic surface need be polished. The pupil centre must be accurately marked on the clear shell so that it is correctly located in the prosthetic duplicate, otherwise a squinting appearance may inadvertently be introduced. The iris colour and pattern, as well as the scleral colour and conjunctival blood vessel pattern, are matched with the other eye from a set of coloured buttons or a coloured chart. Careful measurements of iris and pupil size must be made. Fincham (1947) has reproduced iris colours and patterns very satisfactorily by taking a positive black and white transparency of the good eye and backing it with black plastics suitably painted to render correct colouring. This is incorporated in the cosmetic lens or shell. A black background alone gives a blue or grey 'iris' colour dependent on the fineness of the iris pattern and the amount of light scattered.

Methods of manufacture vary; but basically, the iris is usually painted on a layer of black plastics from which a small circular central portion is removed and replaced by clear material if the optic is to be sighted. In the case of sclerals, the black plastics may continue over the haptic portion if light is to be prevented from entering the eye as, for example, through a poorly pigmented choroid. This black layer is then covered by a layer of white plastics. Otherwise, the iris button is surrounded by a layer of white or opal plastics on which a blood vessel pattern is painted or fine strands of red silk or cotton are stuck to simulate conjunctival blood vessels. The whole is then embedded in clear plastics, which is pressed over a cast of the correctly fitting shell and polymerized by boiling. Great care is taken in this process to ensure complete polymerization.

If it is not necessary to have an artificial 'sclera', the iris button alone may be incorporated in the clear plastics material. The effect of an anterior chamber is achieved by making the clear optic portion in front of the painted iris thicker than the haptic portion of the lens, which has a total thickness of about 1.00 mm with a minimum of 0.50 mm.

The thickness of the prosthetic scleral lens or shell may cause the eye to appear to protrude slightly as the palpebral aperture size is increased relative to the other eye. Additional spectacles incorporating a negative lens of about −5.00 D on that side renders this appearance less noticeable. The prosthetic scleral lens must be suitably sighted to allow for this.

When fitting squinting eyes, a clear scleral shell is made to fit the eye in the normal way and the position of the iris pattern and pupil are marked on this so that the visual axes will appear parallel. It may be possible to leave a gap in the iris pattern of the prosthetic shell opposite the actual pupil in order to prevent complete loss of the visual field of this eye.

In the case of corneal lenses, there are two different types available. These are the older type with an iris pattern, with or without clear pupil, embedded in clear material – like scleral lenses, and the newer type in which the iris pattern consists of a tinted material distributed in the form of a pattern in the clear material, the clear and tinted materials being fused together by a baking process. The latter type are mainly used for cosmetic purposes where people wish to change their eye colour. The older type has the advantage that the real iris pattern cannot be seen through the lens, but the disadvantage of making it impossible to check the fit with fluorescein. A clear lens is therefore made for fitting purposes and adjusted to allow maximum wearing time. The final prosthetic lens is then made to the same adjusted back surface specification but is usually thicker (about 0.50 mm in thickness), and may therefore behave differently on the eye. For this reason a thick clear fitting lens should be used where possible.

Prosthetic corneal lenses have another disadvantage in that they have to be large to cover the existing iris pattern. The size may curtail normal metabolism and thereby restrict the wearing time. This also applies to the newer cosmetic type of lens, although its construction permits a thinner lens which aids metabolism, and being partially clear the fluorescein picture can be studied through the lens allowing the fit of the final lens to be checked *in situ*. It is recommended that the latter type be fitted some 1–2 mm smaller than the cornea, but this must be related to the lower lid position as it is essential that the clear centre of the lens should cover the pupil area. A small BCOD of about 7.00 mm is recommended with gradually flattening peripheral curves to permit maximum tears exchange. A lenticular construction permits such large lenses to be kept as thin and lightweight as possible and allows better control of edge thickness.

Prosthetic soft lenses are available either as corneal sized lenses, or in semi-scleral size with transparent haptic portion, the latter tending to be more stable on the eye. Both may be made either as sighted lenses or with a black opaque 'pupil' area. They are very satisfactory in practice and except where the sclera is disfigured or there is a pronounced squint they are to be preferred to scleral lenses. They are also usually more comfortable than corneal lenses, and generally are more satisfactory cosmetically because of their relative stability as compared to a corneal lens. They are made rather like a prosthetic scleral lens. The iris pattern is painted on to a thin dehydrated hydrophilic 'lens'. This is then completely immersed in hydrophilic monomer with appropriate cross-linking agents added. The whole is polymerized to form a hydrophilic button with embedded iris pattern. The button is then allowed to dehydrate and the clear outer portion is cut and polished to the required specification for the patient, and then rehydrated. Such lenses are somewhat thicker than normal soft lenses and their oxygen transmission is said to be reduced by the presence of the painted iris pattern. However, in practice they work very well, possibly because they are often fitted to scarred corneas which have an additional oxygen supply via associated corneal blood vessels. The selection of the iris pattern and colour is made from a set of cards, and the pupil and iris size are chosen to correspond with the other eye.

PROTECTIVE LENSES

Radiation Treatment

For malignant tumours of the orbital region, the eye itself may be protected by a plastics-covered lead scleral shell. Where the tumour is ocular, a partial lead shell may be specially constructed to cover all of the anterior eye except the part to be irradiated.

Albinos and Aniridics

These patients require protection from excessive light in order to get satisfactory visual acuity. In the albino, the retinal image is spoiled by light scattered through the iris and choroid. In aniridics, the aberrations of the entire cornea and crystalline lens cause optical distortion of the retinal image. Both also usually suffer from nystagmus due to poor visual acuity. It is therefore advisable that babies with albinism or aniridia should be fitted with contact lenses as early in life as possible. This is usually done by the impression technique (often under general anaesthesia) and the parents are taught how to handle the lenses. Visual acuity may then develop normally and nystagmus may possibly be prevented.

Albinos may be catered for with a pair of prosthetic scleral lenses in which the white haptic portion has a black backing to prevent light entering the eye via the sclera and choroid – the latter being deficient in pigment. An opaque iris pattern is essential for the same reason – so that light may enter the eye only via the artificial pupil.

Aniridics require only an opaque iris with normal-size pupil. Since the aniridic eye appears to have a black iris anyway, the same appearance may be maintained by employing a black-painted iris in the final lens. Visual acuity may be improved in both cases, although the improvement is not necessarily immediate. Scleral lenses may help to reduce any nystagmus by virtue of restricting eye movement.

Cosmetic soft lenses may also be used, but are less helpful in albinism than aniridia. Chapter 21, page 614 gives more detail.

Fenestrated Scleral Lenses

These may be used for protective purposes where patients suffer entropion and/or trichiasis and the lashes are liable to damage the cornea. In ectropion and lagophthalmos, where the cornea is unduly exposed, a scleral lens has a protective function in that it keeps the cornea moist.

The same application for scleral lenses occurs in cases where the lacrimal output is deficient, for example, in Sjögren's syndrome. It may then be necessary to employ a non-fenestrated lens and use it with a solution of artificial tears (see Chapter 3, Volume 1). Scleral lenses may also be employed as protection against small flying particles (such as dental surgeons experience) and as protection against exposure in very cold and windy atmospheres.

Tonometry

Soft lenses may be used to protect the cornea during tonometry. Reliable readings are said to be obtained without the need for a local anaesthetic (Deluca, Forgacs and Skolnick, 1974).

APEX LENSES

Apex lenses are similar to FLOM lenses (Chapter 10, Volume 1) and have been used successfully for fitting aphakics. The difficulty of fitting the haptic portion is removed as this is only about 2 mm wide. Fitted in reduced optic form they are considerably lighter in weight than a high positive scleral lens. Because they are fitted to touch the cornea, they are apt to give rise to corneal abrasions. Bagshaw, Gordon and Stanworth (1966) have described their fitting and uses.

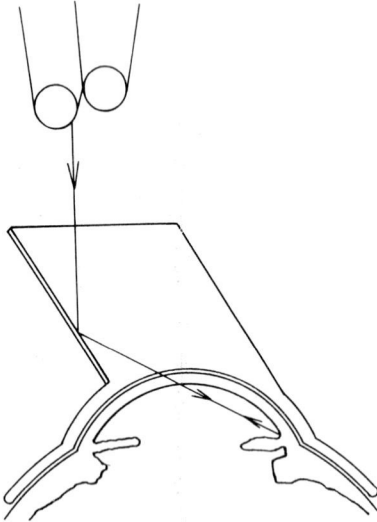

Figure 24.9–Cross-section of a Goldmann gonioscopy lens. Light from a slit lamp is reflected, as shown, into the anterior chamber angle, and returns along the same path to be viewed through the microscope

DIAGNOSTIC LENSES

A number of special contact lenses has been developed to assist observation of the internal eye in diagnosing eye disease.

GONIOSCOPY CONTACT LENSES

Observation of the angle of the anterior chamber has been made possible by the use of contact lenses which either partially or completely neutralize the power of the cornea, thus enabling observation of the anterior chamber angle directly or by means of mirror devices.

Most modern gonioscopy lenses are based on the designs introduced by Koeppé (1919), Uribe Troncoso (1921) and Goldmann (1938). The Goldmann lens incorporates a mirror and is used in conjunction with a slit lamp biomicroscope (*Figure 24.9*). The angle of the anterior chamber is seen by reflection.

To see the entire angle, the lens must be rotated on the eye and the slit beam rotated with it but perpendicular to it, a horizontal slit being used when the mirror is vertical and vice versa. Magnification is given by the biomicroscope. The need for all but small amounts of rotation of the lens has been overcome by the use of multiple mirrors, as in the Lovac six-mirror goniolens, the pyramid gonioscope of van Beuningen (1953), and the Zeiss pyramid gonioscope (*Figures 24.10, 24.11* and *24.12*). The principle employed by Koeppé and Uribe Troncoso was to use a spherical contact lens and observe by looking perpendicular to the anterior lens surface (*Figure 24.13*). This allows observation of the entire angle of the anterior chamber without rotation of the lens. Although the narrow focal beam from a slit lamp is to be preferred, illumination without a slit

Figure 24.10–The 'Lovac' six-mirror goniolens giving a composite image of the entire anterior chamber angle. The central fundus can be viewed through the centre of the lens (reproduced by kind permission of Medical Workshop, Holland)

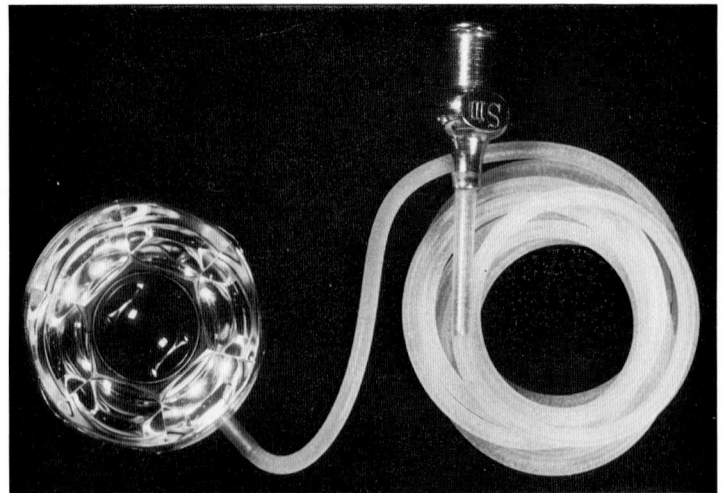

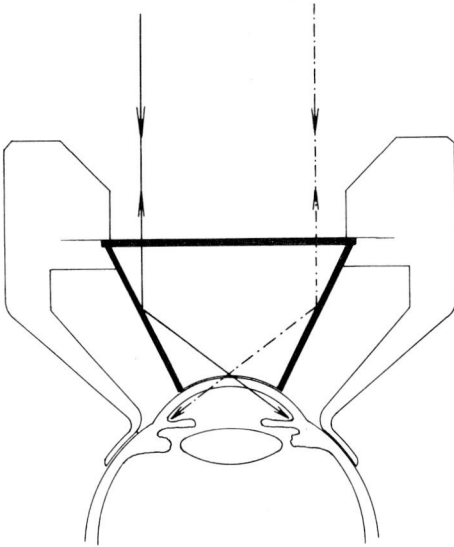

Figure 24.11–The pyramid gonioscope of van Beuningen. The pyramid goniolens is held in place by a support which rests on the sclera

lens, which is filled with saline prior to insertion. As soon as the lens touches the eye, the end of this cannula is lowered, thereby creating a negative hydrostatic pressure. This prevents the lens dropping out and prevents the formation of bubbles behind the lens – problems common with other types of goniolens. However, if left in place for too long (more than about 15 minutes) corneal oedema sufficient to disrupt the observer's view, may result (Sabell, 1970).

A further type of goniolens is the Lovac Direct Goniolens as shown in *Figure 24.15*. The anterior chamber angle is viewed directly without reflection through the flat surface of the goniolens, which is angled at about 45 degrees to the patient's visual axis. This allows about half the entire anterior chamber angle to be viewed at one time and readily permits goniophotography.

Lenses employing similar optical principles to the various gonioscopy lenses are also used in the surgical technique known as goniotomy. The Barkan lens, originally developed in 1936 (Barkan, 1936), is shown in *Figure 24.16* and the Medical Workshop prismatic goniotomy lens is shown in *Figure 24.17*.

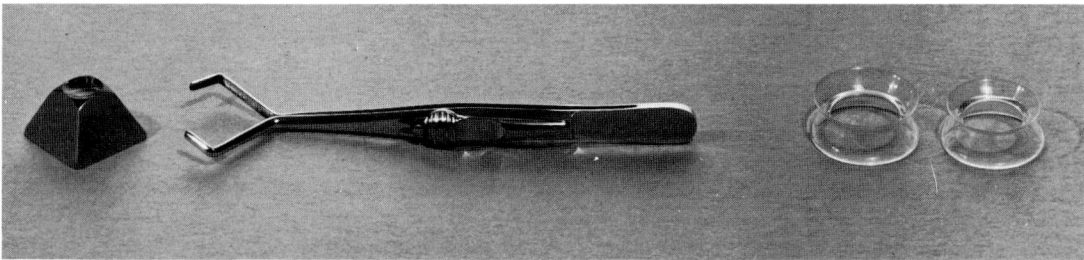

Figure 24.12–The Zeiss pyramid gonioscope with special forceps, and scleral holders which keep the lids apart (reproduced by kind permission of Carl Zeiss, Oberkochen)

lamp is possible and may be provided by an ophthalmoscope or pen torch. The magnification is about ×2 unaided and may be increased with the aid of a loupe. The disadvantage of this system is the aberration given by the steeply curved spherical front surface of the goniolens.

A modern development of this is the Lovac Double Focus contact lens, which has a small section of convex radius of curvature of 6.00 mm incorporated in the major lens, which has a front surface radius of 8.00 mm (*Figure 24.14*). Magnification of ×15 may be obtained by direct ophthalmoscopy through the steeply curved sector. A stereoscopic appearance is obtained if an indirect binocular ophthalmoscope is used, as in *Figure 24.14*.

The Lovac series of lenses adhere readily to the eye by means of negative pressure afforded by a long cannula running from the back surface of the

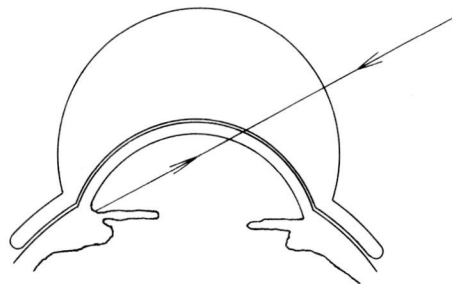

Figure 24.13–Cross-section of a spherical goniolens as used by Koeppé and Uribe Troncoso. Observation and illumination are from the same direction, perpendicular to the front surface. Alternatively, the limbus region may be illuminated by a slit beam from one side

Figure 24.14–Cross-section of the 'Lovac' double-focus goniolens being used with indirect ophthalmoscopy

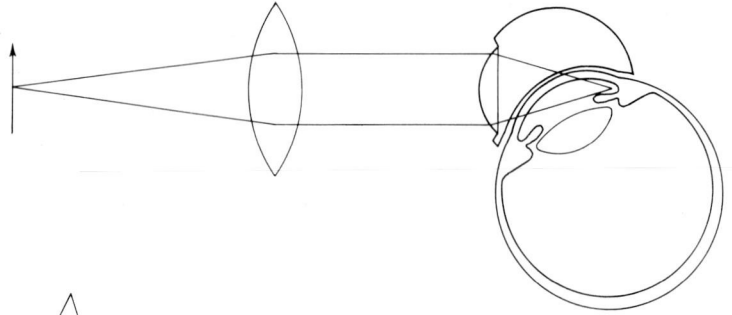

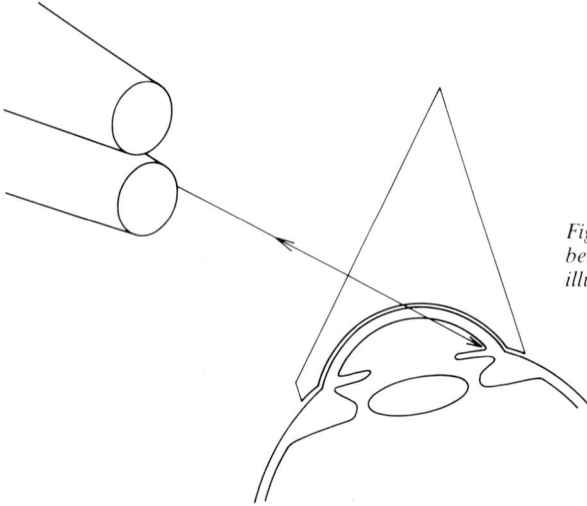

Figure 24.15–Cross-section of the 'Lovac' direct goniolens being used with the biomicroscope. The direction of illumination and observation are the same

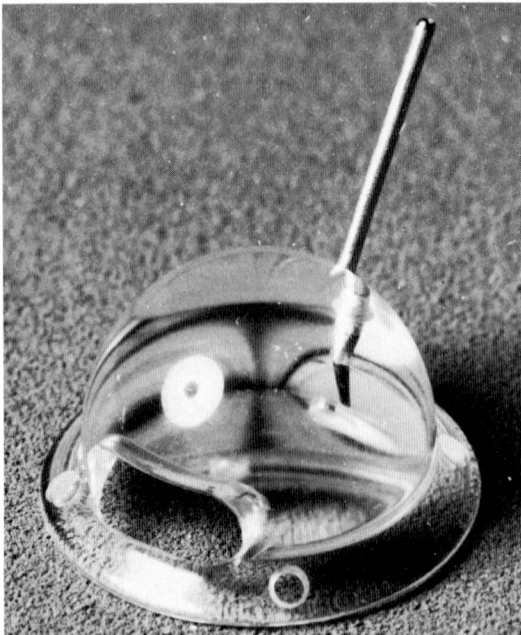

Figure 24.16–The Barkan goniotomy lens giving ×2 magnification. This has a small haptic portion with four perforations, as well as a lateral window and a cannula (reproduced by kind permission of Medical Workshop, Holland)

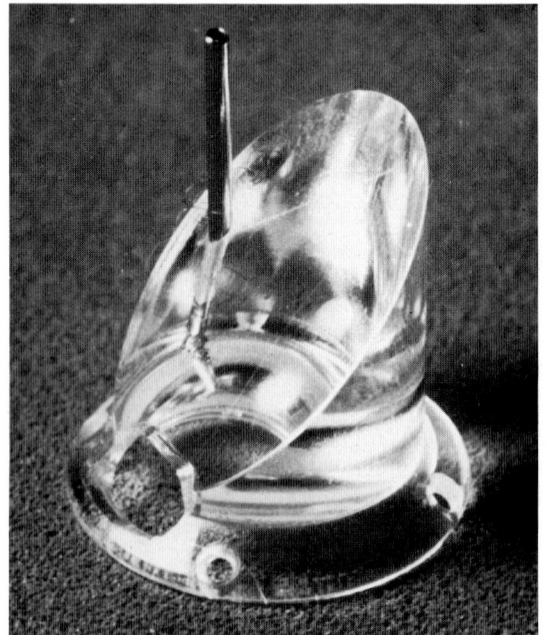

Figure 24.17–The Medical Workshop prismatic goniotomy lens which is used in conjunction with an operating microscope (reproduced by kind permission of Medical Workshop, Holland)

THE ANTERIOR CHAMBER ANGLE

Gonioscopy permits observation of the angle of the anterior chamber. The essential features of the angle are illustrated in *Figure 24.18a*. On the corneal side of the angle these are as follows.

Schwalbe's line which is the termination of the corneal endothelium and Descemet's membrane. Sometimes this is visible using ordinary direct illumination and slit lamp biomicroscopy, because the endothelium may terminate in a small tag of tissue which projects into the aqueous. This is then known as posterior embryotoxon or embryotoxin and if it occurs all round the entire angle it adds to the risk of angle closure glaucoma. It delineates the anterior end of the *corneo-scleral trabecular meshwork*. This is the sponge-like tissue separating the aqueous from the *canal of Schlemm*. The latter becomes visible in gonioscopy if filled with blood. The rear of the corneo-scleral trabecular tissue is

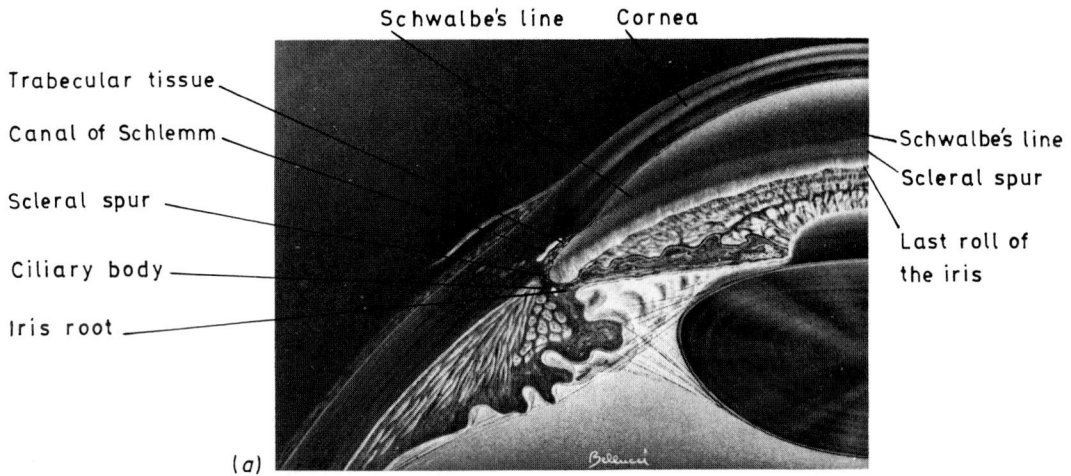

(a)

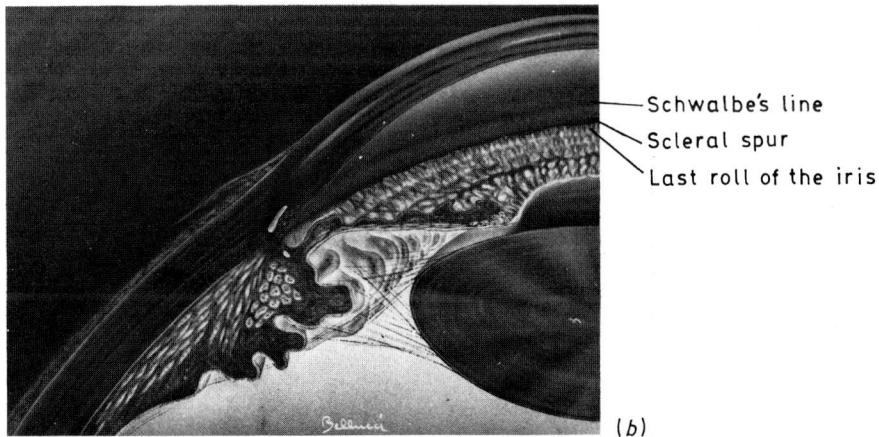

(b)

Figure 24.18–(a) Cross-section and gonioscopic appearance of an open angle. Both the trabecular meshwork (between Schwalbe's line and the scleral spur) and the ciliary body (between the scleral spur and iris) appear wide, so the classification is 3-A. (b) Cross-section and gonioscopic appearance of an angle classified as 3-0. Such an angle might close completely during mydriasis as the last roll of the iris could move forward blocking the aqueous outlet via the trabecular tissue. This could occur with or without pupil block and its resultant iris bombé (reproduced from Becker (1972) by his kind permission and that of The C. V. Mosby Company)

demarcated by the *scleral spur* which is scleral tissue projecting forward as far as the angle at this point. It can be said to represent the mid-point of the angle as seen by gonioscopy.

Beyond the scleral spur on the iris side of the angle is first the *ciliary body* and then the *root of the iris* at the apex of the angle and just beyond. Then the iris tissue itself takes over and the *last roll of the iris* is seen.

Becker (1972) has devised a goniogram (*Figure 24.19*) to illustrate the state of the anterior chamber angle as seen by gonioscopy, which also relates to his classification of the angle. The goniogram consists of seven concentric circles, the central one denoting the scleral spur. The outer three circles are used to denote the apparent width of the trabecular tissue, that is, the relative distance of Schwalbe's line from the scleral spur. If the trabecular tissue appears wide (classification 3) then Schwalbe's line

is marked in on the outermost circle, if medium (2) on the next circle, and if narrow (1) on the innermost of these three outer circles. The apparent width of this trabecular tissue depends on the angle at which it is viewed. This in itself depends on the narrowness of the anterior chamber angle. If the latter is very narrow, the angle of view to see into it is so tangential to the trabecular meshwork that it appears forshortened (1).

The three inner circles of the goniogram are used to denote the position of insertion of the iris root into the ciliary body relative to the scleral spur. The iris root is marked on the innermost circle if it is inserted posteriorly (classification C) allowing a good view of the ciliary portion of the angle; on the next circle if the iris is inserted in a mid-position (B) and on the third circle in if the iris insertion is anteriorly placed (A) indicating a narrow angle, with hardly any of the ciliary body visible.

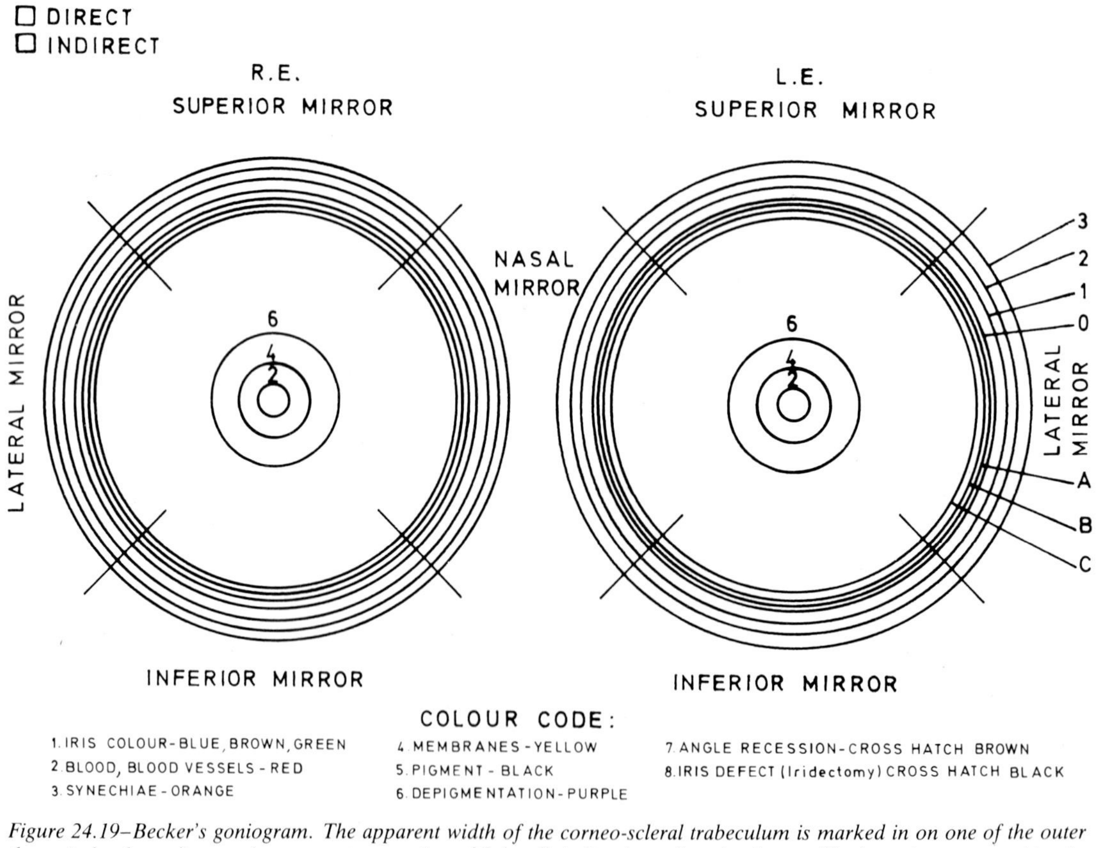

Figure 24.19–Becker's goniogram. The apparent width of the corneo-scleral trabeculum is marked in on one of the outer three circles depending on the apparent separation of Schwalbe's line from the scleral spur. The latter is represented by the heavy central circle. Likewise, the width of the ciliary body seen between the scleral spur and iris is marked on the inner three circles. Other features may be drawn in as indicated. The pupil size and characteristics may also be recorded (reproduced from Becker (1972) by his kind permission and that of The C. V. Mosby Company)

Thus, the angle of the anterior chamber is denoted by first a number (0, 1, 2 or 3) and then a letter (O, A, B or C) enabling a description of both 'sides' of the angle. An O indicates that the structure is not visible and OO indicates complete closure. All four quadrants of the angle can be drawn in on the goniogram as indicated, so that variations can be seen and pigmentation and other features such as iris processes can be marked in. The upper quadrant usually has the narrowest portion of the anterior chamber angle, and the angle is at its widest in the lower quadrant.

Other methods of classification include the Shaffer (1962) system which relates the grade to the angle made by the iris with the ciliary body and trabecular tissue. Grade O is a closed angle. Grade 1 is 10 degrees or less – an extremely narrow angle. Grade 2 is 20 degrees – a narrow angle. Grade 3 is 20–35 degrees and Grade 4 is 35–45 degrees – both wide open angles. Angle closure is thought to be impossible in Grades 3 and 4, possible in 2 and probable in 1.

Prior to this, Scheie (1957) used a grading system to denote angle width and pigmentation.

Considerable experience is required for correct interpretation of the anterior chamber angle. *Figure 24.18a* shows an open angle (classification 3-C), and *Figure 24.18b* shows a narrower angle (3-0) with potential for closure if pupil block should occur during mydriasis with resultant iris bombé pushing the last roll of the iris forward to close the angle.

Greater detail of gonioscopy and the appearances seen is available in Becker's work.

CONTACT LENSES FOR EXAMINATION OF THE FUNDUS

Any high-negative-powered contact lens assists observation of the fundus of the high myope during ophthalmoscopy by reducing the magnification and enlarging the field of view.

Observation of the ocular fundus employing the slit-lamp is useful as it allows detection of changes in level of the fundus (by bending and alteration in focus of the slit) and permits a binocular view with

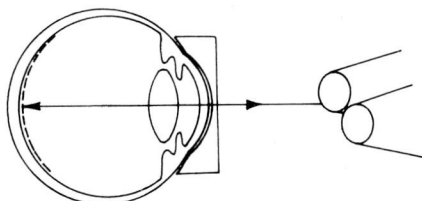

Figure 24.20–Fundus observation with the biomicroscope, by means of a contact lens with a flat front surface

magnification. Such observation is aided by the use of special contact lenses having flat front surfaces which eliminate refraction due to the cornea (*Figure 24.20*). The central (macula) region of the fundus may be observed directly with such a high negative lens, and mirrors may be employed to observe the mid-periphery and extreme periphery of the fundus. A dilated pupil is necessary. The Zeiss Three-Mirror contact lens allows all these methods of observation

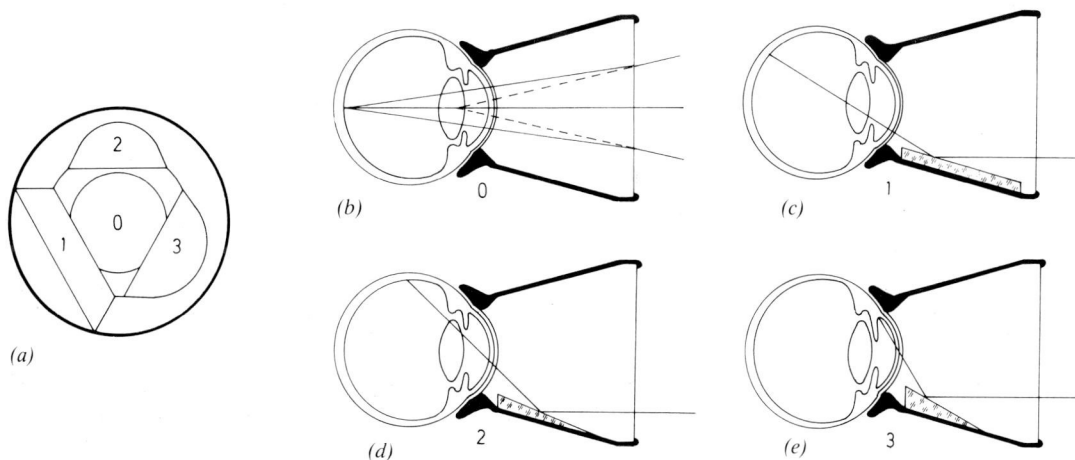

Figure 24.21–(a) Location of mirrors in the Zeiss three-mirror goniolens. 0 gives direct viewing as in (b). 1, 2 and 3 are mirrors inclined as in (c), (d) and (e). (b) The central fundus viewed directly through portion 0, without utilizing a mirror. (c) Observation of the mid-peripheral fundus using mirror 1. (d) Observation of the peripheral fundus using mirror 2. (e) Observation of the anterior chamber angle using mirror 3

as well as gonioscopy (*Figure 24.21a–e*). A lens similar to the Lovac Direct Goniolens (*Figure 24.15*), known as the Lovac Peripheral Fundus Contact Lens, also allows direct observation of the peripheral fundus. The lens must be rotated to see the entire peripheral fundus and a scleral depressor is used to view the ora serrata. Schirmer (1965) has described a modification of the Troncoso goniolens using either plane or concave facets. These may

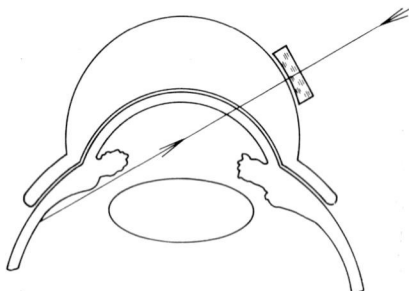

Figure 24.22–Observation of the ora serrata by means of a Troncoso goniolens with negative additional lens

form part of the lens or may be additions adhering to the lens with methyl cellulose, and thus movable over its surface. The fundus may be inspected through these facets by means of a special gonio slit lamp suspended from above. These facets have enabled observation as far round as the ora serrata and pars plana of the ciliary body (*Figure 24.22*). Better viewing, with a bigger field of view, is obtained if the facet is cut with its surface as near to the pupil as possible (*Figure 24.23*).

Goldmann and Schmidt (1965) have also described a contact lens which allows observation of the ciliary body and ora serrata with the assistance of scleral depression.

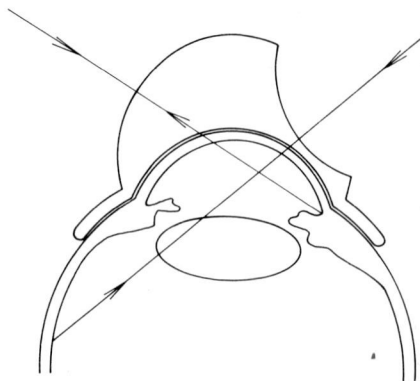

Figure 24.23–A negative facet cut into a Troncoso goniolens to allow observation of the peripheral fundus as well as the anterior chamber angle

Fundus examination contact lenses, employing a suction effect to keep the eye steady, are used in conjunction with a modified slit lamp, during laser treatment of certain retinal disorders such as detachments and haemorrhages, and the growth of new blood vessels.

FOREIGN BODY LOCATOR

Metallic intra-ocular foreign bodies show up on radiographs, but their relative position is difficult to decide on without adequate reference marks on the radiograph.

These reference marks may be provided by lead pellets incorporated in a scleral contact lens. Typically, four to six lead pellets are used (*Figure 24.24*), and radiographs taken in different planes allow the

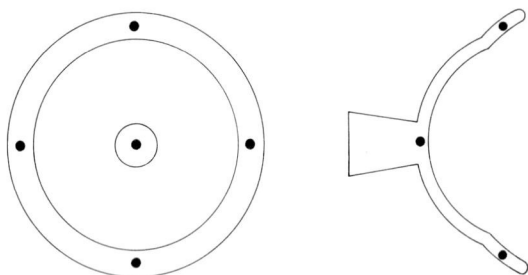

Figure 24.24–A foreign body locator with a handle attached to the front surface, showing lead reference pellets. (a) Direct view. (b) Cross-section

metallic intra-ocular foreign body to be located with respect to these. This method has been and is still being used satisfactorily to locate foreign bodies. Their removal is then effected with a strong magnet from the nearest position to the foreign body. However, this method of localization is now being superseded by the use of ultrasonic apparatus.

EXOPHTHALMOMETRY

Contact lenses incorporating a metallic insert at the central optic have been used with radiographs to make measurements for both relative and absolute exophthalmometry. Silva (1967) has described the latest techniques.

DIAGNOSIS OF CORNEAL ABNORMALITIES

Any ordinary sighted contact lens may be used to assist in the diagnosis of suspected keratoconus. If visual acuity during refraction with a contact lens in place is markedly better than visual acuity with the best possible spectacle correction and keratoconus is suspected, its diagnosis may be confirmed. Suspected corneal dystrophies also show a similar improvement in visual acuity with contact lenses, as do many other conditions of corneal irregularity.

The presence of a contact lens also permits abnormal corneal conditions to be studied more easily with the slit lamp, for the contact lens gets rid of unwanted reflections from the irregular corneal surface.

By largely removing the corneal irregularities, a contact lens permits ophthalmoscopic or slit lamp examination of the media and fundus, thereby making easier the diagnosis of internal eye conditions in patients having an irregular cornea. The fundus of the high myope is also more easily observed if viewed through a high minus contact lens which reduces the excessively high magnification obtained in direct ophthalmoscopy of these patients.

ASSESSMENT OF CORNEAL THICKNESS

Friedman (1967) has developed a corneal lens having a stepped front surface to give a central portion 0.8 mm thick, an intermediate portion 0.6 mm thick and an outer portion 0.4 mm thick. Used with a narrow slit beam corneal thickness can be estimated by comparison with the lens, prior to surgery (*see* Measurement of Corneal Thickness, Chapter 5, Volume 1, page 150, and Pachometry, Chapter 7, Volume 1, page 173).

THERAPEUTIC LENSES

Contact lenses are often helpful in treating certain eye conditions. They fall into several categories.

BANDAGE LENSES

Hydrophilic contact lenses, of the order of 0.08 mm thickness (for example, the Bausch and Lomb Plano T lens), have been very successfully used as corneal bandage lenses for severe corneal ulceration, following keratoplasty and in the management of bullous keratopathy (Petropoulou, 1975; Aquavella, 1976). In the latter case they are often used in conjunction with hypertonic saline drops. Levinson, Weissman and Sachs (1977) report the successful use of thicker lenses (averaging 0.18 mm) of HEMA material for cases of bullous keratopathy and following corneal grafts and burns. But in neuroparalytic keratitis and in the dry-eye syndrome difficulty was experienced

with lenses drying out and falling off the eye, as well as becoming contaminated with biochemical deposits. They also point out the necessity for in-patient hospital supervision of many of these patients because the risk of infection is so high. The presence of the bandage lens aids regular corneal healing and prevents the eyelid from rubbing the damaged cornea. Aphakic continuous wear hydrophilic lenses have also been successfully applied at the time of operation for cataract extraction, acting as a splint and bandage, as well as permitting immediate good vision post-operatively (Kersley, 1975). All these types of lens are dealt with, in detail, in Chapter 21.

MEDICAL APPLICATORS

The use of hydrophilic lenses as medical applicators is now well established (Hillman, 1976). As stated in Chapter 21, page 613, they have been used in the application to the eye of antibiotics, mydriatics, local anaesthetics and particularly the miotic pilocarpine in the treatment of glaucoma. The lens is soaked in the drug for about 2 hours so that it becomes saturated. When placed on the eye there is a slow release of the drug into the conjunctival sac over the following 2 hours. Hillman reports that high water content material is slightly more efficient than low water content material, and with pilocarpine treatment best results have been obtained using a solution of 1 per cent strength rather than the higher strengths which are usually used in drop form. Hillman also reports the introduction into the United Kingdom of the Ocusert which is shaped to be placed in the lower or upper fornix and consists of a hydrophilic core, soaked in pilocarpine, 2 per cent or 4 per cent, surrounded by a hydrophobic membrane to delay drug release. This provides continuous delivery of the drug for 7 days, at which time it is replaced.

Other medical applicators are still sometimes used in intensive drug therapy when it is necessary to

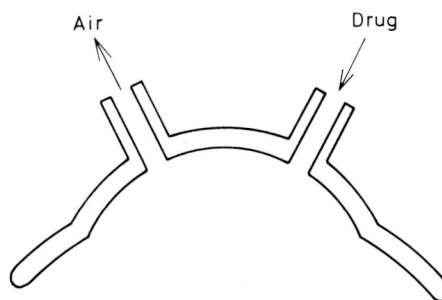

Figure 24.25–The Klein applicator

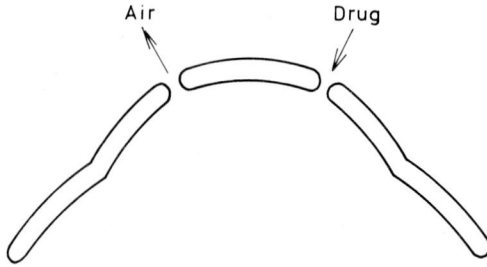

Figure 24.26–The Anderson medicator

keep antibiotic or other drugs in constant contact with the eye. Two examples are the Klein applicator (Klein, 1949) and the Anderson medicator (Anderson, 1952), shown in *Figures 24.25* and *24.26*. Both basically consist of modified scleral contact lenses. The Anderson medicator has two holes, through one of which the drug is instilled and out of the other air escapes. The optic portion gives ample corneal clearance, and this acts as a reservoir for the drug. The Klein applicator is similar but has two tubes extending from the optic in place of the holes. This is easier for nurses to handle but a little less comfortable to wear than the Anderson medicator as the lids cannot close over it.

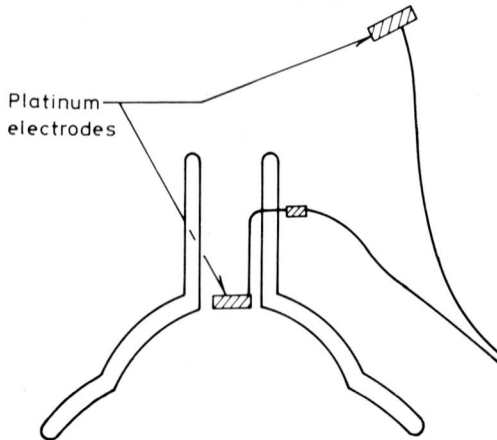

Figure 24.27–An iontophoresis contact lens used for application of drugs to the eye, seen in cross-section

Another, more elaborate, lens is one containing a platinum electrode which almost touches the cornea. Another electrode is attached to the cheek, or elsewhere on the body, and a continuous low voltage electric current is passed. This serves to make the cornea more permeable. Drugs administered via the tube and holes around the electrode gain more rapid entry to the cornea and thence into the aqueous. The lens is illustrated in section in *Figure 24.27*.

SPLINTS

In the emergency departments of hospitals, scleral shells are frequently applied to the eye following facial burns. The shell prevents the lids sticking to the globe (symblepharon). Another type of shell can be used to prevent the lids sticking together (ankyloblepharon). The shells are left in place during the healing process so that the fornices remain formed, otherwise the conjunctival sac might become almost non-existent. As an alternative, large soft lenses may be used (*see* Chapter 21, page 606). Scleral or soft lenses may have to be worn during

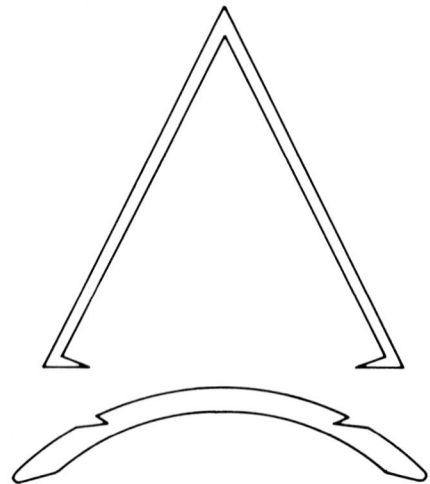

Figure 24.28–A contact lens splint and toothed forceps in cross-section

attacks of Stevens–Johnson syndrome, when all bodily mucous membranes become severely irritated: in the eye, the bulbar and palpebral conjunctivae may adhere unless a scleral or large soft lens is used to prevent it (*see* also Chapter 21, page 609).

Splints, in the form of large corneal lenses, are also used to hold corneal grafts in place following keratoplasty and to hold the cornea in position following cataract extraction. In both cases, the front surface of the cornea is not held by stitches, which tend to encourage irregular healing, but by the smooth spherical back surface of the contact lens. Good optical results have been achieved with this method of supporting the healing tissue. The splint itself may be held by stitches to the bulbar conjunctiva. When these are cut, the splint is removed by special toothed forceps which fit into small slots on the front surface of the splint (*Figure 24.28*).

ORTHOPTIC USES

A contact lens may be used as a cosmetic occluder in cases of intractable binocular diplopia. Any type of contact lens may be used. Usually, complete occlusion can only be achieved by having an opaque iris pattern and opaque pupil, but an opaque pupil in an otherwise clear lens may be sufficient.

In squint treatment, contact lens occluders have been used before the better eye to assist in eliminating amblyopia. Rather than fitting an opaque prosthetic type of shell, adequate occlusion may be achieved with a high negative lens or a very high positive lens (Catford and Mackie, 1968).

Partial occlusion with contact lenses has also been used in the treatment of suppression.

The fitting of anisometropic amblyopes with contact lenses has brought about some dramatic improvements in visual acuity and assisted in the orthoptic treatment of squints in such cases.

CONTROL OF REFRACTIVE ERRORS

It is well known that contact lenses can prevent the advancement of keratoconus, and they may thus be considered to be of therapeutic value in that condition.

It has been suggested that contact lenses prevent the progression of myopia. Most contact lens practitioners have noticed the apparent stabilization of myopia from the time when contact lenses are first worn, and there are many reports of such instances. Most, such as Dickinson (1957), Morrison (1958), Neill (1962) and Nolan (1964), attribute the stabilization directly to the contact lenses; and stabilization of myopia has been reported where no flattening of the cornea occurs, although the latter can obviously bring about reduction in myopia. On the other hand, Bailey (1966) has shown that the apparent halt in the increase in myopia which occurs when contact lenses are worn can be explained by alterations in corneal curvature being neutralized by the liquid lens, by too much negative power being used to start with to minimize the blur due to residual astigmatism, and by other factors such as flattening of the contact lens itself.

Kelly and Butler (1964, 1971), Baldwin *et al.* (1969), and others, including the author, are currently investigating this apparent stabilization of myopia. Controlled studies are being undertaken in an attempt to produce positive proof of the therapeutic value of contact lenses on myopia. The latest results (Stone, 1976) show that conventionally fitted hard corneal lenses, fitted wth BCOR just steeper than the flattest keratometer reading, have brought about a slowing down of the rate of progress of myopia in a group of contact-lens-wearing children, as compared to a similar group of spectacle-wearing children. About half of the reduction in rate of progress could be attributed to corneal flattening by the contact lenses (*see* Chapter 17), but the remainder can only be explained on the basis that wearing corneal lenses has some retarding effect on axial elongation.

The technique of orthokeratology is a purposeful attempt to reduce the refractive error of an eye by changing the corneal curvature with contact lenses – usually corneal lenses. The change in corneal curvature is normally brought about in gradual stages, by progressively changing the back surface radii of curvature of the lens fitted. The technique has certain uses in helping recruits achieve suitable standards of visual acuity to gain entry to the armed services or other occupations, and it has permitted many ametropes to obtain adequate visual acuity without any form of optical correction for at least part of the time. In some cases myopia is reduced but contact lenses still have to be worn to permit maximum visual acuity; in other cases emmetropia is achieved and may last for a few hours, days, weeks or months but then retainer lenses must be resorted to for varying periods of time. To reduce myopia the aim is to fit lenses which slightly flatten the cornea, but do not cause distortion, oedema or tissue damage. Once a flatter corneal curvature has been achieved and this remains stable, a slightly flatter lens is fitted to flatten the cornea a little more, and again on stabilization a flatter lens still is fitted, and so on. The cost to the patient is obviously high, but for some people the reward justifies the expense. Further details of the methods used have been described by Jessen (1964) and more recently by Nolan (1969) and by Grant and May (1972). Kerns (1977), in a carefully controlled study of orthokeratological procedures, found that whilst the technique is predictable in as far as flattening of corneal curvature and reduction of myopia is concerned, the magnitude of this change is not predictable. He also concluded that changes in the vertical meridian of the cornea could not be predicted and he noted that the corneas of young people are more likely to be flattened than those of older patients. His study is continuing.

AS AN AID TO DEFECTIVE COLOUR VISION

A red contact lens worn in one eye only has been recommended by La Bissoniere (1974) in an attempt to overcome certain red-green colour deficiencies, by allowing a comparison of the different contrasts then perceived by the two eyes. The method is only of very limited use.

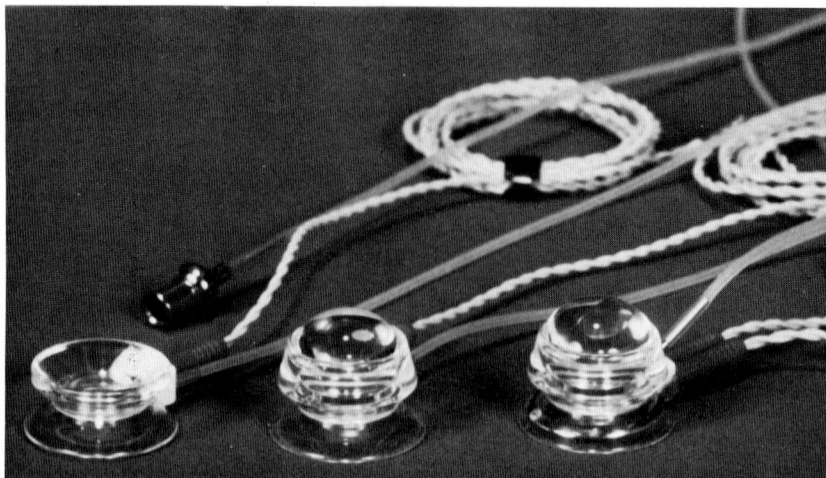

Figure 24.29–'Lovac' electroretinography lenses. These are lightweight electrode bearing contact lenses used in ERG studies. Each has a small haptic portion and a blepharostatic cone which takes different colour filters and diaphragms. A circular silver electrode in the limbal region is connected to a tiny permanently attached electric flex leading to the electroretinograph (reproduced by kind permission of Medical Workshop, Holland)

CONTACT LENSES USED FOR RESEARCH INTO VISUAL FUNCTION

Contact lenses are a means of holding suitable objects in contact with the eye for research purposes. Such objects may be electrodes, thermisters, oxygen probes, mirrors or telescopic devices, all of which have been incorporated in contact lenses at various times.

ELECTRODES

An electrode incorporated in a contact lens may be used in iontophoresis for therapeutic purposes, as already mentioned. For research purposes, the most frequent use of electrodes in contact lenses is in ERG (electro-retinography) studies. Most electrical activity in the eye region takes place in the retina, and the potential difference in the retina may be measured – as different light stimuli are applied – by means of one electrode attached to the nearby skin and one touching the eye, the two electrodes being connected to a suitable meter, amplifier and pen-recorder. Typical contact lenses for this purpose are illustrated in *Figure 24.29*. The conical front surface projection is to prevent eyelid closure and to prevent any discomfort from the eyelids contacting the electrode. Electrodes are usually of silver or platinum. Small scleral lenses have been most frequently used in the past. A good description of the method of making these lenses has been given by Fletcher (1966) under the pseudonym Haptos.

More recently, a flexible glycolmethacrylate corneal lens has been described by Bornschein, Wichterle and Wündsch (1966). This incorporates a silver spherical electrode in its front surface. The lens itself is electrically conducting. A corneal contact lens using a silver electrode has also been described by Ruedmann and Noell (1961).

ERG studies by Alvis (1966) have suggested that this may, in future, form an additional diagnostic test in glaucoma.

Other more complicated types of electrode are used for measurement of temperature and gas exchange at the eye's surface and are described in the appropriate sections below.

EYE MOVEMENTS

Studies of voluntary and involuntary eye movements have been made by mounting a small mirror on a contact lens and reflecting light from a stationary source. The angular movement of the reflected image is then double the angular movement of the eye. However, the method has been largely superseded by cine-photography of reflections from the anterior surface of the cornea.

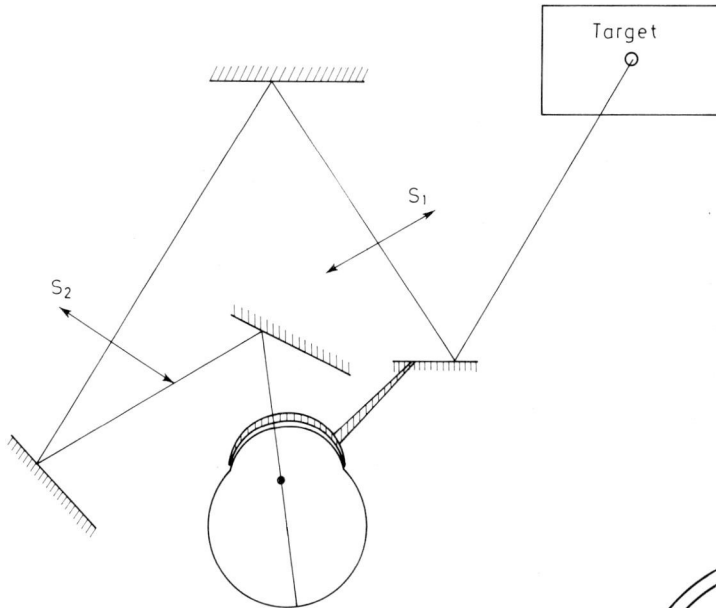

Figure 24.30–A contact lens with projecting stalk and mirror attached, used to produce a stabilized retinal image by means of a mirror and lens system (after Millodot, 1965)

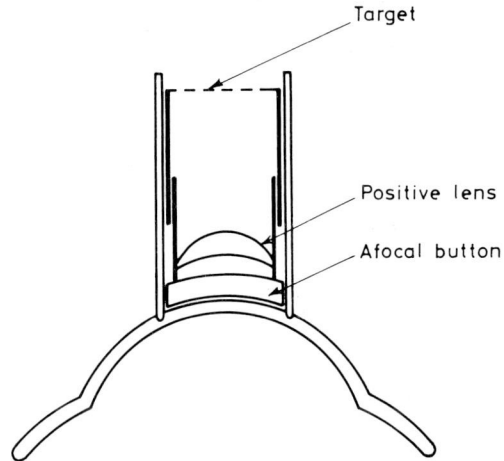

Figure 24.31–A contact lens incorporating a small telescopic device, used in the study of stabilized retinal images. The target is in the focal plane of a positive lens. Sliding supports allow some latitude in focusing. The positive lens is separated from the eye by an afocal button

STABILIZED RETINAL IMAGES

A better understanding of the physiological and psychological aspects of seeing has been achieved by studying what happens when the retinal image of an object remains stationary on the retina, that is, when small movements of the retinal image, due to saccadic movements of the eye, are prevented. This may be done by flash exposure of short duration or by means of contact lenses, which, because they move with the eye, may be used to overcome the effects of eye movements in the formation of the retinal image.

Two basic systems have been employed. One utilizes a tightly fitting contact lens with a protruding stalk on the end of which is a plane mirror. The mirror is used to reflect light from a target through a compensating optical system into the eye. Such a system was originally devised by Ditchburn and Ginsborg (1952). A more recent system (Millodot, 1965) is depicted in *Figure 24.30*.

Any movement of the eye causes a corresponding movement of the mirror, and the reflected image of the target is moved through twice this angle. To compensate for this doubling of angular movement, lenses S_1 and S_2 give a reduction in magnification of a half. Thus, light passing through the optical system is always imaged on the same portion of the retina, regardless of eye movements.

The other system, used by Evans and Piggins (1963), is to incorporate a small telescopic device into the contact lens itself, as shown in *Figure 24.31* and as described by Evans (1965). A suitably illuminated target is placed approximately in the anterior focal plane of a high positive lens, which is itself separated from the contact lens by an afocal button. The whole optical system is contained in aluminium tubing, and the target and positive lens are movable relative to each other to facilitate accurate focusing on the retina.

In attempts to provide contact lenses which did not lag behind the eye during eye movements, rubber contact lenses with attached pressure bulbs to obtain suction have been used in the past. These were liable to cause damage to the eye. Best results seem to have been achieved with small scleral lenses (17 mm back haptic size) for the telescopic type of device, and a 14 mm overall size, single curve corneal lens, fitted tightly, for the type incorporating a mirror.

The results obtained with these devices suggest that perception comprises multiple pattern recognition.

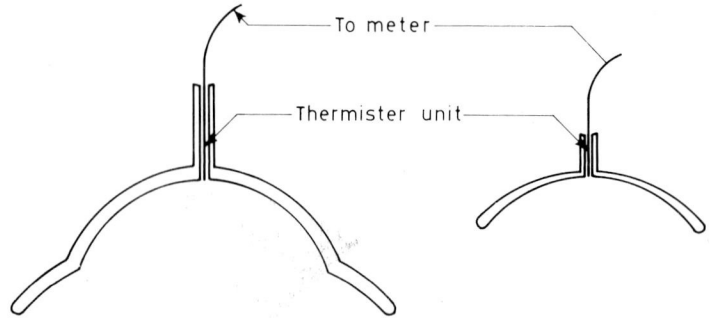

Figure 24.32–A scleral and a corneal lens, each incorporating a thermister for temperature measurement

TEMPERATURE MEASUREMENT

In studying ocular changes due to contact lenses, the effects of lid aperture size, lid closure, eye position and the very presence of the contact lens itself cause temperature changes of the cornea, sometimes to an extent beyond which normal corneal metabolism can no longer continue.

These temperature changes can be monitored, using a thermister – a tiny electrical device sensitive to temperature changes. Thermisters can be incorporated in both scleral and corneal lenses. Typical lenses are shown in *Figure 24.32*. Hill and Leighton (1965) have described their findings on temperature changes of the eye when using a scleral contact lens containing one of these devices, and they have shown how the rise in temperature behind a lens affects the corneal metabolism.

GAS EXCHANGE OF THE CORNEA DURING CONTACT LENS WEAR

In order to hold an oxygen probe against the cornea, scleral lenses were used at first. Hill and Fatt (1966) have described such a lens which is depicted in *Figure 24.33a*. The probe is a polaragraphic oxygen electrode covered by an oxygen-containing membrane. As the oxygen from this is lost to the corneal cells or surrounding liquid, the current in the electrode is lowered. A similar system has since been used in a corneal lens (Fatt and Hill, 1970) as pictured in *Figure 24.33b*.

Similar systems allow the output of carbon dioxide by the corneal epithelium to be recorded.

Figure 24.33–(a) A scleral contact lens incorporating a probe for recording oxygen tension (after Hill and Fatt, 1966). (b) A corneal lens used for measurement of oxygen uptake (after Fatt and Hill, 1970)

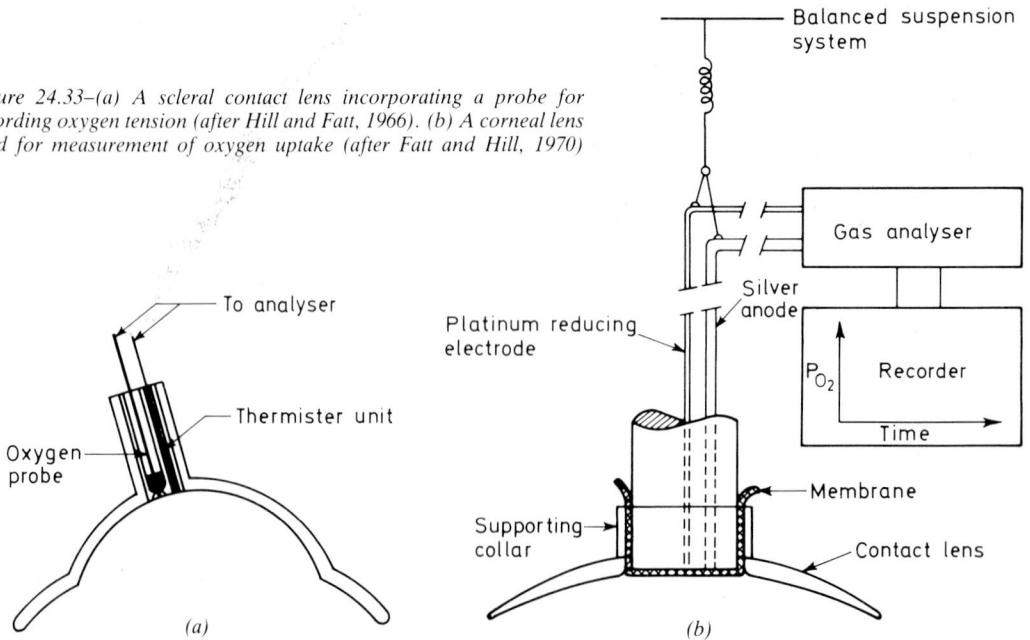

LENSES FOR ANIMALS

Many experiments are carried out on animals prior to being carried out on humans, and special lenses have been constructed for monkeys, rabbits, cats, squirrels, octopi and other creatures to assess various aspects of visual function.

The contact lens has become a major tool in visual research, both from the physiological and psychological aspects. There is no doubt that it will find further uses in addition to those described above.

LENSES FOR SPORTS PURPOSES

Because of the ease with which corneal lenses are lost or misplaced during vigorous contact sports, it is desirable that lenses should be specially designed for sports. Good vision is important, and bubbles and transitions crossing the pupil area should be avoided.

The criteria to be satisfied if contact lenses are to be worn for sports purposes are: the lens must not be capable of being misplaced on the eye due to accidental foreign pressure; the optic must remain centred; the tears lens must remain completely free of bubbles in front of the pupil area; and corneal metabolism should not be interfered with during the period required for the game.

Several types of lens have been designed with these criteria in mind.

HYDROPHILIC LENSES

All types of soft lens are fairly stable on the eye, but particularly the semi-scleral variety which are less easily dislodged than the corneal-sized lenses. If they are to be worn only for sports purposes, and not all day, they can be fitted fractionally steeper than if intended for all-day wear. For example, a BOR 0.2–0.3 mm steeper, or an OS 0.5 mm larger than would be fitted for daily wear lenses, can usefully be employed to give extra stability, without causing any visual disturbance. Soft lenses are now in most cases the lens of choice for sports purposes.

SCLERAL LENSES, SEALED, CHANNELLED AND FENESTRATED

A correctly fitted scleral lens, with minimum apical clearance and no fenestration hole, is ideal for sports purposes and is not difficult to fit. If the corneal clearance is kept to a minimum and the haptic portion is not steep, normal tears exchange prevents veiling for long periods and, in some instances, it is possible for this type of lens to be worn all day. To avoid trapping air bubbles behind the lens during insertion, the lens must be inserted filled with a suitable solution (*see* Chapter 3, Volume 1). Too much corneal clearance may mean that the normal tears exchange is inadequate to renew the liquid lens at a rate sufficient to prevent the cornea from being deprived of oxygen. However, 3–4 hours' wear may normally be achieved, even with excessive corneal clearance.

The lens which is minimally apically clear is easier to insert free of bubbles than is the lens which has a lot of clearance. A non-fenestrated lens is ideal as no bubbles are contained behind the optic and there is therefore no risk of interference to vision at a crucial stage of the game. Channelled lenses permit long wearing times, up to all-day, and usually allow bubble-free wearing to be maintained. Many designs of channel in the haptic portion of the lens have been tried. One of the most successful seems to be the S-bend channel described by McKay Taylor (1969), where an S-shaped channel connects the back optic to the edge of the lens at both top and bottom of the lens.

Some less violent sports (such as croquet) are unlikely to involve vigorous eye movements and, in such cases, fenestrated scleral lenses may be eminently suitable. A quick method of fitting fenestrated scleral lenses has been described by Lewis (1970). Keratometry, refraction through a trial contact lens, and impressions are carried out. Casts are made and the lenses are ordered with an annular transition, 3.5 mm wide and 1 mm deep at the centre of the annulus. The back optic is made double curved with BCOR fitted to the nearest 0.25 mm flatter than the flattest keratometer reading, and the BPOR is 1.25 mm flatter than the BCOR. The BCOD is 7.0 mm and the BPOR blends into the transition. The manufacturers are instructed to obtain the necessary back optic clearance from the cast by first trueing the back optic with a tool of the required BCOR and then grinding out a further 0.10 mm with this tool. The BPOR and transition are then made. On receipt of the lenses they are tried in and fenestrated first after checking that there is no rotation. The fit is then examined and usually the only modification necessary is a possible reduction in overall size, but the lens should be left as large as possible.

SMALL SCLERAL LENSES

A lens having a single curve back optic surface and a haptic portion which is about 2 mm in width, so that the overall size is 16–18 mm, has proved satisfactory for sports purposes for short periods of wear. It is fitted like a FLOM (*see* Chapter 10, Volume 1) but not fenestrated, although it is worn without solution.

Disadvantages are the introduction of bubbles and a propensity for the lens to become misplaced. This has led to the introduction of a special type of large corneal lens, described below.

SPECIAL CORNEAL LENSES

Levey (1964) has described what he calls a 'microscleral' lens which is 14–18 mm in overall size. The central 10 mm of the back surface is designed in much the same way as the back surface of a corneal lens, with successive curves flattened by 0.5 mm in radius and 0.5 mm in width. Beyond 10 mm in diameter, the back surface radii and widths vary according to the central optic radius. For optic radii steeper than 7.5 mm, the radii continue to flatten by 0.5 mm and are 1.0 mm in width; for optic radii between 7.5 and 8.0 mm, the radii flatten by 1.0 mm and are 1.0 mm wide; and for optic radii over 8.0 mm, the radii flatten by 1.5 mm and are 1.5 mm wide. Smaller overall sizes are generally fitted to steeper corneas. These lenses are fitted with multiple fenestrations and minimum thickness consistent with adequate edge thickness – which means that they are about the same thickness as the average scleral lens.

A similar lens has been described by Jessen (1966). This is 18 mm in overall size, has multiple fenestrations and is designed with a back central optic diameter of 8.5 mm, with progressive flattening beyond this. The optic and 'haptic' portions are fitted independently, and the lens is intended to be apically clear but bubble-free. Wearing time is limited to 4 hours.

CONVENTIONAL CORNEAL LENSES

These are suitable for many non-contact sports but may have to be fitted slightly larger and/or steeper to prevent excessive movement. In that case corneal metabolism is likely to be slightly upset and a reduced wearing time must be accepted, but this is normally adequate for the period of the game.

LENSES FOR SKIN DIVING

Under water, the power of the eye is reduced by approximately 42 D. This is due to water replacing air in front of the cornea. If the front surface of the cornea is assumed to have a radius of curvature of 8.0 mm, then the reduction in power is as follows.

$$\frac{\text{Power of front surface}}{\text{of cornea, in air}} - \frac{\text{Power of front surface}}{\text{of cornea, in water}}$$

$$\frac{(1.376 - 1)1000 \text{ D}}{8.0} - \frac{(1.376 - 1.333)1000 \text{ D}}{8.0}$$

$$= 41.5 \text{ D}$$

The emmetropic eye therefore becomes hypermetropic to this extent. This power loss may be replaced in two ways, as follows.

(1) A contact lens may be worn which incorporates a steeply curved high refractive index glass button (*Figure 24.34*). The additional power is

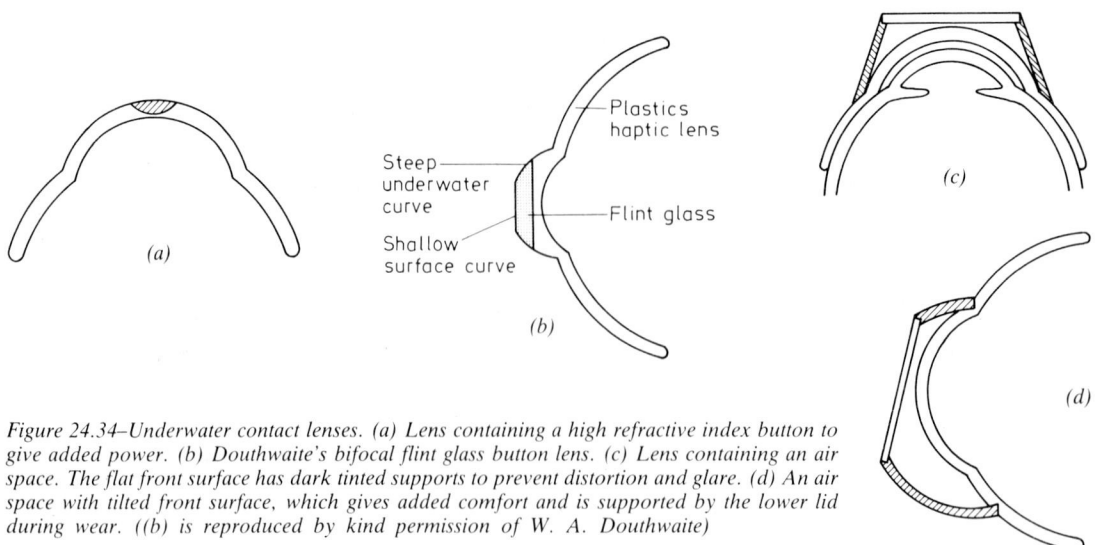

Figure 24.34–Underwater contact lenses. (a) Lens containing a high refractive index button to give added power. (b) Douthwaite's bifocal flint glass button lens. (c) Lens containing an air space. The flat front surface has dark tinted supports to prevent distortion and glare. (d) An air space with tilted front surface, which gives added comfort and is supported by the lower lid during wear. ((b) is reproduced by kind permission of W. A. Douthwaite)

achieved by the difference of refractive indices, these being 1.6 and 1.333 at the front surface as compared to 1.49 and 1.333 for the carrier portion, and 1.6 and 1.49 at the interface. It is necessary to incorporate the button in a fairly thick scleral lens.

The button may be made very small so that it only partially covers the pupil. This allows vision through the carrier portion of the lens when in air as the carrier portion can be correctly sighted to allow for the wearer's normal refractive error.

Such a lens has been reported by Ward (1961). It suffered from two main disadvantages, namely, that it was extremely difficult to locate the button so that vision both above and below water was possible, and it was difficult to find a suitable cement which did not dissolve in sea water to attach the button to the carrier portion.

These problems appear to have been overcome by Douthwaite (1971) who described a similar type of lens in which a flint glass button was fused by the 'Uniseal' method to a plastics scleral lens, the interface between the two being plane (*Figure 24.34b*). The same concentric principle is employed but the outer steep curve on the front of the flint button permits vision under water where the illumination is low and the pupil dilated, and the central flatter front surface curve caters for vision in air when the pupil is likely to be more constricted in daylight. The type of bifocal lens described is less noticeable than the air-cell type of lens described below, is more comfortable to wear, does not give rise to the magnification effect nor to the distortion encountered with the air-cell lens. It gives a full, unrestricted field of view. Its disadvantages are slight displacement on the eye which can cause a loss of vision above water, and also the out-of-focus image formed by the peripheral portion in air may give rise to a haze which reduces contrast and affects visual acuity.

Douthwaite also suggested a bifocal underwater lens similar to a solid spectacle bifocal lens, the lower part being used for vision above water when the wearer is likely to be looking in a relatively downwards direction while treading water, and the upper part being used for underwater vision when the gaze is usually relatively upwards as the diver swims along in a horizontal direction. He also pointed out that direction of gaze can vary considerably which would then make this type of lens difficult to wear.

The air-cell type of lens is one which has a plane front surface enclosing an air space in front of a conventional scleral lens sighted to correct the wearer's normal refractive error. This type of lens is, as it were, a tiny 'face mask' worn in front of the eye only (*Figure 24.34c*). The optical effect is the same as looking through any plane surface into water.

Refraction of light from water to air causes objects to appear at three-quarters of their real distance, giving a magnification of $\times 1.333$. Due to total internal reflection at the plane face, the visual field is restricted to 97.2 degrees in air and approximately 55–60 degrees in water (Cockell, 1967). If the side supports are left transparent, there is considerable distortion of the peripheral visual field.

Mossé (1964) described a lens in which the front plane face is tilted, as in *Figure 24.34d*, and in which the supports are opaque, eliminating the distortion of the peripheral field. The tilt of the plane face makes upper lid movement more comfortable and prevents the lens from sagging as it is better supported by the lower lid.

The mode of attachment of the plane face to the lens is important so that the air chamber does not collapse in the pressures experienced under water. *Figure 24.34d* shows the system used in France, and *Figure 24.35* shows Cockell's construction in which

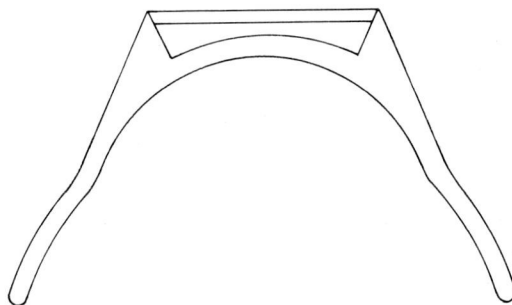

Figure 24.35–Cockell's underwater contact lens (developed at the City University, London)

all but the plane face is made from one solid piece of plastics material.

Attempts have been made to fill the space with air under pressure. The incorporation of a little silica gel in the air space prevents condensation. The plane face should be as close as possible to the front optic surface of the scleral lens, but not sufficiently close to cause interference fringes.

The advantage of such a lens is that it gives adequate vision both above and below water without allowing the diver to be seen from afar, which happens due to reflections when a plane face mask is worn. (This is an important function in times of war, when skin divers need to remain as invisible as possible – especially on surfacing). This type of lens can be worn satisfactorily for periods of about 4 hours.

LENSES FOR THE PARTIALLY SIGHTED

Partially sighted people need additional magnification in order to be able to see detail. Such magnification may be provided in the form of a Galilean telescope device, in which a contact lens forms the eyepiece and a conventional spectacle lens the objective. The optical system is depicted in *Figure 24.36*.

Since the eyepiece contacts the cornea, the magnification (for an emmetropic eye) is given directly by

$$\frac{w_2}{w_1} = \frac{f_1'}{f_2'} = \frac{f_1'}{f_1' - d} = \frac{1}{1 - dF_1'} \ (d \ \text{in metres}).$$

With a typical power for F_1' of +25 D and a vertex distance, d, of 12 mm,

$$\text{Magnification} = \frac{1}{1 - 3/10} = \frac{1}{0.7} \div \quad \times 1.4$$

The powers of the two lenses and their separation must be such as to correct the patient's refractive error, K, where

$$K = \frac{F_1'}{1 - dF_1'} + F_2' \quad (d \ \text{in metres}).$$

only, as is often the case. The patient then has a normal visual field with one eye, whilst the other eye receives the magnified image for detailed vision, in a reduced visual field (Moore, 1964). However, this does require the facility of alternate suppression by the patient, or else alternate occlusion of the eyes to avoid confusion. It is surprising how well patients with low visual acuity are able to adapt to such a system so long as it provides an obvious benefit to them.

The magnification reduces the visual field and can cause disorientation, but this may be minimized to some extent by magnifying only a small central portion of the visual field. This may be done by using a carefully fitted contact lens worked to correct the refractive error but with the front central portion made quite flat, giving a high negative power centrally. The diameter of this portion must be about two-thirds of the pupil diameter in normal illumination; and according to Filderman (1964), it is typically between 3.5 and 4.0 mm, and of about −50 D power. This is the high negative eyepiece of power F_2' which is used in conjunction with a positive segment of about 10 mm diameter and +25 D power, cemented on to the back surface of an afocal spectacle lens of 12 D base. Below this, a near

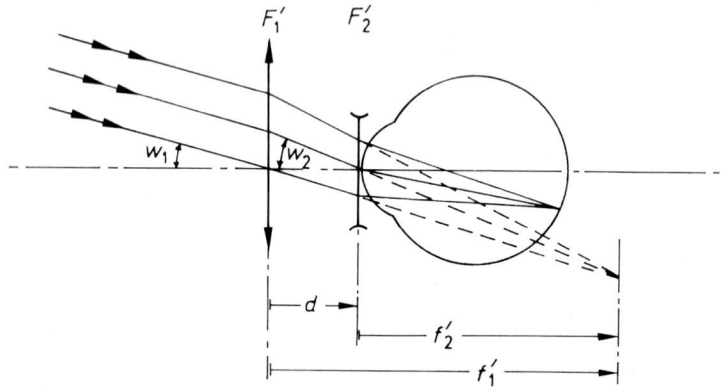

Figure 24.36–A Galilean telescope system incorporating a contact lens of power F_2' as eyepiece, and a spectacle lens of power F_1' as objective

This system has been used with soft, scleral and corneal lenses forming the eyepiece, soft and scleral lenses being generally more satisfactory as they are more stable. The advantages over the telescopic type of spectacle aid are the reduction in weight and the psychological benefit of improved cosmetic appearance. The weight of the high positive spectacle lens can be further relieved by the use of a Fresnel press-on lens as utilized and recommended by Gerstman and Levene (1974). The disadvantage is that contact lenses cannot be removed as quickly and conveniently as spectacles. This is less of a disadvantage when the system is worn by one eye

addition may be cemented on to the carrier lens (*Figure 24.37*). Fresnel press-on segments may be used as an alternative to cemented segments.

F_2' depends on the thickness and back optic radius of the contact lens. Since

$$K = \frac{F_1'}{1 - dF_1'} + F_2'$$

and since d is known, or can be measured, F_1' may be determined. The magnification may then be computed from

$$\frac{1}{1 - dF_2'}$$

Filderman described a small corneal lens fitted to rest on the lower lid and ballasted to keep it down, with the optic displaced to put it in front of the pupil and the upper edge of the lens only just above the upper pupil margin. He also stated that best results were obtained with scleral lenses, but soft lenses may now supersede them (Stone and Breakspear, 1977).

Such lenses cannot be fitted to old people. Not only do they have pupils which are too small but also the disorientation is usually too great to be tolerated by them. Young people can usually cope with these difficulties.

An attempt has been made by Feinbloom (1961) to incorporate both positive objective and negative eyepiece in one scleral lens with an air space

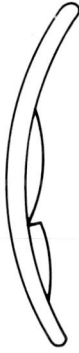

Figure 24.37–A spectacle lens used as the objective for a Galilean telescope system, having separate portions for distance and near vision, cemented on to an afocal carrier lens

between the two. While being theoretically possible, lenses so far made have been very thick and heavy, making them uncomfortable to wear and unsightly.

Drasdo (1970) has developed a similar lens to be used in conjunction with a spectacle lens, which he described as a 'feedback corrected' lens system since it gives magnification without altering the angular amount of movement of the eye required to take up fixation of peripheral objects. It therefore overcomes one of the major disadvantages of disorientation.

A reversed telescope system has been mentioned by Bier (1960b) for people with loss of peripheral vision, and the author, with others, has also successfully fitted one for a person with homonymous hemianopia. A high positive scleral lens used with a high negative spectacle lens, suitably designed to give minimum aberrations, gives a reduction in magnification (and, incidentally, a reduced visual acuity) but allows more to be seen in the existing visual field.

OXYGEN PERMEABLE LENSES

The hydrophilic materials described in Chapter 13 are very slightly permeable to oxygen and carbon dioxide, and transmit more when the lens is thin and the material is of a high water content. However, besides these there are other materials being used for contact lenses, which are of sufficiently high gas permeability to alleviate some of the corneal oedema problems associated with polymethyl methacrylate lenses and even to be considered for continuous or extended wear. They are therefore potentially of considerable interest.

SILICONE RUBBER SOFT FLEXIBLE LENSES

Silicone rubber is an internally plasticized material of hydrocarbon substituted polysiloxane rubber, flexible like hydrophilic soft lens material (Sarwar and Fydelor, 1966). It is non-toxic and chemically inert (Breger, 1971). Although flexible, the material is highly elastic and lenses deformed during blinking rapidly spring back to their original shape. Like lenses of hydrophilic material, silicone rubber lenses tend to wrap themselves to conform to the shape of the cornea. Very little corneal astigmatism can therefore be corrected with spherical lenses. The material absorbs less fluid than polymethyl methacrylate, that is, there is virtually no uptake of water, so that there are no problems of alterations in vision as occur with soft hydrophilic lenses when they dry on the eye. Also, there are thus no curvature changes with hydration and dehydration. However, storage in solution is recommended in order to maintain the best possible wetting properties. Soaking solutions cannot be absorbed into the lens to leach out onto the eye later, so there is no risk of the 'red eye' reaction which results when this happens with hydrophilic lenses.

In the United States of America a patent was filed in 1962 for transparent silicone rubber contact lenses (Becker, 1966). Work by Hill (1966) and by Hill and Schoessler (1967) showed that the permeability to oxygen of silicone rubber corneal lenses was sufficiently great to allow normal corneal oxygen uptake to be maintained during a 90-second period of static corneal lens wear. Further research (Fatt, Bieber and Pye, 1969; Fatt and St. Helen, 1971) has shown that both during waking and sleeping conditions the silicone rubber lens permits sufficient oxygen to reach the cornea, for normal corneal oxygen uptake to be maintained. Hill (1974) has studied diurnal variations in corneal curvature during the wearing of silicone rubber lenses, and found a mean horizontal and vertical variation of less than 0.25 D. This lack of corneal curvature change is comparable with the small changes in curvature found during hydrophilic lens wear, and in the case of silicone rubber is due to the lack of corneal oedema directly attributable to the gas permeability of the material which is permeable to carbon dioxide as well as oxygen. The lack of corneal curvature change while wearing these lenses is a distinct advantage compared to polymethyl methacrylate lenses, as it means that there is very little spectacle blur with all its attendant problems. Unlike some hydrophilic materials the material has very good tear strength, and as it is also biologically inert, it is very safe to wear.

The early lenses were more difficult to adapt to than hydrophilic lenses and caused some lid sensation, possibly because the thickness of the lens required to give it sufficient rigidity meant that a large lens had to be fitted. According to Breger (1971), the early lenses were moulded between dies and then vulcanized or cured. The peripheral curves were moulded at the same time, and edges mechanically produced. All negative lenses were lenticular to reduce edge thickness, and high positive lenses were also made lenticular. Because of their thickness (average centre thickness of 0.3 mm) these lenses tended to drop, and were therefore made large, with OS of 10.0 mm, or more often of 10.5 mm. The BCOD was 9.0 mm with three gradually flattening peripheral curves. The fitting technique recommended by Breger was to fit the BCOR approximately in alignment with the flattest keratometer reading.

According to Danker (1976) silicone rubber lenses, because of their high gas permeability, are suitable for extended wear, with weekly removal for cleaning. Their main drawback in the past has been the problem of poor surface wetting and adherence of mucus to the lenses. Various laboratories have attempted to use surface coating and other techniques to convert the surface from hydrophobic to hydrophilic, and recent attempts have been very successful.

The most recent lenses are just larger than the cornea, and are as flexible as the 40 per cent water content hydrophilic lenses. They are made with very thin edges and cause a minimum of lid sensation, but care has to be taken in fitting so as not to irritate the limbal region. Only clear material is so far available. The lenses are fitted using fluorescein, the fitting techniques being described in Chapter 14, page 463.

HARD LENS MATERIALS

The most well known of the oxygen permeable hard materials is cellulose acetate butyrate, known as CAB. It is very slightly permeable to oxygen (Fatt and Lin, 1977) and to carbon dioxide and nitrogen.

According to Stahl, Reich and Ivani (1974), at a thickness of 0.15 mm it transmits five times the oxygen necessary for the metabolism of the cornea, but this has proved to be mistaken as Hill (1977) as well as Fatt and Lin have shown. The oxygen permeability of Hartflex CAB lenses (manufactured by Wöhlk Contact Lenses in Germany) is given as 4.2×10^{-11} $(cm^2/sec)(ml\ O_2/ml\ mm\ Hg)$, as stated by Gasson (1978). Stahl and his colleagues gave all the properties of the material. They gave a refractive index of 1.52, but there are a number of CAB materials available, and two English contact lens manufacturers give figures of 1.48 (Madden, 1975) and 1.47 (Nissel, 1976a). Like PMMA it is basically hydrophobic, but despite this it has a water absorption of up to 3.5 per cent, and it has a contact angle of 30 degrees (Madden, 1975), a specific gravity of 1.20–1.22 and a light transmission of 92 per cent. It is softer than polymethyl methacrylate and more flexible. It is not brittle but once deformed it is slow to return to its original curvature. Reich (1975) states that it is non-irritating, non-toxic and non-flammable. Both Pearson (1977) and Stone (1978) have shown that lathe-cut CAB lenses are unstable in curvature, especially high negative lenses. It appears to be a good material for low powered hard corneal lenses and there are reports of CAB lenses having been successfully worn continuously for 6 months, being removed once a week for cleaning (Danker, 1976). CAB lenses have also been successfully fitted to eyes with keratoconus and recurrent corneal abrasions (Reich, 1975).

Clear and tinted materials are available and lenses are manufactured in the same way as conventional polymethyl methacrylate lenses, some by lathe-cutting and some by injection moulding. Modifications may also be carried out in a similar manner to conventional lenses. Fitting is done in the same way as for normal hard lenses, and fluorescein is used similarly. It is recommended that these lenses are kept in soak when not being worn due to the large variations in curvature during hydration and dehydration. The slight gas permeability seems to make them useful for patients who suffer corneal oedema with polymethyl methacrylate lenses, as O'Leary (1976) and Reich (1976) have shown. Like silicone rubber lenses they cause minimal corneal curvature changes (Reich, 1976).

Besides instability of curvature one other disadvantage at first was that the otherwise most suitable available CAB material for contact lenses, contained an ultra-violet inhibitor which could cause dermatitis (Nissel, 1976b). However, as there are over one hundred types of CAB material made, and some specifically for contact lens manufacture without this inhibitor are now available, this should no longer be a problem.

Other materials include one which is a combination of hydroxy-ethyl methacrylate (HEMA) and a modified silicone, one which is produced by the DuPont Corporation in the United States of America and which has a significantly higher oxygen permeability than CAB, as assessed by its 'equivalent oxygen performance' (Hill, 1977), and others marketed under the names Boston and Polycon, also both from America. Westerhout (1977) reports excellent results with the latter material in cases of intractable corneal oedema with conventional hard lenses. Similar results have been reported with the Toyo material, Mericon O_2.

It is obvious that there may shortly be a major breakthrough in obtaining a hard lens material which is gas permeable as well as being stable, non-toxic and having good wetting properties. Indeed, the material may already be available but still being subjected to stringent testing by the Food and Drugs Administration Bureau in the United States.

SPECIAL SCLERAL LENSES

Several unusual methods of fitting scleral lenses have been developed but have not been dealt with in Chapters 9 and 10, Volume 1. Lewis's (1970) method of fitting impression scleral lenses has been described on page 681, and McKay Taylor's (1969) use of S-bend channels mentioned on pages 664 and 681. A brief description of some other methods follows.

FLUSH-FITTING LENSES

Occasionally, a cornea is so irregular that a better optical result may be achieved by aligning the back surface of the plastics contact lens with the irregularities rather than fitting a regular spherical back surface which allows collections of bubbles or mucus in the corneal irregularities, thus interfering with vision. This flush-fitting technique has been advocated by Ridley (1954) and has met with great success in these extremely irregular eyes. Lenses of this type have also been used to assist healing of corneal wounds, the lenses being altered to remain flush-fitting as healing progresses (Girard, Soper and Sampson, 1966). They are also beneficial in neurotrophic keratitis (Gould, 1967). In all cases, the method of lens manufacture is to mould a shell over a cast of the eye impression; then the front optic surface only is worked to optical quality, as described in Chapter 20, page 594.

A modification of this method has been used successfully by Miller, Holmberg and Carroll (1968). Their technique is to take a cast of the eye impression and remove a central core of 6 mm diameter, replacing it by a metal rod which is flush with the corneal portion of the cast and finely polished to a radius best following the corneal profile. A shell is then pressed out over this, which results in it having a back central optic portion of optical quality. Then, by working the front surface, a lens of known power and BCOR can be made which is still more or less flush with the cornea.

DALLOS 'TYPE' SHELLS

Dallos (1932), the first person to perfect the eye impression technique, made so many eye impressions and shells from casts of these that he was able to look at an eye and, from its shape, pick out a suitable shell from his collection. He classified his shells into types, according to size and shape, and built up a fitting set of 'preformed' lenses based on them.

The technique has been used by a number of contact lens fitters; but owing to the vast experience required before being able to pick out a type of shell likely to be a good fit on a particular eye, this method of fitting has not been widely adopted.

GRATICULE LENSES

McKay Taylor (1966) has described a method of preformed scleral lens fitting which uses single curve corneal lenses of 10 mm overall size to assess the optic fit. These have back optic radii in 0.1 mm steps, from 7.4 to 9.1 mm. Fenestrated transitional shells with an overall size of 13–16 mm and radii of 9–12 mm are used to assess the fit of the transition region. These lenses have a back optic radius of 7 mm, designed to give adequate central corneal clearance, and have an engraved ring of 10 mm diameter at the junction between the back optic and transition curves.

The haptic portion is assessed by means of 'graticule' lenses which are fenestrated and engraved radially at 30 degree intervals in red, black and green. The geometrical centre is marked with a cross to allow the optic displacement to be gauged. The fit of all three portions – optic, transition and haptic – is independently assessed, the graticule lenses allowing location of tight and loose areas.

TRUHAP LENSES

These are similar to the BSD lenses described in Chapter 10, Volume 1. They have a double curve temporal haptic portion and a conical transition with a flattened nasal haptic portion. The temporal haptic curves are worked about an axis with centre offset nasally as compared to the optic and nasal haptic portions. For a preformed scleral lens, these lenses come as close as possible to the normal shape of the globe (Jackson, 1970).

ANIMALS' LENSES

At various times, contact lenses have been used for animals. Most fall into two categories as follows.

Experimental Lenses

Lenses used for research purposes have already been mentioned earlier in this chapter.

Utilitarian Lenses

Chickens and turkeys have been provided with opaque and coloured contact lenses to reduce their acuity and so prevent featherpecking (Anon, 1967).

MISCELLANEOUS LENSES

Certain lenses or types of lens do not fall into any of the above categories, and yet some mention of them should be made.

TINTED LENSES

The reasons for prescribing tinted lenses have already been dealt with. Tinted lenses are available in a large number of different hues usually denoted by a number (*see Table 22.1*, page 642), their spectral transmission curves being available from the plastics or contact lens manufacturers.

Two main dangers arise in the use of tinted lenses. The first, as has been pointed out by Estevez (1967), is their possible toxicity to ocular tissues – particularly if soluble dyes or surface dyeing is used for colouration. In Great Britain, only Perspex CQ, made by I.C.I., has been proven by clinical trials to be non-toxic to ocular tissues. This is available in clear and neutral grey tints, (9042 and 9043, previously 911 CQ and 912 CQ) the latter tinting being achieved by the use of inert fine carbon particles dispersed in the monomer before polymerization. The pigment is thus locked in the molecular chain. The fine carbon particles are visible in the material when the contact lenses are observed on the eye with the biomicroscope.

Although Estevez states that pigments incorporated in this way are solid particles and therefore may reduce the transparency of the material (except where fine carbon particles are used), contact lenses tinted with such insoluble dyes have proved satisfac-tory in wear. Capelli (1966) has shown that no dye leached out of 20 different coloured samples boiled for 80 hours. A minute non-coloured residue was obtained after boiling, which was slightly less from tinted lenses (33.5 μg) than from clear lenses (40.0 μg). The fact that these lenses have been worn so satisfactorily by many wearers suggests that the toxicity problem and the transparency problem are both small ones.

Soft lenses may be tinted by the use of vegetable dyes. Some of these dyes leach out of the lens during wear and the patient can renew the tint by the application of a few drops of dye to the lens each day. Other dyes are more stable but may be removed from the lens during one of the stringent cleaning processes, such as the Ren-O-Gel (*Alcon*) system.

The second danger has been outlined by Fletcher and Nisted (1963), who have shown that some tinted lenses raise the light threshold, thereby worsening dark adaptation. Also, by their selective spectral transmission, they can be potentially dangerous when used in certain near monochromatic illumination. For example, certain blue-tinted lenses used in sodium lighting could severely reduce visibility, and green lenses could reduce the visibility of red traffic lights and rear lights.

Another hazard, which is not confined to tinted lenses but applies equally to clear lenses, has been suggested by Ball (1964). He postulated that some of the photophobia experienced by new contact lens wearers may be due to increased ultra-violet radiation reaching the cornea. The cornea is most sensitive to a radiation of 288 nm, and most plastics (tinted or otherwise) have a cut-off at 290 nm. An alternative explanation for increased photophobia with contact lenses was given by Fletcher (1964), who showed that significantly more light is admitted to the eye by a clear lens of approximately 0.3 mm thickness and this increase is offset by tinting. He attributes the increase to the optical effect of moving the entrance pupil forward, which increases its size and thereby admits more light into the eye. However, the entrance pupil size would only be increased by a positive contact lens system. Its size would be decreased by a negative lens (Stone, 1968). This factor would therefore only be of significance in causing photophobia if positive lenses are worn, as in aphakia. In all probability, most photophobia is due to corneal oedema during the adaptation period (*see* Chapter 16, page 513).

SURFACE COATING

Some contact lens wearers have problems because their lenses do not wet properly. The contact angle may be reduced (that is, surface wetting improved) by coating the surfaces of the lenses chemically or by deposition of a thin metal compound. In either case, the surface of the lens is converted from a hydrophobic to a hydrophilic one.

The former method, of chemical coating, was developed by Erb (1961) and is known as the Erb method. The lens is thoroughly cleaned and dipped in a solution of titanium dioxide. This improves the wetting properties of the lens; but if the lens becomes greasy, the effect is spoiled. Eventually, the coating deteriorates due to wear. A thin film of silica, applied by treating the surface with water and silicon tetrachloride vapour, has since proved more reliable (Blue, 1966).

Vacuum coating is the other method, which is also of rather a temporary nature because plastics material, for obvious reasons, has to be coated in a cold state. The method, apart from the difference in temperature, is essentially that used to put an anti-reflection coating on glass lenses.

Both methods must be carried out on a finally finished contact lens, when all modifications to the fit have been made. In both cases, greasing of the lenses is minimized; but if it does occur, the wetting properties are spoiled until the grease is removed.

Another vacuum method of converting the surface to hydrophilic has been described by Gesser, Funt and Warriner (1965). It is claimed that about half the surface molecular groups are changed in chemical composition by removal of hydrogen atoms. Lenses are placed in a vacuum discharge tube in the presence of ammonia but out of the path of the discharge glow. An electrical discharge causes a chemical action to take place on the surface of the plastics material. The altered molecules are hydrophilic instead of hydrophobic. Lenses treated in this way wet well, and there is minimal build up of grease and oil on their surfaces.

MATERIALS WITH LOWERED WETTING ANGLE

Besides the special surface coatings and treatments mentioned above, several materials for hard lenses are now available made of polymethyl methacrylate in which the cross-linking agents have been changed to reduce the surface wetting angle (Harris *et al.*, 1973). Such materials are, for example, the Aqua-Lens made by Morgan Optics in the United States, BP-flex made by Burton Parsons which is PMMA with an added methacrylic component, and the Hydro-15 lens marketed by Madden Contact Lenses in England. These materials are very useful for patients who suffer greasing problems with conventional polymethyl methacrylate lenses. Goldberg

(1975) found such a material very good for patients having corneal oedema with conventional lenses. He attributes the reduction of oedema with this material to better transport of tears and therefore of gaseous exchange behind the lens, due to less frictional resistance and by allowing more oxygen to be present in the tears at the lens–cornea interface. He also found the same effect with the CAB material described on page 686. The latter material also has a lower wetting angle than polymethyl methacrylate. The fluorescein pattern with a Hydro-15 lens must be viewed with blue light as the material does not transmit the appropriate ultra-violet wavelength.

LENSES OF HIGH AND LOW REFRACTIVE INDEX

Lenses of low refractive index have already been described, namely, hydrophilic and silicone rubber lenses.

Lenses of high refractive index were tried, with varying degrees of success. The higher refractive index allows a thinner lens to be made, which is useful for lenses of high power. Hyfrax, a material produced in the United States, has been described by Morrison (1962). It has a refractive index of 1.568 and is lighter in weight than polymethyl methacrylate. Some difficulties have been experienced with its wetting properties. Although the contact angle is smaller than with polymethyl methacrylate, the material is somewhat lipophilic (fat attracting). It absorbs less water than polymethyl methacrylate and, correspondingly, contact lenses made from Hyfrax have a more constant curvature.

Similar high refractive index plastics are now being used, often with the addition of a fluorescent dye, for the segments of bifocal contact lenses. The addition of the dye, though invisible in normal light, renders fitting more easy when viewed by ultra-violet illumination.

The experimental use of synthetic sapphire material has been reported by Nissel (1969). This has a very high refractive index of about 2.

LENSES INCORPORATING BACTERICIDES

The material for such contact lenses has been developed in the United States (Torgerson, 1964). These lenses have a significant effect in inhibiting bacterial growth as compared with normal lenses, the degree of inhibition depending on the contact time (Mote, Schoessler and Hill, 1969; Mote and Hill, 1970). Conversely, Chalkley, Sarnat and Shock (1966) had previously found lenses of this material to be of no apparent value.

This concludes the details of special contact lenses; but it is anticipated that, in the near future, there will be many more special types of lens and special uses for contact lenses in the fields of scientific research, where expansion continues at a phenomenal rate.

ACKNOWLEDGMENTS

I am indebted to my father, Mr R. G. Stone, for drawing the diagrams, and to Miss Carolyn Christie of The Belgravia Optical Co. Ltd., and Miss Stella Dampier of The City University, London, for typing assistance.

REFERENCES

Alvis, D. L. (1966). 'Electroretinographic changes in controlled open angle glaucoma.' *Am. J. Ophthal.* **61,** 121–131

Anderson, J. M. (1952). *Contact Lenses, Clinical and Other Observations*, p. 33. Brighton: Courtenay Press

Anon (1967). 'Contact lenses for turkeys – report.' *Optician* **154,** 575

Aquavella, J. V. (1976). 'New aspects of contact lenses in ophthalmology. In *Advances in Ophthalmology*, 32, pp. 2–34, ed. by Roper-Hall, M. J., Sautter, H. and Streiff, E. B. Basel: Karger

Bagshaw, J., Gordon, S. P. and Stanworth, A. (1966). 'A modified corneal contact lens: binocular single vision in unilateral aphakia.' *Br. orthopt. J.* **23,** 19–30

Bailey, N. J. (1966). 'Do contact lenses control myopia?' *Optica International* **3,** 25–30

Baldwin, W. R., West, D., Jolley, J. and Reid, W. (1969). 'Effects of contact lenses on refractive, corneal and axial length changes in young myopes.' *Am. J. Optom.* **46,** 903–911

Ball, G. V. (1964). 'Characteristics of tinted contact lenses.' *Br. J. physiol. Optics* **21,** 219–223

Barkan, O. (1936). 'New operation for chronic glaucoma: restoration of physiological function by opening Schlemm's canal under direct magnified vision.' *Am. J. Ophthal.* **19,** 951

Becker, S. C. (1972). *Clinical Gonioscopy.* St. Louis, Missouri: Mosby

Becker, W. E. (1966). 'Corneal contact lens fabricated from transparent silicone rubber.' Filed June 29, 1962, *U.S. Patent Office Official Gazette* (3,228,741), p. 609, January 11, 1966

Bier, N. (1957). *Contact Lens Routine and Practice*, pp. 49–52, 2nd ed. London: Butterworths

Bier, N. (1960a). *Correction of Subnormal Vision*, p. 100. London: Butterworths

Bier, N. (1960b). *Correction of Subnormal Vision*, p. 87. London: Butterworths

Blackstone, M. (1966). 'Hydrophilic lenses: some practical experiments.' *Optician* **151,** 5–6

Blue, H. D. (1966). 'Method of producing permanent wettability on plastic contact lenses.' *J. Am. optom. Ass.* **37,** 678–681

Bornschein, H., Wichterle, O. and Wündsch, L., (1966). 'A contact lens electrode for comparative E.R.G. studies.' *Vision Res.* **6,** 773–774

Breger, J. L. (1971). 'The silicone rubber lens.' *Optician* **162**(4189), 12–14

Capelli, Q. A. (1966). 'Water extractives from coloured contact lenses – a report.' *Opt. J. Rev. Optom.* **103,** 32

Catford, G. V. and Mackie, I. A. (1968). 'Occlusion with high plus corneal lenses.' *Br. J. Ophthal.* **52,** 342–345

Chalkley, T., Sarnat, L. and Shock, D. (1966). 'Evaluation of "bacteriostatic" contact lenses.' *Am. J. Ophthal.* **61,** 866–869

Chiquiar Arias, V., Liberatore, J. C., Voss, E. H. and Chiquiar Arias, M. (1959). 'A new technique of fitting contact lenses on keratoconus.' *Contacto* **3,** 393–415

Chiquiar Arias, V. (1963a). 'The correction of keratoconus with contact lenses.' *Optician* **146,** 447–451, 474–477, 501–505, 527–530, 553–559

Chiquiar Arias, V. (1963b). 'The C. A. dynamic fluoroscopic technique.' *Contacto* **7,** 3–15

Clifford Hall, K. G. (1963). 'A comprehensive study of keratoconus.' *Br. J. physiol. Optics* **20,** 215–256

Cockell, R. R. (1967). 'A survey of underwater visual problems.' Paper read to The Contact Lens Society, January, 1967

Dallos, J. (1932). 'Ueber den Einfluss der Form der Haftglässer auf ihren Korrektionswert.' *Klin. Mbl. Augenheilk.* **89,** 108

Danker, F. (1976). 'The present state of silicone lenses and cellulose acetate butyrate lenses in the United States.' Paper read at meeting of International Society of Contact Lens Specialists, Fuschl, Austria, Sept., 1976, and reported in *Optician* **172**(4453), 15–16

Deluca, T. J., Forgacs, L. S. and Skolnick, S. D. (1974). 'The use of the Bausch & Lomb Soflens^IM in tonometry.' *J. Am. optom. Ass.* **45,** 1028–1038

Dickinson, F. (1957). 'The value of microlenses in progressive myopia.' *Optician* **133,** 263–264

Ditchburn, R. W. and Ginsborg, B. L. (1952). 'Vision with a stabilized retinal image.' *Nature* **170,** 36–37

Douthwaite, W. A. (1971). 'Bifocal underwater contact lenses.' *Ophthal. Optician* **11,** 10–14

Drasdo, N. (1970). 'The effect of high powered contact lenses on the visual fixation reflex.' *Br. J. physiol. Optics* **25,** 14–22

Erb, R. A. (1961). *Method for Producing Wettable Surfaces on Contact Lenses by Chemical Formation of Inorganic Films*, U.S. Dept. of Commerce, Office of Technical Services, Government Research Report AD-257290

Evans, C. R. and Piggins, D. J. (1963). 'A comparison of the behaviour of geometrical shapes when viewed under conditions of steady fixation, and with apparatus for producing a stabilized retinal image.' *Br. J. physiol. Optics* **20,** 261–273

Evans, C. R. (1965). 'A universally fitting contact lens for the study of stabilized retinal images.' *Br. J. physiol. Optics* **22,** 39–45

Estevez, J. M. J. (1967). 'Poly(methyl methacrylate) for use in contact lenses.' *Contact Lens* **1**, 19–26

Fatt, I., Bieber, M. T. and Pye, S. D. (1969). 'Steady state distribution of oxygen and carbon dioxide in the *in vivo* cornea of an eye covered by a gas-permeable contact lens.' *Am. J. Optom.* **46**, 3–14

Fatt, I. and Hill, R. M. (1970). 'Oxygen tension under a contact lens during blinking – a comparison of theory and experimental observation.' *Am. J. Optom.* **47**, 50–55

Fatt, I. and Lin, D. (1977). 'Oxygen tension under a hard, gas-permeable contact lens.' *Am. J. Optom.* **54**, 146–148

Fatt, I. and St. Helen, R. (1971). 'Oxygen tension under an oxygen-permeable contact lens.' *Am. J. Optom.* **48**, 545–555

Feinbloom, W. (1961). 'Feinbloom miniscope contact lens.' Described by Allan Isen, *Encyclopaedia of Contact Lens Practice III*, Supplement 13, Appendix B, 53–55, South Bend, Indiana: International Optics Publishing Corporation

Filderman, I. P. (1964). 'The spectacle lens – contact lens system.' *Br. J. physiol. Optics* **21**, 195–196

Fincham, E. F. (1947). 'Some recent developments in artificial eyes.' *Optician* **113**, 551–556

Fletcher, R. J. (1964). 'A study of the total light flux admitted to the interior of the eye through contact lenses.' *Br. J. physiol. Optics* **21**, 134–146

Fletcher, R. J. ['Haptos'] (1966). 'Electrode-bearing contact lenses.' *Contact Lens* **1**(1), 19

Fletcher, R. J. and Nisted, M. (1963). 'A study of coloured contact lenses and their performance.' *Ophthal. Optician* **3**, 1151–1154, 1161–1163, 1203–1206, 1212–1213

Friedman, B. (1967). 'A contact lens for estimating corneal thickness.' *Eye Ear Nose Throat Mon.* **46**, 344–345

Gasson, A. P. (1978). 'Clinical appraisal of Hartflex CAB lenses.' *Optician* **175**(4521), 20, 22

Gerstman, D. R. and Levene, J. R. (1974). 'Galilean telescope for the partially sighted.' *Br. J. Ophthal.* **58**, 761–765

Gesser, H. D., Funt, B. L. and Warriner, R. E. (1965). 'A method of improving the wettability of contact lenses by free radical treatment.' *Am. J. Optom.* **42**, 321–324

Girard, L. J., Soper, J. W. and Sampson, W. G. (1966). 'Therapeutic uses of flush-fitting scleral contact lenses.' Paper read at Symposium on Contact Lenses of 20th International Congress of Ophthalmology, Munich, published in *Contact Lenses*, Karger, Basle, 1967, pp. 109–111

Goldberg, J. B. (1975). 'Must the gas go through?' *Optom. Wkly* **66**(34), 15–16

Goldmann, H. (1938). 'Zur Technik der Spaltlampenmikroskopie.' *Ophthalmologica* **96**, 90

Goldmann, H. and Schmidt, T. (1965). 'Ein Kontaktglas zur Biomikroskopie der Ora Serrata und der Pars Plana.' *Ophthalmologica* **149**, 481–483

Gould, H. L. (1967). 'Treatment of neurotrophic keratitis with scleral contact lenses.' *Eye Ear Nose Throat Mon.* **46**, 1406–1414

Grant, S. C. and May, C. H. (1972). 'Orthokeratology – the control of refractive errors through contact lenses.' *Optician* **163**(4214), 8–11

Harris, M. G., Oye, R., Hall, K. and Fatt, I. (1973). 'Contact angle measurements on hard contact lenses.' *Am. J. Optom.* **50**, 446–451

Hill, J. F. (1974). 'Diurnal variations in corneal curvature after wearing silicone contact lenses.' *Am. J. Optom.* **51**, 61–65

Hill, R. M. (1966). 'Effects of a silicone rubber contact lens on corneal respiration.' *J. Am. optom. Ass.* **37**, 1119–1121

Hill, R. M. (1977). 'Oxygen permeable contact lenses: how convinced is the cornea?' *Internat. Contact Lens Clin.* **4**(2), 34–36

Hill, R. M. and Leighton, A. J. (1965). 'Temperature changes of human cornea and tears under a contact lens, I, II & III.' *Am. J. Optom.* **42**, 9–16, 71–77, 584–588

Hill, R. M. and Fatt, I. (1966). 'Oxygen measurements under a contact lens.' *Am. J. Optom.* **43**, 233–237

Hill, R. M. and Schoessler, J. (1967). 'Optical membranes of silicone rubber.' *J. Am. optom. Ass.* **38**, 480–483

Hillman, J. S. (1976). 'The use of hydrophilic contact lenses.' *Optician* **172**(4458), 9–11

Jackson, J. (1970). Personal communication

Jessen, G. N. (1964). 'Contact lenses as a therapeutic device.' *Am. J. Optom.* **41**, 429–435

Jessen, G. N. (1966). 'Baseball and contact lenses – possible solution to the problem.' *Am. J. Optom.* **43**, 320–324

Kelly, T. S-B. and Butler, D. (1964). 'Preliminary report on corneal lenses in relation to myopia.' *Br. J. physiol. Optics* **21**, 175–186

Kelly, T. S-B. and Butler, D. (1971). 'The present position of contact lenses in relation to myopia.' *Br. J. physiol. Optics* **26**, 33–48

Kerns, R. L. (1977). 'Research in orthokeratology. Part VI: Statistical and clinical analyses.' *J. Am. optom. Ass.* **48**, 1134–1147

Kersley, H. J. (1975). 'Continuous wear lenses after aphakic operation.' *Optician* **170**(4393), 12–18

Klein, M. (1949). 'Contact shell applicator for use as a corneal bath.' *Br. J. Ophthal.* **33**, 716–717

Koeppé, L. (1919). 'Die Theorie und Anwendung der Stereomikroskopie des lebenden menschlichen Kammerwinkels in fokalen Lichte der Gullstrandschen Nernstspaltlampe.' *München. med. Wehnsch.* **66**, 708

La Bissonierre, P. E. (1974). 'The x-chrom lens.' *Internat. Contact Lens Clin.* **1**(4), 48–55

Levey, E. M. (1964). 'The sports wearer of contact lenses – a new approach.' *Br. J. physiol. Optics* **21**, 197–199

Levinson, A., Weissman, H. A. and Sachs, U. (1977). 'Use of the Bausch & Lomb Soflens[TM] plano T contact lens as a bandage.' *Am. J. Optom.* **54**, 97–103

Lewis, E. M. T. (1970). 'A haptic lens design.' *Ophthal. Optician* **10**, 56–60, 86

Madden, P. (1975). Technical Bulletin – The Super Comfort Lens. St. Leonards-on-Sea, Sussex: Madden Contact Lenses

McKay Taylor, C. (1966). 'A new method of fitting haptic lenses.' *Optician* **152**, 529–530

McKay Taylor, C. (1969). 'The s-bend and other channelled haptic lenses.' *Ophthal. Optician* **9**, 1256–1258

Miller, D., Holmberg, A. and Carroll, J. M. (1968). 'A flush fitting optical scleral contact lens.' *Archs Ophthal.* **79**, 311–314

Millodot, M. (1965). 'Stabilized retinal images and disappearance time.' *Br. J. physiol. Optics* **22**, 148–152

Moore, L. (1964). 'The contact lens for subnormal visual acuity.' *Br. J. physiol. Optics* **21**, 203–204

Morrison, R. J. (1958). 'Observations on contact lenses and the progression of myopia.' *Contacto* **2**, 20–25

Morrison, R. J. (1962). 'A new substance for contact lenses.' *Am. J. Optom.* **39**, 252–256

Moss, H. (1959). 'The contour principle in corneal contact lens prescribing for keratoconus.' *J. Am. optom. Ass.* **30**, 570–572

Mossé, P. (1964). 'Underwater contact lenses.' *Br. J. physiol. Optics* **21**, 250–255

Mote, E. M., Schoessler, J. P. and Hill, R. M. (1969). 'Lens incorporated germicides: I.' *J. Am. optom. Ass.* **40**, 291–293

Mote, E. M. and Hill, R. M. (1970). 'Lens incorporated germicides: II.' *J. Am. optom. Ass.* **41**, 260–262

Neill, J. C. (1962). 'Contact lenses and myopia.' *Pen. State Alumni Bulletin* **16**, 109–116

Nissel, G. (1969). Unpublished report to The Contact Lens Society

Nissel, G. (1976a). 'Cellulose acetate butyrate.' Technical bulletin published by G. Nissel & Co., Hemel Hempstead, Herts.

Nissel, G. (1976b). 'Comments on CAB material.' Paper read at meeting of International Society of Contact Lens Specialists, Fuschl, Austria, Sept., 1976,, and reported in *Optician* **172**(4453), 15–16

Nolan, J. A. (1964). 'Progress of myopia and contact lenses.' *Contacto* **8**, 25

Nolan, J. A. (1969). 'Approach to orthokeratology.' *J. Am. optom. Ass.* **40**, 303–305

O'Leary, D. J. (1976). 'Treatment of corneal lens-induced oedema.' *Optician* **172**(4458), 19–21

Petropoulou, N. (1975). 'The soft lens as a therapeutical dressing.' *Optician* **169**(4380), 6–11

Pearson, R. M. (1977). 'Dimensional stability of certain hard contact lens materials.' Paper read at meeting of Am. Acad. of Optom., London, and awaiting publication in *Am. J. Optom.*

Reich, L. A. (1975). 'Clinical application of a new gas-permeable contact lens to pathological corneas – case reports.' *J. Am. optom. Ass.* **46**, 284–289

Reich, L. A. (1976). 'Clinical comparison of identically designed contact lenses of PMMA vs. Rx-56 materials.' *Internat. Contact Lens Clin.* **3**(2), 52–56

Ridley, F. (1954). 'The contact lens in investigation and treatment.' *Trans. Ophthal. Soc.* **74**, 377–410

Ruedmann, A. D., Jr. and Noell, W. K. (1961). 'The electroretinogram in central retinal degeneration.' *Trans. Am. Acad. Ophthal. & Otolaryngol.* **65**, 576–594

Sabell, A. G. (1970). 'Some notes on diagnostic contact lenses.' *Ophthal. Optician* **10**, 1160–1162, 1173–1178

Sarwar, M. and Fydelor, P. J. (1966). 'Materials for implantation in or on to ocular tissue.' *Ophthal. Optician* **6**, 221–223

Scheie, H. G. (1957). 'Width and pigmentation of the angle of the anterior chamber.' *A.M.A. Archs Ophthal.* **58**, 510–512

Schirmer, K. E. (1965). 'Faceted contact lens with a modified viewing device for fundus examination.' *Archs Ophthal.* **74**, 465–469

Shaffer, R. N. (1962). *Stereoscopic Manual of Gonioscopy.* St. Louis, Missouri: Mosby

Silva, D. (1967). 'Radiographic exophthalmometry examination with the use of contact lenses.' *Contacto* **11**, 57–60

Stahl, N. O., Reich, L. A. and Ivani, E. (1974). 'Report on laboratory studies and preliminary clinical application of a gas-permeable plastic contact lens.' *J. Am. optom. Ass.* **45**, 302–307

Stone, J. (1968). 'The effects of contact lenses on heterophoria and other binocular functions.' *Contact Lens* **1**(7), 5–8, 26, 32

Stone, J. (1976). 'The possible influence of contact lenses on myopia.' *Br. J. physiol. Optics* **31**, 89–114

Stone, J. (1978). 'Changes in curvature of cellulose acetate butyrate lenses during hydration and dehydration.' *J. Br. contact Lens Ass.* **1**, 22–35

Stone, J. and Breakspear, H. R. (1977). 'Two interesting cases of low visual acuity seen at The London Refraction Hospital.' *Contact Lens J.* **6**(3), 3–4, 6

Torgerson, J. T. (1964). 'Antimicrobial activity of contact lenses incorporating disinfectants through a process of polymerization.' National Eye Research Foundation Report. *Contacto* **8**, 9–26

Uribe Troncoso, M. (1921). 'Gonioscopy with the electric ophthalmoscope.' New York Academy of Medicine, referred to in *Gonioscopy*, by Troncoso, Davis Company, Philadelphia, 1947

van Beuningen, E. G. A. (1953). 'Das Pyramidengonioskop.' *Klin. Mbl. Augenheilk.* **122**, 172–178

Ward, B. (1961). Personal communication, Unpublished report, The City University, Department of Ophthalmic Optics, London

Westerhout, D. (1977). Personal communication

Index